Clinical Sports Nutrition

FOURTH EDITION

Clinical Sports Nutrition

Louise Burke PhD, APD, OAM
Head, Department of Sports Nutrition
Australian Institute of Sport
Visiting Professor of Sports Nutrition,
Deakin University, Melbourne

Vicki Deakin MSc, APD
Senior Lecturer & Acting Head, Nutrition and Dietetics
University of Canberra

The McGraw-Hill Companies

Sydney New York San Francisco Auckland
Bangkok Bogotá Caracas Hong Kong
Kuala Lumpur Lisbon London Madrid
Mexico City Milan New Delhi San Juan
Seoul Singapore Taipei Toronto

The **McGraw·Hill** Companies

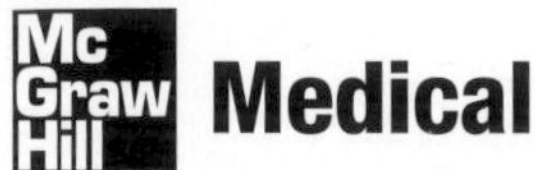

NOTICE

Medicine is an ever-changing science. As new research and clinical experience broaden our knowledge, changes in treatment and drug therapy are required. The editors and the publisher of this work have checked with sources believed to be reliable in their efforts to provide information that is complete and generally in accord with the standards accepted at the time of publication. However, in view of the possibility of human error or changes in medical sciences, neither the editors, nor the publisher, nor any other party who has been involved in the preparation or publication of this work warrants that the information contained herein is in every respect accurate or complete. Readers are encouraged to confirm the information contained herein with other sources. For example, and in particular, readers are advised to check the product information sheet included in the package of each drug they plan to administer to be certain that the information contained in this book is accurate and that changes have not been made in the recommended dose or in the contraindications for administration. This recommendation is of particular importance in connection with new or infrequently used drugs.

National Library of Australia Cataloguing-in-Publication data:
Clinical sports nutrition / editors, Louise Burke, Vicki Deakin.
4th ed.
Includes index. Bibliography.
ISBN 978 0 070 27720 5 (pbk.)
1. Athletes—Nutrition. 2. Physical fitness—Nutritional aspects. 3. Exercise—Physiological aspects.
I. Burke, Louise. II. Deakin, Vicki.
613.2088796

Published in Australia by
McGraw-Hill Australia Pty Ltd
Level 2, 82 Waterloo Road, North Ryde NSW 2113
Publisher: Elizabeth Walton
Editorial Coordinator: Fiona Richardson
Senior Production Editor: Yani Silvana
Copy Editor: Rosemary Moore
Art Director: Astred Hicks
Cover design: Tom Wall
Internal design: Patricia McCallum
Typesetter: diacriTech
Proofreader: Anne Savage
Indexer: Russell Brooks
Printed in China on 80 gsm matt art by 1010 Printing International Ltd

CONTENTS

CONTENTS

PREFACE

If only *Rocky* had known about state-of-the-art sports nutrition, he would have been able to get stronger with each sequel. McGraw-Hill has nutured *Clinical Sports Nutrition* into its fourth edition, knowing that the both the science and practice of sports nutrition continue to grow in rigour and credibility. Sports Dietitians Australia, who gave birth to the original book, has unveiled a career pathway for their members (www.sportsdietitians.com.au). At the international level, the Diploma in Sports Nutrition from the International Olympic Committee grows in strength and numbers, and Professionals in Nutrition for Sports and Exercise has been launched to assist in the global networking of sports dietitians and sports nutritionists. (www.sportsoracle.com)

This fourth edition of *Clinical Sports Nutrition* contines to update the science and practice of sports nutrition in this unique format, which combines the viewpoints of two sports nutrition experts:

- the scientific principles underpinning each issue are reviewed by an internationally recognized nutritionist with extensive research experience
- a sports dietitian summarises the practice tips that can be drawn from these principles.

Topics include nutritional assessment of athletes, measuring physique, weight loss and weight making, post-exercise recovery, nutritional strategies before and during competition, iron depletion, micronutrient needs, eating disorders in athletes, supplements and sports foods, and requirements for special athletic populations and environments (e.g. children, vegetarians and Masters athletes).

The new edition includes the latest information in sports nutrition, including updates in the position stands and consensus viewpoints from international bodies such as the International Olympic Committee and the American College of Sports Medicine. Our new features are commentaries on antioxidant needs of athletes, the Female Athlete Triad and nutritional strategies to reduce the risk of illness in athletes.

This textbook is aimed at students interested in a career in sports nutrition, and sports nutrition professionals who need to translate science into their practice with athletes and coaches. We wish all of you excellence in your endeavours and hope that *Clinical Sports Nutrition* can assist you on this pathway.

Thank you to our authors who contributed further expertise and experience in updating this edition of the book. Once again, we have had to shut ourselves away from the daily needs of our families, friends and workplaces to make this project happen. We thank many people for being understanding about this—and in particular, the men in our lives—Lachlan Deakin, and John and Jack Hawley.

Thank you to Elizabeth Walton and Yani Silvana at McGraw-Hill, and to freelance copyeditor Rosemary Moore, for helping us to meet tight deadlines without too much nagging.

As usual, thank you to our work colleagues. The team in the Department of Sports Nutrition at the Australian Institute of Sport undertakes a large variety of inspiring activities each day. To that we have added writing book chapters. All things are possible with the best team in the world.

Finally we thank all the coaches and athletes with whom we have worked, and who continue to challenge us to bring out the best in them and ourselves through good nutrition.

ABOUT THE EDITORS

LOUISE BURKE, PHD, BSC, GRAD DIP DIET, FSMA, FACSM, OAM, APD

Louise has been the Head of the Department of Sports Nutrition at the Australian Institue of Sport since 1990 and has nearly 30 years of experience in counselling and educating athletes. She has been appointed as a Visiting Professor of Sports Nutrition at Deakin University in Melbourne, and is a Director of the International Olympic Committee's Diploma in Sports Nutrition. Her research interests include dietary periodisation for training and competition performance, post-exercise recovery, nutritional ergogenic aids, carbohydrate and fat metabolism during exercise, and fluid needs in sport. She has produced a number of education resources for athletes, coaches, students and practitioners, including best selling books. She was appointed as the Dietitian to the Australia Olympic Team for the 1996, 2000, 2004 and 2008 Olympic Games, and is a Fellow of Sports Dietitians Australia, Sports Medicine Australia and the American College of Sports Medicine. In 2009 she received a Citation Award from the American College of Sports Medicine and Membership of the Order of Australia (OAM) from the Australian Government in recognition of her work in sports nutrition.

VICKI DEAKIN, MSC, BSC, DIP T, GRAD DIP NUTR DIET, APD

Vicki is an Associate Professor and Head of Nutrition and Dietetics at the University of Canberra, where she initiated the undergraduate and postgraduate courses in Nutrition and Dietetics and Sports Nutrition. Sports nutrition is available to students as part of the undergraduate and postgraduate course in Nutrition and is also compulsory component of the new Master of Exercise Science. She is a member of the research team for the Centre for Research and Action in Public Health in the Faculty of Health and Head Dietitian with the ACT Academy of Sport in Canberra. Her involvement with elite athletes dates back to her initiation of the nutrition services at the Australian Institute of Sport in 1985. She is passionate about enhancing professional education opportunities in sports nutrition for coaches and has embedded sports nutrition as an integral part of formal coach education in Australia. Her research interests include iron deficiency, dietary survey methods, and determining barriers and facilitators that affect food choice and physical activity behaviours in different population groups.

EDITORS AND CONTRIBUTORS

EDITORS

Louise Burke
PhD, APD, FACSM
Head, Department of Sports Nutrition
Australian Institute of Sport
PO Box 176
Belconnen ACT 2616
and
Visiting Professor of Sports Nutrition
Deakin University
Melbourne
AUSTRALIA

Vicki Deakin
MSc, BSc, Dip T, Grad Dip Nutr Diet, APD
Head Dietitian, ACT Academy of Sport
Sports Dietitian
Associate Professor
Faculty of Health
University of Canberra
ACT 2616
AUSTRALIA

CONTRIBUTORS

Timothy R Ackland
PhD
Associate Professor
Biomechanics, Ergonomics and Applied Anatomy
School of Human Movement and Exercise Science
The University of Western Australia
35 Stirling Highway
Crawley WA 6009
AUSTRALIA

Kylie Andrew
BSc, M Nutr & Diet
Sports Dietitian
Victorian Institute of Sport
PO Box 12608
Melbourne Vic 8006
AUSTRALIA

Shona Bass
BAppSci, MSc, PhD
School of Health Sciences
Deakin University
221 Burwood Highway
Burwood Vic 3125
AUSTRALIA

Katherine A Beals
PhD, RD, FACSM
Adjunct Professor and Nutrition Clinic Director
Division on Nutrition
University of Utah
Salt Lake City UT 84112
USA

Kim Bennell
BAppSci (Physio), PhD
Professor, Centre for Sports Medicine Research and Education
School of Physiotherapy
University of Melbourne
Parkville Vic 3052
AUSTRALIA

Elizabeth Broad
BSc, Dip Nutr Diet, MAppSc, PhD
Manager, Clinical Services
Department of Sports Nutrition
Australian Institute of Sport
PO Box 176
Belconnen ACT 2616
AUSTRALIA

Louise Burke
PhD, APD, FACSM
Head, Department of Sports Nutrition
Australian Institute of Sport
PO Box 176
BelconnenACT 2616 and
Visiting Professor of Sports Nutrition
Deakin University
Melbourne
AUSTRALIA

Glenn Cardwell
BSc, Grad Dip Diet, Grad Dip App Sc, APD
Sports Dietitian
PO Box 1035
Bentley DC WA 6983
AUSTRALIA

Ian Caterson
AM MB BS, BSc (Med), PhD, FRACP
Boden Professor of Human Nutrition
Head, School of Molecular and Microbial Biology
University of Sydney
NSW 2006
AUSTRALIA

Gabrielle Cooper
B Pharm, DHP, PhD
Associate Professor of Pharmacy
Division of Health, Design and Science
University of Canberra
University Drive
Belconnen ACT 2601
AUSTRALIA

Michelle Cort
BAppSc, Grad Dip Nutrition and Diet MHSc
Sports Performance Dietitian
Cricket Australia Centre of Excellence
Po Box 122 Albion
Brisbane Qld 4010
AUSTRALIA

Greg Cox
BHMS, Grad Dip Nutr Diet, MHSc (Nutrition)
Senior Sports Dietitian
Department of Sports Nutrition
Australian Institute of Sport
PO Box 176
Belconnen ACT 2616
AUSTRALIA

Ruth Crawford
BSc (Nutr), MND, Grad Dip Ed (Adult), APD
Consultant Dietitian
Bnython ACT 2905
AUSTRALIA

Nicola K Cummings
BSc (Nutr & Food Sci), Grad Dip Diet
Consultant Dietitian
St John of God Medical Clinic Murdock
Murdock WA 6150
AUSTRALIA

Belinda Dalton
BApp Sci, Grad Dip Nutr & Diet, Grad Cert Sports Nutrition, APD
Director
The Oak House
PO Box 210
Surrey Hills VIC 3127
AUSTRALIA

Vinni Dang
MSc (Nutr & Diet), BSc (Nutr), BIT (Eng)
Food Service Dietitian
Department of Sports Nutrition
Australian Institute of Sport
PO Box 176
Belconnen ACT 2616
AUSTRALIA

Vicki Deakin
MSc, BSc, Dip T, Grad Dip Nutr Diet, APD
Head Dietitian, ACT Academy of Sport
Sports Dietitian
Associate Professor
Faculty of Health
University of Canberra
ACT 2616
AUSTRALIA

Ben Desbrow
PhD, BSc, Grad Dip Nutr & Diet, Grad Dip Sc (HMS)
Nutrition Unit, Griffith University
Gold Coast
PMB50 GCMC 9726

Christine Dziedzic
APD
Sports Dietitian—Gatorade Fellow
Department of Sports Nutrition
Australian Institute of Sport
PO Box 176
Belconnen ACT 2616
AUSTRALIA

Kieran Fallon
MD, MBBS (Hons), MSpExSc, MHEd, FRACGP, FACSP
Associate Professor
Head, Department of Sports Medicine
Australian Institute of Sport
PO Box 176
Belconnen ACT 2616
AUSTRALIA

Mark A Febbraio
PhD
NHMRC Principal Research Fellow Professor of Cell Biology
Head, Cellular and Molecular Metabolism Laboratory
Baker IDI Heart and Diabetes Institute
Melbourne Vic
AUSTRALIA

Mikael Fogelholm
DSc
Director, Health Research Unit
Academy of Finland
POB 99, 00501 Helsinki
FINLAND

Peter Fricker
OAM, MBBS, FACSM, FASMF, FACSP
Adjunct Professor, Director
Australian Institute of Sport
PO Box 176
Belconnen ACT 2616
AUSTRALIA

Lorna Garden
BSc, Dip Diet, APD
Sports Dietitian
PO Box 365
Noosaville Qld 4566
AUSTRALIA

Stephen Gurr
Sports Dietitian—Nestle Fellow
Department of Sports Nutrition
Australian Institute of Sport
PO Box 176
Belconnen ACT 2616
AUSTRALIA

Mark Hargreaves
PhD
Department of Physiology
The University of Melbourne
Parkville Vic 3010
AUSTRALIA

John Hawley
PhD, MA, Cert Ed, BSc (Hons), FACSM
Professor, Department of Human Biology and Movement Science
RMIT University
Bundoora Campus
PO Box 71
Bundoora Vic 3083
AUSTRALIA

Linda Houtkooper
PhD, RD, FACSM
Professor and Head
Department of Nutritional Sciences
PO Box 210038
Univeristy of Arizona
Tucson Arizona 85721-0038
USA

Karen Inge
BSc, Dip Diet, FSMA, APD
Coordinator Nutrition Services
Victorian Institute of Sport
PO Box 148
Canterbury Vic 3126
AUSTRALIA

Deborah Kerr
BSc, Grad Dip Diet, MSc, PhD
Senior Lecturer
School of Public Health
Curtin University of Technology
Perth WA 6001
AUSTRALIA

Karim Khan
MD, PhD, FACSP, FACSM
Associate Professor
Dept of Family Practice and
School of Human Kinetics
Centre for Hip Health
University of British Columbia
2150 Western Parkway
Vancouver V6T 1V6
CANADA

Benita Lalor
Peformance Dietitian
Essendon Football Club
PO Box 17
Essendon Vic 3040
AUSTRALIA

Melinda M Manore
PhD, RD, CSSD, FACSM
Professor and Extension Nutrition Specialist
Department of Nutrition/
Exercise Sciences
108 Milam Hall
2520 SW Campus Way
Oregon State University
Corvallis OR 97331
USA

David Martin
PhD, CSCS
Senior Sport Physiologist
Sport Science Coordinator
Cycling Australia
Australian Institute of Sport
Department of Physiology
PO Box 176
Belconnen ACT 2616
AUSTRALIA

Ron Maughan
BSc, PhD
Professor of Sport and Exercise Nutrition
School of Sport and Exercise Sciences
Loughborough University
Loughborough
Leicestershire LE11 3TU
UNITED KINGDOM

Michelle Minehan
BAppSc, MND
Lecturer, Division of Health, Design and Science
University of Canberra
University Drive
Belconnen ACT 2601
AUSTRALIA

Helen O'Connor
PhD
Senior Lecturer
University of NSW
Cumberland College
Lidcombe NSW 2141
AUSTRALIA

Fiona Pelly
BSc, Grad Dip Nutr Diet, PhD
Snr Lecturer Nutrition and Dietetics
School of Health and Sport Sciences
University of the Sunshine Coast
Maroochydore DC QLD 4558
AUSTRALIA

David Pyne
PhD, FACSM
Sports Physiologist
Department of Physiology
Australian Institute of Sport
PO Box 176
Belconnen ACT 2616
AUSTRALIA

Peter Raeburn
BHMS (Ed) (Hons), PhD
School of Health and Human Performance
Central Queensland University
Rockhampton QLD 4702
AUSTRALIA

Gary Slater
PhD, BSc, Grad Dip Nutr Diet
Senior Lecturer in Nutrition and Dietetics
School of Health and Sport Sciences
Faculty of Science, Health and Education
University of the Sunshine Coast
Maroochydore DC QLD 4558
AUSTRALIA

Greg Shaw
Sports Dietitian
Department of Sports Nutrition
Australian Institute of Sport
PO Box 176
Belconnen ACT 2616

Nikki Shaw
BN&D (Hons), APD
Sports Dietitian
Department of Sports Nutrition
Australian Institute of Sport
PO Box 176
Belconnen ACT 2616
AUSTRALIA

Lisa Sutherland
B App Sci (Human Movement), MND, GradCert (Sports Nutrition)
Sports Dietitian and Fitness Consultant
Victorian Institute of Sport
Olympic Park, Swan Street
Melbourne Vic 3000
PO Box 12608 A'Beckett Street
Melbourne Vic 8006

Mark Tarnopolsky
MD, PhD, FRCP(C)
Professor of Pediatrics and Medicine
Hamilton Hospitals Assessment Center Endowed Chair in Neuromuscular Disorders
Director of Neuromuscular and Neurometabolic Clinic
McMaster University Medical Center
1200 Main Street W
Hamilton, Ontario L8N 3Z5
CANADA

Janice L Thompson
PhD, FACSM
Professor and Head
The University of Bristol
Department Exercise, Nutrition & Health Sciences
Tyndall Avenue
Bristol UK
BS8 1TP, UK

Janet Walberg Rankin
PhD
Professor, Human Nutrition and Foods Department
Drill Field
215 War Memorial Hall
Virginia Tech
Blacksburg VA 24061-0351
USA

Trent Watson
BHSc (N&D), PhD, APD
Consultant Dietitian (Clued on Food)
Unit D, 10 Bradford Close
Kotara NSW 2289
AUSTRALIA

Dennis Wilson
BSc (Hons), MBBAO, BCh (Hons), MD, FRCP, FRACP
Clinical Associate Professor
Director, Endocrinology
The Canberra Hospital
PO Box 11
Woden ACT 2606
AUSTRALIA

Nick Wray
BAppSc, Grad Dip Hum Nutr, MND
Senior Dietitian
Nutrition and Dietetics Dept
Flinders Medical Centre
Bedford Park SA 5042
AUSTRALIA

CHAPTER 1

Exercise physiology and metabolism

MARK HARGREAVES

Introduction

1.1

Physical exercise requires a coordinated physiological response involving the interplay between systems responsible for increased energy metabolism, supply of oxygen and substrates to contracting skeletal muscle, removal of metabolic waste products and heat, and the maintenance of fluid and electrolyte status. Knowledge of these responses is important for an understanding of the potential mechanisms by which nutrition can influence exercise and sports performance. It is beyond the scope of this chapter to summarize all of these responses in great detail, and readers are referred to various exercise physiology texts and the cited review papers for a more thorough discussion. Nevertheless, this chapter attempts to identify important aspects of the physiological and metabolic responses to exercise.

Skeletal muscle

1.2

Skeletal muscle can account for as much as 45% of the total body mass. It is the tissue responsible for the generation of the forces required for joint movement during exercise. By virtue of its mass and metabolic capacity, skeletal muscle has a major impact on whole-body metabolism in health and disease. Factors influencing the ability of muscle to produce force include total cross-sectional area, fiber type, number of active motor units, motor neuron firing frequency, muscle length and velocity of contraction. The sequence of events involved in muscle contraction is summarized as follows:

1. motor cortical activation and excitation of alpha motor neuron
2. arrival of electrical impulse at neuromuscular junction
3. propagation of muscle action potential across sarcolemma
4. excitation–contraction (EC) coupling:
   a. conduction of excitation in t-tubules
   b. release of calcium from sarcoplasmic reticulum
   c. action of calcium on actin myofilament

5. actin-myosin cross-bridge formation and tension development (sliding filament theory)
6. re-uptake of calcium by sarcoplasmic reticulum (SR) and muscle relaxation

The chemical energy required for skeletal muscle to undertake mechanical work is provided by the hydrolysis of adenosine triphosphate (ATP), and this reaction is catalyzed by myosin ATPase. Since the intramuscular stores of ATP are relatively small (approximately 5–6 mmol/kg wet weight), other metabolic pathways responsible for the resynthesis of ATP must be activated in order to maintain contractile activity. These energy pathways are summarized in Figure 1.1. Creatine phosphate (CrP) is a high-energy compound, stored in greater amounts (approximately 20 mmol/kg) in skeletal muscle, and can be broken down quickly during intense exercise to provide energy for ATP resynthesis. In addition, ATP can be formed from adenosine diphosphate (ADP) in a reaction catalyzed by adenylate kinase. These reactions form what is called the alactic or phosphagen system. The other non-oxidative energy system is the lactacid system or 'anaerobic' glycolysis, in which glucose units, derived primarily from intramuscular glycogen reserves, are broken down to lactate. These two energy systems are maximally active during high-intensity exercise of short duration. During prolonged exercise, the aerobic system becomes the predominant provider of energy for contracting skeletal muscle, the major oxidative substrates being carbohydrate (CHO) and lipid.

One aspect of muscle physiology that has received great attention over the years is the potential link between skeletal muscle fiber composition and exercise performance (Zierath & Hawley 2004). Human skeletal muscle is composed of two main fiber types: slow twitch (ST) and fast twitch (FT). The FT fibers have been further divided into FTa and FTb on the basis of differences in their glycolytic and oxidative potential. The fiber types differ in their contractile, morphological and metabolic characteristics, and are usually differentiated using histochemical staining for myosin ATPase (Saltin & Gollnick 1983). The ST fibers rely primarily on oxidative metabolism, are well supplied by capillaries and are fatigue resistant. Not surprisingly, they are well suited to prolonged, low-intensity activity. In contrast, FT fibers have a higher glycolytic capacity (FTb > FTa), a lower oxidative capacity (FTb < FTa) and are more fatigable. They are more suited to high-intensity exercise. During

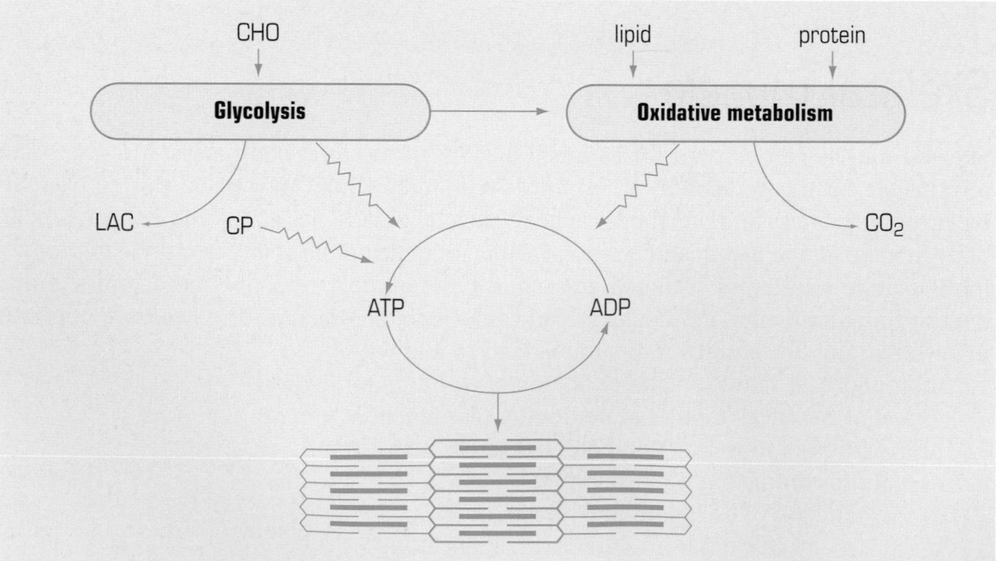

FIGURE 1.1 Metabolic pathways and sources of ATP generation in skeletal muscle

progressive exercise, ST fibers are involved at the lower intensities and as exercise intensity increases there is progressive recruitment of more ST and FT fiber populations.

This general pattern of muscle fiber recruitment during exercise has been confirmed in humans using histochemically determined glycogen depletion patterns as an index of fiber involvement. During prolonged, submaximal exercise, the ST fibers are preferentially recruited, although there may be involvement of FTa fibers in the latter stages (Vøllestad et al. 1984).

As exercise intensity increases, the FT fibers are recruited so that during maximal exercise all fiber types are involved (Vøllestad & Blom 1985; Vøllestad et al. 1992). These patterns of recruitment have resulted in interest in the link between muscle fiber composition and exercise performance in specially trained athletes. Indeed, elite endurance athletes possess a high percentage of ST muscle fibers (70–90%), while sprint and explosive athletes possess relatively more FT fibers (Costill et al. 1975; Saltin & Gollnick 1983). This appears to be due to a combination of genetic factors and possible training-induced alterations in muscle fiber composition (Saltin & Gollnick 1983; Schantz 1986).

Exercise metabolism

1.3

During high-intensity, dynamic exercise (such as sprinting, track cycling and interval training), the breakdown of ATP and CrP and the degradation of glycogen to lactic acid are the major sources of energy. These substrates are also important during static exercise, particularly above 30–40% maximum voluntary contraction (MVC), since an increase in intramuscular pressure will impair muscle blood flow, thereby reducing oxygen and substrate delivery to contracting skeletal muscle. Activation of muscle phosphagen and glycogen degradation occurs with the onset of exercise. Although the capacity for ATP generation is greater for the glycolytic system (190–300 mmol ATP/kg dry muscle) than for the phosphagen system (55–95 mmol ATP/kg), the power output is lower (4.5 mmol ATP/kg/s compared with 9 mmol/kg/s). For this reason, when the levels of CrP decline with maximal exercise, the rate of anaerobic turnover cannot be sustained (see Fig. 1.2 overleaf), and this contributes to the decline in power output that is observed during all-out exercise.

During prolonged exercise, the oxidative metabolism of CHO and lipid provides the vast majority of ATP for muscle contraction. Although amino acid oxidation occurs to a limited extent during exercise, CHO and lipid are the most important oxidative substrates. The relative contribution of CHO and lipid is influenced by exercise intensity and duration, preceding diet and substrate availability, training status and environmental factors.

Muscle glycogen is the important substrate during both intense, short-duration exercise and prolonged exercise. Its rate of utilization is most rapid during the early part of exercise and is related to exercise intensity (Vøllestad et al. 1984; Vøllestad & Blom 1985; Vøllestad et al. 1992). As muscle glycogen declines with continued exercise, blood glucose becomes more important as a CHO fuel source. Muscle glucose uptake increases in both an exercise-intensity and duration-dependent manner. This is a consequence of increased sarcolemmal glucose transport, due to translocation of the GLUT-4 glucose transporter isoform to the plasma membrane, activation of the metabolic pathways responsible for glucose metabolism and enhanced glucose delivery due to increased skeletal muscle blood flow (Hargreaves 2000). Accompanying the increased muscle glucose uptake is an increase in liver glucose output, so that blood glucose levels usually remain at, or slightly above, resting levels. Liver glycogenolysis supplies the majority of liver glucose output; however, during the latter stages of prolonged exercise, when liver glycogen levels are

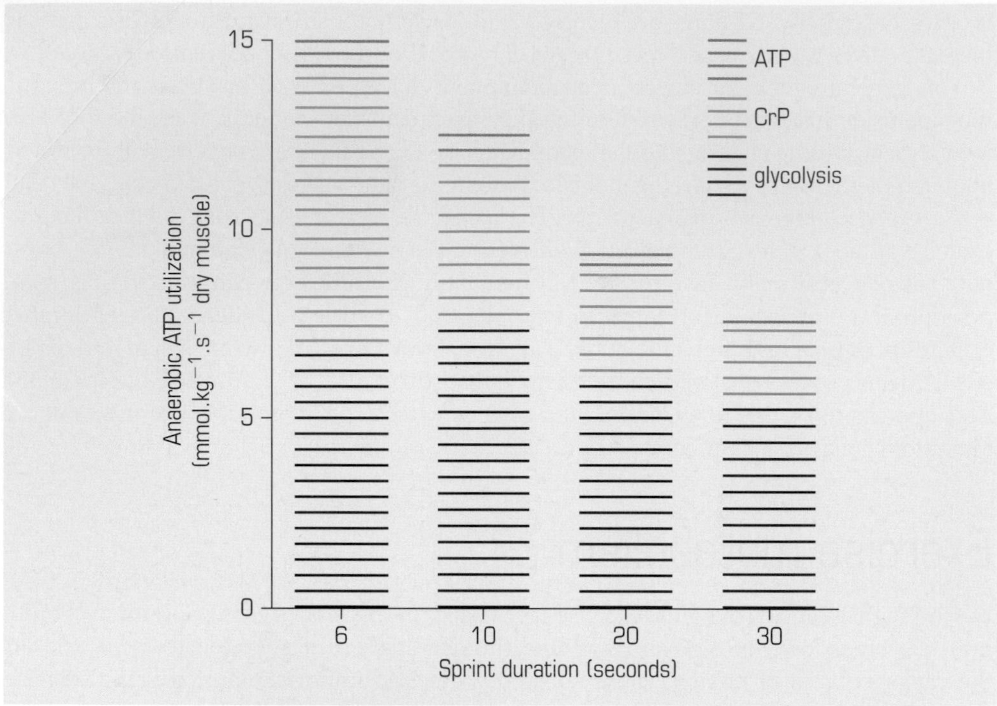

FIGURE 1.2 Anaerobic ATP utilization during maximal cycling exercise of varying duration (From ME Nevill, GC Bogdanis, LH Boobis, HKA Lakomy and C Williams, 1996, Chapter 19: Muscle metabolism and performance during sprinting. In *Biochemistry of exercise IX*, edited by RJ Maughan and SM Shirreffs, page 249, Figure 19.3 © 1996 by Human Kinetics Publishers, Inc. Reprinted with permission from Human Kinetics (Champaign, IL).)

low, gluconeogenesis is an important source of glucose. Under such circumstances, liver glucose output may fall behind muscle glucose uptake, resulting in hypoglycemia. Fatigue during prolonged exercise is often, but not always, associated with muscle glycogen depletion and/or hypoglycemia (Hargreaves 1999). Thus considerable attention has focused on CHO nutrition and exercise performance, and athletes are encouraged to adopt nutritional strategies that maximize CHO availability before, during and after exercise (Hargreaves 1999; Hawley et al. 1997). These strategies are reviewed in Chapters 12, 13 and 14. There is increasing evidence that lactate, derived from contracting and inactive muscle, is an important oxidative and gluconeogenic precursor and is a valuable metabolic intermediate, rather than simply being a waste product of anaerobic glycolysis (Brooks 1986).

Contracting skeletal muscle also derives energy from the ß-oxidation of plasma free fatty acids (FFA), derived from adipose tissue lipolysis. Plasma FFA levels usually peak after 2–4 hours of exercise, at which time they are a major substrate for muscle (Coyle 1995). The muscle uptake and utilization of FFA is determined, in part, by the arterial FFA concentration and the ability of the muscle to take up and oxidize FFA. Increasing plasma FFA availability and utilization may reduce the reliance on muscle glycogen and blood glucose, and this has resulted in interest in strategies designed to enhance FFA oxidation (e.g. high-fat diets, caffeine lipid ingestion and carnitine supplementation), although results in the literature remain equivocal (Hawley et al. 1998). These strategies are reviewed in greater detail in Chapter 15.

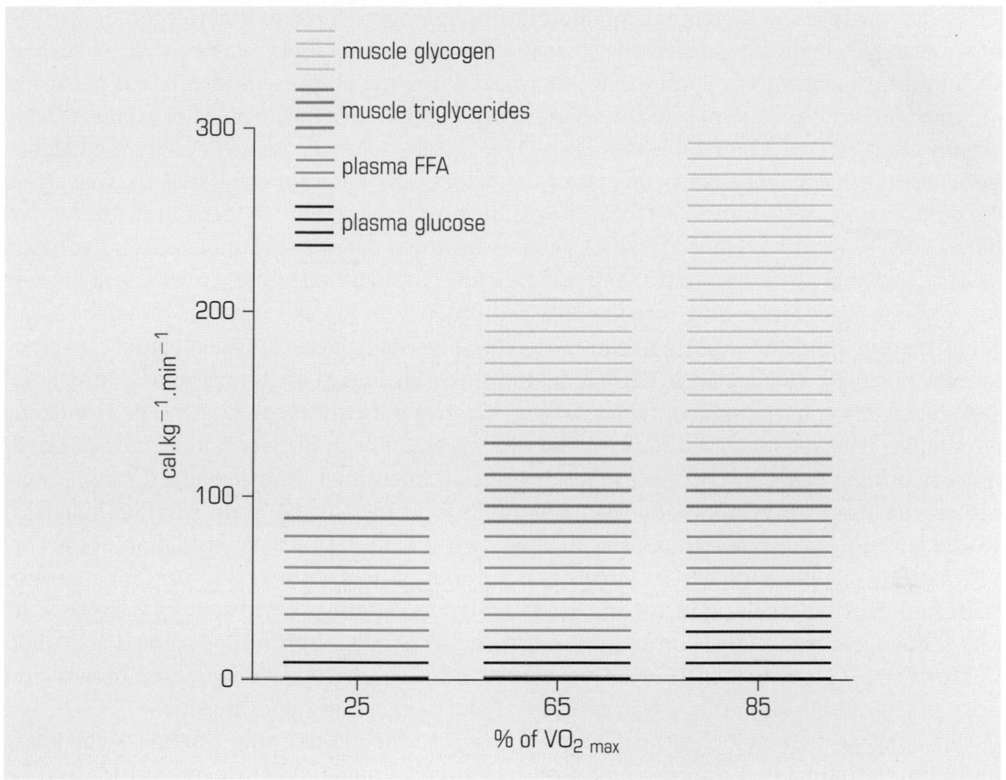

FIGURE 1.3 Relative contributions of the various CHO and lipid substrates for oxidative metabolism during exercise of increasing intensity in trained men (from Romijn et al. 1993)

It should be noted that a major metabolic adaptation to endurance training is an increased capacity for lipid oxidation. Muscle triglyceride stores can also be used by contracting muscle (Van Loon 2004; Watt et al. 2002) and are believed to be more important early in exercise and during exercise at higher intensities where mobilization of FFA from adipose tissue is inhibited (see Fig. 1.3; Coyle 1995). During high-intensity exercise, mitochondrial oxidation of FFA derived from both adipose tissue and muscle triglycerides is reduced and CHO, predominantly muscle glycogen, is the main fuel.

Amino acids, particularly the branched-chain amino acids, can also be oxidized during prolonged exercise, but their overall contribution is small. The contribution from amino acids is enhanced when CHO reserves are low. This is particularly important for athletes in heavy training, who are likely to place a large stress on their endogenous CHO reserves and in whom the training-based adaptations (e.g. increased metabolic enzymes, myofibrillar mass and buffer capacity) are protein dependent. Protein requirements for exercise are reviewed in Chapter 4.

Oxygen transport system

1.4

The increased oxidative metabolism during exercise is dependent upon the adequate delivery of oxygen to active skeletal muscle and, thus, upon the functional capacities of the cardiovascular and respiratory systems. The most widely accepted measure of aerobic fitness is maximal oxygen uptake ($VO_{2\ max}$), and over the years there has been considerable interest in the physiological determinants of $VO_{2\ max}$.

The cardiovascular system is regulated during exercise to ensure that oxygen delivery to contracting skeletal and cardiac muscle is increased, that metabolic waste products such as CO_2 and heat are removed, and that mean arterial blood pressure and cerebral perfusion are maintained. Skeletal muscle vasodilation occurs rapidly with the onset of exercise and is closely coupled to the metabolic demands. Muscle blood flow is determined by the balance between neural activity (vasoconstrictor) and local vasodilation mediated by vasoactive substances released from contracting skeletal muscle, vascular endothelium and/or red blood cells (Clifford & Hellsten 2004). Such substances include ATP, potassium, hydrogen ions, adenosine, nitric oxide (NO) and prostanoids. No single substance can account entirely for exercise hyperemia and considerable redundancy exists (Clifford & Hellsten 2004). Mean arterial pressure (MAP) is maintained, despite the decrease in skeletal muscle vascular resistance, by an increase in cardiac output (increased heart rate and stroke volume) and vasoconstriction in the splanchnic, renal and inactive muscle vascular beds. The cutaneous circulation receives increased flow for the dissipation of heat, although it becomes a target of sympathetic vasoconstriction at higher exercise intensities. Active skeletal muscle may also be a target for sympathetic vasoconstriction in order to maintain MAP as maximal cardiac output approaches (Calbet et al. 2004; Saltin et al. 1998). The regulation of the cardiovascular response to exercise involves a number of neurohumoral factors. The general pattern of cardiovascular effector activity is set by descending neural activity from the cardiovascular centre (central command), increased in parallel with motor cortical activation of skeletal muscle (Mitchell 1990). This activity is influenced by feedback from muscle and arterial chemoreflexes, arterial baroreflexes, hypovolemia and hyperthermia.

An increase in pulmonary ventilation is essential for maintaining arterial oxygenation and eliminating carbon dioxide, produced by oxidative metabolism in contracting muscle. During incremental exercise, ventilation increases in proportion to the increases in oxygen consumption and carbon dioxide production; however, at higher intensities a point is reached where there is an abrupt increase in ventilation. This is often referred to as the ventilatory or anaerobic threshold and it has been suggested that it arises from stimulation of the peripheral chemoreceptors by increased carbon dioxide, due to bicarbonate buffering of lactic acid produced by contracting skeletal muscle (Wasserman et al. 1986). There is considerable debate and controversy in the literature regarding the mechanisms of lactate production during exercise, and the link between hyperventilation and blood lactate accumulation (Brooks 1986; Wasserman et al. 1986; Katz & Sahlin 1988). Despite the controversy, measurement of lactate threshold and lactate/ventilatory variables remains commonplace in endurance athlete assessment, given the strong links between such variables and endurance exercise performance (Coyle et al. 1988). The ventilatory responses to exercise are regulated by a number of neural and humoral factors. These include carbon dioxide flux to the lung, descending activity from respiratory neurons in the hindbrain, increased body temperature, alterations in arterial H^+, K^+ and adrenaline levels, and feedback from muscle chemoreceptors and proprioceptors.

The ability of the muscles to consume oxygen in metabolism, and the combined abilities of the cardiovascular and respiratory systems to deliver oxygen to the muscle mitochondria, are reflected in $VO_{2\,max}$, the most widely accepted measure of aerobic fitness. Values for $VO_{2\,max}$ range from 30–40 mL/kg/min in inactive sedentary individuals to as high as 80–90 mL/kg/min in highly trained endurance athletes. Such high values reflect a combination of genetic endowment and vigorous physical training. There has been much interest in the physiological factors that limit $VO_{2\,max}$ (see Fig. 1.4), with reasonably general agreement that it is oxygen supply to muscle that represents the major limiting factor (Richardson 2003; Saltin & Rowell 1980). It is likely that all components

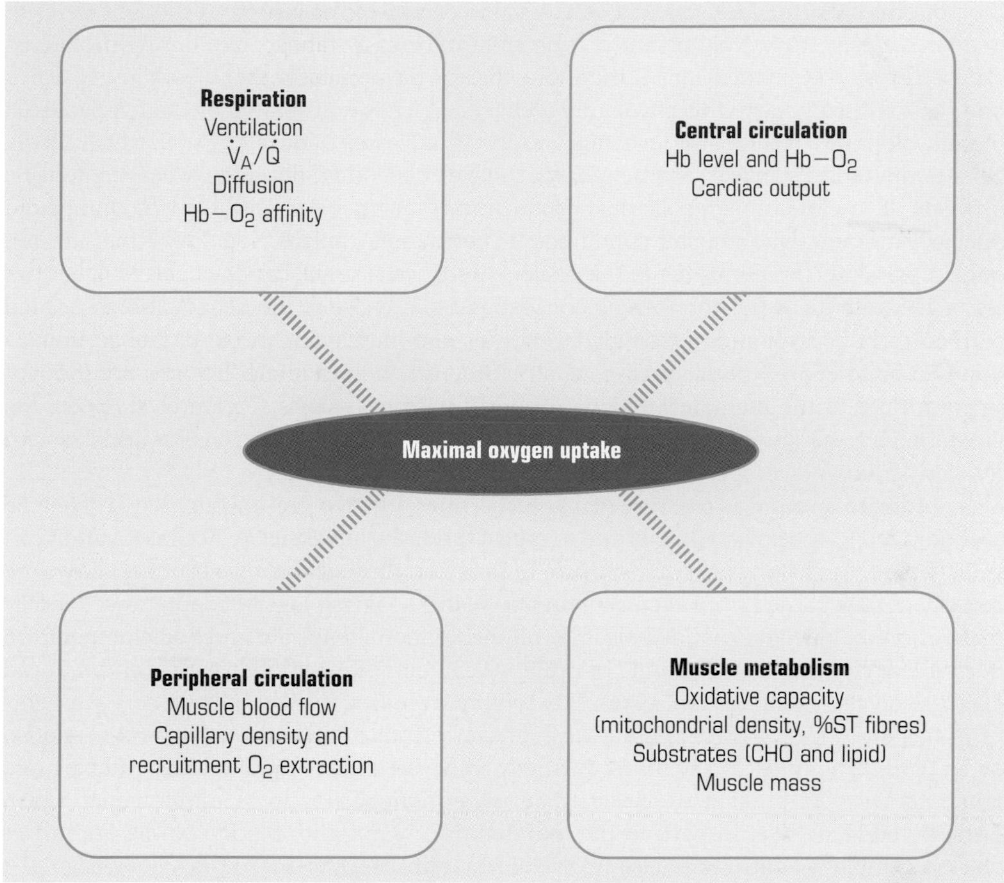

FIGURE 1.4 Physiological determinants of maximal oxygen uptake

of the oxygen transport system, by influencing either oxygen delivery to muscle or tissue diffusion of oxygen, will play a role in determining $VO_{2\,max}$ (Richardson 2003). Strategies (like blood doping and erythropoietin supplementation) designed to increase red blood cell mass and arterial hemoglobin, and therefore arterial oxygen-carrying capacity, have received attention from endurance athletes over the years. Furthermore, since iron is an important component of hemoglobin, myoglobin and the cytochromes within the respiratory chain, there has been much interest in the iron status of endurance athletes and the potential effects of iron deficiency, and subsequent supplementation, on endurance exercise performance. Iron requirements for training are reviewed in Chapter 10.

Temperature regulation and fluid balance 1.5

The metabolic heat that is produced during exercise must be dissipated so as to avoid hyperthermia. During exercise in air, as much as 75% of this heat loss is achieved by the evaporation of sweat, with approximately 580 kcal of heat being dissipated for each liter of sweat evaporated. Sweat rates can be as high as 1–2 L/h during prolonged exercise and under extreme conditions may reach 2–3 L/h for short periods. The transfer of heat to the skin is achieved by vasodilation of the cutaneous circulation, thereby displacing blood to the periphery (Fortney & Vroman 1985). A fall in central blood volume is thought to result in a decrease in stroke volume and a concomitant increase in heart rate during prolonged exercise or exercise in the heat. Furthermore, there is the possibility that blood flow to active muscle is reduced due to this 'circulatory conflict', which is exacerbated by the hypovolemia that develops as a result of the sweating-induced fluid losses (González-Alonso et al. 1998). Core temperature stabilizes at a new, elevated level, depending upon the exercise intensity; however, if the rate of metabolic heat production is maintained, or if heat loss is impaired due to extreme environmental conditions, hyperthermia can develop. Hyperthermia not only impairs exercise performance (González-Alonso et al. 1999; Parkin et al. 1999), but can also have potentially life-threatening consequences. Exercise in the heat is also associated with accelerated liver and muscle glycogenolysis and muscle and blood lactate accumulation (Febbraio et al. 1994; Hargreaves et al. 1996). Although CHO depletion is not thought to contribute to the premature fatigue observed with heat stress (Parkin et al. 1999), the greater CHO use during exercise in the heat has nutritional implications for athletes who regularly train and compete in hot environments (see Chapter 23).

In order to minimize the risk of hyperthermia, athletes are encouraged to become acclimatized to hot environments and to ingest fluids during exercise. Acclimatization can be achieved, in part, by passive exposure to heat and through exercise training; however, most benefit is gained from exercising in the heat. The physiological adaptations to acclimatization include an expanded plasma volume, reduced heart rate and body temperature during exercise, increased volume of dilute sweat, earlier onset of sweating and reduced glycogenolysis (Febbraio et al. 1994). Pre-cooling, resulting in a lower body core temperature, has also been shown to enhance exercise tolerance in the heat (González-Alonso et al. 1999). The ingestion of fluids during exercise attenuates the increases in heart rate and body temperature that are observed during prolonged exercise (Hamilton et al. 1991). This seems to be due, in part, to the maintenance of a higher blood volume and lower plasma osmolality during exercise (Coyle & Montain 1992).

There has been debate on the optimal volume and composition of rehydration solutions during exercise (Hargreaves 1996). Since sweat is hypotonic, replacement of fluid is a priority; however, during prolonged exercise the inclusion of CHO and a small amount of electrolyte is recommended (Coyle & Montain 1992; Gisolfi & Duchman 1992). The effects of fluid ingestion appear to be graded in proportion to the volume of fluid ingested (Coyle & Montain 1992). Thus athletes should be encouraged to drink as much as is required to minimize exercise-induced body weight loss; however, this is often a difficult task, since fluid is not always readily available and ingestion of large fluid volumes can result in gastrointestinal distress. Although the body has hormonal mechanisms for restoring water and electrolyte levels following exercise, fluid ingestion during recovery should be encouraged to facilitate rehydration. Solutions containing a small amount of CHO and electrolyte appear to provide an advantage over plain water (Maughan et al. 1997). Fluid and CHO intake during exercise is reviewed in detail in Chapter 13.

1.6 Fatigue

Fatigue is defined as a reduction in the force or power-generating capacity of muscle. The sites of fatigue include the central nervous system and motor outflow (Gandevia 2001) and peripheral sites such as the sarcolemma, t-tubule system, SR and myofilaments within skeletal muscle (Fitts 1994). These peripheral sites reflect the processes of membrane excitation,

EC coupling and uncoupling, cross-bridge formation and metabolic energy supply. While central fatigue occurs during exercise, most attention has focused on peripheral mechanisms of fatigue. It is unlikely that a single mechanism can explain fatigue under all circumstances, but possible mechanisms include ionic disturbances, impaired EC coupling, accumulation of metabolites and substrate depletion.

Loss of potassium from contracting skeletal muscle has been implicated in fatigue during both intense and prolonged exercise (McKenna 1992). Potassium efflux, which is most pronounced during intense, short-duration exercise, results in reduced membrane excitability and contributes to intracellular acidosis. Intense exercise is also associated with accumulation of H^+, ADP and inorganic phosphate. Acidosis has been linked to fatigue via a number of mechanisms. These include effects on myofilament force production and ATP generation within skeletal muscle. Ingestion of oral alkalizing agents (such as bicarbonate) has been employed to minimize these effects of acidosis and is associated with improved high-intensity exercise performance in many investigations (see Chapter 16). Increases in inorganic phosphate and ADP are also believed to inhibit muscle force generation.

A failure of EC coupling is also likely to be involved in the fatigue process (Allen et al. 1995; Favero 1999). Possible mechanisms include reduced calcium release from the SR and impaired myofibrillar calcium sensitivity (Allen et al. 1995). Impaired SR calcium release could be due to a reduction in ATP supply in the region of the calcium release channel (Chin & Allen 1997), increased metabolite/ion (e.g. Ca^{2+}, Mg^{2+}, H^+, lactate, inorganic phosphate) accumulation (Westerblad et al. 2002), or modification by free radicals (Favero 1999). In addition, reduced SR calcium uptake and calcium ATPase activity following both intense (Li et al. 2002) and prolonged (Leppik et al. 2004) exercise suggest impairment of SR function.

Alterations in energy supply may also be an important factor in fatigue during exercise (Sahlin et al. 1998). Muscle ATP levels usually fall only about 30–50% during intense exercise; in contrast, CrP levels can be totally depleted following intense exercise (Söderlund & Hultman 1991) and this could contribute to the reduced power output associated with fatigue during such exercise. Dietary creatine supplementation is a potential intervention to increase skeletal muscle CrP availability and enhance high-intensity exercise performance (Greenhaff 1997) (see Chapter 16). During prolonged exercise, muscle glycogen depletion and/or hypoglycemia are often associated with fatigue (Hargreaves 1999). Increased CHO availability, either by muscle glycogen loading prior to exercise (see Chapter 12) or CHO ingestion before (see Chapter 12) and during exercise (see Chapter 13), is associated with enhanced endurance exercise performance (Hargreaves 1999; Hawley et al. 1997). Other factors contributing to fatigue during prolonged, strenuous exercise include dehydration and hyperthermia (see Chapter 13), and impaired SR and mitochondrial function (possibly as a consequence of oxidative damage due to increased free radical activity). Thus, in recent years, interest has focused on the potential relationship between anti-oxidant (vitamins C and E) supplementation and endurance performance, although definitive evidence of their ergogenic benefits is still required (see Chapters 11 and 16).

Summary 1.7

This chapter provides only a brief overview of the physiological and metabolic responses to exercise. Nevertheless, it should be apparent that nutrition can have a major impact on many physiological aspects of exercise. The specific nutritional strategies designed to optimize exercise and sports performance are described in detail in the following chapters.

PRACTICE TIPS

NICK WRAY

- A sound knowledge of the physiology and practice of sport is critical to the understanding of nutritional strategies that can enhance exercise performance. A good comprehension of the specific energy systems used in a sport and the factors limiting performance are essential before appropriate nutritional advice can be given.
- To determine this information, it is necessary to establish the characteristics of the athlete's training and competition schedule. A better understanding of the specific physiological requirements and challenges faced by each athlete allows dietary advice to be tailored to the athlete and to the situation. The practical aspects of achieving nutritional goals also need to be considered. Important information for the sports dietitian to collect to assess the specific nutrition demands and challenges faced by an athlete is summarized in Tables 1.1 (training) and 1.2 (competition).

TABLE 1.1 NUTRITION FOR OPTIMAL TRAINING

This list of questions may help to identify the nutritional requirements and challenges involved in optimizing the effectiveness of the athlete's training program.

- What are the typical exercise requirements of the athlete's training schedule? Type of training sessions? Frequency? Duration? Intensity? How are training sessions periodized over the week, month, season and year? What total energy and fuel requirements do such exercise patterns set?
- What is the environment in which training sessions are undertaken? What are the typical sweat losses and fuel requirements of training sessions? What opportunities are available to consume fluid or foods during the session? How are such foods or fluids made available?
- What are the opportunities to practice competition intake strategies in a training session?
- What are the typical exercise patterns during the off-season or during an injury break?
- How important are body mass and composition to performance in this sport? What are the typical characteristics of the physique of elite performances in this sport—body mass, lean body mass, body fat levels? What is the current physique of the athlete, and what is their history of physique changes? What is the range of physique characteristics that should allow the athlete to achieve optimal training, and then competition performances? Will these physique goals be achieved as a result of genetics and training or must a special dietary program be organized to assist gain of muscle mass and/or loss of body fat?
- What is the typical domestic situation in which the athlete lives? Where does the athlete eat most of their meals? Who does the cooking?
- What are the typical dietary intakes and practices of athletes (or a particular athlete) in this sport?
- What is the risk of the athlete developing any of the following problems:
  - iron deficiency (low iron intake, increased iron requirements, increased iron losses)
  - menstrual dysfunction
  - compromised bone status
  - disordered eating
  - other nutrient deficiencies
- Does the athlete undertake special training programs (e.g. altitude training and/or heat acclimatization)?
- Is there direct or indirect evidence that supplementation with ergogenic aids (e.g. creatine, caffeine and anti-oxidant vitamins) enhances training adaptation and performance?
- What are the practical considerations or difficulties in arranging food intake during a typical training day?
- At what times does the athlete train?
- What other activities need to be timetabled into the day?

TABLE 1.1 (continued)

- What factors limit access to food during the day?
- Do gastrointestinal considerations or appetite limit food intake, particularly at strategic times?
- How often or how far does the athlete need to travel to fulfill training commitments?
- Is the athlete's nutrition influenced by other factors such as financial constraints, or religious or social customs?
- What are the current nutritional beliefs of athletes from this sport?
- Where do athletes in this sport commonly seek their dietary advice or information?
- What is the typical level of nutrition awareness of athletes in this sport?

Source: Burke 2007

TABLE 1.2 NUTRITION FOR COMPETITION PERFORMANCE

This list of questions may help to identify the nutritional strategies that will help to optimize the athlete's competition performance.

- What are the exercise requirements of competition? What is the frequency? Duration? Intensity of the specific activity? Is this specialized into individual events or different playing positions/styles?
- Is competition undertaken as a single event or a series of activities? For example, is it a tournament, schedule of heats and finals, multi-day stages, or a weekly fixture?
- What are the typical environmental conditions in which competition is undertaken? What is the temperature? Humidity? Airflow?
- How often is major competition undertaken by the athlete?
- Are there competition weight limits that dictate the class of competition or overall eligibility to compete? How often does the athlete need to weigh in? What is the time interval between weigh-in and competition?
- What is the indirect or direct evidence that any of the following factors might limit competition performance:
  - dehydration
  - CHO availability
  - gastrointestinal problems
- What is the indirect or direct evidence that sports nutrition strategies such as the following may affect competition performance:
  - CHO loading
  - CHO refueling before or between events
  - CHO intake in the 1–4 hours before the event
  - fluid intake during the event
  - CHO intake during the event
  - hydration strategies before the event
  - hydration strategies between events
  - acute use of supplements such as caffeine, bicarbonate or creatine
  - strategies to promote fat availability and utilization
- What time of day does competition occur?
- Are the athletes in familiar surroundings or have they traveled to undertake competition? What is the food availability in these surroundings?

(continued)

PRACTICE TIPS

TABLE 1.2 (continued)

- What other practical considerations affect competition nutrition strategies? Is the athlete's nutrition affected by financial constraints, or religious or social practices?
- Do gastrointestinal problems commonly occur? Are these affected by pre-exercise intake? Is hydration status markedly affected during exercise? What amount and type of fluid and/or food might be needed during exercise?
- What opportunities does the athlete have to consume fluid and foods during the event? How is such food/fluid made available? What strategies can be undertaken to improve availability and opportunity?
- What factors interfere with post-exercise eating? How can foods and fluids be made available to the athlete?
- What are the current nutritional beliefs of athletes in this sport?
- What are the current competition practices of the athletes, or a particular athlete, in this sport?
- Where do athletes in this sport commonly seek their nutrition information and advice?

Source: Burke 2007

- Information to provide answers to the questions raised in the tables may be obtained directly from the athlete or coach. However, there are other resources that allow the sports dietitian to learn more about the physiological requirements and practical challenges of specific sports. Many books have been written about individual sports, including texts that may specifically address physiological and training issues. Encyclopedias of sports are very useful in providing a brief summary of the main rules and features of the vast array of competitive and recreational sports. The Internet provides websites prepared by the governing bodies of various sports. In Australia, a directory of national sporting organizations can be obtained from the Australian Sports Commission. Direct contact with the executive or coaching directors of a sport can be useful and provide contacts with other sports nutrition, medicine or science professionals who are involved closely with that sport. There are also numerous reviews, textbooks and journal articles that address the applied physiology of individual sports. The resources listed at the end of the chapter provide useful information about the physiological and nutritional demands of selected sports.
- The following example illustrates how a sound understanding of the nutritional requirements and practical challenges of a sport can assist the sports dietitian to provide relevant and accurate dietary advice to an athlete.

An Ironman triathlete requests information about the amounts of energy, CHO and fluid intake he needs to consume during a race, providing the sports dietitian with information about his event (3.8 km swim, 180 km cycle and 42.2 km run). More detailed knowledge about the energy costs of the race, likely sweat losses and available race supplies (such as foods and drinks available at aid stations) would enable the sports dietitian to provide the athlete with specific and practical advice. Kimber and colleagues (2002) investigated the nutritional needs and practices of triathletes participating in an Ironman race and reported that males expended around 10 000 kcal (42 MJ) over the race, but only consumed around 4000 kcal (16.8 MJ). Over 70% of this energy intake occurred during the cycle stage of the race. The observed intake of CHO during the race was about 1.3 g/kg body mass per hour during the cycle leg and 0.8 g/kg/h during the run from a range of foods and drinks. This information provides the sports dietitian with some approximate fuel intake targets to achieve during the race, and highlights the importance of the cycle stage to maximize nutrient intake and provide fuel for the marathon run.

BIBLIOGRAPHY OF REVIEWS OF APPLIED PHYSIOLOGY OF SPORTS

Anderson RE, Montgomery DL. Physiology of alpine skiing. Sports Med 1988;6:210–21.

Bangsbo J. Team sports. In: RJ Maughan, ed. Nutrition in sport. Oxford: Blackwell Science, 2000:574–87.

Benardot D. Gymnastics. In: RJ Maughan, ed. Nutrition in sport. Oxford: Blackwell Science, 2000: 588–608.

Bentley DJ, Cox GR, Green D, Laursen PB. Maximising performance in triathlon: applied physiological and nutritional aspects of elite and non-elite competitions. J Sci Med Sport 2008; 11:407–16.

Berg K. Endurance training and performance in runners. Sports Med 2003;33:9–73.

Burke LM. Court and indoor team sports. In: Practical sports nutrition. Champaign, Illinois: Human Kinetics Inc, 2007:221–39.

Burke LM. Field-based team sports. In: Practical sports nutrition. Champaign, Illinois: Human Kinetics Inc, 2007:185–219.

Burke LM. Gymnastics. In: Practical sports nutrition. Champaign, Illinois: Human Kinetics Inc, 2007:313–33.

Burke LM. Middle and long distance running. In: Practical sports nutrition. Champaign, Illinois: Human Kinetics Inc, 2007:109–39.

Burke LM. Nutritional practices of male and female endurance cyclists. Sports Med 2001;31:521–32.

Burke LM. Practical sports nutrition. Champaign, Illinois: Human Kinetics Inc, 2007.

Burke LM. Racket sports. In: Practical sports nutrition. Champaign, Illinois: Human Kinetics Inc, 2007:241–64.

Burke LM. Road cycling and the triathlon. In: Practical sports nutrition. Champaign, Illinois: Human Kinetics Inc, 2007:71–108.

Burke LM. Sprinting and jumping. In: Practical sports nutrition. Champaign, Illinois: Human Kinetics Inc, 2007:169–84.

Burke LM. Strength and power sports. In: Practical sports nutrition. Champaign, Illinois: Human Kinetics Inc, 2007:265–87.

Burke LM. Swimming and rowing. In: Practical sports nutrition. Champaign, Illinois: Human Kinetics Inc, 2007:141–67.

Burke LM. Weight-making sports. In: Practical sports nutrition. Champaign, Illinois: Human Kinetics Inc, 2007:289–312.

Burke LM. Winter sports. In: Practical sports nutrition. Champaign, Illinois: Human Kinetics Inc, 2007:335–58.

Burke LM, Cox G. The complete guide to food for sports performance. Third edition. Sydney: Allen and Unwin, 2010.

Douda HT, Toubekis AG, Avloniti AA, Tokmakidis SP. Physiological and anthropometric determinants of rhythmic gymnastics performance. Int J Sports Physiol Perform. 2008;3:41–54.

Duthrie G, Pyne DB, Hooper S. Applied physiology and game analysis of rugby union. Sports Med 2003; 33:973–1001.

Ebert TR. Nutrition for the Australian Rules football player. J Sci Med Sport 2000;3:369–82.

Eisenman PA, Johnson SC, Bainbridge CN, Zupan MF. Applied physiology of cross-country skiing. Sports Med 1989;8:67–79.

Ekblom B. Applied physiology of soccer. Sports Med 1986;3:50–60.

Ekblom B, Bergh U. Cross-country skiing. In: RJ Maughan, ed. Nutrition in sport. Oxford: Blackwell Science, 2000:656–62.

Ekblom B, Williams C, eds. Foods, nutrition and soccer performance. J Sports Sci 1994;12 (special issue).

Faria IE. Applied physiology of cycling. Sports Med 1984;1:187–204.

Gabbett T. Science of rugby league football: a review. J Sports Sci 2005; 23:961–76.

Gabbett T, King T, Jenkins D. Applied physiology of rugby league. Sports Med 2008;38:119–38.

Groppel JL, Robert EP. Applied physiology of tennis. Sports Med 1992;14:260–8.

Hagerman FC. Applied physiology of rowing. Sports Med 1984;1:303–26.

Hargreaves M. Racquet sports. In: RJ Maughan, ed. Nutrition in sport. Oxford: Blackwell Science, 2000:632–6.

Hausswirth C, Brisswalter J. Strategies for improving performance in long duration events: Olympic distance triathlon. Sports Med. 2008;38: 881–91.

Hawley JA, Schabort EJ, Noakes TD. Distance running. In: RJ Maughan, ed. Nutrition in sport. Oxford: Blackwell Science, 2000:550–61.

Hoff J, Helgerud J. Endurance and strength training for soccer players. Sports Med 2004;34:165–78.

Hoffman JR. The applied physiology of American Football. Int J Sports Physiol Perform 2008;3:387–92.

Horswill CA. Applied physiology of amateur wrestling. Sports Med 1992;14:114– 43.

Jeukendrup AE. Cycling. In: RJ Maughan, ed. Nutrition in sport. Oxford: Blackwell Science, 2000: 562–73.

Jeukendrup AE, Craig NP, Hawley JA. The bioenergetics of world class cycling. J Sci Med Sport 2000;3:414–33.

Jeukendrup AE, Jentjens RL, Moseley L. Nutritional considerations in triathlon. Sports Med 2005;35: 163–81.

Kimber NE, Ross JJ, Mason SL, Speedy DB. Energy balance during an ironman triathlon in male and female triathletes. Int J Sport Nutr Exerc Metab 2002;12:47–62.

Lamb DR, Knuttgen HG, Murray R. Perspectives in exercise science and sports medicine.Vol 7: Physiology and nutrition for competitive sport. Carmel: Cooper Publishing Group, 1994.

Lavoie J, Montpetit R. Applied physiology of swimming. Sports Med 1986;3:165–89.

Lees A. Science and the major racket sports: a review. J Sports Sci 2003;21:707–32.

Lin YC. Applied physiology of diving. Sports Med 1988;5:74–98.

Lucia A, Earnest C, Arribas C. The Tour de France: a physiological review. Scand J Med Sci Sports 2003;13:275–83.

Maestu J, Jurimae J, Jurimae T. Monitoring of performance and training in rowing. Sports Med 2005;35:597–617.

Maughan RJ, Horton ES, eds. Current issues in nutrition in athletics. J Sports Sci 1995;13(special issue).

Mendez-Villanueva A, Bishop D. Physiological aspects of surfboard riding performance. Sports Med 2005;35:55–70.

Meyer NL, Parker-Simmons S. Nutrition for winter sports. In: Burke LM, Practical sports nutrition. Champaign, Illinois: Human Kinetics Inc, 2007:335–58.

Montgomery DL. Physiology of ice hockey. Sports Med 1988;5:99–126.

Montpetit RR. Physiology of squash. Sports Med 1990;10:31–41.

Mujika I, Padilla S. Physiological and performance characteristics of male professional road cyclists. Sports Med 2001;31:479–87.

Nicholas CW. Sprinting. In: RJ Maughan, ed. Nutrition in sport. Oxford: Blackwell Science, 2000: 535–49.

O'Toole ML, Douglas PS. Applied physiology of triathlon. Sports Med 1995;19:251–67.

O'Toole ML, Douglas PS, Hiller WBD. Applied physiology of triathlon. Sports Med 1989;8:201–25.

Rehrer NJ. Fluid and electrolyte balance in ultra-endurance sport. Sports Med 2001;31:701–15.

Reilly T, Borrie A. Physiology applied to field hockey. Sports Med 1992;14:10–26.

Reilly T, Drust B, Clarke N. Muscle fatigue during football match-play. Sports Med 2008;38(5):357–67.

Reilly T, Secher N, Snell P, Williams C, eds. Physiology of sports. London: E & FN Spon, 1990.

Rogozkin VA. Weightlifting and power events. In: RJ Maughan, ed. Nutrition in sport. Oxford: Blackwell Science, 2000:621–31.

Sharp RL. Swimming. In: RJ Maughan, ed. Nutrition in sport. Oxford: Blackwell Science, 2000:609–20.

Shephard RJ. Science and medicine of canoeing and kayaking. Sports Med 1987;4:19–33.

Smith HK. Applied physiology of water polo. Sports Med 1998;26:317–34.

Snyder AC, Faster C. Skating. In: RJ Maughan, ed. Nutrition in sport. Oxford: Blackwell Science, 2000:646–55.

Sparling RB, Nieman DC, O'Connor PJ. Selected scientific aspects of marathon racing. Sports Med 1993;15:116–32.

Stolen T, Chamari K, Castagna C, Wisloff U. Physiology of soccer: an update. Sports Med 2005;35: 501–36.

Townes DA. Wilderness medicine: strategies for provision of medical support for adventure racing. Sports Med 2005;35:557–64.

Tumilty D. Physiological characteristics of elite soccer players. Sports Med 1993;16:80–96.

Wilmore JH. Weight category sports. In: RJ Maughan, ed. Nutrition in sport. Oxford: Blackwell Science, 2000:637–45.

References

Allen DG, Lännergren J, Westerblad H. Muscle cell function during prolonged activity: cellular mechanisms of fatigue. Exp Physiol 1995;80:497–527.

Brooks GA. The lactate shuttle during exercise and recovery. Med Sci Sports Exerc 1986;18:360–8.

Burke LM. Practical sports nutrition. Champaign, Illinois: Human Kinetics Inc, 2007.

Calbet JAL, Jensen-Urstad M, Van Hall G, Holmberg H-C, Rosdahl H, Saltin B. Maximal muscular vascular conductances during whole body upright exercise in humans. J Physiol 2004;558:319–31.

Chin E, Allen DG. Effects of reduced muscle glycogen concentration on force, Ca^{2+} release and contractile protein function in intact mouse skeletal muscle. J Physiol 1997;498:17–29.

Clifford PS, Hellsten Y. Vasodilatory mechanisms in contracting skeletal muscle. J Appl Physiol 2004;97:393–403.

Costill DL, Daniels J, Evans W, Fink WJ, Krahenbuhl G, Saltin B. Skeletal muscle enzymes and fibre composition in male and female track athletes. J Appl Physiol 1975;40:149–54.

Coyle EF. Substrate utilization during exercise in active people. Am J Clin Nutr 1995;61 (4 Suppl):968S–79S. Review.

Coyle EF, Coggan AR, Hopper MK, Walters TJ. Determinants of endurance in well-trained cyclists. J Appl Physiol 1988;64:2622–30.

Coyle EF, Montain SJ. Benefits of fluid replacement with carbohydrate during exercise. Med Sci Sport Exerc 1992;24(Suppl):324S–30S.

Favero TG. Sarcoplasmic reticulum Ca^{2+} release and muscle fatigue. J Appl Physiol 1999;87:471–83.

Febbraio M, Snow RJ, Hargreaves M, Stathis CG, Martin IK, Carey MF. Muscle metabolism during exercise and heat stress in trained men: effect of acclimation. J Appl Physiol 1994;76:589–97.

Fitts RH. Cellular mechanisms of muscle fatigue. Physiol Rev 1994;74:49–94.

Fortney S, Vroman NB. Exercise, performance and temperature control: temperature regulation during exercise and implications for sports performance and training. Sports Med 1985;2:8–29.

Gandevia SC. Spinal and supraspinal factors in human muscle fatigue. Physiol Rev 2001;81;1725–89.

Gisolfi CV, Duchman SM. Guidelines for optimal replacement beverages for different athletic events. Med Sci Sports Exerc 1992;24:679–87.

González-Alonso J, Calbet JAL, Nielsen B. Muscle blood flow is reduced with dehydration during prolonged exercise in humans. J Physiol 1998;513:895–905.

González-Alonso J, Teller C, Andersen SL, Jensen F, Hyldig T, Nielsen B. Influence of body temperature on the development of fatigue during prolonged exercise in the heat. J Appl Physiol 1999; 86:1032–9.

Greenhaff PL. The nutritional biochemistry of creatine. Nutr Biochem 1997;8:610–18.

Hamilton MT, González-Alonso J, Montain SJ, Coyle EF. Fluid replacement and glucose infusion during exercise prevents cardiovascular drift. J Appl Physiol 1991;71:871–7.

Hargreaves M. Carbohydrate metabolism and exercise. In: Garrett WE, Kirkendall DT, eds. Exercise and sport science. New York: Lippincott Williams & Wilkins, 2000:3–8.

Hargreaves M. Metabolic responses to carbohydrate ingestion: effects on exercise performance. In: Lamb DR, Murray R, eds. Perspectives in exercise science and sports medicine. Vol 12: The metabolic bases of performance in sport and exercise. Carmel: Cooper Publishing Group, 1999:93–119.

Hargreaves M. Physiological benefits of fluid and energy replacement during exercise. Aust J Nutr Diet 1996;53(Suppl 4):3S–7S.

Hargreaves M, Angus D, Howlett K, Marmy-Conus N, Febbraio M. Effect of heat stress on glucose kinetics during exercise. J Appl Physiol 1996;81:1594–7.

Hawley JA, Brouns F, Jeukendrup AE. Strategies to enhance fat utilisation during exercise. Sports Med 1998;25:241–57.

Hawley JA, Schabort EJ, Noakes TD, Dennis SC. Carbohydrate-loading and exercise performance: an update. Sports Med 1997;24:73–81.

Katz A, Sahlin K. Regulation of lactic acid production during exercise. J Appl Physiol 1988;65:509–18.

Kimber NE, Ross JJ, Mason SL, Speedy DB. Energy balance during an ironman triathlon in male and female triathletes. Int J Sport Nutr Exerc Metab 2002;12:47–62.

Leppik JA, Aughey RJ, Medved I, Fairweather I, Carey MF, McKenna MJ. Prolonged exercise to fatigue in humans impairs skeletal muscle Na^+-K^+-ATPase activity, sarcoplasmic Ca^{2+} release and Ca^{2+} uptake. J Appl Physiol 2004;97:1414–23.

Li JL, Wang XN, Fraser SF, Carey MF, Wrigley TV, McKenna MJ. Effects of fatigue and training on sarcoplasmic reticulum Ca^{2+} regulation in human skeletal muscle. J Appl Physiol 2002;92:912–22.

Maughan RJ, Leiper JB, Shirreffs SM. Factors influencing the restoration of fluid and electrolyte balance after exercise in the heat. Br J Sports Med 1997;31:175–82.

McKenna MJ. The role of ionic processes in muscular fatigue during intensive exercise. Sports Med 1992;13:134–45.

Mitchell JH. Neural control of the circulation during exercise. Med Sci Sports Exerc 1990;22:141–54.

Nevill ME, Bogdanis GC, Boobis LH, Lakomy HKA, Williams C. Muscle metabolism and performance during sprinting. In: Maughan RJ, Shirreffs S, eds. Biochemistry of exercise IX. Champaign, Illinois: Human Kinetics Inc, 1996:243–59.

Parkin JM, Carey MF, Zhao S, Febbraio MA. Effect of ambient temperature on human skeletal muscle metabolism during fatiguing submaximal exercise. J Appl Physiol 1999;86:902–8.

Richardson RS. Oxygen transport and utilization: an integration of the muscle systems. Adv Physiol Educ 2003;27:183–91.

Romijn JA, Coyle EF, Sidossis LS, et al. Regulation of endogenous fat and carbohydrate metabolism in relation to exercise intensity and duration. Am J Physiol 1993;265:E380–91.

Sahlin K, Tonkonogi M, Söderlund K. Energy supply and muscle fatigue in humans. Acta Physiol Scand 1998;162:261–6.

Saltin B, Gollnick PD. Skeletal muscle adaptability: significance for metabolism and performance. In: Peachy LD, Adrian RH, Geiger SR, eds. Handbook of physiology, skeletal muscle. Bethesda: American Physiological Society, 1983:555–631.

Saltin B, Rådegran G, Koskolou MD, Roach R. Skeletal muscle blood flow in humans and its regulation during exercise. Acta Physiol Scand 1998;162:421–36.

Saltin B, Rowell LB. Functional adaptations to physical activity and inactivity. Fed Proc 1980;39: 1506–13.

Schantz P. Plasticity of human skeletal muscle. Acta Physiol Scand 1986;128(Suppl):558S.

Söderlund K, Hultman E. ATP and phosphocreatine changes in single human skeletal muscle fibres after intense electrical stimulation. Am J Physiol 1991;261:737–41.

Van Loon LJC. Use of intramuscular triacylglycerol as a substrate source during exercise in humans. J Appl Physiol 2004;97:1170–87.

Vøllestad NK, Blom PCS. Effect of varying intensity on glycogen depletion in human muscle fibres. Acta Physiol Scand 1985;125:395–405.

Vøllestad NK, Tabata I, Medbo JI. Glycogen depletion in different human muscle fibre types during exhaustive exercise of short duration. Acta Physiol Scand 1992;144:135–41.

Vøllestad NK, Vaage O, Hermansen L. Muscle glycogen depletion patterns in type I and subgroups of type II fibres during prolonged severe exercise in man. *Acta Physiol Scand* 1984;122:433–41.

Wasserman K, Beaver WL, Whipp BJ. Mechanisms and patterns of blood lactate increase during exercise in man. Med Sci Sports Exerc 1986;18:344–52.

Watt MJ, Heigenhauser GJF, Spriet LL. Intramuscular triacylglycerol utilization in human skeletal muscle during exercise: is there a controversy? J Appl Physiol 2002;93:1185–95.

Westerblad H, Allen DG, Lännergren J. Muscle fatigue: lactic acid or inorganic phosphate the major cause? News Physiol Sci 2002;17:17–21.

Zierath JR, Hawley, JA. Skeletal muscle fibre type: influence on contractile and metabolic properties. PLoS Biology 2004;2:E348.

CHAPTER 2

Measuring nutritional status of athletes: clinical and research perspectives

VICKI DEAKIN

2.1 Introduction

Nutritional status measurements provide an indicator of health and a benchmark to monitor athletes' responses to training from a dietary perspective. A nutritional status assessment of an individual athlete by a sports dietitian, in combination with a medical check-up, a musculo-skeletal assessment and a psychological assessment, have now become routine for many sporting organizations at the start of a training season. Each health professional plays a role in screening athletes and detecting potential short- and long-term problems and helping the athlete to maximize his or her training capacity. Many national and professional sports now provide such a team of sports science and medicine professionals to assess, treat and educate their athletes. Clearly, the focus for nutrition intervention has moved from a therapeutic to a preventive approach.

The purpose of nutrition assessment is to identify athletes at risk of diet-related problems. Coaches and athletes now recognize that symptoms such as lethargy, fatigue, poor performance capacity, poor concentration and slow recovery can be nutrition-related. Increased incidence of injury and infection and excessive gains or losses in body mass (BM) are also nutrition-related. Early detection of these symptoms and early dietary intervention can help prevent many problems. The goals of nutrition assessment are to:

- identify athletes who require nutritional support to restore or maintain nutritional status
- provide appropriate nutrition therapy (e.g. dietary intervention or education or behavioral change)
- monitor the progress and efficacy of dietary therapy

Measuring nutritional status is not just an evaluation of what a person eats and drinks, but involves a combination of several diagnostic procedures including social, medical and psychological influences on food choices; dietary analysis, physique and skinfold assessment; and an evaluation of biochemical measures of blood and urine.

The more information gathered, the more accurate the nutrition assessment will be. For example, an individual may have a history of an inadequate intake of dietary iron, but may not necessarily be anemic. Iron deficiency is confirmed in individuals when biochemical indicators in combination with clinical symptoms and history are evident.

This chapter focuses on the applications, strengths and limitations of methods used for measuring nutritional status in clinical practice and in research studies, and their relevance to athletes.

Dietary measurement 2.2

In clinical practice, dietary assessment involves collecting information on dietary intakes and then interpreting food or nutrient intakes against reference measures. Collecting dietary intake data and appropriately applying any population reference measure is not a simple process (as it may appear to the untrained observer), but one that requires care, precision and a high degree of skill and knowledge at all stages. The limitations of the methods of collecting and interpreting dietary intake data are not always fully appreciated or described in either clinical practice or journals. The focus of this section is not to consider in detail which method of measuring dietary intake is best suited to a clinical or research situation, but rather to focus on some of the key pitfalls and issues that should be considered when:

- collecting dietary intake data from individuals or groups of individuals, with particular emphasis on an athletic population
- interpreting or analyzing dietary data using population references

Data collection methods and nutrient reference standards for evaluating food or nutrient intakes may need to be modified when applying to an athlete population. Although athletes may have similar eating habits to non-athletes, their requirements for some nutrients and volume of food consumed may be higher. For example, standard serve sizes and predetermined serves on food frequency questionnaires (FFQs) are likely to be too small for an adolescent athlete who consumes large volumes of food. A dietitian should be aware of the eating habits, food quantities consumed, and the food attitudes and beliefs of different groups of athletes; all of these are important for providing nutrition intervention targeted to the specific needs and behaviors of each group. Such background data are also crucial to conduct quality research on dietary intakes, dietary attitudes and beliefs in any population group.

Why measure dietary intake? 2.3

Table 2.1 overleaf defines the broad uses and applications of measuring dietary intakes in athletes.

In research 2.4

The main method used to assess dietary/food/nutrient intakes of athletes has been food records using household measures, which are best suited to small samples (Burke et al. 2001, 2003). When assessing dietary intakes of groups, qualitative measures of food consumption can be used where ranking of foods or nutrient intake is the objective. Qualitative assessments (such as less fat, more carbohydrate, more meat and more fruit) are also useful when assessing the relative differences in dietary beliefs and attitudes in groups of athletes.

TABLE 2.1 USES AND APPLICATION OF MEASURING DIETARY INTAKES

USE	APPLICATION
Determining nutritional status	Calculating average nutrient intakes in population groups of athletes Comparing apparent adequacy of group nutrient intake with population nutrient standards Combining dietary intake assessment with other parameters (e.g. biochemical, anthropometric and medical) to assess nutritional status of individuals and groups
Assessing the links with performance, diet and health status	Comparing and contrasting indices of nutritional status with the incidence and prevalence of health problems or performance measures in groups
Evaluating nutrition education and intervention	Providing feedback on the efficacy of dietary intervention programs in individuals or groups of athletes
Assessing the effect of different dietary regimens on performance measures or metabolic responses	Determining potential ergogenic effects of diets, components of diets or supplements
Assessing the effect of different training periods or intensities on dietary intake	Determining the turnover of nutrient requirements at different training intensities and duration in combination with other parameters

FFQs, although more suitable than food records for surveying larger samples, have been infrequently used in dietary surveys of athletes. Where FFQs have been used, researchers have mostly adapted questionnaires that have been validated in other population groups, to match the eating habits of the athletes surveyed (for more detail, see Fogelholm & Lahti-Koski 1991; Hinton et al. 2004; Ward et al. 2004; and section 2.9).

There is a real need to develop and validate dietary assessment tools specifically for use in athletes in both clinical practice and research. Rather than developing and validating new FFQs or rapid dietary assessment methods, most researchers use modifications of previously validated dietary survey instruments, such as FFQs. Ideally any previously validated FFQ or rapid dietary assessment tool that has subsequently been modified for use in another population, such as athletes, should be re-validated in that population, particularly if changes to the original food list are substantial. However, the difficulties inherent in collecting accurate information on food intake in human subjects and the logistics and cost associated with the design, sampling and implementation of any validity study probably preclude the development and validation of new FFQs in athletes. A large sample size is needed.

2.5 In clinical practice

Collecting dietary intake data on individuals in clinical practice has several objectives: to assess the probability of inadequate nutrient intakes or inappropriate food choices, for intervention of risk-related dietary behaviors or to evaluate dietary intervention. The outcome of dietary assessment provides a benchmark to target appropriate food choice and dietary habits to achieve a desired change and assist in diagnosing diet-related problems.

2.6 How many days are needed to measure nutrient intakes with reliability?

The number of days needed to provide an estimate of average intake of nutrients with statistical confidence varies for different nutrients and also between individuals and groups. Based on 1 year of diet records in twenty-seven subjects (not athletes), a minimum of 3 days was required to capture usual intake of energy from the group, compared with an average of 27 days for individuals within that group (Basiotis et al. 1987). In the same study, protein, fat and carbohydrate (CHO) required 4, 6 and 5–6 days of recording food intake, respectively, to estimate average intake of the group. Estimating macronutrient intake in individuals and micronutrient intakes for a group or individuals requires much longer. Approaches and estimates for calculating the number of days required to determine or estimate micronutrient intakes are beyond the scope of this chapter and vary for different populations (for reviews, see Marr & Heady 1986; Basiotis et al. 1987; Buzzard 1998; Lee & Nieman 2002).

2.7 Techniques for measuring dietary intakes

Techniques for measuring dietary intake are categorized into two main types: current dietary intakes and past dietary intakes (retrospective short- or long-term recall of foods consumed) and have been reviewed elsewhere (see Marr 1971; Block 1982; Bingham et al. 1994; Lee & Nieman 2002). The main methods and their applications are summarized in Table 2.2. Sources of errors associated with these methods are found in section 2.11.

TABLE 2.2 APPLICATIONS, STRENGTHS AND LIMITATIONS OF DIETARY INTAKE METHODS FOR MEASURING DIETARY INTAKES IN GROUPS AND INDIVIDUALS

DATA COLLECTION METHOD	APPLICATION	STRENGTHS	LIMITATIONS
	CURRENT FOOD CONSUMPTION		
FOOD RECORDS			
Weighed method using scales or computerized approaches	Assess food choices and eating habits mostly from 1 to 7 days[a,b,c] with some exceptions (e.g. 1 year[c])	Is considered an accurate method[d,e]	Is time-consuming to conduct and analyze Requires trained personnel Requires literate and cooperative respondents Distorts food choice[b,k]
Estimated method using household measures	Acceptable for research because of better compliance than weighed method[g,h]	Provides information about eating habits Is fairly valid up to 5 days[h] Provides detailed information	Compliance is poor after four days[i,j] Is not representative of usual diet, unless repeated[l,m] Underestimates energy intake by 20–50%[f,k]

(continued)

TABLE 2.2 *(continued)*

DATA COLLECTION METHOD	APPLICATION	STRENGTHS	LIMITATIONS
	CURRENT FOOD CONSUMPTION		
FOOD RECORDS			
Duplicate food collections	Uses duplicate meals/ foods for direct chemical analysis	Is the most accurate method	Has high respondent burden Is expensive to analyze Distorts food choice Under-reporting[n] Other biases are poorly documented
FOOD CONSUMPTION IN THE PAST (RECALL METHODS)			
24-hour recall	Used mainly to rank food or nutrient intakes of groups of people	Allows for minimal distortion of food intake Has low respondent burden Has good response rate	Is not representative of usual intake of individuals unless repeated at random[o]
	Can be used to rank food and nutrient intakes of individuals, if food recording methods are repeated at random	Has low administration cost	Has memory/recall bias Underestimates total energy intakes[s]
Food frequency questionnaire	Used mainly for ranking usual food or nutrient intakes of groups of people in qualitative or semi-quantitative terms Used as a screening tool to detect, measure or rank specific nutrients or food intakes in groups or individuals Used as an adjunct to educating, documenting and modifying dietary behavior of individuals in clinics	Provides similar advantages to the 24-hour recall Measures usual diet and may be more representative of 'usual' intake than repeated diet records[g] Is quick to administer Is cost-effective	Has similar limitations to the 24-hour recall Is less accurate than food recording methods List of foods may not fully represent foods consumed by respondents Is difficult to quantify portion sizes Overestimates at low energy intake and in long-term studies[t,u] and underestimates at high energy intakes[j,p,q,r]
Dietary history	Combines a 24-hour diet recall and a FFQ Provides assessment of usual intakes of individuals in clinical practice	Provides comprehensive assessment of the usual nutrient intake, including seasonal changes	Is time-consuming to conduct Is dependent on a highly trained interviewer Is dependent on memory and cooperation of the respondent Tends to overestimate nutrient intakes[h]

Sources: [a]Block 1989; [b]Pekkarinen 1970; [c]Willett et al. 1987; [d]Marr 1971; [e]Bingham 1985; [f]Rutishauser 1988; [g]Lee & Neiman 2002, pp. 53–4, 58–9; [h]Bingham et al. 1988; [i]Daniels 1984; [j]Gersovitz et al. 1978; [k]Stockley 1985; [l]Willett 1998, p. 53; [m]Block 1989; [n]Lee-Han et al. 1989; [o]Sempos et al. 1992; [p]Stunkard & Waxman 1981; [q]Carter et al. 1981; [r]Faggiano et al. 1992; [s]Krall & Dwyer 1987; [t]Sorenson et al. 1985; [u]Larkin et al. 1989

Dietary intakes in the present (food record methods)

Where current diet is of interest, diet records (either weighed measures or estimated measures, using household measures) are mainly used.

Diet records

In research

Although there is no truly accurate measure of current dietary intake, except in a controlled environment, a diet record is considered the most accurate and feasible method for research (Bingham 1985). A weighed record is the gold standard against which other or new methods are compared or validated (Bingham 1987). Diet records, however, are not representative of usual diet unless repeated several times, usually 2 to 3 months apart, using non-consecutive random days (including weekends) and conducted over different seasons (Block 1989; Buzzard 1998).

Self-reported diet records involve weighing all foods and beverages consumed (including wastage) or estimating weights using standard household measures. One-to-seven-day periods are mostly used in population surveys (Block 1989), although surveys of up to 12 months of continuous diet recording have been conducted (Willett et al. 1987). In a review of dietary surveys of athletes by Burke and colleagues (2001), 3- or 4-day diet records using household measures were predominantly the method of choice. The number of days of data collection affects accuracy of responses. Periods longer than 3 to 4 days of food records reduce compliance and accuracy, and have a high drop-out rate (Daniels 1984; Krall & Dwyer 1987).

The main disadvantages of diet records as a research tool are that they take a long time to complete, and require a literate and cooperative respondent and a trained interviewer (Marr 1971). For a 4-day food record, the time required for collecting data equates to a 1-hour respondent training session, 30 min/d to complete and an additional 20-minute interview for review (Kristal et al. 1990).

Weighed food records are more accurate for measuring food intake than household measures, providing respondents are trained and motivated. Even in motivated subjects, poor compliance and a distortion of food choice limits their usefulness in providing a valid measure (Dennis & Shifflet 1985). Although records using household measures are less accurate, they have acceptable validity for use in research and are more representative of what people actually eat than weighed records (Lee & Nieman 2002). To enhance accuracy and decrease respondent error, it is essential to provide standard measuring cups and spoons and/or calibrated scales, or use grids, photographs of food or food models, rather than relying on respondents' perceptions (Rutishauser 1988).

A novel recording method using mobile phones with cameras is currently being refined as an alternative method for measuring current dietary intake (Weiss 2009). Such devices will provide objective dietary assessment that reduces the burden of recording and the bias of under-reporting. The images from digital photographs can be downloaded or marked with a variety of input methods to estimate the amount of food or beverage consumed. Early validation and reliability studies of these devices has shown promise, especially in measuring food intake in children (Martin et al. 2007).

In clinical practice

For assessment of food choices and eating patterns, 3 or 4 days of diet records, using estimated food record measures taken over consecutive days, are traditionally used.

Unfortunately, respondent inaccuracy in describing food portions is high and can deviate between 20% and 50% below the true weight (Rutishauser 1988), so an under-estimation of amounts consumed is an inherent problem.

Nevertheless, the advantages of using diet record methods in clinical practice are mainly to:

- raise awareness of eating habits
- provide a benchmark for evaluating diet and follow-up counseling
- provide a self-monitoring tool
- avoid the problems of memory bias

2.9 Dietary intakes in the past (recall methods)

24-hour recall

For a 24-hour recall, respondents are asked to remember and describe quantities of food and beverages consumed in the previous 24 hours (i.e. yesterday) and may include information on the timing of meals and snacks, eating environment and food preparation. Usually a 24-hour recall is administered by face-to-face or telephone interview or the respondent records the information in an open-ended format.

In research

Short-term recalls such as the 24-hour recall are used mainly in epidemiological research to estimate group rather than individual nutrient or food intakes. When 24-hour recalls are repeated a number of times at random (multi-pass method), they can be used to measure usual nutrient intake; this is the method of choice for large population surveys such as national surveys (Sempos et al. 1992; Holmes et al. 2008). Repeated application over multiple days of data collection also adjusts for individual variation in day-to-day nutrient intake (Sempos et al. 1985). Repeated 24-hour recalls are valuable aids in classifying dietary intake in groups of people and can provide an accurate assessment of an individual's food intake, if sufficient numbers of recalls are obtained. To date there are no data published using such repeated measures in large groups of athletes.

In 2005, the National Cancer Institute in the US began development of the 24-hour recall method into a web-based, automated, self-administered tool. This tool, called ASA24, which is based on using the multi-pass method used by the US National Health and Nutrition Surveys, will reduce the burden and cost of using trained professionals for data collection (Subar et al. 2009). It will be available free for professional use in the near future. Another similar web-based program for collecting 24-hour recall data, specifically designed for children, called the Food Intake Recording Software System or FIRSSt4, is also being refined in collaboration with the National Cancer Institute tool (Baranowski 2009), so may also be available for research use in the near future.

In clinical practice

Where usual dietary intake is erratic or inconsistent, which is not uncommon in adolescents and young adults, a 24-hour recall is useful and forms the basis for pursuing a broader or more detailed assessment of usual intake using a diet history.

Food frequency questionnaires

FFQs contain a predetermined food list, with or without portion sizes, plus a frequency response option for respondents to report how often (e.g. per day, week or month) each food was eaten. The questionnaire usually provides an opportunity for respondents to report on other foods not on the list and about food preparation, supplement use and other food-related behaviors. In its early form, the FFQ was designed as a qualitative method, seeking information on the frequency of consumption of specific food items without specification of the actual serve sizes consumed. Later forms of FFQs allowed more quantitative analyses using portion sizes, although the effect of this on improving accuracy is still equivocal.

In research

FFQs have been designed and validated in different population groups to retrospectively assess intakes of nutrients, specific foods or selected food groups consumed in the recent or distant past (24 hours to 20 years). The most common use is to measure usual diet of groups over 6 to 12 months.

FFQs have been adapted and validated for new and different uses in research other than to gain a picture of usual intake (e.g. as screening tools to detect or rank intake of one or several nutrients, foods or selected food groups). FFQs are infrequently used as a survey method in athletes despite their utility and widespread use in epidemiological research. The limited number of FFQs used in dietary surveys of athletes have used modifications of previously validated questionnaires (see Fogelholm & Lahti-Koski 1991; Hinton et al. 2004; Ward et al. 2004). Fogelholm and Lahti-Koski (1991) used a modified version of an FFQ by Pietinen and colleagues (1988) to measure intakes of selected micronutrients in 427 physically active young Finnish men. The modified version showed good agreement at the group level when validated against a 7-day food record in another population of eighty-four male athletes, but poor agreement in individuals (Fogelholm & Lahti-Koski 1991). More recently, Hinton and colleagues (2004) used a previously validated FFQ, the Youth Assessment Questionnaire, to measure the nutrient intakes of 345 college-aged athletes in the US. Only minor modifications were made to the original questionnaire so an independent reproducibility or validity study of the revised questionnaire was not undertaken or considered necessary. Ideally both reliability and validity of a FFQ should be tested with another similar population group rather than the test population, although this is not always feasible. Cade and colleagues (2004) have provided an excellent review of FFQs published between 1980 and 1999. From this work, and in collaboration with other experts, these authors have provided recommendations to assist researchers to improve the design, application and validation of new FFQs or to modify existing FFQs for use in different population groups (see Cade et al. 2004). For a detailed description of the basis for these recommendations, see Cade and colleagues (2002).

In clinical practice

FFQs are used in clinical practice for several purposes including:

- to evaluate the impact of dietary intervention counseling or intervention programs
- as an education resource, for self-help intervention
- to monitor compliance with diet intervention
- as a rapid screening tool or rapid assessment method for selected nutrients
- for a variety of clinical situations (such as recent large loss/gain of BM) where there is a need to gather dietary information over a short period of time
- to generate inexpensive and rapid behavioral feedback to an individual on dietary intake

Diet history

A diet history, originally described by Burke in 1947, involves a combination of a 24-hour recall and a FFQ to determine usual eating patterns. The original method also included a 3-day record, which Burke suggested was the least valuable component of the diet history (Burke 1947).

In research

Although a diet history provides a comprehensive assessment of the usual diet and can include seasonal influences, it is time-consuming, dependent on a skilled interviewer and relies on memory and the cooperation of the respondent (Block 1989). These factors limit its use in research.

In clinical practice

A modification of the original diet history, which takes about 20 minutes to complete, is the technique of choice used by most dietitians in clinical practice to assess usual dietary intake in individual athletes. Apart from assessing dietary intakes, a diet history provides an opportunity to explore the social, behavioral and medical influences on food choice and investigate an athlete's knowledge, beliefs and attitudes as well as their main sources of nutrition information.

2.10 Sources of error in dietary measurement

Error or bias is inherent in all dietary survey methods. Recognizing and reducing error when collecting and analyzing dietary intake data is crucial in both research and clinical practice. In research, the magnitude of errors should be addressed in dietary intake studies, although all too frequently this is overlooked (for review, see Beaton et al. 1997; Kipnis et al. 2002).

2.11 Sources of error common to all methods of dietary intake data collection

The largest source of error in collecting dietary intake data is respondent inaccuracy in either recalling or reporting actual food intake (Block 1989). The ability of any respondent, including athletes, to provide accurate dietary intake data depends on their motivation, literacy, memory, communication skills and awareness of food intake. The perception of foods eaten, both in type and quantity, is crucial to the success of data collection. Athletes are likely to give biased responses because they may not want to reveal inappropriate food choice to the coach or dietitian, or because they want to impress. Biased reporting towards socially desirable foods (such as fresh fruits and vegetables) rather than sweet or fatty foods is common in surveys of the general population (Worsley et al. 1984) and is likely to be similar or even more pronounced in athletes. The process of collecting dietary intake data also substantially distorts usual eating behavior (Marr 1971). Also the personality of the dietitian, the way questions are asked, possibly poor communication skills, and failure to develop rapport or gain the confidence of the athlete introduce response bias.

Most dietary survey methods, except the dietary history, under-estimate energy and nutrient intakes (see Table 2.2). Techniques used to check the magnitude of under-reporting that can be applied to a research or clinical situation are discussed in section 2.13.

Errors using food records 2.12

Few respondents are experts at recording food intake and providing accurate food records. Motivated and educated volunteers provide the most accurate and reliable food intake data (Black et al. 1991). Athletes are unlikely to be motivated or see the relevance of recording food intakes if someone else (such as a concerned coach or parent) has sent them to see a dietitian. Also, self-recording food intake changes eating behavior. It discourages snacking and inhibits spontaneous food selection and consumption of mixed meals, and consequently distorts true food intake. In one study, over 50% of respondents completing weighed food records freely admitted altering their intake because of inconvenience, being self-conscious or being ashamed (Macdiarmid & Blundell 1997). Athletes are usually far too busy to collect weighed records, especially if they perceive nutrition as a low priority and have not sought dietary assistance of their own accord.

Estimates of dietary intakes using household measures are more appropriate than weighed diet records for the busy athlete, although training athletes to quantify serve sizes and then cross-check these for accuracy after completion is warranted because of the difficulties in accurately reporting household measures.

Under-reporting, either intentionally or unintentionally, is highest using food records compared to other methods in surveys of the general population (Buzzard 1998). Similar under-reporting also occurs in athletes, although few studies have applied measures to check this. Based on the Goldberg equation (see section 2.18), under-estimates of energy (and hence nutrient) intake using food records have been reported in female endurance athletes (Haggarty et al. 1988; Schoeller 1995), in female gymnasts (Jonnalagadda et al. 2000), in cyclists in the Tour de France (Westerterp et al. 1986) and in Australian rugby players (Lundy et al. 2006).

Based on validity studies of energy intakes in the general population, under-reporting is highest in adolescents, women and in both sexes who are obese/overweight, conscious about their weight, and regularly follow weight-restriction diets (Livingstone & Black 2003). Under-reporting of up to 50% of energy intake has been reported in obese subjects (Lichtman et al. 1992) and is higher in African-Americans and Hispanics than Caucasians (Neuhouser et al. 2008). In elite athletes preoccupied with weight or in those who need to maintain a lean BM for their sport, distortion of energy intake is also likely to be high, although there is little research on athletes' responses to recording food intakes to confirm this assumption. In one study, 61% of gymnasts were classified as under-reporters (Jonnalagadda et al. 2000), which is not surprising for this sport.

Errors in recall methods 2.13

Recall methods tend to over-estimate the intakes of those with low energy intakes and underestimate intakes of those with high energy intakes compared with the food records (Gersovitz et al. 1978). Barr (1987) suggests that error could be a problem in athletes who consume habitually very low or very high energy intakes (such as ballet dancers and footballers). However, validity studies of recall methods used in athletes to confirm or refute this claim have not been undertaken.

FFQs that measure nutrients in the usual diet have been criticized for their lower accuracy compared with diet records and 24-hour recalls. Recall bias and varying abilities of respondents to remember past intake and quantify foods accurately are the main reasons for this. Respondents consistently have difficulty quantifying foods, particularly meat and breakfast cereals that are not presented in packaged serves (Willett 1998). Athletes are reported to be no different from the general population in this respect (Fogelholm & Lahti-Koski 1991). I have also observed large discrepancies in athletes' perceptions of weights of foods and volumes of beverages compared to actual weights and volumes, irrespective of age and gender.

2.14 Errors and limitations in converting foods into nutrients using food composition data

The conversion of food into nutrients is another major source of error in dietary surveys and is a reflection of the skills and knowledge of the researcher, the method of data collection and the food composition database. Translating foods into nutrients is not simply about multiplying the amount of food eaten by the nutrient for that food. A sound knowledge of food composition and skill in data collection and analysis is essential to undertake this task. Lack of specificity in the description of food or quantities consumed, together with insufficient knowledge about common preparation methods, edible portions, weight for volume and how to select foods that are not instantly matched by the food composition database, compound the error.

Food composition data do not contain the large number of foods that are consumed in real life, so inappropriate food substitutes, omission of foods and guesswork substantially distort accuracy. Defining a coding and food substitute protocol to address these issues is crucial for minimizing error before data analysis, especially in research.

Although researchers usually report the food composition database used in a study, few acknowledge other factors that might influence the accuracy of the nutrient analysis in their publications. When interpreting nutrient data derived from food composition data and entering food intake data for nutrient analysis, the following limitations should be recognized.

(a) Food composition data are only estimates of nutrient composition

Nutrient intakes calculated from food composition data are estimates only. Nutrient composition of any given food is not constant in a single raw food grown in the same environment. This variation is highest for micronutrients, especially ß-carotene, vitamin C and selenium, and also varies considerably for foods produced within the same country of origin (Cashel 1990). Natural, biological, geographical and agricultural factors affect the nutrient composition of raw foods, and different cooking and processing technologies introduce wider differences (Food Standards Agency 2002). Additives and brand names are not included, although some databases include commercial foods (e.g. take-aways and some standard recipes typical of the country of origin). In Australia and New Zealand, food composition data are based on foods as purchased.

(b) Food composition data are specific to the country of origin

Nutrient values documented in the Australian and New Zealand food composition database (Food Standards Australia New Zealand 2006), for example, are not appropriate for use in other countries because of differences in biological variants, agricultural practices and food regulations. Some data in this database are imported from the UK. Hence using food composition data from one country to analyze dietary intakes of athletes living in another country is unacceptable.

(c) Information on nutrients and foods is incomplete

Food composition data rapidly evolve because of changes to plant and animal breeding and to food regulation and processing techniques, and so do not contain all foods available for consumption in the country of origin or all nutrients in the foods selected for testing within that country. The cost of testing a rapidly changing food supply precludes comprehensive testing.

(d) Food composition data may require substitute foods

Where a specific food or ingredient is unavailable in the food composition tables, substitutes have to be made. When several substitutes are made, inaccuracy is compounded. No food should be assigned a blank or zero value in nutrient analysis, so an imputed substitute is mandatory and is a better approximation of the truth than a zero value (Willett & Buzzard 1998). Adding nutrient information from food labels to food composition data is not acceptable because labels do not have a complete representation of the nutrient composition of the food.

(e) Serve sizes are difficult to standardize

Athletes (and most people) do not necessarily eat the serve sizes described on food labels or specified in dietary analysis programs. Therefore use of the default serve size is inappropriate and requires manual changes to food weights/volumes on the program to avoid systematic error.

(f) There may be errors in coding

Inexperienced and untrained people can introduce many errors when coding and entering foods for nutrient analysis. Large differences in entering foods are also a problem for trained people. Even when using experienced sports dietitians to enter foods into a food composition database, substantial differences were reported between coders in a study designed to measure the magnitude of variability between coders who analyzed nutrient intakes from self-reported dietary intake records collected from Australian athletes in the 1996 Olympic team (Braakhuis et al. 2003). The coders were given no formal instructions or coding protocols when entering data, although strict protocols were given to respondents when recording food intake. Errors in coding were attributed to different interpretations of foods and food substitutes. The outcome of this study highlights the importance of developing coding protocols and cross-checking for translation error.

Methods used to measure under-reporting of dietary intakes 2.15

Misreporting is inherent in almost every dietary survey method. Most methods demonstrate a high frequency of under-reporting energy intakes (and hence nutrient intakes) when validated against more accurate measures. Several external measures or criteria are used to determine the extent of under-reporting of dietary intakes. These include the doubly labeled water method, biochemical indices and EI:BMR (see overleaf). For a comprehensive review of these external methods and their application see Livingston & Black (2003).

2.16 The doubly labeled water method for validating total energy intakes

The doubly labeled water (DLW) ($^{2}H_2{}^{18}O$) method is considered the gold standard for measuring free-living energy expenditure and validating other methods for assessing energy intake. Subjects drink water containing a load dose of stable isotopes (deuterium $^{2}H_2$ and oxygen ^{18}O) and provide periodic urine samples to measure the rate of elimination of these isotopes. The uses and limitations of this technique are described in section 5.14. This method is expensive, as it requires specialized equipment and investigator training, and is not suitable for use in large dietary studies.

2.17 Validation of protein

The 24-hour urinary nitrogen test, a measure of nitrogen balance and hence protein balance, is well accepted for external evaluation of the validity of habitual food intake against the more accurate DLW method (Black et al. 1991; Bingham 1994). This test has been used extensively in clinical studies to verify protein intake. When agreement between urinary nitrogen excretion and estimated protein intake is acceptable, then intake of other nutrients is assumed to be fairly well represented (Lee & Nieman 2002). The validity of this test has not been established in athletes and theoretically could be distorted by the catabolic effects of training on nitrogen balance or use of protein supplements.

2.18 The ratio of energy intake to basal metabolic rate (EI:BMR)

A less expensive method to validate energy intakes than DLW and urinary nitrogen is reported energy intake (EI) divided by basal metabolic rate (BMR), originally described by Goldberg and colleagues in 1991. The final EI:BMR ratio determines whether reported energy intakes using a food record method are consistent with energy intakes required for a person to live a normal (not bed-bound) lifestyle (McLennan & Podger 1998). This ratio is represented by minimum cut-off values derived from whole body calorimetry and DLW measurements for determining energy expenditure (Goldberg et al. 1991). The cut-off limits for the EI:BMR ratio are adjusted for sample size and duration of measurement of dietary intakes (Goldberg et al. 1991). These researchers defined two categories for cut-off values: those based on habitual or usual intake (cut-off 1) and those based on actual intake over a specified measurement period as used in food records (cut-off 2). For example, a sample size for one individual using a 3-day diet record can be assessed using cut-off 2. BMR is estimated using predictive equations. For athletes, the Cunningham equation is the best predictor where lean body mass (LBM) or fat-free mass (FFM) is available. Where only height and BM are available, the Harris–Benedict equation is recommended (see Chapter 5).

In summary, although the EI:BMR ratio is crude and dependent on estimates of BMR, which are themselves inaccurate, this method is well accepted in research and clinical practice for checking under-reporting of dietary intakes in individuals and groups.

2.19 Criteria for interpreting dietary intakes

Several criteria are used to interpret dietary intake data. The criteria chosen depend on the objectives for collecting data. Dietary guidelines and food guides provide a qualitative means of evaluating diet as well as educating both athletes and the general population about food choice. Population nutrient references can be applied to interpreting dietary intakes of athletes in most circumstances, although for some nutrients there are specific and absolute benchmarks, which are described in sections 2.20–2.24 below.

Nutrient targets/goals for athletes 2.20

Absolute quantitative amounts (in grams: g) of CHO and protein intakes are now accepted as a benchmark for recommending and assessing nutrient intakes in athletes. These values can be adjusted for BM and type, intensity and duration of physical activity (see Chapters 4 and 13).

In dietary surveys of athletes, CHO (and other macronutrient intakes) have been reported in numerous ways: from absolute amounts usually g/d, percent of energy from macronutrient to total energy in the diet, and more recently in g CHO/kg or in nutrient density terms (g CHO/1000 kJ). Adjusting for energy and BM standardizes these values and makes comparison between athletes and controls more meaningful.

Dietary guidelines 2.21

Dietary guidelines are qualitative, individual statements relating to the diet that describe the major areas of dietary change needed to help people achieve an improvement in food choice and lifestyle (e.g. eat plenty of vegetables, legumes and fruits; be physically active; and eat according to your energy needs). Dietary guidelines translate nutritional recommendations into practical advice to consumers about food choice. Most western-style countries have devised dietary guidelines for this purpose. The rationale for dietary guidelines is to improve the nutritional health of the population by helping to reduce the risk of chronic nutrition-related diseases.

Revised dietary guidelines have been released in Australia for adults, and children and adolescents (NHMRC 2003a, 2003b), Canada (Health Canada 2009), and the US in January 2005 (see http://www.healthierus.gov/dietaryguidelines/). The Australian dietary guidelines are currently under revision and due for release in late 2010 (see http://www.nhmrc.gov.au/your_health/healthy/nutrition/index.htm).

Dietary guidelines provide a baseline for consistent nutrition education messages to the consumer. These same messages are appropriate for nutrition education of athletes and are used by dietitians in combination with food guides when assessing the nutrient density of the diet and advising athletes about food choice.

Food guides 2.22

Food guides are nutrition education tools and guides for consumers that build a diet from food groups that are similar in origin and nutrient content. These food groups contain recommendations for a suggested number of serves from each group, and can assist consumers to plan and select a nutritionally desirable diet consistent with the dietary guidelines. Most countries have devised food selection guides specific to the food supply, nutrient recommendations and cultural needs of their population. Examples of food guides used in Australia are the Nutrition Foundation's food pyramid/core food groups (Cashel & Jeffreson 1995) and *The Australian guide to healthy eating* (Smith et al. 1998), currently under revision. Similar food guides are used in other countries, for example, *MyPyramid*

(US) (http://www.mypyramid.gov) and *Food guide for healthy eating* (Canada) (http://www.hc-sc.gc.ca/fn-an/food-guide-aliment/index-eng.php).

2.23 Food composition data

The most recent version of the Australia and New Zealand food composition analytical database (Food Standards Australia New Zealand 2006) is available online. Another online food composition database called AUSNUT 2007 contains compilation data from several sources including NUTTAB 2006 as well as earlier NUTTAB data, imported data from the US and data from commercial foods and recipes. This database was developed for estimating nutrient intakes in the 2007 National Children's Nutrition and Physical Activity Survey in Australia but is not as accurate as the primary database NUTTAB 2006.

Errors and limitations of using food composition data were discussed in section 2.14 and are important to consider when interpreting nutrient intakes. For example, lack of specificity in the description of food and quantities, and the use of substitutes for missing foods on the database, decrease accuracy. Considerable food knowledge by users of food composition data is important for entering the most representative food.

2.24 Population nutrient standards: are they relevant to athletes?

Population nutrient standards termed Nutrient Reference Values (NRV) in Australia and New Zealand and Dietary Reference Intakes (DRI) in the US and Canada are available for essential macro- and micronutrients (Commonwealth Department of Health and Ageing et al. 2006; Institute of Medicine 2000a). In the past, one nutrient standard was used to represent the amount of a nutrient needed to prevent deficiency and meet the nutrient requirements of most (97–98%) of the population (Institute of Medicine 2000b). This standard was termed Recommended Dietary Intake (RDI) in Australia and New Zealand, Recommended Dietary Allowance (RDA) in the US and Recommended Nutrient Intake (RNI) in Canada. The revised nutrient reference values (i.e. DRI/NRV) are broader in scope and application than RDA/RDI/RNI and include multiple levels of nutrient standards based on four nutrient-based reference values: Estimated Average Requirements (EAR); Adequate Intake (AI); and Upper Level of Intake (UL) in Australia and New Zealand, or Upper Intake Level (UIL) in the US and Canada. The objective of these new levels is to shift the emphasis from preventing nutrient deficiency to decreasing the risk of chronic diet-related diseases in the population.

Irrespective of these multiple levels of nutrient standards and differences in terminology between countries, the applications are similar (see Table 2.3).

For an individual and group, the EAR is considered the best estimate of a nutrient requirement (Institute of Medicine 2000b; Murphy & Poos 2002). Although EARs may not be applicable for athletes without some adjustment, they can serve as a benchmark to examine the probability that usual nutrient intake is 'inadequate' or 'adequate' for an individual athlete or for groups of athletes (Institute of Medicine 2000b). Where an EAR is unavailable for a nutrient, AI is used for individual assessment. The RDI or AI is used to indicate the intake at which, or above which, there is a low probability of inadequacy (Commonwealth Department of Health and Ageing et al. 2006). The AI is of limited

TABLE 2.3 RECOMMENDED USES OF DRI/NRV FOR ASSESSING INDIVIDUALS AND GROUPS

FOR AN INDIVIDUAL	FOR A GROUP
EAR: Examines the probability that usual intake of a nutrient is inadequate	**EAR:** Estimates the prevalence of inadequate nutrient intake within a group
RDA/RDI: Usual intake of a nutrient at or above this level has a low probability of inadequacy	**RDA/RDI:** Do not use to assess nutrient intake of groups
AI: Usual intake of a nutrient at or above this level has a low probability of nutrient inadequacy	**AI:** Mean usual intake at or above this level implies a low prevalence of inadequate nutrient intakes
UL/UIL: Usual nutrient intake above this level may place an individual at risk of adverse effects from excessive nutrient intake	**UL/UIL:** Estimates the percentage of the population at potential risk of adverse effects from excessive nutrient intake

DRI = Dietary Reference Intakes (US and Canada), NRV = Nutrient Reference Values (Australia & New Zealand), EAR = Estimated Average Requirements, RDA = Recommended Dietary Allowance, RDI = Recommended Dietary Intake, AI = Adequate Intake, UIL = Tolerable Upper Intake Level (US/Canada), UL = Upper Level of Intake (Australia)
Source: Adapted from Institute of Medicine 2000b

value in assessing nutrient adequacy and should not be used to assess the prevalence of inadequacy (Murphy & Poos 2002). For detailed information about the derivation, use, limitations and interpretation of the DRI for use in assessing nutrient adequacy in research or clinical practice, see the Institute of Medicine report (2000a). For a summary of these applications for use in dietary assessment, see Murphy & Poos (2002) and Murphy and colleagues (2006).

Using the DRI/NRV for *planning* diets for individuals and groups is more complex and requires a different approach. Providing guidelines to plan diets for groups or individual athletes using these benchmarks is beyond the scope of this chapter. For reviews and guidelines, see Murphy and Barr 2005) and Institute of Medicine (2003).

There are further limitations to applying population nutrient reference values for assessing apparent nutrient inadequacy in an athlete population, if the physical characteristics and energy demands of the athlete group deviate substantially from the general population. Athletes involved in strenuous endurance training or with a large BM, for example, are likely to need higher intakes of micronutrients than suggested by population EAR values, although definitive recommendations have not yet been established. Recent evidence supports a slight increase in some micronutrient requirements for athletes involved in strenuous endurance training compared to non-athletes, to compensate for high nutrient turnover and increases in free radical formation induced by exercise (see Chapter 11). However, this evidence is based mainly on biochemical and physiological indices of micronutrients, which are highly variable between individual athletes and often difficult to interpret. Of the micronutrients investigated, nutrient requirements (not recommendations) for antioxidant vitamins (C, E and ß-carotene), B group vitamins, magnesium, zinc and iron may need to be slightly higher in athletes than non-athletes, but are unlikely to exceed RDAs/RDIs. More research is needed on large groups of athletes participating in different sports to allow micronutrient recommendations to be quantified.

Evidence for slightly higher macronutrient requirements (protein and CHO) for endurance athletes compared to non-athletes is well documented (see Chapters 4 and 13). Definitive quantitative targets are specified for these nutrients for those athletes involved in endurance and power sports and are recommended for use in preference to population nutrient standards or population goals and targets.

In summary, the DRI/NRV for micronutrients are appropriate for most athletes, because of the wide safety margins for nutrient recommendations (American College of Sports Medicine et al. 2000). Adjustment may need to be made for some nutrients in athletes with very high energy expenditures or diets that have poor nutrient bioavailability (such as vegetarian diets). For example, the EAR for iron is 1.3–1.7 times higher for athletes and 1.8 times higher for vegetarians (non-athletes) to account for low bioavailability (Institute of Medicine 2000a).

2.25 Clinical examination and medical history

The purpose of a clinical examination is to uncover any medical condition or physiological factors that interfere with food intake, digestion and metabolism. Recent or chronic illness, anxiety, depression and some drugs interfere with absorption of nutrients and thus affect nutritional status. Diarrhea, loss of appetite, gastrointestinal disturbances and BM loss could be associated with an underlying illness. Psychosocial stress also affects appetite and eating behavior. However, loss of appetite is a normal physiological response for some athletes for up to 1 to 2 hours after hard workouts. Some athletes also experience discomfort or nausea when food is consumed before strenuous exercise, and may avoid eating anything for 2 or more hours before training. This behavior can certainly affect an athlete's recovery and ability to meet daily nutrient and energy requirements.

2.26 Biochemical analysis

Although biochemical tests are objective and used as external criteria for validating dietary intake methods, they are not necessarily diagnostic of nutrient depletion or deficiency (for review see Lee & Nieman 2002).

Low blood levels of some micronutrients may reflect low dietary intake, defective absorption, increased utilization or excretion. As well, biomarkers for many nutrients have large diurnal variations (e.g. serum iron) or are under such strict homeostatic control (e.g. calcium) that interpretation is misleading (Fogelholm 1995). Biochemical indices and their interpretation in an athletic population are discussed in detail in other chapters: vitamins and minerals (see Chapter 11), iron (see Chapter 10), protein (see Chapter 4) and calcium (see Chapter 9).

Population reference ranges for biochemical indicators are still used in clinical practice and research studies of athletes. These standards may be inapplicable for athletes involved in strenuous training with high turnover or losses of some nutrients, and therefore need some adjustment.

Several diagnostic criteria should be investigated to establish the micronutrient status of an individual in a clinical situation. A single biochemical analysis representing a nutrient imbalance may not necessarily be diagnostic of a clinical or even subclinical condition. Use of several biochemical tests rather than one test gives more reliable information about individuals and may reveal trends. Nutrient depletion or deficiency from biochemical tests is confirmed in individuals when large deviations from their usual level or from the population reference level are seen.

Anthropometric assessment 2.27

Anthropometry involves the application of physical measurements to appraise human size, shape, proportion, body composition, maturation and gross function. These measurements are useful to reflect both growth and development of children and adolescents and give some indication of body composition in adults. They are also useful as an indication of moderate to severe under-nutrition or overweight or obesity.

Physical measurements, including height, BM, skinfolds, mid-arm muscle circumference, girth and frame size, are well-recognized measures used by dietitians and kinanthropometrists. These are used indirectly to estimate body composition and predict estimates of energy requirements. Comparison of height and BM parameters with 'ideal' or reference standards such as the body mass index (BMI) (height (m)/weight (kg)^2) is inappropriate for many athletes. Those athletes with a large muscle bulk are categorized by these standards as overweight or, in some cases, obese, despite having low body fat. BMI and growth charts for children and adolescents can be useful for showing very lean athletes that they are not overweight. These measures provide no true or reliable indication of body composition.

The sum of skinfold measures is a practical, inexpensive and reliable method to estimate body fat or to monitor changes in body composition of athletes over time, so it is particularly useful in a clinical situation. Other methods for measuring body composition are described in Chapter 3. Using absolute values for skinfolds, such as the sum of six to eight skinfold sites, is preferable to using the numerous equations that calculate body fat percentage used extensively in the past. Because these equations are derived from cadavers and assume that the fat mass (FM) has the same density as the FFM—an invalid assumption—they are no longer favored. Chapter 3 provides normative skinfold data on elite athletes for comparison.

Summary 2.28

The collection of nutritional status measures in sportspeople is critical to our understanding of the association between nutrition, health and sports performance. Data collection of such measures requires highly trained people who are familiar with the protocols for data collection and limitations in collecting and interpreting these data.

In dietary assessment of groups or individuals, only estimates of food or nutrient intakes of athletes are possible. Therefore techniques chosen for evaluating food or nutrient intakes are related to the intended purpose of the dietary assessment and the data collection method used.

To improve accuracy when collecting food intake data, researchers and dietitians need to be familiar with the dietary habits of athletes so that appropriate serves and quantities of food likely to be consumed can be better quantified. Despite the use of food models and other techniques for improving accuracy of data collection (such as training and standardized household measures), under-reporting and misreporting is a major problem in all dietary survey methods, although under-reporting can quickly be checked against the ratio EEI:BMR (see section 2.18).

Population standards for nutrients and biochemical indices can be applied to athletes, with caution, and with few exceptions. Because of the extensive research on CHO and protein intakes in athletes, specific recommended values for average daily intakes of these nutrients are available. More research is needed in varying groups of athletes before such recommendations can be made for micronutrient intakes, except perhaps iron. The recommended nutrient values for CHO, protein and iron represent the upper limits as they are derived from laboratory or field studies of mostly elite or semi-elite athletes involved in regular and often intensive training programs. Athletes involved in less rigorous training programs, or those involved in intermittent training, such as in team sports, are unlikely to need these upper limits.

Normative data on physique and skinfold measures in elite international- and national-level athletes involved in different sports are available elsewhere for comparative purposes (see Chapter 3). Again, comparison of these data with similar measurements of individuals needs to be interpreted with caution because of the large standard deviations observed. Clearly a large standard deviation between and within sports indicates a high variability in individual differences. Individuals may not fit within these normative data or have optimum physiques for their chosen sport but can still become world champions. Therefore, such values should not be the basis for prescriptive targets for BM and skinfolds, impossible for many individuals to attain.

In conclusion, assessment of nutrient adequacy or recommendations for nutrient requirements for any individual (or group) is imprecise and must be interpreted cautiously and in combination with biomedical and medical information.

PRACTICE TIPS

VICKI DEAKIN

COLLECTING INFORMATION

- The more information one has from a variety of sources (such as family, biochemical and medical) about an individual's eating behavior and about factors influencing eating behavior, the more reliable the assessment. Such comprehensive nutritional assessments are not always appropriate, necessary or feasible. Nutritional assessment can involve minimal to comprehensive screening, and can be tailor-made for an individual athlete or team.

DIETARY ASSESSMENT OF AN INDIVIDUAL ATHLETE

- Identify the athlete's reasons for dietary consultation early in the interview.
- Find out the athlete's attitude and beliefs about nutrition (e.g. have they been sent by the coach? Do they consider nutrition important in their training program?). Often their beliefs are based on the testimony from other athletes or convictions of their coaches.
- Make a preliminary assessment of expected outcomes of the dietary assessment—knowing what they expect to gain by seeing a dietitian is always helpful.
- Enquire about the type, intensity and duration of their training program and determine the influence of training on eating habits, timing of meals and food preparation (e.g. early-morning training sessions may mean that the athlete skips breakfast; late afternoon or early evening sessions are associated with a reliance on take-away foods). Allocating a scheduled time for shopping and cooking to fit in with the training program is a worthwhile strategy.
- Assessment of daily fluid intake is a critical factor and requires investigation even in cold climates. Cramps, for instance, are associated with low fluid intakes or high sweat rates. School-aged athletes often do not drink enough fluid at school and before training, and then tend to drink large volumes during and after training to compensate. Hydration kits are useful for checking urine color and hydration status and are routinely used at elite training centers.
- The use of vitamin and mineral supplements and other sports food supplements needs to be investigated during the interview. Often they are unnecessary and used inappropriately.
- Specific nutritional assessment forms (e.g. diet record sheets, FFQs and self-assessment checklists for specific nutrients) facilitate the interview process. In clinical practice, dietary histories are the most frequently used method for assessing diet. A 3- to 7-day diet record accompanied by a training diary is often necessary to gain a full understanding of training commitments, timing of meals and dietary practices. Comprehensive instruction and a data collection protocol are needed to make the diet record worthwhile, especially if dietary analysis is expected. Compliance in reporting intake accurately for as long as 7 days needs to be encouraged. Although dietary intake can be distorted or under-reported (see section 2.11), it is useful for providing a window into eating habits, especially in an athlete who eats erratically.

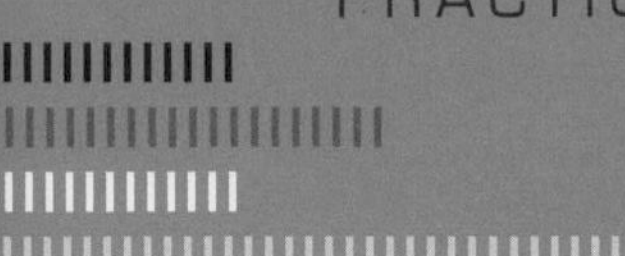

PRACTICE TIPS

- Athletes need specific training and instructions on how to handle a range of issues when recording food intakes, for example weighing or estimating serve size of individual foods, quantifying components of mixed dishes and recipes, reporting wastage and foods eaten, and how to report foods eaten away from home. The necessity for precision in all aspects of recording needs to be explained clearly. Including instructions about cooked or uncooked foods, type of cooking (e.g. grilled or baked), level of fat trimming, use of added sugar, brand name, food descriptor (e.g. reduced or modified fat), type and quantity of oil/fat in cooking and beverages is important for improving accuracy. Determining the day of the week and the number of days of data collection should also be clearly specified.
- Serve sizes on commercial foods are useless for athletes. A standard bowl of breakfast cereal could be a pudding basin for an athlete! It is not uncommon for athletes to have three or more serve sizes of breakfast cereal at one sitting. When collecting information using household measures, distribute standardized measuring devices rather than relying on an athlete's perceived version of a cup or tablespoon.
- Concurrent interaction with computer software for dietary analysis during an interview raises an athlete's awareness of food composition and demonstrates the effects of modifications to usual eating habits. This is especially useful for follow-up consultations.
- An assortment of sports supplements and sports foods is useful as an education tool. However, displaying these openly in a consulting room can be counterproductive and detract from the interview. Such displays can inappropriately influence athletes who are looking for that 'extra edge' or quick fix.
- The factorial method can be used to estimate average energy requirements (see Chapter 5). This involves estimating BMR and assigning an activity factor or PAL (physical activity level) value represented as a ratio to BMR. (See Commonwealth Department of Health and Ageing et al. 2006 or Institute of Medicine 2002 for PAL ratios.) As this calculation is a crude estimate, it should be used only as a guideline.
- Nutrient reference standards (DRI/NRV) should be used with caution in some groups of athletes, when used to assess the probability of nutrient 'adequacy' or inadequacy'. The EAR/RDA cut-offs may not be applicable to athletes with large BM and very high energy expenditure. Protein, calcium and iron cut-offs may need some adjustment when planning diets or assessing intakes (see Chapters 4, 9 and 10).

CLINICAL OBSERVATION AND MEDICAL HISTORY

- Despite the availability of medical records or medical referrals in some dietetic practices, confirmation of clinical symptoms is warranted. Athletes often do not mention their low-grade symptoms to their doctors. It is not uncommon for athletes to reveal chronic gastrointestinal symptoms, post-training loss of appetite, recurring mild infections, nausea, headache, fatigue and bowel or menstrual problems to a dietitian without seeking medical attention.

BIOCHEMICAL MEASUREMENTS

- Interpretation of nutrient status from a single blood test can be misleading, especially if the athlete is dehydrated when tested and the nutrient tested is under homeostatic control. Dehydration is associated with hemoconcentration, resulting in falsely high readings.

ANTHROPOMETRIC MEASURES

- Techniques and standards for assessing body composition are found in Chapter 3. In clinical practice, height, BM and sometimes body frame and skinfolds are measured. Measuring skinfolds in young or adolescent athletes, who are rapidly growing, especially prior to menstruation, is not recommended. A sudden increase in skinfolds can have devastating psychological effects on an adolescent female. She may think she is suddenly getting very fat, when it is natural for girls to increase skinfolds at this time. When used appropriately and conducted by a trained kinanthropometrist, skinfolds are more reliable than weight measurement for setting realistic weight targets, which vary between sports. Average values or ranges for skinfolds or weights for elite national and international athletes are not necessarily applicable or realistic for some individuals (see Chapter 3) and are better suited as targets for teams.
- Many elite athletes are preoccupied with BM and body composition. Having a BMI chart prominently displayed can be unnecessarily stressful for large-framed muscular athletes, who should be reassured that many athletes do not fit into the usual population reference standards. A BMI chart can be useful for showing very lean athletes of slight build, who perceive themselves as overweight, that they are not overweight.
- One technique that is useful for discouraging a preoccupation with daily weighing is to ask athletes to record their BM before and after each training session for 1 or 2 weeks. It is not unusual to see fluctuations of one or more kilograms before and after training sessions and large fluctuations between continuous training days and rest days. Athletes soon realize that large diurnal and weekly BM fluctuations occur and that interpretation of changes in BM is difficult and may not be due to food ingestion alone.

SUMMARY

- If dietitians in both clinical practice and research used standardized methods for anthropometry and biochemical indices, and adopted rigorous protocols for collecting and analyzing food intake data, then data could be compared more reliably across studies. There is a real need to collect and analyze dietary data on sufficient numbers of athletes in different sports at varying levels to allow micronutrient recommendations for athletes to be quantified. A dietitian in clinical practice is in an ideal situation to collect and publish longitudinal data on athletes. Tracking studies of nutritional status of athletes, particularly children and adolescents, and retiring athletes are scarce. Such studies will provide health professionals with a better insight into the association between physical activity, diet and health outcomes and help quantify micronutrient recommendations for elite athletes.

Useful websites

http://www.mypyramid.gov
US food guide, 2005

http://www.healthierus.gov/dietary guidelines/
Dietary guidelines for Americans, 2005

http://www.nhmrc.gov.au/publications/synopses/dietsyn.htm
Dietary guidelines for adult Australians and children and adolescents in Australia, 2003

http://www.health.gov.au/pubhlth/strateg/food/guide
Australian guide to healthy eating, 1998

References

American College of Sports Medicine, American Dietetic Association, Dietitians of Canada. Nutrition and athletic performance. Med Sci Sports Exerc 2000;32:2130–45.

Baranowski T. Food intake recording software system—version 4 (FIRSSTt4) 24-hour dietary recalls in children: adapting the ASA24. Lisbon, Portugal: International Society of Behavioral Nutrition and Physical Activity, 2009.

Barr SI. Women, nutrition and exercise: A review of athletes; intakes and a discussion of energy balance in active women. Prog Food Nutr Sci 1987;11:307–61.

Basiotis PP, Welsh SO, Cronin FJ, Kelsay JL, Mertz W. Number of days of food intake records required to estimate individual and group nutrient intakes with defined confidence. J Nutr 1987;117:1638–41.

Beaton GH, Burema J, Ritenbaugh C. Errors in interpretation of dietary assessments. Am J Clin Nutr 1997;65(Suppl):1100S–7S.

Bingham S. Aspects of dietary survey methodology. British Nutrition Foundation, Nutrition Bulletin 1985;44:90–103.

Bingham SA. The dietary assessment of individuals; methods, accuracy, new techniques and recommendations. Nutr Abst Rev 1987;57:705–43.

Bingham SA. The use of the 24-hr urine sample and energy expenditure to validate dietary assessments. Am J Clin Nutr 1994;59;275–315.

Bingham SA, Gill C, Welch A, et al. Comparison of dietary assessment methods in nutritional epidemiology: weighed records versus 24-h recalls, food-frequency questionnaires and estimated diet records. Br J Nutr 1994;72:619–43.

Bingham SA, Nelson M, Paul AA, Haraldsdottir J, Bjorge-Loken E, van Staveren WA. Methods for data collection at an individual level. In: Cameron ME, Van Staveren WA, eds. Manual on methodology of food consumption studies. NY: Oxford University Press, 1988:53–106.

Black AE, Goldberg GR, Jebb S, Livingstone MBE, Cole TJ, Prentice AM. Critical evaluation of energy intake data using fundamental principles of energy physiology: 2. Evaluating the results of published surveys. Eur J Clin Nutr 1991;45:583–99.

Block G. A review of validations of dietary assessment methods. Am J Epidemiol 1982;115:492–505.

Block G. Human dietary assessment: methods and issues. Prev Med 1989;18:653–60.

Braakhuis AJ, Meredith K, Cox GR, Hopkins WG, Burke LM. Variability in estimation of self-reported dietary intake data from elite athletes resulting from coding by different sports dietitians. Int J Sports Nutr & Exerc Metabol 2003;13:152–65.

Burke BS. The dietary history as a tool in research. Am Diet Assoc 1947; 23:1041–6.

Burke LM, Cummings NK, Desbrow B. Guidelines for daily carbohydrate intake: do athletes achieve them? Sport Med 2001;31;267–99.

Burke LM, Slater G, Broad EM, et al. Eating patterns and meal frequency of elite Australian athletes. Int J Sport Nutr & Exerc Metabol 2003;13:521–38.

Buzzard M. 24-hour dietary recall and food record methods. In: Willett WC, ed. Nutritional epidemiology. Second edition. New York: Oxford University Press, 1998;32–56.

Cade J, Thompson R, Burley V, Warm D. Development, validation and utilisation of food-frequency questionnaires—a review. Pub Health Nutr 2002;5:567–87.

Cade JE, Burley VJ, Warm DL, Thompson RL, Margetts BM. Food-frequency questionnaires: a review of their design, validation and utilisation. Nutr Res Rev 2004;17:5–22.

Carter RL, Sharbough CO, Stapell CA. Reliability and validity of the 24-hour recall. J Am Diet Assoc 1981;79:5472–7.

Cashel K. Compilation and scrutiny of food composition data. In: Greenfield H, ed. Uses and abuses of food composition data. Food Aust 1990;42(Suppl):21S–4S.

Cashel K, Jeffreson S. The core food groups. The scientific basis for developing nutrition education tools. Canberra: Australian Government Publishing Service, 1995.

Commonwealth Department of Health and Ageing (Aust), Ministry of Health (NZ) and National Health and Medical Research Council. Nutrient Reference Values Australia and New Zealand. Canberra: NHMRC, 2006.

Daniels L. Collection of dietary data from children with cystic fibrosis: some problems and practicalities. Hum Nutr Appl Nutr 1984;38(2):110–18.

Dennis B, Shifflett PA. A conceptual and methodological model for studying dietary habits in the community. Ecol Food and Nutr 1985;17:253–62.

Faggiano F, Vineis P, Cravanzola D, et al. Validation of a method for the estimation of food portion size. Epidemiol 1992;3:379–83.

Fogelholm M. Indicators of vitamin and mineral status in athletes' blood: a review. Int J Sport Nutr 1995;5:267–86.

Fogelholm M, Lahti-Koski M. The validity of a food use questionnaire in assessing the nutrient intake of physically active young men. Eur J Clin Nutr 1991;45:267–72.

Food Standards Agency, McCance and Widdowson's. The composition of foods. Sixth summary edition. Cambridge: Royal Society of Chemistry, 2002.

Food Standards Australia New Zealand. AUSNUT 2007. At http://www.foodstandards.gov.au/monitoringandsurveillance/foodcompositionprogram/ausnut2007/index.cfm (accessed 24 April 2009).

Food Standards Australia New Zealand. NUTTAB 2006. At http://www.foodstandards.gov.au/monitoringandsurveillance/nuttab2006/onlineversionintroduction/onlineversion.cfm (accessed 24 April 2009).

Gersovitz M, Madden JP, Smiciklas-Wright H. Validity of the 24-hour dietary recall and a seven-day record for group comparisons. J Am Diet Assoc 1978;73:48–55.

Goldberg GB, Black AE, Jebb SA, et al. Critical evaluation of energy intake data using fundamental principles of energy physiology. I. Derivation of cut-off limits to identify under-recording. Eur J Clin Nutr 1991;45(12):569–81.

Haggarty P, McGraw BA, Maughan RJ, Fenn C. Energy expenditure of elite female athletes measured by the doubly-labelled water method. Proc Nutr Soc 1988;47:35A.

Health Canada. Office of Nutrition Policy and Promotion, Nutrition Recommendations for Canadians, 20 April 2009. At http://www.hc-sc.gc.ca/fn-an/nutrition/pol/action_healthy_eating-action_saine_alimentation-02-eng.php (accessed April 2009).

Hinton PS, Sanford TC, Davidson MM, Yakushko OF, Beck NC. Nutrient intakes and dietary behaviors of male and female collegiate athletes. Int J Sport Nutr & Exerc Metabol 2004;14:389–405.

Holmes, B, Dick K, Nelson M. A comparison of four dietary assessment methods in materially deprived households in England. Pub Health Nutr 2008;11:444–5.

Institute of Medicine. Dietary Reference Intakes for energy, carbohydrates, fibre, fat, protein and amino acids (macronutrients). Food and Nutrition Board. Washington DC: National Academies Press, 2002.

Institute of Medicine. Dietary Reference Intakes for vitamin A, vitamin K, arsenic, boron, chromium, copper, iodine, iron, manganese, molybdenum, nickel, silicon, vanadium and zinc. Food and Nutrition Board. Washington DC: National Academies Press, 2000a.

Institute of Medicine. Dietary Reference Intakes: applications in dietary assessment. A report of the subcommittee on interpretation and uses of Dietary Reference Intakes and the Standing Committee on the Scientific Evaluation of Dietary Reference Intakes. Food and Nutrition Board, Washington DC: National Academies Press, 2000b.

Institute of Medicine. Dietary Reference Intakes: applications in dietary planning. A report of the subcommittee on interpretation and uses of Dietary Reference Intakes and the Standing Committee on the Scientific Evaluation of Dietary Reference Intakes. Food and Nutrition Board, Washington DC: National Academies Press, 2003.

Jonnalagadda SS, Benardot D, Dill MN. Assessment of under-reporting of energy intake by elite female gymnasts. Int J Sport Nutr Exerc Metabol 2000;10:315–25.

Kipnis V, Midthune D, Freedman L, et al. Bias in dietary-report instruments and its implications for nutritional epidemiology. Pub Health Nutr 2002;5:915–23.

Krall EA, Dwyer JT. Validity of a food frequency questionnaire and a food diary in a short term recall situation. J Am Diet Assoc 1987;87:1374–7.

Kristal AR, Shattuck AL, Henry HJ, Fowler AS. Rapid assessment of dietary intake of fat, fiber and saturated fat: validity of an instrument suitable for community intervention research and nutritional surveillance. Am J Health Prom 1990;4:288–95.

Larkin FA, Metzner HL, Thompson FE, Flegal KM, Guire KE. Comparison of estimated intakes by food frequency and dietary records in adults. J Am Diet Assoc 1989;89:215– 23.

Lee RD, Nieman DC. Measurement of diet. In: Lee RD, Nieman DC, eds. Nutritional assessment. Third edition. Iowa: WC Brown Comm Inc, 2002.

Lee-Han H, McGuire V, Boyd NF. A review of the methods used by studies of dietary measurement. J Clin Epidemiol 1989;42:269–79.

Lichtman SW, Pisarska K, Berman ER, et al. Discrepancy between self-reported and actual caloric intake and exercise in obese subjects. New Eng J Med 1992;327:1893–8.

Livingstone MBE, Black AE. Markers of the validity of reported energy intake. J Nutr 2003;133(Suppl): 895S–920S.

Lundy B, O'Connor H, Pelly F, Caterson I. Anthropometric characteristics of competition dietary intakes of professional rugby players. Int J Sport Nutr Exerc Metabol 2006;16:199–213.

Macdiarmid JI, Blundell JE. Dietary under-reporting: what people say about recording their food intake. Eur J Clin Nutr 1997;51:199–200.

Marr JW. Individual dietary surveys: purposes and methods. World Rev Nutr Diet 1971;13:105–64.

Marr JW, Heady JA. Within- and between-person variation in dietary surveys: Number of days needed to classify individuals. Hum Nutr Appl Nutr 1986;40(5):347–64.

Martin CK, Newton RL Jr, Anton SD, et al. Measurement of children's food intake with digital photography and the effects of second servings upon food intake. Eat Behav 2007;8:148–56.

McLennan W, Podger A. Australian Bureau of Statistics/Commonwealth Department of Health and Family Services. National Nutrition Survey: selected highlights Australia, 1995. Canberra: Australian Bureau of Statistics, Cat. No. 4802, 1998.

Murphy S, Barr SI. Challenges in using the dietary reference intakes to plan diets for groups. Nutr Rev 2005;63:267–7.

Murphy S, Guenther P, Kretsch M. Using the dietary reference intakes to assess intakes of groups: pitfalls to avoid. J Amer Diet Assoc 2006;October:1550–3.

Murphy SP, Poos MI. Dietary Reference Intakes. Summary of applications in dietary assessment. Pub Health Nutr 2002;5:843–9.

Neuhouser, ML, Tinker L, Shaw PA, et al. Use of recovery biomarkers to calibrate nutrient consumption self-reports in the Women's Health Initiative. Amer J Epidemiol 2008;167(10):1247–59.

National Health and Medical Research Council (NHMRC). Food for health. Dietary guidelines for children and adolescents in Australia. A guide to healthy eating. Canberra: National Health and Medical Research Council, 2003a.

National Health and Medical Research Council (NHMRC). Food for health. Dietary guidelines for Australian adults. A guide to healthy eating. Canberra: National Health and Medical Research Council, 2003b.

Pekkarinen M. Methodology in the collection of food consumption data. World Rev Nutr Diet 1970;12:145–71.

Pietinen P, Hartman AM, Haapa E, et al. Reproducibility and validity of dietary assessment instruments. I. A self-administered food use questionnaire with a portion size picture booklet. Am J Epidemiol 1988;128:655–66.

Rutishauser I. Making measurements: diet. Melbourne: Menzies Technical Report No. 3 1988;89–120.

Schoeller DA. Limitations in the assessment of dietary energy intake by self-report. Metab 1995;44(Suppl):18S–22S.

Sempos CT, Briefel RR, Flegal KM, Johnson CL, Murphy RS, Woteki CE. Factors involved in selecting a dietary survey methodology for national nutrition surveys. Aust J Nutr Diet 1992;9:96–100.

Sempos CT, Johnson NE, Smith EL, Gilligan C. Effects of intraindividual and interindividual variation in repeated dietary records. Am J Epidemiol 1985;121:120–30.

Smith A, Kellett E, Schmerlaib Y. The Australian guide to healthy eating. Adelaide: Children's Health Development Foundation, 1998.

Sorenson AW, Caulkins BM, Connolly MA, Diamond E. Comparison of nutrient intake determined by four dietary instruments. J Nutr Educ 1985;17:92–8.

Stockley L. Changes in habitual food intake during weighed inventory surveys and duplicate diet collections. A short review. Ecol Food Nutr 1985;17:263–9.

Stunkard AJ, Waxman M. Accuracy of self-reports of food intake. J Am Diet Assoc 1981;79:547– 51.

Subar A, Thompson F, Zimmerman R, et al. Development of an automated self-administered 24-hour recall (ASA24). Lisbon, Portugal: International Society of Behavioral Nutrition and Physical Activity, 2009.

Ward K, Hunt KM, Burstyne Berg M, et al. Reliability and validity of a brief questionnaire to assess calcium intake in female collegiate athletes. Int J Sport Nutr Exerc Metabol 2004;14:209–21.

Weiss R. Automatic identification and volume computation of food using a mobile phone. Lisbon, Portugal: International Society of Behavioral Nutrition and Physical Activity, 2009.

Westerterp KR, Saris WH, van Es M, ten Hoor F. Use of the doubly labeled water technique in humans during heavy sustained exercise. J Appl Physiol 1986;61:2162–7.

Willett WC. Nutritional epidemiology. Second edition. New York: Oxford University Press, 1998;74–100.

Willett WC, Buzzard IM. Foods and nutrients. In: Willett WC. Nutritional epidemiology. Second edition. New York: Oxford University Press, 1998;18–32.

Willett WC, Reynolds RD, Cottrell-Hoehner MS, Sampson L, Browne MS. Validation of a semi-quantitative food frequency questionnaire: Comparison with a 1-year diet record. J Am Diet Assoc 1987;87:43–7.

Worsley A, Baghurst KI, Leitch DR. Social desirability response bias and dietary inventory responses. Hum Nutr Appl Nutr 1984;38(1):29–35.

CHAPTER 3

Kinanthropometry: physique assessment of the athlete

DEBORAH KERR AND TIM ACKLAND

3.1 Introduction

Kinanthropometry is a term used to describe the appraisal of human physique, which includes the size, shape, proportion and tissue composition of the individual (Ross & Marfell-Jones 1991). This appraisal allows the interpretation and monitoring of sports performance and growth. Studies of world-class and Olympic athletes indicate there are specific physique requirements for certain sports (DeRose et al. 1989; Carter & Ackland 1994; Ackland et al. 1997a, 1997b, 1998, 2001, 2003). Even within a sport, the position of the player may require unique physique characteristics. Changes in rules or technique can alter the anthropometric characteristics required for successful performance.

In sports where the body mass (BM) must be transported a distance, a lean physique can offer a competitive advantage (Tittel 1978). These sports include gymnastics, distance running or jumping types of sports where the assessment of body composition and body fat is of primary interest. The same assessment is also important for weight category and aesthetic sports (such as rhythmic gymnastics) where a low level of body fat is also desirable (McArdle et al. 1999). An understanding of kinanthropometry is necessary to be able to interpret anthropometric data in relation to performance. A cooperative relationship between the sports dietitian, exercise scientist and coach is essential. But physique is only one of many factors that will determine sports performance. Athletes can still achieve competence in their chosen sports without having the optimal physique for those sports.

3.2 Physique assessment in athletes

The choice of method for assessing physique depends largely on available resources, testing conditions, and the application of the results as a clinical and research outcome. On most occasions, an estimation of the subcutaneous adipose tissue mass, or body fat as it is commonly known, is all that is required. The assessment of physique in sports science has four fundamental applications:

1. to identify physique characteristics of elite performers
2. to assess and monitor growth
3. to monitor training programs
4. to determine optimal body composition for weight category sports

3.3 Identifying physique characteristics

Athletes who reach Olympic or world-class standard represent the optimum combination of ethnicity, heredity and environment to produce peak performance (Carter 1984). Kinanthropometry relates to the structure of the athletic body to the specialized function needed for various tasks and can help us to understand the limitations of such relationships (Carter 1984). For example, world championship swimmers have a larger arm span than their height (Carter & Ackland 1994). This information is of interest to the exercise scientist and coach and can be used in the identification of athletic potential (Ross & Marfell-Jones 1991). The methods used to identify physique differences are somatotyping (Carter & Honeyman Heath 1990) and proportionality assessment (Ross & Wilson 1974).

Somatotyping is a combined shape–body-composition method, which provides a description of the physique by means of a three-number rating representing the components of endomorphy (adiposity), mesomorphy (muscularity) and ectomorphy (linearity). Somatotyping has been used extensively to describe the shape characteristics of athletes. Some sports are less tolerant of size and shape variance (e.g. gymnastics), whereas others display a wider distribution. In the latter group of sports, factors other than physique are dominant. A detailed description of the method of somatotyping is given by Carter and Honeyman Heath (1990).

Proportionality is described as the relationship of body parts to one another or to the whole body (Ross & Marfell-Jones 1991). The methodology proposed by Ross and Wilson (1974) makes use of a unisex reference human, or 'phantom', as a calculation device. It is not a normative system, but enables proportional differences in anthropometric characteristics within and between athletes to be quantified (Ross & Ward 1984). Using this method, which scales anthropometric data to a common stature, proportional differences can be assessed between athletes in different sports and events, and between males and females.

3.4 Assessing and monitoring growth

Investment in competitive sport can begin at or prior to puberty. This is a time of rapid changes in size, shape and body composition for both sexes. The time of onset of puberty varies considerably between individuals. For example, the difference in age between an early-maturing girl and a late-maturing boy may be as much as 6 years (Ross & Marfell-Jones 1991). This difference in maturation has important implications for sporting ability, as the late-maturing boy will not be as strong as early-maturing boys, as the spurt in strength will follow the spurt in height (Ackland et al. 1994). In girls, late maturation is an advantage in sports where low BM and narrow hips assist movement such as in gymnastics, ballet and distance running (Ackland et al. 2003).

3.5 Changes in adipose tissue during growth

During pubertal growth, the relative gain in adipose tissue drops markedly for both males and females, which is a response to an increase in energy requirements at this time. The absolute amount of adipose tissue declines in adolescent males (He et al. 2004) compared to females, who show increased fat deposition after puberty. It is important that coaches and young female athletes are aware of these normally expected body composition changes associated with maturation, especially in sports where a petite build or small BM is expected.

3.6 Changes in muscle tissue during growth

A growth spurt in muscle mass occurs during the adolescent growth period. Males under the influence of testosterone show a more marked increase in muscle mass than females. Muscle mass reaches a level greater than 40% of total BM in adult males, compared with a maximum of 39% in females (Bloomfield et al. 2003).

3.7 Monitoring training programs

Assessment of body composition is an important component of the ongoing monitoring of athletes. Monitoring of skinfolds indicates changes in adipose tissue mass in response to changes in training and energy intake. The body mass index (BMI), or population index of weight status, is not sensitive to changes in body composition (Ross et al. 1988) and should not be used for monitoring athletes. Girths and corrected girths can be used to monitor changes in muscularity. The skinfold-corrected arm girth is calculated by the following formula (Ward et al. 1989):

skinfold-corrected arm girth (AGRsc) = AGR – (3.14 × TPSK)

where:

AGR = relaxed arm girth (cm)

TPSK = tricep skinfold (cm)

Usually, the skinfold reading will be in millimeters and must therefore be converted to centimeters for the calculation. The skinfold-corrected girths are used in the O-scale and Oz-scale systems (see section 3.19).

3.8 Determining optimal body composition for weight-category sports

In weight-category sports, athletes attempt to gain a competitive advantage by making the lowest weight category possible. These sports include the combative sports such as judo, wrestling, boxing, weightlifting and lightweight rowing. Aesthetic sports such as gymnastics, diving, ballet and figure-skating are in essence weight-category sports, as a low BM is a requirement. In distance running, a lower BM has been shown to offer a competitive advantage when competing in warm and humid environments (Marino et al. 2000).

The assessment of body composition, in particular body fat, can be useful in identifying whether the desired weight category is realistic. If an athlete already has low body fat, as assessed by the skinfold sum (seven or eight sites), then significant weight loss could be achieved only by loss of fat-free mass (FFM). It is important that this issue is discussed with the coach and athlete before weight loss is undertaken, as loss of FFM can compromise strength and endurance capacity.

Methodologies for assessing body composition 3.9

Martin and Drinkwater (1991) have suggested three approaches to body composition assessment. The first approach is the direct assessment or Level I method, which is based on cadaver analysis. All body composition methodologies available to assess athletes provide an indirect assessment of body composition. Therefore all other approaches are indirect (Level II methods) or doubly indirect (Level III methods). Level II and III approaches must make certain assumptions to be able to predict the body composition and are, therefore, termed indirect methods of assessing body composition. For comprehensive reviews on body composition, see Martin and Drinkwater (1991), Roche and colleagues (1996), Brodie and colleagues (1998) and Ellis (2000).

Direct assessment of body composition (Level I) 3.10

The German anatomists reported the earliest data on direct body composition analysis over 100 years ago (Keys & Brozek 1953). Until the 1980s there had been only eight complete adult dissections (Mitchell et al. 1945; Forbes et al. 1956), when Clarys and colleagues (1984) undertook a study to compare surface anthropometry with anatomically dissected cadavers. Twenty-five cadavers sampled from an elderly Belgian population were dissected into the gross tissue masses of skin, adipose tissue, muscle, bone and organs. Comprehensive comparisons were made between the gross tissue weights and the surface anthropometry. This study provided important data which questioned many of the commonly held assumptions in the techniques for measuring body composition. A review of the adult dissection data has been reported by Clarys and colleagues (1999).

Indirect assessment (Level II) 3.11

Historically, the interest in body composition arose from a desire to measure body fat. The work of Behnke and colleagues (1942) on naval divers was the first time body density had been used to estimate body fat. Researchers assume that the body is composed of two compartments—fat mass (FM) and fat-free mass (FFM)—and the densities of each compartment are known and the same for all individuals. This is the basis of predicting the percentage of fat from body density. Hydrodensitometry, or underwater weighing as it is also known, was considered the criterion method or the 'gold standard' for validating other methods of body composition analysis.

Now other techniques, including total body water (TBW), total body potassium (TBK) and dual energy X-ray absorptiometry (DXA), have been put forward as criterion methods. Multi-component chemical methods that use more than one method are particularly useful in research applications in body composition assessment (Heymsfield et al. 1990; Friedl et al. 1992; Shen et al. 2005). As all Level II methods indirectly assess body composition, none is absolutely accurate. All methods have assumptions and it is important to be alert to conditions where the assumptions may be violated.

In practice, the assessment of body composition should be inexpensive, safe and non-invasive. Therefore, most Level II methods, although safe, are not suitable for everyday use in athletes, mainly because they require sophisticated and expensive equipment. Level II methods have a research application and are used to validate Level III methods. The applications of hydrodensitometry and DXA are outlined below. These methods are covered in detail, as they are the most commonly used in sports science. The other Level II methods (TBK, TBW and magnetic resonance imaging) are outside the scope of this chapter and are limited to research applications. Excellent reviews of their applications are found in Jebb and Elia (1993), Roche and colleagues (1996) and Ellis (2000).

3.12 Hydrodensitometry (underwater weighing)

Hydrodensitometry is a technique for the assessment of body density, which is extrapolated to compute the relative fat content of the body. It is based on the principle of buoyancy or relative floatability, a principle first observed by Archimedes (287–212 BC). When the mass and density of an object and the densities of its constituent parts are known, the mass of each can be calculated.

Using hydrodensitometry or volume displacement techniques, with the appropriate corrections for the buoyant force of lung and visceral entrapped air, the density of the body can be determined. One must then assume constant densities of fat (0.90 g/mL) and non-fat (1.10 g/mL) to translate the obtained density value into percent body fat. The most commonly used equations are the Siri (1961) and Brozek (1960) equations. The review article 'Body fat in adult man' (1953) by Keys and Brozek outlines the historical development of these equations. Anatomical evidence from the Brussels Study (Clarys et al. 1984) questioned the assumptions underpinning hydrodensitometry. Measurement error involved in hydrodensitometry has also been a problem. The two primary sources of error include the use of air trapped in the lungs and gastrointestinal tract. In 1995, a commercially available air-displacement method, known as the BOD POD™ (made by Life Measurement, Inc, Concord, CA) became available (Dempster & Aitkens 1995). The BOD POD is based on the principles of hydrodensitometry, but uses an air displacement plethysmograph to measure body volume. To minimize measurement error, a standard testing protocol should be followed with subjects dressed in minimal, skin-tight clothing (Fields et al. 2000; Hull & Fields 2005). As this method does not require submersion in water it is more practical for a wider range of subjects, including children and the elderly. Fields and colleagues (2002) have reviewed this method in detail.

3.13 Dual energy X-ray absorptiometry

Dual energy densitometers were primarily developed to estimate bone mineral content—BMC (g)—and bone mineral density—BMD (g/cm^2)—of regions of the skeleton and for the whole body. The development of DXA whole body scan, based on a sealed X-ray source with dual energy photons, allowed body composition assessment as well (Mazess et al. 1984). Soft tissue can be distinguished from bone by the difference in the attenuation co-efficient of the X-ray beam over soft tissue compared to that over bone. The relative attenuation of the photons in soft tissue changes in proportion to the fat content over the soft tissue being scanned (Lohman 1992).

Studies that have compared DXA with chemical analysis in pigs have shown DXA is able to measure soft-tissue (fat and lean tissue) composition accurately (Svendsen et al. 1993; Van Loan et al. 1995; Mitchell et al. 1998; Mitchell et al. 2000). Whereas several studies have shown close correlation between DXA and other criterion methods generally, there are systematic differences between the methods and the machine used to measure DXA (Van Loan & Mayclin 1992; Van Loan et al. 1995; Norcross & Van Loan 2004; Schoeller et al. 2005). There are several different commercial machines available (from Lunar Corporation, Madison, WI, US; Hologic, Waltham, MA, US; Norland Corporation, Ft Atkinson, WI, US), which all differ slightly in how body composition is determined. In very heavy subjects (over 120 kg, depending on the commercial machine), the machine can fail to scan. Also subjects more than 2 m in stature may not fit within the scanning region. There is also a small radiation dose associated with whole-body DXA scans, so female athletes must be scanned very early in their menstrual cycle and avoid being scanned if pregnant. Currently the interpretation of the body composition data is difficult because no normal range data exists for athletes, which is not the case for anthropometric measures such as skinfolds. Although the radiation dose is low, this still makes this method unsuitable for routine monitoring of athletes, especially female athletes. DXA is best considered a research tool rather than a routine method of assessment for athletes.

Doubly indirect (Level III) methods 3.14

Level III methods have been referred to by Martin and Drinkwater (1991) as 'doubly indirect' as they require validation against Level II methods to determine percentage body fat. Therefore assumptions of the Level II method must also be considered when interpreting data. This is in addition to the assumptions of the Level III method itself. Body fat estimated by either skinfolds or bioelectrical impedance methods should therefore be interpreted with caution when assessing individual athletes.

Bioelectrical impedance analysis 3.15

Bioelectrical impedance analysis (BIA) is based on the differing dielectrical properties of fat and lean tissues of the body, where body fluids are highly conductive and fat and bone are not (Segal et al. 1985). An estimate of the FFM is calculated after normalizing for stature. FM is derived from the total BM by the subtraction of estimated FFM. The leg-to-leg Tanita BIA™ (from Tanita Corporation, Arlington Heights, IL, US) is gaining popularity as it includes a weighing scale. Like skinfold equations, BIA equations require validation against a Level II criterion method, and are therefore population-specific. Factors that affect the recorded electrical resistance in the BIA technique have been outlined by Baumgartner (1996). Variations in diet, hydration, ethnicity and disease states affect the body's electrolyte balance, which in turn influences the FM estimate (Malina 1987). In athletes, it is important to control for testing conditions such as hydration (Segal 1996). To date, most studies have evaluated the precision and accuracy of BIA under standard conditions of normal hydration, which is not always possible in the athletic setting (Clark et al. 2004). A comparison of estimation of body fat in wrestlers by DXA, height and weight (HW), skinfolds and BIA with a four-component criterion method found excellent precision with HW and skinfolds (Clark et al. 2004). An additional issue with BIA is a lack of comprehensive normal range data on a variety of sports, so the method is not useful for comparative purposes.

How skinfolds are used to predict body fat 3.16

Skinfold calipers are commonly used in sports science because they are non-invasive, inexpensive and accessible to most sports scientists and dietitians. A skinfold caliper reading measures the compressed thickness of a double layer of skin and the underlying subcutaneous adipose tissue. The sums of skinfold measures have been used to predict FM and percent body fat from several predictive equations. Norton (1996) has summarized the prediction equations specific to different population groups. However, the application and interpretation of these equations require considerable caution and are frequently misinterpreted and misused.

The observation that skinfolds were correlated with criterion techniques such as underwater weighing (UWW) has led to a proliferation of regression equations to predict body fat. Since 1950, more than 100 equations to predict body fat from skinfolds have been reported in the literature (Lohman 1981). The problem is that these equations are population-specific and should be used only on a similar population to that from which the particular equation was developed (Johnston 1982; Norton 1996). Predicting body fat from skinfold measures also requires the acceptance of the assumption of these equations—that the densities of the FM and FFM are the same between individuals—which is not a valid assumption. Extensive training is required to become a reliable and accredited measurer of skinfold sites. Even in trained anthropometrists, other errors can be introduced. The major source of error in skinfold measures is skinfold compressibility, which varies considerably between and within individuals and at different skinfold sites on the same person. The repeated use of a skinfold caliper on a specific site causes a decrease in the reading after the initial application (Martin et al. 1985). The important implication, however, is that two individuals may have identical skinfold values, but very large differences in uncompressed adipose tissue thickness.

3.17 Indices of height and weight

Weight–height indices have been used for many years in an attempt to determine the 'ideal weight' for an individual. The best known of these is the BMI: weight (kg) ÷ height (m^2). All indices provide a measure of ponderosity, which is not the same as measuring adiposity. For an individual of any given stature, BM will vary according to the amount and density of lean body mass (LBM) or FFM as well as the adipose tissue mass. The rationale for the use of the BMI as an indicator of relative fatness lies in the fact that it seems to dissociate height; that is, it is maximally correlated with weight and minimally correlated with height. The BMI does not distinguish the body composition or structure of individuals, so misclassification is a problem, especially in sportspeople with a muscular physique (Ross et al. 1988).

3.18 Interpreting anthropometric data

Anthropometric data have been used in a variety of ways to estimate body composition size and structure. To estimate body fat, a skinfold sum is determined and compared to normative data published on elite athletes (see Tables 3.1 and 3.2) or is monitored over time. This approach is preferable to using percentage body equations, which are not reliable for individual predictions. As suggested more than two decades ago by Johnston (1982), it is better to use anthropometry itself and changes in absolute measures in individuals rather than making predictions of percent body fat based on questionable assumptions.

When interpreting anthropometric data, it is important to recognize the variability in physique between athletes. The physique and level of adiposity that equates to optimal

TABLE 3.1 NORMATIVE DATA FOR INTERNATIONAL AND NATIONAL LEVEL FEMALE ATHLETES

SPORT	LEVEL	POSITION/EVENT	NUMBER OF SUBJECTS	SKINFOLD SUM (mm)* MEAN	RANGE
Athletics[a]	National	SASI Jumps	4	61.1 ± 12.7	41.7–72.8
		SASI Throws	9	95.3 ± 49.4	53.0–203.7
		SASI Sprint	7	60.3 ± 11.9	45.1–83.9
		SASI Middle distance	20	59.2 ± 19.6	37.4–110.6
		SASI Long distance	6	51.3 ± 8.8	40.4–68.3
Basketball[b]	International	Guard	64	76.6 ± 22.2	36.4–143.5
		Forward	65	76.0 ± 20.1	40.9–131.7
		Centre	47	88.0 ± 21.1	45.7–146.8
Cricket[a]	National		27	90.8 ± 19.7	55.9–141.1
Cycling, Road[a]	National		32	61.9 ± 12.0	33.8–89.5
Diving[c]	International		39	65.6 ± 17.0	32.1–114.3
Gymnastics[a]		SASI Elite	68	37.9 ± 6.1	27.4–57.6
Hockey[a]		SASI Senior	57	87.4 ± 18.5	48.1–140.3
Netball[a]		SA Senior	33	83.4 ± 17.3	51.5–124.0
Rowing[d]	International	Lightweight	14	59.5 ± 11.9	40.1–77.9
	International	Heavyweight	74	89.0 ± 23.2	46.0–145.0
Slalom Canoe/ Kayak[d]	International		12	68.9 ± 13.9	45.8–99.0
Sprint Paddlers/ Kayak[d]	International		23	78.5 ± 16.8	52.9–103.7
Swimming[c]	International		170	72.6 ± 19.6	37.9–147.1
Synchronized swimming[c]	International		137	81.7 ± 22.1	37.5–145.8
Triathlon[e]	International		19	62.8 ± 13.4	40.3–98.4
Volleyball[a]		SASI Senior	29	90.5 ± 25.1	35.8–147.1
Waterpolo[c]	International		109	89.8 ± 23.8	39.7–151.6

*Sum of seven skinfolds (unless otherwise indicated) = triceps, subscapular, biceps, supraspinale, abdominal, front thigh, medial calf; SA = South Australia

Sources: [a]Adapted with permission from the South Australian Sports Institute (SASI) and published previously by Woolford et al. 1993; [b]Ackland et al. 1997a; [c]Sum of six skinfolds from Carter & Ackland 1994 = triceps, subscapular, supraspinale, abdominal, front thigh, medial calf; [d]Sum of eight skinfolds from Ackland et al. 2001 = triceps, subscapular, biceps, iliac crest, supraspinale, abdominal, front thigh, medial calf; [e]Sum of eight skinfolds from Ackland et al. 1998 = triceps, subscapular, biceps, iliac crest, supraspinale, abdominal, front thigh, medial calf

performance in one athlete may not be the same for another athlete. Genetic variability in body composition (Bouchard et al. 1988; Bouchard & Tremblay 1997) means that some athletes can maintain a low level of adiposity without having to restrict their energy intake, whereas others may have more difficulty in maintaining a lower body fat.

TABLE 3.2 NORMATIVE DATA FOR INTERNATIONAL AND NATIONAL LEVEL MALE ATHLETES

				SKINFOLD SUM (mm)*	
SPORT	LEVEL	POSITION/EVENT	NUMBER OF SUBJECTS	MEAN	RANGE
Athletics[a]	State	SASI Pole	3	46.8 ± 0.3	46.4–47.1
		SASI Sprint	4	56.1 ± 2.2	53.9–58.3
		SASI Middle distance	9	38.6 ± 12.0	25.8–68.2
		SASI Long distance	4	49.8 ± 6.4	41.3–56.4
Australian Rules Football[a]	National	Under 17 years	20	67.2 ± 6.9	44.7–104.1
Boxing[a]	State		13	57.5 ± 17.7	34.2–95.2
Cricket[a]	National		22	77.8 ± 23.0	52.3–135.2
Cycling[a]	State	Road	24	58.1 ± 11.9	42.9–85.0
	National	Track	83	53.9 ± 12.7	26.4–85.3
Diving[b]	International		43	45.9 ± 11.4	28.0–79.7
Gymnastics[a]	State	SASI Elite	41	41.6 ± 7.2	27.5–59.1
Hockey[a]	State	Under 21 squad	22	59.4 ± 17.0	38.7–107.2
Kayaking[a]	State	SASI Senior	64	58.0 ± 14.0	37.4–96.7
Rowing[d]	International	Lightweight	57	44.8 ± 7.9	29.8–65.0
	International	Heavyweight	151	65.7 ± 17.2	35.4–122.7
Slalom Canoe/ Kayak[d]	International		31	52.7 ± 10.7	32.4–73.7
Sprint Paddlers/ Kayak[d]	International		60	55.4 ± 16.2	55.4–116.1
Rugby Union[a]	State	SASI Senior	58	92.2 ± 32.9	50.6–2223.2
Triathlon[c]	International		19	48.3 ± 10.2	36.8–85.9
Swimming[b]	International		231	45.8 ± 9.5	26.6–99.9
Volleyball[a]	State	SASI Senior	17	56.8 ± 13.2	36.9–79.6
Weightlifting[a]	State	SASI Squad	47	74.9 ± 34.4	33.9–190.2
Waterpolo[b]	International		190	62.5 ± 17.7	27.9–112.1

*Sum of seven skinfolds (unless otherwise indicated) = triceps, subscapular, biceps, supraspinale, abdominal, front thigh, medial calf
Sources: [a]Adapted with permission from the South Australian Sports Institute (SASI) and published previously by Woolford et al. 1993; [b]Sum of six skinfolds from Carter & Ackland 1994 = triceps, subscapular, supraspinale, abdominal, front thigh, medial calf; [c]Sum of eight skinfolds from Ackland et al. 1998 = triceps, subscapular, biceps, iliac crest, supraspinale, abdominal, front thigh, medial calf; [d]Sum of eight skinfolds from Ackland et al. 2001 = triceps, subscapular, biceps, iliac crest, supraspinale, abdominal, front thigh, medial calf

The O-scale and Oz-scale systems

3.19

The O-scale system (Ward et al. 1989) provides a method of comparing individual skinfold results with a normative database categorized by age and gender. The databases were constructed from 1236 children and over 19000 adults from the YMCA Life Project (Bailey et al. 1982). The measures recorded in this system were age, gender, height, weight and six skinfolds (triceps, subscapular, supraspinale, abdominal, front thigh and medial calf). From these data, the adiposity (A) and proportional weight (pwt) ratings can be calculated as shown below.

The A rating is determined from the sum of six skinfolds (S6SF) and compared to the appropriate age/sex norm. The S6SF is dimensionally scaled to account for individuals of varying size using the equation:

$$pSFSF = S6SF\ (170.18 \div ht)$$

where:

*p*SFSF = the proportional sum of six skinfolds (mm)

ht = the subject's height (cm)

The A rating is then determined by reference to normative data shown in Tables 3.3 and 3.4 (Ward et al. 1989).

The W rating is determined by geometrically scaling the subject's weight to a common height in order to produce a proportional weight (pwt) as follows:

$$pwt = wt\ (170.18 \div ht)^3$$

where:

wt = the subject's weight (kg)

ht = the subject's height (cm)

The W rating is then determined by reference to normative data.

When used in combination, the A and W ratings provide a significant description of the physique and composition of the individual. The A rating indicates 'fatness' with respect to the same age and gender and may be used for intra-individual comparisons over time. The W rating is a ponderosity index and together with the A rating may be used to indicate musculo skeletal development.

The Oz-scale system is based on the O-scale system (see Tables 3.3 and 3.4) but uses Australian normative data and some differences in scaling procedures (Norton & Olds 1996). The data required for this system are six skinfolds (triceps, subscapular, biceps, supraspinale, abdominal and calf skinfolds), height, weight, relaxed arm girth, hip girth and waist girth. The LifeSize™ software package (Olds et al. 1994) is available for personal computers and includes calculation of somatotype, percentage body fat and technical error of measurement, in addition to the Oz-scale printout.

Summary

3.20

When evaluating the indirect methodologies available to assess body composition in athletes, a value judgement needs to be made as to the 'best' technique for the particular application. Clearly, indices of height and weight are not appropriate for assessing athletes. In most instances (for those with the required level of skill), anthropometry will provide a

TABLE 3.3 O-SCALE SYSTEM ADIPOSITY RATINGS FOR FEMALE SUBJECTS

	STANINE THRESHOLD VALUES[a]							
AGE (YEARS) 1	2	3	4	5	6	7	8	9
6	46.8[b]	56.1	61.7	69.5	77.9	96.7	128.6	144.0
7	44.3	47.4	60.2	68.3	76.1	91.8	113.2	140.0
8	43.7	49.2	63.9	69.8	81.4	94.5	111.7	143.2
9	45.5	53.4	66.1	73.2	87.7	98.6	111.7	143.3
10	49.2	59.6	67.6	78.6	98.3	109.7	143.2	173.5
11	51.9	56.4	66.5	75.6	96.4	108.8	150.0	173.4
12	53.0	59.3	66.5	77.8	98.7	111.4	153.0	175.6
13	46.7	56.9	67.9	77.4	97.7	114.9	153.0	165.5
14	46.7	60.9	69.0	81.9	99.6	113.4	147.4	164.8
15	49.4	62.6	72.4	85.4	99.6	113.2	145.3	162.1
16	53.8	65.0	76.2	90.3	101.1	112.0	142.4	158.1
17	62.1	69.4	78.3	92.8	106.5	117.6	141.4	156.4
18–19	63.4	70.5	78.5	90.2	103.4	118.2	135.9	155.7
20–25	64.0	72.5	81.2	92.0	104.2	118.9	138.0	164.0
25–30	64.0	74.1	82.2	93.0	107.9	122.9	141.0	169.2
30–35	64.1	72.0	81.9	94.6	108.0	126.0	144.3	172.2
35–40	64.5	73.9	85.5	97.9	112.1	131.7	148.0	178.4
40–45	69.5	80.5	90.3	102.4	120.7	140.9	161.1	187.3
45–50	72.5	83.2	97.7	110.5	125.7	141.8	165.1	194.0
50–55	70.0	84.5	96.2	112.5	127.8	144.8	168.3	196.5
55–60	76.9	90.1	102.6	115.7	130.5	152.8	169.9	198.2
60–65	78.3	85.3	96.8	114.6	130.6	146.4	166.0	194.0
65–70	74.3	84.8	97.0	110.4	130.7	140.7	153.4	164.6

[a]Individual adiposity ratings are determined from nine standard intervals (stanines), which provide divisions at the percentile equivalents of P4, 11, 23, 40, 60, 77, 89 and 96; [b]Proportional sum of six skinfolds (mm)
Source: Ward et al. 1989

useful method of monitoring body composition. These values should not be transformed into estimates of percentage body fat using regression equations since they were based on selected population groups and can only reliably be applied to that group. The individual skinfold values can be summed and compared to normative data of athletes. When interpreting any anthropometric or body composition data it is important to be aware of the underlying assumptions and the limitations.

TABLE 3.4 O-SCALE SYSTEM ADIPOSITY RATINGS FOR MALE SUBJECTS

	STANINE THRESHOLD VALUES[a]							
AGE (YEARS) 1	2	3	4	5	6	7	8	9
6	43.0[b]	47.4	57.4	63.0	70.0	80.9	92.7	121.0
7	40.2	44.6	51.2	59.0	70.9	83.0	99.5	131.0
8	41.2	45.7	50.7	56.8	65.4	77.6	99.5	137.9
9	43.6	47.1	50.9	55.9	64.2	77.7	105.2	172.4
10	45.1	47.1	53.7	59.1	65.4	83.7	129.1	183.2
11	41.5	45.1	50.8	58.4	68.3	90.9	154.7	193.2
12	37.6	43.1	47.0	53.4	65.7	89.3	126.6	188.9
13	34.8	40.2	44.9	51.7	62.7	86.1	116.4	166.5
14	34.7	37.2	43.4	49.3	57.3	70.9	103.5	146.1
15	33.5	35.7	42.1	47.0	55.9	69.0	100.8	146.1
16	32.3	35.4	40.4	44.6	53.3	63.1	79.4	126.7
17	32.3	35.4	39.5	44.7	53.3	62.4	79.4	107.8
18–19	31.5	34.3	41.7	47.6	57.0	70.3	87.3	109.3
20–25	35.0	40.9	48.1	57.8	71.5	89.0	109.0	130.0
25–30	38.3	45.5	54.5	66.8	81.8	99.5	119.3	144.0
30–35	41.9	49.8	60.3	72.2	87.3	103.9	121.3	145.5
35–40	43.9	53.0	62.3	73.9	88.1	102.5	121.9	143.0
40–45	46.0	53.9	64.2	74.6	87.5	102.5	121.0	142.5
45–50	44.7	55.2	64.8	76.3	90.5	106.8	123.4	147.0
50–55	47.2	56.3	66.3	75.7	87.8	105.0	121.0	140.0
55–60	46.9	56.8	65.8	76.4	87.5	101.1	115.9	136.0
60–65	47.3	53.9	64.8	74.5	87.2	98.3	116.8	134.3
65–70	43.0	53.0	60.5	71.6	84.3	92.9	104.8	121.5

[a]Individual adiposity ratings are determined from nine standard intervals (stanines) which provide divisions at the percentile equivalents of P4, 11, 23, 40, 60, 77, 89 and 96; [b]Proportional sum of six skinfolds (mm)
Source: Ward et al. 1989

PRACTICE TIPS

DEBORAH KERR AND TIM ACKLAND

ASSESSING PHYSIQUE

- It is essential that the anthropometrist is sensitive to the potential psychological impact of anthropometric assessment on the athlete. Many athletes are preoccupied with their BM and skinfolds and sensitive to comments about their BM from coaches, parents and especially peers. For this reason, anthropometric assessment should be done in private. Some athletes can be psychologically devastated by either the measurement process itself or the results of the total sum of skinfolds. Some athletes are overly concerned about the results, which could be an indication of body image disturbances or a more serious underlying eating disorder. When discussing the interpretation of these results with athletes, focus on the effects on athletic performance and physiological expectations rather than body composition issues. Individual data should be kept confidential and not discussed or displayed publicly.

CHOICE OF METHOD TO ASSESS PHYSIQUE AND BODY COMPOSITION

- Dietitians and coaches are mostly interested in assessing changes in body composition in athletes in response to training and dietary intervention rather than physique assessment. For individuals, anthropometry measures (including height, BM, skinfolds, girths and wrist circumferences) are often used. Skinfold measures and the O-scale technique are used routinely in elite sports programs to provide an estimate of the subcutaneous adipose tissue mass and monitor relative changes in body composition of individual athletes. Usually seven skinfold sites (but preferably eight) are taken (tricep, subscapular, biceps, supraspinale, abdominal, front thigh and medial calf). Girths and skinfold-corrected girths provide an estimate of relative muscularity, and are useful to measure body composition changes in athletes at the beginning and end of a strength training or weight-loss program.

PROTOCOL AND ACCREDITATION IN ANTHROPOMETRY

- The recommended measurement protocol is that endorsed by the International Society for the Advancement of Kinanthropometry (ISAK). Definitions of the anthropometric sites and standard protocols have been published by Norton and Olds (1996) and Bloomfield and colleagues (2003). For dietitians wishing to take skinfolds on athletes, accreditation by ISAK and undertaking courses though this organization is recommended (see http://www.isakonline.com).

EQUIPMENT

- *Skinfold calipers*: the Harpenden skinfold caliper is the instrument of choice, although the inexpensive Slimguide™ calipers have the same jaw pressure as the Harpenden caliper and produce almost identical results (Schmidt & Carter 1990).
- *Anthropometry tapes*: the Lufkin™ (W606PM) is the preferred tape. This is a flexible metal tape calibrated in centimeters with automatic retraction.

MINIMIZING ERROR IN ANTHROPOMETRY

- With training and continual practice, anthropometry can provide accurate and useful data on physique. A minimum of two sets (ideally three) of measurements should be taken and the mean of two scores or median (of three) scores recorded. Determining the technical error of measurement (TEM) and comparing it to the recommended measurement tolerances, as outlined by Norton and Olds (1996), allows an assessment of measurement error. Anthropometrists can minimize measurement error by:
  - undertaking accredited training in anthropometry
  - using a standard protocol
  - repeating measurements (double or triple measures)
  - using standard equipment
  - assessing measurement error (TEM)

ASSESSING AND INTERPRETING ANTHROPOMETRIC DATA

- Interpretation of anthropometric data requires caution and an understanding of the specific performance expectations of the sport or team position and current phase of training. Changes in body composition should always be monitored in relation to performance increments or decrements. Combining anthropometric data and dietary intake/nutritional assessment data are important to determine whether an individual athlete's body composition goals are realistic and achievable, based on weight history, physique and genetic makeup. Most athletes have a preferred competition weight or skinfold level. It is unrealistic and unnecessary to attempt to maintain this level throughout the year; large fluctuations in BM, however, should be avoided. An athlete may already have reduced their energy intake under the guidance of the dietitian, but still not achieved the desired reduction in the skinfold sum. If this occurs, adjusting the aerobic output may be warranted, but any increase in activity should be discussed with the coach and exercise scientist to avoid overtraining and potential injury.
- The skinfold sum is often compared to normative data, but giving this information to a weight-sensitive athlete can be psychologically traumatic and is best avoided. Individual skinfold values are more useful in clinical practice when tracked over time. The O-scale computer program or LifeSize™ (see section 3.19) provides a printout of comparisons with normative data as well as changes in individual scores over time, so is a useful education resource.

TARGETS FOR SKINFOLDS

- Published values for skinfolds of elite athletes should be used as a guide only and not used to determine a specific skinfold 'cut-off' for an individual athlete. Such definitive values do not account for individual genetic variability and may not be applicable to recreational athletes. For those athletes who do not meet elite skinfold values, providing assurance that body composition is only one factor contributing to performance helps

PRACTICE TIPS

diminish concern about body image. For some athletes, the 'ideal' skinfold sum can never be achieved.

- The rate of weight loss in relation to reduction in skinfold sum shows individual variation. As a general guide, at higher skinfolds (>80 mm for the sum of seven sites) a 1 kg weight loss will be equivalent to a 10 mm loss from the total skinfold sum. At lower skinfold sum (<80 mm for sum of seven sites) a 1 kg weight loss is approximately equivalent to 5 mm of fat loss. This can be used as a guide in determining if a particular weight category is possible. It should be remembered, however, that not all athletes will follow this pattern. Changes in skinfold compressibility may occur with weight loss and athletes may lose body fat from sites not identified with skinfold calipers.

ANTHROPOMETRIC EQUIPMENT AND SOFTWARE

- Rosscraft Division of Batchelor's Datamedia Limited
- rosscraft@datamedia.ca or tel 604-324-9400 or fax 604-324-4998
- http://www.rosscraft.ca
- LifeSize™ computer package is available from Human Kinetics
- http://www.humankinetics.com

References

Ackland T, Elliott B, Richards J. Growth in body size affects rotational performance in women's gymnastics, Sports Biomech 2003;2:163–76.

Ackland T, Kerr D, Hume P, et al. Anthropometric normative data for Olympic rowers and paddlers. In: Conference of Science and Medicine in Sport, 23–27 October 2001. Perth: Sports Medicine Australia, 2001:157.

Ackland TR, Blanksby BA, Bloomfield J. Physical growth and motor performance of adolescent males. In: Blanksby BA, Bloomfield J, Ackland JR, Elliott BC, Morton AR, eds. Athletics, growth and development in children: the University of Western Australia Study. Chur, Switzerland: Harwood Academic Press, 1994:200–15.

Ackland TR, Blanksby BA, Landers G, Smith D. Anthropometric profiles of elite triathletes. J Sci Med Sport 1998;1:52–6.

Ackland TR, Schreiner A, Kerr DA. Technical note: anthropometric normative data for female international basketball players. Aust J Sci Med Sport 1997a;29:22–4.

Ackland TR, Schreiner AB, Kerr DA. Absolute size and proportionality characteristics of World Championship female basketball players. J Sports Sci 1997b;15:485–90.

Bailey DA, Carter JE, Mirwald RL. Somatotypes of Canadian men and women. Hum Biol 1982;54:813–28.

Baumgartner RN. Electrical impedance and total body electrical conductivity. In: Roche AR, Heymsfield SB, Lohman TG, eds. Human body composition. Champaign, Illinois: Human Kinetics, 1996:790–807.

Behnke AR Jr, Feen B, Welham WC. The specific gravity of healthy men. J Am Med Assoc 1942;118:495–8.

Bloomfield J, Ackland TR, Elliot BC. Applied anatomy and biomechanics in sport. Carlton, Victoria: Blackwell Scientific Publications, 2003.

Bouchard C, Perusse L, Leblanc C, Tremblay A, Theriault G. Inheritance of the amount and distribution of human body fat. Int J Obes 1988;12:205–15.

Bouchard C, Tremblay A. Genetic influences on the response of body fat and fat distribution to positive and negative energy balances in human identical twins. J Nutr 1997;127:5(Suppl):943S–7S.

Brodie D, Moscrip V, Hutcheon R. Body composition measurement: a review of hydrodensitometry, anthropometry, and impedance methods. Nutr 1998;14:296–310.

Brozek J. The measurement of body composition. In: Montagu MFA, ed. A handbook of anthropometry. Springfield, Illinois: Charles C. Thomas, 1960.

Carter JE, Ackland TR, eds. Kinanthropometry in aquatic sports. Champaign, Illinois: Human Kinetics, 1994.

Carter JEL, ed. 1984, Physical structure of Olympic athletes: Part II, Kinanthropometry of Olympic athletes. Basel, Switzerland: Karger, 1984.

Carter JEL, Honeyman Heath B. Somatotyping—development and applications. Cambridge, Great Britain: Cambridge University Press, 1990.

Clark RR, Bartok C, Sullivan JC, Schoeller DA. Minimum weight prediction methods cross-validated by the four-component model. Med Sci Sports Exerc 2004;36:639–47.

Clarys JP, Martin AD, Drinkwater DT. Gross tissue weights in the human body by cadaver dissection. Hum Biol 1984;56:459–73.

Clarys JP, Martin AD, Marfell-Jones MJ, Janssens V, Caboor D, Drinkwater DT. Human body composition: a review of adult dissection data. Am J Hum Biol 1999;11:167–74.

Dempster P, Aitkens S. A new air displacement method for the determination of human body composition. Med Sci Sports Exerc 1995;27:1692–7.

DeRose EH, Crawford SM, Kerr DA, Ward R, Ross WD. Physique characteristics of Pan American Games lightweight rowers. Int J Sports Med 1989;10:292–7.

Ellis KJ. Human body composition: in vivo methods. Physiol Rev 2000;80:649–80.

Fields DA, Goran MI, McCrory MA. Body-composition assessment via air-displacement plethysmography in adults and children: a review. Am J Clin Nutr 2002;75:453–67.

Fields DA, Hunter GR, Goran MI. Validation of the BOD POD with hydrostatic weighing: influence of body clothing. Int J Obes Relat Metab Disord 2000;24:200–5.

Forbes RM, Cooper AR, Mitchell HH. The composition of the adult human body as determined by chemical analysis. J Biol Chem 1956;203:359–66.

Friedl KE, DeLuca JP, Marchitelli LJ, Vogel JA. Reliability of body-fat estimations from a four-compartment model by using density, body water, and bone mineral measurements. Am J Clin Nutr 1992;55:764–70.

He Q, Horlick M, Thornton J, et al. Sex-specific fat distribution is not linear across pubertal groups in a multiethnic study. Obes Res 2004;12:725–33.

Heymsfield SB, Lichtman S, Baumgartner RN, et al. Body composition of humans: comparison of two improved four-compartment models that differ in expense, technical complexity, and radiation exposure. Am J Clin Nutr 1990;52:52–8.

Hull HR, Fields DA. Effect of short schemes on body composition measurements using air-displacement plethysmography. Dyn Med 2005;4:8.

Jebb SA, Elia M. Techniques for the measurement of body composition: a practical guide. Int J Obes Relat Metab Disord 1993;17:611–21.

Johnston FE. Relationships between body composition and anthropometry. Hum Biol 1982;54:221–45.

Keys A, Brozek J. Body fat in adult man. Physiol Rev 1953;33:245–325.

Lohman TG. Advances in body composition assessment. Champaign, Illinois: Human Kinetics Publishers, 1992.

Lohman TG. Skinfolds and body density and their relation to body fatness: a review. Hum Biol 1981;53:181–225.

Malina RM. Bioelectric methods for estimating body composition: an overview and discussion. Hum Biol 1987;59:329–35.

Marino FE, Mbambo Z, Kortekaas E, et al. Advantages of smaller body mass during distance running in warm, humid environments. Pflugers Arch 2000;441:359–67.

Martin AD, Ross WD, Drinkwater DT, Clarys JP. Prediction of body fat by skinfold caliper: assumptions and cadaver evidence. Int J Obes 1985;9(Suppl 1):31S–9S.

Martin AD, Drinkwater DT. Variability in the measures of body fat. Assumptions or technique? Sports Med 1991;11:277–88.

Mazess RB, Peppler WW, Gibbons M. Total body composition by dual-photon (153Gd) absorptiometry. Am J Clin Nutr 1984;40:834–9.

McArdle WD, Katch FI, Katch VL. Body composition assessment and sport-specific observations. In: McArdle WD, Katch FI, Katch VL. Sports and exercise nutrition. Baltimore, Maryland: Lippincott Williams & Wilkins, 1999:372–425.

Mitchell AD, Scholz AM, Conway JM. Body composition analysis of pigs from 5 to 97 kg by dual energy X-ray absorptiometry. Appl Radiat Isot 1998;49:521–3.

Mitchell AD, Scholz AM, Pursel VG. Dual-energy X-ray absorptiometry measurements of the body composition of pigs of 90- to 130-kilograms body weight. Ann NY Acad Sci 2000;904:85–93.

Mitchell HH, Hamilton TS, Steggerda FR, Bean HW. The chemical composition of the adult human body and its bearing on the biochemistry of growth. J Biol Chem 1945;158:625–37.

Norcross J, Van Loan MD. Validation of fan beam dual energy X-ray absorptiometry for body composition assessment in adults aged 18–45 years. Br J Sports Med 2004;38:472–6.

Norton K. Anthropometric estimation of body fat. In Norton K, Olds T, eds. Anthropometrica. Sydney: University of New South Wales Press, 1996:172–98.

Norton K, Olds T, eds. Anthropometrica. Sydney: University of New South Wales Press, 1996.

Olds TS, Ly SV, Norton K. LifeSize computer software. Champaign, IL: Human Kinetics, 1994.

Roche AR, Heymsfield SB, Lohman TG, eds. Human body composition. Champaign, IL: Human Kinetics, 1996.

Ross WD, Crawford SM, Kerr DA, Ward R, Bailey DA, Mirwald RM. Relationship of the body mass index with skinfolds, girths, and bone breadths in Canadian men and women aged 20–70 years. Am J Phys Anthropol 1988;77:169–73.

Ross WD, Marfell-Jones MJ. Kinanthropometry. In: MacDougall D, Wenger HA, Green HJ, eds. Physiological testing of the high-performance athlete. Second edition. Champaign, Illinois: Human Kinetics Books, 1991:223–308.

Ross WD, Ward R. Proportionality of Olympic athletes. In: Carter JEL, ed. Physical structure of Olympic athletes: Part II, Kinanthropometry of Olympic athletes. Basel, Switzerland: Karger 1984:110–43.

Ross WD, Wilson NC. A stratagem for proportional growth assessment. Acta Paediatr Belg 1974;28(Suppl):169S–82S.

Schmidt PK, Carter JE. Static and dynamic differences among five types of skinfold calipers. Hum Biol 1990;62:369–88.

Schoeller DA, Tylavsky FA, Baer DJ, et al. QDR 4500A dual-energy X-ray absorptiometer underestimates fat mass in comparison with criterion methods in adults. Am J Clin Nutr 2005;81:1018–25.

Segal KR. Use of bioelectrical impedance analysis measurements as an evaluation for participating in sports. Am J Clin Nutr 1996;64(Suppl):469S–71S.

Segal KR, Gutin B, Presta E, Wang J, Van Itallie TB. Estimation of human body composition by electrical impedance methods: a comparative study. J Appl Physiol 1985;58:1565–71.

Shen W, St-Onge MP, Pietrobelli A, et al. Four-compartment cellular level body composition model: comparison of two approaches. Obes Res 2005;13:58–65.

Siri WE. Body composition from fluid spaces and density: analysis of methods. In: Brozek J, Henschel A, eds. Techniques for measuring body composition. Washington DC: National Academy of Sciences, 1961.

Svendsen OL, Haarbo J, Hassager C, Christiansen C. Accuracy of measurements of body composition by dual-energy X-ray absorptiometry in vivo. Am J Clin Nutr 1993;57:605–8.

Tittel K. Tasks and tendencies of sport anthropometry's development. In: Landry F, Orban WA, eds. Biomechanics of sport and kinanthropometry. Miami: Symposia Specialists, 1978:283–96.

Van Loan MD, Mayclin PL. Body composition assessment: dual-energy X-ray absorptiometry (DEXA) compared to reference methods. Eur J Clin Nutr 1992;46:125–30.

Van Loan MD, Keim NL, Berg K, Mayclin PL. Evaluation of body composition by dual-energy X-ray absorptiometry and two different software packages. Med Sci Sports Exerc 1995;27:587–91.

Ward R, Ross WD, Leyland AJ, Selbie S. The advanced O-scale physique assessment system. Burnaby, Canada: Kinemetrix Inc, 1989.

Woolford S, Bourdon P, Craig N, Stanef T. Body composition and its effects on athletic performance. Sports Coach 1993;16:24–30.

CHAPTER 4

Protein and amino acid needs for training and bulking up

MARK TARNOPOLSKY

Introduction 4.1

Traditionally, athletes and coaches have believed that very high dietary protein intakes are required to maximize net protein accretion during resistance-exercise training. Given that human skeletal muscle is predominately composed of protein, it is easy to understand how this belief became so pervasive. This concept can even be traced to ancient Greece, where records from the Olympics indicated that athletes consumed large amounts of meat to maximize strength/power performance (Harris 1966). Eventually, the importance of lipid and carbohydrate (CHO) oxidation in muscle metabolism were realized and a central role for protein oxidation in the supply of energy to muscle waned (Cathcart 1925). During much of the past 50 years, there has been ongoing debate as to whether physical activity of any type alters the dietary requirement for protein (Tarnopolsky 2004; Tipton & Wolfe 2004; Phillips 2006; Tipton & Witard 2007). This chapter will review the pathways of protein metabolism in skeletal muscle with emphasis on the effect(s) of exercise on metabolic and anabolic pathway regulation. I shall then examine methods to assess the adequacy of dietary protein intakes and review studies that have attempted to determine whether athletes require dietary protein intakes higher than those for sedentary individuals. Throughout the chapter I shall broadly classify exercise as either 'endurance' or 'resistance' to highlight the two major classifications of exercise that are at the opposite ends of the metabolic-demand spectrum. For example, most people involved in resistance-type exercise desire increases in strength, power and muscle mass as outcomes, whereas endurance athletes seek metabolic adaptations that enhance long-duration power output, such as increased oxygen consumption and reduced body fat. A particular sport (e.g. football, volleyball or rugby) may have different proportions of strength and endurance and the athlete and coach must decide how the literature review and recommendations put forth in this chapter are to be applied in each individual case.

4.2 Protein metabolism

Proteins are molecules that serve important structural and regulatory functions. Structural proteins include cytoskeletal proteins such as dystrophin, titin, sarcoglycan, vimentin, desmin and connective tissue proteins such as collagen; regulatory proteins include enzymes such as lactate dehydrogenase, citrate synthase or carbonic anhydrase. Proteins are comprised of amino acids (AA)—compounds containing an amino group ($-NH_2$), a carboxylic acid group (-COOH) and a radical group (different for each of the amino acids). There are twenty amino acids that are found as constituents of proteins or present as free amino acids. Of these amino acids, nine are considered essential or 'indispensable' (histidine, isoleucine, leucine, lysine, methionine, phenylalanine, threonine, tryptophan and valine), and arginine is sometimes considered as being conditionally essential (Pellet 1990). The essential amino acids must come from the diet and/or from endogenous protein breakdown. Since proteins serve such a critical role in the function of the organism, it is not surprising that their metabolism is complex, tightly regulated and generally conserved. A detailed examination of protein metabolism per se would require an entire dedicated textbook; consequently, I shall focus on the basics of protein turnover, which will allow for a conceptual understanding of protein metabolism and nutrition during exercise.

4.3 Protein synthesis

Protein synthesis starts with a signal (e.g. nutrient, hormone or mechanical) that induces gene expression. In general, it is considered that each gene ultimately directs the synthesis of one protein, although alternative splicing can generate homologous proteins with polymorphic differences in structure and function. Gene expression begins when a signal is sensed and transduced to the nucleus of the cell though a transcription factor that, in turn, binds to regulatory regions on DNA that are in close proximity to the gene (promotor sequence). Promoters and enhancers initiate a process called transcription, where a messenger RNA (mRNA) is formed from the gene template. Transcription is initiated with a start codon and terminated with a stop codon. The primary transcript is modified by splicing out non-coding regions of the gene called introns with a splicesome complex, and is further processed by capping at the 5′ end and poly-adenylation at the 3′ end. Each amino acid in a given protein is ultimately derived from a 3-nucleotide mRNA sequence called a codon. The mature mRNA is exported through nuclear pores to the cytosol. Once in the cytosol, the mRNA is translated into a protein through the process of translation by the ribosomes, which are free in the cytosol or bound to rough endoplasmic reticulum. The process of translation requires a second form of RNA, called transfer RNA (tRNA). The tRNAs are combined with their respective amino acids via specific tRNA syntheses to form amino-tRNA complexes (e.g. leucyl-tRNA and histidinyl-tRNA). Within the ribosome 'scaffolding', the mRNA codons are 'read' by the specific tRNA anti-codon to form an amino acid. The process of translation requires three distinct steps called initiation, elongation and termination.

There has been an explosion of data regarding the control of translation in muscle and how it is regulated by nutrition and muscle contraction. In general, adenosine monophosphate-activated kinase (AMPK) is considered a signaling molecule that senses cellular energy charge and increases in activity (phosphorylation) when cellular energy charge is low (i.e. high AMP content).

Activated AMPK in turn leads to an increase in lipid oxidation and glucose transport and can increase mitochondrial biogenesis (Hardie 2004; Jorgensen et al. 2006; Richter & Ruderman 2009). Activated AMPK also leads to a reduction in protein and lipid synthesis (Matsakas & Patel 2009; Richter & Ruderman 2009). The opposite effect is mediated by the mammalian target of rapamycin (mTOR) pathway that activates protein synthesis when phosphorylated by upstream kinases including the insulin signaling pathway (Matsakas & Patel 2009).

More recent work has also shown a role for mTOR in mediating mitochondrial biogenesis (Cunningham et al. 2007). In general the mTOR pathway and the AMPK pathway work in opposite directions and activation of AMPK can inhibit mTOR signaling (Deldicque et al. 2005). When mTOR is activated by amino acids (primarily leucine) or insulin there is an activation of downstream kinases including p70S6K1 and rpS6 (Glover et al. 2008). Resistance and endurance exercise can activate the Akt-mTOR-p70S6K1 pathway in the hours following exercise and this effect is enhanced in the presence of proteins (Glover et al. 2008; Hulmi et al. 2009). Activation of this pathway leads to a reduction in the phosphorylation of epsilon subunit of eukaryotic initiation factor 2B (eIF2Bepsilon) that activates this initiation factor of the translation process.

The protein synthetic processes can be broadly classified into four sites of potential regulation: transcriptional (e.g. promoter region binding), post-transcriptional/pre-translational (e.g. mRNA stability, poly-adenylation), translational (e.g. tRNA charging, speed and efficiency of translation) and post-translational (e.g. nascent protein stability, glycosylation, protein degradation). Exercise is a potent physiological stress that ultimately results in an adaptive response by the cell to prevent future threats to homeostasis. In the case of a bodybuilder, the increase in contractile proteins allows for a greater absolute force output, whereas an increase in mitochondrial volume allows the endurance athlete to run for hours. Although this divergence in the adaptive response to exercise is well known to any bodybuilder or runner, the fundamental regulation of these processes is complex and only just being better characterized at the signaling level (Coffey et al. 2006; Wilkinson et al. 2008).

When the entire process of mixed muscle protein synthesis is considered, there are many references that have shown early (hours), robust and similar increases after both endurance (Tipton et al. 1996; Bolster et al. 2005) and resistance (Chesley et al. 1992; Phillips et al. 1997, 1999; Tipton et al. 2001; Miller et al. 2003) exercise.

The site of regulation and how this generalized protein synthetic response is fine-tuned to allow for phenotypical divergence is just becoming known. We have used micro-array technology and found that over 200 mRNA species are already differentially expressed by 3 hours after endurance exercise (Mahoney et al. 2005), and we have recently shown that the transcriptome expression pattern is different following lengthening/eccentric contractions (Mahoney et al. 2008). Others have found phosphorylation of proteins such as p70S6k, 4E-BP1, eIF-2B, AMPK and eEF2 in response to different contraction patterns in skeletal muscle (Atherton et al. 2005; Wilkinson et al. 2008). Together, these data show that there are changes at multiple levels (e.g. transcription and translation) within the protein synthetic pathway that simultaneously respond to exercise to modulate the ultimate phenotypic response to a given pattern of muscle contraction. Another important factor to consider in evaluating the role of transcriptional and translational regulation of protein turnover is the state of training of an individual. At the whole-body level, there is an attenuation of the acute exercise-induced increase in fractional synthetic rate, with a higher basal/resting level (Phillips et al. 1999; Kim et al. 2005). Exercise training also alters the transcriptome profile in human skeletal muscle (Timmons et al. 2005). Finally, aging has an important influence on the activation of protein turnover in human muscle and its response to feeding (Smith et al. 2008; Kumar et al. 2009).

4.4 Amino acid oxidation/protein breakdown

Human skeletal muscle can oxidize at least eight amino acids (alanine, asparagine, aspartate, glutamate, isoleucine, leucine, lysine and valine) (Goldberg & Chang 1978). During endurance exercise, it appears that the branched-chain amino acids (BCAA: isoleucine, leucine, and valine) are preferentially oxidized (Goldberg & Chang 1978; Wolfe et al. 1984); however, lysine can also be oxidized (Lamont et al. 2001a). Given the predominance of BCAA oxidation during exercise, it is important to understand the regulation of this pathway. BCAA are transaminated to their ketoacid analogues by branched-chain aminotransferase (BCAAT), and the resultant ketoacid is oxidized by branched-chain oxo-acid dehydrogenase enzyme (BCOAD) (Khatra et al. 1977; Boyer & Odessey 1991). In the cytosol, the amino-N group is usually transaminated with α-ketoglutarate to form glutamate, which is in turn transaminated with pyruvate to form alanine (Wolfe et al. 1984), or aminated via glutamine synthase to form glutamine. Some of the amino-N may end up as free ammonia released from muscle; however, during high-intensity contractions most of the ammonia comes from the myoadenylate deaminase pathway (Wagenmakers et al. 1991; Tarnopolsky et al. 2001a).

The BCOAD enzyme is rate-limiting for BCAA oxidation (Khatra et al. 1977; Boyer & Odessey 1991). At rest, the proportion of BCOAD in the active form is about 5–8% and this increases to 20–25% during exercise (Wagenmakers et al. 1989; McKenzie et al. 2000). This activation is thought to be related to a decrease in the ATP/ADP ratio, an increase in intramuscular acidity and a depletion of muscle glycogen (Kasperek 1989; Wagenmakers et al. 1991). The inverse correlation between BCOAD percent activation and muscle glycogen concentration (Wagenmakers et al. 1989; Wagenmakers et al. 1991), provides a theoretical basis for CHO loading to attenuate BCOAD-mediated amino acid oxidation during endurance exercise. The latter findings may partly explain a lower amino acid oxidation during exercise with CHO supplementation (Riddell et al. 2003), and why amino acid release was greater (proteolysis) from a leg with glycogen depletions during one-legged exercise (Blomstrand & Saltin 1999). The total amount of BCOAD protein and activity does increase with endurance-exercise training (McKenzie et al. 2000; Howarth et al. 2007), and this may increase the overall capacity for amino acid oxidation in highly trained endurance athletes (see below).

Protein degradation is the process of breaking down proteins into their constituent amino acids. These amino acids contribute to the intracellular free amino acid pool, which may be exported into the plasma, directly oxidized, or re-incorporated back into tissue protein (synthesis). Although most athletes think only of maximizing protein synthesis, it is equally logical to try to attenuate degradation, for net protein balance is a function of synthesis minus degradation. Therefore, a bodybuilder could achieve net protein retention by decreasing degradation even without a change in synthesis.

The three main pathways for protein degradation in human skeletal muscle include the lysosomal and non-lysosomal (ubiquitin and calpain) pathways. The lysosomal pathway degrades endocytosed proteins, some cytosolic proteins, hormones and immune modulators (Mitch & Goldberg 1996). The lysosomal pathway is not a major contributor to human skeletal muscle protein degradation (Lowell et al. 1986), except when there is significant muscle damage and inflammation such as in muscualr dystrophy (Tidball & Spencer 2000). The two major non-lysosomal pathways in human skeletal muscle are the adenosine triphosphate (ATP)-dependent ubiquitin pathway (Mitch & Goldberg 1996; Lecker et al. 2004), and the calcium-activated neutral protease or calpain pathway (Belcastro et al. 1998; Bartoli & Richard 2005).

The calpain pathway is felt to play a role in skeletal muscle proteolysis during exercise (Belcastro et al. 1998). The ubiquitin pathway is activated after the targeting of proteins for degradation (e.g. oxidative modification). Following targeting, ubiquitin molecules are linked to lysine residues through a series of pathways catalyzed by three enzymes, termed E1, E2 and E3, and are then degraded by the 26S proteosome into peptides (Mitch & Goldberg 1996). This pathway is strongly activated during starvation and muscle atrophy (Gomes et al. 2001; Jagoe et al. 2002), and may be involved in the remodeling of skeletal muscle (Murton et al. 2008). Recent evidence suggests that activation of apoptotic pathways, particularily caspase 3, is a prerequisite for initiation of ubiquitin-proteosome mediated proteolysis (Du et al. 2004).

Models and measurement of protein turnover 4.5

The amino acids found in the plasma can come from dietary intake (I), protein breakdown (B) and, in the case of non-essential amino acids, de novo synthesis. Amino acids can be removed from the plasma, either for protein synthesis (S), oxidation (O), or incorporation into other metabolic pathways after transamination/deamination. For an essential amino acid such as leucine, the only sources to enter the body are from I or B. Leucine is also completely oxidized in the human body to CO_2, allowing the measurement of O as well. Therefore, if an amino acid such as leucine is used to study metabolism, the flux (Q) is equal to intake + breakdown, which is in turn equal to synthesis + oxidation ($Q = I + B = S + O$). This simple model is helpful in the measurement of protein turnover/flux, since amino acid tracers can be used to measure Q and O, and if intake equals zero, then $Q = B$, and by subtraction, $S = Q - O$ (Tarnopolsky et al. 1992). Although useful, this model is very simplistic in that there are multiple amino acid pools turning over at very different rates. Isotopic studies are used to derive these variables of protein turnover.

Isotopes are molecules that share the same atomic number (protons), yet have different numbers of neutrons (atomic mass). Stable isotopes occur naturally and do not emit ionizing radiation, whereas radioactive isotopes undergo spontaneous decay. For these reasons stable isotopes have become very popular in exercise research (Wolfe et al. 1984; McKenzie et al. 2000; Tipton et al. 2001; Hartman et al. 2006; Wilkinson et al. 2007).

There are many other models of protein turnover at the whole body and tissue level. At the most basic level, the balance between all protein intake and excretion would provide a net balance measurement. This protein balance can be measured using nitrogen balance (NBAL) methods. With the NBAL method, measurements are completed of all sources of nitrogen intake (diet and intravenous) and output (urine, feces, sweat, and miscellaneous) and a balance is calculated. If the balance is positive, the person is in a state of net retention and if it is negative, the person is in a state of net depletion. The measurement of nitrogen is based upon the fact that proteins are about 16% nitrogen by weight

(Tarnopolsky et al. 1988). Using arteriovenous catheters, one can also measure the amino acid balance across a limb, and measurements of amino acid transport, muscle protein synthesis and breakdown can be made by simultaneously using stable isotopes (Biolo et al. 1995; Tipton et al. 1999). Another method to measure protein synthesis is the fractional synthetic rate (FSR) method. This requires the infusion of an isotope and the measurement of the incremental increase in isotopic enrichment within a tissue or specific protein over time. We, and others, have used muscle biopsies to look at mixed skeletal muscle FSR after exercise with this method (Phillips et al. 1999; Bolster et al. 2005; Wilkinson et al. 2007). Myofibrillar and mitochondrial FSR can also be determined using stable isotopic tracer incorporation in combination with a gel separation of the component proteins (Balagopal et al. 1997), or differential centrifugation (Wilkinson et al. 2008). A recent development has been the measurement of collagen synthesis in both muscle and tendons using the FSR method (De Boer et al. 2007). This appears to be responsive to acute exercise but not nutrient provision (Babraj et al. 2005).

A significant limitation to our understanding of protein turnover has been the lack of a good method to measure muscle protein breakdown. Initially, there was much enthusiasm for the use of 3-methylhistidine (3-MH), which is a post-translational modification of histidine residues in the actin and myosin of skeletal muscle (Young & Munro 1978). This method requires accurate urinary collections and assumes that most of the 3-MH arises from skeletal myofibrillar proteolysis and that the proportional contribution from other sources relative to muscle remains constant under varying physiological situations (Young & Munro 1978).

These limitations are not so concerning in crossover studies where the subject is his or her own control, yet the collection issues are still important. More recently, microdialysis has been used to measure 3-MH directly in the interstitial fluid of skeletal muscle to show higher rates of proteolysis in older versus younger adults (Trappe et al. 2004). A method for the determination of mixed muscle fractional breakdown rate (FBR) using a stable isotopic decay kinetic method has been developed in the laboratory of Wolfe and colleagues (Phillips et al. 1997), and we have used this method to show that FBR is not altered following resistance training in the fed state (Phillips et al. 2002).

It is important to understand the theories and limitations of the model that is used in any study of protein metabolism during exercise. In this way, the reader can understand the validity of the conclusions drawn from the results. A more detailed examination of the limitations of protein and tracer methodology can be found in reviews and texts (Wolfe 1984; Wolfe & George 1993).

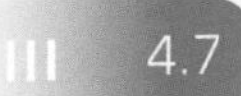

4.6 The effect of exercise on protein metabolism

4.7 The effect of acute endurance exercise on amino acid oxidation

The majority of the energy for endurance exercise is derived from the oxidation of lipid and CHO (Table 4.1). As mentioned above, skeletal muscle has the metabolic capacity to oxidize certain amino acids for energy. It is counterproductive to oxidize proteins during

TABLE 4.1 ENERGY REQUIREMENTS DURING A ONE-HOUR RUN AT 65–75% OF $VO_{2\ MAX}$

ENERGY	(KCAL/H)	% FAT	% PROTEIN	% CHO
Males	*816 (122)	24 (19)	5 (3)	71 (24)
Females	603 (45)	38 (17)	2 (2)	60 (18)

*Males are different from females for all variables ($p < 0.01$). Values are mean (SD) from forty-one females and forty males using pooled data (Tarnopolsky et al. 1990; Phillips et al. 1993; Tarnopolsky et al. 1995; Tarnopolsky et al. 1997; McKenzie et al. 2000; Riddell et al. 2003)

exercise, since they serve either a structural or functional role. Amino acid oxidation may also be required for exchange reactions in the tricarboxylic acid cycle, and this may increase their net utilization (Gibala et al. 1998; Gibala 2001).

Earlier studies evaluated urea excretion as an indicator of protein oxidation (urea is a breakdown product formed in the liver following amino acid oxidation). Several studies found that urinary urea excretion was higher following endurance exercise as compared to rest (Dolny & Lemon 1988; Tarnopolsky et al. 1988). Studies have also shown that a significant amount of urea is excreted in the sweat during exercise (Lemon & Yarasheski 1985; Tarnopolsky et al. 1988). Therefore, a person exercising in high ambient temperatures and/or humidity would be expected to have a high urea sweat loss that may contribute to a more negative protein balance. Studies of urea excretion provide only indirect evidence for amino acid oxidation and in some cases do not correlate well with direct measures of amino acid oxidation (Wolfe et al. 1984).

A number of studies have shown that endurance exercise increases leucine oxidation (Phillips et al. 1993; Lamont et al. 1995, 2001a; Bowtell et al. 2000; McKenzie et al. 2000; Hamadeh et al. 2005). Leucine oxidation during endurance exercise increases with higher exercise intensities (Lamont et al. 2001b). Leucine oxidation (Phillips et al. 1993; McKenzie et al. 2000), and plasma urea content (Haralambie & Berg 1976), also increase with exercise duration. Finally, leucine oxidation increases with glycogen depletion, which may partly explain the increase with exercise duration (Wagenmakers et al. 1991; Blomstrand & Saltin 1999). Acutely following endurance exercise, there is a rapid return towards baseline of the elevated leucine oxidation (Phillips et al. 1993). There may be a slight increase in leucine oxidation that persists for up to 10 days following eccentric exercise (Fielding et al. 1991). This may partly explain why nitrogen balance is negative at the onset of unaccustomed endurance exercise, yet becomes more positive as the person adapts to the stress (Gontzea et al. 1968). Endurance-exercise training (McKenzie et al. 2000; Howarth et al. 2007), and the acute consumption of CHO (Riddell et al. 2003), attenuate the exercise-induced increase in leucine oxidation during exercise.

Clearly, there is an increase in amino acid oxidation during endurance exercise that can be modified by training and diet manipulation. This may account for 1–6% of the total energy cost for an endurance-exercise session at about 65% $VO_{2\ max}$ (see Table 4.1).

The increase in amino acid oxidation with exercise has been shown with both leucine and lysine tracers (McKenzie et al. 2000; Lamont et al. 2001a). These results cannot be extrapolated to other amino acids or an intact protein. If only a few of the amino acids are oxidized during endurance exercise, then the predicted effect on protein requirements may be minimal. Conversely, an increase in an essential amino acid oxidation (e.g. leucine and lysine) may affect protein requirements, since they can only come from dietary intake and/or protein breakdown.

4.8 The effect of acute resistance exercise on protein synthesis and breakdown

In contrast to endurance exercise, we have shown that acute, whole-body resistance exercise does not alter leucine oxidation (Tarnopolsky et al. 1991; Tarnopolsky et al. 1992). In this same study we also did not find an effect of acute resistance exercise on whole-body protein synthesis, either during exercise or for up to two hours post-exercise (Tarnopolsky et al. 1991). We hypothesized that since muscle protein synthesis (MPS) accounted for only 25% of whole-body synthesis (Nair et al. 1988), changes in MPS may be either not measurable, or would be negated by a reciprocal change in the synthesis of another protein such as in the gastrointestinal tract.

To measure the acute effect of resistance exercise on muscle protein synthesis, several groups have used the FSR tracer incorporation method described above. Chesley and colleagues (1992) and others have also shown an increase in muscle protein synthesis for between 24 and 48 hours following an acute bout of resistance exercise using the FSR method (Phillips et al. 1997; Miller et al. 2003; Kim et al. 2005) and arteriovenous balance method (Biolo et al. 1995). Investigators have also found an increase in FSR in older adults after an acute bout of resistance exercise (Welle et al. 1995; Yarasheski et al. 1999).

Studies have also measured protein breakdown after resistance exercise using the intracellular tracer dilution (Phillips et al. 1997), and the arteriovenous balance or tracer (Biolo et al. 1995) methods. Phillips and colleagues (1997) demonstrated that fractional protein breakdown (FBR) was increased after resistance exercise, yet the magnitude of the increase was less than for FSR (e.g. the muscle was in a more positive balance). Furthermore, they showed that FBR returned to baseline values before FSR. Biolo and colleagues (1995) found that muscle synthesis and breakdown were increased following an acute bout of resistance exercise. The net balance (synthesis minus degradation) was negative prior to exercise and was more positive (but still net negative) after exercise, as the subjects were in the fasted state. Taken together, these data indicate that muscle FSR and FBR are increased in the post-exercise period following resistance exercise. In the fasted state, net protein balance is negative, and resistance exercise renders the muscle in a less negative balance. Therefore, the post-exercise time period may be an important time for the delivery of nutrients, as discussed in section 4.10.

4.9 The effect of exercise training on protein metabolism

Chronic endurance-exercise training might be expected to achieve adaptations that would attenuate the oxidation of protein for energy. This would be predicted based on the sparing of muscle glycogen that accompanies chronic endurance training (causing lower BCOAD activation). Early work by Gontzea and colleagues (1968) showed that untrained persons who started endurance training were in a negative nitrogen balance, but as they continued to train, the nitrogen balance became less negative. Animal data have yielded conflicting results, with some studies showing that training increased amino acid oxidation (Dohm et al. 1977; Henderson et al. 1985), and another finding a reduction in the contribution of leucine to total energy consumption (Hood & Terjung 1987).

To date, human data have not yielded a consistent answer to this issue. Following endurance-exercise training, whole-body protein synthesis is higher in the basal state and there is a greater proportion of leucine flux diverted towards oxidation in the untrained versus trained athlete (Lamont et al. 1990). However, differences in leucine turnover between trained and untrained subjects disappeared when the data were expressed relative to lean mass (Lamont et al. 1999). These findings are not consistent with the biochemical expectation that endurance-exercise training should attenuate glycogen use and spare protein oxidation. For this reason, we designed an experiment to train sedentary individuals for a period of 38 days and to measure their leucine oxidation and BCOAD activation during exercise, before and after training (McKenzie et al. 2000). We found that leucine oxidation during exercise was lower after training, as was BCOAD activation. However, consequent to the increase in total mitochondrial content, the *total* capacity of BCOAD enzyme activity was higher in the trained state (McKenzie et al. 2000).

Our findings were confirmed in a more recent study that showed that resting BCOAD content was higher and that activation was lower due to a higher protein content for BCOAD kinase (inactivates BCOAD) (Howarth et al. 2007). Furthermore, another study found that whole-body amino acid oxidation was lower after endurance-exercise training (Gaine et al. 2005). Taken together, data from the above studies are all consistent with the fact that chronic endurance training results in a sparing of amino acid oxidation. With the greater amount of total BCOAD activity/content after endurance-exercise training (McKenzie et al. 2000; Howarth et al. 2007), it is possible that the capacity for amino acid oxidation would be higher in the trained state; however, it is likely that only top sport athletes training for long hours and at a high relative intensity could ever stress their metabolic capacity such that amino acid oxidation would exceed that in the untrained or moderately trained individual.

Although there are fewer studies concerning resistance training, it is logical that protein requirements/synthesis would be greater in the early stages of adaptation when the initial hypertrophy is achieved, compared to a long-term maintenance phase (assuming no compensatory changes in re-utilization). We demonstrated that whole-body protein synthesis and degradation were greater in resistance-trained athletes compared to sedentary controls (Tarnopolsky et al. 1992), and that basal FSR was higher after a period of resistance-exercise training (Phillips et al. 2002; Kim et al. 2005). Furthermore, there is an attenuation of the acute exercise induced increase in mixed muscle FSR after a period of resistance-exercise training (Phillips et al. 2002; Kim et al. 2005). These latter findings would theoretically predict that a trained weightlifter could have either a lower (reduced post-exercise pulse) or a higher (elevated basal FSR) protein requirement. The elevation in basal mixed FSR after training is consistent with the finding of a higher whole-body protein synthesis in well-trained strength athletes as compared to sedentary controls (Tarnopolsky et al. 1992). However, protein requirements appear to be lower for well-trained strength-trained athletes (Tarnopolsky et al. 1988), as compared to those starting a training program (Lemon et al. 1992), but both are still higher than requirements for sedentary people (Tarnopolsky et al. 1988). A study of resistance training in older adults suggested that protein efficiency was enhanced following a resistance-training program (Campbell et al. 1995).

Diet and protein turnover 4.10

It is obvious that diet has an effect on protein metabolism. For example, in starvation there is a clear net negative protein balance that results in cachexia. Conversely, there is a point at which dietary protein becomes optimal for the growth and maintenance of an organism and above this there is a 'plateau' in synthesis, with amino acids being diverted into oxidative (e.g. leucine) or other pathways (e.g. phenylalanine is not oxidized in skeletal muscle). For years it has been known that both dietary energy and CHO intake have a net positive effect on nitrogen balance (Welle et al. 1989; Krempf et al. 1993). The positive effects of CHO on net protein balance are probably due to an insulin-mediated permissive effect on protein synthesis and an attenuation of protein breakdown (see section 4.11). A high CHO intake per se has positive effects on protein balance (Welle et al. 1989; Krempf et al. 1993). CHO loading has been shown to attenuate plasma and sweat urea excretion following endurance exercise (Lemon & Mullin 1980). Furthermore, CHO supplementation increases whole-body protein synthesis (Welle et al. 1989), and attenuates proteolysis (Krempf et al. 1993). Interestingly, the sparing effect of CHO intake on leucine oxidation during endurance exercise is apparent only when dietary protein intakes are at the average intake for men (1.8 g/kg/d) as opposed to a suboptimal amount of protein (0.7 g/kg/d) (Bowtell et al. 2000). Habitual dietary protein intake can also influence mixed muscle FSR, for lower rates were seen in endurance athletes consuming 3.6 g of protein/kg/d as compared to 0.8 g of protein/kg/d (Bolster et al. 2005).

There are a number of athletes who feel that the human body has an infinite capacity to increase synthesis in response to protein and energy intake and often consume an inordinate amount of each in their diet. If this were the case, everyone could become a world-class bodybuilder just by eating a huge amount of energy and protein. A number of dietary supplement companies have marketed products based on this premise for years. We have not infrequently recorded dietary protein intakes in the range of 3–4 g/kg/d in bodybuilders and Varsity level football players. We evaluated one professional American football player consuming a daily intake of 80 egg whites, 4 L of milk and 250 g of protein powder per day during a pre-season training camp! It is not uncommon to see young strength athletes spending over US$40 per week on amino acid and protein supplements.

We have shown that the provision of dietary protein at levels above requirement (e.g. 2.8 versus 1.8 g/kg/d) resulted in an exponential increase in amino acid oxidation with no further increase in protein synthesis (Tarnopolsky et al. 1992). In addition, Lemon and colleagues found that the provision of dietary protein at 2.6 g/kg/d during resistance-exercise training in young males did not confer any strength or mass benefits compared to a diet supplying 1.35 g/kg/d (Lemon et al. 1992). During and after endurance exercise, the provision of extra protein (beyond requirement) resulted in an increase in leucine oxidation (Bowtell et al. 1998; Forslund et al. 1998) and actually attenuated muscle FSR (Bolster et al. 2005). Taken together, these data indicate that protein consumed in excess of need is oxidized as energy and does not have a net anabolic effect per se. However, there is a lower limit of protein intake where a further reduction in protein intake will have a negative impact on protein synthesis. It is the determination of these points that ultimately will determine the optimal protein intake for a given type of exercise (see section 4.15).

There has been an interest in the timing of nutrient delivery and the effects on recovery. The effects of co-ingestion of protein with CHO on post-exercise glycogen synthesis are covered in detail in Chapter 14. Given the known beneficial effects of CHO intake on protein metabolism, we became interested in determining whether there were beneficial effects of immediate post-resistance exercise glucose supplements on 24-hour protein balance (Roy et al. 1997). We compared the effect of CHO supplementation (1 g/kg) given immediately and an hour after resistance exercise to the same supplement given with breakfast in eight men. The post-exercise CHO supplement resulted in a more positive nitrogen balance and an attenuation of 3-MH excretion (myofibrillar proteolysis). It is important to note that this post-exercise strategy had a net positive effect on nitrogen balance over a 24-hour period and not just in the immediate post-exercise period (Roy et al. 1997). It has also been shown that an insulin infusion decreases protein degradation following resistance exercise (Biolo et al. 1999), which supports the idea that the effects of the post-exercise glucose drink were mediated by insulin. The convenience and relative inexpense of CHO supplementation makes this an attractive strategy to favorably alter net protein balance in resistance sports.

In addition to CHO, there has been interest in whether amino acids per se stimulate net protein balance (e.g. increase synthesis and/or decrease degradation). There is good evidence that an intravenous amino acid infusion has a stimulatory effect on muscle protein synthesis (Castellino et al. 1987; Tessari et al. 1987; Svanberg et al. 1996; Biolo et al. 1997; Svanberg 1998), independent of the insulin effect (Castellino et al. 1987). Furthermore, the essential and branched-chain amino acids seem to increase the sensitivity of the muscle to the protein stimulatory effects of insulin (Garlick & Grant 1988), especially leucine (Garlick 2005). On the other side of the equation, amino acids appear to have equivocal effects on protein degradation (Castellino et al. 1987; Tessari et al. 1987; Svanberg et al. 1996). The problem with this body of literature is that it does not directly answer the question about protein requirements, for it is impossible to determine whether the amino acids acted to stimulate protein synthesis during a state of deficiency, as compared to a situation of adequate protein status.

In parallel to the effect of timing of CHO intake on glycogen re-synthesis, there also appears to be a potentiation of amino acid transport into muscle after an acute bout of training (Zorzano et al. 1986; Biolo et al. 1997). Following resistance exercise, the stimulatory effects of hyperaminoacidemia (achieved by intravenous amino acids) have been shown to further enhance amino acid transport and muscle protein synthesis (Biolo et al. 1997). Net balance only becomes positive with feeding and several studies have found that it is the essential amino acids that are critical to this response (Tipton et al. 1999; Borsheim et al. 2002).

Complete proteins that contain high biological value amino acids (whey and casein) also stimulate post-resistance exercise net protein anabolism without a difference between the two sources (Tipton et al. 2004). Our group has also shown that milk has a more stimulatory effect on net protein balance and muscle protein synthesis as compared to soy (Wilkinson et al. 2007), and that over time this acute effect is reflected in greater lean mass accretion during training (Hartman et al. 2007). We have also conducted a dose-response study to intake of high-quality protein in the immediate recovery from resistance training in male athletes, and found that ~20 g of protein is sufficient to elicit a maximal response on muscle FSR; protein intake greater than this only served to increase protein oxidation (Moore et al. 2009).

CHOs have an interactive effect with amino acids in that amino acids appear to increase protein synthesis, whereas CHOs reduce protein breakdown (Miller et al. 2003; Borsheim et al. 2004).

The addition of protein (0.4 g/kg/h) to a CHO (1.2 g/kg/h) supplement did lead to a higher rate of muscle FSR and whole-body protein balance, but did not enhance glycogen resynthesis following endurance exercise (Howarth et al. 2009). In contrast, others have found that the addition of CHO in varying amounts to the same amount of protein (0.3 g/kg/h × 5 h = 1.5 g/kg protein) did not enhance whole-body protein kinetics or muscle FSR following acute exercise (Koopman et al. 2007). One study found that the provision of CHO and essential amino acids *before* a bout of resistance exercise increased amino acid (phenylalanine) uptake to a greater extent than when provided immediately after and that this was due to a greater delivery of amino acids (Tipton et al. 2001). Finally, a more positive protein balance mediated by a reduction in breakdown and an increase in FSR was seen when CHO + protein + leucine was given as compared to CHO or CHO + protein following resistance exercise in young men (Koopman et al. 2005) but not older men (Koopman et al. 2008).

Taken together, the aforementioned observations suggest that the immediate post-exercise period, or at the onset or during exercise, is an important time for the resistance athlete to consume protein and CHO. This may have an impact on protein requirements and permit optimal muscle adaptive gains (myofibrillar accretion) for any given protein intake. For the endurance athlete, the immediate provision of CHO is not as critical to glycogen resynthesis over the ensuing 24 hours, provided that CHO intake is high (~10 g/kg/d) and the addition of protein does not appear to enhance glycogen storage in the first few hours post-exercise as long as CHO intake is at least 1 g/kg/h. The addition of CHO to a high protein intake (at least 0.3 g/protein/kg/h) following endurance exercise does not further enhance muscle FSR or whole-body protein retention. From a performance perspective, there is some evidence that very high protein intake following intensive endurance activity on repeated days does enhance performance in men (Rowlands et al. 2008). Finally, the provision of CHO + protein + fat early following endurance exercise improves performance after a simulated training camp in young women (Roy et al. 2002).

4.11 Hormones and protein turnover

There are many hormones that directly and indirectly affect protein turnover, including insulin, cortisol, testosterone, growth hormone and insulin-like growth factor. A complete examination of these effects would require at least a dedicated chapter. Therefore, I will focus briefly on only two of these, namely insulin and testosterone.

I will mention testosterone only because of the significant controversy surrounding its unethical use in sporting events and its potent effects on protein metabolism. For years it was assumed that testosterone had stimulatory effects on net protein synthesis, based on observations of male/female differences in lean mass as well as the increases noted for those who supplemented with pharmacological doses. Only recently have there been proper investigations into the metabolism and efficacy of testosterone administration (Griggs et al. 1989; Bhasin et al. 1996; Ferrando et al. 1998). Even without resistance exercise, testosterone administration can increase lean body mass (Griggs et al. 1989; Bhasin et al. 1996); however, the effects are magnified with a resistance-exercise training program (Bhasin et al. 1996). At the muscle level, testosterone acts by increasing protein synthesis and intracellular amino acid re-utilization and not degradation (Ferrando et al. 1998). It should be kept in mind that acute resistance exercise also increases plasma testosterone concentration (Volek et al. 1997; Kraemer et al. 1998), and no studies have yet compared optimal nutritional intervention to testosterone in a comparative study. Another interesting finding that may serve to reduce the enthusiasm for very high protein intakes was the negative correlation between protein intake and plasma testosterone concentration (Volek et al. 1997).

Another key hormone that is important in protein metabolism and is the major factor in the efficacy of CHO–protein nutrition is insulin. Insulin has a net stimulatory effect upon muscle protein synthesis (Biolo et al. 1999), primarily through a reduction in muscle proteolysis (Castellino et al. 1987; Tessari et al. 1987). The effect of insulin on protein synthesis appears to depend on whether or not there is an abundance of amino acids (Biolo et al.

1999). Several studies have not found a stimulation of insulin on muscle protein synthesis (Castellino et al. 1987; Tessari et al. 1987; McNurlan et al. 1994); however, it is likely that the hypoaminoacidemia that results from insulin inhibits the stimulatory effect of insulin on protein synthesis (Biolo et al. 1997, 1999). When amino acids are provided simultaneously with insulin (to prevent hypoaminoacidemia), there appears to be a stimulation of protein synthesis (Castellino et al. 1987; Tessari et al. 1987; Moller-Loswick et al. 1994). Other studies have found that hyperinsulinemia stimulates both muscle FSR and amino acid transport (Biolo et al. 1995). Finally, the effects of insulin on protein metabolism are different before and after resistance exercise (Biolo et al. 1999). In the resting state, insulin induces a more positive protein balance by increasing synthesis and increasing amino acid transport; after exercise there was no effect on synthesis, yet there was a significant reduction in degradation and a threefold increase in amino acid transport (Biolo et al. 1999). These findings provide the theoretical basis for the provision of protein and CHO in the early post-exercise period in athletes performing resistance-type exercise, a finding confirmed by Miller and colleagues (2003).

Determining the adequacy of protein intake (dietary requirements) during exercise 4.12

Nitrogen balance 4.13

As defined above, NBAL is the method whereby the investigator determines all of the protein that enters a person (e.g. diet or intravenous) and all of the nitrogen that is excreted (Pellet 1990). Since the body excretes nitrogenous compounds rather than whole proteins and since proteins are ~16% nitrogen by weight, the technique involves measurement of the total nitrogen intake (N_{in}) and the total nitrogen excretion (N_{out}), through urine, feces, sweat and miscellaneous (e.g. menstrual loss, hair, semen and skin). If the person is in a state of net anabolism, then there is a positive NBAL, whereas if the person is losing protein then there is a negative NBAL. The protein intake requirement for a given physiological state (e.g. exercise, pregnancy and lactation) is determined by feeding the person varying protein intakes and determining the NBAL at each level of intake. From this, one can calculate a regression equation from which a zero NBAL can be interpolated. In order to account for inter-individual variability in the development of general guidelines, two standard deviations are added to the zero estimate. In this way, the 'safe' protein intake level is estimated to cover 97% of the given population. It is important to note that the NBAL experiment must indicate the biological value of the dietary protein used in the study. For example, a protein requirement of 1.0 g/kg/d based on egg white and milk protein would have to be higher than for a diet based on lower biological value proteins such as grains. Most countries in the world base their dietary protein intake recommendations relative to a biological value estimated to be the mean for the population (Pellet 1990).

In studies of athletes, it is important to recall that CHO and total energy intake can positively affect NBAL (Todd et al. 1984; Pellet 1990). Therefore, athletes with low CHO and energy intakes may require more protein than those with adequate intakes. These dietary interactions between protein, energy and CHO may have implications for those athletes who habitually consume low energy intakes or diets that encourage a very low CHO intake (which were massively promoted to the public in North America in the early 2000s).

One of the problems with the NBAL method is that the protein requirement estimates may under-estimate what is required for 'optimal' functioning. This concern comes from the fact that as protein intake decreases there is an increase in the efficiency of amino acid re-utilization and a lower overall amino acid flux (Young et al. 1987, 1989; Pellet 1990; Tarnopolsky et al. 1992). Therefore, NBAL may be achieved with a compromise in some physiologically relevant processes. For example, an endurance athlete may slow the induction of aerobic enzyme activity or a resistance athlete may not achieve the same degree of skeletal muscle hypertrophy over a period of training.

4.14 Tracer methods

Because of the limitations in the NBAL method, Young and colleagues have been instrumental in devising a conceptual framework from which to determine optimal protein intakes using stable isotopic tracers. They have coined the terms 'nutrient deficiency', 'accommodation', 'adaptation' and 'nutrient excess' (Young et al. 1987, 1989). In a state of protein deficiency, there would be a maximal reduction in amino acid oxidation and a reduction in protein synthesis to all but the essential organs (e.g. the brain), which ultimately would result in muscle wasting (negative NBAL). The state of accommodation would be the state where NBAL would be achieved with a decrease in a physiologically relevant process. The state of adaptation would be the dietary intake that provided for optimal rates of protein synthesis for growth, inter-organ amino acid exchange and immune function. Finally, the state of protein excess would be defined as that intake where amino acids are oxidized for energy or used in fat storage, and protein synthesis is not further stimulated by a further increase in intake.

The four states above can be determined using amino acid tracers during studies at varied protein intakes. The optimal protein intake would be that where amino acid oxidation starts to increase exponentially and protein synthesis starts to plateau. There have only been a few of these studies performed in athletes (Tarnopolsky et al. 1992; Forslund et al. 1998; Bolster et al. 2005).

Ultimately, the best method to determine the dietary requirements for athletes would be to provide a large group of sedentary individuals with a variety of graded protein intakes over a prolonged period of training and determine which was the optimal intake to achieve maximal improvements in several physiological outcome variables (e.g. $VO_{2\,max}$, muscle strength and muscle mass). Furthermore, one would also want to determine that the optimal protein intake resulted in optimal function in other critical areas such as resistance to infections. Unfortunately, this approach would be prohibitively expensive and time-consuming and as such is not likely to ever be completed.

4.15 Dietary protein requirements for athletes

4.16 The habitual intakes of athletes—a story of deficiency and excess

Athletes are a group of individuals who are constantly striving for optimal performance. Because of this, many of them may fall victim to false or unsubstantiated claims concerning diet and nutrient supplements. For example, the protein and amino acid supplement market in the US is a multi-million-dollar industry sustained by a motive to sell product rather than to encourage optimal nutrition through food. It is common to observe individuals consuming protein and amino acid intakes that would clearly be considered to be a gross nutrient excess. Another problem of many supplements is that they replace other components of the diet that may have known (e.g. vitamins, minerals, fiber and anti-oxidants) or as yet unknown factors that are critical for optimal body functioning. There may be a role for limited supplement use, such as when an athlete is traveling to a foreign country and the availability of familiar foods may be limited. In addition, there may be cases where an individual is on a weight-restrictive diet and protein intake may not be adequate to meet the needs of a rigorous training program. Even in such instances it should be possible to take advantage of factors such as timing of nutrient intake (see above) to optimize protein balance. For the most part, however, the problem of protein excess is predominantly one affecting strength athletes and not endurance athletes. In general, resistance-training athletes, who are not energy restricting, consume protein that is already in excess of their protein requirement (see Table 4.3, p. 77).

In contrast, some individuals may suffer from protein deficiency where chronically low intakes may lead to a compromise of function and ultimately to a loss of body protein (atrophy). This is clearly evident in the extreme case of anorexia nervosa and possibly in sports where weight categories are assigned. In the latter case, athletes may use extreme measures such as sweating and severe fluid and energy restriction to attain the lowest possible weight category (Brownell et al. 1987; Tarnopolsky et al. 1996). This situation is discussed in Chapter 7. There are four groups of athletes who appear to be at highest risk from protein and energy deficiency: amenorrheic female runners (Marcus et al. 1985; Drinkwater et al. 1990), male wrestlers (Brownell et al. 1987; Tarnopolsky et al. 1996), male and female gymnasts and female dancers (Short & Short 1983; Brownell et al. 1987). As seen in Table 4.2 overleaf, most groups of athletes consume adequate amounts of protein and energy. It is important to remember that these nutrition surveys are mean intakes for a group and the range can be wide within a group. For example, in one study, the mean energy and protein intake reported by male gymnasts was 2080 kcal and 1.1 g/kg/d respectively; however, some athletes reported intakes as low as 568 kcal and 0.16 g/kg/d (Short & Short 1983). Similarly, in a study of female runners, Deuster and colleagues (1986) found that the mean reported energy and protein intake was 2397 kcal and 1.56 g/kg/d respectively, yet the lowest reported intakes were 1067 kcal and 0.53 g/kg/d. It is also important to note that there is often under-reporting of dietary intake by female athletes in weight-dependent activities such as lightweight rowing (Hill & Davies 2002). Nevertheless, there are still disturbing numbers of women with disordered eating, and an increasing recognition of the issue in men, to the point that some athletes may compromise function and body mass (including bone density) through low energy and protein and micronutrient intakes.

In summary, the majority of strength and endurance athletes consume adequate protein and energy to meet their needs. Even when one takes into account the modest increases required by certain athletes (see section 4.18), most athletes are still above these levels. It appears that the human body homeostatically adapts to exercise by matching protein and energy intakes to cover any increase in demand from the activity in question. In some groups there are extrinsic pressures to restrict intake for weight class or aesthetic reasons. In fact, certain groups may not even be attaining the recommended intake levels for sedentary individuals and it is attention to the 'extremes' that requires intervention

TABLE 4.2 HABITUAL PROTEIN INTAKES OF MEN AND WOMEN ENDURANCE ATHLETES

		PROTEIN	
REFERENCE	SUBJECTS	(g/kg/d)	(%E_{IN})
Zalcman et al. 2007	*n* = 6 women	2.0	18
	n = 18 men	1.9	18
Petersen et al. 2006	*n* = 24 women	1.3	13
Carter et al. 2001	*n* = 8 men	1.7	16
	n = 8 women	1.3	17
Tarnopolsky et al. 1997	*n* = 8 men	1.9	17
	n = 8 women	1.2	14
Tarnopolsky et al. 1995	*n* = 7 men	1.8	15
	n = 8 women	1.0	12
Tarnopolsky et al. 1988	*n* = 6 men	1.5	11
Phillips et al. 1993	*n* = 6 men	1.9	15
	n = 6 women	1.0	13
Tarnopolsky et al. 1990	*n* = 6 men	1.2	12
	n = 6 women	1.7	13
Saris et al. 1989	*n* = 5 men	2.2	15
Deuster et al. 1986	*n* = 51 women	1.6	13
Nelson et al. 1986	*n* = 17 EUM	1.0	15
	n = 11 AMEN	0.7	15
Marcus et al. 1985	*n* = 6 EUM	1.3	17
	n = 11 AMEN	1.0	15
Drinkwater et al. 1984	*n* = 13 EUM	1.1	13
	n = 14 AMEN	1.2	16
Mean values	Men	1.8 (0.4)	14 (2)
	Women	1.3 (0.4)	14 (2)

Values are mean (SD); EUM = eumenorrheic; AMEN = amenorrheic women; E_{in} = Energy intake

by nutritionists and allied health care professionals. Consequently, each athlete must be considered as an individual when determining the adequacy of dietary protein and energy intakes. The identification of the 'at-risk' groups above may help the nutritionist or coach to be aware of those who may need special nutrition counseling (Hinton et al. 2004). Even elite male athletes may be in negative energy balance, especially when preparing for competitions (Fudge et al. 2006).

4.17 Protein requirements for endurance sports

In most countries there are no specific allowances for an effect of physical exercise on protein requirements. It is sometimes stated that these are not required because all athletes

TABLE 4.3 HABITUAL PROTEIN INTAKES OF RESISTANCE ATHLETES

REFERENCE	PARTICIPANTS	PROTEIN (g/kg/d)	PROTEIN ($\%E_{IN}$)
Roy & Tarnopolsky 1998	*n* = 10 men (trained*)	1.6	18
Tarnopolsky et al. 1992	*n* = 7 men (footballers)	1.8	16
Lemon et al. 1992	*n* = 12 men (bodybuilders)	1.4	14
Chesley et al. 1992	*n* = 12 men (bodybuilders)	1.6	17
Tarnopolsky et al. 1988	*n* = 6 men (bodybuilders)	2.7	17
Faber et al. 1986	*n* = 76 men (bodybuilders)	2.4	22
Short & Short 1983	*n* = 30 men (footballers)	2.5	18
	n = 6 men (bodybuilders)	2.3	20
Burke et al. 1991	*n* = 18 men (weightlifters)	1.9	18
Burke & Read 1988	*n* = 56 men (footballers)	1.5	15
Bazzarre et al. 1990	*n* = 8 women (bodybuilders)	2.8	37
	Mean values	2.0 (0.5)	19 (6)

Values are mean (SD); *trained = weight-trained four times per week for more than two years

consume more energy and subsequently achieve adequate protein intakes. Others have argued that moderate exercise does not increase the requirement for dietary protein (Butterfield & Calloway 1984; Campbell et al. 1995; El-Khoury et al. 1997), and therefore there is no need to provide specific protein requirements for athletes. However, these studies were undertaken using exercise intensities that would be considered recreational by most standards. Clearly, an elite athlete is performing daily exercise at a much higher intensity and for a longer duration than the novice. Therefore, it is critical to quantify the state of training and the daily volume for any study looking at protein requirements in athletes. Although most athletes consume enough protein to cover any potential increase in dietary need, there are individuals who may not even meet minimal requirements and it is for this group that a knowledge of protein requirements is useful. For example, a person who is performing regular, strenuous activity while on an energy-restrictive diet may wish to know the minimal protein intake for optimal functional status.

Given that amino acids can be oxidized as energy during exercise, it is theoretically possible that this may affect the need for extra dietary protein. The determination of dietary protein requirements for endurance athletes is a function of the duration and intensity of exercise, gender, age, training status, and habitual energy and CHO intake. To determine the effect of endurance-exercise training on amino acid oxidation, we measured leucine oxidation in six males and six females during endurance exercise at 60% $VO_{2\ peak}$ both before and after a 38-day training program (McKenzie et al. 2000). We found that leucine oxidation and BCOAD activation were significantly attenuated following the training period, yet the total BCOAD maximal activity was increased (McKenzie et al. 2000). This study suggested that at the same absolute exercise intensity there was a training-induced sparing of protein use, yet the capacity existed to oxidize more protein under the period of energy deficiency, CHO depletion and during high-intensity workouts. The results of these studies demonstrate the importance of indicating the training status of the group of subjects being studied and also their current training regime.

In a simplistic approach to determining protein requirements, it is possible to calculate the estimated need for dietary protein by an athlete from first principles. For example, if a 70 kg male was running for 1.5 hours at 70% $VO_{2\,peak}$ and protein accounted for 5% of the total energy, he would oxidize about 15 g of protein. If his basal protein requirement was 0.86 g/kg/d (60 g), this would represent an additional 25% increase in his daily protein requirement (1.07 g/kg/d). Most male and female athletes habitually consume more protein than this (see Table 4.3). These calculations are only rough estimates and most studies have used NBAL to try to quantify dietary protein requirements for endurance athletes.

Two often-quoted studies determined NBAL following the initiation of an endurance-exercise program on a constant protein intake and while consuming two different protein intakes (Gontzea et al. 1962, 1968). In a group of males starting an endurance-exercise program they found that a protein intake of 1.5 g/kg/d was adequate to maintain a positive NBAL, whereas 1.0 g/kg/d was inadequate (Gontzea et al. 1968). In addition, they also found that the subjects on a constant protein intake showed progressive adaptation to the moderate exercise program by improving NBAL over the course of about one week (Gontzea et al. 1962). These latter findings suggested that there were adaptive changes to the stress of exercise (e.g. an increase in amino acid re-utilization efficiency) and therefore an increased protein intake was needed only at the initiation of an endurance-exercise program. This is similar to our findings in men and women following a modest training program (McKenzie et al. 2000). An improvement in NBAL with moderate-intensity endurance-exercise training is due to a lower resting (Gaine et al. 2005) and exercise-induced (McKenzie et al. 2000) amino acid oxidation.

With moderate-intensity endurance exercise (≤50% $VO_{2\,peak}$), there does not appear to be an increase in protein requirements (Butterfield & Calloway 1984; Todd et al. 1984). At these modest exercise intensities, protein utilization is enhanced (Butterfield & Calloway 1984), and energy deficits are better tolerated (Todd et al. 1984). In another study of endurance exercise at moderate intensity (46% $VO_{2\,peak}$), El-Khoury and colleagues (1997) used a combined isotopic tracer and nitrogen excretion method and found that a protein intake of 1 g/kg/d was adequate for young males. The improvement in NBAL observed by Gaine and colleagues (2005) occurred in men and women with modest aerobic capacity (39 mL/kg/min) after 4 weeks of modest exercise training (4–5 X/wk @ 65–85% max heart rate).

Likely the most comprehensive study of endurance-exercise training and protein metabolism was completed by Forslund and colleagues (1998). They studied leucine oxidation, protein, CHO fat and energy balance over a 24-hour period in men performing low/moderate-intensity exercise (90 minutes @ 45–50% $VO_{2\,peak}$) while consuming a higher (2.5 g/kg/d) and lower (1.0 g/kg/d) protein intake. Whole-body protein balance was slightly negative on the 1.0 g/kg/d diet, and positive on the 2.5 g/kg/d diet. These results suggest that people performing modest-intensity exercise do not require an increase in dietary protein intake or at most it is only marginally above 1.0 g/kg/d (Forslund et al. 1998). However, most athletes exercise at intensities of 65–85% of $VO_{2\,peak}$ where there may be a negative impact on protein homeostasis and NBAL. A final observation that requires further study is the fact that fat oxidation and CHO storage were higher on the higher-protein diet in the Forslund study (Forslund et al. 1998), and these findings could be of significance in an endurance athlete.

In contrast, there does appear to be an increase in protein requirements for well-trained endurance athletes (Tarnopolsky et al. 1988; Brouns et al. 1989; Friedman & Lemon 1989; Meredith et al. 1989; Phillips et al. 1993) (for review see Tarnopolsky 2004). One study used NBAL to determine the protein requirements in a group of endurance-trained males who were young (27 y; $VO_{2\ peak}$ = 65 mL/kg/min) or middle-aged (52 y; $VO_{2\ peak}$ = 55 mL/kg/min) (Meredith et al. 1989). These researchers found that a protein intake of 0.94 g/kg/d was required for NBAL, and whole-body protein synthesis (glycine tracer) increased with increasing protein intakes (0.61 > 0.92 > 1.21 g/kg/d). When accounting for inter-individual variability by adding two standard deviations to the zero NBAL intercept, the estimated protein requirement for these males was about 1.28 g/kg/d (Meredith et al. 1989). A study performed in our laboratory found that both male ($VO_{2\ peak}$ = 59 mL/kg/min) and female ($VO_{2\ peak}$ = 55 mL/kg/min) endurance athletes were in negative NBAL while consuming a dietary protein intake that was close to the Canadian, US and Australian recommended intake for sedentary individuals (males = 0.94 g/kg/d; females = 0.80 g/kg/d) (Phillips et al. 1993).

There are three studies using NBAL methodology to examine the protein requirements of elite endurance-trained athletes (Tarnopolsky et al. 1988; Brouns et al. 1989; Friedman & Lemon 1989). We performed an NBAL experiment in six elite male endurance athletes ($VO_{2\ peak}$ = 76.2 mL/kg/min, training >12 h/wk) to determine what we considered to be close to the upper limit of protein requirements for endurance athletes (Tarnopolsky et al. 1988). We determined the safe protein intake for the elite athletes to be 1.6 g/kg/d, whereas the estimate for a sedentary control group (n = 6) was 0.86 g/kg/d, which was very close to Canadian and US recommendations (Tarnopolsky et al. 1988). In a simulated Tour de France cycling study, Brouns and colleagues (1989) found that well-trained cyclists ($VO_{2\ peak}$ = 65.1 mL/kg/min) required protein intakes of 1.5–1.8 g/kg/min to maintain NBAL. In a final study, Friedman and Lemon (1989) calculated the protein requirement for five well-trained runners to be about 1.49 g/kg/d, using NBAL.

To summarize the available data, it appears that low- and moderate-intensity endurance exercise does not result in an increase in dietary protein requirements. At the initiation of an endurance-exercise program there may be a transient increase in dietary protein need, yet the body rapidly adapts to the increase in need. For the well-trained athlete (training 4 to 5 days per week for >45 min @ >60% VO_{max}), there appears to be an increase of about 20–25% in dietary protein requirements. In the elite athlete, the increase in dietary protein intake may be as high as 1.6 g/kg/d (or nearly twice the recommended intake for sedentary persons). Given that the $VO_{2\ peak}$ of the Tour de France riders (Brouns et al. 1989) and of the athletes in our study (Tarnopolsky et al. 1988) are among the highest reported, I feel that this is probably the highest requirement needed for endurance athletes. Clearly, there may be some more demanding events; however, the day-to-day training is not likely to exceed that reported for the athletes in these studies (Tarnopolsky et al. 1988; Brouns et al. 1989). In spite of these elevated requirements, there is no need for supplementation with a mixed diet of adequate energy intake providing 15% of the energy from protein. For example, with an energy intake of about 3500 kcal/d (which is still modest), this would amount to about 125 g protein/d or ~1.6–1.8 g/kg/d.

One final point about protein requirements for endurance athletes is the possibility of a gender difference. We first found a gender difference in protein metabolism in 1990 (Tarnopolsky et al. 1990), with men showing increased urinary urea excretion on an exercise compared to rest day, whereas women did not. We concluded that this was due to a glycogen-sparing effect seen in the women. In the study where we found that the Canadian recommended intake for protein was inadequate for well-trained endurance athletes, we also found that the females were in a less negative NBAL and their basal leucine oxidation was lower compared to the males (Phillips et al. 1993). In a subsequent study, we also found that females had lower leucine oxidation both at rest and during

TABLE 4.4 ESTIMATED PROTEIN REQUIREMENTS FOR ATHLETES

GROUP	PROTEIN INTAKE (G/KG/D)
Sedentary men and women	0.80–1.0
Elite male endurance athletes	1.6
Moderate-intensity endurance athletes[a]	1.2
Recreational endurance athletes[b]	0.80–1.0
Football, power sports	1.4–1.7
Resistance athletes (early training)	1.5–1.7
Resistance athletes (steady state)	1.0–1.2
Female athletes	~10–20% lower than male athletes

[a]Exercising approximately four to five times per week for 45–60 min; [b]Exercising four to five times per week for 30 min at <55% $VO_{2\,peak}$

exercise before and after a 38-day training program compared to males (McKenzie et al. 2000). These findings may indicate that the dietary protein recommendations for endurance athletes (see Table 4.4) may be 10–20% lower for females than males.

4.18 Protein requirements for strength sports

In contrast to endurance exercise, resistance exercise results in muscle hypertrophy (Lemon et al. 1992; Tarnopolsky et al. 2001b), rather than an increase in amino acid oxidation and mitochondrial biogenesis (McKenzie et al. 2000; Howarth et al. 2007). If there are no changes in efficiency of amino acid retention (see below), there must, at some point, be a protein intake in excess of basal requirements to provide the amino acids required for anabolism. The extent of this increased need is again a function of the basal state of training, the duration and the intensity of the training program.

An early study used NBAL and lean mass measurements to estimate the protein requirements during an isometric-exercise training program (Torun et al. 1977). Torun and colleagues found that a daily protein intake of 1.0 g/kg (egg white and milk) was required to maintain positive NBAL and lean mass accretion in males performing isometric exercise for 75 min/d (Torun et al. 1977). The equivalent protein intake from a mixed source would be about 1.2 g/kg/d. Similar results were found in young males performing circuit training with both endurance and resistance exercise where even after a 40-day adaptation period, protein requirements were ~1.4 g/kg/d (Consolazio et al. 1975).

Modest-intensity resistance-exercise programs can attenuate nitrogen loss at protein intakes close to the US and Canadian recommended protein intake levels in older adults (Campbell et al. 1995). Although there may be the ability to achieve NBAL (through increased nitrogen utilization efficiency) with modest resistance exercise, this may be indicative of accommodation and not adaptation, because at the lower protein intake (~0.8 g/kg/d) Campbell and colleagues (1995) also found that whole-body protein synthesis was lower than for the group who consumed protein intakes of 1.6 g/kg/d. This is another example of the utility of amino acid kinetics to provide more information on the physiological adequacy of a given protein intake.

We performed an NBAL experiment in six well-trained bodybuilders (>2 years training experience) and six sedentary individuals and found that the protein requirement for the trained bodybuilders was only 12% greater than for the sedentary controls (Tarnopolsky et al. 1988). We also found that the bodybuilders in this study were habitually consuming protein intakes of ~2.7 g/kg/d (Tarnopolsky et al. 1988). The error of the NBAL method was demonstrated in this study; if the positive NBAL on the high protein intake was extrapolated to net protein retention (assuming no change in breakdown), there would have been a 200 g/d increase in lean body mass each day! Some lay reports have used these data in support of the high protein intakes consumed by the bodybuilders. However, the magnitude of the positive NBAL cannot be directly extrapolated to an increase in lean mass, for two reasons. First, there is an inherent error in the technique, which over-estimates NBAL at high nitrogen intakes (Young et al. 1987), and second, protein synthesis and breakdown change in parallel (Phillips et al. 1997).

We followed up on our observations with two studies to more accurately characterize the impact of resistance training on dietary protein needs. In the first we reasoned that the protein requirements would be highest during the early adaptation period to unaccustomed training, since most of the myofibrillar protein accretion occurs within the first several months following the initiation of a resistance-exercise program. Therefore, we exposed twelve young males to 2 months of a supervised resistance-exercise program (6 days per week, 2 hours per day, 70–85% 1RM [maximum repetition]) and measured NBAL, muscle mass, muscle protein and strength before and after a 1-month period where they were randomized to receive protein at 1.44 and 2.6 g/kg/d.

We calculated the estimated protein requirement during this period to be ~1.65 g/kg/d (Lemon et al. 1992). Strength, muscle protein and lean mass gains following training were not different between the two protein intakes (Lemon et al. 1992). We went on to use the conceptual framework put forth by Young and Bier (1987) and studied the protein kinetic response to graded protein intakes in young males who were performing weight-training and high-intensity sprinting/power activities (e.g. football and rugby) (Tarnopolsky et al. 1992). In this study we randomly allocated six sedentary males and seven athletes to receive a diet supplying protein at each of three levels (Canadian recommended intake ~0.86 g/kg/d; moderate ~1.4 g/kg/d; and high ~2.4 g/kg/d). We measured NBAL, whole-body protein synthesis, leucine oxidation and protein breakdown, and calculated the estimated safe protein intake to be 0.89 g/kg/d for the sedentary group and 1.76 g/kg/d for the athletes (Tarnopolsky et al. 1992). The whole-body protein synthesis was greater for the athletes as compared to the sedentary controls at all protein intakes. Furthermore, whole-body protein synthesis was lower at 0.86 g/kg/d as compared to 1.4 and 2.8 g/kg/d, and appeared to plateau at around 1.4 g/kg/d for the strength-trained athletes. At protein intakes of 2.8 g/kg/d, leucine oxidation increased nearly twofold, which provided evidence that protein intake above the requirement is merely oxidized for energy (Tarnopolsky et al. 1992).

Potential side effects of excessive protein intake 4.19

In general, there are probably few side effects arising from daily protein intakes under 2.0 g/kg/d in healthy people. Perhaps the most definite effect of a very-high-protein diet would be the cost of protein supplements or protein-rich foods. Even with dietary protein, the ultimate cost to produce a kilogram of beef is more than an isoenergetic amount of wheat. Furthermore, most meat products also contain significant amounts of fat, which, if taken at a high enough level, may render the diet atherogenic. Again, these are not likely to be a problem with protein intakes below 2.0 g/kg/d.

Although it is probable that most people can safely maintain very high protein intakes for long periods of time, there are several caveats that must be considered. First, a high-protein diet can increase urinary calcium excretion (from the sulphur-containing amino acids) (Whiting et al. 1997), which may be a concern for the female athlete with a low energy intake and amenorrhea; however, recent studies have demonstrated that higher protein diets (20% of E_{in}) are associated with higher calcium absorption, which compensates for the slightly higher excretion (Hunt et al. 2009).

Second, high protein intakes in conjunction with pre-existing renal disease may accelerate the progression of the disease (Brenner et al. 1982); however, there is no evidence at all that a diet supplying 1.8 g of protein/kg/d has any deleterious effects. Third, rodents fed very high protein intakes have been found to exhibit morphological changes in liver mitochondria (Zaragoza et al. 1987); however, the relative amount of protein is much larger than any amount reasonably consumed by humans, and hepatic toxicity in rodents cannot be directly applied to humans (Tarnopolsky et al. 2003). Finally, some problems may occur if the protein is taken as an amino acid supplement. One possible problem relates to contamination of purified amino acids, as in the case of L-tryptophan supplements that were manufactured in Japan and caused a life-threatening disorder called eosinophilic myalgia syndrome (EMS) (Hertzman et al. 1990). Evidence suggests that this occurred due to a high pressure liquid chromatography (HPLC) purified contaminant present from a bacterial processing method (Yamaoka et al. 1994).

In addition to the expense involved, large doses of purified amino acids could potentially be carcinogenic and mutagenic. Such warnings are noted on the Materials Safety Data Sheets (MSDS) labels of purified chemical-grade laboratory amino acids, although these problems have not been substantiated in humans. Even if purified amino acids are safe, they are expensive and their efficacy has not been established in spite of many studies. Although essential amino acids appear to be the most potent in stimulating post-exercise protein synthesis (Borsheim et al. 2002), this response does not appear to be greater than that seen with the consumption of high biological value proteins (Tipton et al. 2004), including milk (Wilkinson et al. 2007).

Furthermore, the consumption of a drink containing exclusively essential amino acids may exclude amino acids that could enhance other aspects of the adaptation to exercise (such as proline for connective tissue adaptations or arginine and glycine for creatine synthesis).

4.20 Summary

Protein is an important component of the diet and is involved in almost every structural and functional component of the human body. In general, endurance exercise may affect the need for dietary protein by increasing the oxidation of amino acids. Resistance exercise may also have an impact through the need for amino acids to support muscle hypertrophy. At the onset of an endurance-exercise program there is a negative effect on NBAL, yet with time the body adapts to the stress and NBAL and leucine oxidation are attenuated. After endurance-exercise training, the amount of amino acid oxidized at the same absolute exercise intensity is reduced, yet the capacity of the body to oxidize amino acids is increased. However, only in the elite athlete (who is training very hard every day) is there a significant impact upon dietary protein requirements, with a maximal requirement of ~1.6 g/kg/d. For the resistance-trained athlete, there also appears to be a homeostatic adaptation to the stress of the exercise, where very well-trained athletes require only marginally more protein than sedentary persons and those in the early stages of very intensive resistance exercise may require up to 1.7 g/kg/d. A dietary protein intake that represents 15% of the total energy intake with an energy-sufficient diet should easily cover the requirements for nearly all strength and endurance athletes. Given the increase in energy intake by most athletes, there is no need to use protein supplements to attain these levels. However, athletes on a low-energy diet and/or a low-CHO diet could have an inadequate protein intake to cover their needs. The timing of nutrient delivery appears to be important for resistance and endurance athletes, where an immediate post-exercise (or pre/during exercise) intake of CHO and protein will lead to a more positive protein NBAL, probably by reducing protein breakdown (CHO) and stimulating synthesis (protein).

PRACTICE TIPS

GARY SLATER

- Bulking up can be an important outcome in the development of many athletes. For most, the intent to bulk up or increase weight is a desire to increase muscle mass and strength. Few athletes intentionally plan to increase fat mass. To ensure gains in muscle mass are prioritized, the combination of a well-designed overall training program that incorporates resistance exercise, plus an energy-dense, strategically planned diet is required.
- If gains in muscle mass are a priority, a hypertrophy phase needs to be incorporated into the athlete's yearly training schedule. This period should include consistent allocation of resistance-training sessions each week with a concurrent reduction in overall training volume, especially conditioning sessions, which can limit the potential for gains in muscle mass. The off-season and early pre-season are ideal times to prioritize muscle mass gains. Too often, athletes identified as too weak or small mid-season are placed on a hypertrophy program that is destined to fail—not because of a lack of commitment from the athlete, but because of the high energy demands of routine training/competition during that phase of the season.
- The sports dietitian should ensure that short and long-term weight gain goals are realistic. An increase in body mass of 0.25–0.5 kg per week may be possible but will depend on genetics and the resistance-training history of the athlete—significant prior gains inevitably ensure only smaller future gains are possible. Significantly greater rates of gain are likely to include increments in body fat stores that may have to be reduced at a later stage. It is also important to ensure overall body composition goals are realistic. Far too many athletes want to increase muscle mass and decrease body fat simultaneously. This is not achievable for most athletes as the two goals are mutually exclusive: one demands an increase in energy availability while the other requires a reduction in energy availability. Priorities must be set and dietary intervention applied accordingly.
- Monitoring body composition during a hypertrophy phase is an important tool for assessing progress. It helps identify if the meal plan is supporting gains in muscle mass and may alleviate fears of body fat gain for those athletes who are weight-focused. Regular monitoring of body mass and body fat stores provides an accurate indication of any changes in body composition. See Chapter 3 for a closer examination of physique assessment tools.
- Meeting the increased protein needs of both strength and endurance athletes in hard training is essential if adaptation and recovery are to be optimized. Fortunately, the higher food intake of most athletes ensures a generous protein intake, usually well above requirements typically prescribed (a daily intake of 1.2–1.7 g/kg BM). As energy intake increases to meet the additional energy demands of training, extra protein requirements can be achieved from a meal plan providing ~15% of total energy as protein. However, some athletes are at risk of inadequate protein intake. These include athletes involved in weight restriction or aesthetically judged sports as well as athletes with disordered or restrictive eating patterns and those following fad diets. Failure to consume sufficient protein may result in a reduction in muscle mass and compromise training adaptations and immune function.

- It may be too simplistic to assess the adequacy of an athlete's dietary protein intake through total daily intake alone. Recent research suggests that for any given protein intake, the metabolic response is dependent on other factors, including the timing of ingestion in relation to exercise, the composition of ingested amino acids, co-ingestion of other nutrients (especially CHO), total energy intake and the rate of protein digestion. Future research will help to ascertain the importance of these factors in optimizing chronic adaptations to training. The type of training undertaken, desired outcomes of training and training status of the athlete should also be considered when assessing protein needs.
- The timing of protein intake may be just as important as total protein intake over the day. As consumption of large amounts of protein at any one time merely stimulates protein oxidation, the inclusion of small amounts of protein-rich food at each meal and snack may result in enhanced muscle recovery and hypertrophy goals. The meal plans in Table 4.5 illustrate both a poorly distributed protein intake (emphasizing the majority of daily protein intake at the evening meal, common among many athletes) and a more evenly distributed protein intake across the day.

TABLE 4.5 TWO MEAL PLANS WITH SIMILAR TOTAL NUTRITIONAL VALUE BUT DIFFERING IN THEIR DISTRIBUTION OF PROTEIN THROUGHOUT THE DAY (FOR AN 80 KG ATHLETE, PROTEIN NEEDS ARE EASILY ACHIEVED WITHOUT THE USE OF EXPENSIVE PROTEIN SUPPLEMENTS)

ADEQUATE PROTEIN—POOR DISTRIBUTION		ADEQUATE PROTEIN—WELL DISTRIBUTED	
MEAL	**PROTEIN**	**MEAL**	**PROTEIN**
Breakfast 2½ cups cereal, low-fat milk 2 slices toast, jam	32	Breakfast 2½ cups cereal, low-fat milk 2 slices toast, jam	32
Morning tea 2 cereal bars	6	Morning tea 200 g low-fat yoghurt	11
Lunch 2 ham, cheese, salad rolls Orange juice	32	Lunch 2 ham, cheese, salad rolls Orange juice	32
Afternoon tea 2 slices fruit loaf	5	Afternoon tea Milk shake	15
Training Water, sports drink	0	Training Water, sports drink	0
Post-training	0	Post-training 300 ml low-fat flavored milk	10
Dinner 250 g lean steak 2 cups steamed rice, vegetables Reduced-fat custard, banana	75	Dinner 120 g lean steak 2 cups steamed rice, vegetables Reduced-fat custard, banana	50
Total protein (g)	150 (1.9 g/kg)	Total protein	150 (1.9 g/kg)

PRACTICE TIPS

- Consuming a protein-and-CHO-containing snack both before and immediately after resistance exercise can help maximize training adaptations by increasing the production of anabolic hormones, reducing protein breakdown and supplying amino acids for muscle building. There is some evidence that the response is strongest when protein is consumed with CHO rather than alone. Muscle growth is stimulated only in the presence of an adequate amino acid supply, so spreading protein intake throughout the day optimizes amino acid availability. Post-training snacks rich in CHO and protein can also help enhance recovery of energy reserves (especially for athletes following low-CHO and/or low-energy meal plans) and should be planned after all training sessions. The amount of protein required acutely in recovery is quite small (within the range of 10–20 g) and thus should be achievable even for athletes on tight energy budgets. Suitable recovery snacks include a tub of yoghurt or creamed rice, glass of flavored milk or smoothie, cereal with milk, or lean meat/cheese sandwich. However, meticulous planning of pre- and post-training snacks will not compensate for inadequacies in an athlete's meal plan throughout the remainder of the day.
- Any evaluation of an athlete's protein requirements should also consider the energy content of their diet. For any given protein intake, increasing energy density of the meal plan will enhance nitrogen balance. In fact, the most important dietary component of a weight-gain program is an increase in energy density. For some athletes this can be a real challenge. Frequent and/or prolonged training sessions can limit opportunities for meals and snacks while intense training may suppress an athlete's appetite. Novel strategies like an increased reliance on energy-dense snacks and drinks may be required to overcome such obstacles. The following tips may help to increase energy density of a meal plan:
  - Increase meal or snack frequency. Intestinal tolerance is generally higher when the frequency of meals is increased rather than the size of existing meals and snacks. Eating frequently should become a priority, even during busy days. Meal plans with five or six or more meals and snacks (including pre- and post-training snacks) throughout the day should be encouraged.
  - Make use of energy-dense drinks (such as smoothies, milk shakes, powdered liquid meal supplements, UHT packs of flavored milk, fruit juice, cordial, soft drink and sports drinks) and other energy-dense foods (e.g. low-fat dairy snacks like yoghurt and custard, cereal or sports bars, fruit bread, dried fruit and nuts or trail mix). Commercial liquid meal supplements are a convenient option for athletes on the run; products fortified with vitamins and minerals plus a combination of both CHO and protein (in a ratio of 2–3:1) are most suitable. Alternatively, homemade milk drinks can be fortified with skim milk powder to add an extra protein and energy boost. These drinks can be particularly useful for athletes unable to tolerate solid food before and/or after training or those with small appetites.
  - While increasing overall energy consumption, intake of high-satiety/high-fiber foods may need to be tempered. Low-energy fruit and vegetables, while a great source of nutrients, may also need to be moderated, allowing more room for energy-dense, nutrient-rich options.

  - Athletes may need reminding that the period of increased energy density is not an excuse for gluttony and junk food, rather a period where well-planned, frequent-eating occasions of nutritious foods and fluids are prioritized.
- While the energy surplus required to support a 1 kg gain in muscle mass is likely to vary between individuals (depending on current training and diet, genetic profile, etc.), a conservative 1500–2000 kJ (360–480 kcal) increase in daily energy intake for an athlete with a stable body mass (and thus presumably in energy balance) is a sensible starting point. However, more aggressive increments in daily energy intake of 4000 kJ (960 kcal) or more may be warranted for some athletes, especially if the energy cost of resistance training has to be accounted for (e.g. if the athlete has not previously been undertaking regular resistance training). Regular body mass and composition monitoring will provide invaluable feedback on the requirement for further adjustments in energy intake to support muscle hypertrophy.
- Foods rich in protein are shown in Table 4.6. While high biological value proteins like meat, poultry, seafood and dairy products provide ~50% of protein intake in a typical western diet, other sources, such as cereals and cereal products like bread, pasta, rice, legumes and breakfast cereals, also contribute significant amounts of protein as well as other important nutrients. Ideally, a mixture of protein sources should be included in the diet. However, if low biological value protein sources predominate in the meal plan, total protein intake goals should be adjusted towards the upper range of guidelines. Similarly, athletes following low-energy meal plans may require a proportionally higher protein intake. Aiming for the upper range of guidelines may be advisable but will depend on total available energy budget and consideration of other nutrients essential for fueling and recovery.
- Athletes should be guided to choose meal combinations that match protein requirements with other nutrient needs, for example three or more serves of low-fat dairy foods daily for protein and calcium, and one or two serves of lean meat, seafood, poultry or vegetarian alternatives daily for protein, iron and zinc.

TABLE 4.6 COMMON FOOD SOURCES OF PROTEIN: EACH OF THE FOLLOWING FOODS PROVIDES ~10 G OF PROTEIN; THESE FOODS HAVE LOW TO MODERATE FAT CONTENTS AND ARE RICH IN OTHER NUTRIENTS

ANIMAL FOODS	PLANT FOODS
35 g cooked lean beef/ pork/ lamb	4 slices bread
40 g skinless cooked chicken	3 cups wholegrain cereal
50 g cooked fish or canned tuna/ salmon	2 cups cooked pasta
1 cup low-fat milk	3 cups cooked rice
200 g low-fat yoghurt	¾ cup cooked lentils/ kidney beans
30 g (1.5 slices) reduced-fat cheese	120 g tofu
70 g cottage cheese	60 g nuts or seeds
2 small eggs	1 cup soy milk

PRACTICE TIPS

- While most athletes readily ingest 1.2–2.0 g protein per kilogram body mass each day, some athletes eat more than 4 g/kg, believing this will further enhance gains in muscle mass. Current research suggests such extreme diets are neither necessary nor beneficial, as excess dietary protein does not have an anabolic effect and will simply be oxidized for energy production. However, routine consumption of a high-protein diet does not appear to negatively impact renal function in healthy individuals, nor have a significant impact on hydration status or bone health. A likely disadvantage for the athlete is that a high protein intake may displace other important nutrients necessary to support their training/competition demands, add to their weekly shopping bill and potentially be a major source of saturated fat.
- Many athletes will require advice about lifestyle and time management to allow them to achieve adequate time for eating, sleeping, training and their other daily commitments. Planning the day's intake—what and when—may assist some athletes in ensuring suitable foods and drinks are on hand when required. A ready supply of non-perishable snacks in a locker or training bag can be a great idea, for example Tetra™ packs of ultra-high-temperature (UHT) flavored milk/fruit juice, cereal bars, powdered liquid meal supplements and sports drinks. The sports dietitian should assess the potential of the athlete's environment for purchasing suitable foods, or for storing snacks brought from home.
- As resistance training influences protein metabolism for upwards of 48 hours afterwards, athletes should be encouraged to follow these muscle building strategies throughout the week, not just on training days.
- Emotive labeling on products promoted in many gyms, sporting magazines and health food stores ensures dietary supplements are very popular among athletes attempting to increase muscle mass. Athletes can be confronted by a huge array of products from protein powders and amino acid formulas to proclaimed growth enhancers and 'pre-training stimulators'. Some products may be of benefit to certain athletes in specific situations (by meeting specific nutrient needs or offering a degree of convenience) but the claims of most supplements do not hold up to the scrutiny of scientific research. Athletes must be reminded that the core of a successful hypertrophy program is a suitably designed training program and well-structured meal plan—supplements are not essential! Chapter 16 provides a detailed review of the most commonly promoted dietary supplements, including products (such as liquid meal supplements, sports bars and creatine) that may be of benefit to athletes attempting to increase muscle mass.

References

Atherton PJ, Babraj J, Smith K, Singh J, Rennie MJ, Wackerhage H. Selective activation of AMPK-PGC-1alpha or PKB-TSC2-mTOR signaling can explain specific adaptive responses to endurance or resistance training-like electrical muscle stimulation. FASEB J 2005;19:786–8.

Babraj JA, Cuthbertson DJ, Smith K, Langberg H, Miller B, Krogsgaard MR, Kjaer M, Rennie MJ. Collagen synthesis in human musculoskeletal tissues and skin. Am J Physiol Endocrinol Metab 2005;289:E864–9.

Balagopal P, Ljungqvist O, Nair KS. Skeletal muscle myosin heavy-chain synthesis rate in healthy humans. Am J Physiol 1997;272:E45–50.

Bartoli M, Richard I. Calpains in muscle wasting. Int J Biochem Cell Biol 2005;37:2115–33.

Bazzarre TL, Kleiner SM, Litchford MD. Nutrient intake, body fat, and lipid profiles of competitive male and female bodybuilders. J Am Coll Nutr 1990;9:136–42.

Belcastro AN, Shewchuk LD, Raj DA. Exercise-induced muscle injury: a calpain hypothesis. Mol Cell Biochem 1998;179:135–45.

Bhasin S, Storer TW, Berman N, Callegari C, Clevenger B, Phillips J, Bunnell TJ, Tricker R, Shirazi A, Casaburi R. The effects of supraphysiologic doses of testosterone on muscle size and strength in normal men. N Engl J Med 1996;335:1–7.

Biolo G, Maggi SP, Williams BD, Tipton KD, Wolfe RR. Increased rates of muscle protein turnover and amino acid transport after resistance exercise in humans. Am J Physiol 1995;268:E514–20.

Biolo G, Tipton KD, Klein S, Wolfe RR. An abundant supply of amino acids enhances the metabolic effect of exercise on muscle protein. Am J Physiol 1997:273;E122–9.

Biolo G, Williams BD, Fleming RY, Wolfe RR. Insulin action on muscle protein kinetics and amino acid transport during recovery after resistance exercise. Diabetes 1999;48:949–57.

Blomstrand E, Saltin B. Effect of muscle glycogen on glucose, lactate and amino acid metabolism during exercise and recovery in human subjects. J Physiol 1999;514(Pt 1):293–302.

Bolster DR, Pikosky MA, Gaine PC, Martin W, Wolfe RR, Tipton KD, Maclean D, Maresh CM, Rodriguez NR. Dietary protein intake impacts human skeletal muscle protein fractional synthetic rates after endurance exercise. Am J Physiol Endocrinol Metab 2005;289:E678–83.

Borsheim E, Cree MG, Tipton KD, Elliott TA, Aarsland A, Wolfe RR. Effect of carbohydrate intake on net muscle protein synthesis during recovery from resistance exercise. J Appl Physiol 2004;96:674–8.

Borsheim E, Tipton KD, Wolf SE, Wolfe RR. Essential amino acids and muscle protein recovery from resistance exercise. Am J Physiol Endocrinol Metab 2002;283:E648–57.

Bowtell JL, Leese GP, Smith K, Watt PW, Nevill A, Rooyackers O, Wagenmakers AJ, Rennie MJ. Effect of oral glucose on leucine turnover in human subjects at rest and during exercise at two levels of dietary protein. J Physiol 2000;525(Pt 1):271–81.

Bowtell JL, Leese GP, Smith K, Watt PW, Nevill A, Rooyackers O, Wagenmakers AJ, Rennie MJ. Modulation of whole body protein metabolism, during and after exercise, by variation of dietary protein. J Appl Physiol 1998;85:1744–52.

Boyer B, Odessey R. Kinetic characterization of branched chain ketoacid dehydrogenase. Arch Biochem Biophys 1991;285:1–7.

Brenner BM, Meyer TW, Hostetter TH. Dietary protein intake and the progressive nature of kidney disease: the role of hemodynamically mediated glomerular injury in the pathogenesis of progressive glomerular sclerosis in aging, renal ablation, and intrinsic renal disease. N Engl J Med 1982;307:652–9.

Brouns F, Saris WH, Stroecken J, Beckers E, Thijssen R, Rehrer NJ, ten Hoor F. Eating, drinking, and cycling. A controlled Tour de France simulation study, Part I. Int J Sports Med 1989;10(1 Suppl):32S–40S.

Brownell KD, Steen SN, Wilmore JH. Weight regulation practices in athletes: analysis of metabolic and health effects. Med Sci Sports Exerc 1987;19:546–56.

Burke LM, Gollan RA, Read RSD. Dietary intakes and food use of groups of elite Australian male athletes. Int J Sport Nutr 1991;1:378–94.

Burke LM, Read RSD. A study of dietary patterns of elite Australian football players. Can J Sport Sci 1988;13:15–19.

Butterfield GE, Calloway DH. Physical activity improves protein utilization in young men. Br J Nutr 1984;51:171–84.

Campbell WW, Crim MC, Young VR, Joseph LJ, Evans WJ. Effects of resistance training and dietary protein intake on protein metabolism in older adults. Am J Physiol 1995;268:E1143–53.

Carter SL, Rennie C,Tarnopolsky MA. Substrate utilization during endurance exercise in men and women after endurance training. Am J Physiol Endocrinol Metab 2001;280:E898–907.

Castellino P, Luzi L, Simonson DC, Haymond M, DeFronzo RA. Effect of insulin and plasma amino acid concentrations on leucine metabolism in man. Role of substrate availability on estimates of whole body protein synthesis. J Clin Invest 1987;80:1784–93.

Cathcart EP. Influence of muscle work on protein metabolism. Physiol Rev 1925;5:225–43.

Chesley A, MacDougall JD, Tarnopolsky MA, Atkinson SA,Smith K. Changes in human muscle protein synthesis after resistance exercise. J Appl Physiol 1992;73:1383–8.

CoffeyVG, Zhong Z, Shield A, Canny BJ, Chibalin AV, Zierath JR, Hawley JA. Early signaling responses to divergent exercise stimuli in skeletal muscle from well-trained humans. FASEB J 2006;20:190–2.

Consolazio CF, Johnson HL, Nelson RA, Dramise JG, Skala JH. Protein metabolism during intensive physical training in the young adult. Am J Clin Nutr 1975;28:29–35.

Cunningham JT, Rodgers JT, Arlow DH,Vazquez F, MoothaVK, Puigserver P. mTOR controls mitochondrial oxidative function through a YY1-PGC-1alpha transcriptional complex. Nature 2007;450:736–40.

De Boer MD, Selby A, Atherton P, Smith K, Seynnes OR, Maganaris CN, Maffulli N, Movin T, Narici MV, Rennie MJ. The temporal responses of protein synthesis, gene expression and cell signalling in human quadriceps muscle and patellar tendon to disuse. J Physiol 2007;585:241–51.

Deldicque L, Theisen D, Francaux M. Regulation of mTOR by amino acids and resistance exercise in skeletal muscle. Eur J Appl Physiol 2005;94:1–10.

Deuster PA, Kyle SB, Moser PB, Vigersky RA, Singh A, Schoomaker EB. Nutritional survey of highly trained women runners. Am J Clin Nutr 1986;44:954–62.

Dohm GL, Hecker AL, Brown WE, Klain GJ, Puente FR, Askew EW, Beecher GR. Adaptation of protein metabolism to endurance training. Increased amino acid oxidation in response to training. Biochem 1977;164:705–8.

Dolny DG, Lemon PW. Effect of ambient temperature on protein breakdown during prolonged exercise. J Appl Physiol 1988;64:550–5.

Drinkwater BL, Bruemner B, Chesnut 3rd CH. Menstrual history as a determinant of current bone density in young athletes. JAMA 1990;263:545–8.

Drinkwater BL, Nilson K, Chesnut 3rd CH, Bremner WJ, Shainholtz S, Southworth MB. Bone mineral content of amenorrheic and eumenorrheic athletes. N Engl J Med 1984;311:277–81.

Du J, Wang X, Miereles C, Bailey JL, Debigare R, Zheng B, Price SR, Mitch WE. Activation of caspase-3 is an initial step triggering accelerated muscle proteolysis in catabolic conditions. J Clin Invest 2004;113:115–23.

El-Khoury AE, Forslund A, Olsson R, Branth S, Sjodin A, Andersson A, Atkinson A, Selvaraj A, Hambraeus L, Young VR. Moderate exercise at energy balance does not affect 24-hour leucine oxidation or nitrogen retention in healthy men. Am J Physiol 1997;273:E394–407.

Faber M, Benade AJ, van Eck M. Dietary intake, anthropometric measurements, and blood lipid values in weight training athletes (body builders). Int J Sports Med 1986;7:342–6.

Ferrando AA, Tipton KD, Doyle D, Phillips SM, Cortiella J, Wolfe RR. Testosterone injection stimulates net protein synthesis but not tissue amino acid transport. Am J Physiol 1988;275:E864–71.

Fielding RA, Meredith CN, O'Reilly KP, Frontera WR, Cannon JG, Evans WJ. Enhanced protein breakdown after eccentric exercise in young and older men. J Appl Physiol 1991;71:674–9.

Forslund AH, Hambraeus L, Olsson RM, El-Khoury AE, Yu YM, Young VR. The 24-hour whole body leucine and urea kinetics at normal and high protein intakes with exercise in healthy adults. Am J Physiol 1998;275:E310–20.

Friedman JE, Lemon PW. Effect of chronic endurance exercise on retention of dietary protein. Int J Sports Med 1989;10:118–23.

Fudge BW, Westerterp KR, Kiplamai FK, Onywera VO, Boit MK, Kayser B, Pitsiladis YP. Evidence of negative energy balance using doubly labelled water in elite Kenyan endurance runners prior to competition. Br J Nutr 2006;95:59–66.

Gaine PC, Viesselman CT, Pikosky MA, Martin WF, Armstrong LE, Pescatello LS, Rodriguez NR. Aerobic exercise training decreases leucine oxidation at rest in healthy adults. J Nutr 2005;135:1088–92.

Garlick PJ. The role of leucine in the regulation of protein metabolism. J Nutr 2005;135(Suppl):1553S–6S.

Garlick PJ, Grant I. Amino acid infusion increases the sensitivity of muscle protein synthesis in vivo to insulin. Effect of branched-chain amino acids. Biochem J 1988;254:579–84.

Gibala MJ. Regulation of skeletal muscle amino acid metabolism during exercise. Int J Sport Nutr Exerc Metab 2001;11:87–108.

Gibala MJ, MacLean DA, Graham TE, Saltin B. Tricarboxylic acid cycle intermediate pool size and estimated cycle flux in human muscle during exercise. Am J Physiol 1998;275:E235–42.

Glover EI, Oates BR, Tang JE, Moore DR, Tarnopolsky MA, Phillips SM. Resistance exercise decreases eIF2Bepsilon phosphorylation and potentiates the feeding-induced stimulation of p70S6K1 and rpS6 in young men. Am J Physiol Regul Integr Comp Physiol 2008;295:R604–10.

Goldberg AL, Chang TW. Regulation and significance of amino acid metabolism in skeletal muscle. Fed Proc 1978;37:2301–7.

Gomes MD, Lecker SH, Jagoe RT, Navon A, Goldberg AL. Atrogin-1, a muscle-specific F-box protein highly expressed during muscle atrophy. Proc Natl Acad Sci USA 2001;98:14440–5.

Gontzea I, Sutzesco P, Dumitrache S. Influence of adaptation to effort on nitrogen balance in man. Arch Sci Physiol (Paris) 1962;16:127–38.

Gontzea I, Sutzesco P, Dumitrache S. Research on the influence of muscular activity on nitrogen metabolism and on the protein requirement of man. Ann Nutr Aliment 1968;22:183–236.

Griggs RC, Kingston W, Jozefowicz RF, Herr BE, Forbes G, Halliday D. Effect of testosterone on muscle mass and muscle protein synthesis. J Appl Physiol 1989;66:498–503.

Hamadeh MJ, Devries MC, Tarnopolsky MA. Estrogen supplementation reduces whole body leucine and carbohydrate oxidation and increases lipid oxidation in men during endurance exercise. J Clin Endocrinol Metab 2005;90:3592–9.

Haralambie G, Berg A. Serum urea and amino nitrogen changes with exercise duration. Eur J Appl Physiol Occup Physiol 1976;36:39–48.

Hardie DG. AMP-activated protein kinase: a key system mediating metabolic responses to exercise. Med Sci Sports Exerc 2004;36:28–34.

Harris HA. Nutrition and physical performance. The diet of Greek athletes. Proc Nutr Soc 1966;25:87–90.

Hartman JW, Moore DR, Phillips SM. Resistance training reduces whole-body protein turnover and improves net protein retention in untrained young males. Appl Physiol Nutr Metab 2006; 31:557–64.

Hartman JW, Tang JE, Wilkinson SB, Tarnopolsky MA, Lawrence RL, Fullerton AV, Phillips SM. Consumption of fat-free fluid milk after resistance exercise promotes greater lean mass accretion than does consumption of soy or carbohydrate in young, novice, male weightlifters. Am J Clin Nutr 2007;86:373–81.

Henderson SA, Black AL, Brooks GA. Leucine turnover and oxidation in trained rats during exercise. Am J Physiol 1985;249:E137–44.

Hertzman PA, Blevins WL, Mayer J, Greenfield B, Ting M, Gleich GJ. Association of the eosinophilia-myalgia syndrome with the ingestion of tryptophan. N Engl J Med 1990;322:869–73.

Hill RJ, Davies PS. Energy intake and energy expenditure in elite lightweight female rowers. Med Sci Sports Exerc 2002;34:1823–9.

Hinton PS, Sanford TC, Davidson MM, Yakushko OF, Beck NC. Nutrient intakes and dietary behaviors of male and female collegiate athletes. Int J Sport Nutr Exerc Metab 2004;14:389–405.

Hood DA, Terjung RL. Effect of endurance training on leucine metabolism in perfused rat skeletal muscle. Am J Physiol 1987;253:E648–56.

Howarth KR, Burgomaster KA, Phillips SM, Gibala MJ. Exercise training increases branched-chain oxoacid dehydrogenase kinase content in human skeletal muscle. Am J Physiol Regul Integr Comp Physiol 2007;293:R1335–41.

Howarth KR, Moreau NA, Phillips SM, Gibala MJ. Coingestion of protein with carbohydrate during recovery from endurance exercise stimulates skeletal muscle protein synthesis in humans. J Appl Physiol 2009;106:1394–1402.

Hulmi JJ, Tannerstedt J, Selanne H, Kainulainen H, Kovanen V, Mero AA. Resistance exercise with whey protein ingestion affects mTOR signaling pathway and myostatin in men. J Appl Physiol 2009;106:1720–9.

Hunt JR, Johnson LK, Roughead ZF. Dietary protein and calcium interact to influence calcium retention: a controlled feeding study. Am J Clin Nutr 2009;89:1357–65.

Jorgensen SB, Richter EA, Wojtaszewski JF. Role of AMPK in skeletal muscle metabolic regulation and adaptation in relation to exercise. J Physiol 2006;574:17–31.

Kasperek GJ. Regulation of branched-chain 2-oxo acid dehydrogenase activity during exercise. Am J Physiol 1989;256:E186–90.

Khatra BS, Chawla RK, Sewell CW, Rudman D. Distribution of branched-chain alpha-keto acid dehydrogenases in primate tissues. J Clin Invest 1977;59:558–64.

Kim PL, Staron RS, Phillips SM. Fasted-state skeletal muscle protein synthesis after resistance exercise is altered with training. J Physiol 2005;568:283–90.

Koopman R, Beelen M, Stellingwerff T, Pennings B, Saris WH, Kies AK, Kuipers H, van Loon LJ. Coingestion of carbohydrate with protein does not further augment postexercise muscle protein synthesis. Am J Physiol Endocrinol Metab 2007;293:E833–42.

Koopman R, Verdijk LB, Beelen M, Gorselink M, Kruseman AN, Wagenmakers AJ, Kuipers H, van Loon LJ. Co-ingestion of leucine with protein does not further augment post-exercise muscle protein synthesis rates in elderly men. Br J Nutr 2008;99:571–80.

Koopman R, Wagenmakers AJ, Manders RJ, Zorenc AH, Senden JM, Gorselink M, Keizer HA, van Loon LJ. Combined ingestion of protein and free leucine with carbohydrate increases postexercise muscle protein synthesis in vivo in male subjects. Am J Physiol Endocrinol Metab 2005;288:E645–53.

Kraemer WJ, Hakkinen K, Newton RU, McCormick M, Nindl BC, Volek JS, Gotshalk LA, Fleck SJ, Campbell WW, Gordon SE, Farrell PA, Evans WJ. Acute hormonal responses to heavy resistance exercise in younger and older men. Eur J Appl Physiol Occup Physiol 1998;77:206–11.

Krempf M, Hoerr RA, Pelletier VA, Marks LM, Gleason R, Young VR. An isotopic study of the effect of dietary carbohydrate on the metabolic fate of dietary leucine and phenylalanine. Am J Clin Nutr 1993;57:161–9.

Kumar V, Selby A, Rankin D, Patel R, Atherton P, Hildebrandt W, Williams J, Smith K, Seynnes O, Hiscock N, Rennie MJ. Age-related differences in the dose-response relationship of muscle protein synthesis to resistance exercise in young and old men. J Physiol 2009;587:211–17.

Lamont LS, McCullough AJ, Kalhan SC. Beta-adrenergic blockade heightens the exercise–induced increase in leucine oxidation. Am J Physiol 1995;268:E910–16.

Lamont LS, McCullough AJ, Kalhan SC. Comparison of leucine kinetics in endurance-trained and sedentary humans. J Appl Physiol 1999;86:320–5.

Lamont LS, McCullough AJ, Kalhan SC. Gender differences in leucine, but not lysine, kinetics. J Appl Physiol 2001a;91:357–62.

Lamont LS, McCullough AJ, Kalhan SC. Relationship between leucine oxidation and oxygen consumption during steady-state exercise. Med Sci Sports Exerc 2001b;33:237–41.

Lamont LS, Patel DG, Kalhan SC. Leucine kinetics in endurance-trained humans. J Appl Physiol 1990;69:1–6.

Lecker SH, Jagoe RT, Gilbert A, Gomes M, Baracos V, Bailey J, Price SR, Mitch WE, Goldberg AL. Multiple types of skeletal muscle atrophy involve a common program of changes in gene expression. FASEB J 2004;18:39–51.

Lemon PW, Mullin JP. Effect of initial muscle glycogen levels on protein catabolism during exercise. J Appl Physiol 1980;48:624–9.

Lemon PW, Tarnopolsky MA, MacDougall JD, Atkinson SA. Protein requirements and muscle mass/strength changes during intensive training in novice bodybuilders. J Appl Physiol 1992;73:767–75.

Lemon PW, Yarasheski KE. Feasibility of sweat collection by whole body washdown in moderate to high humidity environments. Int J Sports Med 1985;6:41–3.

Lowell BB, Ruderman NB, Goodman MN. Evidence that lysosomes are not involved in the degradation of myofibrillar proteins in rat skeletal muscle. Biochem J 1986;234:237–40.

Mahoney DJ, Parise G, Melov S, Safdar A, Tarnopolsky MA. Analysis of global mRNA expression in human skeletal muscle during recovery from endurance exercise. FASEB J 2005;9:1498–1500.

Mahoney DJ, Safdar A, Parise G, Melov S, Fu M, MacNeil L, Kaczor J, Payne ET, Tarnopolsky MA. Gene expression profiling in human skeletal muscle during recovery from eccentric exercise. Am J Physiol Regul Integr Comp Physiol 2008;294:R1901–10.

Marcus R, Cann C, Madvig P, Minkoff J, Goddard M, Bayer M, Martin M, Gaudiani L, Haskell W, Genant H. Menstrual function and bone mass in elite women distance runners. Endocrine and metabolic features. Ann Intern Med 1985;102:158–63.

Matsakas A, Patel K. Intracellular signalling pathways regulating the adaptation of skeletal muscle to exercise and nutritional changes. Histol Histopathol 2009;24:209–22.

McKenzie S, Phillips SM, Carter SL, Lowther S, Gibala MJ, Tarnopolsky MA. Endurance exercise training attenuates leucine oxidation and BCOAD activation during exercise in humans. Am J Physiol Endocrinol Metab 2000;278:E580–7.

McNurlan MA, Essen P, Thorell A, Calder AG, Anderson SE, Ljungqvist O, Sandgren A, Grant I, Tjader I, Ballmer PE, et al. Response of protein synthesis in human skeletal muscle to insulin: an investigation with L-[2H5]phenylalanine. Am J Physiol 1994;267:E102–8.

Meredith CN, Zackin MJ, Frontera WR, Evans WJ. Dietary protein requirements and body protein metabolism in endurance-trained men. J Appl Physiol 1989;66:2850–6.

Miller SL, Tipton KD, Chinkes DL, Wolf SE, Wolfe RR. Independent and combined effects of amino acids and glucose after resistance exercise. Med Sci Sports Exerc 2003;35:449–55.

Mitch WE, Goldberg AL. Mechanisms of muscle wasting. The role of the ubiquitin-proteasome pathway. N Engl J Med 1996;335:1897–905.

Moller–Loswick AC, Zachrisson H, Hyltander A, Korner U, Matthews DE, Lundholm K. Insulin selectively attenuates breakdown of nonmyofibrillar proteins in peripheral tissues of normal men. Am J Physiol 1994;266:E645–52.

Moore DR, Robinson MJ, Fry JL, Tang JE, Glover EI, Wilkinson SB, Prior T, Tarnopolsky MA, Phillips SM. Ingested protein dose response of muscle and albumin protein synthesis after resistance exercise in young men. Am J Clin Nutr 2009;89:161–8.

Murton AJ, Constantin D, Greenhaff PL. The involvement of the ubiquitin proteasome system in human skeletal muscle remodelling and atrophy. Biochim Biophys Acta 2008;1782:730–43.

Nair KS, Halliday D, Griggs RC. Leucine incorporation into mixed skeletal muscle protein in humans. Am J Physiol 1988;254:E208–13.

Nelson ME, Fisher EC, Catsos PD, Meredith CN, Turksoy RN, Evans WJ. Diet and bone status in amenorrheic runners. Am J Clin Nutr 1986;43:910–16.

Pellet PL. Protein requirements in humans. Am J Clin Nutr 1990;51:723–37.

Petersen HL, Peterson CT, Reddy MB, Hanson KB, Swain JH, Sharp RL, Alekel DL. Body composition, dietary intake, and iron status of female collegiate swimmers and divers. Int J Sport Nutr Exerc Metab 2006;16:281–95.

Phillips SM. Dietary protein for athletes: from requirements to metabolic advantage. Appl Physiol Nutr Metab 2006;31:647–54.

Phillips SM, Atkinson SA, Tarnopolsky MA, MacDougall JD. Gender differences in leucine kinetics and nitrogen balance in endurance athletes. J Appl Physiol 1993;75:2134–41.

Phillips SM, Parise G, Roy BD, Tipton KD, Wolfe RR, Tamopolsky MA. Resistance-training-induced adaptations in skeletal muscle protein turnover in the fed state. Can J Physiol Pharmacol 2002;80:1045–53.

Phillips SM, Tipton KD, Aarsland A, Wolf SE, Wolfe RR. Mixed muscle protein synthesis and breakdown after resistance exercise in humans. Am J Physiol 1997;273:E99–107.

Phillips SM, Tipton KD, Ferrando AA, Wolfe RR. Resistance training reduces the acute exercise-induced increase in muscle protein turnover. Am J Physiol 1999;276:E118–24.

Richter EA, Ruderman NB. AMPK and the biochemistry of exercise: implications for human health and disease. Biochem J 2009;418:261–75.

Riddell MC, Partington SL, Stupka N, Armstrong D, Rennie C, Tarnopolsky MA. Substrate utilization during exercise performed with and without glucose ingestion in female and male endurance trained athletes. Int J Sport Nutr Exerc Metab 2003;13:407–21.

Rowlands DS, Rossler K, Thorp RM, Graham DF, Timmons BW, Stannard SR, Tarnopolsky MA. Effect of dietary protein content during recovery from high-intensity cycling on subsequent performance and markers of stress, inflammation, and muscle damage in well-trained men. Appl Physiol Nutr Metab 2008;33:39–51.

Roy BD, Luttmer K, Bosman MJ, Tarnopolsky MA. The influence of post-exercise macronutrient intake on energy balance and protein metabolism in active females participating in endurance training. Int J Sport Nutr Exerc Metab 2002;12:172–88.

Roy BD, Tarnopolsky MA. Influence of differing macronutrient intakes on muscle glycogen resynthesis after resistance exercise. J Appl Physiol 1998;84:890–6.

Roy BD, Tarnopolsky MA, MacDougall JD, Fowles J, Yarasheski KE. Effect of glucose supplement timing on protein metabolism after resistance training. J Appl Physiol 1997;82:1882–8.

Saris WH, van Erp-Baart MA, Brouns F, Westerterp KR, ten Hoor F. Study on food intake and energy expenditure during extreme sustained exercise: the Tour de France. Int J Sports Med 1989;10(1 Suppl):26S–31S.

Short SH, Short WR. Four-year study of university athletes' dietary intake. J Am Diet Assoc 1983;82:632–45.

Smith GI, Atherton P, Villareal DT, Frimel TN, Rankin D, Rennie MJ, Mittendorfer B. Differences in muscle protein synthesis and anabolic signaling in the postabsorptive state and in response to food in 65–80 year old men and women. PLoS ONE 2008;3:E1875.

Svanberg E. Amino acids may be intrinsic regulators of protein synthesis in response to feeding. Clin Nutr 1998;17:77–9.

Svanberg E, Moller-Loswick AC, Matthews DE, Korner U, Andersson M, Lundholm K. Effects of amino acids on synthesis and degradation of skeletal muscle proteins in humans. Am J Physiol 1996;271:E718–24.

Tarnopolsky LJ, MacDougall JD, Atkinson SA, Tarnopolsky MA, Sutton JR. Gender differences in substrate for endurance exercise. J Appl Physiol 1990;68:302–8.

Tarnopolsky M. Protein requirements for endurance athletes. Nutrition 2004;20:662–8.

Tarnopolsky MA, Atkinson SA, MacDougall JD, Chesley A, Phillips S, Schwarcz HP. Evaluation of protein requirements for trained strength athletes. J Appl Physiol 1992;73:1986–95.

Tarnopolsky MA, Atkinson SA, MacDougall JD, Senor BB, Lemon PW, Schwarcz H. Whole body leucine metabolism during and after resistance exercise in fed humans. Med Sci Sports Exerc 1991;23:326–33.

Tarnopolsky MA, Atkinson SA, Phillips SM, MacDougall JD. Carbohydrate loading and metabolism during exercise in men and women. J Appl Physiol 1995;78:1360–8.

Tarnopolsky MA, Bosman M, Macdonald JR, Vandeputte D, Martin J, Roy BD. Postexercise protein-carbohydrate and carbohydrate supplements increase muscle glycogen in men and women. J Appl Physiol 1997;83:1877–83.

Tarnopolsky MA, Bourgeois JM, Snow R, Keys S, Roy BD, Kwiecien JM, Turnbull J. Histological assessment of intermediate- and long-term creatine monohydrate supplementation in mice and rats. Am J Physiol Regul Integr Comp Physiol 2003;285:R762–9.

Tarnopolsky MA, Cipriano N, Woodcroft C, Pulkkinen WJ, Robinson DC, Henderson JM, MacDougall JD. Effects of rapid weight loss and wrestling on muscle glycogen concentration. Clin J Sport Med 1996;6:78–84.

Tarnopolsky MA, MacDougall JD, Atkinson SA. Influence of protein intake and training status on nitrogen balance and lean body mass. J Appl Physiol 1988;64:187–93.

Tarnopolsky MA, Parise G, Gibala MJ, Graham TE, Rush JW. Myoadenylate deaminase deficiency does not affect muscle anaplerosis during exhaustive exercise in humans. J Physiol 2001a;33:881–9.

Tarnopolsky MA, Parise G, Yardley NJ, Ballantyne CS, Olatinji S, Phillips SM. Creatine-dextrose and protein-dextrose induce similar strength gains during training. Med Sci Sports Exerc 2001b;33:2044–52.

Tessari P, Inchiostro S, Biolo G, Trevisan R, Fantin G, Marescotti MC, Iori E, Tiengo A, Crepaldi G. Differential effects of hyperinsulinemia and hyperaminoacidemia on leucine-carbon metabolism in vivo. Evidence for distinct mechanisms in regulation of net amino acid deposition. J Clin Invest 1987;79:1062–9.

Tidball JG, Spencer MJ. Calpains and muscular dystrophies. Int J Biochem Cell Biol 2000;32:1–5.

Timmons JA, Larsson O, Jansson E, Fischer H, Gustafsson T, Greenhaff PL, Ridden J, Rachman J, Peyrard-Janvid M, Wahlestedt C, Sundberg CJ. Human muscle gene expression responses to endurance training provide a novel perspective on Duchenne muscular dystrophy. FASEB J 2005;19:750–60.

Tipton KD, Elliott TA, Cree MG, Wolf SE, Sanford AP, Wolfe RR. Ingestion of casein and whey proteins result in muscle anabolism after resistance exercise. Med Sci Sports Exerc 2004;36:2073–81.

Tipton KD, Ferrando AA, Phillips SM, Doyle D Jr, Wolfe RR. Postexercise net protein synthesis in human muscle from orally administered amino acids. Am J Physiol 1999;276:E628–34.

Tipton KD, Ferrando AA, Williams BD, Wolfe RR. Muscle protein metabolism in female swimmers after a combination of resistance and endurance exercise. J Appl Physiol 1996;81:2034–8.

Tipton KD, Rasmussen BB, Miller SL, Wolf SE, Owens-Stovall SK, Petrini BE, Wolfe RR. Timing of amino acid-carbohydrate ingestion alters anabolic response of muscle to resistance exercise. Am J Physiol Endocrinol Metab 2001;281:E197–206.

Tipton KD, Witard OC. Protein requirements and recommendations for athletes: relevance of ivory tower arguments for practical recommendations. Clin Sports Med 2007;26:17–36.

Tipton KD, Wolfe RR. Protein and amino acids for athletes. J Sports Sci 2004;22:65–79.

Todd KS, Butterfield GE, Calloway DH. Nitrogen balance in men with adequate and deficient energy intake at three levels of work. J Nutr 1984;14:2107–18.

Torun B, Scrimshaw NS, Young VR. Effect of isometric exercises on body potassium and dietary protein requirements of young men. Am J Clin Nutr 1977;30:1983–93.

Trappe T, Williams R, Carrithers J, Raue U, Esmarck B, Kjaer M, Hickner R. Influence of age and resistance exercise on human skeletal muscle proteolysis: a microdialysis approach. J Physiol 2004;554:803–13.

Volek JS, Kraemer WJ, Bush JA, Incledon T, Boetes M. Testosterone and cortisol in relationship to dietary nutrients and resistance exercise. J Appl Physiol 1997;82:49–54.

Wagenmakers AJ, Beckers EJ, Brouns F, Kuipers H, Soeters PB, van der Vusse GJ, Saris WH. Carbohydrate supplementation, glycogen depletion, and amino acid metabolism during exercise. Am J Physiol 1991;260:E883–90.

Wagenmakers AJ, Brookes JH, Coakley JH, Reilly T, Edwards RH. Exercise-induced activation of the branched-chain 2-oxo acid dehydrogenase in human muscle. Eur J Appl Physiol Occup Physiol 1989;59:159–67.

Welle S, Matthews DE, Campbell RG, Nair KS. Stimulation of protein turnover by carbohydrate overfeeding in men. Am J Physiol 1989;257:E413–17.

Welle S, Thornton C, Statt M. Myofibrillar protein synthesis in young and old human subjects after three months of resistance training. Am J Physiol 1995;268:E422–7.

Whiting SJ, Anderson DJ, Weeks SJ. Calciuric effects of protein and potassium bicarbonate but not of sodium chloride or phosphate can be detected acutely in adult women and men. Am J Clin Nutr 1997;65:1465–72.

Wilkinson SB, Phillips SM, Atherton PJ, Patel R, Yarasheski KE, Tarnopolsky MA, Rennie MJ. Differential effects of resistance and endurance exercise in the fed state on signalling molecule phosphorylation and protein synthesis in human muscle. J Physiol 2008;586:3701–17.

Wilkinson SB, Tarnopolsky MA, Macdonald MJ, Macdonald JR, Armstrong D, Phillips SM. Consumption of fluid skim milk promotes greater muscle protein accretion after resistance exercise than does consumption of an isonitrogenous and isoenergetic soy-protein beverage. Am J Clin Nutr 2007;85:1031–40.

Wolfe RR. Tracers in metabolic research: radioisotope and stable isotope/mass spectrometry methods. Lab Res Methods Biol Med 1984;9:1–287.

Wolfe RR, George S. Stable isotopic tracers as metabolic probes in exercise. Exerc Sport Sci Rev 1993;21:1–31.

Wolfe RR, Wolfe MH, Nadel ER, Shaw JH. Isotopic determination of amino acid-urea interactions in exercise in humans. J Appl Physiol 1984;56:221–9.

Yamaoka KA, Miyasaka N, Inuo G, Saito I, Kolb JP, Fujita K, Kashiwazaki S. 1,1′-Ethylidenebis(tryptophan) (Peak E) induces functional activation of human eosinophils and interleukin 5 production from T lymphocytes: association of eosinophilia-myalgia syndrome with a L tryptophan contaminant. J Clin Immunol 1994;14:50–60.

Yarasheski KE, Pak-Loduca J, Hasten DL, Obert KA, Brown MB, Sinacore DR. Resistance exercise training increases mixed muscle protein synthesis rate in frail women and men >/=76 yr old. Am J Physiol 1999;277:E118–25.

Young VR, Bier DM. A kinetic approach to the determination of human amino acid requirements. Nutr Rev 1987;45:289–98.

Young VR, Bier DM, Pellett PL. A theoretical basis for increasing current estimates of the amino acid requirements in adult man, with experimental support. Am J Clin Nutr 1989;50:80–92.

Young VR, Gucalp C, Rand WM, Matthews DE, Bier DM. Leucine kinetics during three weeks at submaintenance-to-maintenance intakes of leucine in men: adaptation and accommodation. Hum Nutr Clin Nutr 1987;41:1–18.

Young VR, Munro HN. Ntau-methylhistidine (3-methylhistidine) and muscle protein turnover: an overview. Fed Proc 1978;37:2291–300.

Zalcman I, Guarita HV, Juzwiak CR, Crispim CA, Antunes HK, Edwards B, Tufik S, de Mello MT. Nutritional status of adventure racers. Nutrition 2007;23:404–11.

Zaragoza R, Renau-Piqueras J, Portoles M, Hernandez-Yago J, Jorda A, Grisolia S. Rats fed prolonged high protein diets show an increase in nitrogen metabolism and liver megamitochondria. Arch Biochem Biophys 1987;258:426–35.

Zorzano A, Balon TW, Goodman MN, Ruderman NB. Insulin and exercise stimulate muscle alpha-aminoisobutyric acid transport by a Na^+-K^+-ATPase independent pathway. Biochem Biophys Res Commun 1986;134:1342–9.

CHAPTER 5

Energy requirements of the athlete: assessment and evidence of energy efficiency

MELINDA M MANORE AND JANICE L THOMPSON

5.1 Introduction

Most individuals, including athletes, maintain a stable body mass over long periods of time, while paying little attention to the amount of energy consumed or expended each day. However, energy balance is of primary concern to the athlete who wants to alter body mass and/or composition to improve their exercise performance or meet a designated weight requirement for their sport. When energy consumption is insufficient to match that expended, much of the effort of training can be lost, since both fat and muscle will be used for energy. In addition, if energy intake is limited or restricted, the ability to obtain other essential nutrients (such as carbohydrate, protein, fat, vitamins and minerals) necessary for optimal sport performance and good health will also be compromised.

Many athletes, especially female athletes, feel pressured by their coaches, parents, peers and themselves to reduce body mass. To maintain a low body mass, these athletes restrict energy intake even though their energy expenditure is high. Athletes of any age must consume enough energy to cover the energy costs of daily living, the energy cost of their sport, and the energy costs associated with building and repairing muscle tissue. Females of reproductive age must also cover the costs of menstruation, whereas younger athletes must cover the additional costs of growth. What are the consequences of restricting energy intake when energy expenditure is high? It has been hypothesized that one consequence of this behavior is an increased energy efficiency, thus decreasing the amount of energy actually required to maintain body mass.

This chapter will briefly review the concept of energy and macronutrient balance and the factors that contribute to energy balance in an athlete or active individual. Manipulating the energy balance equation for either gain or loss of body mass for an individual athlete is covered in other sections of this book (see Practice Tips in Chapter 4 for body mass gain and Chapters 6 and 7 for body mass loss). We will then discuss the concept of energy efficiency and the research evidence for and against this phenomenon in the athlete.

Energy and macronutrient balance

For body mass to be maintained, energy in (total kilojoules or kilocalories consumed and those drawn from body stores) must equal energy expended. Under these conditions an individual is considered to be in energy balance. This concept can be stated using the equation below. In this simple equation, 'energy in' means 'metabolizable energy' (energy intake minus energy lost in feces and urine). For most individuals, metabolizable energy is about 90–95% of energy intake (Jéquier & Tappy 1999).

Energy balance occurs when:

$$E_{in} = E_{out}$$

where:

E_{in} = energy in (kJ/d or kcal/d)
E_{out} = energy expended (kJ/d or kcal/d)

If an athlete is trying to increase body mass, then E_{in} must exceed E_{out}. Conversely, if an athlete is trying to reduce body mass, E_{out} must exceed E_{in}. Thus, inducing an imbalance between E_{in} and E_{out} will result in the most dramatic changes in body mass. Although a number of popular diets (like high-protein, high-fat/low-carbohydrate) claim to induce weight loss by just altering diet composition, body mass will not be lost unless E_{out} is more than E_{in}. In addition, these types of diets are often detrimental to the serious athlete. Diet composition will influence long-term changes in body mass and composition only when there is an imbalance between E_{in} and E_{out} (Melby & Hill 1999). In addition to diet composition, maintenance of body mass and composition are influenced by a number of factors, including physiological, environmental, behavioral and genetic (Jéquier & Tappy 1999).

We now know that the maintenance of body mass and composition over time requires that $E_{in} = E_{out}$ and that intakes of protein, carbohydrate (CHO), fat and alcohol equal their oxidation rates (Jéquier & Tappy 1999). Therefore macronutrient balance occurs when:

$$protein_{in} = protein_{oxidation}$$
$$CHO_{in} = CHO_{oxidation}$$
$$fat_{in} = fat_{oxidation}$$
$$alcohol_{in} = alcohol_{oxidation}$$

where:

$protein_{in}$ = the amount of protein intake (g/d)
$protein_{oxidation}$ = the amount of protein oxidized (g/d)

These same notations apply to CHO, fat and alcohol.

The energy and macronutrient balance equations are both dynamic and time-dependent, and allow for the effect of changing energy stores on energy expenditure over time. The following example, given by Swinburn and Ravussin (1993), illustrates this point. What would happen if an individual decided to consume an extra 413 kJ (100 kcal) a day for 40 years? The amount of extra energy consumed in this time would equal about 6 million kJ or 1.5 million kcal. If one assumes that there are 31 786 kJ/kg (7700 kcal/kg) of body fat, the theoretical gain in body mass would equal 190 kg over this 40-year period, yet the actual gain would be about 2.7 kg. After a period of positive energy balance, extra energy intake would cause a gain in body mass (both fat and lean tissue). The larger body size would cause an increase in energy expenditure that would eventually balance the extra energy consumed. Of course, the actual gain in body mass will depend on the amount of extra energy consumed, and to a lesser extent on the composition of this energy (the amount of fat, CHO, protein or alcohol) and overall energy expenditure. Therefore a gain in body mass is the consequence of an initial positive energy balance, but can also be a mechanism whereby energy balance is eventually restored at a higher body mass and energy requirement.

5.3 Macronutrient balance

As indicated earlier, alterations in either energy intake or expenditure are the primary determinants of body mass. However, changes in the type and amount of macronutrients consumed (protein, fat, CHO and alcohol) and the oxidation of these macronutrients within the body must be considered when examining long-term weight maintenance (Flatt 2001). Under normal physiological conditions, CHO, protein and alcohol are not easily converted to body fat (Swinburn & Ravussin 1993; Prentice 1998). Thus, increases in the intake of non-fat nutrients stimulate their oxidation rates proportionally. Conversely, an increase in dietary fat intake does not immediately stimulate fat oxidation, thus increasing the probability that excess dietary fat will be stored as adipose tissue (Abbott et al. 1988; Westerterp 1993; Prentice 1998; Saris & Tarnopolsky 2003; Schutz 2004a). In this way, the type of food eaten can play a role in the amount of energy consumed and expended each day (Acheson et al. 1984; Swinburn & Ravussin 1993; Schutz 2004a).

5.4 Carbohydrate balance

Under energy balance conditions, CHO balance is precisely regulated such that CHO intake matches oxidation (Acheson et al. 1984; Flatt 2001; Jebb et al. 1996; Prentice 1998; Saris 2003). The ingestion of CHO stimulates both glycogen storage and glucose oxidation, and inhibits fat oxidation. Glucose not stored as glycogen is oxidized directly in almost equal balance to that consumed (Flatt et al. 1985). The conversion of excess dietary CHO and protein to triglycerides (de novo lipogenesis or DNL) is very limited in normal-weight humans except under non-physiological situations (Schutz 2004b; Hellerstein et al. 1991). However, if large amounts of CHO are consumed over several consecutive days, and E_{in} exceeds E_{out}, fat in the form of triglyceride is synthesized (Acheson et al. 1988). Schutz (2004b) has reviewed DNL in detail and discusses how CHO intake influences fat balance and DNL.

5.5 Protein balance

As with CHO, the body adjusts to a wide range of protein intakes by altering the rate of oxidation of dietary protein. After body protein needs are met, the carbon skeletons of any excess amino acids are diverted into the energy substrate pool and used for energy. The adequacy of total energy intake, and CHO intake in particular, appear to affect this process dramatically. Inadequate intakes of either energy or CHO result in negative protein balance (Krempf et al. 1993). Conversely, excess intake of either energy or CHO will spare protein. This protein is then available to support brief periods of protein accumulation until the protein pool is expanded to a new balance point. At this point, the degradation of endogenous protein matches the available exogenous protein. The excess protein consumed or the protein made available through protein sparing may contribute indirectly to fat storage by diverting dietary fat for storage. Thus protein will be used for energy preferentially over fat, leaving the excess dietary fat to be stored as adipose tissue.

Fat balance 5.6

Fat balance is not as precisely regulated as CHO and protein balance (Prentice 1998; Schutz 2004a). As dietary fat intake increases, the short-term oxidation of fat does not increase proportionately (Astrup et al. 1994; Schrauwen et al. 1997). In addition, when energy expenditure is fixed and protein held constant, there is a precise inverse relationship between CHO and fat oxidation. Under these conditions, the greater the proportion of CHO oxidized, the less fat is oxidized (Schutz 2004a, 2000b). Over the long term, a positive fat balance, due to excess energy intake from a palatable high-fat diet, will lead to a progressive increase in total body-fat stores as the body attempts to achieve energy balance (Melby & Hill 1999; Schutz 2004a). It has been hypothesized that increases in body-fat stores are due to low rates of fat oxidation relative to fat intake (Flatt 1995, 2001). As fat stores expand, they increase the free fatty acid concentrations in the blood as a consequence of the constant flux of triglycerides occurring in these stores. This increase in circulation of free fatty acids may increase fat oxidation slightly; thus, the larger adipose tissue mass promotes increased fat oxidation. When the new rate of fat oxidation equals the rate of fat intake, the individual will again achieve fat balance (and hence energy balance), but at a significantly higher body weight (Schutz 2004a).

Alcohol balance 5.7

Alcohol consumption causes a rapid rise in alcohol oxidation until all the alcohol is cleared from the body. Thus alcohol is used preferentially as an energy source over other substrates and can suppress the oxidation of fat and, to a lesser degree, that of protein and CHO (Shelmet et al. 1988; Suter 2005). Alcohol is not converted to triglycerides and stored as adipose tissue, nor can it contribute to the formation of muscle or liver glycogen. It may, however, indirectly divert dietary fat to storage by providing an alternative and preferred energy source for the body (Sonko et al. 1994; Suter 2005). Alcohol has an energy density of about 29 kJ/g (7 kcal/g) and thus can contribute significantly to total daily energy intake. A current review of the impact of alcohol on energy intake by Yeomans (2004) found that all the research to date failed to show a reduction in food intake in response to alcohol ingestion either before or with a meal. Therefore individuals who consume alcohol must reduce their consumption of energy from other dietary components in order to maintain energy balance. See Suter (2005) for a complete review of the effect of alcohol on weight gain and obesity.

Energy expenditure 5.8

Determining energy balance requires the direct measurement or estimate of energy in (energy intake from the diet and from stored energy) and energy expended. This section reviews the various components of energy expenditure and how these components are measured, and discusses how physical activity may influence these components. We will also cover methods for predicting energy expenditure based on age, gender and body size.

5.9 Components of energy expenditure

The components of total daily energy expenditure are generally divided into three main categories (see Fig. 5.1):

1. basal energy expenditure or basal metabolic rate (BMR)
2. the thermic effect of food (TEF)
3. energy expended in planned physical activity and non-exercise activity thermogenesis (NEAT), which, when combined, cover the thermic effect of activity (TEA). The energy expended in fidgeting, which is also called spontaneous physical activity (SPA), would also be included in the total TEA.

BMR is the energy required to maintain the systems of the body and to regulate body temperature at rest. BMR is measured in the morning after an overnight fast, while the individual is resting in a bed. The individual must be comfortable and free from stress, medications or any other stimulation that would increase metabolic activity. In addition, the room where BMR is measured needs to be quiet, temperature-controlled and free of distractions. Because assessment of BMR requires the individual to stay overnight in the laboratory, many researchers measure resting metabolic rate (RMR) instead. Assessment of RMR usually means that the individual slept at home and drove or was driven to the research laboratory, where they rested for a period of time before metabolic rate was assessed. Like BMR, subjects need to have fasted overnight, refrained from strenuous exercise the day before assessment, and be measured in a quiet, temperature-controlled

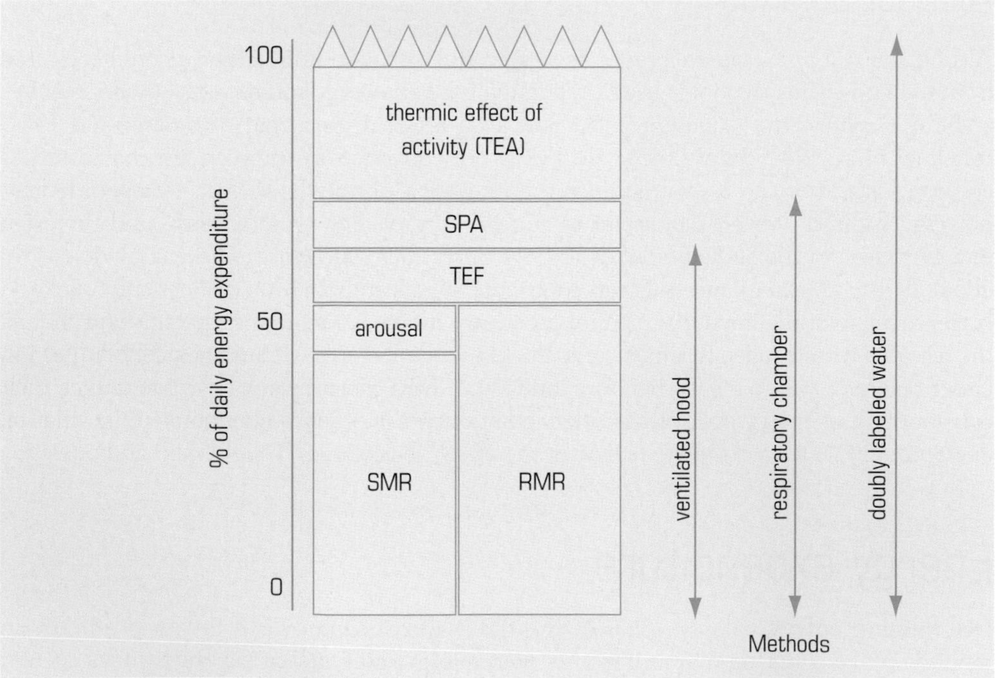

FIGURE 5.1 Components of daily energy expenditure in humans (adapted from Ravussin & Swinburn 1993). SPA = spontaneous physical activity; TEF = thermic effect of food; SMR = sleep metabolic rate; RMR = resting metabolic rate

room. In general, BMR and RMR usually differ by less than 10%. In this chapter, we will use the term RMR (except when a research study specifically reports that BMR was measured), since it is more frequently measured. Dietitians frequently use these terms interchangeably, when in fact they are measured differently.

RMR accounts for approximately 60–80% of total daily energy expenditure in most sedentary healthy adults (Ravussin et al. 1986; Ravussin & Bogardus 1989, 2000). However, in an active individual this percentage will vary greatly. Many elite athletes easily expend 4100–8300 kJ/d (1000–2000 kcal/d) in sport-related activities. For example, Thompson and colleagues (1993) reported that RMR represented only 38–47% of total daily energy expenditure in twenty-four elite male endurance athletes, while Beidleman and colleagues (1995) found in ten female endurance runners that RMR represented only 42% of total energy expenditure. During days of repetitive, heavy competition, such as ultramarathons, RMR may represent less than 20% of total energy expenditure (Rontoyannis et al. 1989).

TEF—sometimes called diet-induced thermogenesis (DIT)—is the increase in energy expenditure above RMR that results from the consumption of food throughout the day. TEF includes the energy cost of food digestion, absorption, transport, metabolism and storage within the body. TEF usually accounts for ~6–10% of total daily energy expenditure. However, TEF for an individual will vary, depending on the energy content of the meal or the food eaten over the day, the types of foods consumed, composition of the diet and the degree of obesity (Stock 1999; Westerterp et al. 1999). Although TEF is frequently used interchangeably with the thermic effect of a meal (TEM), the terms are not synonymous. TEM represents the increase in metabolic rate above RMR after eating a meal. Most researchers measure TEM instead of TEF because of the difficulties in trying to assess the cumulative energy cost of all foods consumed within a day. Thus, most of the research literature examining the energy costs of active individuals reports TEM, unless a metabolic chamber is used to collect data.

TEA is the most variable component of energy expenditure in humans. It includes the energy cost of daily activities above RMR and TEF, such as planned exercise events (like running, swimming or weightlifting) and activities such as walking or bike riding. TEA also includes purposeful activities of daily living (such as dressing, shopping, cooking and standing). These types of daily life activities are also called non-exercise activity thermogenesis or NEAT. Research now suggests that for some individuals, the energy expended in NEAT may play a significant role in helping to maintain energy balance (Levine et al. 2005, 2007). Finally, TEA includes the energy cost of involuntary muscular activity or SPA such as shivering and fidgeting. TEA may be only 10–15% of total daily energy expenditure in sedentary individuals, but may be as high as 50% in active individuals. Levine (2004a, 2004b) provides an in-depth review of NEAT and the environmental and biological factors that influence it. Donahoo and colleagues (2004) have reviewed the variability in total energy expenditure and its components.

A number of factors can increase energy expenditure above normal baseline levels, such as cold, heat, fear, stress and various medications or drugs (e.g. caffeine, alcohol and smoking) (Manore et al. 2009). The thermic effect of these factors is frequently referred to as adaptive thermogenesis (AT). AT represents a temporary increase in thermogenesis that may last for hours or even days, depending on the duration and magnitude of the stimulus. In athletes, a serious physical injury, the stress associated with an upcoming event, going to a higher altitude, performance or training in extreme environmental temperatures, or the use of certain medications, may all increase RMR above normal levels. Wijers and colleagues (2009) have reviewed the impact that individual differences in AT may play in contributing to weight gain and obesity.

5.10 Factors that influence RMR

A variety of factors can influence RMR for a given individual on any given day; however, some factors appear to have more of an influence than others. It is well documented that RMR is influenced by age, sex and body size, including the size of an individual's fat-free mass (FFM) and fat mass (FM). In fact, these factors are usually included in prediction equations for RMR. Three of these variables (age, sex and FFM) generally explain about 80% of the variability in RMR (Bogardus et al. 1986). Since FFM, especially organ tissue, is very metabolically active, any change in FFM can dramatically influence RMR (Sparti et al. 1997; Henry 2000). In general, males have larger RMRs than females because of an increased size and greater FFM; however, there may be other contributing factors to the differences in RMR besides gender (Blanc et al. 2004). Ferraro and colleagues (1992) report that females have a lower BMR than males (413 kJ or 100 kcal/d less), even after controlling for differences in FFM, FM and age. Conversely, Blanc and colleagues (2004) found no difference in RMR when comparing elderly men and women (aged 70–79 years) after controlling for FFM. Age is known to influence BMR, with an estimated decline in BMR of about 1–2% per decade from the second through to the seventh decade of life (Keys et al. 1987). Part of this decrease in RMR is attributed to the decline in quantity and the metabolic activity of FFM that occurs with aging, especially if an individual leads a more sedentary lifestyle (Henry 2000). However, the reduction of brain weight that occurs with aging may be a more significant contributor to the decrease in RMR than the decrease in FFM, as the brain is much more metabolically active than muscle mass (Henry 2000).

RMR also has a genetic component, which means that individuals within families may have similar RMRs. For example, Bogardus and colleagues (1986) found that family membership explained 11% of the variability in RMR ($p < 0.0001$) when they examined 130 non-diabetic adult south-western Native Americans from fifty-four families. Bouchard and colleagues (1989) also found that heritability explained approximately 40% of the variability in RMR in twins and parent–child pairs after adjusting for age, gender and FFM.

Phases of the menstrual cycle may also influence RMR and total energy balance. Although the current research is equivocal, some studies report that RMR values are lowest during the follicular phase of the cycle (beginning of the cycle) and highest during the luteal phase (end of the cycle) (Solomon et al. 1982; Bisdee et al. 1989). The difference in RMR between these two phases is estimated to be approximately 413–1238 kJ/d (100–300 kcal/d); however, adaptations in energy intake appear to mimic the changes in RMR. A study by Barr and colleagues (1995) found that females consumed approximately 1238 kJ/d (300 kcal/d) more during the luteal phase of the menstrual cycle compared with the follicular phase. Thus, the increased energy expenditure, due to a higher RMR during the luteal phase, is compensated for by an increase in energy intake during this period. Additional evidence supporting the impact of menstrual cycle on RMR comes from studies examining the impact of menstrual dysfunction on energy expenditure. Lebenstedt and colleagues (1999) found that RMR was significantly lower (about 460 kJ or 111 kcal/d) in female athletes with menstrual dysfunction (nine periods per year) compared to active controls (twelve periods per year), while Myerson and colleagues (1991) found amenorrheic runners had significantly lower RMRs than eumenorrheic runners and inactive controls. Conversely, Weststrate (1993) and Li and colleagues (1999) found no effect of menstrual cycle on RMR, and Piers and colleagues (1995) found no effect of menstrual cycle phase on RMR or energy intake. Thus, until these issues are resolved, menstrual status and the phase of the menstrual cycle should be documented using some type of hormonal data and/or recorded when measuring RMR or energy intake in females, especially active females.

There are a number of ways that exercise might indirectly or directly change RMR. First, exercise may increase RMR indirectly by increasing an individual's FFM, which is a strong determinant of RMR. It is well documented in the research literature that active individuals, especially elite athletes, are leaner (lower percentage body fat) and have greater FFM than their sedentary counterparts. Thus, for a given body mass, an athlete with a lower percentage of body fat and higher percentage of FFM will have a higher RMR. Second, it has also been hypothesized that exercise training influences RMR; however, data comparing RMR in exercise-trained and sedentary controls have not shown consistent increases in RMR when subjects (athletes and controls) are matched for size and FFM (Manore et al. 2009). The discrepancies in these results may be due to a number of factors, including level of fitness, type of exercise training program, methods used to measure RMR, and level of energy flux (the amount of energy expended in exercise compared with the amount of energy consumed each day) (Bullough et al. 1995; Manore et al. 2009). Third, strenuous exercise may cause muscle tissue damage that requires building and repair after exercise is over, thus indirectly causing an increase in RMR.

An acute bout of strenuous exercise has also been hypothesized to directly influence RMR. It has been observed that RMR is increased for a period of time (minutes or hours) after strenuous exercise; this phenomenon is termed excess post-exercise oxygen consumption (EPOC). How quickly oxygen consumption returns to baseline after exercise is over may depend on a number of factors including level of training, age, environmental conditions, and intensity and duration of the exercise. It appears that to produce a significant increase in EPOC, exercise intensity must be high and/or the duration of exercise must be long. A normal exercise bout of 30–60 minutes of moderate intensity (50–65% $VO_{2\,max}$) does not appear to significantly elevate EPOC for any appreciable amount of time after the exercise is over (Manore et al. 2009). After this type of exercise, oxygen levels usually return to normal within 1 hour. However, if exercise (either aerobic or strength training) is of high intensity and/or of long duration, EPOC appears to be elevated for hours after exercise (Chad & Quigley 1991; Melby et al. 1993; Gillette et al. 1994).

Factors that influence the thermic effect of food 5.11

A number of factors can influence how our bodies respond metabolically when we consume food. TEF can last for several hours after a meal and depends on the energy content of the meal consumed and the composition of the meal (percentage of energy from protein, fat and CHO). In general, the thermic effect of a mixed meal is estimated to be 6–10% of total daily energy intake; however, the total TEF will also depend on the macronutrient composition of the diet. For example, the thermogenic effect of glucose is 5–10%, fat is 3–5% and protein is 20–30% (Flatt 1992). The lower thermic response for fat is due to the lower energy requirement to store fat as triglyceride as compared to the synthesis of proteins from amino acids or glycogen from CHO.

Measurement of total daily energy expenditure 5.12

Total daily energy expenditure or its components can be measured in the laboratory or estimated using prediction equations. The following section discusses the most commonly used laboratory techniques for measuring the components of energy expenditure. When laboratory facilities are not available, prediction equations can be used to estimate total daily energy expenditure.

5.13 Indirect calorimetry

Energy expenditure in humans is commonly assessed using indirect calorimetry, which measures the rate of oxygen consumption (L/min) and carbon dioxide production (L/min) either at rest or during exercise. The ratio between the volume of carbon dioxide produced (VCO_2) and the volume of oxygen consumed (VO_2) can be calculated (VCO_2/VO_2). This ratio, when considered at the cellular level, is termed the non-protein respiratory quotient (RQ) and represents the ratio between oxidation of CHO and lipid. By knowing the amount of each energy substrate oxidized and the amount of oxygen consumed and carbon dioxide produced, total energy expenditure can be estimated using various published formulae. In general, the consumption of one liter of oxygen results in the expenditure of approximately 19.86 kJ (4.81 kcal) if the fuels oxidized represent a mixture of protein, fat and CHO. Since RQ cannot be directly determined at the cellular level in humans, an indirect measurement is taken by measuring gas exchange at the mouth. The relationship of VCO_2/VO_2 measured by this means is termed the respiratory exchange ratio (RER). RER is considered an accurate reflection of RQ under steady-state conditions. Using the indirect calorimetry method, one can measure total daily energy expenditure in a metabolic chamber, or measure RMR by using a mask, hood or mouthpiece in which gases are collected and analyzed for a specified period of time. Reviews by Schoeller and Racette (1990), Webb (1991), Westerterp (1993) and Montoye and colleagues (1996) provide additional information on the methods of indirect calorimetry.

RER values depend on the substrate being utilized, ranging from values of 0.7 (oxidation of fat only) to 1.0 (oxidation of pure CHO). Most individuals consuming a mixed diet of protein, fat and CHO will have an RER value of 0.82–0.87 at rest. However, during times of high exercise intensity, RER will increase and be closer to 1.0, while during times of fasting or low energy intake RER will decrease and be closer to 0.7. Thus, RER depends on the composition of the foods consumed, the energy demands placed on the body and whether body mass is being maintained.

5.14 Doubly labeled water

Because indirect calorimetry requires that an individual be confined to a laboratory setting or a metabolic chamber, it is difficult to measure an individual's free-living energy expenditure. The development of the doubly labeled water (DLW) ($^2H_2{}^{18}O$) method for use in humans has become a valuable tool in determining free-living energy expenditure (Speakman 1998). This method was first developed for use in animals (Lifson et al. 1955) and eventually applied to humans (Schoeller et al. 1986). The DLW method is a form of indirect calorimetry based on the differential elimination of deuterium ($^2H_2$) and ^{18}oxygen (^{18}O) from body water, following a load dose of water labeled with these two stable isotopes. The deuterium is eliminated as water, while the ^{18}O is eliminated as both water and carbon dioxide. The difference between the two elimination rates is a measure of carbon dioxide production (Coward & Cole 1991; Speakman 1998; Schoeller 2002). This method differs from traditional indirect calorimetry in that it only measures carbon dioxide production and not oxygen consumption. One advantage of this method is that it can be used to measure energy expenditure in free-living subjects for 3 days to 3 weeks, and only requires the periodic collection of urine for measurement of the isotope elimination rates. Another advantage is that it is free of bias, and subjects can engage in normal daily activities and sports without the interruption of writing down activities or wearing a heart-rate monitor. This method has become a valuable tool for the validation of other, less expensive field methods of measuring energy expenditure, such as accelerometers (Schoeller & Racette 1990; Ainslie et al. 2003). The major disadvantage of this technique is expense. Another disadvantage is that it has a five-times greater potential for error in estimating energy expenditure because it uses only the energy equivalent of carbon dioxide instead of the energy equivalent of oxygen (Jéquier et al. 1987). Finally, the experimental variability of the DLW technique in adult humans appears to be high (5–8.5%) (Speakman 1998; Ainslie et al. 2003). This variability is high both when repeating the technique in the same individual and between individuals (Goran et al. 1994; Scagliusi et al. 2008).

Predicting total daily energy expenditure 5.15

When laboratory facilities are not available for assessing total energy expenditure, it can be estimated by applying prediction equations to estimate RMR, then multiplying RMR by an appropriate activity factor. A number of prediction equations for estimating RMR have been developed for different populations that vary in age, gender, level of obesity and activity level (see Table 5.1). In general, it is best to use a prediction equation that is the most representative of the population or group of individuals with whom you are working. Table 5.1 summarizes some of the commonly used RMR prediction equations and the populations from which they were derived (Manore et al. 2009). It should be noted that most of the prediction equations have been developed using sedentary individuals. In an effort to determine which of these equations works best for active individuals and athletes, Thompson and Manore (1996) compared the actual RMR values measured in the laboratory with predicted RMR values, using equations listed in Table 5.1. They found that for both active males and active females the Cunningham (1980) equation best predicted RMR in this population, with the Harris–Benedict (1919) equation being the next best predictor. Figures 5.2a and 5.2b graphically show how close these equations actually predicted RMR in a group of endurance-trained males and females. Because the Cunningham (1980) equation requires the measurement of lean body mass (LBM) or FFM in kilograms, the Harris–Benedict (1919) equation is easier to use in settings where FFM cannot be directly measured.

Once RMR has been estimated, total daily energy expenditure can then be estimated by a variety of different factorial methods. These methods vary in how labor-intensive they are to use, and the level of subject burden. Manore and colleagues (2009) provide a detailed description of these methods. The easiest method for assessing total energy expenditure multiplies RMR by an appropriate activity factor, with the resulting value representing total daily energy expenditure. This factor may range from as low as 10–20% (0.10–0.20) of RMR for a bedridden individual to >100% (>1.0) for a very active individual. Although many laboratories establish their own activity factor for their particular research setting, factors of 1.3–1.6 are commonly used with sedentary individuals or individuals doing only light activity. With the activity factor methods, RMR is multiplied by a designated physical activity level or PAL (see Table 5.2). One activity factor can be applied to the whole day or a weighted activity factor can be determined. This activity factor is then multiplied by the RMR to provide a total daily energy expenditure. For example, if

TABLE 5.1 EQUATIONS FOR ESTIMATING RESTING METABOLIC RATE (RMR) IN HEALTHY ADULTS

HARRIS–BENEDICT (1919)[a]					
Males: RMR = 66.47 + 13.75 (wt) + 5 (ht) – 6.76 (age)					
Females: RMR = 655.1 + 9.56 (wt) + 1.85 (ht) – 4.68 (age)					
OWEN ET AL. (1986)[b]					
Active females: RMR = 50.4 + 21.1 (wt)					
Inactive females: RMR = 795 + 7.18 (wt)					
OWEN ET AL. (1987)[c]					
Males: RMR = 290 + 22.3 (LBM)					
Males: RMR = 879 + 10.2 (wt)					
MIFFLIN ET AL. (1990)[d]					
RMR = 9.99 (wt) + 6.25 (ht) – 4.92 (age) + 166 (sex: male = 1, female = 0) – 161					
CUNNINGHAM (1980)[e]					
RMR = 500 + 22 (LBM)					
WORLD HEALTH ORGANIZATION (1985)[f]					
Sex and age (years) range equation to derive RMR in kcal/d:					
Males	18–30	(15.3 × wt) + 679	Females	18–30	(14.7 × wt) + 496
	30–60	(11.6 × wt) + 879		30–60	(8.7 × wt) + 829
	>60	(13.5 × wt) + 487		>60	(10.5 × wt) + 596

wt = weight (kg), ht = height (cm), age = age (yr), LBM = lean body mass (kg)

[a]Harris and Benedict (1919) based on 136 men (mean age 27 ± 9 years; mean wt 64 ± 10 kg) and 103 women (mean age 31 ± 14; mean wt 56.5 ± 1.5) (n = 239 subjects). Included trained male athletes. Research indicates equation frequently over-predicts RMR by >15% (Frankenfield et al. 2005). Units of measurement expressed as basal energy expenditure (BEE), but the methods used were that of RMR;

[b]Owen et al. (1986) used forty-four lean and obese women; eight women were trained athletes (ages 18–65 years; weight range 48–143 kg). No women were menstruating during the study; all were weight-stable for at least 1 month;

[c]Owen et al. (1987) used sixty lean and obese men (ages 18–82 years; weight range 60–171 kg). All were weight-stable for at least 1 month. No athletes were included;

[d]Mifflin et al. (1990) used 498 healthy lean and obese subjects (247 females and 251 males) (ages 18–78 years; weight ranged from 46–120 kg for the women and 58–143 kg for the men). Physical activity levels were not reported. This equation is more likely to estimate RMR to within 10% of measured values in both obese and non-obese individuals (Frankenfield et al. 2005);

[e]Cunningham (1980) used 223 subjects (120 males and 103 females) from the 1919 Harris and Benedict database. They eliminated sixteen males who were identified as trained athletes. In this study, LBM accounted for 70% of the variability of BMR. The age variable did not add much because group age range was narrow. LBM was not calculated in the Harris–Benedict equation, so they estimated LBM based on body mass (kg) and age;

[f]World Health Organization (1985) derived these equations from BMR data.

Source: Adapted from Manore MM, Thompson JL. Sport nutrition for health and performance. Champaign, Illinois: Human Kinetics, 2000.

an individual has a RMR of 6192 kJ/d (1500 kcal/d) and an activity factor of 1.5, then the daily energy expenditure would be 50% above RMR or 9288 kJ/d (2250 kcal/d) (6192 kJ × 1.5 = 9288 kJ/d).

The Food and Nutrition Board of the Institute of Medicine (2002) has also published equations of Estimated Energy Requirements (EER) to predict total daily energy expenditure. These equations are:

$$\text{adult males: EER} = 662 - (9.53 \times \text{age}) + \text{PA} \times (15.91 \times \text{wt} + 539.6 \times \text{ht})$$
$$\text{adult females: EER} = 354 - (6.91 \times \text{age}) + \text{PA} \times (9.36 \times \text{wt} + 726 \times \text{ht})$$

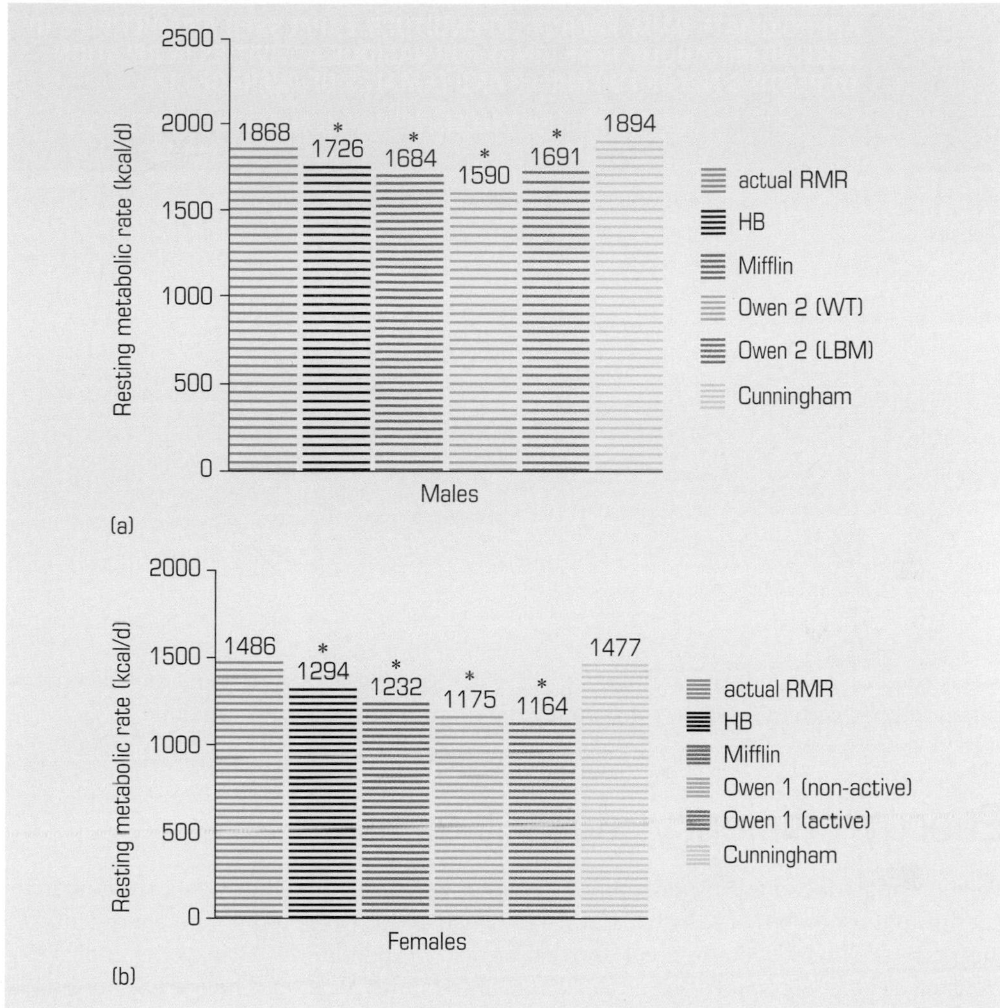

FIGURE 5.2 Mean group differences between actual and predicted resting metabolic rate (RMR) for twenty-four male (a) and thirteen female (b) highly trained endurance athletes (adapted from Thompson & Manore 1996)

*Indicates values were significantly different from actual measured RMR ($p < 0.05$). HB = Harris–Benedict equation (1919); Mifflin = Mifflin et al. equation (1990); Owen 1 = Owen et al. equation (1986) for active and non-active women; Owen 2 = Owen et al. equation (1997) for men using either body weight (wt) or lean body mass (LBM); and Cunningham = Cunningham (1980) equation. Equations are listed in Table 5.1

where:

age = age (yr)
PA = the physical activity quotient based on the person's PAL
wt = weight (kg)
ht = height (m)

PA is equal to 1.0 if PAL is 1.0 to 1.39, 1.11 if PAL is 1.4 to 1.59, 1.25 if PAL is 1.6 to 1.89, and 1.48 if PAL is 1.9 to 2.49.

Regardless of the method used to calculate energy expenditure, it should be noted that all values are estimates. How accurate these values are depends on how accurately activity

TABLE 5.2 APPROXIMATE DAILY ENERGY EXPENDITURE, EXPRESSED AS MULTIPLES OF RESTING METABOLIC RATE (RMR), FOR VARIOUS ACTIVITIES IN RELATION TO RESTING NEEDS FOR MALES AND FEMALES OF AVERAGE SIZE

	REPRESENTATIVE VALUES FOR PHYSICAL ACTIVITY LEVEL (PAL) MALES		FEMALES	
ACTIVITY LEVEL	AVERAGE	RANGE	AVERAGE	RANGE
Bed rest	1.2	1.1–1.3	1.2	1.1–1.3
Very sedentary	1.3	1.2–1.4	1.3	1.2–1.4
Sedentary/maintenance	1.4	1.3–1.5	1.4	1.3–1.5
Light	1.5	1.4–1.6	1.5	1.4–1.6
Light moderate	1.7	1.6–1.8	1.6	1.5–1.7
Moderate	1.8	1.7–1.9	1.7	1.6–1.8
Heavy	2.1	1.9–2.3	1.8	1.7–1.9
Very heavy	2.3	2.0–2.6	2.0	1.8–2.2

Source: National Health and Medical Research Council. Recommended dietary intakes for use in Australia. Part 4, Appendix II. 2001. At http://www.nhmrc.gov.au/publications/diet/n6p4.htm (accessed June 2005)

is recorded or reported, the accuracy of the database that is used to generate the energy expended per activity, and how accurately the required calculations are done.

5.16 Energy efficiency: does it exist?

The potential for energy efficiency among athletes was brought to the attention of researchers through a number of research studies in which active women reported energy intakes that appeared inadequate to meet total daily energy expenditures (Drinkwater et al. 1984; Deuster et al. 1986; Kaiserauer et al. 1989; Dahlstrom et al. 1990; Mulligan & Butterfield 1990; Myerson et al. 1991; Wilmore et al. 1992; Beidleman et al. 1995; Kopp-Woodroffe et al. 1999; Beals & Manore 1998). In these studies, active women (running 20–60 miles per week, or participating in gymnastics, swimming, triathlons or dancing) were reported to be consuming ≤147 kJ (35 kcal) per kg body mass. Despite these low energy intakes and apparent energy deficits, these individuals reported the maintenance of body mass over relatively long periods of time.

There are a number of possible explanations for an athlete's ability to maintain body mass despite the discrepancy between reported energy intake and energy expenditure. First, this discrepancy may be due to inaccuracies in reported estimates of energy expenditure or energy intakes, particularly due to athletes' under-reporting or under-consuming their usual intake during the period of monitoring (Dahlstrom et al. 1990; Wilmore et al. 1992; Schulz et al. 1992). A second explanation is that active individuals become more sedentary during non-exercising portions of the day, thus expending less energy than estimated (Gorsky & Calloway 1983). Finally, these differences may be due to increased metabolic efficiency (Mulligan & Butterfield 1990; Myerson et al. 1991; Thompson et al. 1993, 1995). If metabolic efficiency is present, then the actual energy requirements of these athletes are lower than those estimated by traditional means and would partly explain their ability to maintain body weight despite a seemingly low energy intake. Thus they may expend less energy—at rest, while performing various daily tasks and during exercise—than those whose energy intake appears adequate.

Evidence for

5.17

Thompson and colleagues (1993) reported evidence of energy efficiency in twenty-four male endurance athletes. In this study, the low-energy-balance athletes reported eating 6150 kJ/d (1490 kcal/d) less than the adequate-energy-balance athletes, while the estimated activity level of both groups was similar. Despite these energy intake differences, both groups had similar FFM and had been weight-stable for at least 2 years. RMR was significantly lower in the low-energy-intake group compared with the adequate-energy-intake groups (about 4.9 versus 5.3 kJ/FFM/h or 1.19 versus 1.29 kcal/FFM/h, respectively).

A second study was completed on another group of male endurance athletes classified as having either low or adequate energy intakes (Thompson et al. 1995). This study aimed to determine if there were differences in 24-hour energy expenditure, sleep energy expenditure, RMR and SPA, with these measurements being determined in a respiratory chamber. All subjects were of similar body size and composition. The low-energy-intake athletes reported a daily energy intake of 6446 ± 2163 kJ (1535 ± 524 kcal) less than estimated energy expenditure. The daily 24-hour energy expenditure, RMR, sleep energy expenditure and SPA of the low-energy-intake athletes were significantly lower than the adequate-energy-intake athletes. Thus part of the ability of the low-energy-intake athletes to maintain body mass on a seemingly low energy intake appears to be due to a lower daily sedentary energy expenditure.

Myerson and colleagues (1991) found that amenorrheic runners had a significantly lower RMR than eumenorrheic runners and inactive controls, and the energy intake of these runners was similar to the inactive controls despite higher activity levels. Lebenstedt and colleagues (1999) studied eumenorrheic and oligomenorrheic active women (runners and triathletes). The menstrual function of the women was determined by assessing salivary progesterone levels, and the women were classified as having either normal menstrual function (twelve periods per year) or menstrual disturbances (nine or fewer periods per year). Although the reported energy intake and activity level of these women was not different, the women with menstrual disturbances had a significantly lower RMR and reported significantly higher restrained eating scores. More recent work by De Souza and colleagues (2007) indicated that physically active women (exercising more than 2 hours per week) who also reported a high drive for thinness had significantly lower RMR values and were at a greater risk for menstrual dysfunction than active women or sedentary women reporting a normal drive for thinness, despite all three groups reporting similar levels of energy intake and being of similar body weight. The results of these studies suggest that amenorrheic women and women with menstrual disturbances exhibit energy efficiency, which may be either a cause or a consequence of menstrual cycle disturbances.

Nattiv and colleagues (2007) propose that the mechanism explaining the increased energy efficiency observed in active females with menstrual dysfunction is due to reduced energy availability. Energy availability is defined as the amount of dietary energy remaining to support other body functions after exercise training. When energy availability is too low to support all body functions in addition to exercise, the amount of energy expended for maintaining cellular function, thermoregulation, growth and reproduction is reduced.

This compensation in energy expenditure (or increased energy efficiency) restores energy balance and maintenance of body weight and promotes survival, but can negatively affect health.

Finally, some evidence from the obesity and dieting for weight loss research supports increased energy efficiency in formerly obese subjects. A meta-analysis of this research literature by Astrup and colleagues (1999) found that formerly obese subjects have a 3–5% lower relative RMR value compared to control subjects. More recent evidence reported by Rosenbaum and colleagues (2008) indicated that total daily energy expenditure, NEAT and RMR were significantly lower in healthy men and women who had either maintained a ≥10% weight loss after recent (5–8 wk) completion of weight loss or maintained this same amount of weight loss after sustained (>1 yr) completion of weight loss as compared to those maintaining their usual weight.

5.18 Evidence against

The results of a number of studies of female athletes do not support the existence of energy efficiency. Wilmore and colleagues (1992) and Schulz and colleagues (1992) found that female athletes reported significantly lower energy intakes than expected for their activity level, but measuring energy expenditure showed no evidence of energy efficiency, indicating they under-reported their energy intake. Beidleman and colleagues (1995) also found large differences between reported energy intake and energy expenditure in female distance runners, but could not attribute these differences to metabolic efficiency (lower RMR and energy expenditure during exercise) as compared to untrained controls. However, the data collection period was very brief (3 days), and may not have been long enough to detect true differences. Fogelholm and colleagues (1995) found that gymnasts reported a significantly lower energy balance (energy intake minus energy expenditure) than sedentary controls and soccer players, but the RMR was similar between all groups of athletes.

In most of these studies, metabolic efficiency was examined by comparing the RMR, total daily energy expenditure or energy expenditure during exercise of female athletes to sedentary controls. One criticism is that there was no attempt to compare the athletes who reported significant energy deficits to the athletes within the group who reported an adequate energy intake. A second criticism is that energy expenditure was not measured at the same time during the menstrual cycle in all studies (Schulz et al. 1992; Wilmore et al. 1992). RMR can change over the menstrual cycle, and is reported to be lowest in the follicular phase and highest in the luteal phase (Bisdee et al. 1989; Solomon et al. 1982; Barr et al. 1995). Failure to compare women during the same phase of the menstrual cycle or to clearly document and hormonally assess menstrual status could mask any differences in energy expenditure that may exist. Finally, only four studies (Mulligan & Butterfield 1990; Myerson et al. 1991; Beidleman et al. 1995; Lebenstedt et al. 1999) verified ovulation in eumenorrheic athletes, and only Myerson and colleagues (1991) and Lebenstedt and colleagues (1999) screened for eating disorders. As demonstrated in the study by Lebenstedt and colleagues (1999), active females may report regular menstrual bleeding and still have some type of menstrual dysfunction, a condition that may decrease energy expenditure if hormone responses are blunted (Dueck et al. 1996).

Recent evidence from the weight loss literature suggests that regular physical activity may prevent the increased energy efficiency that results from inadequate energy intakes resulting in weight loss. Redman and colleagues (2009) reported a significant decrease in total daily energy expenditure in free-living healthy individuals losing an average of 10–14% body weight through caloric restriction over 6 months, but those in the treatment group, who combined caloric restriction with structured aerobic exercise five times per week, experienced no decrease in total daily energy expenditure, despite losing the same amount of weight as those in the caloric-restriction-only groups. Although the participants in this study were not active individuals or competitive athletes, these results suggest that becoming physically active during a period of weight loss may protect some individuals from the increased energy efficiency that occurs as a result of energy restriction.

Summary

5.19

This chapter has discussed the components that determine energy balance, both those on the energy input side (dietary energy plus the contribution of energy stores within the body) and the energy expenditure side. In addition, we have covered how the various components of energy expenditure can be measured. It appears that some athletes may have an increased energy efficiency which can influence the energy intake needed to maintain body mass. For any one individual the factors that influence energy balance may be numerous, including gender, age, family history, dietary choices, level of daily activity and stress level. If an individual wishes to permanently change body size, then one or more of the components of energy balance needs to be altered over an extended time. Methods for doing this are discussed in Chapters 4 and 6.

References

Abbott WGH, Howard BV, Christin L, et al. Short-term energy balance: relationship with protein, carbohydrate, and fat balances. Am J Physiol 1988;255:E332–7.

Acheson KJ, Schutz Y, Bessard T, Anantharaman K, Flatt JP, Jéquier E. Glycogen storage capacity and de novo lipogenesis during massive carbohydrate overfeeding in man. Am J Clin Nutr 1988;48:240–7.

Acheson KJ, Schutz Y, Bessard T, Ravussin E, Jéquier E, Flatt JP. Nutritional influences on lipogenesis and thermogenesis after a carbohydrate meal. Am J Physiol 1984;246:E62–70.

Ainslie PN, Reilly T, Westerterp KR. Estimating human energy expenditure: a review of techniques with particular reference to doubly labeled water. Sports Med 2003;33:683–98.

Astrup A, Buemann B, Christensen NJ, Toubro S. Failure to increase lipid oxidation in response to increasing dietary fat content in formerly obese women. Am J Physiol 1994;266:592–9.

Astrup A, Gotzsche PC, van de Werken K, Ranneries C, Toubro S, Raben A, Beumann B. Meta-analysis of resting metabolic rate in formerly obese subjects. Am J Clin Nutr 1999;69:1117–22.

Barr SI, Janelle KC, Prior JC. Energy intakes are higher during the luteal phase of ovulatory menstrual cycles. Am J Clin Nutr 1995;61:39–43.

Beals KA, Manore MM. Nutritional status of female athletes with subclinical eating disorders. J Am Diet Assoc 1998;98:419–25.

Beidleman BA, Puhl JL, De Souza MJ. Energy balance in female distance runners. Am J Clin Nutr 1995;61:303–11.

Bisdee JT, James WPT, Shaw MA. Changes in energy expenditure during the menstrual cycle. Br J Nutr 1989;61:187–99.

Blanc S, Schoeller DA, Bauer D, Danielson ME, Tylavsky F, Simonsick EM, et al. Energy requirements in the eighth decade of life. Am J Clin Nutr 2004;79:303–10.

Bogardus C, Lillioja S, Ravussin E, et al. Familial dependence of the resting metabolic rate. New Eng J Med 1986;315:96–100.

Bouchard C, Tremblay A, Nadeau A, et al. Genetic effect in resting and exercise metabolic rates. Metabolism 1989;38:364–70.

Bullough RC, Gillette CA, Harris MA, Melby CL. Interaction of acute changes in exercise energy expenditure and energy intake on resting metabolic rate. Am J Clin Nutr 1995;61:473–81.

Chad KE, Quigley BM. Exercise intensity: effect on postexercise O_2 uptake in trained and untrained women. J Appl Physiol 1991;70:1713–19.

Coward WA, Cole TJ. The doubly labeled water method for the measurement of energy expenditure in humans: risks and benefits. In: Whitehead RG, Prentice A, eds. New techniques in nutritional research. San Diego, CA: Academic Press, Inc, 1991;139–76.

Cunningham JJ. A reanalysis of the factors influencing basal metabolic rate in normal adults. Am J Clin Nutr 1980;33:2372–4.

Dahlstrom M, Jansson E, Nordevange E, Kaijser L. Discrepancy between estimated energy intake and requirements in female dancers. Clin Physiol 1990;10:11–25.

De Souza MJ, Hontscharuk R, Olmsted M, Kerr G, Williams NI. Drive for thinness score is a proxy indicator of energy deficiency in exercising women. Appetite 2007;48:359–67.

Deuster PA, Kyle SB, Moser PB, Vigersky RA, Singh A, Schoomaker EB. Nutritional intakes and status of highly trained amenorrheic and eumenorrheic women runners. Fertil Steril 1986;46:636–43.

Donahoo WT, Levine JA, Melanson EL. Variability in energy expenditure and its components. Curr Opin Clin Nutr Metab Care 2004;7:599–605.

Drinkwater BL, Nilson K, Chesnut 3rd CH, Bremner WJ, Shainholtz S, Southworth MB. Bone mineral content of amenorrheic and eumenorrheic athletes. N Engl J Med 1984;311:277–81.

Dueck CA, Manore MM, Matt KS. Role of energy balance in athletic menstrual dysfunction. Int J Sport Nutr 1996;6:165–90.

Ferraro R, Lillioja S, Fontvieille AM, Rising R, Bogardus C, Ravussin E. Lower sedentary metabolic rate in women compared to men. J Clin Invest 1992;90:780–4.

Flatt JP. The biochemistry of energy expenditure. In: Bjorntrop P, Brodoff BN, eds. Obesity. New York: JB Lippincott Co, 1992:100–16.

Flatt JP. Use and storage of carbohydrate and fat. Am J Clin Nutr 1995;61(Suppl):952S–9S.

Flatt JP. Macronutrient composition and food selection. Obesity Research 2001;9(4 Suppl):256S–62S.

Flatt JP, Ravussin E, Acheson KJ, Jequier E. Effects of dietary fat on post-prandial substrate oxidation and on carbohydrate and fat balance. J Clin Invest 1985;76:1019–24.

Fogelholm GM, Kukkonen-Harjula TK, Taipale SA, Sievänen HT, Oja P, Vuori IM. Resting metabolic rate and energy intake in female gymnasts, figure-skaters and soccer players. Int J Sport Med 1995;16:551–6.

Food and Nutrition Board, Institute of Medicine. Dietary Reference Intakes for energy, carbohydrates, fiber, fat, protein and amino acids (macronutrients). Washington DC: The National Academy of Sciences, 2002.

Frankenfield DC, Roth-Yousey L, Compher C. Comparison of predictive equations for resting metabolic rate in health nonobese and obese adults: a systematic review. J Am Diet Assoc 2005;105:775–89.

Gillette CA, Bullough RC, Melby CL. Post-exercise energy expenditure in response to acute aerobic or resistive exercise. Int J Sport Nutr 1994;4:347–60.

Goran MI, Poehlman ET, Danforth E. Experimental reliability of the doubly labelled water technique. Am J Physiol 1994;266:E510–15.

Gorsky RD, Calloway DH. Activity pattern changes with decreases in food energy intake. Hum Biol 1983;55:577–86.

Harris JA, Benedict FG. A biometric study of basal metabolism in man. Carnegie Inst Wash Pub No. 279. Philadelphia: FB Lippincott Co., 1919:227.

Hellerstein MK, Christiansen M, Kaempfer S, et al. Measurement of de novo hepatic lipogenesis in humans using stable isotopes. J Clin Invest 1991;87:1841–52.

Henry CJK. Mechanisms of changes in basal metabolism during ageing. Eur J Clin Nutr 2000;54 (3 Suppl):77S–91S.

Jebb SA, Prentice AM, Goldberg GR, Murgatroyd PR, Black AE, Coward WA. Changes in macronutrient balance during over and under feeding assessed by 12-day continuous whole-body calorimetry. Am J Clin Nutr 1996;64:259–66.

Jéquier E, Acheson K, Schutz Y. Assessment of energy expenditure and fuel utilization in man. Ann Rev Nutr 1987;7:187–208.

Jéquier E, Tappy L. Regulation of body weight in humans. Physiological Reviews 1999;79:451–79.

Kaiserauer S, Snyder AC, Sleeper M, Zierath J. Nutritional, physiological, and menstrual status of distance runners. Med Sci Sports Exerc 1989;21:120–5.

Keys A, Taylor HL, Grande F. Basal metabolism and age of adult man. Metabolism 1987;22:5979–87.

Kopp-Woodroffe SA, Manore MM, Dueck CA, Skinner JS, Matt KA. Energy and nutrient status of amenorrheic athletes participating in a diet and exercise training intervention program. Int J Sport Nutr 1999;9:70–88.

Krempf M, Hoerr RA, Pelletier VA, Marks LM, Gleason R, Young VR. An isotopic study of the effect of dietary carbohydrate on the metabolic fate of dietary leucine and phenylalanine. Am J Clin Nutr 1993;57:161–9.

Lebenstedt M, Platte P, Pirke K-M. Reduced resting metabolic rate in athletes with menstrual disorders. Med Sci Sports Exerc 1999;31:1250–6.

Levine RA. Non-exercise activity thermogenesis (NEAT). Nutr Rev 2004a;62(7 Pt 2Suppl):82S–97S.

Levine RA. Non-exercise activity thermogenesis (NEAT): environment and biology. Am J Physiol Endocrinol Metab 2004b;286:E675–85.

Levine JA. Nonexercise activity thermogenesis—liberating the life-force. J Intern Med 2007;262: 273–87.

Levine RA, Lanningham-Foster L, McCrady SK, Krizan AC, Olsen LR, Kane PH, Jensen MD, Clark MM. Interindividual variation in posture allocation: possible role in human obesity. Science 2005;307:584–6.

Li ETS, Tsang LBY, Lui SSH. Resting metabolic rate and thermic effects of a sucrose-sweetened soft drink during the menstrual cycle in young Chinese women. Can J Physiol Pharmacol 1999;77:544–50.

Lifson N, Gordon GB, McClintock R. Measurement of total carbon dioxide production by means of doubly labelled water. J Appl Physiol 1955;7:704–10.

Manore MM, Meyer NL, Thompson JL. Sport nutrition for health and performance. Second edition. Champaign, Illinois: Human Kinetics, 2009.

Melby C, Scholl C, Edwards G, Bullough R. Effect of acute resistance exercise on post-exercise energy expenditure and resting metabolic rate. J Appl Physiol 1993;75:1847–53.

Melby CL, Hill JO. Exercise, macronutrient balance, and body weight regulation. Sports Sci Exchange 1999;112:1–6.

Mifflin MD, St. Jeor S, Hill LA, Scott BJ, Daugherty SA, Koh YO. A new predictive equation for resting energy expenditure in healthy individuals. Am J Clin Nutr 1990;51:241–7.

Montoye HJ, Kemper HCG, Saris WHM, Washburn RA. Measuring physical activity and energy expenditure. Champaign, Illinois: Human Kinetics Publisher, 1996.

Mulligan K, Butterfield GE. Discrepancies between energy intake and expenditure in physically active women. Br J Nutr 1990;64:23–36.

Myerson M, Gutin B, Warren MP, et al. Resting metabolic rate and energy balance in amenorrheic and eumenorrheic runners. Med Sci Sports Exerc 1991;23:15–22.

Nattiv A, Loucks AB, Manore MM, et al. The female athlete triad. Position Stand of the American College of Sports Medicine (ACSM). Med Sci Sports Exerc 2007;39:1867–82.

Owen OE, Holup JL, D'Alessio DA, et al. A reappraisal of the caloric requirements of men. Am J Clin Nutr 1987;46:875–85.

Owen OE, Kavle E, Owen RS, et al. A reappraisal of caloric requirements in healthy women. Am J Clin Nutr 1986;44:1–19.

Piers LS, Diggavi SN, Rijskamp J, van Raaij JMA, Shetty PS, Hautvast JGAJ. Resting metabolic rate and thermic effect of a meal in the follicular and luteal phases of the menstrual cycle in well-nourished Indian women. Am J Clin Nutr 1995;61:296–302.

Prentice AM. Manipulation of dietary fat and energy density and subsequent effects on substrate flux and food intake. Am J Clin Nutr 1998;67(Suppl):535S–41S.

Ravussin E, Lillioja S, Anderson TE, Christin L, Bogardus C. Determinants of 24-hour energy expenditure in man: methods and results using a respiratory chamber. J Clin Invest 1986;78:1568–78.

Ravussin E, Bogardus C. Relationship of genetics, age and physical fitness to daily energy expenditure and fuel utilization. Am J Clin Nutr 1989;49:968–75.

Ravussin E, Swinburn BA. Energy metabolism. In: Stunkard AJ, Wadden TA, eds. Obesity: theory and therapy, Second edition. New York: Raven Press Ltd, 1993:98.

Ravussin E, Bogardus C. Energy balance and weight regulation: genetics versus environment. British J Nutr 2000;83(1Suppl):17S–20S.

Redman LM, Heilbronn LK, Martin CK, et al. Metabolic and behavioral compensations in response to caloric restriction: implications for the maintenance of weight loss. PLoS ONE 2009;4:E4377.

Rontoyannis GP, Skoulis T, Pavlou KN. Energy balance in ultramarathon running. Am J Clin Nutr 1989;49:976–9.

Rosenbaum M, Hirsch J, Gallagher DA, Leibel RL. Long-term persistence of adaptive thermogenesis in subjects who have maintained a reduced body weight. Am J Clin Nutr 2008;88:906–12.

Saris WH. Sugars, energy metabolism and body weight control. Am J Clin Nutr 2003;78(Suppl):850S–7S.

Saris WH, Tarnopolsky MA. Controlling food intake and energy balance: which macronutrient should we select? Curr Opin Clin Nutr Metab Care 2003;6:609–13.

Scagliusi FB, Ferriolli E, Pfrimer K, Laureano C, Cunha CS, Gualano B, Lourenco BH, Lancha AH. Underreporting of energy intake in Brazilian women varies according to dietary assessment: A cross-sectional study using doubly labeled water. J Am Diet Assoc 2008;108:2031–40.

Schoeller DA. Validation of habitual energy intake. Public Health Nutrition. 2002;5(6A):883–8.

Schoeller DA, Racette SB. A review of field techniques for the assessment of energy expenditure. J Nutr 1990;120:1492–5.

Schoeller DA, Ravussin E, Schutz Y, Acheson KJ, Baertschi P, Jequier E. Energy expenditure by doubly labeled water: validation in humans and proposed calculations. Am J Physiol 1986;250:823–30.

Schrauwen P, Lichtenbelt WDV, Saris WHM, Westerterp KR. Changes in fat oxidation in response to a high-fat diet. Am J Clin Nutr 1997;66:276–82.

Schulz LO, Alger S, Harper I, Wilmore JH, Ravussin E. Energy expenditure of elite female runners measured by respiratory chamber and doubly labeled water. J Appl Physiol 1992;72:23–8.

Schutz Y. Concept of fat balance in human obesity revisited with particular reference to de novo lipogenesis. Int J Obesity. 2004b;28(Suppl):3S–11S.

Schutz Y. Dietary fat, lipogenesis and energy balance. Physiology & Behavior. 2004a;83:557–64.

Shelmet JJ, Reichard GA, Skutches CL, Hoeldtke RD, Owen OE, Boden G. Ethanol causes acute inhibition of carbohydrate, fat, and protein oxidation and insulin resistance. J Clin Invest 1988;81:1137–45.

Solomon SJ, Kurzer MS, Calloway DH. Menstrual cycle and basal metabolic rate in women. Am J Clin Nutr 1982;36:611–16.

Sonko BJ, Prentice AM, Murgatroyd PR, Goldberg GR, van de Ven MLHM, Coward WA. Effect of alcohol on postmeal fat storage. Am J Clin Nutr 1994;59:619–25.

Sparti A, DeLany JP, de la Bretonne JA, Sanders GE, Bray GA. Relationship between resting metabolic rate and the composition of the fat-free mass. Metabolism 1997;46:1225–30.

Speakman JR. The history and theory of the doubly labeled water technique. Am J Clin Nutr 1998;68(Suppl):932S–8S.

Stock MJ. Gluttony and thermogenesis revisited. Int J Obesity 1999;23:1105–17.

Suter PM. Is alcohol consumption a risk factor for weight gain and obesity? Crit Rev Clin Lab Sci 2005;42:197–227.

Swinburn B, Ravussin E. Energy balance or fat balance? Am J Clin Nutr 1993; 57(Suppl):766S–71S.

Thompson JL, Manore MM. Predicted and measured resting metabolic rate of male and female endurance athletes. J Am Diet Assoc 1996;96:30–4.

Thompson JL, Manore MM, Skinner JS. Resting metabolic rate and thermic effect of a meal in low- and adequate-energy intake in male endurance athletes. Int J Sport Nutr 1993;3:194–206.

Thompson JL, Manore MM, Skinner JS, Ravussin E, Spraul M. Daily energy expenditure in male endurance athletes with differing energy intakes. Med Sci Sports Exerc 1995;27:347–54.

Webb P. The measurement of energy expenditure. J Nutr 1991;121:1897–901.

Westerterp KR. Food quotient, respiratory quotient, and energy balance. Am J Clin Nutr 1993;57(Suppl):759S–65S.

Westerterp KR, Wilson SAJ, Rolland V. Diet induced thermogenesis measured over 24 hours in a respiration chamber: effect of diet composition. Int J Obesity 1999;23:287–92.

Weststrate JA. Resting metabolic rate and diet-induced thermogenesis: a methodological reappraisal. Am J Clin Nutr 1993;58:592–601.

Wilmore JH, Wambsgans KC, Brenner M, et al. Is there energy conservation in amenorrheic compared with eumenorrheic distance runners? J Appl Physiol 1992;72:15–22.

Wijers SL, Saris WH, van Marken Lichtenbelt WD. Recent advances in adaptive thermogenesis: potential implications for the treatment of obesity. Obes Rev 2009;10:218–26.

World Health Organization (WHO). Energy and protein requirements. Report of a Joint FAO/WHO/UNU Expert Committee. Technical Report Series 724. World Health Organization, Geneva. 1985:206. (Reprinted in the 1989 RDAs National Research Council.)

Yeomans MR. Effects of alcohol on food and energy intake in human subjects: evidence for passive and active over-consumption of energy. Br J Nutr 2004;92(Suppl):31S–4S.

CHAPTER 6

Weight loss and the athlete

HELEN O'CONNOR AND IAN CATERSON

6.1 Introduction

The stereotype of the lean, toned and strong athlete paints a picture of a population that controls its weight and body composition within tight limits with relative ease. This is not necessarily the case, with many studies providing evidence of athletes experiencing difficulty achieving and controlling desired levels of body weight and fat (Walberg-Rankin 1998). In most cases, the perceived excess weight or fat does not place the athlete at an increased health risk. Usually, the desired level of fatness is less than that which would be considered healthy or normal within the context of public health guidelines.

Athletes and coaches are open to just as much misinformation about weight loss and dieting as the rest of the community. In some cases, the methods used to reduce weight, and/or the level of reduction achieved or desired, become dangerous, increasing the likelihood of decreased performance and increasing the risk of detrimental health or psychological effects. This chapter covers a range of issues related to weight loss in athletes. Specific diets and problems related to 'making weight' for competition are covered in Chapter 7.

6.2 Justification for weight loss in athletes

Weight or fat reduction in athletes is generally motivated by a desire either to achieve a pre-designated weight in order to compete in a specific weight class or category (e.g. in horse racing, lightweight rowing, boxing and weightlifting) or to optimize performance by improving power to weight ratio (e.g. in jumping events, distance running, triathlon and road cycling). In aesthetic sports like gymnastics, diving and figure skating, attainment of desired body composition and physical appearance is considered important. Adding to these performance issues are current societal trends that encourage the pursuit of leanness for both men and women (Ballor & Keesey 1991). There is an unrealistic community perception and expectation, of female body size in particular, which is at odds with reality (Craig & Caterson 1990; Cash et al. 1994). Unfortunately, this has become an increasingly important issue in sports where an image of physical attractiveness is created for promotion or advertising. Athletes, or the sport itself, frequently derive significant financial rewards for delivering an image and wearing clothing accentuating physique.

Despite the apparent preoccupation with body weight and fat levels in many sporting groups, there is little empirical evidence of their effect on performance. This is partly due to the difficulty in teasing out the influence of physique compared with other factors that also impact on performance, such as diet and training. At the elite level, body fatness ranges are often quite narrow, and studies therefore have to be carefully designed using measures sensitive enough that they can accurately attribute any performance effects to an alteration in body fat. The relative importance and challenge associated with achieving a particular body or fat mass varies between sports and can be generally assessed by considering how different the desired characteristics are from the general or 'source' population.

Body mass and fatness may differ from the source population mean or have a tighter coefficient of variation (CV). The body mass of winners in the Boston Marathon (the oldest annual marathon race) is tightly clustered and has remained static over many decades despite a substantial increase in the body mass of the source population, suggesting low body mass is critical to success; see review by O'Connor and colleagues (2007). Competitive gradients or 'best' versus the 'rest' analysis (international versus state level performers) demonstrating clear trends in mass and fatness across athletic caliber is also evidence that is particularly (but sometimes inappropriately) used by coaches and athletes.

Experimentally, a high level of body fat has been shown to have an adverse effect on performance from the perspectives of heat exchange (O'Connor et al. 2007), mechanics (Cureton & Sparling 1980) and energy cost (Dempsey et al. 1966). Using a mathematical model, Olds and colleagues have estimated that an increased fat mass of 2 kg would increase 4000 m pursuit cycling performance by about 1.5 s (20 m) and a 40-km time trial by about 15 s (180 m) (Olds et al. 1993). The energy cost is also altered by the additional body mass increasing the rolling resistance. Although it has been suggested that moderate body fatness may actually enhance swimming performance by improving buoyancy, this has not been shown experimentally (Stager & Cordain 1984), and at the elite level of swimming there is currently a good deal of emphasis placed on maintaining low body-fat levels, especially for competition (Hawley & Burke 1998).

In sports where leanness is desired for aesthetic reasons, the reduction of body fat to extremely low levels may not actually benefit performance per se. However, coaches and athletes believe that an appropriate level of leanness is assessed by the 'trained eye' of the judges and that this then influences the score for artistic impression. Regardless of the reason, athletes and coaches, even at the recreational level, frequently place great importance on the attainment of desired body weight and fat levels. Yet even in athletes, as in the general population, the distribution and amount of fat are influenced by genetic and environmental factors as well as the training schedule, the sport and any attempts at weight control or reduction.

6.3 Factors influencing the ability to achieve optimal body weight and composition in athletes

6.4 Genetic factors

A significant proportion of the inter-individual variance in human fatness is attributable to genetic factors. Estimates of the heritability of body fatness and composition from epidemiological studies are varied; however, a trend in the size of estimates is apparent, with those based on twin studies showing the greatest heritability (80%), and those from adoption studies the lowest (10–30%) (Bouchard 1993). Overall it has been suggested that 25–40% of adiposity is due to genetic factors, though this may be up to 70% in some environments (Bouchard 1994). Short- and long-term intervention studies examining energy balance in pairs of identical twins suggest that body weight and fat gains in response to overfeeding are under significant genetic control, evidenced by a threefold higher between-pair (compared to within-pair) variance in weight and fat gain (Bouchard et al. 1990). Comparable results are found in the converse situation with similar losses of adiposity in twin pairs subjected to a period of relative underfeeding and increased activity (Bouchard & Tremblay 1997).

Twin studies have also shown a greater similarity in dietary intake and food preference in monozygotic compared with dizygotic twins, suggesting genetic factors contribute to dietary intake (Heller et al. 1988; Perusse et al. 1988). However, high correlations in dietary variables are observed in individuals sharing the same environment. When expressed as a percentage of total energy intake, carbohydrate (CHO) and fat were characterized by a genetic effect of 20%, while cultural transmission and environmental effects explained 10% and 70% of their intake respectively (Perusse et al. 1988). Twin studies may under-estimate the effect of environment on the food choices of athletes as it is likely that they are strongly influenced by the culture of the sport in which they participate, and by the focus on the role of nutrition on sports performance or physique.

A number of genes are known to be associated and/or linked with human obesity. These appear to be 'susceptibility genes', which increase the risk for obesity, but not necessarily its expression. An individual with deficient or unfavorable alleles at a large number of susceptibility genes will be at a higher risk of developing greater levels of body fatness, while a person with a smaller number will be more resistant (Bouchard 1993). Recently, a number of single gene mutations producing obesity have been discovered. These include mutations of the melanocortin-4 receptor (MCR-4), of leptin, and of pro-hormone convertase. These mutations tend to be associated with gross obesity and hypogonadotrophic hypogonadism. These are rare, but the MCR-4 mutation is the most common and has been described in 2–5% of those with morbid obesity in some studies. Other such genes are likely to be discovered.

The gap between gene discovery and the application of this knowledge to obesity in humans is demonstrated by our current knowledge of the protein leptin. In 1973, mouse studies demonstrated the presence of a circulating factor that appeared to be a satiety factor (Coleman 1973). Some animals (ob/ob mice) appeared to be deficient in this factor and became obese; others appeared to be insensitive to the factor and also became obese (db/db mice). In 1994, leptin, a protein corresponding to this satiety factor, was described (Zhang et al. 1994). It is produced by the adipocyte, and serum levels in both rodents and humans correlate closely with percent body fat and body mass index (Considine et al. 1996; Rosenbaum et al. 1996). Serum levels appear to act as a signal of adequacy of energy stores. Leptin binds to receptors in the hypothalamus, influences energy intake and increases activity in the mouse (Weigle et al. 1995). Despite hopes to the contrary (that obese humans might be deficient in leptin and therefore leptin replacement would become a treatment for obesity), serum leptin levels are elevated in obese humans and, except in a very few individuals who are lacking this factor (Montague et al. 1997), leptin deficiency is not a cause of obesity. Leptin levels are higher in females than males (Considine et al. 1996), and are elevated by increasing energy intake and particularly by increasing CHO intake (Jenkins et al. 1997).

In the human, it appears that, rather than being a satiety factor, leptin acts as a signal of nutritional adequacy and protection against famine. It signals the level of fat stores and is important in the initiation of puberty and in fertility. Leptin levels are low in anorexia nervosa sufferers (Grinspoon et al. 1996); similarly, in those sports where low levels of body fatness are desired, it would be expected that leptin would be low. The long-term effect on reproductive potential, or on eating and activity, of such suppressed leptin is not yet known. Human obesity is characterized by resistance to insulin action. It is evident from studies that leptin does have effects on peripheral metabolism, in particular the rates at which fats are mobilized and oxidized (Ahima & Lazar 2008). In athletes, leptin levels appear consistent with reduced body fat, although animal studies suggest there may be an independent effect of exercise in reducing leptin (Kowlalska et al. 1999). After a marathon, leptin levels are further reduced, and it has been suggested that major changes in energy expenditure (as in marathon running) may also alter leptin levels (Leal-Cerro et al. 1998).

Specific metabolic risk factors associated with increased weight gain in certain populations (Ravussin et al. 1988; Ravussin & Swinburn 1993)—such as a low resting metabolic rate (RMR) relative to that predicted for body size, a high 24-hour respiratory quotient (RQ) indicating a high rate of CHO relative to fat oxidation (Zurlo et al. 1990), and a lower rate of spontaneous physical activity (Ravussin et al. 1986)—almost certainly have a genetic basis. However, the relative contribution of genetic versus environmental factors still remains a point of debate. The rapid increase of obesity prevalence throughout the world—in western countries, economies in transition and in the third world—highlights the importance of the interaction between genes and the environment in the development of excess body fatness and obesity.

Another factor that needs to be considered when weight loss is attempted or contemplated is the fact that body weight and composition tend to remain stable in most people for significant periods (years). This suggests that body weight is regulated and that there are a series of set points for an individual's body weight throughout life. Reductions or increases in weight away from the current baseline, or set point, result in metabolic alterations that resist the maintenance of a new weight and promote weight loss or gain towards the set point.

Although most athletes exhibit lower levels of fatness than the general population, genetic factors still influence the relative effort that might be required to attain the desired body composition and weight. Genetics ultimately influences athletes' ability to successfully and safely achieve and maintain these desired levels.

6.5 Environmental factors

6.6 Energy intake and macronutrient selection

For many years there was a consensus that a stable body weight was maintained by a tight control of energy balance, and that each kilojoule had the same value in this balance, independent of whether it came from protein, fat, CHO or alcohol. In this view, excesses of CHO or protein would be converted into lipid and then stored as adipose tissue through the process of de novo lipogenesis. For some time it has been widely accepted that de novo lipogenesis does not occur to any great extent in humans (Acheson et al. 1988). This was thought to be partly because lipogenesis is an energetically expensive process and also because net de novo lipogenesis requires forced overfeeding and does not occur under the conditions of ad libitum eating (eating at any time) in normal individuals (Astrup & Raben 1992). However, there is evidence in healthy, sedentary, male subjects that habitual high-CHO diets induce enzymes in the de novo lipogenesis pathway (Aarsland et al. 1997). In one study, massive overfeeding of CHO (2.5 times energy expenditure) resulted in net fat synthesis of 170 g per day, of which 98% occurred in adipose tissue. Although this amount of CHO is extreme, even for athletes, it does demonstrate that a high-CHO diet alters metabolism with the potential to allow greater fat storage, particularly in sedentary individuals.

Dietary macronutrient composition is currently one of the most hotly debated areas in weight management. Although earlier work strongly favored the need to maintain tight regulation over CHO requirements to ensure energy balance (Jebb et al. 1996), there is emerging evidence for the critical role of protein or the so-called 'protein leverage hypothesis'; see review by Simpson & Raubenheimer (2005). Central to this hypothesis is that protein, not CHO, is the most tightly regulated nutrient. When faced with unbalanced diets, humans (and evidence exists for other vertebrates) prioritize protein. Over-consumption of energy occurs when fat and/or CHO are more accessible, affordable or available in highly desirable, palatable varieties. This results in passive, excess consumption of CHO and fat to obtain the obligatory requirement for protein. As protein intake constitutes a smaller proportion of dietary energy, a small decrease in the percentage of dietary protein drives additional feeding until the protein requirement is satisfied: the so-called 'protein leverage effect'. It is theoretically possible that increased protein needs of athletes (see Chapter 4) further influence this leverage effect but additional research is required to confirm its existence.

In western countries, avoiding an energy-dense, nutrient-poor diet requires discipline and dedication, even for athletes. Despite efforts to educate athletes about the health and performance benefits of a balanced diet intake, surveys suggest that athletes typically follow diets that conform to cultural and population norms (Brotherhood 1984). Recently, increased intake of manufactured CHO (e.g. high-fructose corn syrup products) has also been highlighted in the obesity literature, particularly with the explosion of low-fat, high-CHO 'diet' products that have relatively high energy density (Van Baak & Astrup 2009). Many sports foods are modeled on these criteria and are necessarily energy-dense to provide fuel in a compact form suitable for consumption during and around training sessions. For some athletes, the convenience of these products within a hectic training schedule results in regular and possibly over-consumption of these energy-dense, often protein- and nutrient-poor carbohydrates. This may result in energy imbalance (see section 6.14).

Although some athletes are protected from weight and fat gain by virtue of adaptations associated with aerobically based training such as increased oxygen delivery through improved capillarisation (Andersen & Henriksson 1977), greater density of mitochondria (Hoppeler et al. 1973) and elevated concentrations of enzymes are required for fat metabolism (Henriksson & Reitman 1976). Others, despite training for many hours each day, may not elevate fat oxidation substantially. Athletes in sports such as gymnastics, diving and figure skating fall into this category as their training is mainly skill-based, providing little opportunity to enhance fat oxidation or even substantially elevate energy expenditure. Even after a low-fat, low-energy intake, some of these athletes face a constant struggle with body weight and fat to achieve the desired physique requirements of their sport. To a degree, the struggle with weight is partly offset at the elite level, where there is selective survival of individuals with the genetic propensity to be extremely light and/or lean. However, even those more suited to a sport's physique requirements usually need to limit both fat and energy consumption as the desired levels of leanness, at least in females, are below what is biologically natural.

6.7 Exercise training and appetite

Evidence suggests that exercise has an important role in weight management (American College of Sports Medicine 2009a). However, the extent to which exercise affects appetite, energy intake, energy balance and ultimately weight or body fat loss is not completely understood. Energy intake post-exercise has been reported to result in partial, complete and even over-compensation of the energy expended during exercise. Post-exercise energy intake has been reported to be affected by numerous factors, such as the intensity, duration or mode of exercise. Early studies by King and colleagues (1994) suggest only a weak, short-term coupling between energy expenditure and energy intake. These studies demonstrated a short-term suppression of hunger and relative energy intake (relative to the energy used during the exercise bout) only after longer duration (60-minute versus 30-minute) intense exercise (cycling at 70% $VO_{2\ max}$ versus 30% $VO_{2\ max}$). Short-term, exercise-induced suppression of appetite may be related to elevated body temperature (Andersson & Larson 1961), increased levels of lactic acid (Baile et al. 1970) or even higher concentrations of tumor necrosis factor (Grunfield & Feingold 1991). There is also a complex interplay between hormones and neuropeptides (leptin, ghrelin, glucagon-like peptide-1, pancreatic polypeptide); see review by Martins and colleagues (2008). Most short-term (1–2 days) and medium-term (7–16 days) studies demonstrate that men and women can tolerate a substantial negative energy balance from exercise. Compensation for energy expended tends to be partial and incomplete up to around 2 weeks but there appears to be a difference between individuals, with some more able to compensate for the expended energy than others; see review by King and colleagues (2007). Differential compensatory responses to exercise make some individuals more susceptible to weight loss through physical activity while others are resistant. The reasons for this are not understood (see Martins et al. 2008) but dietary restraint and body weight/fat levels appear to play a role (King et al. 2007). Variability in the hedonic response or implicit wanting for food may explain why some individuals over-compensate for energy expenditure after exercise when compared to non-compensators; this is not explained by differences in subjective feelings of hunger (Finlayson et al. 2009). Although not specifically demonstrated in athletic populations, habitual exercisers demonstrate more sensitivity and accuracy in regulation of energy intake (King et al. 2007). In athletes this finding may be challenged by periodized programs or the seasonality of sport, where habitual activity can be highly variable.

Few studies have investigated the effect of mode of exercise. King and Blundell (1995) compared treadmill with cycling exercise and failed to observe a difference. Although there is anecdotal evidence of an increase in appetite after swimming, there are no studies directly comparing swimming to other modes of exercise. However, a more recent study reported that cycling submerged in cold (20°C) versus neutral (33°C) water temperatures stimulated greater post-exercise energy intake, so there may be an effect of temperature that influences appetite in some sports (White et al. 2005).

There is some evidence that exercise alters macronutrient selection, stimulating the drive for CHO, theoretically to aid replenishment of limited glycogen stores. Tremblay and colleagues reported a relationship between exercise-induced changes in RQ and energy intake, whereby individuals with the greatest reduction in RQ during exercise show the smallest increase in post-exercise energy intake (Tremblay et al. 1985).

Taken a step further, feeding a low-fat versus high-fat diet after exercise has been shown to result in negative energy balance, with a positive balance occurring after the high-fat diet (Tremblay et al. 1985; King & Blundell 1995). This may be due to alterations in appetite associated with the composition of the fuel mix oxidized or, alternatively, due to passive over-consumption as a result of the high palatability and energy density of the low-CHO diet, which is known to have a weak effect on satiation (King & Blundell 1995). In more recent research by Melby and colleagues (2002), consumption of 45 g of CHO when sedentary or during moderate (65% $VO_{2\ peak}$) exercise by normal-weight, physically active women resulted in significantly lower energy intake over the rest of the day and only modest suppression of fat oxidation during exercise. This finding provides additional support to the notion that post-exercise appetite may relate to the drive to replenish CHO stores; however, no study has investigated this from the protein leverage viewpoint.

Gender may also influence the energy intake in response to exercise training, with evidence of a higher compensatory increase in women than men which may be explained by differential baseline body fat levels; see review by King and colleagues (2007). These findings may help to explain gender differences in the capacity for body-fat losses and may arise from biologically based evolutionary differences (Tremblay et al. 1984; King et al. 1997).

6.8 Physical activity and energy expenditure

The amount of energy expended during exercise depends on variables attributable to the individual (e.g. body weight and efficiency of performing a particular activity), and those related to the activity itself (e.g. frequency, duration and intensity). Greater body mass increases the work required to perform weight-bearing activities, while skills developed in training reduce the energy cost of exercise by improving efficiency. The frequency, intensity and duration of exercise determine the overall energy expended during activity. However, exercise intensity in particular affects the magnitude of the post-exercise elevation in metabolic rate (Bahr & Sejersted 1991). Post-exercise energy expenditure may be significantly elevated in athletes who perform high-intensity, long-duration exercise, even though this component of expenditure is considered to be trivial for most non-athletes (Freedman-Akabas et al. 1985). Genetic predisposition is also important as it ultimately dictates an individual's aerobic capacity and potential to perform sustained, moderate- to high-intensity activity. The interaction of genetic factors with the type, intensity and magnitude of training influences the capacity to oxidize fat and the potential for fat loss through exercise.

Total physical activity includes the athlete's regular training or exercise, plus any other activity occurring in non-training hours. Levine and Miller (2007) developed the concept of non-exercise activity thermogenesis or NEAT, which they define as energy expenditure from sleeping, eating and unplanned exercise programs. Elite athletes may experience a decrease in NEAT due to the incorporation of daytime rest and the limitation of work and leisure activities to accommodate training. Reduction in NEAT has been observed in the elderly after an increase in organized training (Goran & Poehlman 1992), but typically not in other groups (Meyer et al. 1991)—again, this has not been formally assessed in athletes.

Another factor to consider is the seasonal nature of many sports, which may also coincide with Christmas or winter, where there appears to be a significant trend for weight gain (Almeras et al. 1997). Injury or illness will also decrease total energy expenditure and this influences weight control. One of the aims in any off-season or off-training time should be the prevention of excess weight or fat accumulation. Assessment of energy expenditure in athletes therefore requires an understanding of their energy expenditure both during and outside of training.

Effect of physical activity on resting metabolic rate and the thermic effect of food

Elevation in resting metabolism has been observed in elite athletes with high energy expenditures and intakes (Poehlman et al. 1989). It has been suggested that this increase is an adaptation to a chronic high energy flux, but may be due to exercise-related gains in lean body mass (Sharp et al. 1992) or changes in energy intake or balance (Melby et al. 1998). Physical activity, such as would be used in a typical prescription for weight loss in the general community, appears less likely to have an impact on resting metabolism (Melby et al. 1998).

A number of studies have focused on the impact of exercise training on the thermic effect of food (TEF); see review by Melby and colleagues (1998). This accounts for about 10–15% of daily energy expenditure and is small compared to RMR and the potential contribution of physical activity (Reed & Hill 1996). Small deficits in TEF are considered unlikely to contribute significantly to weight gain (Ravussin & Swinburn 1992). Despite a number of studies of both obese and trained populations, there is no consistent evidence that physical activity has a biologically important effect on TEF (Melby et al. 1998).

Physical activity and substrate utilization

The intensity of exercise determines which fuel is used to supply energy to the working muscle. Plasma free fatty acids are the predominant fuel during low-intensity exercise (<50% $VO_{2\ max}$) (Romijn et al. 1993). As intensity increases there is a greater reliance on muscle glycogen and plasma glucose (Coyle et al. 1986). The amount of CHO utilized during exercise also depends on the training status of the individual. Well-trained athletes oxidize more fat than the untrained due to improved mitochondrial density (Hoppeler et al. 1973; Davis et al. 1981) and an increased concentration of oxidative enzymes (Henriksson & Reitman 1976; Oscai et al. 1982). In addition, transport of fatty acids into the mitochondria may be enhanced (Kiens 1977), and at a given submaximal workload well-trained athletes have lower levels of circulating catecholamines (Deuster et al. 1989). These adaptations, along with a greater capillary density (Andersen & Henriksson 1977) and an increase in intramuscular triglyceride (Hurley et al. 1986), enhance the delivery of oxygen and improve the ability to utilize fat, especially during low-intensity to moderate-intensity exercise. Although training also results in adaptations that enhance CHO utilization, such as an increase in glucose transport and insulin sensitivity, it is the enhanced fat utilization that mostly aids in weight control. Endurance exercise rather than high-intensity exercise has been associated with most of the exercise-related adaptations mentioned above, but recent research provides evidence that high-intensity exercise may promote greater fat oxidation during recovery (Yoshioka et al. 2001). Although relatively few studies have investigated the effect of resistance exercise, there is some evidence that it also supports greater fat oxidation during recovery from both a single bout (Melby et al. 1993) and a 16-week strength-training program (Treuth et al. 1995). Despite this, resistance training studies in the general population do not support the idea that this form of training significantly adds to weight/body-fat loss in overweight individuals (American College of Sports Medicine 2009a). Further research is required in athletes, who typically have much higher levels of resistance exercise than that prescribed to participants in weight-management studies. Except in a few sports (e.g. weightlifting and bodybuilding), most athletes habitually combine resistance training with some component of aerobic conditioning that has clearly been established as an effective approach for reducing body fat (American College of Sports Medicine 2009a).

6.9 Social and behavioral factors

Eating behaviors are important in the maintenance of desired body weight (Wing & Jeffery 1979). Food may be a form of recreation, release or reward for athletes, who tend to have regimented lifestyles that revolve around training and competition schedules. The sporting environment may also expose athletes to cafeteria or buffet-style eating. This has been associated with over-consumption in other populations (Stunkard & Kaplan 1977), especially when the food is high in fat and palatable. Pressure to perform or achieve a particular weight or body fat may result in rebellion against a dietary regimen designed to control body composition. Alternatively, obsession with weight loss may result in disordered eating (Thornton 1990). Typically, adolescent or young adults demonstrate age-related diet preferences that lean towards high-fat, fast and take-away foods (Truswell & Darnton-Hill 1981). During this period of life alcohol consumption often begins, and there is potential for over-consumption, particularly in team sports, where alcohol use may be seen as part of a 'team bonding' experience (Burke & Read 1987).

6.10 Growth and pubertal changes

Restriction of dietary energy to control body weight and fat levels may retard and possibly stunt growth in young athletes (Daly et al. 2002). Pubertal development in girls may influence their ability to achieve physique requirements in sports that require extreme leanness. The effect of energy restriction and weight loss on growth, maturation, health and performance in young athletes is covered in Chapters 7 and 8.

6.11 Tapering for competition

Tapered training to facilitate physical recovery and restoration of fuel reserves may result in a reduction in energy expenditure and increase the risk for lean mass loss and fat gain (McConell et al. 1993; Margaritis et al. 2003). Anecdotally, weight gain during this time is often reported in different groups of athletes, yet a number of studies (Houmard et al. 1990; Flynn et al. 1994; Dressendorfer et al. 2002) investigating various physiological and metabolic effects of tapering report relative weight stability. Unfortunately, these studies failed to measure body composition changes. Acutely imposing a sedentary routine of 1.4 times RMR versus a habitual 1.8 times RMR in young lean males while in a whole body, indirect calorimeter for 7 days with an ad libitum medium-fat diet failed to induce a compensatory reduction in energy intake and resulted in a significant positive energy balance (Stubbs et al. 2004). An inability to compensate energy intake after acute reductions in energy expenditure during tapering may also be complicated in athletes by the need to travel to competition, where dietary intake is more difficult to control. Practical strategies for managing this situation are covered in the practice tips at the end of the chapter.

Approaches to weight and fat loss in athletes 6.12

Dietary approaches for weight and fat loss 6.13

A number of dietary approaches have been studied for weight and fat loss.

Energy versus fat reduction and energy density 6.14

Ad libitum reduction in fat intake results in a modest decrease in both energy intake and body weight and fat mass in obese individuals; see review by Astrup and colleagues (2000). A large cohort study of women also found this approach induced spontaneous weight loss over a period of 7 years when compared to a normal fat control diet (Howard et al. 2006). Although not specifically studied in athletes, ad libitum low-fat eating typically produces a satisfactory result in those who have long-term, modest weight or fat reduction goals, particularly when energy expenditure is high. Clearly, this approach is less restrictive and avoids jeopardizing CHO and micronutrient intake.

However, ad libitum low-fat eating will not produce the energy deficit required for those athletes desiring more extreme losses of body weight or fat. When planned energy restriction is required, careful dietary design is required to optimize nutrient intake and prevent insufficient energy availability (American College of Sports Medicine 2009b). The least energy restriction that will achieve the desired result is recommended and a deficit of 2100 kJ (500 kcal) from theoretical requirements (American College of Sports Medicine 2001) may be a useful guide. However, gradual energy reduction of 10% or 20% may be a better initial approach and prevent the athlete from feeling too hungry. Erratic dieting or weight cycling, more commonly reported in 'making weight' sports (Chapter 7), should also be minimized as it may be associated with adverse health risks, including obesity, in later life (Saarni et al. 2006).

Diets that emphasize nutrient-rich, low-energy-density foods are also recommended. In an elegant series of studies, initial relative over-consumption demonstrated in participants fed 40% and 60% compared to 20% fat diets while living in a 24-hour calorimeter was attributable to energy density, not fat content (Prentice & Poppit 1996). Redesign of the study diets employing identical density resulted in abolition of energy over-consumption associated with the higher-fat diets (Stubbs et al. 1995a, 1995b). This effect has been termed 'passive over-consumption': eating more energy in a similar weight of food.

This principle should be upheld via the thoughtful use of sports foods (e.g. sports drinks, energy bars and gels) for athletes on an energy-restricted diet.

Although these foods are a compact and convenient means of replacing energy during and around exercise, they are energy-dense, less satiating and are often micronutrient-poor and over-consumed. Strategic timing of usual meals and snacks around exercise sessions may be preferable for energy-restricted athletes so they can obtain the nutrition they need to support training and recovery.

6.15 Reduced-carbohydrate diets

Reduced-CHO diets popular with athletes include those promoted in *The Zone: a dietary road map* (Sears 1995) and *Doctor Atkins' new diet revolution* (Atkins 1992). Both of these diets base their success around the reduction of insulin secretion, which is stimulated by eating CHO. Sears claims that eating in the 'Zone' (40% of energy from CHO, 30% from protein and 30% from fat) balances the insulin to glucagon ratio, which increases lipolysis and controls eicosanoid regulation. Some of these eicosanoids control blood flow and oxygen delivery to the muscle. Eating in the 'Zone' is also claimed to increase the intake of precursor fatty acids required for 'good' eicosanoid production. Unfortunately, eicosanoid metabolism is complex, with little predictability. Often the theoretical changes expected do not occur in response to dietary manipulation (Stone et al. 1978). Although Sears bases some of his claims on plausible scientific theory, there are many flaws in the arguments and the diet itself contains contradictory information (e.g. misclassification of the glycemic index of some foods). The claim that a reduction in CHO intake to 40% of energy—based mainly around low to moderate glycemic index foods—will significantly decrease plasma insulin levels is misleading, as a reduction in CHO intake to less than 25% of energy is required before insulin levels are significantly reduced (Coulston et al. 1983).

In practice, eating the 'Zone' diet is impractical as all meals and snacks need to be reorganized to comply to the 40:30:30 ratio. This is quite different from the way most athletes eat and a number of recipes in the book do not conform to the set ratio. When the diet is followed precisely it is low in energy, typically providing between 4200 and 8400 kJ/d (1000–2000 kcal/d), so it is not surprising that followers lose weight on the program, particularly if undertaking heavy exercise. For reviews see Cheuvront (1999, 2003). Evidence that eating in the 'Zone' results in superior exercise performance or weight loss is lacking (Jarvis et al. 2002; Bosse et al. 2004).

Surpassing the popularity of the Zone and most other popular diets is the Atkins diet, the book of which has sold over 45 million copies in the past 40 years (Astrup et al. 2004). The most rigorous version of this diet provides only 30 g of CHO; however, it is not energy-restricted. The diet permits unlimited quantities of high-protein/high-fat foods, providing they contain no or minimal CHO. This induces ketosis, which Atkins claims is critical to promote substantial weight loss and to assist with appetite control. This diet has been evaluated by a number of randomized controlled trials in obese adults (Foster et al. 2003; Samaha et al. 2003; Stern et al. 2004; Yancy et al. 2004; Dansinger et al 2005; Gardner et al. 2007). Weight loss at 3 and 6 months is typically higher in the Atkins-style diet compared to a conventional low-fat diet. However, weight loss at 12 or 24 months is modest and not differential (Foster et al. 2003; Stern et al. 2004; Sacks et al. 2009) except for one study (Gardner et al. 2007). Typically the greatest weight loss is achieved at 3 or 6 months followed by regain in the subsequent 6 to 18 months of follow-up (Foster et al. 2003; Stern et al. 2004; Sacks et al 2009). Losses on the Atkins diet were not superior to programs that include professional support and behavioral therapy (Wadden & Foster 2000), although they were often achieved with minimal professional intervention. Greater short-term weight loss with low-CHO diets has been related to satiety (Skov et al. 1999), thermogenesis (Nair et al. 1983), energy expenditure (Dauncey & Bingham 1983), and even diet simplicity/monotony (Foster et al. 2003). A reduction in glycemic load may also be a factor (Ebbeling et al. 2003). As the degree of ketosis has not been associated with extent of weight loss, it is considered unlikely that this is a key factor (Foster et al. 2003). Probably the most important factor in weight loss success is dietary adherence. Although this is not often reported, the results of three dietary comparison studies including reduced-CHO diets concluded that attendance or adherence was associated with more successful weight loss than diet composition (Dansinger et al. 2005; Alhassan et al. 2008; Sacks et al. 2009).

One concern with low-CHO diets is their effect on lean mass loss. However, some studies report preservation of lean tissue (Parker et al. 2002; Layman et al. 2003). It has been suggested that weight loss and body composition changes with higher-protein or higher-CHO diets may be a function of insulin sensitivity. One small study found better weight loss and normalization of insulin levels on a high-protein compared to a high-CHO diet (Torbey et al. 2002). Loss of lean mass in particular would be a negative result for athletes and, due to their higher energy and CHO needs, the mobilization of lean mass via gluconeogenesis would be a concern. However, there is evidence in studies of athletes 'making weight' (see Chapter 7) that a higher protein diet may enhance retention of lean mass when energy intake is restricted, although typically these diets are not as low in CHO as the Atkins diet.

No studies have evaluated the Atkins diet in athletes. Firstly, it is extremely low in CHO and even studies using low-CHO diets designed to enhance fat oxidation (via fat adaptation) to promote improved endurance do not usually find this strategy enhances performance (reviewed in Chapter 15). In the short term, induction diet side effects, including headaches, fatigue and nausea (Sumithran & Proietto 2008), are unlikely to promote high-quality training sessions.

There is still insufficient evidence to support the safety of low-CHO diets in the long-term. Ketosis is potentially harmful, with possible long-term sequelae including hyperlipidemia, impaired neutrophil function, optic neuropathy and osteoporosis, as well as alterations in cognitive function (Denke 2001; Sumithran & Proietto 2008). Although improvement in cardiovascular risk factors has recently been reported in obese populations on reduced-CHO diets, this may be primarily due to weight loss, and elevation of low density lipoprotein is often reported (Sumithran & Proietto 2007). In athletes, high activity levels may be protective and attenuate cardiovascular disease risk (Sarna & Kaprio 1994).

Nutritional adequacy is another concern. A review of twenty popular diets demonstrates that the Atkins induction diet phase is below the male adult Recommended Dietary Intake (RDI) for fiber (13% RDI), vitamins B1 and B2 (47 and 77% RDI), vitamin C (72% RDI), calcium (89% RDI), magnesium (54% RDI) and iron (72% RDI). The Atkins ongoing weight loss and maintenance diets fare better, but are still below the RDI for some nutrients (Williams & Williams 2003). Although it is difficult to ensure 100% of the RDI for all nutrients when planning energy-restricted diets, and dietary supplements can be taken to correct these deficiencies, the limiting of dairy, grains, fruit and starchy vegetables also decreases the intake of phytochemicals, substances acknowledged as having important health-protection benefits (Ralph & Provan 2000).

Low-CHO diets may help athletes with short-term weight loss, but they will result in glycogen depletion and, as a consequence, fatigue, delayed recovery and possibly a reduction in lean mass and immune function. Nutrient intake will almost certainly be inadequate and, if followed in the longer term, there may be serious health risks. Early performance improvement due to weight loss from these diets always needs to be balanced with the longer-term picture, which will inevitably include at least some of these negative effects. For these reasons, low-CHO diets for weight loss in athletes are not recommended.

6.16 Manipulation of the glycemic index (GI)

Evidence supporting (McMillan-Price & Brand Miller 2006) and questioning (Sloth & Astrup 2006) the effectiveness of low-GI diets for weight management is available. A recent meta-analysis of glycemic index on weight reduction indicates it has a small positive effect in promoting weight loss (Thomas et al. 2009). The effect of low-GI diets on satiety may be particularly helpful for 'hungry' athletes or those needing to chronically restrict energy intake (e.g. jockeys, ballet dancers and gymnasts). Satiety effects have not been specifically investigated in athletes, but have been observed in a number of studies; for review see McMillan-Price & Brand Miller (2006). Unlike restriction of CHO, reduction of dietary GI is not associated with negative health consequences, although the impact on glycogen storage and performance in athletes has not been evaluated. More medium- to long-term studies, including those on athletes, need to be performed.

6.17 Role of calcium and dairy products in weight management

Data from several large populations—including the National Health and Nutrition Examination Survey (NHANES), and Quebec Family, Heritage and CARDIA studies—support an inverse relationship between dietary calcium/dairy intake and body mass index (BMI), body fat and incidence of obesity. The CARDIA study also provides evidence of a negative association between dairy product intake and the incidence of insulin resistance; for review see Major and colleagues (2008). Although much of the early evidence for calcium and dairy was observational, recent clinical trials now provide further support for the beneficial role of calcium and dairy products in weight management. In one such trial, designed to evaluate the effect of calcium and dairy intake on weight and fat loss in obese subjects on a hypocaloric diet (2000 kJ or 500 kcal/d deficit), those on the control diet (0–1 servings of dairy food and 400–500 mg supplemental calcium a day) lost 6.5% of their body weight over 24 weeks (Zemel et al. 2004).

This loss was increased by 26% using the same diet with 800 mg/d supplemental calcium and, remarkably, to 70% (loss of 10.9% initial body weight) in a high dairy product diet (3–4 servings of dairy, providing 1200–1300 mg calcium a day). Although fat loss followed a similar trend, fat loss in the trunk region represented 19% of the total fat loss in the low calcium (control) diet group and up to 50% and 66% in the diets high in supplemental calcium or high in dairy calcium respectively. The authors concluded that an increase in calcium from suboptimal to optimal can improve the efficacy of weight and fat loss on energy-restricted diets in obese subjects and that these effects are even greater when dairy foods rather than supplemental calcium are consumed. There is emerging evidence that benefits may be limited to, or more pronounced in, individuals with habitually low (below 500–600 mg calcium per day) compared to high (>800 mg/d) calcium intakes and there may be additional benefit with vitamin D supplementation; for review see Major and colleagues (2008).

Unfortunately, seemingly to their detriment, athletes striving to remain lean or reduce weight or fat are often reported to consume inadequate calcium (Barr 1987).

The biological mechanisms underpinning weight-loss benefits are uncertain but several plausible biological mechanisms have been proposed (Major et al. 2008). These include the role of intracellular calcium in the regulation of adipocyte lipid metabolism and triglyceride storage (Zemel 2003). Further, as intracellular calcium can be regulated by calcitrophic hormones, including parathyroid hormone and 1,25-dihydroxyvitamin D, a theoretical basis for the additional anti-obesity effects of dairy products is also available

(Bell et al. 1985; Shi et al. 2002). Calcium itself, with its capacity to stimulate lipolysis, inhibit fatty acid synthase and de novo lipogenesis, may also mediate beneficial effects through an *increase* in uncoupling protein 2 expression, which is thought to influence fat cell apoptosis, increase fat oxidation and attenuate the decline in thermogenesis that occurs with energy restriction (Shi et al. 2001). High dietary calcium has also been observed to increase fecal fat excretion (Major et al. 2008). One study (Lorenzen et al. 2006) demonstrated a 2.5 fold increase in daily fecal fat (~14 g loss of fat equivalent to 350 kJ) after consumption of a higher dairy diet. This effect, while useful, still fails to explain the magnitude of the weight and fat loss benefits observed in clinical weight loss trials. Evidence also exists for a positive influence of calcium/dairy on reducing appetite; see review by Major and colleagues (2008).

Other popular diets 6.18

In their evaluation of twenty popular diets, Williams and Williams (2003) scored diets based on their nutritional adequacy, flexibility, physical activity and supplement recommendations in addition to scientific support. Popular diets with point scores below 50 out of a total of 100 points included 'Slim Forever' (32), 'Dr Atkins' New Diet Revolution' (35), 'Eat Right for Your Type' (36), 'Sugar Busters' (40), 'The Fit for Life Diet' (41), 'The Zone and Liver Cleansing Diet' (42), 'The Carbohydrate Addicts Diet' (43), 'The Complete Scarsdale Medical Diet' (44) and 'Diet Signs—The Health Signs Diet' (45). Top-scoring diets included 'The Volumetrics Weight Control Plan' (97), 'Licence to Eat' (96), 'Fat Loss for Life' (87), 'The Diet that Works', 'Eat More Weigh Less' (85) and 'The Fat Stripping Diet' (80).

Adaptation to high-fat diets and 'train low' strategies 6.19

Adaptation to high-fat diets has been used to delay fatigue in endurance exercise by enhancing fat oxidation and sparing CHO stores (Lambert et al. 1994). Although not typically employed to promote weight loss, athletes have been interested in the notion that fat adaptation might result in a permanent up-regulation of fat metabolism and subsequent improvement in body-fat control. Similarly there is anecdotal evidence of athletes using 'train low' strategies to enhance weight/body-fat loss, although this has not been systematically assessed in any of the available literature. See Chapter 15 for further information.

Very low energy diets (VLEDs) 6.20

Very low energy (VLEDs) or very low calorie diets (VLCDs) diets provide 1600–2400 kJ (400–600 kcal) and less than 100 g CHO/d in the form of a liquid meal (such as Modifast™ or Optifast™) with added vitamins and minerals to levels approximating the RDI (Brodoff & Hendler 1992). Weight loss induced by VLEDs is large and rapid (1.5–2 kg per week) (Donnelly et al. 1991), but often not sustained (see review by Saris 2001). These diets are therefore a short-term strategy for the very obese, though when used appropriately they may produce a sustained weight loss. Rather than just being used as a 'total' meal replacement system, programs now may rely on a period of total replacement but follow this with a long-term plan where one or perhaps two meals a day may be replaced to help maintain loss while providing the necessary vitamins and micronutrients (Ditschuneit et al. 1999). Side effects of VLEDs include nausea, halitosis (bad breath), hunger (which may decrease after the initiation of ketosis), headaches, hypotension, light-headedness and precipitation of gout (Brodoff & Hendler 1992). Other effects, including glycogen depletion, loss of lean body mass, dehydration, electrolyte imbalance and hypotension, make VLEDs unsuitable and dangerous for athletes.

6.21 Weight loss groups and centers

These groups or centers (such as Weight Watchers and Jenny Craig) are designed for the general public, to provide support for weight loss. Many have professional input from dietitians, psychologists and medical practitioners to aid in keeping their programs safe, effective and relevant for clients. The programs are not designed specifically for athletes; however, some have the facility to provide additional energy and CHO in their meal plans or diet meals. Athletes seeking to use this method of weight loss need to choose an accredited program that has professional input and the capacity to cater for their special needs.

6.22 Exercise prescriptions for weight and fat loss

6.23 High- versus low-intensity exercise for fat loss

Although it would seem logical for athletes to try to increase the volume of low- to moderate-intensity activity to maximize lipid oxidation, low-intensity activity may not be the most efficient prescription for fat loss in fit individuals. While the proportion of fat utilized is greater at low to moderate intensities, well-trained athletes still oxidize substantial proportions of fat at higher intensities, providing this is less than their anaerobic threshold. The effectiveness of high- versus low-intensity training on body fatness and skeletal muscle metabolism was first investigated by Tremblay and colleagues (1994). In this study, young adults (eight men and nine women) were randomized to either high- or low-intensity, intermittent or endurance training for 15 or 20 weeks respectively. The mean cost of the high-intensity program (57.9 MJ) was significantly lower than that of the endurance training (120.4 MJ). However, despite its lower energy cost, the high-intensity exercise program produced a ninefold greater reduction in skinfold measurements of subcutaneous fat. In addition, the high-intensity program resulted in a greater increase in 3-hydroxyacyl coenzyme A dehydrogenase (HAD), a marker of β-oxidation. In a more recent study, higher-intensity exercise was observed to produce a greater post-exercise, post-prandial oxygen consumption and lipid oxidation than a low-intensity stimulus, an effect that the authors suggest is possibly mediated by β-adrenergic stimulation (Yoshioka et al. 2001). These data are also consistent with a clinical trial conducted by the same research group that demonstrated that reduced-obese individuals who adhered to a high-intensity exercise program were more able to maintain body weight and even accentuate fat loss (Doucet et al. 1999). A recent study in young women provides further evidence of a benefit of high-intensity training on body fat reduction (Trapp et al. 2008).

Although a lower proportion of fat is utilized in the fuel mix oxidized at higher exercise intensities, a greater energy deficit occurs in less time and this results in a higher total fat utilization (Romijn et al. 1993). As mentioned above, fat oxidation may also be greater in the post-exercise recovery period and there are potentially other benefits, including an increase in RMR and the TEF (see section 6.8) and possibly a decrease in appetite (see section 6.7). The efficiency of high-intensity exercise may also be attractive to many athletes who have little time to incorporate extra training that expends 800–2000 kJ (200–500 kcal) just for fat loss. Interestingly, a recent study by Knechtlet and colleagues (2008) reported a significant association between race intensity and body-fat loss (measured by skinfold thicknesses) during an Ironman triathlon. Unfortunately, energy intake during the race was not assessed. As with the study by Trapp and colleagues (2008) (preferential abdominal fat loss), there was a suggestion that fat loss was site-specific (higher in the upper body), something that athletes often desire but for which evidence is clearly lacking.

Mode of exercise and fat loss 6.24

Weight-bearing exercise, in particular running, is often used to promote weight and fat loss in athletes. Apart from running being practical, runners tend to be leaner and lighter than other highly trained athletes in aerobically based sports such as swimming or cycling. Flynn and colleagues (1990) demonstrated that swimming utilized similar energy to running, but proposed that the higher proportion of body fat in swimmers may be due to differences in post-exercise energy expenditure or appetite. It is also possible that control of thermoregulation and the recovery from the impact of running contribute to higher post-exercise energy expenditure. Although there is as yet no explanation for the superior weight control benefits of running, it is frequently used for this purpose. The choice of other modes of exercise is often due to factors such as avoidance of the high impact and injury risk associated with running, because use of different muscle groups is required and/or because running is not preferred by the athlete.

Negative aspects of weight control in athletes 6.25

Menstrual and endocrine disturbance 6.26

Inadequate energy intake adopted to induce loss of body weight and fat may produce menstrual dysfunction and osteopenia in female athletes. The risks and consequences associated with this are outlined in Commentary A (see p. 193).

Reduced lean body mass and resting metabolic rate 6.27

Weight loss brought about by dieting usually results in a reduction in metabolic rate, making future weight loss more difficult (Jeffery et al. 1984; Leibel et al. 1995). As exercise promotes the increase or maintenance of lean body mass, there is interest in whether athletes experience reductions in RMR with dieting as the obese do. Although there is limited evidence, athletes appear to lose lean body mass with dieting, even with heavy resistance training as in bodybuilding (Heyward et al. 1989). Greater reductions are observed in the athletes who consume the least energy. Lean mass loss may be reduced by maintaining an adequate protein intake (Walberg-Rankin et al. 1994) and allowing the body to adapt to energy restriction, as lean body mass loss appears to decline over time.

Repeated cycles of weight loss and gain theoretically decrease lean mass and increase fat mass over time. This is because with each weight loss cycle, lean mass, and hence resting metabolic rate, is reduced, facilitating a gain in body fat when energy restriction ceases. Although there is some evidence to support this theory from cross-sectional studies, longitudinal studies do not support this view. In fact, there is good evidence that metabolic rate returns to a level appropriate for a person's lean body mass after the acute effects of dieting have been lifted, even though this may take some months. In a prospective study designed specifically to test the effects of repeated weight loss–weight regain cycles in an obese population using VLEDs, basal metabolic rate was not suppressed significantly after three weight loss cycles (Jebb et al. 1991). In an extensive review of both animal and human research, including large-scale population studies, Wing concluded that there was little evidence to support a permanent fall in metabolic rate with cycles of dieting (Wing 1992) if overall weight loss has not been achieved. Studies of weight cycling in athlete populations have mainly been performed in wrestlers. While a cross-sectional study suggested RMR was lower than in non-weight-cycling counterparts (Steen et al. 1988), these results were not verified in a longitudinal study (Melby et al. 1990). A recent, large, population-based study investigating mortality from intentional weight cycling in middle-aged to older women did not support that this increased all-cause or cardiovascular mortality (Field et al. 2009). However, a study of retired athletes suggests that weight cycling associated with athletic involvement may increase the risk of weight gain and obesity in later life (Saarni et al. 2006) (for further information see Chapter 7).

6.28 Illness and immunity

There is a popular perception that dieting increases the risk for illness. This is partly due to the potential inadequacy in energy, protein or vitamin and mineral intake while food is restricted. Inadequate micronutrient intake in athletes on restricted diets has been reported in a number of studies, especially in female athletes in sports where leanness is emphasized (Barr 1987). The importance of adequate CHO and n 3 fatty acids for the maintenance of immunity has also been highlighted; see review by Pedersen and colleagues (1999). Adequate CHO appears to attenuate the cortisol and growth hormone response to exercise, resulting in fewer perturbations in blood immune cell counts (Nieman et al. 1997). There also appears to be a role for fat intake, as shifting the ratio of n-6 to n-3 fatty acids towards a higher proportion of n-3s has been shown in animal research to counteract the production of a prostaglandin hormone (PGE_2) and subsequent suppression of the cellular immune system (Johnson et al. 1993, cited in Pedersen et al. 1999). It is possible that dieting may result in an inadequate CHO and fat intake and that this has an impact on immunity. For further information see Commentary C (see p. 501).

Intake of anti-oxidants is also considered important for optimal immune function (Peters et al. 1993). Modest energy-restricted diets based on public health guidelines recommend generous consumption of fruit and vegetables, so anti-oxidant intake may even be increased with these diets. Unfortunately, CHO-restricted diets limit intake of most fruit and starchy vegetables, decreasing the anti-oxidant intake from these sources. For further information see Commentary B (see p. 205).

6.29 Psychological effects and disordered eating

Energy restriction may induce a dysphoric mood and increase the risk of disordered eating. Mood disturbance after dieting has been reported in the overweight (Leon & Chamberlain 1973) and in athletes (Horswill et al. 1990). A higher prevalence of disordered eating is usually reported in sports where leanness is prized (Davis & Cowles 1989). Dieting is one of the known triggers for disordered eating and this, together with other factors such as performance pressure and age-related body image issues, may significantly increase the risk of eating problems (for further information see Chapter 8).

Performance 6.30

Studies investigating the effects of dieting on performance have concentrated mainly on acute weight loss where athletes need to make weight. These effects are discussed in Chapter 7.

Adjunctive agents for weight and fat loss 6.31

Dietary supplements 6.32

A number of dietary supplements have been touted as assisting with weight control; these include L-carnitine, chromium picolinate, hydroxy-methyl-butarate (HMB) and pyruvate. The basis of these claims and an assessment of their efficacy related to weight loss are covered in Chapter 16. The general lack of efficacy of other over-the-counter supplements touted to assist weight loss, including cellasene, chitosan, St John's wort, brindleberry, capsaicin, and grapeseed extract have been reviewed elsewhere (Egger et al. 1999; Dwyer et al. 2005).

Pharmacological agents 6.33

Pharmacological agents may be used to regulate or alter weight in the short term and the medium–long term. Many of these agents are not permitted by sports drug agencies and should be used only in the appropriate situation under medical supervision.

Drugs for short-term weight loss or weight control 6.34

Diuretics are the drugs used for this purpose, but they are not permitted for use by athletes under anti-doping codes as they can be 'masking agents' for other proscribed drugs. As the name implies, they cause a diuresis of extra fluid and some electrolytes by the kidneys. They produce short-term weight loss, but weight (fluid) is rapidly regained once they are ceased. Their effect lasts from hours to a day. Side effects include hypokalemia (which may affect muscle functioning and produce weakness), hyponatremia, hypotension and dehydration. These agents should not be taken in hot environments without adequate fluid and electrolyte replacement being at hand.

Drugs that produce weight loss in the medium term 6.35

These drugs can act either locally (on the gastrointestinal tract) or centrally (on appetite control or thermogenic mechanisms).

Drugs acting on the gastrointestinal tract

Drugs used previously were generally bulking agents, providing a sense of fullness and therefore satiety. Methylcellulose is the only such agent that has been shown to be effective in a controlled trial (Enzi et al. 1980). Acarbose, a glucosidase inhibitor that prevents the breakdown of sucrose, and therefore the absorption of sugar, has helped obese patients maintain lower body weight, when it was given in high doses (Caterson 1990). There are many other agents in this category, with no evidence of effectiveness (Egger et al. 1999).

Orlistat is a gastrointestinal lipase inhibitor that prevents fat breakdown in the gut and therefore its absorption. Some 30% of ingested fat is malabsorbed and passed through the bowel when a person is on a course of orlistat. This loss of energy from fat in the diet results in weight loss. Orlistat is given at a dosage of 120 mg three times a day. Because of the fat loss in the stool, a low-fat diet must be prescribed (and adhered to) with orlistat, otherwise diarrhea and anal fat or oil loss may result. Over a 6- to 12-month period, some 10 kg is lost with orlistat treatment compared to 6 kg on placebo (Sjostrom et al. 1998). The side effects of treatment are abdominal discomfort, diarrhea, anal leakage and the potential to have loss of fat-soluble vitamins (to date this has not been demonstrated, though levels decline over a 2-year course of treatment). Orlistat has been used for 4 years (the XENDOS trial) and has helped maintain weight loss over this period, with no significant side effects (Torgerson et al. 2004). Other beneficial effects of orlistat include a lowering of serum cholesterol, reduction in blood pressure, and better control of diabetes. In part this latter effect is due to the loss of fat from the bowel, with fewer circulating fatty acids and a reduction in insulin resistance (Kelley et al. 2004). Orlistat is now marketed over the counter in many countries and is available in a lower dose formulation. A newer agent in this class, cetilistat, is being trialed. It is said to produce similar weight loss but to have fewer gastrointestinal side effects.

There are no data available on the use of orlistat in athletes. It has the potential benefit of reducing fat absorption while allowing normal CHO absorption, and so should not interfere with the accumulation of muscle glycogen. As athletes are not at a health risk through excess weight, it becomes an ethical question as to whether drugs like orlistat should be used, even though they are permitted by sports drug agencies.

Drugs acting centrally or on thermogenesis to produce weight loss

Ephedrine and caffeine have been and are used for weight reduction in obese patients. Ephedrine is a sympathomimetic drug and acts on the catecholamine receptors. In addition to its other properties and actions, such as bronchodilation, it can suppress appetite and increase thermogenesis (Astrup & Raben 1992). Ephedrine at a dose of 150 mg daily can produce weight loss (Astrup et al. 1992), but best results are produced with the ephedrine (20 mg/d)–caffeine (200 mg/d) combination in conjunction with a reduced-energy diet (Astrup et al. 1992, 1996; Astrup & Toubro 1993). Caffeine, though used for weight loss, does not seem to be effective alone and even the combination therapy is not much utilized worldwide. The side effects of ephedrine are tremor and nervousness, elevated blood pressure, increased heart rate and arrhythmias. Although useful for those with asthma, ephedrine should not be used by those with diabetes, hypertension or hyperthyroidism. Ephedrine alone, or the combination of ephedrine–caffeine, is effective in producing weight loss (1.7 kg and 3.8 kg more than placebo over 24 weeks respectively). These drugs have been shown to be effective in obese patients—a total weight loss of some 16 kg in 24 weeks when used with a reduced energy intake (Astrup & Raben 1992). In lean subjects, ephedrine and caffeine (together with theophylline) have been shown to increase thermogenesis and energy expenditure, but there are no data on weight loss using these agents in athletes. It should be noted that ephedrine is banned under anti-doping codes.

Nicotine too may suppress appetite and increase resting energy expenditure. Smokers have higher resting energy expenditure at night and for a short while post-smoking (Audrain et al. 1995). Smokers tend to be thinner and certainly there is weight gain on the cessation of smoking (Flegal et al. 1995; Rasky et al. 1996). This being said, the health consequences of smoking (particularly vascular disease and cancer) and the effect of smoking on athletic performance make this an inappropriate way for athletes to attempt to lose weight.

Older appetite suppressant agents, including phentermine, benzphetamine, phendimetrazine, mazindol and diethylpropion, are still available. They are effective in producing weight loss over a period of months when used with a lifestyle program including diet and exercise (Atkinson & Hubbard 1994). Again, most of the experience is in obese subjects, and there is little experience of the use of these drugs in athletes for weight control as they are not permitted by sports drug agencies. They are amphetamine derivatives and tend to have stimulatory side effects on the central nervous and cardiovascular systems. Another older drug, phenylpropanolamine, is available in some countries in over-the-counter preparations for weight loss. It is related to both noradrenalin and the amphetamine derivatives. It can be effective, but has the potential to stimulate the cardiovascular and central nervous systems.

Fluoxetine is a member of a newer class of antidepressants, the selective serotonin reuptake inhibitors (SSRIs). It acts by increasing serotonin levels locally in the central nervous system. In depressed patients, it can produce weight loss and may be useful, at higher than normal doses, in producing weight loss in non-depressed individuals. Sibutramine, which is both a SSRI and a SNRI (selective noradrenaline reuptake inhibitor), is an effective weight loss agent. Because of its mode of action, it has both serotonergic (appetite suppressant) and noradrenergic (thermogenic) effects. At a dose of 10–15 mg/d, combined with an appropriate lifestyle program of diet and exercise, it produces significant weight loss (some 12 kg compared to 6 kg on placebo), which can be maintained for 2 years (James et al. 2000). This drug does increase the pulse rate marginally (by two to three beats per minute) and, with treatment and weight loss, blood pressure may not fall as much as it does on placebo. It also produces a significant rise in HDL cholesterol (protective cholesterol), which, combined with the weight loss produced, benefits diabetes control and other serum lipid levels. There are no reports of its use for weight control in athletes. A trial of its long-term effectiveness on hard cardiovascular outcomes is nearing completion and will be the first trial to study international weight loss and outcomes.

There are effective pharmacologic measures available for reducing weight, but there is little if any information about the use of such agents in athletes. The use of such drugs by athletes must be considered carefully and raises an ethical question. These drugs were designed to assist those at health risk, not young, fit individuals. It is better that they not be used except where there is a risk to health of excess weight. It should also be remembered that some of these drugs (such as ephedrine) are banned under anti-doping codes.

Guidelines for fat loss

6.36

Recommendations for safe weight loss in non-athletes are in the vicinity of 0.5–1 kg per week. These guidelines seem reasonable for many athletes. Loss of this weight equates to an approximate energy deficit of 2100–4200 kJ (500–1000 kcal). This deficit can be achieved by diet, training or both. Moderate energy restriction without compromising CHO or nutrient intake is optimal and best achieved by the implementation of diet low in fat (15–25% of energy), and moderate to high in CHO (6–8 g/kg body weight per day). Protein intake should be approximately 1.5–2 g/kg body weight per day with the upper level recommended if energy restriction is substantial, as this may assist with satiety and maintenance of lean body mass. Foods high in fiber and/or of low glycemic index may assist with appetite control. Calcium intake at or above the RDI, ideally from dairy foods, may also assist with weight management.

Exercise complements dietary approaches to weight loss by increasing energy expenditure and inducing negative energy balance. Although lower-intensity, aerobically based exercise has been recommended as 'best' for fat loss, this prescription may not be the most efficient in athletes. Higher-intensity exercise that can be maintained for a reasonable duration (30–60 min/d), in addition to an athlete's standard training, may be a useful and perhaps even better approach to weight loss (see section 6.23). However, careful consideration of the risk of fatigue, injury and the mode of additional exercise is important. Exercise prescriptions should be tailored to an athlete's individual needs.

6.37 Summary

Athletes may attempt to lose weight to improve power to weight ratio, attain a desired body composition in a sport that has an aesthetic ideal or make a pre-designated weight in order to compete. Most will not need to lose weight for health reasons.

Body weight and composition are determined by many factors, both biological and environmental. Genes have a significant influence on the susceptibility for weight or fat gain and indeed the potential to attain a particular physique. Genes may act through food preferences and appetite, through energy expenditure or through metabolic factors such as substrate partitioning (selecting which fuel is oxidized).

Currently, alteration in environmental or lifestyle factors is the only way to manipulate body weight and composition. The two major factors influencing energy balance are energy intake and expenditure. Approaches that manipulate dietary intake to facilitate weight or fat loss range from modest reductions in dietary fat and energy intake through to severe reductions in total energy and CHO consumption. Interventions focusing on reduction of fat intake are sufficient to produce the desired weight or fat loss in most athletes. This approach is in line with public health guidelines and is also less likely to result in glycogen depletion. Some athletes, however, will also need to restrict their total energy intake to achieve their desired goals. To maintain satiety, adequate protein intake and the use of low-GI CHOs may be beneficial. Emerging evidence also supports the importance of adequate calcium intake, particularly from dairy sources, for promoting optimal weight loss.

Diets advocating CHO restriction are currently popular in the community and with athletes. Unfortunately, greater weight loss in the short-term (1–6 months) in obese subjects is not maintained at 12 months. There are significant side effects and potential health risks of reduced-CHO diets, which have not been evaluated in the long term. The effectiveness of reduced-CHO weight-loss diets in athletes and their impact on exercise performance and recovery have not been adequately evaluated.

Physical activity directly increases energy expenditure during exercise and indirectly through potential alterations in RMR and TEF. Although it is assumed that additional exercise will result in an energy and fat deficit, it is possible that an individual may compensate, partly or even fully, for increased energy expenditure by consuming more food. This may occur through changes in appetite, but the precise nature of the effect of exercise on appetite is yet to be established, particularly over the medium to long term. There appears to be an acute, post-exercise suppression of appetite and, in some studies, an increase in the preference for CHO. Incomplete dietary compensation for the energy expended in exercise may persist for around 2 weeks. Athletes may be susceptible to weight gain when physical activity ceases or decreases, especially during the off-season or through periods of illness or injury. Careful planning of food intake and the maintenance of some physical activity is important to help prevent weight or fat gain at these times.

Exercise prescriptions for weight loss in athletes are similar to those designed for the overweight, incorporating low-intensity (50% $VO_{2\ max}$), medium-duration (60 minutes) aerobic activity. This prescription may not be the most efficient for fat loss in fit individuals. Exercise regimens using shorter-duration, medium- to high-intensity exercise and possibly in combination with resistance-training components may also be effective in reducing excess body fat. This latter approach may be attractive to many athletes because of the limited time available to incorporate extra training for the specific purpose of weight or fat reduction.

Athletes and coaches are open to just as much misinformation about weight loss and dieting as the rest of the community. Unfortunately this often results in the use of unbalanced dietary regimens, nutrition supplements and drugs that lack scientific support or that are not permitted by sports drug agencies. Such approaches may result in decreased performance and have negative health consequences. The promotion of safe and effective weight-loss strategies is an important role of the sports medicine team.

PRACTICE TIPS

HELEN O'CONNOR AND IAN CATERSON

These tips are designed to assist practitioners with assessment and management of the athlete presenting for weight or fat loss.

ASSESSMENT OF THE NEED TO LOSE WEIGHT OR FAT

- The initial assessment for weight or fat loss in an athlete should include measurement of weight, stature, adiposity and muscularity using a standardized measurement protocol. Surface anthropometry is frequently used as it is portable, inexpensive and non-invasive. Anthropometric measures should be performed in duplicate by an accredited anthropometrist using an appropriate protocol (the International Society for the Advancement of Kinanthropometry protocol is recommended; see Chapter 3). Other methods of assessing body composition and their relative benefits and pitfalls are discussed in Chapter 3. (For adolescents and children see Chapter 16.)
- Error associated with body composition measurement should be explained to the athlete. This is especially important for interpreting change when serial measurements are performed.
- Body composition assessment should be complemented with a history of personal and family weight patterns and methods of weight management previously used. Any goals set need to be realistic.
- Information should be gathered regarding past and current medical history (including injuries), signs of disordered eating, and menstrual cycle (for females). Recent biochemical, hematological and bone density results should also be considered.
- The athlete's goals need to be evaluated within the context of their history, current body composition and the optimal ranges of weight and fat in their sport.
- Goals for weight and fat loss need to be realistic, ideally not greater than 0.5 kg per week or for body fat a maximum of 5 mm reduction in total skinfold (over seven or eight sites) per week. The goal of weight or fat loss should not compromise health or performance.

DIETARY ASSESSMENT

- Dietary assessment should focus on recent eating patterns. A dietary history and food frequency checklist is ideal for this purpose. Food diaries can complement this information.
- Dietary histories of athletes presenting for weight or fat loss need to include questions related to eating away from home, strategies used when travelling, cooking skills, comfort or stress eating, hunger and use of alcohol.
- Direct measurement of RMR or estimation using prediction equations (see Chapter 5) should be considered for athletes experiencing difficulty with weight loss. The ratio of energy intake to RMR would be expected to be greater than 1:3 as ratios less than this are implausible even for sedentary individuals (Goldberg et al. 1991). Ratios greater than 1:5 would typically be expected and in very heavy training may be close to 3.

If under-reporting is suspected, issues of body image or other stressors need to be explored. Discussing the implausible nature of reported food intake with the athlete may help to reveal the practical or psychological issues impeding weight or fat loss.

- Athletes experiencing great difficulty with weight loss may be better to direct their energies towards sports where the physique requirements are less extreme.

TRAINING, EXERCISE AND PHYSICAL ACTIVITY ASSESSMENT

- An athlete's daily energy expenditure can be estimated from prediction equations (see Chapter 5), tables of energy expenditure for different sporting activities, and activity history or diaries. Accelerometers or heart-rate monitors can also be used. These methods provide approximate estimates that can guide meal planning. Alternatively, an estimate can be obtained from the athlete's current energy intake. Although assessment of energy intake is notoriously inaccurate, it is often the most immediate and practical method in a clinical setting.
- Ideally an approximate training program for the following 12-month period is available. Although weight- or fat-loss goals may be more immediate, it is critical to adjust the diet for different training phases, including tapering for competition and the off-season. In some sports, weight- or body-fat levels can be effectively periodized, allowing an athlete to be strategic about when they need to be at their lightest or leanest. This is helpful when physique requirements are quite rigorous or extreme yet training can still be optimized without constant physique maintenance. Large swings in body weight or fat are not recommended, but for many athletes, periodizing weight or fat tapers help them to consume a more enjoyable, less restricted and balanced diet at other less-critical times.

DIETARY APPROACH

- It is preferable to start most athletes on a low-fat diet that is only moderately (10–20%) reduced in energy. This should produce a gradual weight loss (0.5–1 kg per week at most).
- More rigorous restriction of energy intake may be required when extreme leanness is necessary or when an athlete needs to 'make weight' for competition. Careful planning of meals is important to ensure the diet is nutrient-dense and delivers adequate CHO.
- Inclusion of a protein choice at each meal and snack may assist with satiety. High-fiber, low-glycemic-index CHOs may also help to satisfy the appetite of a hungry athlete. Regular consumption of nutrient-rich, lower-energy-dense meals and snacks is recommended to prevent the build-up of hunger over the day. Organization is important as impulse eating is often a problem, especially for the busy athlete.
- Planning meals or snacks to follow training sessions will promote recovery using nutritious and satiating food choices within the athlete's daily kilojoule budget. Energy-dense sports foods/beverages, while convenient, may not be the most nutritious or

PRACTICE TIPS

satisfying snack or recovery choice for hungry athletes on a daily basis. Use of sports foods and beverages can be planned to coincide with longer, more strenuous sessions or during competition where consumption of lower kilojoule, bulkier foods is less effective or acceptable.

- Emerging evidence supports a beneficial role for dairy foods/calcium, particularly in those with habitual low intakes. It is therefore recommended that athletes consume at least their RDI of calcium (ideally from dairy food sources) each day. Supplemental calcium should be considered if this is not possible.
- Dietary consultations should assess the athlete's (or their parent's/guardian's) shopping and cooking skills. Shopping trips and cooking classes provide a practical and enjoyable form of athlete education. A list of suitable cookbooks and resources is also useful.

TRAINING, EXERCISE AND PHYSICAL ACTIVITY

- Additional training or physical activity is a means of creating an energy deficit. Additional exercise should be combined with a sensible eating plan to offset any increase in appetite that could negate the energy deficit. Assessment of appetite and desire to eat using visual analogue scales is also useful.
- Additional exercise of medium to longer duration (60 minutes), at low to moderate intensity (50–60% $VO_{2\ max}$) is usually recommended as the best choice for weight or fat loss. Medium-duration (30–60 minutes), higher-intensity activity (65–70% $VO_{2\ max}$ or below anaerobic threshold) uses similar or more kilojoules and fat (even though the proportion of fat oxidized appears less). Higher-intensity exercise can therefore be an effective and time-efficient means of enhancing daily energy expenditure in athletes.
- Resistance training may increase lean body mass and therefore RMR. These benefits should be considered within the context of the exercise program devised.
- The best mode of exercise is generally determined by considering issues of access, time, injury risk and propensity for overuse of certain muscle groups. While running or weight-bearing activity appears (at least anecdotally) to produce superior weight loss results, other forms of aerobic exercise, such as swimming or cycling, may be selected as they result in less impact on the skeleton.

PSYCHOLOGICAL ASPECTS AND BEHAVIOR MODIFICATION

- Approaches used to examine food behavior—including food diaries and visual analogue scales to measure hunger, emotional eating and food cravings—can help athletes identify triggers to inappropriate eating. Behavior modification techniques can then be used to manage, control or avoid problem eating behaviors.
- Referral to a clinical or sports psychologist is often integral to the success of weight-loss programs as the mental approach is a major factor in the client's confidence and subsequent compliance.

TRAVELING AND SPECIAL ATHLETE CONSIDERATIONS

- Traveling may disrupt weight loss, as appropriate food is not always available and the daily routine is interrupted. Strategies that may assist include the organization of low-fat, low-energy or athlete meals on airline flights, and the development of a traveling meal plan and shopping list (if meals are self-catered), or a menu plan for professional caterers. A list of best choices from restaurants or take-away outlets is also useful. Avoidance of inappropriate snacks is easier if nutritious alternatives have been pre-organized.
- A meal plan to maintain energy balance when training is reduced (e.g. tapered) or interrupted due to injury, illness or during the off-season is beneficial to athletes prone to weight gain at these times.
- Athletes are exposed to buffet-style eating, especially in athlete villages and residential dining halls. Buffets encourage over-consumption and inclusion of foods that might not be typically consumed. Weight gain and 'buffet boredom' can be offset by advising the athlete to avoid sampling every dish on offer at each meal. Rather, they should select a protein, CHO and several vegetable options as would be typical of a home-prepared meal. Within a menu cycle, they will eventually sample most options on the menu.
- Fad or unscientific dietary regimens often appeal to athletes because they promise quick, effective weight loss. Athletes need to be advised on sound diet and training approaches to facilitate weight loss, and these need to be supported by their coach or trainer and (where appropriate) their parent, guardian or partner. The use of the sports medicine team, including a sports dietitian, is essential.
- The use of supplements and/or drugs to assist weight loss is a major temptation for athletes. Despite claims, dietary supplements promoted for weight loss lack scientific support. Although a number of drugs have proven efficacy for weight loss, these are either deemed illegal by sports drug agencies or their use would seem unethical or unsafe in athletes who are not at a medical risk because of excess weight.

References

Aarsland A, Chinkes D, Wolfe R. Hepatic and whole-body fat synthesis in humans during carbohydrate overfeeding. Am J Clin Nutr 1997;65:1774–82.

Acheson KJ, Schutz Y, Bessard T, et al. Glycogen storage capacity and de novo lipogenesis during massive carbohydrate overfeeding in man. Am J Clin Nutr 1988;48:240–7.

Ahima RS, Lazar MA. Adipokines and the peripheral and neural control of energy balance. Molecular Endocrinology 2008;22:1023–31.

Alhassan S, Kim S, Bersamin et al. Dietary adherence and weight loss success among overweight women: results from the A to Z weight loss study. Int J Obes 2008;32:985–991.

Almeras N, Lemieux S, Bouchard C, Tremblay A. Fat gain in female swimmers. Physiolog Behav 1997;61:811–17.

American College of Sports Medicine. Appropriate physical activity intervention strategies for weight loss and prevention of weight regain for adults. Med Sci Sports Exerc 2009a;41:459–71.

American College of Sports Medicine. Nutrition and athletic performance. Med Sci Sports Exerc 2009b;41;709–31.

Andersen P, Henriksson J. Capillary supply of the quadriceps femoris muscle of man: adaptive response to exercise. J Physol 1977;270:677–90.

Andersson B, Larson B. Influence of local temperature changes in the preoptic area and rostral hypothalamus in the regulation of food and water intake. Acta Physiol Scand 1961;52:75–89.

Astrup A, Breum L, Toubro S, Hein P, Quaade F. The effect and safety of an ephedrine–caffeine compound compared to ephedrine, caffeine and placebo in obese subjects on an energy restricted diet: a double blind trial. Int J Obes 1992;16:269–77.

Astrup A, Grunwald GK, Melanson EL, et al. The role of low-fat diets in body weight control: a meta analysis of ad libitum dietary intervention studies. Int J Obes 2000;24:1545–52.

Astrup AD, Hansen DL, Toubro S. Ephedrine and caffeine in the treatment of obesity. Int J Obes 1996;20:1–3.

Astrup A, Larsen T, Harper A. Atkins and other low carbohydrate diets: hoax or an effective tool for weight loss? Lancet 2004;364:897–9.

Astrup A, Raben A. Obesity: an inherited metabolic deficiency in the control of macronutrient balance? Eur J Clin Nutr 1992;46:611–20.

Astrup A, Toubro S. Thermogenic, metabolic and cardiovascular responses to ephedrine and caffeine in man. Int J Obes 1993;17(Suppl):41S–3S.

Atkins RC. Doctor Atkins' new diet revolution. New York: Avon Books, 1992.

Atkinson RL, Hubbard VS. Report on the NIH workshop on pharmacological treatment of obesity. Am J Clin Nutr 1994;60:153–6.

Audrain JF, Klesges RC, Klesges LM. Relationship between obesity and the metabolic effect of smoking in women. Health Psychol 1995;14:116–32.

Bahr R, Sejersted OM. Effect of intensity of exercise on excess postexercise oxygen consumption. Metabolism 1991;40:836–41.

Baile CA, Zinn WN, Mayer J. Effects of lactate and other metabolites on food intake of monkeys. Am J Physiol 1970;219:1606–13.

Ballor DL, Keesey RE. A meta-analysis of factors affecting exercise-induced changes in body mass, fat mass and fat-free mass in males and females. Int J Obes 1991;15:717–26.

Barr S. Women, nutrition and exercise: a review of athletes' food intakes and a discussion of energy balance in active women. Prog Food Nutr Sci 1987;11:307–61.

Bell NH, Epstein S, Greene A, et al. Evidence for the alteration of the vitamin D-endocrine system in obese subjects. J Clin Invest 1985;76:370–3.

Bosse MC, Davis SC, Puhl SM, et al. Effects of Zone Diet macronutrient proportions on blood lipids, blood glucose, body composition, and treadmill exercise performance. Nutr Res 2004;24:521–30.

Bouchard C. Recent advances in the molecular and genetic basis of human obesity. In: Aihaud G, Guy-Grand B, Lafontan M, Ricquier D, eds. Obesity in Europe 93. London: John Libbey, 1993:1–8.

Bouchard C. Genetics of obesity: overview and research directions. In: Bouchard C, ed. The genetics of obesity. Boca Raton: CRC Press, 1994:223–33.

Bouchard C, Tremblay A. Genetic influences on the response of body fat and fat distribution to positive and negative energy balances in human identical twins. J Nutr 1997;127(5 Suppl):943S–7S.

Bouchard C, Tremblay A, Déspres J-P, et al. The response to long-term overfeeding in identical twins. N Engl J Med 1990;322:1477–82.

Brodoff BN, Hendler R, eds. Very low calorie diets in obesity. Philadelphia, USA: Lippincott, 1992.

Brotherhood JR. Nutrition and sports performance. Sports Med 1984;1:350–89.

Burke LM, Read RSD. Alcohol use by elite Australian Rules football players (abst). Proc Nutr Soc Aust 1987;12:127.

Cash TF, Novy PL, Grant JR. Why do women exercise? Factor analysis and further validation of the reasons for exercise inventory. Perc Motor Skills 1994;78:539–44.

Caterson ID. Management strategies for weight control: eating, exercise and behaviour modification. Drugs 1990;30(Suppl):20S–32S.

Cheuvront SN. The Zone Diet and athletic performance. Sports Med 1999;27:213–28.

Cheuvront SN. The Zone Diet phenomenon: a closer look at the science behind the claims. J Am Coll Nutr 2003;22:9–17.

Coleman DL. Effects of parabiosis of obese mice with diabetes and normal mice. Diabetologia 1973;9:294–8.

Considine RV, Sinha MK, Heiman MK, et al. Serum immunoreactive-leptin concentrations in normal-weight and obese humans. N Engl J Med 1996;334:292–5.

Coulston AM, Liu GC, Reaven GM. Plasma glucose, insulin and lipid responses to high-carbohydrate, low-fat diets in normal humans. Metabolism 1983;32:52–6.

Coyle EF, Coggan AR, Hemmett MK, Ivy JL. Muscle glycogen utilization during prolonged strenuous activity when fed carbohydrate. J Appl Physiol 1986;61:165–72.

Craig PL, Caterson ID. Weight and perception of body image in women and men in a Sydney sample. Community Health Stud 1990;14:373–83.

Cureton KJ, Sparling PB. Distance running performance and metabolic responses to running in men and women with excess weight experimentally equated. Med Sci Sports Exerc 1980;2:288–94.

Daly RM, Bass S, Caine D, Howe W. Does training affect growth? Answers to common questions. Phys Sports Med 2002;30:21–9.

Dansinger ML, Gleason JA, Griffith JL, Selkjer HP, Schaefer EJ. Comparison of the Atkins, Ornish, Weight Watchers and Zone diets for weight loss and heart disease risk reduction. A randomized trial. JAMA 2005;293:43–53.

Dauncey MJ, Bingham SA. Dependence of 24-hour energy expenditure in man on the composition of nutrient intake. Br J Nutr 1983;50:1–13.

Davis C, Cowles M. A comparison of weight and diet concerns and personality factors among female athletes and non-athletes. J Psychosoma Res 1989;33:527–36.

Davis KJ, Packer L, Brooks GA. Biochemical adaptation of mitochondria, muscle and whole-animal respiration to endurance training. Arch Biochem Biophys 1981;209:539–54.

Dempsey JA, Reddan W, Baike B, Walberg-Rankin J. Work capacity determinants and physiologic cost of weight-supported work in obesity. J Appl Physiol 1966;22:181–5.

Denke M. Metabolic effects of high-protein, low carbohydrate diets. Am J Cardiol 2001;88:59–61.

Deuster PA, Chrousos GP, Luger A, et al. Hormonal and metabolic responses of untrained, moderately trained and highly trained men to three exercise intensities. Metabolism 1989;38:141–8.

Ditschuneit HH, Fletchner-Mors M, Johnson TD, Alder G. Metabolic and weight-loss effects of a long term dietary intervention in obese patients. Am J Clin Nutr 1999;69:198–204.

Donnelly JE, Jakicic J, Gunderson S. Diet and body composition: effect of very low calorie diets and exercise. Sports Med 1991;12:237–49.

Doucet E, Imbeault P, Alaméras N, Tremblay A. Physical activity and low-fat diet: is it enough to maintain weight stability in the reduced obese individual following weight loss by drug therapy and energy restriction? Obes Res 1999;7:323–33.

Dressendorfer RH, Petersen SR, Moss Lovshin SE, et al. Performance enhancement with maintenance of resting immune status after intensified cycle training. Clin J Sport Med 2002;12:301–7.

Dwyer JT, Allison DB, Coates PM. Dietary supplements in weight reduction. JADA 2005;105(Suppl): 80S–6S.

Ebbeling CB, Leidig MM, Sinclair KB, Hangen JP, Ludwig DS. A reduced glycaemic load diet in the treatment of adolescent obesity. Arch Pediatr Adolesc Med 2003;157:773–9.

Egger G, Cameron-Smith D, Stanton R. The effectiveness of popular, non-prescription weight loss supplements. Med J Aust 1999;171:604–8.

Enzi G, Inelman EM, Crepaldi G. Effect of hydrophilic mucilage in the treatment of obese patients. Pharmatherapeutica 1980;2:421–8.

Field AE, Malspeis S, Willett WC. Weight cycling and mortality among middle-aged or older women. Arch Int Med 2009;169:881–6.

Finlayson G, Bryant E, Blundell JE, King NA. Acute compensatory eating following exercise is associated with implicit hedonic wanting for food. Phys Behav 2009;97:62–7.

Flegal KM, Troiano RP, Pamuk ER, Kuczmarski RJ, Campbell SM. The influence of smoking cessation on the prevalence of overweight in the United States. N Engl J Med 1995;333:1165–70.

Flynn MG, Costill DL, Kirwan JP, et al. Fat storage in athletes: metabolic and hormonal responses to swimming and running. Sports Med 1990;11:433–40.

Flynn MG, Pizza FX, Boone Jr JB, et al. Indices of training stress during competitive running and swimming sessions. Int J Sports Med 1994;15:21–6.

Foster GD, Wyatt HR, Hill JO, et al. A randomized trial of a low-carbohydrate diet for obesity. NEJM 2003;348:2082–90.

Freedman-Akabas S, Colt E, Kissileff HR, Pi Sunyer FX. Lack of sustained increase in VO_2. Am J Clin Nutr 1985;41:545–9.

Gardner CD, Kiazand A, Alhassan S, et al. Comparison of the Atkins, Zone, Ornish, and LEARN diets for change in weight related risk factors among overweight premenopausal women: the A to Z Weight Loss Study: a randomized trial. JAMA 2007;297:969–77.

Goldberg GR, Black AE, Jebb SA, et al. Critical evaluation of energy intake data using fundamental principles of energy physiology: 1. Derivation of cut-off limits to identify under-recording. Eur J Clin Nutr 1991;45:569–81.

Goran MI, Poehlman ET. Endurance training does not enhance energy expenditure in healthy elderly persons. Am J Physiol 1992;263:E950–7.

Grinspoon S, Gulick T, Askari H, et al. Serum leptin levels in women with anorexia nervosa. J Clin Endocrinol Metab 1996;81:3861–3.

Grunfield C, Feingold KR. The metabolic effects of tumour necrosis factor and other cytokines. Biotherap 1991;3:143–58.

Hawley J, Burke L. Changing body size and shape. In: Peak performance: training and nutritional strategies for sport. Sydney: Allen & Unwin, 1998:233–60.

Heller RF, O'Connell DL, Roberts DCK, et al. Lifestyle factors in monozygotic and dizygotic twins. Genet Epidemiol 1988;5:311–21.

Henriksson J, Reitman JS. Quantitative measures of enzyme activities in type I and type II muscle fibres of man after training. Acts Physiol Scand 1976;97:392–7.

Heyward VH, Sandoval WM, Colville BC. Anthropometric, body composition, and nutritional profiles of body builders during training. J Appl Sports Sci Res 1989;3:22–9.

Hoppeler H, Luthi P, Claasen H, Weibel ER, Howald H. The ultrastructure of the normal human skeletal muscle: a morphometric analysis on untrained men, women and well-trained orienteers. Pflugers Arch 1973;344:217–32.

Horswill CC, Hickner RC, Scott JR, Costill DL, Gould D. Weight loss, dietary carbohydrate modifications, and high intensity physical performance. Med Sci Sports Exerc 1990;22:470–7.

Houmard JA, Costill DL, Mitchell JB, et al. Reduced training maintains performance in distance runners. Int J Sports Med 1990;131:46–52.

Howard B, Howard BV, Manson JE, et al. Low fat dietary pattern and weight change over 7 years: the Women's Health Initiative Dietary Modification trial. JAMA 2006;296:39–49.

Hurley BF, Nemeth PM, Martin WH, et al. Muscle triglyceride utilization during exercise: training effect. J Appl Physiol 1986;60:562–7.

James WPT, Astrup A, Finer N, et al. Effect of sibutramine on weight maintenance after weight loss: a randomized trial. Lancet 2000;356:2119–23.

Jarvis M, McNaughton L, Seddon A, et al. The acute 1 week effects of the Zone Diet on body composition, blood lipid levels, and performance in recreational endurance athletes. J Strength Cond Res 2002;16:50–7.

Jebb SA, Goldberg GR, Coward WA, Murgatroyd PR, Prentice AM. Effects of weight cycling caused by intermittent dieting on metabolic rate and body composition in obese women. Int J Obes 1991;15:367–74.

Jebb SA, Prentice AM, Goldberg G, et al. Changes in macronutrient balance during over and underfeeding assessed by 12-day continuous whole body calorimetry. Am J Clin Nutr 1996;64:259–66.

Jeffery RW, Björnson WM, Rosenthal BS, et al. Correlates of weight loss and its maintenance over two years of follow-up among middle-aged men. Prev Med 1984;13:155–68.

Jenkins AB, Markovic TP, Fleury A, Campbell LV. Carbohydrate intake and short-term regulation of leptin in humans. Diabetologia 1997;40:348–51.

Kelley DE, Kuller LH, McKolanis TM, et al. Effects of moderate weight loss and orlistat on insulin resistance, regional adiposity and fatty acids in type 2 diabetes. Diabetes Care 2004;27:33–40.

Kiens B. Effect of endurance training on fatty acid metabolism: local adaptations. Med Sci Sports Exerc 1977;29:640–5.

King NA, Blundell JE. High-fat foods overcome energy expenditure due to exercise after cycling and running. Eur J Clin Nutr 1995;49:114–23.

King NA, Burley VJ, Blundell JE. Exercise-induced suppression of appetite: effects on food intake and implications for energy balance. Eur J Clin Nutr 1994;48:715–24.

King NA, Cauldwell P, Hopkins M, et al. Metabolic and behavioural compensatory responses to exercise interventions: Barriers to weight loss. Obesity 2007;15:1373–83.

Kowlalska J, Straczkowski M, Gorski J, Kinalska I. The effect of fasting and physical exercise on plasma leptin concentrations in high-fat fed rats. J Physiol Pharmacol 1999;50:309–20.

Knechtlet B, Schwanke M, Knechtlet P, Kohler G. Decrease in body fat during an ultra-endurance triathlon is associated with race intensity. B J Sports Med 2008;42:609–13.

Lambert EV, Speechly DP, Dennis SC, Noakes TD. Enhanced endurance in trained cyclists during moderate intensity exercise following two weeks adaptation to a high fat diet. Eur J Appl Physiol 1994;69:287–93.

Layman DK, Boileau RA, Erickson DJ, et al. A reduced ratio of dietary carbohydrates to protein improves body composition and blood lipid profiles during weight loss in women. J Nutr 2003;133:411–17.

Leal-Cerro A, Garcia-Luna PP, Astorga R, et al. Serum leptin levels in male marathon athletes before and after the marathon run. J Clin Endocrinol Metab 1998;83:2376–9.

Leibel RL, Rosenbaum M, Hirsch J. Changes in energy expenditure resulting from altered body weight. N Engl J Med 1995;332:621–8.

Leon GR, Chamberlain K. Comparison of daily eating habits and emotional states of overweight persons successful or unsuccessful in maintaining weight loss. J Consult Clin Psychol 1973;41:108–15.

Levine JA, Miller JM. The energy expenditure of using a 'walk and-work' desk for office workers with obesity. B J Sports Med 2007;41:558–61.

Lorenzen JK, Molgaard C, Michaelson K, et al. Calcium supplementation for 1 year does not reduce body weight or fat in young girls. Am J Clin Nutr 2006;83:18–23.

Major GC, Chaput J-P, Ledoux M, et al. Recent developments in calcium related obesity research. Obes Rev 2008;9:428–45.

Margaritis I, Palazetti S, Rousseau A-S, et al. Antioxidant supplementation and tapering exercise improve exercise induced antioxidant response. J Am Coll Nutr 2003;22:147–56.

Martins C, Morgan L, Truby H. A review of the effects of exercise on appetite regulation: an obesity perspective. Int J Obes 2008;32:1337–1347.

McConell GK, Costil DL, Widrick JJ, et al. Reduced training volume and intensity maintain aerobic capacity but not performance in distance runners. Int J Sports Med 1993;14:33–7.

McMillan-Price J, Brand-Miller J. Low glycemic index diets and body weight regulation. Int J Obes 2006; 30(Suppl):40S–46S.

Melby CL, Commerford SR, Hill JO. Exercise, macronutrient balance and weight control. In: Lamb D, Murray R, eds. Perspectives in exercise science and sports medicine. Vol 11: Exercise, nutrition and control of body weight. Carmel: Cooper Publishing Group, 1998:1–60.

Melby CL, Osterberg KL, Resch A, et al. Effect of carbohydrate ingestion during exercise on post-exercise substrate oxidation and energy intake. Int J Sport Nut Exerc Metabol 2002;12:294–309.

Melby CL, Schmidt WD, Corrigan D. Resting metabolic rate in weight-cycling collegiate wrestlers compared with physically active, noncycling control subjects. Am J Clin Nutr 1990;52:409–14.

Melby CL, Scholl C, Edwards G, Bullough R. Effect of acute resistance exercise on postexercise energy expenditure and resting metabolic rate. J Appl Physiol 1993;75:1847–53.

Meyer GAL, Janssen GME, Westerterp KR, et al. The effect of a month endurance training programme on physical activity: evidence for a sex-difference in the metabolic response to exercise. Eur J Appl Physiol 1991;62:11–17.

Montague CT, Farooqi IS, Whitehead JP, et al. Congenital leptin deficiency is associated with severe early-onset obesity in humans. Nature 1997;387:903–8.

Nair KS, Halliday D, Garrow JS. Thermic response to isoenergetic protein, carbohydrate, or fat meals in lean and obese subjects. Clin Sci 1983;65:307–12.

Nieman DC, Henson DA, Garner EB, et al. Carbohydrate affects natural killer cell redistribution but not activity after running. Med Sci Sports Exerc 1997;29:1318–24.

O'Connor H, Olds T, Maughan RJ. Physique and performance for track and field events. J Sports Sci 2007;25(1 Suppl):49S–60S.

Olds TS, Norton KI, Craig NP. Mathematical model of cycling performance. J Appl Physiol 1993;75:730–7.

Oscai LB, Caruso RA, Wergeles AC. Lipoprotein lipase hydrolyzes endogenous triacylglycerols in muscle of exercised rats. J Appl Physiol 1982;52:1059–63.

Parker B, Noakes M, Luscombe N, et al. Effect of a high-protein, high-monounsaturated fat weight loss diet on glycemic control and lipid levels in type 2 diabetes. Diabetes Care 2002;25:425–30.

Pedersen BK, Bruunsgaard H, Jensen M, et al. Exercise and the immune system—influence of nutrition and ageing. J Sci Med Sport 1999;2:234–52.

Perusse L, Tremblay A, Leblanc C, et al. Familial resemblance in energy intake: contribution of genetic and environmental factors. Am J Clin Nutr 1988;47:629–35.

Peters EM, Goetzsche JM, Grobbelaar B, Noakes TD. Vitamin C supplementation reduces the incidence of post-race symptoms of upper-respiratory-tract infection in ultramarathon runners. Am J Clin Nutr 1993;57:170–4.

Poehlman ET, Melby CL, Badylak SF, Calles J. Aerobic fitness and resting energy expenditure in young adult males. Metabolism 1989;38:85–90.

Prentice AM, Poppitt SD. The importance of energy density and macronutrients in the regulation of energy intake. Int J Obes 1996;20(2 Suppl):18S–23S.

Ralph A, Provan GJ. Phytoprotectants. In: Garrow JS, James WPT, Ralph A, eds. Human nutrition and dietetics. Tenth edition. London UK: Churchill Livingstone, 2000:417–26.

Rasky E, Stronegger WJ, Freidl W. The relationship between body weight and patterns of smoking in women and men. Int J Epidemiol 1996;25:1208–12.

Ravussin E, Lillioja S, Anderson TE, Christin L, Bogardus C. Determinants of 24-hour energy expenditure in man: methods and results using a respiratory chamber. J Clin Invest 1986;78(6):1568–78.

Ravussin E, Lillioja S, Knowler WC, et al. Reduced rate of energy expenditure as a risk factor for body-weight gain. N Engl J Med 1988;318:467–72.

Ravussin E, Swinburn BA. Pathophysiology of obesity. Lancet 1992;340:404–8.

Ravussin E, Swinburn BA. Metabolic predictors of body weight gain: cross-sectional versus longitudinal data. Int J Obes 1993;17:528–31.

Reed GW, Hill JO. Measuring the thermic effect of food. Am J Clin Nutr 1996;63:164–9.

Romijn JA, Coyle EF, Sidossis L. Regulation of endogenous fat and carbohydrate metabolism in relation to exercise intensity. Am J Physiol 1993;265:E380–91.

Rosenbaum M, Nicholson M, Hirsch M, et al. Effects of gender, body composition and menopause on plasma concentrations of leptin. J Clin Endocronol Metab 1996;81:3424–7.

Saarni SE, Rissaen A, Sarna S, et al. Weight cycling of athletes and subsequent weight gain in middle age. Int J Obes 2006;30:1639–44.

Sacks FM, Bray GA, Carey VJ, et al. Comparison of weight loss diets with different compositions of fat, protein and carbohydrates. NEJM 2009;360:859–73.

Samaha, FF, Iqbal N, Seshadri P, et al. A low-carbohydrate compared with a low fat diet in severe obesity. NEJM 2003;348:2074–81.

Saris WHM. Very low calorie diets and sustained weight loss. Obes Res 2001;9(Suppl):295S–310S.

Sarna S, Kaprio J. Life expectancy of former athletes. Sports Med 1994;17:149–51.

Schlundt DG, Hill JO, Pope-Cordle J, et al. Randomized evaluation of a low fat ad libitum carbohydrate diet for weight reduction. Int J Obes 1993;17:623–9.

Sears B. The Zone: a dietary road map. New York: Harper Collins, 1995.

Sharp TA, Reed GW, Sun M, Abumrad NN, Hill JO. Relationship between aerobic fitness level and daily energy expenditure in weight stable humans. Am J Physiol 1992;263:E121–8.

She H, Dirienzo D, Zemel MB. Effects of dietary calcium on adipocyte lipid metabolism and body weight regulation in energy restricted aP2-agouti transgenic mice. FASEB J 2001;15:291–3.

Shi H, Norman AW, Okamura WH, et al. 1(-25) dihydroxyvitamin D_3 inhibits uncoupling protein 2 expression in human adipocytes. FASEB J 2002;16:1808–10.

Simpson S J, Raubenheimer D. Obesity: the protein leverage hypothesis. Obes Rev 2005;6:133–42.

Sjostrom L, Rissanaen A, Andersen T, et al. Randomised placebo-controlled trial of orlistat for weight loss and prevention of weight regain in obese patients. Lancet 1998;352:167–72.

Skov AR, Toubro S, Rønn B, et al. Randomized trial on protein vs carbohydrate in ad libitum fat reduced diet for the treatment of obesity. Int J Obes 1999;23:528–36.

Sloth B, Astrup A. Low glycemic index diets and body weight. Int J Obes 2006;30(Suppl):47S–51S.

Stager JM, Cordain L. Relationship of body composition to swimming performance in female swimmers. J Swim Res 1984;1:21–4.

Steen SN, Opplinger RA, Brownell KD. Metabolic effects of repeated weight loss and regain in adolescent wrestlers. J Am Med Assoc 1988;260:47–50.

Stern L, Igbal P, Seshadri KL, et al. The effects of low-carbohydrate versus conventional weight loss diets in severely obese adults: one year follow-up of a randomized trial. Ann Intern Med 2004;140:778–85.

Stone KJ, Willis AL, Hart M, et al. The metabolism of dinomo-gamma-linolenic acid in man. Lipids 1978;14:174–80.

Stubbs RJ, Harbron CG, Murgatroyd PR, Prentice AM. Covert manipulation of dietary fat and energy density: effect on substrate flux and food intake in men feeding ad libitum. Am J Clin Nutr 1995a;62:316–29.

Stubbs RJ, Hughes DA, Johnstone AM, King N, Horgan GW, Blundell JE. A decrease in physical activity affects appetite, energy and nutrient balance in lean men feeding ad libitum. Am J Clin Nutr 2004;79:62–9.

Stubbs RJ, Ritz P, Coward WA, Prentice AM. Covert manipulation of the dietary carbohydrate to fat ratio and energy density: effect on food intake and energy balance in free-living men, feeding ad libitum. Am J Clin Nutr 1995b;62:330–7.

Stunkard AJ, Kaplan D. Eating in public places: a review of reports of the direct observation of eating behaviour. Int J Obes 1977;1:89–101.

Sumithran P, Proietto J. Ketogenic diets for weight loss: a review of their principles, safety and efficacy. Obes Res & Clin Pract 2008;2:1–13.

Thomas D, Elliott EJ, Baur L 2007. Low glycaemic index or low glycaemic index load diets for overweight and obesity. Cochrane Database of Systematic Reviews. Issue 18(2). Article No. CD005105.

Thornton J. Feast or famine: eating disorders in athletes. Phys Sports Med 1990;18:116–23.

Torbey N, Hwalla Baba N, Sawaya S, et al. High-protein vs high-carbohydrate hypoenergetic diet in treatment of obese normoinsulinaemic and hyperinsulinaemic subjects. Nutr Res 2002;22:587–98.

Torgerson JS, Hauptman J, Boldrin MN, et al. Xenical in the prevention of diabetes in obese subjects (XENDOS) study: a randomized study of orlistat as an adjunct to lifestyle changes for the prevention of type 2 diabetes in obese subjects. Diabetes Care 2004;27:155–61.

Trapp EG, Chisholm DJ, Freund J, Boutcher SH. The effects of high-intensity intermittent exercise training on fat loss and fasting insulin levels of young women. Int J Obes 2008;32:684–691.

Tremblay A, Déspres J-P, Bouchard C. The effects of exercise-training on energy balance and adipose tissue morphology and metabolism. Sports Med 1985;2:223–33.

Tremblay A, Déspres J-P, Leblanc C, Bouchard C. Sex dimorphism in fat loss in response to exercise training. J Obesity Weight Reg 1984;3:193–203.

Tremblay A, Simoneau JA, Bouchard C. Impact of exercise intensity on body fatness and skeletal muscle metabolism. Metabolism 1994;43:814–18.

Treuth MS, Hunter GR, Weinsier RL, Kell SH. Energy expenditure and substrate utilization in older women after strength training: 24-hour calorimeter results. J Appl Physiol 1995;78:2140–6.

Truswell AS, Darnton-Hill I. Food habits in adolescence. Nutr Rev 1981;39:73–88.

Van Baak MA, Astrup A. Consumption of sugars and body weight. Obes Rev 2009;10(1 Suppl):9–23.

Wadden TA, Foster GD. Behavioural treatment of obesity. Med Clin North Am 2000;84:441–61.

Walberg-Rankin J. Changing body weight and composition in athletes. In: Lamb D, Murray R, eds. Perspectives in exercise and sports medicine. Vol 11: Exercise, nutrition, and control of body weight. Carmel: Cooper Publishing Company, 1998:199–242.

Walberg-Rankin J, Hawkins CE, Fild DS, Sebolt DR. Effect of weight loss and refeeding diet composition on anaerobic performance in wrestlers. Med Sci Sports Exerc 1994;28:1292–9.

Weigle DS, Bukowski TR, Foster DC, et al. Recombinant ob protein reduces feeding and body weight in the ob/ob mouse. J Clin Invest 1995;96:2065–70.

White LJ, Dressendorfer RH, Holland E. Increased caloric intake soon after exercise in cold water. Int J Sports Nutr Exerc Met 2005;15:38–47.

Williams L, Williams P. Evaluation of a tool for rating popular diet books. Nutr Diet 2003;60:185–97.

Wing RR. Weight cycling in humans: a review of the literature. Ann Behav Med 1992;14:113–19.

Wing RR, Jeffery RW. Outpatient treatments of obesity: a comparison of the methodology and clinical results. Int J Obesity 1979;3:261–79.

Yancy WS, Olsen MK, Guyton JR, et al. A low carbohydrate ketogenic diet versus a low-fat diet to treat obesity and hyperlipidaemia: a randomized, controlled trial. Ann Intern Med 2004;140:769–77.

Yoshioka M, Doucet E, St Pierre S, et al. Impact of high-intensity exercise on energy expenditure, lipid oxidation and body fatness. Int J Obes 2001;25:332–9.

Zemel, MB. Role of calcium and dairy products in energy partitioning and weight management. Am J Clin Nutr 2004;79(Suppl):907S–12S.

Zemel, MB. Role of dietary calcium and dairy products in modulating adiposity. Lipids 2003;38:139–46.

Zemel MB, Thompson W, Milstead, et al. Dietary calcium and dairy products accelerate weight and fat loss during energy restriction in obese adults. Obes Res 2004;12:582–90.

Zhang Y, Proenca R, Maffei M, et al. Positional cloning of the mouse obese gene and its human homologue. Nature 1994;372:425–32.

Zurlo F, Lillioja S, Esposito-Del Puente A, et al. Low rate of fat to carbohydrate oxidation as a predictor of weight gain: study of 24-hour RQ. Am J Physiol 1990;259:E650–7.

CHAPTER 7

Making weight in sports

JANET WALBERG RANKIN

Introduction

7.1

Most athletes who compete in weight-category sports reduce weight quickly over one to several days in order to achieve their weight goal. Loss of 5% or more of body weight is not unusual for athletes competing in sports such as wrestling, lightweight rowing or boxing. These athletes must be weighed in the presence of an official prior to their match or competition to compete in their designated weight category. If BM is even slightly higher than the category allows, the athlete will be disqualified from competing. This provides a powerful motivation to achieve the required weight. The most dramatic and unfortunate result of effort to lose weight in wrestling was the death of three collegiate wrestlers in 1997 trying to 'make weight' (American Medical Association 1998).

In order for nutritionists and medical personnel to assist athletes to make weight safely, it is important to be familiar with the rules and specific constraints of the sport regarding weight divisions/restrictions, as well as the typical practices of the athletes to reduce body mass. This chapter will review these issues as well as the research concerning the potential health and performance hazards of rapid loss of body mass. Although body mass (BM) is the correct term, this chapter will use the terms 'weight' or 'body weight' interchangeably with BM, since these are the common terms used by those involved in weight-division sports. Finally, suggestions will be made for safe and effective means of making weight and recovering afterwards, based on the available research.

Sports with weight divisions or restrictions

7.2

A variety of sports involve weight divisions or restrictions for competition purposes, and each has its own procedures for prescribing and monitoring competition weights for its participants. Wrestlers compete in a number of designated weight categories; for example, collegiate wrestling involves ten weight classes (see Table 7.1 in the practice tips). One of the modifications to the wrestling rules from the National Collegiate Athletic Association

(NCAA) in 1998 was to add 6 lb (2.7 kg) to each weight category definition to allow for the overall increased weight of the population. Lightweight rowers must meet restrictions placed on individual competitors as well as the total boat crew: male rowers can weigh no more than 72.5 kg with a crew average of 70.0 kg, while female competitors must be 59.0 kg or less, with a crew average of 57.0 kg. Lightweight football is played at a minority of institutions in the US, but allows participation of individuals who are too light to be competitive on most football teams. Players are required to be less than 71.8 kg (158 lb) two days prior to the game. In horse racing, the body weight of jockeys may be controlled to provide a 'handicap' to the competing horse. The target weight (including the saddle) for flat-race jockeys may be as light as 47.7 kg (105 lb) and for jump jockeys, 60.4 kg (133 lb) (King & Mezey 1987).

The intention of weight categories is to provide an 'even playing field' for sports where the larger individual will have a clear advantage. It would be expected that an athlete who has greater muscle mass and reach can generate more power in strength events, or be more competitive in combative sports, than a smaller and lighter opponent. Thus, matching individuals of similar body weight should theoretically make these sports safer and fairer. The reality is that athletes will dehydrate or otherwise achieve rapid weight loss to make a lower weight division, hoping to recover between the weigh-in and the competition, and compete with an advantage over a smaller opponent.

Most wrestlers believe that weight loss is a critical part of the culture of wrestling. For example, 70% of the high school wrestlers interviewed from nine rural teams claimed that losing weight during the season was 'very important' for winning (Marquart & Sobal 1994). Most of the wrestlers thought making weight was hard; 31% worked 'very hard' while 47% worked 'somewhat hard'. So losing weight clearly adds to the stresses and complexities as well as the risks of competing in sports.

7.3 Methods used to make weight

7.4 Wrestlers

Some of the earliest studies of weight-loss methods of wrestlers were undertaken with high school wrestlers in Iowa in the late 1960s. Eighty-three percent of the 528 wrestlers surveyed claimed they used food restriction to lose weight; 77% used fluid restriction, and 83% increased exercise to lose weight (Tipton & Tcheng 1970). Other surveys of high school wrestlers have uncovered other clearly inappropriate methods used for weight loss including fasting (60%), saunas (45%), rubber suits (26%), laxatives (13%) and vomiting (13%) (Steen & Brownell 1990). The most recent assessment of the weight-loss behavior of high school wrestlers shows that the traditions have not changed much. Alderman and colleagues (2004) studied male wrestlers aged 15–18 years competing at the national championship in international-style wrestling over a 2-year period in 1997 and 1998. Mat-side scales were used to weigh the wrestlers just before competition; the weight gained between weigh-in and the match was assumed to be close to the amount lost for weigh-in. The average weight gain for the over 2600 athletes was 3.4 kg, representing 4.8% of body weight. The range was dramatic in that some athletes gained up to 16.7 kg or 13.4% of their weight. A subset of the athletes agreed to be interviewed concerning the methods they used to lose weight. Although none of the athletes claimed to use purging, a large proportion used additional aerobic exercise (running 91%, swimming 24%, cycling 33%) or some means of dehydration (saunas 55%, exercising in vapor-impermeable suits 49%). Eleven percent used laxatives to hasten weight loss.

Several studies provided an estimate of weight lost by collegiate wrestlers for weigh-in by measuring the weight gain between weigh-in and the match. Two studies of collegiate wrestlers showed an average gain of about 5% following weigh-in (Horswill et al. 1994; Scott et al. 1994). Both of these studies examined the weight-loss behavior of collegiate wrestlers prior to the NCAA rule changes implemented in 1998 to discourage rapid and significant weight loss (specifics of rule changes are discussed below). One study performed the year after implementation of the new rules in 741 collegiate wrestlers from forty-three teams (Oppliger et al. 2003) showed that the weekly average weight lost was 2.9 kg or 4.3% of weight and their off-season weight was an average of 5.5 kg or 8.6% greater than during the season. Inappropriate weight-loss methods were still used (55% fasting, 28% saunas, 27% impermeable suits), but most used more appropriate methods such as gradual dieting (79%) or increased exercise (75%) to lose the weight. They concluded that the weight-loss amount and methods were less extreme than those observed prior to the rule changes. However, the rule changes did not eliminate unsafe practices.

Lightweight rowers 7.5

Many rowers lose a similar magnitude of weight as wrestlers in order to meet the requirements of lightweight competition. Morris and Payne (1996) reported that female lightweight rowers dropped an average of 5.9% of their body weight while men dropped 7.8% of their body weight during the competitive season compared to pre-season. They achieved this most often via additional exercise (73.3%), food restriction (71.4%) and fluid restriction (62.9%).

Slater and colleagues (2005) studied 107 lightweight competitors at a national rowing championship. Most athletes (76% of males and 84% of females in the U23 category) lost weight in order to qualify to compete. The maximum weight loss over the 4 weeks prior to the regatta reported by men was 6 kg and 4.5 kg for women. Most used moderate energy restriction and additional exercise to lose weight, but dehydration was also popular (83%). Female rowers were more likely to use carbohydrate, sodium and fiber restriction to lose weight than males.

Jockeys 7.6

Fourteen jockeys in England responded to a survey distributed to forty-eight stables (King & Mezey 1987). They were an average of 13% below the population weight for their height with the lightest being 21% below average. Jockeys reported that weight control was a priority over most other aspects of their lives during the racing season. They used a variety of methods to reduce their already low body weight—food avoidance, saunas, laxatives, diuretics and appetite suppressants. The use of saunas was especially popular, with jockeys spending up to 4 hours in the sauna in a single session. A fast of up to 6 days was reported by one of the jockeys.

Weight loss and competitive success 7.7

Most athletes in weight-division sports think weight-loss behaviors are important to their success in the sport. Does research verify this? The question has been examined in wrestlers by determining whether the acute weight gain after weigh-in (assumed to reflect weight lost) is predictive of success during the wrestling match. There was no evidence that magnitude of weight gain affected the outcome of the match for eleven collegiate wrestlers over four matches in their season (Utter & Kang 1998) or for 668 wrestlers at an NCAA tournament in the US (Horswill et al. 1994; Scott et al. 1994). However, virtually all the wrestlers were losing weight for the weigh-in and there was only a small range in the weight losses undertaken at competition. Thus, these studies were not able to test whether athletes who did not lose weight for weigh-in would be at a disadvantage upon competition. Ninety-five percent of the wrestlers at the NCAA tournament gained at least 1.4 kg over the 20 hours between weigh-in and match, with the overall average gain of 4.9% of BM.

7.8 Potential negative consequences to weight loss

Most weight-category sports are based on anaerobic energy utilization, with an emphasis on muscle power (e.g. wrestling, boxing, judo, power lifting and lightweight football). A typical race for lightweight rowers is more aerobic, requiring a maximal effort for 6–7 minutes. The goal of all these athletes is to reduce BM through loss of body fat or fluid, rather than lean tissue, and to recover any water loss prior to the competition. In addition, they intend to maintain physical performance and health while making weight, or at least be able to recover their performance to pre-weight loss levels after the weigh-in. There is evidence that at least some athletes do not achieve these goals and, in fact, experience impairment of performance or health. Sections 7.9–7.15 provide information that should be used to educate athletes concerning possible negative outcomes to inappropriate weight loss.

7.9 Plasma volume loss and susceptibility to heat illness

Dehydration played a major role in the weight-loss strategies of the three collegiate wrestlers who died while making weight (American Medical Association 1998). Before their deaths, all had exercised in vapor-impermeable suits and hot environments; one of these individuals had a body temperature of 42°C (108°F) upon death. The acute dehydration coupled with the use of heat and excessive exercise contributed to their deaths as dehydration reduces the ability of the body to produce sweat and therefore increases the risk of heat injury. A large drop in plasma volume may be expected as a result of dehydration strategies. In one study where wrestlers used a sauna to lose 3.8% of body weight, plasma volume fell 7.5% (Greiwe et al. 1998). Collegiate wrestlers who lost about 6% of their weight had a drop in plasma volume of 11% (Yankanich et al. 1998). Thus, use of dehydration can have dramatic effects on plasma volume.

7.10 Lean tissue maintenance or growth

It is difficult to maintain lean tissue mass with dramatic weight loss. Although most of the energy deficit is made up from a reduction in body fat stores, some body protein may be used for gluconeogenesis. Thus, dietary protein needs are higher during periods of low energy consumption. We found that resistance training athletes who lost weight over a week while consuming a formula diet of 75 kJ (18 kcal) per kilogram lost body protein if they were given the Recommended Dietary Allowance (RDA) (0.8 g/kg) for protein, but were in nitrogen balance (no net body protein loss) if the diet contained twice the RDA for protein (Walberg et al. 1988).

Several studies have verified that wrestlers and rowers have less lean tissue than age-matched controls over the competitive season. For example, studies in female lightweight rowers reported a reduction in the fat-free mass during their season compared to pre-season measurements (McCargar et al. 1993) and a lower serum IGF-1 in those who energy-restricted (Slater et al. 2005). Wrestlers had lower increases in arm and thigh muscle cross-sectional areas and reduction in growth-inducing hormones over the wrestling season compared to non-wrestling classmates (Roemmich & Sinning 1997). Fortunately, they found no effect on linear growth and during the off-season the wrestlers showed a rebound in muscle growth and hormonal pattern to bring them up to the average for controls.

Although these changes appeared to be temporary in these older athletes, there is a question of whether a chronic negative energy balance could affect linear growth in younger athletes. Theintz and colleagues (1993) examined the estimated bone age and predicted height in a cross-sectional study of young elite gymnasts and swimmers for over 2 years. Over the period studied they reported stunting of leg length growth, and thus predicted height, in the gymnasts but not in the swimmers. It is important to point out that there were no dietary measures performed in this study. However, the information is provocative and suggests that severe emphasis on body weight in young athletes may have long-term effects on growth.

In summary, athletes practicing repeated weight loss over a season are likely to inhibit lean tissue growth. At least in older athletes, there appears to be catch-up of lean growth during the off-season.

Metabolic rate and weight loss 7.11

Early research noted that wrestlers who reported repeated weight loss and gain (termed 'weight cyclers') had a lower metabolic rate than those who were not weight cyclers (Steen et al. 1988). However, later studies, which used longitudinal measures of metabolic rate in wrestlers over a season and in post-season, did not verify a permanent effect of weight loss on metabolic rate (Melby et al. 1990). However, a drop in metabolic rate during the season will make weight loss more difficult since more restriction in energy intake will be required to cause a negative energy balance. Blood biochemical measures support a drop in metabolic rate with weight loss; lightweight rowers who restricted their diet for weight loss had lower serum thyroxine compared to non-dieters (Slater et al. 2005). In summary, it appears from the literature that resting metabolic rate is likely to drop significantly during energy restriction and will alter the energy intake prescription for weight loss. However, the evidence that these metabolic changes continue after the season is not strong.

Cognitive function 7.12

Not surprisingly, most people do not feel mentally sharp and at their peak while dieting. Even short-term weight loss can have adverse effects on mood and cognitive abilities. Horswill and colleagues (1990a) showed that the rate of perceived exertion during a performance test designed to simulate wrestling was 7% higher when the athletes had lost weight over 4 days. So, wrestling workouts as well as matches will feel more difficult for those trying to lose weight. Another set of fourteen collegiate wrestlers tested for mood and cognitive ability before and after loss of an average of 6.2% of their body weight reported impaired mood (more tension, depression, anger, fatigue and confusion) and poorer short-term memory ability after weight loss (Choma et al. 1998). All these impairments returned to baseline after 72 hours of food and fluid consumption.

In summary, athletes are not likely to feel or perform mental tasks as well during periods of weight loss. There is no research at this point to determine whether particular dieting strategies may dampen these mental disturbances.

7.13 Nutritional status

It is unlikely that a period of brief dieting or weight loss by itself will have a negative effect on nutritional status. Our bodies can typically handle brief periods of low nutrient intake. Several studies confirmed poor intake of various micronutrients in athletes making weight, but none demonstrated abnormal biochemical nutrient status (Folgelholm et al. 1993; Steen & McKinney 1986).

Problems with nutritional status may be more likely in those athletes who are repeatedly restricting their diet for weight loss or are dieting over a prolonged period. Biochemical evidence of nutritional deficiency was observed in athletes who lost weight over a 3-week period, but not for those dieting over just a few days (Fogelholm et al. 1993). Two studies reported reductions in serum pre-albumin, an indicator of protein status, in wrestlers during their season (Horswill et al. 1990b; Roemmich & Sinning 1997).

In summary, the diets of most athletes attempting rapid weight loss are likely to be low in many nutrients. A single weight-loss effort is unlikely to cause problems in nutrient status, but repeated weight loss over a season is more likely to cause a deterioration of nutritional status. More research is required to determine the specific changes expected. Counseling an athlete to choose a higher nutrient density diet with sufficient micronutrients and protein will lessen the likelihood of nutritional deficiencies.

7.14 Bone

Four days of fasting has been reported to cause a 40–50% reduction in markers of bone synthesis and resorption in healthy females (Grinspoon et al. 1995). This lower bone turnover may result in lower bone mass over time. A recent study in lightweight male rowers confirmed that a 24-hour fast influenced markers of bone formation and breakdown (Talbott & Shapses 1998). Serum indicators of bone synthesis and resorption were altered 20–27%. In summary, athletes, particularly females who have menstrual disturbances and therefore have an elevated risk of reduced bone mass, should be educated on the potential effect on bone of repeated weight loss (see Chapter 9).

7.15 Performance

The effect of rapid weight loss on performance appears to depend on the method of weight loss, the magnitude of weight loss and the type of exercise performance test utilized (Folgelholm 1994; Walberg Rankin 1998). The detrimental effect of weight loss on aerobic performance via dehydration is documented, but the effect on muscle power or strength is less clear. One study reported a reduction in muscle strength following weight loss via dehydration (Viitasalo et al. 1987) while another study found no effect of dehydration on muscle isometric strength and endurance (Greiwe et al. 1998).

Adding energy restriction to dehydration, or dieting alone, appears to be more consistent in causing impairments of muscle performance. Muscle strength was reduced in athletes who lost weight using energy restriction alone (Walberg et al. 1988; Walberg-Rankin et al. 1994) and in those who energy-restricted first and then dehydrated (Viitasalo et al. 1987). Addition of energy restriction to dehydration appears to be more likely to cause impairments than dehydration alone.

Tests using intermittent bouts of high-intensity work have been developed to attempt to mimic the pattern of muscle use in sports, including wrestling. Several studies showed that weight loss over several days significantly reduced the amount of work accomplished during an intermittent upper body sprint test (Hickner et al. 1991; Horswill et al. 1990a; Walberg Rankin et al. 1996). It is interesting that many wrestlers perceive their performance to be impaired by their weight-loss efforts. Sixty-three percent of high school wrestlers surveyed reported a depression of muscle strength, 56% speed, 42% agility and 42% concentration as a result of weight loss (Marquart & Sobal 1994). Studies looking at muscle performance of wrestlers over their season have confirmed a depression in muscle strength for adolescent wrestlers compared to their non-wrestling classmates (Roemmich & Sinning 1997).

In summary, acute weight loss in the range of 5% of body weight has been shown in some studies to reduce performance in athletes, particularly in repeated high-intensity sprint tests. A reduction in physical performance over a season of repeated weight loss may be secondary to limited growth of lean tissue. Many of the athletes already believe that weight loss hurts their performance.

Strategies for weight loss 7.16

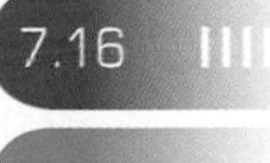

Dehydration 7.17

Since dehydration is banned by the NCAA for wrestlers and some high school wrestling associations (see later discussion), it is not ethical to recommend dehydration as a means of making weight. Athletes involved in sports that do not ban dehydration and who intend to use dehydration for weight loss and who have less than 24 hours to recover are cautioned to not lose more than 2% of BM with this method, as performance, tolerance to heat, and ability to fully rehydrate are probably impaired with greater degrees of dehydration.

Diet 7.18

A few researchers have compared the effects of rapid compared to gradual weight loss in athletes. Fogelholm and colleagues (1993) had judo and wrestler athletes lose 6% of their weight with energy restriction and dehydration over 2.4 days or reduce weight a similar amount but more gradually over 3 weeks. Neither strategy was shown to be superior with regard to changes in performance.

Another study compared the effects of losing similar amounts of weight over either 2 or 4 months in national caliber lightweight rowers (Koutedakis et al. 1994). Six rowers were studied over 2 years; the rapid weight loss strategy (3.8 kg over 2 months) was implemented in the first and the gradual approach (4.7 kg over 4 months) in the next year. Neither method was able to exclusively cause fat loss; about 50% of the weight lost with both strategies was a reduction in fat-free mass. However, the more rapid weight loss was associated with a decline in lactate threshold and leg strength, while these measures as well as $VO_{2\,max}$ and anaerobic power were actually increased during the slower weight loss period. This study suggests that a more gradual weight loss is superior for maintenance or increases in performance, but does not affect body composition.

One study has examined the effect of altering frequency of eating on weight loss in athletes. Boxers ate 5020 kJ (1200 kcal) per day for 2 weeks as either two meals per day or six meals per day (Iwao et al. 1996). The same body-weight loss was noted, but more reduction in lean body mass occurred for the two meals per day pattern.

Several studies have demonstrated the value of CHO in a weight-loss diet. Wrestlers could maintain high-power performance on a high-CHO diet (66–70% of energy respectively), but not when they consumed a modest (41–55%) CHO diet for weight loss (Horswill et al. 1990a; McMurray et al. 1991). A practical suggestion, based on these studies, is to maximize CHO intake within other dietary goals in an energy-restricted diet (e.g. to include at least 60–70% of energy in a weight-loss diet as CHO).

The high CHO intake recommended above should not be at the expense of dietary protein since it has been shown that protein requirements are increased during weight loss using energy restriction (see section 7.11). This research suggests that dietary protein should be at least 1.2 g/kg during weight loss. Since this might contribute up to 20% of energy, this leaves a suitable dietary fat content of weight-loss diets at ≤20%.

7.19 Recovery strategies

7.20 Fluids and electrolytes

Recovery of fluids lost through dehydration may take 24–48 hours, longer than is commonly appreciated by athletes (Costill & Sparks 1973). A loss of 5% of BM, accompanied by a 12.5% reduction in plasma volume, was not eliminated by a 2-hour rehydration period with 1.5 L of water (Burge et al. 1993). Although the traditional recommendation has been to ingest about 1 L of fluid for each kilogram lost due to dehydration, more recent research suggests that increasing this to 150% of the volume of fluid lost due to dehydration is more effective (Shirreffs et al. 1996). Consuming fluid in volumes greater than that lost is preferable due to the loss of some of the fluid ingested via urine production (see Chapter 14).

In the dehydration study with rowers, rehydration was attempted using tap water containing no electrolytes or other nutrients in the water consumed (Burge et al. 1993). Research shows that rehydration will occur more rapidly if electrolytes are included in the fluid consumed (Shirreffs et al. 1996). The benefit of sodium in a rehydration fluid appears to be related to the stimulatory effect of sodium on water absorption in the gut as well as the maintenance of thirst drive. Ingestion of water will reduce the osmolality of the blood and reduce the desire to drink, counterproductive to rehydration (see Chapter 14). Current recommendations are that optimal sodium concentration in a rehydration beverage should be at least 50 mmol/L (Shirreffs & Maughan 2000). Chapter 14 provides a detailed discussion on optimal rehydration strategies.

Few studies have characterized the typical dietary recovery strategy of athletes. Slater and colleagues (2005) questioned lightweight rowers concerning their food and fluid intake during the 1–2 hours between weigh-in and competition. Energy intake varied by gender and competitive category (e.g. U23 or Open) but ranged from 30–53 kJ/kg. The majority of those calories were carbohydrate, with about 15% of energy as protein and 7% as fat for the U23 rowers. Fluid and especially sodium intake (about 8–14 mL/kg fluid and 10–20 mmol/L sodium) were below recommendations for optimal rehydration.

Carbohydrate 7.21

Weight loss in athletes has been associated with reduced muscle CHO storage. Wrestlers losing 5% of their weight with food and fluid restriction had a 54% decline in muscle glycogen (Tarnopolsky et al. 1996). A similar weight loss in rowers over just 24 hours was accompanied by a 30% drop in muscle glycogen content (Burge et al. 1993). Suboptimal muscle glycogen levels can be overcome with time and adequate CHO intake (see Chapter 14), but this may not be realistically achieved between the weigh-in and the start of competition. Wrestlers who lost about 5% of their weight with energy restriction and were re-fed a 50% CHO diet over 5 hours did not recover their performance to baseline levels, while those fed a higher CHO diet (70%) had a performance similar to baseline after the recovery (Walberg Rankin et al. 1996). We found that most collegiate wrestlers consumed a high-CHO diet (66%) between weigh-in and the match, but the range in reported energy intake from CHO during re-feeding was 28–87% (Pesce et al. 1996). Thus, since energy restriction to produce weight loss is likely to cause a drop in muscle and liver glycogen, which may contribute to impairment of performance if recovery time is short, athletes should be counseled to eat a high-CHO diet during recovery from energy restriction to make weight.

No studies have looked at the role of different types of CHO on recovery rate of glycogen following weight-making strategies. However, it is likely that this situation would be similar to that of recovery of muscle glycogen after prolonged endurance exercise (Burke et al. 1993); an enhanced rate of glycogen resynthesis would be likely if CHO-rich foods with a high glycemic index are consumed. Strategies to enhance recovery of muscle glycogen are summarized in greater detail in Chapter 14.

Measures to reduce dangerous weight loss practices 7.22

Introduction 7.23

Many athletes could use assistance to develop a plan for weight loss. When a group of high school wrestlers were asked who helped them plan their weight-loss efforts, 'nobody' was the second highest answer (42%), after coaches (44%) (Marquart & Sobal 1994). Most coaches are not trained in nutrition and thus may not be able to appropriately advise the athletes on safe weight loss. Sossin and colleagues (1997) demonstrated a poor knowledge of issues of making weight in a group of high school wrestling coaches: the percentage of correct answers on a nutrition knowledge survey was 64% for weight loss, 59% for training diets, 57% for dehydration and 52% for body composition. Although this could be improved through coach education, the best approach is to use health professionals for counseling in this area. A minority of the wrestlers used trainers (11%), doctors (7%) or dietitians (3%) (Marquart & Sobal 1994). 'Other rowers' was the most common answer from elite lightweight rowers when they were asked who had a 'very high' influence on their body-weight practices (Slater et al. 2005). Interestingly, about a fifth of the female rowers but few of the male rowers ranked dietitians as 'very influential'.

It is likely that collegiate and especially Olympic-level athletes have greater access to medical and nutrition professionals. However, there may be resistance by some coaches and athletes to use nutritionists for fear they will discourage weight loss. It is important for nutritionists to understand the stresses placed on the athletes and attempt to help them in a way that will be least likely to cause health problems.

7.24 High school wrestlers

One of the first efforts to discourage unhealthy weight-loss practices was in 1989 when the Wisconsin Interscholastic Athletic Association set up a pilot program to reduce unsafe weight loss in high school wrestlers (Oppliger et al. 1995). This program included new rules for determining weight class based on body composition and maximum weight losses based on a minimum of 7% body fat. These rules were paired with development of nutrition education materials to educate the athletes on appropriate weight-loss methods (developed with the help of state nutrition organisations such as the Wisconsin Dietetic Association). Following the pilot year, 1990 was a voluntary year for use of the program with mandatory implementation of the new rules in 1991. The scope of this program can be realized when one knows that more than 9000 body-fat tests were required each year. Change was difficult for athletes and coaches. Originally 60% of coaches opposed the project, but by 1993 95% felt positive about the changes. Some were pleased to be free of the responsibility for choosing the weight class for each athlete.

There is published evidence that this program has significantly reduced inappropriate weight-loss practices. Oppliger and colleagues (1998) examined weight loss in wrestlers a year before and after implementation of this program. The maximum amount of weight loss fell from an average of 3.2–2.6 kg, average weight loss to certify: 2.8–2.4 kg, weekly weight cycled: 1.9–1.6 kg, longest fast: 20.5–16.5 hours and frequency of weight cutting: 6.2–4.7 times per season. Use of fluid restriction and rubber suits also declined. Thus these rule changes reduced but did not totally eliminate inappropriate weight-loss methods. The success of this program was instrumental in the development of similar recommendations in the American College of Sports Medicine position stand concerning weight loss in wrestlers published in 1996 (American College of Sports Medicine 1996).

7.25 Collegiate wrestlers

Although collegiate wrestling governing bodies were slower to implement new rules, the deaths of the college wrestlers in 1997 accelerated the development of programs for safer weight-management practices. In 1998, the NCAA added new rules to wrestling that reflected those begun in Wisconsin in high school wrestlers. Their stated goal was to 'emphasize the competitive element of wrestling and minimize the emphasis on making weight' (*NCAA news*, 2 March 1998). The rule changes recommended by the NCAA wrestling committee include the following features (NCAA press releases, 13 January 1998 and 13 April 1998):

- Prohibition of dehydration. Guidelines to discourage dehydration had been included in the *NCAA sports medicine handbook* since 1985. These guidelines were expanded and changed to rules. Hot rooms (defined as room hotter than 24°C or 79°F), use of vapor-impermeable suits, excessive food or fluid restriction, laxatives and vomiting are now prohibited. There is also prohibition of artificial rehydration techniques (e.g. intravenous hydration).
- An increase in weight allowance of 6 pounds (2.7 kg) to each weight class.
- Limitations for wrestlers to compete only in the weight classes that are based on body composition assessment prior to the start of the season when urine specific gravity is ≤1.020. Wrestlers may not lose more than 1.5% of body weight per week and the minimum wrestling weight is that with body fat of 5%.
- Rescheduling of weigh-ins to be closer to the event, to discourage the potential for recovery after severe weight-making strategies: weigh-ins shall be held no more than 1 hour before the first match in a regular meet. The weigh-in for a multiple day tournament will occur 2 hours before competition on the first day and 1 hour before competition on subsequent days.

Because some athletes will attempt to circumvent or challenge these rules, researchers have compared various methods to estimate body composition (used for the calculation of minimum weight class) and dehydration. For example, NCAA rules require determination of hydration status prior to body composition assessment (euhydration, defined as urine specific gravity ≤1.020 g/mL, is required in order to advance to body composition assessment), but allowed the use of three methods in the 1998 rules. Steumpfle and Drury (2003) tested the urine specific gravity of twenty-one collegiate wrestlers prior to the start of their wrestling season using three methods: refractometry, hydrometry and reagent strips. Neither hydrometry nor reagent strips were reliable or valid. In 1999, use of reagent strips was eliminated as a choice for assessment of hydration status. Bartok and colleagues (2004b) confirmed that the urine specific gravity cutoff of 1.020 g/mL had high specificity and sensitivity to detect dehydration in the 2–6% of body weight range. Her research group also confirmed the importance of verifying euhydration when body composition is assessed (Bartok et al. 2004a). Calculated minimum weight was reduced by an average of 2 kg when athletes were dehydrated.

The NCAA recommends use of hydrodensitometry, skinfold or BOD POD measurement for estimation of body fat in its 2004 wrestling rule book. Several studies have contrasted the validity of various body composition techniques in wrestlers. Clark and colleagues (2003) confirmed that prediction of body composition using the skinfold procedure was as accurate as a more sophisticated four-compartment model that includes dual energy X-ray, total body water measurement with deuterium dilution and hydrodensitometry. Use of leg-to-leg bioelectric impedance had higher error and poorer precision than the other methods and therefore is not recommended (Clark et al. 2004).

7.26 Summary

Athletes competing in sports with weight categories are highly motivated to lose weight acutely prior to weigh-in. Many will use drastic dietary restriction or dehydration to achieve a temporary weight loss. Quick losses of 5% of body weight, typical in many of these sports, have been shown to result in reductions in physical performance, abnormalities of bone metabolism, impairments in cognitive function and increased susceptibility to heat illness. Prolonged or repeated weight-loss attempts are likely to cause nutritional deficiencies and limit lean tissue growth. Gradual weight loss has fewer negative health consequences and should be recommended when weight loss is desirable.

Weight-loss goals and strategies should be determined with the assistance of health care professionals (such as team physicians and nutritionists) to ensure appropriate and safe weight loss. Body composition assessment using skinfold measurement, euhydration validation with urine specific gravity and diet records can be part of the assessment used by professionals to develop a goal weight and strategy for change. Regular monitoring of the health and performance of the athlete will help in making decisions to adjust the weight-loss plan.

More research is needed to compare different dietary strategies for weight loss to determine the method most likely to cause weight loss while maintaining performance and health. The limited research available suggests that modest energy restriction using a high-CHO, moderate-protein and low-fat diet is recommended. Risk of nutrient deficiencies can be reduced by consumption of nutrient-rich foods. Due to the potentially fatal consequences of dehydration, this method should be used modestly or not at all.

Athletes should understand that substantial weight loss through dehydration causes reductions in plasma volume that are difficult to remedy within several hours between weigh-in and competition. Those athletes who lose weight acutely for weigh-in should attempt to recover as rapidly as possible using a fluid adequate in sodium and carbohydrate.

PRACTICE TIPS

GREG COX

- There is no specific set of nutrition guidelines to address weight-management issues for all weight-making sports. When counseling athletes on weight-making strategies, it is essential to consider the physiological requirements specific to their sport, the rules governing weigh-in procedures and the traditions within the sport. The practice tips outlined below reflect current research findings and personal experience gained from dealing with athletes competing in weight-making sports. Counseling such athletes often involves compromising your professional opinion in order to facilitate a working relationship. In many instances, successful counseling is as simple as attempting to minimize the negative impact of the athlete's current weight-making strategies.
- Before any nutrition intervention is commenced, present dietary habits and weight-making strategies of the athlete should be assessed. Many elite athletes in weight-making sports have established strategies to reduce body weight prior to competition. These strategies are often based on personal experience and practices of other athletes in the sport. Be prepared to hear stories of drastic weight-loss techniques such as food and fluid restriction, excessive exercise, and use of saunas, laxatives and diuretics.
- It is useful to develop a yearly weight-management plan with the athlete. This should consider the length of the competition season, the number of times they are expected to compete throughout the year, the type of training they perform and the weigh-in procedures of the sport. Make allowances for their weight to fluctuate between the off-season and competition season, as it is difficult for athletes to maintain their competition weight year-round.
- It is important to understand the rules that govern weigh-in procedures in the various weight-making sports. Be careful to clarify rules governing weigh-in procedures, since these differ between sports and sometimes differ within the same sport (e.g. weigh-in procedures for professional boxing differ from those in amateur boxing; NCAA wrestling weigh-in procedures differ from those of international wrestling). Weight categories, the time between weighing-in and competition, the length of the tournament and the number of occasions athletes are required to weigh-in vary between sports. These factors ultimately determine the nutrition advice provided to these athletes for making weight and should be investigated prior to the interview or during the interview process. Table 7.1 outlines weight categories and issues relevant to making weight in numerous sports.
- Allowances for growth should be considered for adolescent athletes competing in weight-making sports. Many athletes competing in lighter divisions in boxing, wrestling and judo are still in adolescence. It is common for younger athletes competing in open competition to move across weight categories as they mature.
- Many athletes use extreme short-term measures to make weight in the week immediately preceding competition, rather than implementing long-term strategies to reduce body fat and body weight to reach the competition target. The first strategy of these athletes should be to reduce body-fat levels in order to maximize their power to weight ratio and make a given weight category safely. Chapter 6 outlines dietary strategies to promote decreases in body-fat levels.

PRACTICE TIPS

TABLE 7.1 SUMMARY OF SPECIFIC ISSUES IN MAKING WEIGHT FOR WEIGHT-DIVISION SPORTS

SPORT	COMPETITION	WEIGHT CATEGORIES		WEIGH-IN PROCEDURES	PERSONAL INSIGHT
Wrestling—senior international Includes Greco–Roman and freestyle wrestling	1 bout = 3 × 2-minute rounds for international competition and may require an additional ordered hold position lasting a maximum of 30 seconds. Competition sessions last no longer than 3 hours. Each individual weight category is contested over one day. Four or fewer bouts each day of competition.	*Male (kg)* 50–55 <60 <66 <74 <84 <96 96–120	*Female (kg)* <48* <51 <55* <59 <63* <67 <72* *Only four categories at Olympics	Weigh-in on the evening before competition. Weigh-in period lasts 30 minutes. Expected to weigh-in only once at start of competition.	Typically wrestlers undertake minimal aerobic training in their daily training schedule. Therefore, it may be problematic for them to add significant amounts of aerobic activity close to competition in order to make weight.
Boxing—amateur	Each bout is 3 × 3-minute rounds. Competitors box every second day and may be expected to box 4–5 times during the tournament.	*Male (kg)* <48 kg 48–51 51–54 54–57 57–60 60–64 64–69 69–75 75–81 81–91 >91	 Light fly Fly Bantam Feather Light Light welter Welter Middle Light heavy Heavy Super heavy	All competitors must attend general weigh-in on the morning of the first day of competition. The time from the start of the general weigh-in to the start of the first bout should not be less than 6 hours. On the following days only those who are drawn to box shall appear to weigh-in. Boxing shall not commence earlier than 3 hours after the time appointed for the close of weigh-in on these days.	Amateur boxers are required to weigh-in on the morning of each bout. The requirement for further weigh-ins may limit their ability to rehydrate and refuel after a bout. However, with a period of at least 3 hours between weigh-in and competition, boxers have the luxury of implementing appropriate rehydration strategies to replace lost fluid from weight-making activities.

Boxing—professional	Australian National and the various World Association Title fights are fought over 12 × 3-minute rounds. Fights may vary between 4 and 12 × 3-minute rounds. Competitors usually fight 3–4 times per year.	Weight divisions vary from amateur boxing, and may vary slightly between countries and boxing associations. Below are the weight divisions of the World Boxing Association (WBA). Weight categories are expressed in either metric or imperial. <47.63 kg Mini Flyweight 47.63–48.89 kg Light Fly 48.89–50.80 kg Flyweight 50.80–52.16 kg Super Flyweight 52.16–53.52 kg Bantamweight 53.52–55.34 kg Super Bantamweight 55.34–57.15 kg Featherweight 57.15–58.97 kg Super Featherweight 58.97–61.23 kg Lightweight 61.23–63.50 kg Super Lightweight 63.50–66.68 kg Welterweight 66.68–69.85 kg Super Welterweight 69.85–72.57 kg Middleweight 72.57–76.20 kg Super Middleweight 76.20–79.38 kg Light Heavyweight 79.38–86.18 kg Cruiserweight > 86.18 kg Heavy weight	Competition weigh-in procedures vary between professional boxing associations. For WBA world title fights, competitors weigh-in the day prior to the fight, between 4 and 8 pm.	Since boxers typically compete only 3–4 times a year, there is considerable opportunity to overindulge between fights. This pattern of 'on and off' dieting behavior leads to large weight swings.

(continued)

PRACTICE TIPS

TABLE 7.1 *(continued)*

SPORT	COMPETITION	WEIGHT CATEGORIES	WEIGH-IN PROCEDURES	PERSONAL INSIGHT
Horse racing—jockeys	Races are conducted over various distances, usually 1000–2000 m (lasting 1–2 minutes), but may be as long as 3200 m (the Melbourne Cup). Jockeys may have up to 6–8 rides during one racing session, which lasts roughly 5–6 hours.	Minimum weight for any race in Australia as sanctioned by the Australian Rules is 43.5 kg, including saddle and accessories. Minimum weight varies between states and within states (country versus city) for local races. Minimum weight also varies between countries. Horses are weight-handicapped according to ability or age.	All jockeys weigh-in no later than 45 minutes before racing for each race they compete in. Jockeys on horses that earn prize money (plus the next best finisher) have to weigh-in directly after the race.	As jockeys need to weigh-in *after* the race, recovery strategies cannot be employed prior to their event to address any short-term measures exploited in order to make weight.
Olympic weightlifting	Competitors have three lifts in each discipline: clean-and-jerk and snatch. Competition for any one competitor is conducted over 1 day.	*Male (kg)* <56, <62, <69, <77, <85, <94, <105, 105+ *Female (kg)* <48, <53, <58, <63, <69, <75, 75+		With limited aerobic activity in the daily training regimen, these athletes face similar issues to those of wrestlers.
Karate	Have team and individual events—no weight categories in team events. 3-minute bout for males and a 2-minute bout for females. Competitors may be expected to fight 6–8 times, depending on the number of competitors in the tournament. Competition for a weight category is completed over 1 day.	*Male (kg)* <60, <67, <75, <84, >84 *Female (kg)* <50, <55, <61, <68, >68	Usually 1–2 hours between weigh-in and start of competition.	Skill and reach are likely to play a more significant factor in performance compared to the effect of body weight per se.

Lightweight rowing	Race is over 2000 m course. Competition is over 7 days. Expected to compete every second day.	*Male* Average weight of crew shall not exceed 70 kg. No individual shall weigh more than 72.5 kg. A single sculler shall not weigh more than 72.5 kg.	Weigh-in is not less than 1 hour and not more than 2 hours before race start. Competitors are expected to weigh-in each day and for each event they are competing in.	Rowers are required to make weight on the morning of each heat, repecharge and final in a regatta, requiring a decision to either 'stay down' for the duration of the competition, or to make weight repeatedly for races. It may be best to optimize recovery following weigh-in and then return back to weight following each race. However, rowers should find the strategy that works best for them.
		Female Average weight of crew shall not exceed 57 kg. No individual shall weigh more than 59 kg. A single sculler shall not weigh more than 59 kg. *Coxswain* Minimum weight of a coxswain is 55 kg for men and 50 kg for women and mixed crews. To make this weight a coxswain may carry up to 10 kg of dead weight.		

(continued)

PRACTICE TIPS

TABLE 7.1 *(continued)*

SPORT	COMPETITION	WEIGHT CATEGORIES		WEIGH-IN PROCEDURES	PERSONAL INSIGHT
Judo	Each bout for senior competitors is 5 minutes (females and males). Competition is on 1 day only. Can be expected to contest 4–5 bouts during the competition. Minimum of 10 minutes between bouts.	*Male (kg)* <50 <60 <66 <73 <81 <90 <100 >100	*Female (kg)* <48 <52 <57 <63 <70 <78 >78	Weigh-in period is 1 hour on the morning of competition.	It is common for athletes to employ drastic short-term strategies in order to make weight, rather than adopt a long-term approach to making weight.
Taekwondo	Each bout involves 3 × 3-minute rounds with 1 minute between rounds. Competition is on 1 day only.	At Olympic Games there are four weight divisions whereas at World Championships there are eight.			The nature of the event requires aerobically based training. As a result athletes are able to cope with increased aerobic activity in the lead-up to competition in order to make weight.
	Can be expected to contest 5–8 bouts during the competition.	*Male* <58 kg 58–68 68–80 >80	*Female* <49 kg 49–57 57–67 >67		

- In most situations, qualification tournaments are scheduled months in advance of major international tournaments such as World Championships and Olympic Games. When discussing an ideal weight category for an athlete, account for the practicality of maintaining a weight category between these tournaments, particularly in light of potential growth spurts in adolescent athletes. Athletes are eligible to compete only in the weight category for which they originally qualified.
- The motivation of athletes to compete in a given weight category is determined primarily by their current weight. However, they may also be influenced by their likelihood of winning or qualifying in a given weight category or the expectations of coaches, parents or trainers. In some situations, the added pressures may lead to unrealistic weight category goals for these athletes. Objective anthropometric data such as height, weight and body-fat levels should remain important in determining the chosen weight category.
- For some athletes in weight-division sports, the primary purpose for seeking nutritional advice may be to gain weight. Lean athletes with low body-fat levels may recognize the difficulties associated with reducing weight to meet a lower division. However, they may also find themselves at a disadvantage in being at the lower end of the next weight category, and competing against heavier and stronger opponents. Gaining muscle mass and strength may help them to become competitive in this new division. Chapter 4 outlines strategies to increase lean body mass and strength in athletes.
- The harsh reality of weight-division sports is that athletes will usually endeavor to compete in a weight category below their usual weight. Many athletes practice dehydration techniques such as restricting fluids, exercising in sweat-promoting suits, and using saunas in order to make weight. Sometimes these practices start 7 days before competition starts, impairing exercise performance for the entire week leading up to competition. Against these practices, 24 hours of moderate dehydration (<3% body weight), mild food restriction and a low-residue diet on the day immediately prior to competition, combined with appropriate refueling and rehydration strategies between weigh-in and competition, might be less deleterious to health and competition performance. In sports where athletes weigh-in the evening before competition (like international amateur wrestling) or several hours before competition starts (like international amateur boxing), such a technique may be warranted.
- Some athletes find it valuable to consume a low-residue diet over 24 hours before weigh-in, including low-residue, low-fiber food and fluids combined with commercially available meal supplements and replacements. Replacement of normal dietary intake with a low-residue diet may achieve a 'weight' loss of 300–400 g by reducing the usual gastrointestinal contents.
- Many athletes increase their exercise load immediately prior to competition in order to facilitate sweat losses and promote weight loss. Athletes involved in weight-making sports that involve significant aerobic training (such as boxing) are more likely to cope with increased exercise loads immediately prior to competition. Some athletes who

PRACTICE TIPS

do not routinely include aerobic conditioning in their training may struggle to recover from increased exercise loads implemented to facilitate weight loss immediately prior to competition.

- Implementing appropriate nutritional strategies following weigh-in will facilitate recovery for athletes making weight. Use of sports drinks, liquid meal replacements and high-carbohydrate, low-fat foods may all enhance recovery following weigh-in. For athletes who weigh-in on consecutive days of a tournament, careful planning is imperative to maximize recovery and minimize the likelihood of body-weight fluctuations.
- As with any competition nutrition strategy, weight-making tactics should be practiced prior to competition. Athletes should undertake a simulated competition experience in training, with conditions including a suitable weight allowance and the weigh-in and recovery schedule of their sport. For example, amateur boxers might undertake a series of sparring drills mimicking competition demands every second day, with an allowance of 1 kg above their weight division. This practice would allow weight-making practices to be trialed and fine-tuned.

REFERENCES

Alderman BL, Landers DM, Carlson J, Scott JR. Factors related to rapid weight loss practices among international-style wrestlers. Med Sci Sports Exerc 2004;36:249–52.

American College of Sports Medicine. Position stand on weight loss in wrestlers. Med Sci Sports Exerc 1996;28:ix–xii.

American Medical Association. Hyperthermia and dehydration-related deaths associated with intentional rapid weight loss in three collegiate wrestlers—North Carolina, Wisconsin, and Michigan, November-December 1997. JAMA 1998;279:824–5.

Bartok C, Schoeller DA, Clark RR, Sullivan JC, Landry GL. The effect of dehydration on wrestling minimum weight assessment. Med Sci Sports Exerc 2004a;36:160–7.

Bartok C, Schoeller DA, Sullivan JC, Clark RR, Landry GL. Hydration testing in collegiate wrestlers undergoing hypertonic dehydration. Med Sci Sports Exerc 2004b;36:510–17.

Burge CM, Carey MF, Payne WR. Rowing performance, fluid balance, and metabolic function following dehydration and rehydration. Med Sci Sports Exerc 1993;25:1358–64.

Burke LM, Collier GR, Hargreaves M. Muscle glycogen storage following prolonged exercise: effect of the glycemic index of carbohydrate feedings. J Appl Physiol 1993;75:1019–23.

Choma CW, Sforzo GA, Keller BA. Impact of rapid weight loss on cognitive function in collegiate wrestlers. Med Sci Sports Exerc 1998;30:746–9.

Clark RR, Bartok C, Sullivan JC, Schoeller DA. Minimum weight prediction methods cross-validated by the four-component model. Med Sci Sports Exerc 2004;36:639–47.

Clark RR, Sullivan JC, Bartok C, Schoeller DA. Multicomponent cross-validation of minimum weight predictions for college wrestlers. Med Sci Sports Exerc 2003;35:342–7.

Costill DL, Sparks KE. Fluid replacement following thermal dehydration. J Appl Physiol 1973;34:299–303.

Fogelholm GM. Effects of bodyweight reduction on sports performance. Sports Med 1994;18:249–67.

Fogelholm GM, Koskinen R, Laakso J, Rankinen T, Ruokonen I. Gradual and rapid weight loss: effects on nutrition and performance in male athletes. Med Sci Sports Exerc 1993;25:371–7.

Greiwe JS, Staffey KS, Melrose DR, Narve MD, Knowlton RG. Effects of dehydration on isometric muscular strength and endurance. Med Sci Sports Exerc 1998;30:284–8.

Grinspoon S, Baum H, Kim V, Coggins C, Klibanski A. Decreased bone formation and increased mineral dissolution during acute fasting in young women. Clin Endocrinol Metabol 1995;80:3628–33.

Hickner RC, Horswill CA, Welker JM, Scott J, Roemmich JN, Costill DL. Test development for the study of physical performance in wrestlers following weight loss. Int J Sports Med 1991;12:557–62.

Horswill CA, Hickner RC, Scott JR, Costill DL, Gould D. Weight loss, dietary carbohydrate modifications, and high intensity physical performance. Med Sci Sports Exerc 1990a;22:470–7.

Horswill CA, Park SH, Roemmich JN. Changes in protein nutritional status of adolescent wrestlers. Med Sci Sports Exerc 1990b;22:599–604.

Horswill CA, Scott JR, Dick RW, Hayes J. Influence of rapid weight gain after the weigh-in on success in collegiate wrestlers. Med Sci Sports Exerc 1994;26:1290–4.

Iwao S, Mori K, Sato Y. Effects of meal frequency on body composition during weight control in boxers. Scand J Med Sci Sports 1996;6:265–72.

King MB, Mezey G. Eating behaviour of male racing jockeys. Psychol Med 1987;17:249–53.

Koutedakis Y, Pacy PJ, Quevedo RM, et al. The effects of two different periods of weight-reduction on selected performance parameters in elite lightweight oarswomen. Int J Sports Med 1994;15:472–7.

Marquart L, Sobal J. Weight loss beliefs, practices and support systems for high school wrestlers. J Adol Health 1994;15:410–15.

McCargar LJ, Simmons D, Craton N, Taunton JE, Brimingham CL. Physiological effects of weight cycling in female lightweight rowers. Can J Appl Physiol 1993;18:291–303.

McMurray RG, Proctor CR, Wilson WL. Effect of caloric deficit and dietary manipulation on aerobic and anaerobic exercise. Int J Sports Med 1991;12:167–72.

Melby CL, Schmidt WD, Corrigan D. Resting metabolic rate in weight-cycling collegiate wrestlers compared with physically active, non-cycling control subject. Am J Clin Nutr 1990;52:409–14.

Morris FL, Payne WR. Seasonal variations in the body composition of lightweight rowers. Br J Sports Med 1996;30:301–4.

National Collegiate Athletics Association, USA: NCAA News, 2 March 1998.

National Collegiate Athletics Association. USA: NCAA press release, 13 January 1998 and 13 April 1998.

Oppliger RA, Harms RD, Herrmann DE, Streich CM, Clark RR. The Wisconsin wrestling minimum weight project: a model for weight control among high school wrestlers. Med Sci Sports Exerc 1995;27:1220–4.

Oppliger RA, Landry GL, Foster WW, Lambrecht AC. Wisconsin minimum weight program reduces weight-cutting practices of high school wrestlers. Clin J Sport Med 1998;8:26–31.

Oppliger RA, Nelson Steen S, Scott JR. Weight loss practices of college wrestlers. Int J Sport Nutr Ex Metab 2003;13:29–46.

Pesce T, Walberg-Rankin J, Thomas E, Sebolt D, Wojcik J. Nutritional intake and status of high school and college wrestlers prior to and after competition Med Sci Sports Exerc 1996;28(Suppl):91S.

Roemmich JN, Sinning WE. Weight loss and wrestling training: effects on nutrition, growth, maturation, body composition, and strength. J Appl Physiol 1997;82:1751–9.

Scott, JR, Horswill CA, Dick RW. Acute weight gain in collegiate wrestlers following a tournament weigh-in. Med Sci Sports Exerc 1994;26:1181–5.

Shirreffs SM, Maughan RJ. Rehydration and recovery of fluid balance after exercise. Exerc Sport Sci Rev 2000;28:27–32.

Shirreffs SM, Taylor AJ, Leiper KB, Maughan RJ. Post-exercise rehydration in man: effects of volume consumed and drink sodium content. Med Sci Sports Exerc 1996;28:1260–71.

Slater GJ, Rice AJ, Sharpe K, Mujika I, Jenkins D, Hahn AG. Body-mass management of Australian lightweight rowers prior to and during competition. Med Sci Sports Exerc 2005;37:860–6.

Sossin K, Gizis F, Marquart LF, Sobal J. Nutrition beliefs, attitudes, and resource use of high school wrestling coaches. Int J Sport Nutr 1997;7:219–28.

Steen SN, McKinney S. Nutrition assessment of college wrestlers. Phys Sportsmed 1986;14:100–16.

Steen SN, Oppliger RA, Brownell KD. Metabolic effects of repeated weight loss and regain in adolescent wrestlers. J Am Med Assoc 1988;260:47–50.

Steen SN, Brownell KD. Patterns of weight loss and regain in wrestlers: has the tradition changed? Med Sci Sports Exerc 1990;22:762–8.

Stuempfle KJ, Drury DG. Comparison of 3 methods to assess urine specific gravity in collegiate wrestlers. J Athl Train 2003;38:315–19.

Talbott SM, Shapses SA. Fasting and energy intake influence bone turnover in lightweight male rowers. Int J Sport Nutr 1998;8:377–87.

Tarnopolsky MA, Cipriano N, Woodcroft C, Pulkkinen WJ, Robinson DC, Henderson JM, MacDougall JD. Effects of rapid weight loss and wrestling on muscle glycogen concentration. Clin J Sport Med 1996;6:78–84.

Theintz GE, Howald H, Weiss U, Sizonenko PC. Evidence for a reduction of growth potential in adolescent female gymnasts. J Pediatr 1993;122:306–33.

Tipton CM, Tcheng TK. Iowa wrestling study: weight loss in high school students. JAMA 1970;214:1269–74.

Utter A, Kang J. Acute weight gain and performance in college wrestlers. J Strength Cond Res 1998;12:157–60.

Viitasalo JT, Kyrolainen H, Bosco C, Alen M. Effects of rapid weight reduction on force production and vertical jumping height. Int J Sports Med 1987;8:281–5.

Walberg JL, Leidy MK, Sturgill DJ, Hinkle DE, Ritchey SJ, Sebolt D. Macronutrient content of a hypoenergy diet affects nitrogen retention and muscle function in weight lifters. Int J Sports Med 1988;9:261–6.

Walberg Rankin, J. Changing body weight and composition in athletes. In: Lamb D, Murray R, eds. Perspectives in exercise and sports medicine. Vol 11: Exercise, nutrition, and control of body weight. Carmel: Cooper Publishing Company, 1998:199–242.

Walberg-Rankin J, Hawkins CE, Fild DS, Sebolt DR. The effect of oral arginine during energy restriction in male weight trainers. J Strength Cond Res 1994;8:170–7.

Walberg Rankin J, Ocel JV, Craft LL. Effect of weight loss and refeeding diet composition on anaerobic performance in wrestlers. Med Sci Sports Exerc 1996;28:1292–9.

Yankanich J, Kenney WL, Fleck SJ, Kraemer WJ. Precompetition weight loss and changes in vascular fluid volume in NCAA Division I college wrestlers. J Strength Cond Res 1998;12:138–45.

CHAPTER 8

Disordered eating in athletes

KATHERINE A BEALS, LINDA HOUTKOOPER AND BELINDA DALTON

Introduction

8.1

'For women, eating disorders are like steroids for men. You'll get results, but you'll pay for it' (Noden 1994).

These words, spoken by a successful female cross-country runner recovering from anorexia, epitomize the pressure and rewards related to achieving the thin ideal held by participants in her sport.

To be sure, female athletes face considerable pressures to conform to the specific aesthetic requirements and/or performance demands of their sports. In some sports, a certain physique or a low body mass is considered to be essential for optimal performance, leading to the credo that athletes must be 'thin to win'. Such pressure placed upon a vulnerable athlete can lead to the development of disordered eating behaviors, which may eventually develop into a full-blown, clinical eating disorder.

Although current estimates indicate that 90% of clinical eating disorders occur in females, males are not immune to the pressures imposed by sport. A form of body dysmorphic disorder known as 'muscle dysmorphia' has recently been identified in male bodybuilders and weightlifters.

Unfortunately, disordered eating, like the use of performance-enhancing drugs, has become a part of the sport culture. Thus it is important that those who work with athletes have a clear understanding of the nature and scope of disordered eating, including the etiology, health consequences and methods for prevention, intervention and treatment.

This chapter will investigate the prevalence and suggested causes of the range of disordered eating and dysfunctional body image problems in athletes, extending the discussion begun in Chapters 6 and 7 about the challenges of achieving ideal body mass and physique in sport.

8.2 Disordered eating categories/classifications

Although frequently used interchangeably, the terms 'disordered eating' and 'eating disorder' are not one and the same. 'Disordered eating' is a general term used to describe the spectrum of abnormal and harmful eating behaviors that are used in a misguided attempt to lose weight and/or maintain a lower than normal body weight. On the other hand, the term 'eating disorder' refers to one of the three clinically diagnosable conditions—anorexia nervosa, bulimia nervosa, or eating disorders not otherwise specified (EDNOS)—recognized in the fourth edition of the American Psychiatric Association's *Diagnostic and statistical manual of mental disorders* (DSM-IV) (American Psychiatric Association 1994). To be diagnosed with a clinical eating disorder, an individual must meet a standard set of criteria as outlined in the DSM-IV and described in Tables 8.1–8.3.

TABLE 8.1 DIAGNOSTIC CRITERIA FOR ANOREXIA NERVOSA

A	Refusal to maintain body weight over a minimal normal weight for age and height (e.g. weight loss leading to maintenance of body weight 15% below that expected); or failure to make expected weight gain during period of growth, leading to body weight 15% below that expected.
B	Intense fear of gaining weight or becoming fat, even though underweight.
C	Disturbance in the way in which one's body weight, size or shape is experienced, undue influence of body weight or shape on self-evaluation, or denial of the seriousness of the current low body weight.
D	In postmenarcheal females, amenorrhea, that is, the absence of at least three consecutive menstrual cycles. (A woman is considered to have amenorrhea if her periods occur only following hormone administration.)
SPECIFY TYPE:	
	Restricting type: during the current episode of anorexia nervosa, the person has not regularly engaged in binge-eating or purging behavior (i.e. self-induced vomiting or the misuse of laxatives, diuretics, or enemas).
	Binge-eating/purging type: during the current episode of anorexia nervosa, the person has regularly engaged in binge-eating or purging behavior (i.e. self-induced vomiting or the misuse of laxatives, diuretics, or enemas).

Criterion A for the diagnosis of anorexia specifies that a body mass lower than 85% of what is considered normal for a person's age and height is the cut-off for a minimal body mass. This value for minimal body mass can be calculated from the Metropolitan Life Insurance table values for adults or growth charts used for children and youths up to 18 years of age. An alternative measure of minimal body mass used in the International Classification of Diseases-10 Diagnostic Criteria for Research is a body mass index (mass/height^2) of 17.5 kg/m^2 (American Psychiatric Association 1994). Restriction of food intake is the primary means of weight loss for the restricting type of anorexia nervosa. Individuals may start dieting by excluding foods perceived to be high in kilojoules and/or fat, but most eventually follow a very restricted diet that is often limited to only a few foods (American Psychiatric Association 1994). The binge-eating/purging type of anorexia nervosa is distinguished by regular use of binge-eating and purging behaviors such as self-induced vomiting to achieve weight loss (American Psychiatric Association 1994).

Criterion B specifies that the individual with this eating disorder exhibits intense fear of gaining weight or becoming fat, and this fear is not alleviated by weight loss. In fact, distress about weight gain will often increase as body mass continues to decrease (American Psychiatric Association 1994).

The experience and significance of body mass and shape are distorted in individuals with this disorder **(Criterion C)**. While some individuals feel globally overweight, others realize that they are thin, but are still concerned that parts of their body are too fat. The self-esteem of individuals with anorexia is highly dependent on their body mass and shape, and they are obsessive about weighing themselves and measuring body parts. Weight loss is viewed as a sign of an impressive achievement of self-control, whereas weight gain is perceived as an unacceptable failure of self-control. Although some individuals with this disorder may acknowledge being thin, they typically deny the serious health implications of their condition.

Criterion D stipulates that amenorrhea is present in postmenarcheal females, and menarche is delayed in prepubertal females (American Psychiatric Association 1994). In postmenarcheal females with this disorder, amenorrhea is related to abnormally low levels of estrogen secretion that result from a decreased secretion of follicle-stimulating hormone and luteinizing hormone.

Source: Adapted from American Psychiatric Association 1994

TABLE 8.2 DIAGNOSTIC CRITERIA FOR BULIMIA NERVOSA	
A	Recurrent episodes of binge-eating. An episode of binge-eating is characterized by both of the following:
	1. eating, in a discrete period of time (e.g. within any 2-hour period), an amount of food that is definitely larger than most people would eat during a similar period of time and under similar circumstances
	2. a sense of lack of control over eating during the episode (e.g. a feeling that one cannot stop eating or control what or how much one is eating)
B	Recurrent, inappropriate, compensatory behavior in order to prevent weight gain, such as self-induced vomiting; misuse of laxatives, diuretics, enemas or other medications; fasting; or excessive exercise.
C	The binge-eating and inappropriate compensatory behaviors both occur, on average, at least twice a week for 3 months.
D	Self-evaluation is unduly influenced by body shape and weight.
E	The disturbance does not occur exclusively during episodes of anorexia nervosa.
SPECIFIC TYPE:	
Purging type: during the current episode of bulimia nervosa, the person has regularly engaged in self-induced vomiting or the misuse of laxatives, diuretics or enemas.	
Non-purging type: during the current episode of bulimia nervosa, the person has used other inappropriate compensatory behaviors, such as fasting or excessive exercise, but has not regularly engaged in self-induced vomiting or the misuse of laxatives, diuretics, or enemas.	

Source: Adapted from American Psychiatric Association 1994

TABLE 8.3 DIAGNOSTIC CRITERIA FOR EATING DISORDER NOT OTHERWISE SPECIFIED	
This category is for disorders of eating that do not meet the criteria for any specific eating disorder. Examples include:	
A	For females, all of the criteria for anorexia nervosa are met except that the individual has regular menses.
B	All of the criteria for anorexia nervosa are met except that, despite significant weight loss, the individual's current weight is in the normal range.
C	All of the criteria for bulimia nervosa are met except that the binge-eating and inappropriate compensatory mechanisms occur at a frequency of less than twice a week or for less than 3 months.
D	The regular use of inappropriate compensatory behavior by an individual of normal body weight after eating small amounts of food (e.g. self-induced vomiting after the consumption of two cookies).
E	Repeatedly chewing and spitting out, but not swallowing, large amounts of food.
F	Binge-eating disorder: recurrent episodes of binge-eating in the absence of the regular use of inappropriate compensatory behaviors characteristic of bulimia nervosa.

Source: American Psychiatric Association 1994

The clinical eating disorders 8.3

According to the DSM-IV, the clinical eating disorders—anorexia nervosa, bulimia nervosa and EDNOS—are characterized by *severe* disturbances in eating behavior and body image (American Psychiatric Association 1994). It must be emphasized that the clinical eating disorders are psychiatric conditions and, as such, they go beyond simple body weight/shape dissatisfaction and involve more than just abnormal eating patterns and pathogenic weight-control behaviors. Individuals with clinical eating disorders often experience co-morbid psychological conditions, such as obsessive–compulsive disorder, depression and anxiety disorder (Fairburn & Brownell 2001). In addition, they often display intense feelings of insecurity, personal ineffectiveness and worthlessness, have trouble identifying and displaying emotions, and have an underdeveloped or limited sense of identity. Common personality traits seen in people who develop eating disorders, such as perfectionism, obsessiveness, hypervigilance, discipline and achievement-orientation, are also traits that contribute to athletic success.

Athletes with clinical eating disorders resemble their non-athlete counterparts in many ways. They are extremely dissatisfied with their body weight/shape, are obsessed with the desire to be thin, and are willing to go to any lengths (restrictive eating/starvation or binging and purging) in an attempt to achieve their illusive body weight ideal. However, unlike non-athletes with eating disorders, who generally view thinness as the only goal, athletes with eating disorders strive for thinness *and* the improvement in performance that they believe will accompany it. This is particularly (although not exclusively) true for female athletes, especially those participating in sports that emphasize leanness. Although starving and/or bingeing and purging in the name of improved performance may seem counterproductive to the objective eye, the athlete with anorexia and/or bulimia nervosa is not logical when it comes to body weight and often has come to embrace (and embody) the notion that thinner is better (faster, stronger, more pleasing to the judges, and so on), no matter how it is achieved.

8.4 Subclinical eating disorders

The term 'subclinical eating disorder' has frequently been used by researchers and practitioners to describe individuals, both athletes and non-athletes, who present with considerable eating pathology and body weight concerns, but do not demonstrate significant psychopathology and/or fail to meet all of the DSM-IV (American Psychiatric Association 1994) criteria for anorexia nervosa, bulimia nervosa or EDNOS (Bunnell et al. 1990; Beals & Manore 1994, 1999, 2000; Williamson et al. 1995). Indeed, many athletes who report using pathogenic weight-control methods (such as laxatives, diet pills and excessive exercise) do not technically meet the criteria for a clinical eating disorder. Conversely, athletes may use none of these methods, but still have an obvious eating disorder. A more recently recognized eating disorder, binge-eating disorder (BED) also falls into the category of EDNOS (refer Table 8.3).

For example, one collegiate field hockey player reported routinely eating a daily energy intake of ~1200 kcal (~5 MJ) while training for 2–3 hours every day, and 'working out' at the gym regularly in addition to her regular training regimen. She ate similar foods every day and severely limited her fat intake (no more than 20 g/d). Occasionally she would 'binge' by eating a forbidden food (such as a piece of cake or an order of French fries) and she would have to exercise afterward to 'burn off' what she had eaten and restrict her intake more strictly the following day. Although she was openly dissatisfied with her body weight and shape, she did not display any significant psychological disturbance.

This athlete definitely displays disordered eating behaviors; however, she does not meet the diagnostic criteria for either anorexia nervosa or bulimia nervosa. In fact, depending on the context of the evaluation, she might not even meet the criteria necessary for a diagnosis of EDNOS. Nonetheless, her behaviors are not 'normal'. And, more importantly, they have the capacity to have a negative impact on her performance as well as her health.

A prominent researcher in the area of eating disorders in athletes, Jorunn Sundgot-Borgen, has developed a set of criteria to describe a subclinical variant of anorexia nervosa in athletes, which she refers to as 'anorexia athletica' (Sundgot-Borgen 1993). The essential feature of anorexia athletica is an intense fear of gaining weight or becoming fat, even though the individual weighs 5% less than the expected normal weight for age and height. Weight loss is achieved by restriction of food intake, extensive compulsive exercise, or both (Sundgot-Borgen 1993). Frequently the athletes also report bingeing, self-induced vomiting or the use of laxatives or diuretics. It should be noted that the criteria for anorexia athletica were derived largely from a set of criteria used to describe a disorder referred to as 'fear-of-obesity' observed in a small sample of non-athletic adolescents (Pugliese et al. 1983).

Prevalence of disordered eating among athletes 8.5

Because of heightened body awareness and pressures in some sports to maintain a low body weight and/or body-fat level, there has been speculation that an increased risk of eating disorders may occur. Athletes participating in certain sports are considered to be particularly vulnerable. These sports, often referred to as 'thin-build' or 'weight-dependent' sports, can be categorized into three groups: (1) 'aesthetic sports' such as diving, figure skating, gymnastics and synchronized swimming; (2) sports in which low body mass and body-fat levels are considered a physical or biomechanical advantage, such as distance running, road cycling and triathlon; and (3) sports that require weight categories for competition, such as lightweight rowing, weightlifting and wrestling (Beals 2004).

Current estimates of the prevalence of disordered eating among athletes are highly variable, ranging from less than 1% to as high as 62% in female athletes (Brownell & Rodin 1992; Otis et al. 1997; Byrne & McLean 2001), and between 0% and 57% in male athletes (Andersen 1992; Byrne & McLean 2001). This wide range of estimates is due to differences in the screening instruments/assessment tools used, definitions of eating disorders employed and the athlete populations studied.

Most studies examining the prevalence of disordered eating among athletes have utilized one of the many self-report instruments currently available (e.g. Eating Attitudes Test, Eating Disorder Inventory, Three-Factor-Eating Questionnaire). Not only do self-report questionnaires probably under estimate disordered eating prevalence, but the variety of different measures used in these studies render comparisons between studies difficult and inconsistencies in prevalence estimates more likely. Similarly, studies have varied widely in their definitions of the term 'eating disorder'. While some studies adhered to the strict DSM-IV criteria, most used the clinical term 'eating disorder' to characterize a wide range of abnormal eating behaviors that would be more appropriately labeled 'disordered eating'. Of course, using more strict criteria will result in lower prevalence estimates. Finally, studies have varied greatly in the sample populations used, including the type of athlete (e.g. collegiate versus high school athlete, elite athlete versus recreational athlete versus 'physically active' individual) as well as the number of sports studied. In fact, only four studies have used large (n >400), heterogeneous samples of athletes and validated measures of disordered eating (Sundgot-Borgen 1993; Johnson et al. 1999; Beals Manore 2002; Sundgot-Borgen & Torstveit 2004) (see Table 8.4). The remainder had inadequate sample sizes, examined single sports or used incorrect measures of disordered eating, all of which can bias prevalence estimates.

TABLE 8.4 SUMMARY OF POST-1990 STUDIES EXAMINING THE PREVALENCE OF DISORDERED EATING IN ATHLETES PARTICIPATING IN A RANGE OF SPORTS

STUDY	SAMPLE	INSTRUMENT	EATING DISORDER PREVALENCE
Sundgot-Borgen and Torstveit 2004	660 Norwegian elite female athletes	A two-stage screening process including a questionnaire developed by the authors, including subscales of the EDI, weight history, and self-reported history of eating disorders (stage 1) followed by a clinical interview using the EDE (stage 2).	21% ($n = 121$) of the female athletes were classified 'at risk' after the initial screening. Results of the clinical interview indicated that 2% met the criteria for anorexia nervosa, 6% for bulimia nervosa, 8% for eating disorders not otherwise specified (EDNOS) and 4% for anorexia athletica.
Beals and Manore 2002	425 female collegiate athletes	EAT-26 and EDI-BD	3.3% and 2.4% of the athletes self-reported a diagnosis of clinical anorexia and bulimia nervosa, respectively; 15% and 31.5% of the athletes scored above the designated cut-off scores on the EAT-26 and EDI-BD, respectively.
Johnson et al. 1999	562 female collegiate athletes	EDI-2 and questionnaire developed by the authors using DSM-IV criteria	None of the athletes met the DSM-IV criteria for anorexia nervosa, while 1.1% met the criteria for bulimia nervosa. 1.96% and 5.5% of the athletes believed they might have anorexia nervosa and bulimia nervosa, respectively. Subclinical anorexia and bulimia were identified in 2.9% and 9.2% of the women, respectively. 35–38% demonstrated disordered eating behaviors (e.g. binge-eating, vomiting, laxatives, diuretics, diet pills, elevated Drive for Thinness (EDI-DT) subscale score, elevated Body Dissatisfaction score).
Sundgot-Borgen 1993	522 Norwegian elite female athletes	EDI and in-depth interview developed by the author based on DSM-III criteria	1.3%, 8.0% and 8.2% were diagnosed with anorexia nervosa, bulimia nervosa and anorexia athletica, respectively.

EAT-26 = Eating Attitudes Test (Garner et al. 1982); EDI = Eating Disorder Inventory (Garner et al. 1983); EDI-BD = Body Dissatisfaction subscale (Garner et al. 1983); EDI-DT = Drive for Thinness subscale (Garner et al. 1983); EDI-2 = Eating Disorder Inventory-2 (Garner 1991); DSM-IV = *Diagnostic and statistical manual of psychiatric disorders IV* (American Psychiatric Association 1994); EDE = Eating Disorder Examination (Fairburn & Cooper 1993).

Source: Adapted from Beals 2004

8.6 Etiology of disordered eating among athletes

While not all athletes who go on a 'diet' will develop disordered eating, most athletes who have suffered from an eating disorder report that a period of dieting preceded the onset of their disorder. Indeed, according to Andersen (1990), eating disorders typically begin as a voluntary restriction of food intake that progresses by stages in predisposed individuals into increasingly pathogenic eating and weight-control behaviors. What constitutes an individual's 'predisposition' is believed to be a complex interaction between sociocultural, demographic, environmental, biological, psychological and behavioral factors. In addition, research has identified some sport-specific risk factors for the development of disordered eating among athletes (Sundgot-Borgen 1994a).

Sociocultural factors 8.7

Much has been written about the sociocultural pressures placed on women today to be thin and the impact this has had on the incidence of disordered eating. In most modern, developed countries, being thin is equated with beauty, as well as several other positive attributes, including goodness, success and power (Rodin & Larson 1992; Rodin 1993). This belief is both reinforced and perpetuated by the images presented in movies, television and magazines (Harrison & Cantor 1997; Field et al. 1999). Not surprisingly, disordered eating is more prevalent in developed countries and appears to be influenced by the media, leading many to infer an association between societal pressures and disordered eating behaviors.

Female athletes may face even more pressure than non-athletes to achieve or maintain a particular body weight or shape (Sundgot-Borgen 1994b). Indeed, athletes must not only meet the current body-weight ideals held by society in general, but also conform to the specific aesthetic and performance demands of their sport. This pressure may be particularly high for athletes in thin-build sports or activities that require a low body weight or lean physique, such as dance (especially ballet), gymnastics, distance running, triathlon, swimming, diving, figure skating, cheerleading, wrestling and lightweight rowing. This pressure can be particularly strong (rendering the development of an eating disorder much more likely) when there is a discrepancy between the athlete's actual body weight and the perceived ideal body weight for the athlete's particular sport (Brownell & Rodin 1992). For example, a naturally larger athlete who wishes to compete in gymnastics or a naturally heavier wrestler who is trying to compete in a lower weight class may feel especially strong pressure to alter their body weight.

Although women experience the brunt of societal pressure to be thin, men are reacting to body weight and shape pressures with increasing frequency. Little formal research has been done, but indirect evidence and anecdotal reports suggest that men, particularly those engaged in athletics or who are regularly physically active, are becoming increasingly concerned and subsequently dissatisfied with their bodies (Pope et al. 2000). For example, a group of researchers have described a form of body image disturbance in male bodybuilders and weightlifters that they refer to as 'muscle dysmorphia'. Once referred to as 'reverse anorexia' (Pope et al. 1993), muscle dysmorphia is characterized by an inordinate preoccupation and dissatisfaction with body size and muscularity and a perception of being small and frail when reality indicates the exact opposite.

Psychosocial factors 8.8

Family discord, parental indifference and over-protective parenting have all been shown to increase the risk of eating disorders. A family history of depression, substance abuse and other psychological issues may also increase risk. Several studies indicate that a history of sexual abuse and other stressful life events (eg. bullying, grief and loss) are more common among individuals with eating disorders (Striegel-Moore & Bulik 2007).

Such family environments and life events can cause severe psychological and emotional distress, undermine the development of self-esteem and lead to inadequate coping skills, all of which may increase the risk that an eating disorder might develop. For example, an athlete may feel overwhelmed or out of control as a result of an injury, a particularly poor performance or the excessive demands of a coach. Because of a dysfunctional family environment, the athlete may have never developed the coping skills necessary to handle these problems, and thus the athlete concentrates on something that can be managed, such as body weight.

8.9 Biological factors

An inherited tendency appears to exist: there is an increased risk of anorexia nervosa and bulimia nervosa among first-degree biological relatives or individuals with these disorders (American Psychiatric Association 1994). Furthermore, studies of anorexia nervosa in twins have reported concordance rates for identical twins to be significantly higher than those for fraternal twins (Holland et al. 1988).

A biological–behavioral model of activity-based anorexia nervosa was proposed in a series of studies by Epling and colleagues (1983) and Epling and Pierce (1988). These researchers theorized that dieting and exercising initiate the anorexic cycle and claimed that as many as 75% of the cases of anorexia nervosa are exercise-induced. The theory holds that strenuous exercise suppresses appetite, which leads to a decrease in food intake and subsequent reduction in body weight. It should be noted that this research was conducted with rats and has not been replicated in humans (O'Connor & Smith 1999). Additional biological factors that have been implicated in the development of disordered eating include gender (it is estimated that females outnumber males 10 to 1), early onset of menarche (younger than age 12 years) and propensity towards obesity (American Psychiatric Association 1994; Fairburn et al. 1997).

8.10 Psychological and behavioral factors

Personality traits contribute largely to the psychological predisposition for disordered eating. Some of the general personality traits that are characteristic of athletes are similar to those manifested by patients with eating disorders (Garfinkel et al. 1987). For example, both groups tend to be goal-oriented, achievement-driven, independent, persistent, and tolerant of pain and discomfort. In addition, it has been hypothesized that athletes, particularly female athletes, may be more vulnerable to eating disorders than the general female population because of additional stressors associated with the fitness or athletic environment (Sundgot-Borgen 1994b).

8.11 Sport-specific factors

Research indicates that certain inherent pressures and/or demands of the sport setting may serve to 'trigger' the development of an eating disorder in psychologically susceptible athletes (Sundgot-Borgen 1994a; Williamson et al. 1995). In a study investigating risk and trigger factors for the development of eating disorders, Sundgot-Borgen (1994a) found that female athletes suffering from eating disorders often began sport-specific training and dieting at significantly earlier ages than athletes without eating disorders. In addition, prolonged periods of dieting, frequent weight fluctuations, sudden increases in training volume, or traumatic life events such as an injury or a change of coach tended to trigger the development of eating disorders.

Some researchers have proposed that specific sports or physical activities (those that emphasize leanness or require large training volumes) may 'attract' individuals with eating disorders, particularly anorexia nervosa, because these activities provide a setting in which individuals can use or abuse exercise to expend extra energy and hide or justify their abnormal eating and dieting behaviors (Sacks 1990; Sundgot-Borgen 1998). Moreover, the stereotypical standards of body shape in women's sports and physical activities that emphasize leanness make it difficult for observers to notice when an individual has lost too much weight. These common and accepted low weight standards may help active women with disordered eating hide and/or justify their problem and delay intervention (Sundgot-Borgen 1994a; Sacks 1990).

Performance and health consequences of disordered eating 8.12

The effects of disordered eating on an athlete's health and performance can be surprisingly variable, although they are generally reflective of the severity of the disorder as well as how long it has persisted. Some athletes may be able to engage in disordered eating behaviors for extended periods of time with few long-term negative effects (Thompson & Sherman 1993). For most, however, it is simply a matter of time before the food restriction, weight loss and purging practices negatively affect their physical performance and, more importantly, their physical and emotional health.

Health consequences 8.13

The health consequences associated with disordered eating are directly related to the methods of weight control used. Thus the athlete who severely restricts or chronically restricts energy intake will probably suffer macro- and micronutrient deficiencies, anemia, chronic fatigue and an increased risk of infections, injury and/or illnesses (Manore 1996; Beals & Manore 1998). Additional health effects associated with chronic or severe energy restriction and the resulting weight loss are described in more detail in Chapters 6 and 7 and include decreased basal metabolic rate, cardiovascular and gastrointestinal disorders, depression, menstrual dysfunction and decreased bone mineral density (BMD) (Eichner 1992).

Athletes who engage in bingeing and purging often suffer many of the same health consequences as those with anorexia nervosa (e.g. nutrient deficiencies, chronic fatigue, endocrine abnormalities and BMD reductions), with the added complications that accompany the bingeing and purging behaviors.

Bingeing frequently causes gastric distension that, in rare cases, can result in gastric necrosis and even rupture (Pomeroy & Mitchell 1992). Esophageal reflux and subsequent chronic throat irritation are also common and may increase the risk for esophageal cancer (Carney & Andersen 1996).

Purging via diuretics, laxatives, enemas or self-induced vomiting significantly increases an athlete's risk for dehydration (Carney & Andersen 1996). Electrolyte imbalances, particularly hypokalemia (low blood potassium levels) are also common in individuals who engage in purging behaviors and can have debilitating effects on health (Carney & Andersen 1996). Purging can also lead to dangerous disruptions in the body's acid-base balance and life-threatening alterations in the body's pH. Self-induced vomiting typically results in an increase in serum bicarbonate levels and thus leads to metabolic alkalosis (increase in blood pH). On the other hand, individuals who abuse laxatives are more likely to develop metabolic acidosis (decrease in blood pH) secondary to loss of bicarbonate in the stool (Carney & Anderson 1996). Purging via excessive exercise increases the athlete's risk for over-training syndrome and overuse injuries (Beals 2004).

Cardiovascular complications associated with bingeing and purging are usually secondary to the electrolyte imbalances induced by purging. As described earlier, hypokalemia can result in potentially life-threatening cardiac arrhythmias. In addition, individuals who abuse ipecac may have myocarditis (inflammation of the middle layer of the heart muscle) and various cardiomyopathies (Carney & Anderson 1996). The gastrointestinal complications associated with purging depend on the purging methods used and can include throat and mouth ulcers, dental caries, abdominal cramping, diarrhea and hemorrhoids (Pomeroy & Mitchell 1992).

8.14 Effects on performance

Surprisingly, anecdotal evidence (reports from coaches and personal accounts by athletes with disordered eating) suggests that during the early stages of disordered eating some athletes may actually experience an initial, albeit short-lived, improvement in performance (Beals 2004). The reasons for this transient performance enhancement are not completely understood, but are hypothesized to be related to the initial physiological and psychological effects of starvation and purging (Beals 2004).

Both starvation and purging are physiological stressors and, as such, produce an up-regulation of the hypothalamic–pituitary–adrenal axis (the 'fight-or-flight response') and an increase in the adrenal hormones cortisol, epinephrine and norepinephrine. These hormones have a stimulatory effect on the central nervous system that can mask fatigue and evoke feelings of euphoria in the eating-disordered athlete (Beals 2004). In addition, the initial decrease in body weight (particularly before there is a significant decrease in muscle mass) may induce a transient increase in relative maximal oxygen uptake per kilogram of body weight ($VO_{2\ max}$) (Ingjer & Sundgot-Borgen 1991) (see Chapter 6). Moreover, with weight loss, athletes may feel lighter, which may afford them a psychological boost, particularly if they believe that lighter is always better in terms of performance.

Unfortunately, the eating-disordered athlete often equates these temporary performance improvements with the disordered eating behaviors, causing the behaviors to become more entrenched and significantly more difficult to treat. Thus it must be emphasized to the athlete that any initial improvements in performance are transient. Eventually, the energy deficiencies and purging behaviors will cause the body to break down and performance will suffer.

The Female Athlete Triad

8.15

The Female Athlete Triad (Triad) was originally conceived to describe a combination of three disorders including disordered eating, amenorrhea and osteoporosis (Otis et al.1997). It has since become more broadly defined as energy availability, menstrual function and bone strength to represent the spectrum of potential disorders within each category (Nattiv et al. 2007). Regardless of the definitions used, the development of the Triad is hypothesized to follow a characteristic progression. In an attempt to improve performance and/or meet the aesthetic demands of her sport, the female athlete begins to diet. For a variety of reasons (see section 8.6), the dieting becomes increasingly severe and eventually progresses to disordered eating. The energy imbalance and hormonal alterations resulting from the disordered eating lead to menstrual dysfunction, which eventually results in decreased BMD and possibly premature osteoporosis (Nattiv et al. 2007).

Not only is the Triad born out of disordered eating and the resulting energy imbalance as illustrated by the etiological pattern above, but it carries significant health and performance implications for the female athlete. Aside from the health and performance risks associated with disordered eating described above, both menstrual dysfunction and low BMD carry their own unique health complications for the athlete.

The health consequences of menstrual dysfunction are well documented and include infertility and other reproductive problems, decreased immune function and an increase in cardiovascular risk factors. In addition, the altered hormonal environment associated with menstrual dysfunction is a risk factor for the development of impaired bone health and osteoporosis. Osteoporosis in the young female athlete refers to inadequate bone formation and premature bone loss, resulting in low BMD and increased risk of fracture (Van de Loo & Johnson 1995). Studies conducted with female athletes have shown that premature osteoporosis may occur as a result of menstrual dysfunction and may be partially irreversible, despite resumption of menses, estrogen replacement or calcium supplementation (Cann et al. 1984; Drinkwater et al. 1986, 1990; Rencken et al. 1996). An increase in the risk for stress fractures has been reported in athletes with amenorrhea, and this appears to be related to low BMD (Van de Loo & Johnson 1995). This issue is discussed in greater detail in the commentary at the end of this chapter.

Prevention of disordered eating among athletes

8.16

The course and outcome for those with eating disorders are highly variable. Some individuals fully recover after a single bout of anorexia nervosa, others exhibit a fluctuating pattern of weight gain followed by a relapse, and others experience a chronically deteriorating course of the illness over many years. In some cases, hospitalization is required to help restore weight and to manage fluid and electrolyte imbalances. The long-term consequences of intractable anorexia nervosa can be fatal. In the treated, non-athlete population, anorexia nervosa has a 10–18% mortality rate (Ratnasuriya et al. 1991), with death most commonly resulting from starvation, suicide or electrolyte imbalance. The long-term outcome of bulimia nervosa is unknown (American Psychiatric Association 1994). Even in those who have recovered from eating disorders, health problems can persist (Beals 2004). For these reasons then, efforts to combat disordered eating in athletes should focus on prevention.

The prevention of disordered eating involves targeting the risk factors for disordered eating and then trying to eliminate or at the very least modify them. As was previously described, many of the factors that predispose an athlete to disordered eating (such as biological and personality factors, and family environment) are outside of the direct control of coaches, athletic support staff or health professionals. Thus prevention efforts should focus on those predisposing factors that can be controlled, including the overemphasis on body weight and thinness, unrealistic body weight ideals, unhealthy eating and weight-control practices, and stigmatization of disordered eating, which permeate the athletic environment.

8.17 De-emphasize weight and body composition

One of the most widely held misconceptions that continues to permeate the athletic environment is that reducing body weight invariably leads to improved performance. While no one would argue that an extreme or unhealthy excess of body fat will negatively impact performance, that does not mean that a lower body weight is always more advantageous (Wilmore 1992), particularly if that lower body weight is achieved via severe or pathogenic weight-loss methods (see Chapter 7). Moreover, the stress of the 'evaluation process' involved in body weight and composition measurements, placed upon a vulnerable athlete, can be enough to send them into a tailspin of disordered eating behaviors.

There are several ways that coaches, trainers and athletic staff can help de-emphasize body weight and composition among their athletes. The most obvious is to simply eliminate such measurements altogether (Carson & Bridges 2001). Unfortunately, in many sport settings eliminating anthropometric assessments may not be a viable or even the most appropriate solution. In such cases, measurements should be taken by a qualified health professional not connected with the team (not the coach or trainer) who can thoughtfully and objectively interpret and confidentially communicate the results to each individual athlete. In addition, the athletes as well as the coaches and trainers need to be educated as to the limitations and potential errors in the measurements.

8.18 Dispel nutrition myths and promote healthy eating behaviors

Athletes generally suffer from a dearth of nutrition knowledge, particularly as it relates to athletic performance. Moreover, much of the knowledge they do possess is derived from peers and popular fitness and/or sports magazines (Chapman et al. 1997; Jacobson et al. 2001). Thus nutrition education should be provided to all athletes, focusing on dispelling the myths and misconceptions about dieting and the impact of these factors on athletic performance. Equally important is providing accurate and appropriate nutritional information and dietary guidelines to promote optimal health and athletic performance.

To successfully promote healthy eating behaviors among athletes, nutrition education and information must be reinforced by practice. All those involved in the management of athletes must therefore practice what they preach. Coaches are probably in the best position to reinforce nutrition education messages by bringing healthy foods to practice, choosing healthy restaurants before and after competitions and, of course, eating healthily themselves.

Destigmatize eating disorders 8.19

Coaches, trainers, and other athletic personnel can help reduce the stigma of disordered eating by creating an atmosphere in which athletes feel comfortable discussing their concerns about body image, eating and weight control. Athletic personnel should strive to promote understanding and foster trust between themselves and their athletes. The goal is to create an atmosphere in which athletes feel comfortable confiding an eating problem. In short, coaches, trainers and athletic administrators must make it clear that they place the athletes' health and wellbeing ahead of athletic performance.

Management of disordered eating among athletes 8.20

Management of disordered eating in athletes has been described as encompassing the range of intervention tactics beginning with identification, following with referral and treatment, and concluding with post-treatment follow-up (Thompson & Sherman 1993). Each of these will be described briefly below.

Identification 8.21

The shame and secrecy that often shrouds disordered eating makes identifying those who suffer from it often difficult at best. It is rare that an athlete will willingly admit to a disorder and agree to treatment. Thus it is up to others to recognize the signs and symptoms of disordered eating and initiate intervention.

There are a number of different assessment tools that have been developed to screen for disordered eating. Some of the most common are described in Table 8.5 overleaf. It is important to recognize that none of the instruments listed in Table 8.5 were originally designed to make clinical diagnoses of eating disorders. Rather, they were developed for use in non-clinical settings as screening devices to assess attitudes and behaviors exhibited by individuals who met the clinical diagnoses of anorexia nervosa or bulimia nervosa (Leon 1991). In addition, the self-report nature of the questionnaires renders them susceptible to untruthful or biased responses. Finally, most are of questionable use with athletes as they have not been sufficiently validated in athletic populations.

Because of the limitations imposed by self-report questionnaires, many researchers and practitioners have suggested that interviewing athletes may be a more accurate and effective method of identifying disordered eating behaviors (Sundgot-Borgen 1993). As was the case with screening tools, there are a number of structured interviews available for identifying disordered eating. The most commonly used is the Eating Disorder Examination (EDE) (Cooper & Fairburn 1987; Fairburn & Cooper 1993). The EDE is a semi-structured interview for assessing the symptoms associated with anorexia and bulimia nervosa. It contains four subscales: (1) dietary restraint; (2) eating concern; (3) shape concern; and (4) weight concern. The items derived from the interview are converted into twenty-three symptom ratings made by the interviewer. Although it has been used to identify disordered eating in athletes (Sundgot-Borgen 1993; Beals & Manore 2000) it has not been formally validated in an athlete population. Moreover, it requires a qualified professional to conduct the interview and interpret the results.

TABLE 8.5 COMMON SELF-REPORT SURVEYS AND QUESTIONNAIRES FOR IDENTIFYING DISORDERED EATING

INSTRUMENT	DESCRIPTION
Bulimia Test-Revised (BULIT-R) (Thelen et al. 1991)	A 28-item multiple-choice questionnaire designed to assess the severity of symptoms and behaviors associated with bulimia nervosa (e.g. weight preoccupation and bingeing and purging frequency). Respondents rate each item on a five-point Likert scale in which higher scores are more indicative of bulimia nervosa.
Eating Attitudes Test, 40 items (EAT-40) (Garner & Garfinkel 1979)	A 40-item inventory designed to assess the thoughts, feelings and behaviors associated with anorexia nervosa. Items are scored on a six-point Likert scale ranging from *never* to *always*. A score of ≥30 indicates risk of anorexia nervosa.
Eating Attitudes Test, 26 items (EAT-26) (Garner et al. 1982)	A shortened (26-item) version of the EAT-40 that also identifies thoughts, feelings and behaviors associated with anorexia nervosa. Uses a 6-point Likert scale ranging from *rarely* to *always*. A score of ≥20 indicates risk of anorexia nervosa.
Eating Disorder Inventory (EDI) (Garner et al. 1983)	A 64-item questionnaire with eight subscales. The first three subscales (Drive for Thinness, Bulimia and Body Dissatisfaction) assess behaviors regarding body image, eating and weight-control practices. The remaining five subscales (Interpersonal Distrust, Perfectionism, Interoceptive Awareness, Maturity Fears and Ineffectiveness) assess the various psychological disturbances characteristic of those with clinical eating disorders. Items are answered using a six-point Likert scale ranging from *always* to *never*.
Eating Disorder Inventory-2 (EDI-2) (Garner 1991)	A 91-item multidimensional inventory designed to assess the symptoms of anorexia nervosa and bulimia nervosa. The EDI-2 contains the same eight subscales as the EDI and adds three additional subscales (27 more items): Asceticism, Impulse Regulation and Social Insecurity. Items are answered using a six-point Likert scale ranging from *always* to *never*.
Three-Factor Eating Questionnaire (TFEQ) (Stunkard 1981)	A 58-item true/false and multiple-choice questionnaire that measures the tendency towards voluntary and excessive restriction of food intake as a means of controlling body weight. The questionnaire contains three subscales: Restrained Eating (e.g. 'I often stop eating when I am not full as a conscious means of controlling my weight'), Tendency towards Disinhibition (e.g. 'When I feel lonely, I console myself by eating') and Perceived Hunger (e.g. 'I am always hungry enough to eat at any time').

Source: Adapted from Beals 2004

Sometimes simply observing the athlete's behavior can be the most simple and effective method for identifying disordered eating behaviors. Individuals who have daily contact with athletes (e.g. coaches, trainers, team-mates, family, and friends) are in the best position to recognize behaviors that are consistent with disordered eating. Table 8.6 lists some of the common warning signs and symptoms. Research supports early identification and intervention for better outcomes and shorter timeframes for recovery from an eating disorder.

8.22 Referral and treatment

The preservation of the athlete's health and mental wellbeing is the first goal of treatment (Nattiv & Lynch 1994). A multidisciplinary team involving people experienced in the

TABLE 8.6 WARNING SIGNS FOR EATING DISORDERS

WARNING SIGNS FOR ANOREXIA NERVOSA
• Dramatic weight loss
• A preoccupation with food, calories and weight
• Wearing baggy or layered clothing
• Relentless, excessive exercise
• Mood swings
• Avoiding food-related social activities
WARNING SIGNS OF BULIMIA NERVOSA
• A noticeable weight loss or gain
• Excessive concern about weight
• Bathroom visits after meals
• Depressive moods
• Strict dieting followed by eating binges
• Increased criticism of one's body

management of eating disorders provides the ideal treatment approach (Johnson 1986). Each team member should have a specific role:

- A physician should monitor medical status, rule on athletic participation and often coordinate the care provided by the team.
- A registered dietitian who specializes in eating disorders should provide appropriate nutritional guidance.
- A psychologist, psychiatrist or counselor should address issues of mental wellbeing.
- Trainers, coaches and exercise physiologists should assist with and support training program or performance monitoring as appropriate.
- In the case of young athletes (adolescents 19 years and under) who live at home, family involvement in treatment is essential.

Because eating disorders are psychological disorders, psychological counseling is considered the cornerstone of treatment. A variety of psychological approaches have been used successfully to treat eating disorders, including psychodynamic, cognitive-behavioral and behavioral methods. Additional variables to consider when selecting a treatment approach include the treatment setting (e.g. inpatient versus outpatient) and format (e.g. individual versus group, with or without family). For additional information of psychological treatment, refer to the *Practice guideline for the treatment of patients with eating disorders*, third edition, published by the American Psychiatric Association in 2006.

While psychological counseling aims to uncover and correct the underlying mental and emotional issues fueling the eating disorder, nutrition counseling focuses on changing the disordered eating behaviors (the energy restriction, bingeing and/or purging), treating any nutritional deficiencies, addressing nutrition beliefs and thoughts about food and body, and re-educating the athlete about sound nutritional practices.

In the case of adolescents with anorexia or bulimia, family-based treatment (also known as the Maudsley Approach) is considered best practice in achieving the best outcomes of recovery (Lock et al. 2006). This treatment needs to be delivered with the whole family by a therapist trained in this model, in conjunction with medical monitoring, preferably by a pediatrician. If family-based treatment is not available, family therapy should be included in the multidisciplinary approach for treatment in children and adolescents.

8.23 Post-treatment follow-up

As previously described, recovery from disordered eating can take months or, more typically, years. Thus treatment can continue for at least as long. Nonetheless, active or intensive treatment, particularly if done on an inpatient basis, generally lasts for a more finite period. Managing the transition of the athlete from active treatment back to 'daily' life and to their sport requires careful planning and monitoring. The athlete will probably feel self-conscious and ashamed, convinced of their coach's and team-mates' disappointment. Understanding and reassurance from the coach and team-mates is thus essential for the athlete's successful transition and ultimate recovery.

The issues of returning to training and competing must also be addressed. The decision regarding the degree of training and competition that an athlete may undertake during recovery should be based on their physical, psychological and emotional health as well as their degree of readiness to return to competition. If the athlete is still experiencing lingering physical and/or psychological complications as a result of the eating disorder, competition should be postponed. Similarly, if the athlete refuses to follow post-treatment requirements (such as maintenance of an agreed-upon energy intake or counseling schedule), training and/or competition should be postponed or minimized. A contract that outlines specific terms and conditions under which the athlete may train and/or compete is sometimes helpful to ensure that the athlete returns to their sport in the best psychological and physical shape possible.

8.24 Summary

In the world of athletics, a fraction of a second or one-tenth of a point can mean the difference between winning and losing. These high stakes can place enormous pressure on athletes. Athletes who are pressured to meet a rigid definition of ideal physique, or who lose weight because they think it will improve performance, are at risk of developing dysfunctional eating and exercise practices. Unfortunately, these weight-loss behaviors are often self-defeating. Any initial improvement in performance (as a result of weight loss) is transient. The pathogenic weight-control practices will eventually take their toll on the athlete's health and performance.

Prevention is considered the key to stemming the growing prevalence of disordered eating among athletes. Disordered-eating prevention involves the development of educational programs and strategies designed to dispel the myths and misconceptions surrounding nutrition, dieting, body weight and body composition, and their impact on performance, as well as stressing the role of nutrition in promoting health and optimal physical performance.

Unfortunately, until society in general and sport leaders in particular eliminate the pressures that encourage these behaviors, prevention efforts will probably be largely unsuccessful. Thus there will continue to be a need to recognize and treat disordered eating practices. Early identification and intervention is paramount in limiting the progression and shortening the duration of the disordered eating. Therefore a familiarity with the warning signs and symptoms of disorders is crucial. Treatment for disordered eating involves a combination of psychological and nutritional counseling along with appropriate medical care and family involvement for adolescents. The primary treatment goals for eating disorders in athletes are to normalize eating behaviors and body weight, and identify and correct the underlying psychological issues that initiated and perpetuate the eating disorder.

PRACTICE TIPS

BELINDA DALTON

PRACTICAL TIPS FOR IDENTIFYING ATHLETES WITH EATING DISORDERS

- The DSM-IV criteria are useful when assessing for frank eating disorders; however, the awareness of warning signs may allow the dietitian (or coach or parent) to identify problems at an earlier stage, which often results in better outcomes with treatment (see Table 8.6).
- Many athletes with disordered eating practices gradually reduce the variety of 'allowed' or 'safe' foods in their diets, omitting fatty foods first, then often sugary foods and other foods like meat, dairy, breads and cereals, until only a handful of different foods remain safe. Vegetarianism of recent origin is also common in athletes with disordered eating. For most, this is not true vegetarianism for religious/ethical or environmental reasons. Nor does it usually involve eating a variety of legumes, grains, seeds, nuts and other vegetarian foods. Most simply avoid meat, usually claiming it makes them feel 'heavy' or 'is too hard to digest'. Detailed examination of the rationale for dietary restriction (including beliefs about various foods), and of the adequacy of the variety and quantity of the food intake, may disclose disordered eating practices and inaccurate nutrition knowledge.
- Athletes with eating disorders are often obsessed with quantities of foods and can report exact amounts eaten (measured with cups and spoons or weighed), the energy and fat content of foods and their dietary intakes of these. They also often have rigid timing of food patterns and avoid eating out or in public. When taking a diet history, it is useful to ask the athlete questions that establish if these obsessive behaviors are present.
- It is also useful to question training practices, as these may reveal excessive exercise patterns, obsessive pursuit of training even when fatigued or injured and an obsessive knowledge of the kilojoule expenditure of training sessions.
- Being present when athletes are eating (such as when traveling with teams or conducting cooking classes) provides an ideal opportunity to observe athletes' eating practices.

MANAGING ATHLETES WITH EATING DISORDERS

- The most difficult situations are when:
  - the athlete does not admit to an eating disorder
  - the athlete's coach (or parent) insists on very low body mass or body fat levels
  - body mass has dropped to a level that is inconsistent with heavy training and evidence of side effects (e.g. amenorrhea, stress fractures or anemia) may be present
- Early identification and intervention is essential to promote greater chances of full recovery. Left untreated, eating disorders become chronic, debilitating illnesses that are, in worst cases, fatal.
- A client often presents unwillingly or is ambivalent about treatment. It is necessary to establish rapport and trust with them and show an interest in understanding their

condition. Dietary intake should be increased very gradually (small nutritious snacks six times a day), commencing with the perceived 'safe' foods and progressing to foods and eating situations that create more anxiety for the client. Force-feeding large quantities to someone with an eating disorder is inappropriate and physiologically dangerous. It is safer and easier on the mind and body of the client to encourage slow, consistent weight gain and/or reduce the feeling of fullness that often increases the urge to exercise or purge. Weight gain should not be the focus of treatment unless the client is medically compromised. Regular medical assessment—blood tests, blood pressure (postural drop), heart rate and body temperature—is essential throughout treatment, with hospitalization required for the most severe cases.

- In sports where low body weight or low body fat levels are desirable, some athletes or coaches are sometimes unrealistic in setting goals of body weight and composition. A discussion with the athlete or coach can sometimes be effective in resetting weight and body fat levels to a more realistic and healthy level.

OBJECTIVE INFORMATION FOR ATHLETES WITH EATING DISORDERS AND DISORDERED EATING

- It may be useful to provide athletes, coaches and parents with objective information about the disadvantages of inadequate eating patterns and inappropriate body mass/fat goals. These are summarized in Table 8.7.
- The dietitian may need to justify the nutritional benefit of every food recommended for the athlete to consume, since irrational phobias about some foods may exist.
- Frank explanation of the medical complications of eating disorders is essential.

TABLE 8.7 DISADVANTAGES OF INAPPROPRIATE BODY MASS/BODY FAT GOALS AND METHODS TO ACHIEVE THEM
• Much of the weight loss is due to loss of muscle tissue.
• Training is ineffective and cannot be sustained with low levels of lean body tissue.
• Adequate carbohydrate intake is essential for muscle glycogen stores; inadequate intake will also limit the effectiveness of training.
• Low kilojoule intake and low muscle mass depresses resting metabolic rate.
• Eating disorders may precipitate amenorrhea and increase the risk of bone mass loss and stress fractures.
• Dehydration from the use of laxatives, diuretics and fluid restriction will significantly impair performance.
• Restricted intake of a variety of foods may lead to nutrient inadequacies, affecting health as well as performance.
• The medical complications of severe eating disorders can be fatal.

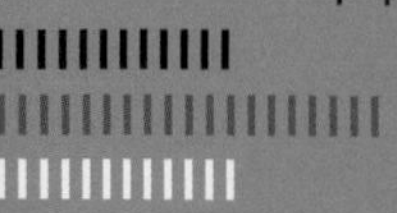

PRACTICE TIPS

FINAL COMMENTS

- It is useful to present case examples of successful athletes who do not follow fad diets and those who have a healthy and happy relationship with their physique and food. It is also helpful to point out that some athletes are successful in spite of, not because of, dietary extremism.
- Personal example is always the best teacher, so it is important that dietitians practice the guidelines of normal, healthy eating, without extremism. This is especially important where dietitians are attached to a team and may be in regular contact with athletes.
- Among athletes, many diets, supplements and fads concerning foods are popular. It is important for a dietitian working with athletes to be familiar with these. Information on dietary supplements and ergogenic aids used by athletes is provided in Chapter 16, and popular fad diets are discussed in Chapter 6.

References

American Psychiatric Association. Diagnostic and statistical manual of mental disorders. Fourth edition. Washington DC: American Psychiatric Association, 1994:539–50.

Andersen AE. A proposed mechanism underlying eating disorders and other disorders of motivated behavior. In: Anderson AE, ed. Males with eating disorders. New York: Brunners/Mazel Publishers, 1990:221–54.

Andersen AE. Eating disorders in male athletes: a special case? In: Brownell KD, Rodin J, Wilmore JH, eds. Eating, body weight and performance in athletes: disorders of modern society. Philadelphia, PA: Lea and Febiger, 1992:72–188.

Beals KA. Disordered eating among athletes: a comprehensive guide for health professionals. Champaign, Ill: Human Kinetics, 2004.

Beals KA, Manore MM. The prevalence and consequences of subclinical eating disorders in female athletes. Int J Sport Nutr 1994;4:175–95.

Beals KA, Manore MM. Nutritional status of female athletes with subclinical eating disorders. J Am Diet Assoc 1998;98:419–25.

Beals KA, Manore MM. Subclinical eating disorders in active women. Topics Clin Nutr 1999;14:14–24.

Beals KA, Manore MM. Behavioral, psychological and physical characteristics of female athletes with subclinical eating disorders. Int J Sport Nutr Exerc Metab 2000;10:128–43.

Beals KA, Manore MM. Disorders of the female athlete triad among collegiate athletes. Int J Sport Nutr Exerc Metab 2002;12:281–93.

Brownell KD, Rodin J. Prevalence of eating disorders in athletes. In: Brownell KD, Rodin J, Wilmore JH, eds. Eating, body weight and performance in athletes: disorders of modern society. Philadelphia: Lea & Febiger, 1992:128–45.

Bunnell DW, Shenker IR, Nussbaum MP, Jacobson MS, Cooper P. Subclinical versus formal eating disorders: differentiating psychological features. Int J Eat Disord 1990;9:357–62.

Byrne S, McLean N. Eating disorders in athletes: a review of the literature. J Sci Med Sport. 2001;4:145–59.

Cann EE, Martin MC, Genant HK, Jaffe RB. Decreased spinal mineral content in amenorrheic women. JAMA 1984;251:626–9.

Carney CP, Andersen AE. Eating disorders: guide to medical evaluation and complications. Psychiatr Clin North Am 1996;19:657–79.

Carson JD, Bridges E. Abandoning routine body composition assessment: a strategy to reduce disordered eating among female athletes and dancers. Canadian Academy of Sport Medicine position statement. Clin J Sports Med 2001;11:280.

Chapman P, Toma RB, Tuveson RV, Jacob M. Nutrition knowledge among adolescent high school female athletes. Adolescence 1997;32:437–46.

Cooper Z, Fairburn CG. The eating disorder examination: a semi-structured interview for the assessment of the specific psychopathology of eating disorders. Int J Eat Disord 1987;6:1–8.

Drinkwater BL, Bruemmer J, Chesnut 3rd CH. Menstrual history as a determinant of current bone density in young athletes. JAMA 1990;263:545–8.

Drinkwater BL, Nilson K, Ott S, Chesnut 3rd CH. Bone mineral density after resumption of menses in amenorrheic athletes. JAMA 1986;256:380–2.

Eichner ER. General health issues of low body weight and undereating in athletes. In: Brownell KD, Rodin J, Wilmore JH, eds. Eating, body weight and performance in athletes: disorders of modern society. Philadelphia: Lea & Febiger, 1992:191–201.

Epling WF, Pierce WD. Activity-based anorexia nervosa. Int J Eat Disord 1988;7:475–85.

Epling WF, Pierce WD, Stefan L. A theory of activity-based anorexia nervosa. Int J Eat Disord 1983;3:27–46.

Fairburn CG, Brownell KD, eds. Eating disorders and obesity: a comprehensive handbook. Second edition. New York, NY: Guilford Press, 2001.

Fairburn CG, Cooper Z. The eating disorder examination. In: Fairburn GC, Wilson GT, eds. Binge eating: nature, assessment and treatment. Twelfth edition. New York, NY: Guilford Press, 1993:3–14.

Fairburn CG, Welch SL, Doll HA, Davies BA, O'Connor ME. Risk factors for bulimia nervosa: a community-based, case-control study. Arch Gen Psychiatry 1997;54:509–17.

Field AD, Cheung L, Wolf AM, Herzog DB, Gortmaker SL, Colditz GA. Exposure to the mass media and weight concerns among adolescent girls. Pediatrics 1999;103:E36.

Garfinkel PE, Garner DM, Goldbloom DS. Eating disorders: implications for the 1990s. Can J Psychiatry 1987;32:624–31.

Garner DM. Eating disorder inventory-2: professional manual. Odessa, Florida: Psychological Assessment Resources, 1991.

Garner DM, Garfinkel PE. The eating attitudes test: an index of the symptoms of anorexia nervosa. Psychol Med 1979;9:273–9.

Garner DM, Garfinkel PE. Handbook of treatment for eating disorders. New York, NY: Guilford Press, 1997.

Garner DM, Olmstead MP, Bohr Y, Garfinkel PE. The eating attitudes test: psychometric features and clinical correlates. Psychol Med 1982;12:871–8.

Garner DM, Olmsted MP, Polivy J. Development and validation of a multidimensional eating disorder inventory for anorexia nervosa and bulimia. Int J Eat Disord 1983;2:15–34.

Harrison K, Cantor J. The relationship between media consumption and eating disorders. Journal of Communication 1997;47:40–67.

Holland AJ, Sicotte N, Treasure J. Anorexia nervosa: evidence for a genetic basis. J Psychosom Res 1988;32:561–71.

Ingjer F, Sundgot-Borgen J. Influence of body weight reduction on maximal oxygen uptake in female elite athletes. Scandinavian Journal of Medicine and Science in Sport 1991;1:141– 6.

Jacobson BH, Sobonya C, Ransone J. Nutrition practices and knowledge of college varsity athletes: a follow-up. J Str Cond Res 2001;15:63–8.

Johnson C. Initial consultation for patients with bulimia and anorexia nervosa. In: Garner DM, Garfinkel PE, eds. Handbook of psychotherapy of anorexia nervosa and bulimia. New York: Guilford Press, 1986:19–33.

Johnson C, Powers PS, Dick R. Athletes and eating disorders: the National Collegiate Athletic Association study. Int J Eat Disord 1999;26:179–88.

Leon GR. Eating disorders in female athletes. Sports Med 1991;12:219–27.

Lock J, le Grange D, Fordsburg S, Hewell K. Is family therapy useful for treating children with anorexia nervosa? Results of a case series. J Am Acad Child and Adolesc Psychiatry 2006;45:1323–38.

Manore MM. Chronic dieting in active women: what are the consequences? Women's Health Issues 1996;6:332–41.

Nattiv A, Lynch L. The female athlete triad: managing an acute risk to long-term health. Phys Sportsmed 1994;22:60–8.

Nattiv A, Loucks AB, Manore MM, Sanborn CF, Sundgot-Borgen J, Warren MP; American College of Sports Medicine. American College of Sports Medicine position stand. The female athlete triad. Med Sci Sports Exerc 2007;39:1867–82.

Noden M. Special report: dying to win. Sports Illustrated 1994;81:52–60.

O'Connor PJ, Smith JC. Physical activity and eating disorders. In: Rippe JM, ed. Lifestyle medicine. Oxford, England: Blackwell Science, 1999:1005–15.

Otis CL, Drinkwater B, Johnson M, Louks A, Wilmore JH. American College of Sports Medicine position stand. The female athlete triad: disordered eating, amenorrhea, and osteoporosis. Med Sci Sports Exerc 1997;29:i–ix.

Pomeroy C, Mitchell JE. Medical issues in the eating disorders. In: Brownell KD, Rodin J, Wilmore JH, eds. Eating, body weight and performance in athletes: disorders of modern society. Philadelphia, PA: Lea and Febiger, 1992:202–21.

Pope HG, Katz DL, Hudson JI. Anorexia nervosa and 'reverse anorexia' among 108 male body builders. Comparative Psychiatry 1993;34:406–9.

Pope HG Jr, Phillips KA, Olivardia R. The Adonis complex: the secret crisis of male body obsession. New York, NY: Free Press, 2000.

Pugliese MT, Lifshitz F, Grad G, Fort P, Marks-Katz M. Fear of obesity. A cause of short stature and delayed puberty. New Engl J Med 1983;309:513–18.

Ratnasuriya RH, Eisler I, Szmukler GI, Russell GF. Anorexia nervosa: outcome and prognostic factors after 20 years. Brit J Psychol 1991;158:495–502.

Rencken ML, Chesnut 3rd CH, Drinkwater BL. Bone density at multiple skeletal sites in amenorrheic athletes. JAMA 1996;276:238–40.

Rodin J. Cultural and psychosocial determinants of weight concerns. Ann Intern Med 1993;119:643–5.

Rodin J, Larson L. Societal factors and the ideal body shape. In: Brownell KD, Rodin J, Wilmore JH, eds. Eating, body weight and performance in athletes: disorders of modern society. Philadelphia: Lea & Febiger, 1992:146–58.

Sacks MH. Psychiatry and sports. Ann Sports Med 1990;5:47–52.

Striegel-Moore RH, Bulik CM. Risk factors for eating disorders. Am Psychol 2007;62:181–98.

Stunkard AJ. 'Restrained eating': what it is and a new scale to measure it. In: Cioffi LA, eds. The body weight regulatory system: normal and disturbed mechanisms. New York: Raven Press, 1981:243–51.

Sundgot-Borgen J. Prevalence of eating disorders in female athletes. Int J Sport Nutr 1993;3:29–40.

Sundgot-Borgen J. Risk and trigger factors for the development of eating disorders in female elite athletes. Med Sci Sport Exerc 1994a;26:414–19.

Sundgot-Borgen J. Eating disorders in female athletes. Sports Med 1994b;17:176–88.

Sundgot-Borgen J. Eating disorders. In: Berning JR, Steen SN, eds. Nutrition for exercise and sport. Gaithsburg, MD: Aspen Publishers, 1998:187–204.

Sundgot-Borgen J, Dlungland M, Torstveit G, Rolland C. Prevalence of eating disorders in male and female elite athletes. Med Sci Sports Exerc 1999;31(Suppl):297S.

Sundgot-Borgen J, Torstveit MK. Prevalence of eating disorders in elite athletes is higher than in the general population. Clin J Sport Med 2004;14:25–32.

Thelen MH, Farmer J, Wonderlich S, Smith M. A revision of the bulimia test: the BULIT-R. J Consult Clin Psychol 1991;3:119–24.

Thompson RA, Sherman RT. Helping athletes with eating disorders. Champaign, Illinois: Human Kinetics, 1993:97–170.

Van de Loo DA, Johnson MD. The young female athlete. Clin Sports Med 1995;14:687–707.

Williamson DA, Netemeyer RG, Jackman LP, Anderson DA, Funsch CL, Rabalais JY. Structural equation modeling for risks for the development of eating disorder symptoms in female athletes. Int J Eat Disord 1995;4:387–93.

Wilmore JH, Wambsgans KC, Brenner M, et al. Is there energy conservation in amenorrheic compared with eumenorrheic distance runners? J Appl Physiol 1992;72:15–22.

The evolution of the Female Athlete Triad

ANNE LOUCKS

COMMENTARY A

Introduction

The Female Athlete Triad was first described as the interrelationship of disordered eating, amenorrhea and osteoporosis (Yeager et al. 1993), and in its initial 1997 position stand on the Female Athlete Triad, the American College of Sports Medicine (ACSM) described the Triad in the same terms (Otis et al. 1997). Since then, a consensus has emerged among scientists investigating the Triad (Nattiv et al. 2007) that:

- the components of the Triad should be redefined as energy availability, menstrual function and bone strength
- each of these components should be understood to span a spectrum from health to disease, with the population of female athletes distributed *and moving* along these spectrums
- an athlete's level of energy availability is the key factor causing her to move in one direction or the other along the other spectrums, and
- the apparent irreversibility of bone loss in premenopausal amenorrheic women warrants the earliest possible intervention to prevent further bone loss

Two discoveries since the publication of the ACSM position stand have most strongly influenced our current understanding of the Triad. First, the cause of athletic amenorrhea has been identified as low energy availability. Amenorrheic and eumenorrheic athletes span a common range of body size and composition (Redman & Loucks, in press). Furthermore, exercise has been found to have no suppressive effect on reproductive function apart from the impact of its energy cost on energy availability (Loucks et al. 1998; Williams et al. 2001b), and even severe stresses involved in military training have been found to have no additional effect (Friedl et al. 2000). Second, low energy availability has been shown to uncouple bone turnover, which can cause irreversible bone loss in bone remodeling units (Compston 2001). In addition to increasing the rate of bone resorption by suppressing estrogen, low energy availability also suppresses the metabolic hormones that promote bone formation (Ihle & Loucks 2004; Zanker & Swaine 1998). While oral contraceptives may prevent further bone loss (Hergenroeder et al. 1997), clinical trials in premenopausal amenorrheic women with low energy availability have found that lost bone is not fully replaced by estrogen replacement (Cumming 1996; Warren et al. 2003), the return of menstrual cycles (Drinkwater et al. 1986; Keen & Drinkwater 1997; Warren et al. 2002, 2003) or weight gain (Soyka et al. 2002). Because bone mass in young adulthood is a major determinant of postmenopausal fractures, prevention is better than any treatment for the Triad, and intervention is better earlier than later. Treatment should be initiated immediately upon the detection of amenorrhea and should not be deferred until athletes satisfy World Health Organization diagnostic criteria for postmenopausal osteoporosis (WHO 1993).

Justification for the Female Athlete Triad

Critics of the Triad have objected to apparently healthy female athletes being singled out as a focus of medical attention. They have argued that the physiological mechanisms involved in the Triad operate in men as well as women, and that publicity about the Triad may discourage girls and women from being more physically active at a time when obesity is a major public health problem. On the contrary, it is appropriate to single out females, because the mammalian dependence of reproductive function on energy availability operates principally in females (Bronson 1985). In addition, it is appropriate to single out athletes, because even though severe dietary restriction alone is sufficient to disrupt reproductive function, the more physically active a woman is, the less dietary restriction is required and, if she expends enough energy in exercise, her reproductive function will be disrupted even though she does not restrict her diet at all (Loucks et al. 1998). Therefore, neither clinical eating disorders nor disordered eating behaviors are necessary to disrupt menstrual function in athletes who expend large quantities of energy in exercise. It is to be emphasized, however, that exercise has no suppressive effect on reproductive function apart from the impact of its energy cost on energy availability, and that the disruption of reproductive function can be prevented and restored by increasing dietary energy intake without any moderation of the exercise regimen (Loucks et al. 1998; Williams et al. 2001a, 2001b). Finally, it is appropriate for apparently healthy female athletes to be the subject of medical attention, because the imperceptible and apparently irreversible bone loss caused by low energy availability predisposes amenorrheic athletes to stress fractures in the near term and to the premature onset of osteoporosis later in life.

Others have questioned how low energy availability can be harmful to women's health, when they have heard so much about how caloric restriction has improved health and longevity in experimental animals. The answer is that it is a matter of degree. The human female reproductive system is not energetically fragile, but there is a limit to the degree of energy deficiency that a woman's body can tolerate before it starts shutting down energy-consuming physiological processes to recover energy balance. Health and longevity have been improved in animal experiments by dietary restrictions of 30% (Kemnitz et al. 1994; Lane et al. 1997; Mattison et al. 2003). In exercising women, reproductive function and bone formation begin to be suppressed when energy availability is reduced by more than 30% (Ihle & Loucks 2004; Loucks & Thuma 2003). Amenorrheic athletes have been reported to practice diet and exercise regimens that reduce energy availability by 65% (Thong et al. 2000)!

The concept of energy availability

Since energy availability is the key component of the Triad, it warrants discussion in some detail. In general, the term 'energy availability' refers to the amount of metabolic fuel in the form of carbohydrates and fats that is available for tissues to oxidize as a source of energy for life-sustaining physiological processes. In mammals, dietary energy is utilized for thermoregulation, cellular maintenance, immunity, growth, reproduction and locomotion. When dietary energy is inadequate for all of these processes, its allocation is prioritized to those that are essential for immediate survival of the individual and away from reproduction, which is essential for survival of the species. In effect, reproduction is deferred until more energy becomes available. Thus the status of the reproductive system is the 'canary in the mine shaft' that indicates the adequacy of energy supplies.

Energy availability is reduced by dietary restriction, of course, but the disruption of reproductive function has also been demonstrated in animal experiments that reduced the cellular availability of metabolic fuels by other types of interventions. These interventions include drugs that block the oxidation of glucose and fatty acids; insulin administration, which diverts blood glucose into storage while inhibiting the mobilization of fat stores; cold exposure, which consumes large quantities of metabolic fuels in thermogenesis; and physical activity, which consumes metabolic fuels in muscular contractions (Wade & Schneider 1992; Wade & Jones 2004). The energy costs of systemic infections and major trauma probably have similar effects.

For athletes, energy availability is usefully defined as dietary energy intake minus exercise energy expenditure. This is the amount of dietary energy remaining after exercise for essential physiological processes. Thus athletes may reduce their energy availability by restricting their dietary energy intake or by increasing their exercise energy expenditure. Many female athletes do both in efforts to reduce fat mass, but those in aesthetic sports tend to emphasise dietary restriction, while high energy expenditure is inherent in endurance sports. In this regard, it is worth noting that the reproductive system is regulated by a small cluster of neurons in the brain. Because fatty acids do not cross the blood–brain barrier, the brain relies on glucose for energy. In humans, the brain is so large and so metabolically active that its daily energy requirement is much greater than can be supplied by liver glycogen (Bursztein et al. 1989). Hence there is a need for humans to replenish liver glycogen stores every day. Moreover, whereas liver glycogen stores are readily available to skeletal muscle, muscle glycogen stores are not available to the brain, because skeletal muscle lacks the enzyme to return glucose stored as muscle glycogen to the bloodstream. Consequently, skeletal muscle competes directly and aggressively against the brain for all dietary carbohydrate. In a marathon race, working muscle consumes as much glucose in 2 hours as the brain requires for a week.

Nutritionists are used to thinking in terms of energy balance (see Chapter 5), but it is important to understand that low energy availability is not synonymous with negative energy balance. In addition to suppressing reproductive hormones, the brain responds to chronic, severe low energy availability by altering a wide spectrum of metabolic hormones that suppress energy-consuming physiological processes (Laughlin & Yen 1996; Loucks & Thuma 2003). This involuntary and imperceptible suppression of energy expenditure tends to restore energy balance, but it is a pathological state of energy balance in which infertility and skeletal demineralization are part of the price paid to preserve essential body protein.

Energy balance is an especially inappropriate standard for the nutrition of athletes, because energy balance is not always the objective of athletic training. Athletic performance is improved, in part, by acquiring an optimum sport-specific (and, in team sports, position-specific) body size, body composition and mix of energy stores. For many women, these objectives include a reduction in fat mass. Thus many female athletes pursue diet and exercise regimens that place their reproductive and skeletal health at risk. The nature of that risk needs to be understood and acknowledged by everyone involved, and then carefully managed so that female athletes achieve their athletic potential without sacrificing their reproductive and skeletal health.

Energy balance is also very difficult and expensive to measure outside of a highly sophisticated residential laboratory. As described above, even when energy balance is accurately determined, it conveys no information about the suppression of physiological processes that may have occurred. Consequently, it is impractical for athletes, trainers and coaches to apply in their daily lives, and it does not provide the information that they need to know. By contrast, energy availability can be calculated by simple methods that are readily available to the lay public, and energy availability is the information that athletes, trainers and coaches need to know. Reproductive function and bone turnover are disrupted in exercising women when energy availability falls below 125 kilojoules per kilogram of fat-free mass per day (30 kilocalories per kilogram of fat-free mass per day) (Loucks & Thuma 2003; Ihle & Loucks 2004).

The methods for calculating energy availability include prospective records of exercise and diet. Many nutritionists have become skeptical of the diet records of female athletes, because studies comparing data from such records to estimations or measurements of energy expenditure have repeatedly found apparently huge negative energy balances, some exceeding 4 MJ/d, in athletes with stable body weights (Mulligan & Butterfield 1990; Wilmore et al. 1992; Edwards et al. 1993; Beidleman et al. 1995; Hill & Davies 2002). Such large discrepancies have been interpreted as indicating that female athletes grossly under-report their dietary intake. Few of these studies have included biochemical measurements to validate this interpretation, however, and under-reporting would not account for biochemical evidence of energy deficiency. In several studies characterizing reproductive disorders in female athletes in which metabolic substrates and hormones have been measured, there is a consistent story of chronic energy deficiency (Myerson et al. 1991; Loucks et al. 1992; Jenkins et al. 1993; Laughlin & Yen 1996; Laughlin & Yen 1997; De Souza et al. 2003). Some female athletes display a whole spectrum of metabolic substrate and hormone abnormalities indicative of a decline in glucose utilization, the mobilization of fat stores and a slowing of metabolic rate, with more extreme abnormalities in amenorrheic athletes and less extreme abnormalities in regularly menstruating athletes. So the available biochemical data not only demonstrate that some female athletes are, indeed, chronically energy deficient, but they also tend to substantiate lower than expected energy intakes while calling into question the accuracy of assumptions made in estimating or measuring their basal metabolic rate.

Prevention and treatment of the Female Athlete Triad

Because research to date has focused on what constitutes and causes the Triad, we have learned more about that than we have learned about how to prevent and treat the Triad. Nevertheless, athletes and their families, coaches, trainers, team physicians and sport-governing bodies all have responsibilities today for protecting the health of athletes. With only hazy guidelines from research for fulfilling these responsibilities, everyone will need to experiment for the next several years with educational programs, training regimens, intervention strategies and rule changes, and to publish the results of these experiments to share lessons learned. Different problems and controversies will probably emerge, requiring different solutions in different sports. It will be instructive in this regard for the governing bodies of women's sports to monitor the results of rule changes introduced to prevent harmful weight-loss practices in US collegiate men's wrestling (Bubb 2004; Dick et al. 2005) and international ski jumping (Fédération Internationale Skiing Media Information on-line; Fédération Internationale Skiing on-line; Quarrell 2005).

In addition to the difficulty of reforming misguided goals and behaviors for modifying body size and composition, part of the challenge in nourishing athletes is that 'there is no strong biological imperative to match energy intake to activity-induced energy expenditure' (Blundell & King 1999). Hunger was actually suppressed briefly by a single bout of intense exercise (Blundell & King 1998), and two bouts of intense exercise in a single day induced no increase in ad libitum (at any time) food intake on that or the following 2 days (King et al. 1997). Whereas food deprivation increased hunger, the same amount of exercise energy expenditure did not (Hubert et al. 1998). Even a 30% increase in energy expenditure during 40 weeks of marathon training induced no increase in energy intake (Westerterp et al. 1992). Together, these findings demonstrate that the body possesses no mechanism for automatically accommodating energy intake to the expenditure of energy by working muscle. In our own laboratory, women say that they have to force themselves to eat far beyond their appetites to consume the amount of food that compensates their dietary energy intake for their exercise energy expenditure and thereby prevents the disruption of their reproductive function (Loucks et al. 1998). Other investigators have had to offer special treats to induce exercising amenorrheic monkeys to increase their energy intake enough to restore their menstrual cycles (Williams et al. 2001b). Thus appetite is not a reliable indicator of an athlete's energy requirements. Athletes must learn to eat by discipline to preserve their reproductive and skeletal health.

Because dietary energy intake and exercise energy expenditure are physiological inputs, everyone wants to be able to measure a single, specific, accurate, inexpensive, convenient, minimally invasive, non-falsifiable physiological output to verify the adequacy of energy availability. We are not aware of any such perfect biomarker, but the best available one may be urinary ketones. This marker signifies the mobilization of fat stores and the production of ketones in the liver as an alternative fuel for the brain during periods of glucose deficiency. Of course, there are limitations to the use of urinary ketones as a universal biomarker of chronic low energy availability. Because ketone production declines when fat stores are nearly exhausted, this biomarker fails when near-term survival is at greatest risk. Chronic habits are also easily concealed by consuming a carbohydrate meal shortly before the test. Apart from those shortcomings, however, urinary ketones do identify glucose-deficient individuals and athletes can monitor them at home using inexpensive dipsticks (Loucks 2004). Such dipsticks may be adequate for prevention purposes.

By contrast, no single measurement of any metabolic hormone accurately discriminates energy-deficient individuals, because the variance between individuals is as large as the effects of energy deficiency (Loucks 2004). Nevertheless, repeated measurements of blood samples for metabolic hormones such as tri-iodothyronine (T_3), the ratio of insulin to cortisol, and the ratio of insulin-like growth factor-I to growth hormone, and of biomarkers of bone formation such as osteocalcin and PICP, should all increase in response to an effective intervention to increase energy availability. Such blood samples should be part of the routine medical diagnosis and treatment of female athletes with menstrual disorders or fractures.

References

Beidleman BA, Puhl JL, De Souza MJ. Energy balance in female distance runners. Am J Clin Nutr 1995;61:303–11.

Blundell JE, King NA. Effects of exercise on appetite control: loose coupling between energy expenditure and energy intake. Int J Obes Relat Metab Disord 1998;22(2 Suppl):22S–9S.

Blundell JE, King NA. Physical activity and regulation of food intake: current evidence. Med Sci Sports Exerc 1999;31(Suppl):573S–83S.

Bronson FH. Mammalian reproduction: an ecological perspective. Biol Reprod 1985;32:1–26.

Bubb RG. 2004 NCAA Wrestling Rules and Interpretations. Available at http://www.ncaa.org/library/rules/2004/2004_wrestling_rules.pdf (accessed 23 June 2005).

Bursztein S, Elwyn DH, Askanazi J, Kinney JM. Fuel utilization in normal, starving, and pathological states. Energy metabolism, indirect calorimetry, and nutrition. Baltimore, MD: Williams & Wilkins, 1989:146.

Compston JE. Sex steroids and bone. Physiol Rev 2001;81:419–47.

Cumming DC. Exercise-associated amenorrhea, low bone density, and estrogen replacement therapy. Arch Intern Med 1996;156:2193–5.

De Souza MJ, van Heest J, Demers LM, Lasley BL. Luteal phase deficiency in recreational runners: evidence for a hypometabolic state. J Clin Endocrinol Metab 2003;88:337–46.

Dick RW, Oppliger RA, Scott JR, Utter AC. Wrestling with weight loss: the NCAA Wrestling Weight Management Policy. Available at http:www.ncaa.org/library/sports_sciences/wrestling_ with_weight_loss.pdf (accessed 23 June 2005).

Drinkwater BL, Nilson K, Ott S, Chesnut 3rd CH. Bone mineral density after resumption of menses in amenorrheic athletes. JAMA 1986;256:380–2.

Edwards JE, Lindeman AK, Mikesky AE, Stager JM. Energy balance in highly trained female endurance runners. Med Sci Sports Exerc 1993;25:1398–404.

Fédération Internationale Skiing. Media Information. Available at http://www.fis-ski.com/data/ document/ vorstandjuni04-e.pdf (accessed 23 June 2005).

Fédération Internationale Skiing. Measurement table for ski length and weight. Available at http:// www.fis-ski.com/data/document/masstabellede.pdf (accessed 23 June 2005).

Friedl KE, Moore RJ, Hoyt RW, Marchitelli LJ, Martinez-Lopez LE, Askew EW. Endocrine markers of semistarvation in healthy lean men in a multistressor environment. J Appl Physiol 2000; 88:1820–30.

Hergenroeder AC, Smith EO, Shypailo R, Jones LA, Klish WJ, Ellis K. Bone mineral changes in young women with hypothalamic amenorrhea treated with oral contraceptives, medroxyprogesterone, or placebo over 12 months. Am J Obstet Gynecol 1997;176:1017–25.

Hill RJ, Davies PS. Energy intake and energy expenditure in elite lightweight female rowers. Med Sci Sports Exerc 2002;34:1823–9.

Hubert P, King NA, Blundell JE. Uncoupling the effects of energy expenditure and energy intake: appetite response to short-term energy deficit induced by meal omission and physical activity. Appetite 1998;31:9–19.

Ihle R, Loucks AB. Dose-response relationships between energy availability and bone turnover in young exercising women. J Bone Miner Res 2004;19:1231–40.

Jenkins PJ, Ibanez-Santos X, Holly J, et al. IGFBP-1: a metabolic signal associated with exercise-induced amenorrhoea. Neuroendocrinology 1993;57:600–4.

Keen AD, Drinkwater BL. Irreversible bone loss in former amenorrheic athletes. Osteoporos Int 1997;7:311–15.

Kemnitz JW, Roecker EB, Weindruch R, Elson DF, Baum ST, Bergman RN. Dietary restriction increases insulin sensitivity and lowers blood glucose in rhesus monkeys. Am J Physiol 1994;266:E540–7.

King NA, Lluch A, Stubbs RJ, Blundell JE. High dose exercise does not increase hunger or energy intake in free living males. Eur J Clin Nutr 1997;51:478–83.

Lane MA, Ingram DK, Ball SS, Roth GS. Dehydroepiandrosterone sulfate: a biomarker of primate aging slowed by calorie restriction. J Clin Endocrinol Metab 1997;82:2093–6.

Laughlin GA, Yen SSC. Nutritional and endocrine-metabolic aberrations in amenorrheic athletes. J Clin Endocrinol Metab 1996;81:4301–9.

Laughlin GA, Yen SSC. Hypoleptinemia in women athletes: absence of a diurnal rhythm with amenorrhea. J Clin Endocrinol Metab 1997;82:318–21.

Loucks AB. Energy balance and body composition in sports and exercise. J Sports Sciences 2004;22:1–14.

Loucks AB, Laughlin GA, Mortola JF, Girton L, Nelson JC, Yen SSC. Hypothalamic-pituitary-thyroidal function in eumenorrheic and amenorrheic athletes. J Clin Endocrinol Metab 1992;75:514–18.

Loucks AB, Thuma JR. Luteinizing hormone pulsatility is disrupted at a threshold of energy availability in regularly menstruating women. J Clin Endocrinol Metab 2003;88:297–311.

Loucks AB, Verdun M, Heath EM. Low energy availability, not stress of exercise, alters LH pulsatility in exercising women. J Appl Physiol 1998;84:37–46.

Mattison JA, Lane MA, Roth GS, Ingram DK. Calorie restriction in rhesus monkeys. Exp Gerontol 2003;38:35–46.

Mulligan K, Butterfield GE. Discrepancies between energy intake and expenditure in physically active women. Br J Nutr 1990;64:23–36.

Myerson M, Gutin B, Warren MP, et al. Resting metabolic rate and energy balance in amenorrheic and eumenorrheic runners. Med Sci Sports Exerc 1991;23:15–22.

Nattiv A, Loucks AB, Manore MM, Sanborn CF, Sundgot-Borgen J, Warren MP; American College of Sports Medicine. American College of Sports Medicine position stand. The female athlete triad. Med Sci Sports Exerc 2007;39:1867–82.

Otis CL, Drinkwater B, Johnson M, Loucks A, Wilmore J. American College of Sports Medicine position stand. The Female Athlete Triad. Med Sci Sports Exerc 1997;29:i–ix.

Quarrell R. New rules for skiing. Available at http:www.sportsbite.com/index.pl?id=000217 (accessed 23 June 2005).

Redman LM, Loucks AB. Menstrual disorders in athletes. Sports Med 35:747–55.

Soyka LA, Misra M, Frenchman A, et al. Abnormal bone mineral accrual in adolescent girls with anorexia nervosa. J Clin Endocrinol Metab 2002;87:4177–85.

Thong FS, McLean C, Graham TE. Plasma leptin in female athletes: relationship with body fat, reproductive, nutritional, and endocrine factors. J Appl Physiol 2000;88:2037–44.

Wade GN, Jones JE. Neuroendocrinology of nutritional infertility. Am J Physiol Regul Integr Comp Physiol 2004;287:R1277–96.

Wade GN, Schneider JE. Metabolic fuels and reproduction in female mammals. Neurosci Biobehav Rev 1992;16:235–72.

Warren MP, Brooks-Gunn J, Fox RP, Holderness CC, Hyle EP, Hamilton WG. Osteopenia in exercise-associated amenorrhea using ballet dancers as a model: a longitudinal study. J Clin Endocrinol Metab 2002;87:3162–8.

Warren MP, Brooks-Gunn J, Fox RP, et al. Persistent osteopenia in ballet dancers with amenorrhea and delayed menarche despite hormone therapy: a longitudinal study. Fertil Steril 2003;80:398–404.

Westerterp KR, Meijer GA, Janssen EM, Saris WH, ten Hoor F. Long-term effect of physical activity on energy balance and body composition. Br J Nutr 1992;68:21–30.

Williams NI, Caston-Balderrama AL, Helmreich DL, Parfitt DB, Nosbisch C, Cameron JL. Longitudinal changes in reproductive hormones and menstrual cyclicity in cynomolgus monkeys during strenuous exercise training: abrupt transition to exercise-induced amenorrhea. Endocrinology 2001a;142:2381–9.

Williams NI, Helmreich DL, Parfitt DB, Caston-Balderrama AL, Cameron JL. Evidence for a causal role of low energy availability in the induction of menstrual cycle disturbances during strenuous exercise training. J Clin Endocrinol Metab 2001b;86:5184–93.

Wilmore JH, Wambsgans KC, Brenner M, et al. Is there energy conservation in amenorrheic compared with eumenorrheic distance runners? J Appl Physiol 1992;72:15–22.

World Health Organization (WHO). Prevention and management of osteoporosis. WHO Technical Report Series 2003;921:1–164

Yeager KK, Agostini R, Nattiv A, Drinkwater B. The female athlete triad: disordered eating, amenorrhea, osteoporosis. Med Sci Sports Exerc 1993;25:775–7.

Zanker CL, Swaine IL. Bone turnover in amenorrhoeic and eumenorrhoeic women distance runners. Scand J Med Sci Sports 1998;8:20–6.

CHAPTER 9

Bone, exercise and nutrition

DEBORAH KERR, KARIM KHAN AND KIM BENNELL

9.1 Introduction

Bone is a dynamic tissue that reflects the biological principle of adaptation of structure to function and the metabolic role of mineral homeostasis. The skeleton is made up of two types of bone. The outer bone is known as cortical and the inner softer core is known as trabecular (the more metabolically active bone). The skeleton is designed to provide the strength needed to withstand the mechanical forces of daily weight-bearing. Structurally, the long bones of the skeleton are often referred to as appendicular bones, and the bones of the trunk as the axial skeleton.

Exercise generates loading within the skeleton, which affects the structure at the skeletal site at which the strain is developed. Physical activity is protective of bone, and studies of athletes show they have a higher bone mass than people who are inactive. In amenorrhea, however, bone loss occurs due to the absence of estrogen. But there is some evidence that if the mechanical load is sufficient, it may be protective of bone mass at the site of loading (Young et al. 1994; Robinson et al. 1995).

Bone is continually being broken down and rebuilt in a process known as remodeling, under the regulation of systemic hormones and local growth factors. The remodeling cycle consists of five successive events: quiescence, activation, resorption, reversal and formation (Parfitt 1984; Raisz 1999). Following resorption of a packet of bone by the osteoclast, new bone is laid down by the osteoblast. When bone resorption exceeds formation, bone loss occurs, which, if prolonged, can lead to osteoporosis and increased risk of fracture. The hormonal status interacts with the mechanical environment to influence bone remodeling. The bone remodeling cycle takes 4 to 6 months to complete in adults (Epstein 1988). This is an important concept when evaluating the bone density literature. Ideally, intervention studies are the best way to study exercise effects on bone, and these studies should be of at least 12 months' duration.

Mechanical loading principles

9.2

Loading of the skeleton occurs from the force induced by the contracting muscle (muscle pull) and the gravity-induced strain. Animal studies have shown that the skeleton is primarily sensitive to short periods of loading (Chambers et al. 1993; Chow et al. 1993) with unusual strain distributions, high peak strain magnitudes and rapid change of strain (Lanyon & Rubin 1984; Rubin & Lanyon 1985; Cullen et al. 2001). In response to the mechanical loading of bone, strain-related potentials are produced. Frost (1990) proposed that there was a minimum effective strain (MES) for bone modeling and remodeling and that only when bone strain exceeds the MES will there be a net gain in bone. More recently however, Turner (1999) proposed that bone cells in weight-bearing sites may be programmed differently from bone cells in non-weight-bearing sites. This theory, termed 'cellular accommodation', proposes that bone cells have a memory for loading patterns, and that this modulates the future response to mechanical loading. It is from these mechanical loading principles that progressive resistance training was first examined as a preventive strategy in osteoporosis research.

The measurement of bone mineral density

9.3

Bone densitometry measures the average bone mineral within the region scanned, known as the bone mineral density (BMD). The sites measured are the hip, forearm and lumbar spine, which are the most common fracture sites. The whole body scan can estimate the total bone density and body composition. The BMD can be measured by dual energy X-ray absorptiometry (DXA) and quantitative computerized tomography. A relatively new technology, peripheral quantitative computed tomography (PQCT), makes it possible to calculate biomechanical parameters such as cross-sectional moment of inertia and strength–strain index (Louis et al. 1995; Augat et al. 1996). PQCT also allows imaging of the three-dimensional trabecular microstructure, which is not possible with DXA. The most common method for routine screening for osteoporosis is DXA, but ultrasound is increasingly being used. Low bone mass is defined in terms of how far the measurement falls below the reference range for the young healthy female. A 'fracture threshold' or a cut-off point is used to define osteoporosis and is based on the range of BMD measurements in the population with vertebral or hip fractures.

Definitions: sports osteopenia and osteoporosis

9.4

Osteoporosis is a condition of low bone mass associated with greater bone fragility and increased risk of fractures (WHO 1994). Clinically, osteoporosis is defined in terms of the BMD that is below the age-adjusted reference range. An individual is considered osteoporotic if their BMD is 2.5 standard deviations (SD) or more below the young adult mean for bone density. Osteopenia is a condition of low bone mass in which the BMD is more than one SD below the young adult mean, but less than 2.5 SD below this value. Sports osteopenia refers to low bone mass, and is seen most commonly in female athletes.

The risk of developing osteoporosis and subsequent fractures is largely determined by the peak bone mass achieved in adolescence and early adulthood. Up to 80% of the variability in bone density has been attributed to genetic factors (Pocock et al. 1987; Krall &

Dawson-Hughes 1993; Nguyen et al. 1998). BMD is strongly linked to bone strength and resistance to fracture.

9.5 Exercise effect on bone in athletes and healthy people

Exercise is critical for maintaining both the architecture and mass of the skeleton. Throughout the skeleton there appears to be different strain thresholds for particular bones, which are genetically coded. Weight-bearing bones appear to require both muscle pull and gravitational forces, whereas bones in the upper limbs, not subject to the forces of weight-bearing, may require only muscle pull for the maintenance of bone mass. In amenorrhea, weight-bearing bones may be partially protected by mechanical loading, whereas non-weight-bearing bones may not (Young et al. 1994; Khan et al. 1996). In a study in ballet dancers with oligomenorrhea, bone loss appeared to occur from all sites (Pearce et al. 1996). As design of these studies is cross-sectional the findings need to be viewed with caution.

9.6 Cross-sectional studies of exercise and bone mass

Studies in athletes have shown the benefits of exercise on bone mass, particularly at weight-bearing sites (Davee et al. 1990; Heinrich et al. 1990; Taaffe et al. 1995; Heinonen et al. 1995). In the non-weight-bearing bones, such as the arm, it is clear that muscle pull has a positive effect on the loaded limb in sports such as tennis and squash (Kannus et al. 1994; Haapasalo et al. 1994; Bass et al. 2002). When comparing athletes with non-athlete controls or different athletic groups, there are often differences in body size. In the study by Heinrich and colleagues (1990), the body builders were significantly heavier than the other athletes and had the highest bone density. A large study of young women aged 18 to 35 years found the best predictors of BMD were weight, age, family history and physical activity (Rubin et al. 1999). Body weight explained over half of the variability in BMD at the hip and spine. These results stress the importance of controlling for body weight in studies of bone mass and exercise. Athletes may already have a higher bone density due to genetic influences before commencing an exercise program or may be able to continue exercising without injury because of a high bone mass (Marcus & Carter 1988).

There may be a variety of load thresholds for different bones (Martin & McCulloch 1987). Weight-bearing bones, such as the calcaneus, may require a much greater load to induce a change in bone mass than non-weight-bearing bones (Harber et al. 1991). Weight-bearing bones are acted on by both gravitational forces and muscular pull, whereas the forces on non-weight-bearing bones are mostly muscle pull. Several studies have examined the effect of weight-supported exercise on bone density. In exercises such as swimming and cycling, muscle pull, but not gravitational force, is in operation.

A study in eumenorrheic elite female athletes compared the effects of swimming and gymnastics on bone density (Taaffe et al. 1995). The gymnasts had a higher bone density at the femoral neck than the swimmers. At the lumbar spine and whole body sites, the spine BMD was higher, when adjusted for body weight, in the gymnasts compared with the swimmers and controls. The femoral neck BMD in the swimmers was less than the controls, even though the swimmers participated in some resistance training. The authors suggested that the amount of time spent in a weight-supported environment may negate the effects of resistance training. However, an intervention study is needed to confirm these findings.

These studies indicate the importance of both gravitational forces and muscle pull in maintaining bone density and confirm that exercise undertaken is specific to the site of loading on the bone. Weight-bearing bones require both muscle pull and gravitational forces and therefore a much greater load threshold compared with non-weight bearing bones, which may require only muscle pull to exert an effect on bone density.

Exercise interventions in children 9.7

The time around puberty is critical for bone mineral accrual. About 26% of adult bone is accumulated during the 2 years around the period of peak bone accrual (Bailey et al. 1999). Exercise interventions have shown beneficial effects on bone mineral accrual in the growing skeleton (Morris et al. 1997; Bradney et al. 1998; Heinonen et al. 2000; Fuchs et al. 2001; MacKelvie et al. 2003). There does appear to be a greater benefit in bone accrual if the exercise is commenced prior to puberty (Bass et al. 1998) and if the activity is high impact such as jumping (Fuchs et al. 2001; Iuliano-Burns et al. 2003). Daly and colleagues (1999) examined the impact loading that occurs during elite gymnastics training and found that young male gymnasts exert up to ten times their body weight during a training session. These studies emphasize the importance of maintaining a range of high-impact weight-bearing activities, such as team and racquet sports and jumping activities, throughout childhood. Whether these gains in bone mineral accrual will be maintained into adulthood and reduce fracture risk later in life is not known. To optimize bone health and other health benefits from exercise, participation in physical activity and sport throughout childhood should be actively encouraged. A systematic review by MacKelvie and colleagues (2002) has examined the evidence for exercise during childhood.

Exercise interventions in adults 9.8

Studies of exercise intervention on bone density have shown variable results, but generally suggest that weight-bearing exercise (such as jogging, walking, running and gymnastics) has a positive effect on bone mass. Intervention studies of weight-bearing exercise in pre- and postmenopausal women have demonstrated a positive effect on bone mass (Snow-Harter et al. 1992; Grove & Londeree 1992; Bassey & Ramsdale 1994; Prince et al. 1995). However, more favorable effects on the skeleton have been found with resistance training in both premenopausal (Snow-Harter et al. 1992; Vuori et al. 1994; Lohman et al. 1995; Friedlander et al. 1995) and postmenopausal women (Nelson et al. 1994; Kerr et al. 1996, 2001). In an 8-month intervention in young women, there was a significant exercise effect at the lumbar spine from running and progressive resistance training (Snow-Harter et al. 1992). The progressive resistance-exercise program consisted of three sets of eight to twelve repetitions, performed three times a week. The running group progressively increased their running so that they were running about 16 km by the end of the study. There was a significant increase in BMD at the lumbar spine for both the running group (1.3–1.6%) and the resistance-trained group (1.2–1.8%), compared with the control group, but no change at the neck of femur site. The number of repetitions from running may have been sufficient to stimulate bone formation equivalent to resistance training. This suggests that, in young women, running may be equally as effective as resistance training in increasing bone mass.

Three randomized studies measuring the effects of resistance training have been conducted on postmenopausal women (Nelson et al. 1994; Kerr et al. 1996, 2001). Nelson and colleagues (1994), in a randomized controlled trial of 1 year of resistance training in postmenopausal women, found a significant effect on BMD at the femoral neck and lumbar spine. In a unilateral exercise study, Kerr and colleagues (1996) compared two resistance-training regimens that differed only in the number of repetitions of the weight lifted. The exercise effects on the skeleton were specific to the site of exercise loading and dependent on the weight lifted. In another 2-year study on another group of postmenopausal women, a significant effect of resistance exercise at the total hip (0.9 ± 2.6%, $p < 0.05$) and intertrochanter hip was observed (1.1 ± 3.0%, $p < 0.01$), compared to the control group (Kerr et al. 2001). The circuit group, who were lifting much lighter weights, did not show any effects on bone mass, nor did the control group.

The effects of resistance training on BMD in men using randomized controlled trials are lacking, so whether similar effects occur in men to those reported in postmenopausal women are still unclear. Studies conducted on men have not been randomized but have been self-selected, and have not been long enough to allow bone density changes to be identified (Williams et al. 1984; Menkes et al. 1993; Ryan et al. 1994; Cohen et al. 1995). The bone remodeling cycle takes 3 to 4 months to complete. Further studies of the exercise effects in men are clearly needed.

In summary, resistance training appears to be effective for both premenopausal and postmenopausal women, in either slowing or preventing bone loss. In men, the lack of well-designed intervention trials makes it difficult to draw similar conclusions. The effects of exercise, however, would be expected to be equally as favorable in men as those seen in women. Men and women of all ages should be encouraged to participate regularly in either weight-bearing activity or progressive resistance training. The American College of Sports Medicine published a position stand on exercise and bone health (Kohrt et al. 2004) and recommends weight-bearing activity three to five times per week, as well as resistance exercise two or three times per week as a target for maintaining BMD. For elderly men and women, specific activities to improve balance and prevent falls should also be included.

9.9 Calcium intake and bone mineral changes at various life stages

The human skeleton retains the rather primitive function of serving as both a depot for the storage of excess calcium and as a reservoir, available to replenish calcium during times of deprivation. This portable supply of calcium, however, is a double-edged sword. When the calcium reserve, our skeleton, is called upon to meet dietary insufficiencies, bone strength is compromised.

Calcium balance is determined by the balance between the dietary intake of calcium, the amount of calcium absorbed from the intestine and the amount excreted in the urine. Plasma calcium levels are tightly regulated by hormonal control. Hence, when negative balance occurs in response to low estrogen levels, demineralization from the skeleton will follow. Dietary calcium recommendations are based on the amount of dietary calcium needed to maintain calcium balance and optimal bone accretion rates.

Calcium balance studies suggest there may be a threshold effect for calcium intake; this means that calcium retention increases up to a threshold, beyond which any additional intake of calcium does not result in increased calcium retention. Calcium absorption from the small intestine occurs by active absorption at low intake levels and by passive absorption at higher calcium intakes. Traditionally calcium requirements and recommendations have been determined from balance studies in which calcium intake and loss are equal. Little is know about calcium requirements for physically active people (Weaver 2000), although calcium balance studies in physically active children and adolescents are in progress (C. Weaver, pers. comm. May 2009).

The revisions to the nutrient reference standards for calcium in the US and Canada used three approaches as the basis of setting the calcium recommendations for different population groups. These were derived from calcium balance studies; from a factorial model using calcium accretion on bone mineral accretion data; and from clinical trials, which investigated the response of change in BMD or fracture rate to varying calcium intakes. In 2006, Australia adopted the US/Canadian recommendations, with a slight modification. The approach used to set recommendations for calcium in Australia was based on the approach used by the Food and Agricultural Organization of the United Nations and World Health Organization in their 2001 revisions (FAO/WHO 2001). The Recommended Dietary Intake (RDI), the Australian equivalent to the RDA (Recommended Dietary Allowance in the US) for both boys and girls (12–18 years) is 1300 mg/d, which is the same as for elderly men and women (>70 years). For both adult men (19–70 years) and women (19–50 years), the RDI is 1000 mg/d (Commonwealth Department of Health and Ageing et al. 2006). Postmenopausal women have slightly higher recommendations. The EAR (Estimated Average Requirement) is less than the RDI for all values (Commonwealth Department of Health and Ageing et al. 2006). See Chapter 2 for guidelines on the application of these new standards. There are currently no specific recommendations for calcium intake for athletes so, until further studies are undertaken, population reference standards can be used as a benchmark for assessing adequacy.

Effect of calcium intake during childhood and adolescence on bone mineral density 9.10

There is a complex homeostatic control between the amount of calcium ingested, the amount retained after obligatory losses from the various sites (digestive tract, skin, nails, hair, sweat and urine) and the amount that is finally incorporated into the skeleton. The amount of calcium retained in bone is called calcium retention.

A longitudinal study of growing children documented calcium retention efficiencies of 33% for boys and 29% for girls (Bailey et al. 2000). Higher calcium efficiencies appear to compensate for low dietary intakes of calcium. In another study, when calcium intakes dropped to 400 mg/d, absorption efficiency rose to 50% (Abrams et al. 1997). This is striking when compared with the calcium retention of 4–8% in the adult with skeletal deficiency. It is, therefore, only in severe cases of dietary restriction that bone mineral accrual is compromised. Such cases are seldom observed in western cultures. In severe cases of calcium restriction, bone growth may proceed at a slower rate and bones are usually of normal shape and size, but have lower than normal bone mineral mass. Bone growth relates directly to the genetic and mechanical (and not the dietary) control of linear growth and periosteal and endosteal expansion.

Against this background of physiology, all the calcium consumed is not directly transferred into the bone reservoir. Randomized, double-blind, placebo-controlled studies of children found that calcium supplementation given during the growing years increased bone mineral by about 1–3%, independently of energy intake or other nutritional factors (Johnston et al. 1992; Lloyd et al. 1993; Lee et al. 1994; Teegarden & Weaver 1994; Bonjour et al. 1997; Nowson et al. 1997; Iuliano-Burns et al. 2003; Cameron et al. 2004; Lau et al. 2004; Chevalley et al. 2005; Matkovic et al. 2005). In most follow-up studies, after withdrawal of supplementation, the benefit achieved by the formerly supplemented group decreased or disappeared (Slemenda et al. 1997; Nowson et al. 1997; Cameron et al. 2004).

One study in prepubertal girls demonstrated a positive effect on BMD when calcium as milk extract was added to food products (Bonjour et al. 1997). One year after supplementation was withdrawn, girls with habitually low dietary calcium intakes, which had previously been supplemented, still had greater increments in bone mineral content (BMC) and BMD in the femoral shaft than the previously unsupplemented children.

Results of calcium intervention studies in adolescent girls are similar to those performed in younger children. Teenage girls (mean age 14 years, range 10–17 years) supplemented with 1000 mg of calcium for 18 months had a 1.5% increase in BMD at both the spine and the total hip. The greatest effect occurred during the first 6 months of supplementation (Nowson et al. 1997).

Exposure to high calcium intakes, even for 3 years prior to puberty, appears then to have no long-term effect on bone mineral. Although seemingly surprising, this finding is consistent with the hypothesis that bone changes following supplementation with dietary calcium are due to reversible changes in bone remodeling (Kanis 1994a). Calcium retention increases with higher calcium intake in children and adolescents (Matkovic & Heaney 1992; Jackman et al. 1997). Increased bone retention of calcium with high calcium intakes in adolescence is attributable to an increase in absorption and a decrease in bone resorption (Wastney et al. 2000). Children appear to have the ability to absorb and retain calcium at levels that at least partially compensate for low levels of dietary calcium (Martin et al. 1997). Thus, although children have enormous skeletal demand for calcium during the years of peak bone mineral accrual, they may be able to meet these demands by a combination of increased calcium absorption efficiency and borrowing calcium from the cortical shell (Parfitt 1994; Bailey et al. 2000). Once peak bone mass is achieved, it is primarily the mechanical forces acting on the skeleton that stimulate bone formation. Combining calcium with exercise during growth can also produce additive effects on bone accrual (Iuliano-Burns et al. 2003). Thus population recommendations directed at encouraging physical activity and meeting calcium recommendations during the growing years have a strong evidence base.

9.11 Effect of calcium intake on BMD during the premenopausal years

During the premenopausal years, when most women are estrogen replete, calcium retention and absorption operate at peak adult efficiency. This results in lower dietary calcium requirements than at any other time during life. A prospective study of young women suggested that bone mineral mass may even be augmented after the cessation of linear growth—perhaps into the third decade (Recker et al. 1992).

There have been few calcium intervention studies in adult premenopausal women. Smith and colleagues (1989) found no effect of 4 years of calcium supplementation on wrist BMC. In longitudinal studies with a large sample size there has been no effect (on BMD or rates of bone loss) in subjects with high or low levels of calcium intake (Riggs et al. 1987; Mazess & Barden 1991). In a study in young adult distance runners, calcium supplementation over 1 year was found to prevent cortical bone loss, but not trabecular bone loss (Winters-Stone & Snow 2004). But longer follow-up is needed in this group to see if this effect is maintained long-term.

As studies comparing BMD in adult communities that have different intakes of calcium do not reveal differences in bone mass, the effect of genetic and other environmental factors on bone mass may be greater than that of dietary calcium (Kanis 1994a, 1994b). Even the strongest proponents of calcium for bone health concede that 'the evidence for a relation between bone density, bone loss and estimated calcium intake in individuals is somewhat inconclusive' (Nordin & Heaney 1990). The difficulties in measuring current and retrospective calcium intakes in free-living people in combination with other nutrients (phosphorus, protein and sodium), and individual differences in obligatory calcium losses, contribute to this uncertainty (Avioli & Heaney 1991).

Effect of calcium intake on BMD during the early postmenopausal years

9.12

It appears that the biological response to calcium differs between women of early postmenopausal years and late postmenopausal years. Thus the data for women in each of these life stages is summarized separately. The term 'perimenopause' describes the years on both sides of the final menstrual period, when the hormonal milieu is in flux.

Evidence for the benefits of calcium during the perimenopausal and early postmenopausal years is either conflicting or non-existent. It is accepted that decreased bone mass at menopause is related to diminished hormone levels, which is akin to raising the bone bending 'set point'. Decreases in bone mass in perimenopausal women, therefore, are not related to nutrient deficiency but to estrogen withdrawal, and are not even substantially influenced by high doses of calcium. There may be a one-time, rapid downward adjustment of bone mass of as much as 15% in peri- and postmenopausal women compared with premenopausal levels (Heaney 1990).

There are several key studies of calcium and bone in this age group. Cumming (1990) performed a meta-analysis of six calcium intervention studies conducted in 'healthy' women with a mean age around 50 years and found a positive effect of calcium on BMD that ranged from 0–1.7%/year increase (mean = 0.8%/year). Based on these studies, 'a calcium supplement of around 1000 mg/d in early postmenopausal women can prevent loss of just under 1% of bone mass per year at all bone sites except at the vertebrae' (Cumming 1990). This effect size is intermediate between hormone replacement therapy and no treatment. Studies published since Cumming's meta-analysis support his conclusions (Dawson-Hughes et al. 1990; Elders et al. 1994).

9.13 Effect of calcium intake during the later postmenopausal years on BMD

Postmenopausal osteoporosis is associated with accelerated remodeling and accelerated bone loss (Heaney et al. 1978). Notably, calcium supplementation in later postmenopausal women is associated with the maintenance, and not gain, of skeletal mass (Dawson-Hughes et al. 1990; Prince et al. 1995; Reid et al. 1995). For example, in healthy women who were more than 5 years postmenopausal and had a dietary calcium intake of less than 400 mg/d, supplementation to 800 mg/d significantly reduced bone loss (Dawson-Hughes et al. 1990). However, no benefit was observed in those women who had moderate intakes of calcium and were not supplemented with additional calcium. Calcium intake significantly above the recommended level of the NRVs of 1000–1300 mg/d is therefore unlikely to achieve additional benefit for bone health (Sanders et al. 2009). This supports the argument that calcium is a 'threshold nutrient'.

Reid and colleagues (1993) and others (Smith et al. 1989; Prince et al. 1991) found that appendicular bone loss slows with calcium supplementation. These authors also found a positive effect of calcium supplementation on axial bone loss in women who had been postmenopausal for an average of 10 years. This is consistent with findings that such supplementation was ineffective in women who had just reached menopause (Ettinger et al. 1987; Riis et al. 1987). Reid demonstrated a positive effect of calcium on BMD at the proximal femur (Reid et al. 1993).

The mechanism whereby calcium attenuates bone loss in postmenopausal women is most likely decreased activation of new remodeling sites, and continuation of early bone formation at the previously existing bone remodeling sites (Kanis 1994b). This phenomenon is known as the 'bone-remodeling transient' (Heaney 1994). Because there is still a deficit between the calcium lost in resorption and the calcium replaced in formation, bone continues to be lost, albeit at a slower rate, despite calcium supplementation.

9.14 Effects of amenorrhea on bone mass

The effects of prolonged amenorrhea on bone health are reviewed in this section. The effects of athletic amenorrhea on bone mass were first identified in the 1980s by several authors (Drinkwater et al. 1984; Linnell et al. 1984; Cann et al. 1984; Marcus et al. 1985). These studies and others indicate that amenorrheic athletes have lower bone mass than eumenorrheic athletes.

Interpreting the results of studies on the effects of amenorrhea on bone mass is difficult, as the sample sizes have been small and the majority of studies have been cross-sectional, which increases the risk of type II errors. Much of the research comes from the 1980s, as today athletic amenorrhea is treated with hormone replacement (Hobart & Smucker 2000). There is considerable evidence to show that body mass (BM) is a significant predictor of bone mass. Therefore it is important to account for size differences, as amenorrheic athletes often weigh less than eumenorrheic athletes (Linnell et al. 1984; Marcus et al. 1985; Harber et al. 1991; Young et al. 1994). Differences in bone mass may be partly explained by differences in BM, but when BM has been controlled for, the results are not consistent. In a study of ballet dancers' bone at non-weight-bearing sites, bone density was similar between dancers and girls with anorexia nervosa, after controlling for BM (Young et al. 1994). The importance of BM was also seen in a study of ballet dancers, where significant effects of amenorrhea on BMD were demonstrated at the spine, wrist and metatarsal (Warren et al. 1991). All effects of amenorrhea were eliminated by controlling for weight.

In a study of 97 young athletes (Drinkwater et al. 1990), there was a significant linear relationship between the current vertebral BMD and the athletes' past and present menstrual patterns. Women who had always had regular menses had the highest vertebral bone mass. In this study, BM was a significant predictor of both vertebral and femur BMD. Once BMD was adjusted for body mass, only the vertebral BMD remained significantly lower by menstrual status.

An early study by Drinkwater and colleagues (1984) showed amenorrheic athletes had a significantly lower vertebral BMD than eumenorrheic athletes. This finding has been confirmed by other researchers (Marcus et al. 1985; Wolman et al. 1990).

There is some evidence that amenorrhea may affect non-weight-bearing bones to a greater extent than weight-bearing bones (Marcus et al. 1985; Young et al. 1994) because exercise may offer some protection at weight-bearing sites. A study that examined the bone mass of gymnasts and runners with a similar prevalence of menstrual disturbances found gymnasts had a higher femoral neck BMD than the runners or controls (Robinson et al. 1995). Higher-impact forces from the gymnastics training were thought to account for the differences.

Bone mass in amenorrheic athletes is, however, well below age-matched normal controls at weight-bearing sites (Cann et al. 1984; Drinkwater et al. 1984; Lindberg et al. 1984). The lumbar spine BMD was significantly lower in amenorrheic athletes compared with eumenorrheic athletes (Lindberg et al. 1984; Drinkwater et al. 1984).

Effects of resumption of menses on bone mass 9.15

The reversibility of bone loss observed with amenorrhea has been a concern due to the long-term consequences on bone mass. Drinkwater and colleagues (1986) followed up athletes with amenorrhea 15.5 months after they regained menses and compared them to eumenorrheic controls. There was a 6% increase in the vertebral BMD in the amenorrheic athletes who had regained menses. The resumption of menses was also associated with an increase in BM and a reduction in exercise level. It was noted at the time that it was premature to assume that the bone mass would return to the same level for their age group.

It was later reported (Drinkwater et al. 1990) that the gain ceased after 2 years, suggesting that the bone mass may never fully recover. When the amenorrheic athletes were followed up after 8 years (Keen & Drinkwater 1997), despite several years of normal menses or use of oral contraceptives, the vertebral BMD remained lower than the athletes who had always had regular menses. Micklesfield and colleagues (1998) noted similar effects in runners. A history of menstrual irregularity is detrimental to the attainment of peak bone mass and early intervention is recommended, in order to minimize the long-term risks of osteoporosis (Keen & Drinkwater 1997).

Mechanisms of low bone mass in amenorrhea 9.16

Low levels of endogenous estrogen are thought to be responsible for the continued bone loss (Cann et al. 1984; Drinkwater et al. 1984; Marcus et al. 1985). Snead and colleagues

(1992) found lower estradiol and progesterone levels in combination with lower lumbar spine BMD in oligomenorrheic and amenorrheic runners, compared with eumenorrheic runners and controls. The view that amenorrhea is related to estrogen deficiency is consistent with the model of ovarian failure and the responses to menopause. More recently, however, it has been suggested that estrogen deficiency may not be the primary cause of bone loss in amenorrheic athletes (Zanker 1999). Evidence for this hypothesis is the poor responsiveness to estrogen therapy observed in studies of bone turnover in amenorrheic athletes (Hergenroeder 1995; Zanker & Swaine 1998).

The mechanism by which low estrogen levels reduce bone mass is by decreasing the rate of bone turnover and has been confirmed in a study of amenorrheic runners whose bone formation markers were below the normal reference range (Zanker & Swaine 1998). These authors suggested that under-nutrition was implicated as the mechanism associated with reduced bone formation because the bone formation markers were lowest in those amenorrheic runners with a body mass index (BMI) less than 17.5 (below the healthy weight range).

A study that compared anorexia nervosa subjects to amenorrheic controls showed a greater incidence of osteopenia in the anorexia nervosa subjects (Grinspoon et al. 1999). These data suggest that nutritional factors, independent of estrogen, are important in determining bone mass.

9.17 Role of calcium and nutritional factors in amenorrhea

Calcium is required for the normal maintenance and development of the skeleton and teeth; therefore requirements are increased during periods of rapid growth, such as during childhood, adolescence, pregnancy and lactation, and in later life.

To date, no randomized control trials have been conducted in amenorrheic athletes to examine the effects of calcium supplementation on slowing bone loss. It is still thought, however, that calcium, if given in sufficient amounts, may modulate the effects of hypogonadism in female athletes. Since calcium deficiency is a stimulus for bone resorption, the effect of calcium deficiency and hypogonadism may be additive (Dalsky 1990). This was supported by the findings of Wolman and colleagues (1992), who reported a linear relationship between calcium intake and trabecular bone density at the lumbar spine in both amenorrheic and eumenorrheic athletes. However, at all levels of calcium intake, bone density was significantly lower in amenorrheic athletes. Therefore, even though amenorrheic athletes with higher calcium intakes can achieve better bone mass than amenorrheic athletes with lower calcium intakes, this still cannot compensate for the effects of amenorrhea on the skeleton.

Although intervention trials are lacking in athletic populations, it is generally agreed that 1500 mg/d is recommended for athletes with amenorrhea (Nattiv & Armsey 1997). This is also consistent with the US National Institutes of Health (NIH 1994) consensus guidelines for postmenopausal women not taking estrogen. The Australian RDIs for calcium are currently under review. Other nutritional factors, such as sodium and protein, can increase urinary calcium losses. Adding 100 mmol of sodium (2.3 g) to the daily diet will result in a calcium loss of 1 mmol (40 mg) (Nordin et al. 1993). The effects of sodium and protein on calcium excretion are greatest when the person is in negative calcium balance (Nordin 1997). High calcium intake with meals can inhibit iron absorption (see Chapter 10). Therefore, in athletes with high iron requirements, calcium supplements, if prescribed, should be taken at bedtime (Hallberg 1998).

Stress fractures in athletes with menstrual disturbances 9.18

A stress fracture is a partial or complete fracture of bone, and results from the bone's inability to withstand non-violent stress that is applied in a repeated, sub-threshold manner (McBryde 1985). It arises from accumulation of bone micro-damage that cannot be adequately repaired by the remodeling process. Any factor that increases the applied load, decreases bone strength or interferes with the repair process has the potential to increase the risk of stress fracture (Bennell et al. 1996). The diagnosis of stress fracture is based on the clinical findings of a history of exercise-related bone pain with local bony tenderness on examination.

Role of menstrual factors in stress fractures 9.19

Menstrual factors may have an effect on stress fracture etiology through the influence of reduced levels of reproductive hormones on bone remodeling and bone density (Heaney et al. 1978; Slemenda et al. 1987). Studies have reported that stress fractures are more common in athletes with current or past menstrual disturbances, with a relative risk for stress fracture that is between two to four times greater than their eumenorrheic counterparts (Lindberg et al. 1984; Marcus et al. 1985; Lloyd et al. 1986; Warren et al. 1986; Carbon et al. 1990; Frusztajer et al. 1990; Myburgh et al. 1990; Grimston et al. 1991; Kadel et al. 1992; Bennell et al. 1995, 1996) (see Fig. 9.1 overleaf). However, most studies have been cross-sectional designs where women are specifically recruited according to certain criteria, either stress fracture history or menstrual status. In these studies, cohorts are often small, categorization of menstrual status is based on number of menses per year rather than on analysis of hormonal levels, and definitions vary. Where hormonal assessment is included, most are single measurements, often non-standardized with respect to menstrual cycle phase.

The relationship between age of menarche and risk of stress fracture is uncertain. Some authors have found that athletes with stress fractures have a later age of menarche (Warren et al. 1986, 1991; Carbon et al. 1990) while others have found no difference (Frusztajer et al. 1990; Myburgh et al. 1990; Kadel et al. 1992). In a prospective study by Bennell and colleagues (1996), the age of menarche was an independent risk factor for stress fracture, with the risk increasing by a factor of 4.1 for every additional year of age at menarche.

Some authors have claimed that the oral contraceptive pill may protect against stress fracture development. Barrow and Saha (1988) found that runners using the oral contraceptive pill for at least 1 year had significantly fewer stress fractures (12%) than non-users (29%). This was supported by the findings of Myburgh and colleagues (1990), but not by others (Kadel et al. 1992). Since these studies are retrospective in nature, it is not known whether the athletes were taking the oral contraceptive pill prior to or following the stress fracture episode. It is not known whether the risk of stress fracture

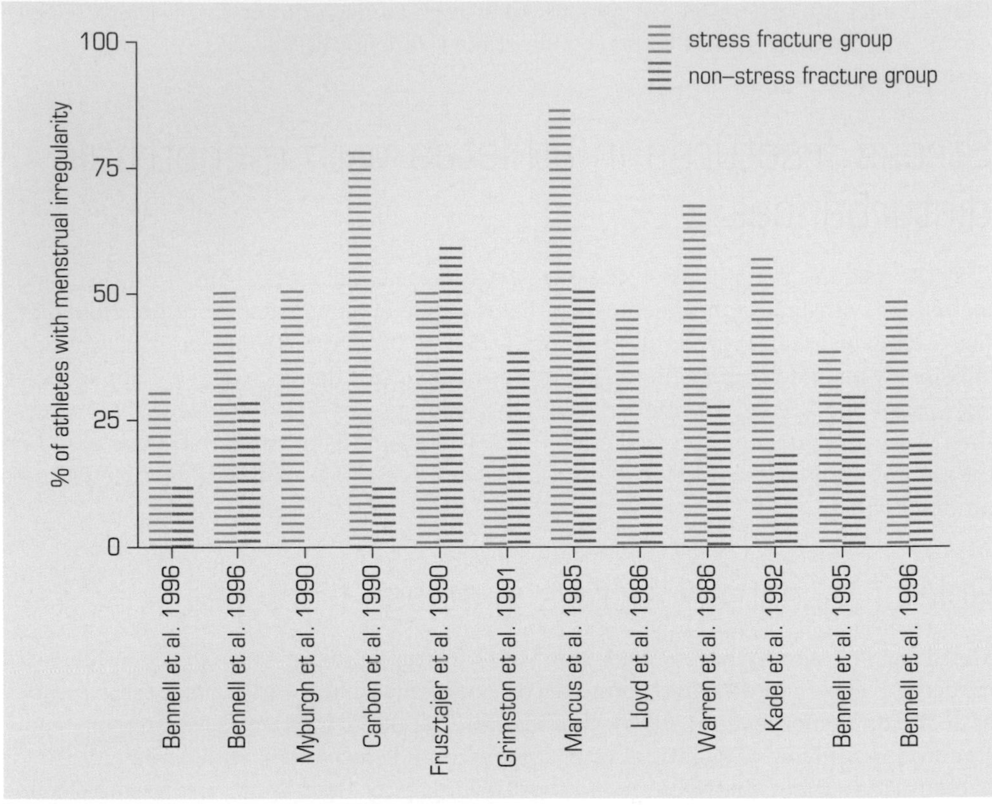

FIGURE 9.1 Studies where the percentage of athletes/recruits with menstrual irregularity could be compared in groups with and without stress fracture (from Brukner et al. 1999, pp. 65–6). Reprinted with permission.

is reduced in athletes with menstrual disturbances who take the oral contraceptive pill after getting a fracture.

Theoretically, low bone density could contribute to the development of a stress fracture by decreasing the fatigue resistance of bone to loading and increasing the accumulation of micro-damage (Carter et al. 1981). A limited number of cross-sectional studies have compared regional bone density in small groups of female athletes with and without stress fractures, but results have been conflicting. This discrepancy may reflect differences in subject characteristics, type of sport, measurement techniques and bone sites tested. However, the findings of the only prospective study to date indicate that lower bone density, assessed by DXA, is a risk factor for stress fractures in female track and field athletes (Bennell et al. 1996). Nevertheless, in this study, the athletes who developed stress fractures still had bone density levels that were similar to or greater than less active subjects. This outcome suggests bone density levels of the bones at risk of stress fractures in these athletes might need to be higher than those of non-athletes.

In summary, there is a higher prevalence of current and past menstrual disturbances in female athletes with stress fractures than in those athletes without stress fractures. A later age of menarche and lower bone density may also contribute to an increased risk of this overuse bone injury. Use of the oral contraceptive pill may afford protection against stress fractures, although this is yet to be fully elucidated.

Summary

9.20

The skeleton represents a complex interaction between the hormonal environment and the stresses and strains placed upon it. Weight-bearing exercise or resistance training has been shown to be effective in slowing or preventing bone loss in both premenopausal and postmenopausal women. In amenorrheic athletes, however, the evidence is not as clear, partly due to the lack of well-designed intervention studies on athletes. Nevertheless, amenorrhea is clearly detrimental to bone health and early intervention is recommended. Adequate calcium intakes are effective in decreasing bone loss, at least in women, and should be increased after menopause or in an athlete with amenorrhea. The prevalence of stress fractures is also higher among athletes who have menstrual disturbances compared with eumenorrheic women. The consequences of untreated menstrual disturbances on bone health are an increased risk of osteopenia and potentially osteoporosis in later life.

PRACTICE TIPS

DEBORAH KERR, KARIM KHAN AND KIM BENNELL

- A key role of the sports dietitian is to raise awareness and educate coaches and athletes about the long-term consequences of amenorrhea, particularly on bone health. Assessing menstrual history is important in an initial consultation with an athlete or when screening groups. The absence of menses for more than 6 months should be referred to a sports physician for assessment.
- The sports dietitian needs to be alert to the possible presence of eating disorders, which can cause serious and irreversible bone loss. Dietary practices known to increase urinary calcium losses (such as excessive intakes of sodium, protein, caffeine and alcohol) should also be assessed. These are of greater importance when dietary calcium intake is low. In this situation, increasing the calcium intake is the priority because at higher calcium intakes (at least >800 mg/d) excessive sodium, protein and caffeine are of less importance. Cigarette smoking also has deleterious effects on bone health.
- There are currently no DRIs/Nutrient Reference Values (NRVs) for calcium for amenorrheic athletes. However, 1500 mg calcium/d has been proposed, which is consistent with the US National Institutes of Health consensus statement for postmenopausal women not taking estrogen. Amenorrheic athletes fit well into the same category. The Australian RDI for calcium is 1000 mg/d (adults) and 1300 mg/d (women >51 years) (or postmenopausal). During adolescence, it is essential that athletes consume adequate calcium as this is the time when peak bone mass occurs.
- What can be done when counseling female athletes who are not consuming enough calcium? Expounding the long-term risk of osteoporosis usually has little impact. However, if an individual has seen the debilitating effects of osteoporosis in their family or friends, they are usually more receptive to preventive strategies. Start by suggesting an increase in calcium intake by dietary means, but if this strategy is not possible or feasible, then a calcium supplement may be required. Referral to a sports physician for a bone density scan can be considered. An athlete with a low calcium intake together with a low bone density may be more receptive to change, once they have seen the results of their bone density scan.
- Female athletes consuming low energy intakes are at high risk of low calcium intakes. There are also many misconceptions in the general population about dairy foods, which are the major source of calcium. Any misinformation about calcium and dairy foods should be addressed in a clinical situation as well as other barriers and facilitators that might affect the choice of calcium-rich foods. Providing practical options for snacks and meals that increase calcium density (e.g. using calcium-fortified foods) is useful.
- Where it is difficult to meet calcium requirements by diet alone, a calcium supplement is warranted. Although bioavailability of calcium from supplements is lower than from dairy sources, taking supplements at bedtime or between meals maximizes absorption and prevents the interference of inhibitory factors found naturally occurring in foods (e.g. phytic acid in cereal grains). Absorption of calcium supplements is most effective in doses of 500 mg or less (Heaney et al. 1975; Heaney et al. 1988). For athletes on 1000 mg calcium/d, however, splitting the dosage into two 500 mg doses (to maximize absorption) reduces compliance, whereas a single dose taken at bedtime enhances

compliance. Commonly prescribed calcium supplement brands are Citracal™ (calcium citrate), Sandocal™ (calcium lactate-gluconate) and Caltrate™ (calcium carbonate).

- Maintaining vitamin D status is also important for bone health. For individuals living in Australia and New Zealand, sunlight exposure is the major source of vitamin D. Suboptimal levels of vitamin D occur in people who are institutionalized or housebound, who actively avoid sunlight exposure. For athletes who train indoors, such as young gymnasts, it is important that they follow the recommendations for safe sun exposure to maintain their vitamin D status (Working Group of the Australian and New Zealand Bone and Mineral Society 2005).
- Pharmacological intervention, biochemical tests of hormone status and bone density assessment may be necessary for female athletes at risk of osteopenia. Situations where medical referral is indicated include:
  - being amenorrheic for longer than 6 months
  - a history of anorexia nervosa
  - occurrence of stress fractures
  - being postmenopausal
  - a strong family history of osteoporosis
- Routine bone density screening of female athletes is not recommended unless indicated, as there is a small radiation dose using DXA.
- Regular weight-bearing activity or weight training has a positive effect on bone density. Weight-bearing activities such as jogging, tennis, aerobics and walking have the greatest effects compared to cycling and swimming. Although these non-weight-bearing activities are excellent for aerobic fitness, they are unlikely to have much effect on bone mass.

USEFUL WEBSITES

http://www.mja.com.au/public/issues/190_06_160309/san10083_fm.html
Calcium and bone health: position statement for the Australian and New Zealand Bone and Mineral Society, Osteoporosis Australia and the Endocrine Society of Australia, 2009

http://www.osteoporosis.org.au/
Osteoporosis Australia

http://www.nof.org/
National Osteoporosis Foundation (US)

http://www.niams.nih.gov/Health_Info/Bone/
National Institutes of Health Osteoporosis and Related Bone Diseases, National Resource Center (US)

http://www.ausport.gov.au/participating/women/issues/osteo
Participating in sport; Female athlete triad/osteoporosis (Australian Sports Commission)

http://www.cdc.gov/nutrition/everyone/basics/vitamins/calcium.html
Calcium and bone health (Centers for Diseases Control and Prevention (US)

References

Abrams SA, Grusak MA, Stuff J, O'Brien KO. Calcium and magnesium balance in 9–14-year-old children. Am J Clin Nutr 1997;66:1172–7.

Augat P, Reeb H, Claes LE. Prediction of fracture load at different skeletal sites by geometric properties of the cortical shell. J Bone Miner Res 1996;11:1356–63.

Avioli LV, Heaney RP. Calcium intake and bone health. Calcif Tissue Int 1991;48:221–3.

Bailey DA, Martin AD, McKay HA, Whiting S, Mirwald R. Calcium accretion in girls and boys during puberty: a longitudinal analysis. J Bone Miner Res 2000;5:2245–50.

Bailey DA, McKay HA, Mirwald RL, Crocker PR, Faulkner RA. A six-year longitudinal study of the relationship of physical activity to bone mineral accrual in growing children: the University of Saskatchewan bone mineral accrual study. J Bone Miner Res 1999;14:1672–9.

Barrow GW, Saha S. Menstrual irregularity and stress fractures in collegiate female distance runners. Am J Sports Med 1988;16:209–16.

Bass S, Pearce G, Bradney M, et al. Exercise before puberty may confer residual benefits in bone density in adulthood: studies in active prepubertal and retired female gymnasts. J Bone Miner Res 1998;13:500–7.

Bass SL, Saxon L, Daly RM, et al. The effect of mechanical loading on the size and shape of bone in pre-, peri-, and postpubertal girls: a study in tennis players. J Bone Miner Res 2002;17:2274–80.

Bassey EJ, Ramsdale SJ. Increase in femoral bone density in young women following high-impact exercise. Osteoporos Int 1994;4:72–5.

Bennell KL, Malcolm SA, Thomas SA, et al. Risk factors for stress fractures in female track-and-field athletes: a retrospective analysis. Clin J Sport Med 1995;5:229–35.

Bennell KL, Malcolm SA, Wark JD, Brukner PD. Models for the pathogenesis of stress fractures in athletes. Br J Sports Med 1996;30:200–4.

Bonjour JP, Carrie AL, Ferrari S, et al. Calcium-enriched foods and bone mass growth in prepubertal girls: a randomized, double-blind, placebo-controlled trial. J Clin Invest 1997;99:1287–94.

Bradney M, Pearce G, Naughton G, et al. Moderate exercise during growth in prepubertal boys: changes in bone mass, size, volumetric density, and bone strength: a controlled prospective study. J Bone Miner Res 1998;13:1814–21.

Brukner P, Bennell K, Matheson G. Stress fractures. Asia: Blackwell Science, 1999.

Cameron MA, Paton LM, Nowson CA, et al. The effect of calcium supplementation on bone density in premenarcheal females: a co-twin approach. J Clin Endocrinol Metab 2004;89:4916–22.

Cann CE, Martin MC, Genant HK, Jaffe RB. Decreased spinal mineral content in amenorrheic women. JAMA 1984;251:626–9.

Carbon R, Sambrook PN, Deakin V, et al. Bone density of elite female athletes with stress fractures. Med J Aust 1990;153:373–6.

Carter DR, Caler WE, Spengler DM, Frankel VH. Uniaxial fatigue of human cortical bone. The influence of tissue physical characteristics. J Biomech 1981;14:461–70.

Chambers TJ, Evans M, Gardner TN, Turner-Smith A, Chow JW. Induction of bone formation in rat tail vertebrae by mechanical loading. Bone Miner 1993;20:167–78.

Chevalley T, Bonjour JP, Ferrari S, Hans D, Rizzoli R. Skeletal site selectivity in the effects of calcium supplementation on areal bone mineral density gain: a randomized, double-blind, placebo-controlled trial in prepubertal boys. J Clin Endocrinol Metab 2005;90:3342–9.

Chow JW, Jagger CJ, Chambers TJ. Characterization of osteogenic response to mechanical stimulation in cancellous bone of rat caudal vertebrae. Am J Physiol Endocrinol Metab 1993;265:E340–7.

Cohen B, Millett PJ, Mist B, Laskey MA, Rushton N. Effect of exercise training programme on bone mineral density in novice college rowers. Br J Sports Med 1995;29:5–8.

Commonwealth Department of Health and Ageing (Aust), Ministry of Health (NZ) and National Health and Medical Research Council. Nutrient Reference Values Australia and New Zealand. Canberra: NHMRC, 2006.

Cullen DM, Smith RT, Akhter MP. Bone-loading response varies with strain magnitude and cycle number. J Appl Physiol 2001;91:1971–6.

Cumming RG. Calcium intake and bone mass: a quantitative review of the evidence. Calcif Tissue Int 1990;47:194–201.

Dalsky GP. Effect of exercise on bone: permissive influence of estrogen and calcium. Med Sci Sports Exerc 1990;22:2:81–5.

Daly RM, Rich PA, Klein R, Bass S. Effects of high-impact exercise on ultrasonic and biochemical indices of skeletal status: a prospective study in young male gymnasts. J Bone Miner Res 1999; 14:1222–30.

Davee AM, Rosen CJ, Adler RA. Exercise patterns and trabecular bone density in college women. J Bone Miner Res 1990;5:245–50.

Dawson-Hughes B, Dallal GE, Krall EA, et al. A controlled trial of the effect of calcium supplementation on bone density in postmenopausal women. N Engl J Med 1990;323:878–83.

Drinkwater BL, Bruemner B, Chesnut 3rd CH. Menstrual history as a determinant of current bone density in young athletes. JAMA 1990;263:545–8.

Drinkwater BL, Nilson K, Chesnut 3rd CH, et al. Bone mineral content of amenorrheic and eumenorrheic athletes. N Engl J Med 1984;311:277–81.

Drinkwater BL, Nilson K, Ott S, Chesnut 3rd CH. Bone mineral density after resumption of menses in amenorrheic athletes. JAMA 1986;256:380–2.

Elders PJ, Lips P, Netelenbos JC, et al. Long-term effect of calcium supplementation on bone loss in perimenopausal women. J Bone Miner Res 1994;9:963–70.

Epstein S. Serum and urinary markers of bone remodeling: assessment of bone turnover. Endocr Rev 1988;9:437–49.

Ettinger B, Genant HK, Cann CE. Postmenopausal bone loss is prevented by treatment with low-dosage estrogen with calcium. Ann Intern Med 1987;106:40–5.

Food and Agricultural Organization of the United Nations (FAO)/World Health Organization (WHO). Human nutrition and mineral requirements. Report of a joint FAO/WHO expert consultation, Bangkok, Thailand. Rome: Food and Agricultural Organization of the United Nations, 2001.

Friedlander AL, Genant HK, Sadowsky S, Byl NN, Gluer CC. A two-year program of aerobics and weight training enhances bone mineral density of young women. J Bone Miner Res 1995;10:574–85.

Frost HM. Skeletal structural adaptations to mechanical usage (SATMU): 2. Redefining Wolff's law: the remodeling problem. Anat Rec 1990;226:414–22.

Frusztajer NT, Dhuper S, Warren MP, Brooks-Gunn J, Fox RP. Nutrition and the incidence of stress fractures in ballet dancers. Am J Clin Nutr 1990;51:779–83.

Fuchs RK, Bauer JJ, Snow CM. Jumping improves hip and lumbar spine bone mass in prepubescent children: a randomized controlled trial. J Bone Miner Res 2001;16:148–56.

Grimston SK, Engsberg JR, Kloiber R, Hanley DA. Bone mass, external loads, and stress fracture in female runners. Int J Sport Biomech 1991;7:293–302.

Grinspoon S, Miller K, Coyle C, et al. Severity of osteopenia in estrogen-deficient women with anorexia nervosa and hypothalamic amenorrhea. J Clin Endocrinol Metab 1999;84:2049–55.

Grove KA, Londeree BR. Bone density in postmenopausal women: high impact vs low impact exercise. Med Sci Sports Exerc 1992;24:1190–4.

Haapasalo H, Kannus P, Sievanen H, et al. Long-term unilateral loading and bone mineral density and content in female squash players. Calcif Tissue Int 1994;54:249–55.

Hallberg L. Does calcium interfere with iron absorption? Am J Clin Nutr 1998;68:3–4.

Harber VJ, Webber CE, Sutton JR, MacDougall JD. The effect of amenorrhea on calcaneal bone density and total bone turnover in runners. Int J Sports Med 1991;12:505–8.

Heaney RP. Estrogen-calcium interactions in the postmenopause: a quantitative description. Bone Miner 1990;11:67–84.

Heaney RP. The bone-remodeling transient: implications for the interpretation of clinical studies of bone mass change. J Bone Miner Res 1994;9:1515–23.

Heaney RP, Recker RR, Hinders SM. Variability of calcium absorption. Am J Clin Nutr 1988;47:262–4.

Heaney RP, Recker RR, Saville PD. Menopausal changes in bone remodeling. J Lab Clin Med 1978;92:964–70.

Heaney RP, Saville PD, Recker RR. Calcium absorption as a function of calcium intake. J Lab Clin Med 1975;85:881–90.

Heinonen A, Oja P, Kannus P, et al. Bone mineral density in female athletes representing sports with different loading characteristics of the skeleton. Bone 1995;17:197–203.

Heinonen A, Sievanen H, Kannus P, et al. High-impact exercise and bones of growing girls: a 9-month controlled trial. Osteoporos Int 2000;11:1010–17.

Heinrich CH, Going SB, Pamenter RW, et al. Bone mineral content of cyclically menstruating female resistance and endurance trained athletes. Med Sci Sports Exerc 1990;22:558–63.

Hergenroeder AC. Bone mineralization, hypothalamic amenorrhea, and sex steroid therapy in female adolescents and young adults. J Pediatr 1995;126:683–9.

Hobart JA, Smucker DR. The female athlete triad. Am Fam Physician 2000;61:3357–64, 3367.

Institute of Medicine. Dietary Reference Intakes for calcium, phosphorus, magnesium, vitamin D, and fluoride. Washington, D.C: National Academy Press, 1997.

Iuliano-Burns S, Saxon L, Naughton G, Gibbons K, Bass SL. Regional specificity of exercise and calcium during skeletal growth in girls: a randomized controlled trial. J Bone Miner Res 2003;18:156–62.

Jackman LA, Millane SS, Martin BR, et al. Calcium retention in relation to calcium intake and postmenarcheal age in adolescent females. Am J Clin Nutr 1997;66:327–33.

Johnston Jr. CC, Miller JZ, Slemenda CW, et al. Calcium supplementation and increases in bone mineral density in children. N Engl J Med 1992;327:82–7.

Kadel NJ, Teitz CC, Kronmal RA. Stress fractures in ballet dancers. Am J Sports Med 1992;20:445–9.

Kanis JA. Calcium nutrition and its implications for osteoporosis. Part I. Children and healthy adults. Eur J Clin Nutr 1994a;48:757–67.

Kanis JA. Calcium nutrition and its implications for osteoporosis. Part II. After menopause. Eur J Clin Nutr 1994b;48:833–41.

Kannus P, Haapasalo H, Sievanen H, Oja P, Vuori I. The site-specific effects of long-term unilateral activity on bone mineral density and content. Bone 1994;15:279–84.

Keen AD, Drinkwater BL. Irreversible bone loss in former amenorrheic athletes. Osteoporos Int 1997;7:311–15.

Kerr D, Ackland T, Maslen B, Morton A, Prince R. Resistance training over 2 years increases bone mass in calcium-replete postmenopausal women. J Bone Miner Res 2001;16:175–81.

Kerr D, Morton A, Dick I, Prince R. Exercise effects on bone mass in postmenopausal women are site-specific and load-dependent. J Bone Miner Res 1996;11:218–25.

Khan KM, Green RM, Saul A, et al. Retired elite female ballet dancers and nonathletic controls have similar bone mineral density at weightbearing sites. J Bone Miner Res 1996;11:1566–74.

Kohrt WM, Bloomfield SA, Little KD, Nelson ME, Yingling VR. American College of Sports Medicine Position Stand: physical activity and bone health. Med Sci Sports Exerc 2004;36:1985–96.

Krall EA, Dawson-Hughes B. Heritable and life-style determinants of bone mineral density. J Bone Miner Res 1993;8:1–9.

Lanyon LE, Rubin CT. Static vs dynamic loads as an influence on bone remodelling. J Biomech 1984;17:897–905.

Lau EM, Lynn H, Chan YH, Lau W, Woo J. Benefits of milk powder supplementation on bone accretion in Chinese children. Osteoporos Int 2004;15:654–8.

Lee WT, Leung SS, Wang SH, et al. Double-blind, controlled calcium supplementation and bone mineral accretion in children accustomed to a low-calcium diet. Am J Clin Nutr 1994;60:744–50.

Lindberg JS, Fears WB, Hunt MM, et al. Exercise-induced amenorrhea and bone density. Ann Intern Med 1984;101:647–8.

Linnell SL, Stager JM, Blue PW, Oyster N, Robertshaw D. Bone mineral content and menstrual regularity in female runners. Med Sci Sports Exerc 1984;16:343–8.

Lloyd T, Andon MB, Rollings N, et al. Calcium supplementation and bone mineral density in adolescent girls. JAMA 1993;270:841–4.

Lloyd T, Triantafyllou SJ, Baker ER, et al. Women athletes with menstrual irregularity have increased musculoskeletal injuries. Med Sci Sports Exerc 1986;18:374–9.

Lohman T, Going S, Pamenter R, et al. Effects of resistance training on regional and total bone mineral density in premenopausal women: a randomized prospective study. J Bone Miner Res 1995; 10:1015–24.

Louis O, Boulpaep F, Willnecker J, Van den Winkel P, Osteaux M. Cortical mineral content of the radius assessed by peripheral QCT predicts compressive strength on biomechanical testing. Bone 1995;16:375–9.

MacKelvie KJ, Khan KM, McKay HA. Is there a critical period for bone response to weight-bearing exercise in children and adolescents? A systematic review. Br J Sports Med 2002;36:250–7; discussion 257.

MacKelvie KJ, Khan KM, Petit MA, Janssen PA, McKay HA. A school-based exercise intervention elicits substantial bone health benefits: a 2-year randomized controlled trial in girls. Pediatrics 2003;112:E447.

Marcus R, Cann C, Madvig P, et al. Menstrual function and bone mass in elite women distance runners. Endocrine and metabolic features. Ann Intern Med 1985;102:158–63.

Marcus R, Carter DR. The role of physical activity in bone mass regulation. In: Grana WA, ed. Advances in sports medicine and fitness. Chicago, Illinois: Year Book Medical Publishers, 1988.

Martin AD, Bailey DA, McKay HA, Whiting S. Bone mineral and calcium accretion during puberty. Am J Clin Nutr 1997;66:611–15.

Martin AD, McCulloch RG. Bone dynamics: stress, strain and fracture. J Sports Sci 1987;5:155–63.

Matkovic V, Goel PK, Badenhop-Stevens NE, et al. Calcium supplementation and bone mineral density in females from childhood to young adulthood: a randomized controlled trial. Am J Clin Nutr 2005;81:175–88.

Matkovic V, Heaney RP. Calcium balance during human growth: evidence for threshold behavior. Am J Clin Nutr 1992;55:992–6.

Mazess RB, Barden HS. Bone density in premenopausal women: effects of age, dietary intake, physical activity, smoking, and birth-control pills. Am J Clin Nutr 1991;53:132–42.

McBryde Jr AM. Stress fractures in runners. Clin Sports Med 1985;4:737–52.

Menkes A, Mazel S, Redmond RA, et al. Strength training increases regional bone mineral density and bone remodeling in middle-aged and older men. J Appl Physiol 1993;74:2478–84.

Micklesfield LK, Reyneke L, Fataar A, Myburgh KH. Long-term restoration of deficits in bone mineral density is inadequate in premenopausal women with prior menstrual irregularity. Clin J Sport Med 1998;8:155–63.

Morris FL, Naughton GA, Gibbs JL, Carlson JS, Wark JD. Prospective ten-month exercise intervention in premenarcheal girls: positive effects on bone and lean mass. J Bone Miner Res 1997;12:1453–62.

Myburgh KH, Hutchins J, Fataar AB, Hough SF, Noakes TD. Low bone density is an etiologic factor for stress fractures in athletes. Ann Intern Med 1990;113:754–9.

National Institutes of Health (NIH). Optimal calcium intake. National Institutes of Health Consensus Statement. Bethesda, MD: National Institutes of Health, 1994.

Nattiv A, Armsey Jr TD. Stress injury to bone in the female athlete. Clin Sports Med 1997;16:197–224.

Nelson ME, Fiatarone MA, Morganti CM, et al. Effects of high-intensity strength training on multiple risk factors for osteoporotic fractures. A randomized controlled trial. JAMA 1994;272:1909–14.

Nguyen TV, Howard GM, Kelly PJ, Eisman JA. Bone mass, lean mass, and fat mass: same genes or same environments? Am J Epidemiol 1998;147:3–16.

Nordin BE. Calcium and osteoporosis. Nutrition 1997;13:664–86.

Nordin BE, Heaney RP. Calcium supplementation of the diet: justified by present evidence. BMJ 1990;300:1056–60.

Nordin BE, Need AG, Morris HA, Horowitz M. The nature and significance of the relationship between urinary sodium and urinary calcium in women. J Nutr 1993;123:1615–22.

Nowson CA, Green RM, Hopper JL, et al. A co-twin study of the effect of calcium supplementation on bone density during adolescence. Osteoporos Int 1997;7:219–25.

Parfitt AM. The cellular basis of bone remodeling: the quantum concept reexamined in light of recent advances in the cell biology of bone. Calcif Tissue Int 1984;36 Suppl 1:S37–45.

Parfitt AM. The two faces of growth: benefits and risks to bone integrity. Osteoporos Int 1994; 4:382–98.

Pearce G, Bass S, Young N, Formica C, Seeman E. Does weight-bearing exercise protect against the effects of exercise-induced oligomenorrhea on bone density? Osteoporos Int 1996;6:448–52.

Pocock NA, Eisman JA, Hopper JL, et al. Genetic determinants of bone mass in adults. A twin study. J Clin Invest 1987;80:706–10.

Prince R, Devine A, Dick I, et al. The effects of calcium supplementation (milk powder or tablets) and exercise on bone density in postmenopausal women. J Bone Miner Res 1995;10:1068–75.

Prince RL, Smith M, Dick IM, et al. Prevention of postmenopausal osteoporosis. A comparative study of exercise, calcium supplementation, and hormone-replacement therapy. N Engl J Med 1991;325:1189–95.

Raisz LG. Physiology and pathophysiology of bone remodeling. Clin Chem 1999;45:1353–8.

Recker RR, Davies KM, Hinders SM, et al. Bone gain in young adult women. JAMA 1992;268:2403–8.

Reid IR, Ames RW, Evans MC, Gamble GD, Sharpe SJ. Effect of calcium supplementation on bone loss in postmenopausal women. N Engl J Med 1993;328:460–4.

Reid IR, Ames RW, Evans MC, Gamble GD, Sharpe SJ. Long-term effects of calcium supplementation on bone loss and fractures in postmenopausal women: a randomized controlled trial. Am J Med 1995;98:331–5.

Riggs BL, Wahner HW, Melton 3rd LJ, et al. Dietary calcium intake and rates of bone loss in women. J Clin Invest 1987;80:979–82.

Riis B, Thomsen K, Christiansen C. Does calcium supplementation prevent postmenopausal bone loss? A double-blind, controlled clinical study. N Engl J Med 1987;316:173–7.

Robinson TL, Snow-Harter C, Taaffe DR, et al. Gymnasts exhibit higher bone mass than runners despite similar prevalence of amenorrhea and oligomenorrhea. J Bone Miner Res 1995;10:26–35.

Rubin CT, Lanyon LE. Regulation of bone mass by mechanical strain magnitude. Calcif Tissue Int 1985;37:411–17.

Rubin LA, Hawker GA, Peltekova VD, et al. Determinants of peak bone mass: clinical and genetic analyses in a young female Canadian cohort. J Bone Miner Res 1999;14:633–43.

Ryan AS, Treuth MS, Rubin MA, et al. Effects of strength training on bone mineral density: hormonal and bone turnover relationships. J Appl Physiol 1994;77:1678–84.

Sanders EM, Nowson CA, Kotowicz MA, et al. Calcium and bone health: position statement for the Australian and New Zealand Bone and Mineral Society, Osteoporosis Australia and the Endocrine Society of Australia. MJA 2009;190:316–20.

Slemenda C, Hui SL, Longcope C, Johnston CC. Sex steroids and bone mass. A study of changes about the time of menopause. J Clin Invest 1987;80:1261–9.

Slemenda CW, Peacock M, Hui S, Zhou L, Johnston CC. Reduced rates of skeletal remodeling are associated with increased bone mineral density during the development of peak skeletal mass. J Bone Miner Res 1997;12:676–82.

Smith EL, Gilligan C, Smith PE, Sempos CT. Calcium supplementation and bone loss in middle-aged women. Am J Clin Nutr 1989;50:833–42.

Snead DB, Weltman A, Weltman JY, et al. Reproductive hormones and bone mineral density in women runners. J Appl Physiol 1992;72:2149–56.

Snow-Harter C, Bouxsein ML, Lewis BT, Carter DR, Marcus R. Effects of resistance and endurance exercise on bone mineral status of young women: a randomized exercise intervention trial. J Bone Miner Res 1992;7:761–9.

Taaffe DR, Snow-Harter C, Connolly DA, et al. Differential effects of swimming versus weight-bearing activity on bone mineral status of eumenorrheic athletes. J Bone Miner Res 1995;10:586–93.

Teegarden D, Weaver CM. Calcium supplementation increases bone density in adolescent girls. Nutr Rev 1994;52:171–3.

Turner CH. Toward a mathematical description of bone biology: the principle of cellular accommodation. Calcif Tissue Int 1999;65:466–71.

Vuori I, Heinonen A, Sievanen H, et al. Effects of unilateral strength training and detraining on bone mineral density and content in young women: a study of mechanical loading and deloading on human bones. Calcif Tissue Int 1994;55:59–67.

Warren MP, Brooks-Gunn J, Hamilton LH, Warren LF, Hamilton WG. Scoliosis and fractures in young ballet dancers. Relation to delayed menarche and secondary amenorrhea. N Engl J Med 1986;314:1348–53.

Warren MP, Brooks-Gunn J, Fox RP, et al. Lack of bone accretion and amenorrhea: evidence for a relative osteopenia in weight-bearing bones. J Clin Endocrinol Metab 1991;72:847–53.

Wastney ME, Martin BR, Peacock M, et al. Changes in calcium kinetics in adolescent girls induced by high calcium intake. J Clin Endocrinol Metab 2000;85:4470–5.

Weaver CM. Calcium requirements of physically active people. Am J Clin Nutr 2000;72(2 Suppl): 579S–84S.

Williams JA, Wagner J, Wasnich R, Heilbrun L. The effect of long-distance running upon appendicular bone mineral content. Med Sci Sports Exerc 1984;16:223–7.

Winters-Stone KM, Snow CM. One year of oral calcium supplementation maintains cortical bone density in young adult female distance runners. Int J Sport Nutr Exerc Metab 2004;14:7–17.

Wolman RL, Clark P, McNally E, Harries M, Reeve J. Menstrual state and exercise as determinants of spinal trabecular bone density in female athletes. BMJ 1990;301:516–18.

Wolman RL, Clark P, McNally E, Harries MG, Reeve J. Dietary calcium as a statistical determinant of spinal trabecular bone density in amenorrhoeic and oestrogen-replete athletes. Bone Miner 1992;17:415–23.

Working Group of the Australian and New Zealand Bone and Mineral Society, Endocrine Society of Australia, Osteoporosis Australia. Vitamin D and adult bone health in Australia and New Zealand: a position statement. Med J Aust 2005;182:281–5.

World Health Organization (WHO). Assessment of fracture risk and its application to screening for post-menopausal women, Technical Report Series No 843, WHO Scientific Study Group. Geneva: World Health Organization, 1994.

Young N, Formica C, Szmukler G, Seeman E. Bone density at weight-bearing and nonweight-bearing sites in ballet dancers: the effects of exercise, hypogonadism, and body weight. J Clin Endocrinol Metab 1994;78:449–54.

Zanker CL. Bone metabolism in exercise associated amenorrhoea: the importance of nutrition. Br J Sports Med 1999;33:228–9.

Zanker CL, Swaine IL. Bone turnover in amenorrhoeic and eumenorrhoeic women distance runners. Scand J Med Sci Sports 1998;8:20–6.

CHAPTER 10

Prevention, detection and treatment of iron depletion and deficiency in athletes

VICKI DEAKIN

10.1 Introduction

Athletes, in particular females and adolescents, are at risk of depleting iron stores. If untreated, iron depletion could eventually develop into iron deficiency anemia (IDA), which severely affects training capacity. Recent findings suggest that maintaining an optimum iron status within the cells and tissues is far more important for athletes than has previously been realized. Even a mild shortfall in tissue iron status appears not only to reduce maximum oxygen uptake and aerobic efficiency, but also to reduce the body's endurance capacity. Any athlete involved in regular high-intensity physical activity has a higher requirement and turnover of iron and can quickly deplete iron stores.

Although iron is widely distributed in foods, inappropriate food combinations can compromise its absorption. High-carbohydrate (CHO) diets recommended for athletes undertaking high levels of physical activity may be high in compounds that inhibit iron absorption. While diet contributes to iron depletion in athletes, physiological and medical factors also play a role. Dietary strategies to help prevent iron depletion should be implemented early in the training program in high-risk individuals. Early detection of depleted iron stores and dietary intervention are warranted. Recovery from depleted or exhausted iron stores is slow; iron stores can take months to replenish.

Different types of anemia are linked to other nutrients such as deficiencies of folate, vitamin B12 and vitamin C and induced by inflammation or chronic disease (i.e. the anemia of inflammation). These types of anemia will not be considered in this chapter.

10.2 Stages of iron depletion

Several commonly used hematological markers are used to categorize iron status in the general population. These are also applied to an athletic population. Although iron depletion is a continuous process, traditionally three categories or stages of iron deficiency have been identified, based on hematological markers as shown in Table 10.1.

TABLE 10.1 POPULATION CUT-OFFS FOR HEMATOLOGICAL MARKERS COMMONLY USED TO EVALUATE IRON STATUS IN CLINICAL PRACTICE

STAGE OF IRON DEFICIENCY	HEMATOLOGICAL MARKERS	DEFICIENCY/OVERLOAD STATE
STAGE 1		
Depleted iron stores	Stainable iron in the bone marrow	Absent
	Total iron binding capacity	>400 µg/dL
	SF	<12 µg/L (>15 years)
STAGE 2		
Early functional iron deficiency	Transferrin saturation	<16% (>10 years)
	Serum transferrin receptor	>8.5 mg/L
STAGE 3		
IDA	Hemoglobin	<130 g/L (males >15 years)
		<120 g/L (females >15 years)
	MCV	<80 fL

IDA = iron deficiency anemia, MCV = mean cell volume, SF = serum ferritin
Sources: Expert Scientific Working Group 1985; INACG 1985; Ferguson et al. 1992; Sauberlich 1999; Food and Nutrition Board 2000a

An additional category unrelated to iron status but common in athletes, called dilutional pseudo-anemia (or sports anemia), has been used to describe a unique physiological response to training in an athletic population (see section 10.14). As iron stores are depleted progressively, iron-containing compounds in the body, including ferritin, hemoglobin, transferrin and myoglobin, also become depleted, but not all compounds are affected at the same time as implied by these three stages. Cut-off values for determining the iron status in children and adolescents are published elsewhere (Looker et al. 1997). Interpreting these indicators in athletes is described in detail in section 10.35.

The terminology and cut-off values for each stage of iron depletion vary considerably, especially in studies on athletes. Terms including marginal iron deficiency, early iron depletion, iron deficiency without anemia and iron deficiency erythropoiesis are often used interchangeably in the literature. Iron deficiency without anemia is the most frequently used term and appears to encompass depleted iron stores and perhaps early functional iron deficiency—normal hemoglobin and low serum ferritin (SF) values. When iron stores are exhausted, the functional iron compartment, which affects the oxidative capacity of the muscle, then becomes affected (Suominen et al. 1998). In the absence of standard reference values for athletes, researchers have set cut-offs for SF (the main indicator of depleted iron stores), ranging from <16 µg/L (Zhu & Haas 1998; Hinton et al. 2000) to <30 µg/L (Telford et al. 1992) to designate iron deficiency without anemia. An SF level of 20 µg/L is the value most frequently used (Malczewska et al. 2000; Friedmann et al. 2001; Brutsaert et al. 2003; Dubnov & Constantini 2004; Deruisseau et al. 2004). These different values confound interpretation of the true effects of different stages of iron status on performance measures or other health outcomes.

SF reflects the magnitude of the storage iron compartment, not the amount of iron available in the tissue or its functional pool. The emergence of a new hematological marker that measures tissue iron status—serum transferrin receptor (sTfR)—has allowed researchers to distinguish between depleted iron stores and functional iron deficiency, and to investigate how inadequate iron in the tissue, compared to low SF, might affect the performance capacity of athletes. Calculating the ratio of sTfR to low SF is a way of combining sTfR and SF and is considered a more reliable determinant of iron status in individuals than either indicator used alone, especially in borderline cases (see section 10.37). These indicators have not yet been characterized in athletes, so there are no standardized cut-offs that represent the point at which low levels of tissue iron might limit performance capacity.

10.3 How common is iron deficiency/iron depletion in athletes?

The estimated prevalence of iron deficiency (including iron depletion) in the US population is highest in female adolescents aged 16–19 years (16.6%), male adolescents aged 12–15 years (4.5%) and adult females aged 20–49 years (13.4%), based on data from the National Health and Nutrition Examination Survey IV (NHANES IV) in the US between 1994 and 2004 (Cardenas et al. 2006).

Three groups of athletes at the highest risk of iron depletion and deficiency are female athletes, distance runners and vegetarians (and those who eat little red meat) (Fogelholm 1995). Adolescent athletes are at high risk if they undertake sports with endurance training, because of the higher iron requirement for growth (Commonwealth Department of Health and Ageing et al. 2006). The true prevalence of iron depletion or deficiency, however, is unknown because reported prevalence data are usually based on SF measures alone and are confounded by the lack of a universal cut-off for ferritin and the inconsistent terminology used for iron depletion. Low SF levels in isolation do not necessarily confirm a diagnosis of iron deficiency or depletion and could be indicative of early iron depletion or even functional iron deficiency, an already common condition in the population.

10.4 Is the prevalence of low iron stores in athletes different from the general population?

Comparison of SF between athletes and control groups shows mixed results. Some authors have reported lower SF levels in athletes (Pate et al. 1993; Constantini et al. 2000; Dubnov et al. 2004), whereas others have reported higher values than untrained controls, especially in males (Balaban 1992; Fogelholm et al. 1992; Schumacher, Schmid, Grathwohl et al. 2002).

In an analytical study of pooled iron status measures of athletes published from 1980 to 1994, lower SF levels were more frequently found in female athletes and in endurance athletes of both sexes (e.g. runners, rowers and swimmers) compared to untrained controls (Fogelholm 1995). However, in a more recent study of 126 female endurance athletes, average SF values of athletes were higher than those of the controls (Malczewska et al. 2000). In this study, average SF levels were higher in females training an average of 2.5 h/d than in untrained controls. Nevertheless, 26% of all female athletes in this study were still considered iron deficient, based on ferritin (<20 μg/L), compared to a 50% incidence of iron deficiency in the untrained controls.

Prevalence of depleted iron stores in athletes 10.5

In athletes, the prevalence of depleted iron stores based on SF levels below reference cut-offs varies according to type of sport, age of the athlete and sex. The highest prevalence occurs in female and adolescent athletes, irrespective of the type of sport and intensity of training (Pate et al. 1993; Malczewska et al. 2000; Constantini et al. 2000; Dubnov & Constantini 2004; Merkel et al. 2005; Fallon 2004, 2008; Fallon & Gerrard 2007).

Male athletes have a lower prevalence than females because of their lower requirements and higher capacity to store iron, except for runners (Dufaux et al. 1981; Fogelholm 1995; Schumacher et al. 2002b). However, in two studies, 45% of male gymnasts (Constantini et al. 2000) and 15% of male basketball players (Dubnov & Constantini 2004) had SF values below 20 µg/L. In a prospective survey of hematological markers of 303 male and 273 female athletes training at the Australian Institute of Sport, 19% of females and 3.3% of males had SF levels below 30 µg/L and were given iron supplements (Fallon 2007). These results are similar to an earlier study of another cohort of Australian Institute of Sport athletes published in 2004 (Fallon 2004).

Prevalence of iron deficiency anemia in athletes 10.6

The prevalence of IDA in athletes is usually quite low (<3%) and similar between adult athletes and untrained controls (Weight et al. 1992; Fogelholm 1995), with some exceptions (Dubnov & Constantini 2004; Merkel et al. 2005; Israeli et al. 2008). The estimated prevalence of IDA in US adults is 0.6% in men aged 16–69 years and 4.7% in women aged 20–49 years; of concern are substantial differences by race and ethnicity, with 12.2% and 7.6% prevalence in African-American and Mexican-American women respectively (Cardenas et al. 2006; Cusick et al. 2008). In younger age groups, the highest prevalence for IDA in the US population, based on the NHANES IV survey, mimics the trend for iron deficiency/depletion: 4.7% in adult women, 3.3% in adolescent girls aged 16–19 years and 0.6% in teenage boys and adult men (Cardenas et al. 2006; Cusick et al. 2008).

Why is iron important to athletes? 10.7

From a performance perspective, iron participates in several biochemical reactions involved in oxidative energy production. Iron is an essential part of the oxygen transport proteins: hemoglobin in red blood cells, which transports oxygen into body cells, and myoglobin, responsible for facilitating oxygen diffusion to the cellular site of energy production, the mitochondria. Within the mitochondria, iron is a component of oxidative enzymes and respiratory chain proteins including cytochromes involved in substrate oxidation to energy. Clearly, iron has a strong functional role in maintaining the energy release needed to support aerobic and endurance capacity.

Other functional roles of iron can also influence an athlete's training capacity and health status independent of its role in energy production. Iron is also needed for erythropoiesis (red blood cell production), for thyroid hormone metabolism (Bothwell et al. 1979), for neural function (Beard & Connor 2003) and for maintaining immune function (Beard 2001). When iron is in excess in the body, which occurs in people with hemochromatosis, it also acts as a catalyst to generate free oxygen radicals, which attack cellular membranes, protein and DNA and can potentially damage tissue and impair immune function (Reddy & Clarke 2004; Gleeson et al. 2001).

The largest component of iron in the body is found in hemoglobin circulating in the blood (60–70% of total iron) and myoglobin in the muscle tissue (10% of total iron) (Nielsen & Natchtigall 1998). Iron is transported through the plasma and extra-vascular fluids in protein carriers called transferrin. The rest is mainly stored as ferritin and hemosiderin in the liver, bone marrow and muscle, ready for erythropoiesis. Although only a small component of iron (around 2%) is used in metabolic systems, inadequate iron in the iron stores, reflected by the levels of SF, can adversely affect the functional role of iron at the cellular level and potentially the oxidative capacity of the muscle (Hinton & Sinclair 2007).

10.8 Effects of iron status on performance and other health outcomes

The effects of iron depletion on performance capacity have been the focus of much research. Other effects of iron depletion, independent of its role in oxidative metabolism—such as fatigue, altered resistance to infection, and muscle and hormone dysfunction—could also limit training capacity. These effects further compound the negative influence of exhausted iron stores on the ability to undertake physical activity. The greater the severity of iron depletion, the greater the effect, although some individuals are more sensitive to these effects than others.

10.9 Does iron deficiency affect athletic performance?

10.10 Effects of iron deficiency anemia on performance

The debilitating effects of IDA on aerobic and endurance capacity, work capacity and energy efficiency in animal and human studies on both untrained and trained subjects have been confirmed in a review by Haas and Brownlie (2001). IDA impairs erythropoiesis so oxygen delivery to the tissue and work rate ($VO_{2\,max}$) is limited (Celsing et al. 1989).

Even a small decrease in hemoglobin of 1–2 g/100 mL can decrease performance by around 20% (Gardner et al. 1977). Disturbances in brain metabolism, muscle metabolism, immunity and temperature control can occur in IDA, depending on severity of the depletion (Bothwell et al. 1979).

10.11 Effects of iron deficiency without anemia on performance

Although it is well established that IDA impairs training capacity, the effects on performance in the early stages of iron depletion have been less clear. Theoretically, with depleted iron stores, only iron stores, not hemoglobin levels, are compromised, so maximal oxygen uptake to the tissue should not be affected.

Given the role of iron at the cellular level however, inadequate tissue iron should reduce oxidative capacity and also impair endurance capacity. Recent evidence shows some support for this theory. With functional iron deficiency without anemia, when both iron stores and tissue stores become limited, the capacity of muscle and other tissue to use oxygen and other iron-containing proteins for the oxidative production of energy may be compromised. The few early studies on athletes with extremely low iron status found significant improvements in aerobic capacity after iron supplementation in previously iron-deficient athletes (Schoene et al. 1983; Fogelholm et al. 1992; LaManca & Haymes 1993), thereby providing some support for this hypothesis.

The evidence supporting a decreased aerobic or endurance capacity in athletes with depleted or exhausted iron stores (low SF values) has been equivocal. No significant improvement in aerobic capacity (using $VO_{2\,max}$ tests) in response to iron supplementation of athletes compared to controls was found in several well-designed randomized, double-blind, placebo-controlled trials (Rowland et al. 1988; Newhouse et al. 1989; Klingshirn et al. 1992; Zhu & Haas 1998; Peeling et al. 2007). Similar findings were reported in these studies measuring endurance capacity, with some exceptions (Rowland et al. 1988; Friedmann et al. 2001). In a more recent study, compared to controls, no significant improvement in endurance capacity (time to exhaustion) or energy efficiency was observed in eight iron-depleted female trained athletes (sTfR = 5.9 mg/L, SF = 19 μg/L) after iron injection using a $VO_{2\,max}$ test and sub-max (70% $VO_{2\,max}$) test, despite substantial increases in iron stores in the injected group (Peeling et al. 2007). The authors suggest that the 10-minute sub-max test at 70% $VO_{2\,max}$ might not be specific enough to detect performance economy changes. Interestingly, in this study no improvement in mean sTfR in the injected group was seen, which implies that the functional role of iron was not yet affected, which could also explain the lack of improvement in aerobic capacity in the supplemented group.

In contrast, studies in people with very depleted iron stores, using both SF and sTfR, suggest that even at stage 1 (depleted iron stores), both aerobic function and endurance capacity could be compromised, if tissue iron is inadequate (Zhu & Haas 1998; Hinton et al. 2000; Hinton & Sinclair 2007). Zhu and Haas (1998) demonstrated an increased energy efficiency in seventeen physically active women with depleted iron stores (sTfR = 6.0 mg/L, SF = <16 μg/L) after 8 weeks on iron supplements compared to controls, although no difference was observed in endurance capacity between the groups. Increased energy efficiency (work rate) means that at the same exercise intensity (83% $VO_{2\,max}$), the iron-supplemented group was able to complete the test, a modified 15 km simulated time trial, at a lower level of physical exertion.

Using similar testing protocols, Hinton and colleagues found a significant improvement in endurance capacity and energy efficiency in forty-one untrained iron-depleted women, after 4 weeks of iron supplements and aerobic training, compared to controls. The mean sTfR value at baseline for all subjects was close to 8 mg/L, indicative of functional iron deficiency. All hematological markers except hemoglobin significantly improved in the iron-supplemented group compared to baseline and controls (Hinton et al. 2000). Further analyses of these data demonstrated that tissue iron deficiency impaired adaptation to endurance capacity (Brownlie et al. 2002) and that the greatest improvement in aerobic capacity was seen in those subjects who were the most depleted (Brownlie et al. 2004). More recently, Hinton and Sinclair (2007) tested the effects of only 30 mg of elemental iron supplements for 6 weeks in twenty recreational iron-depleted athletes (sTfR = 6.58 mg/L, SF = 11.67 μg/L) and found a significant improvement in ferritin, sTfR and aerobic function using a 60-minute sub-max test at 60% $VO_{2\,max}$ compared to controls.

In contrast, no improvement in endurance capacity (time to exhaustion) or energy efficiency was observed in eight iron-depleted female athletes (sTfR = 5.9 mg/L, SF = 19 μg/L) after injections of 100 mg of iron for 10 days using a sub-max test (70% $VO_{2\,max}$), despite substantial increases in ferritin in the injected group (Peeling et al. 2007). The authors suggest that the 10-minute sub-max test at 70% $VO_{2\,max}$ might not be specific or long enough to detect performance economy changes observed in the 30-minute trial at a higher intensity reported in the Zhu and Haas study (1998) and in the 60-minute trial used by Hinton and Sinclair (2007). An interesting finding in this study was no improvement in sTfR in the injected group, which implies that the functional role of iron was not yet affected, so performance was not compromised.

10.12 Limitations in research design of performance studies

Failure of earlier studies to demonstrate a performance disadvantage of early iron depletion may have been attributed to several factors: (1) using varying cut-offs for SF; (2) small sample size and small effect size; (3) the influence of psychological and training effects; (4) lack of a marker for measuring tissue iron depletion; and (5) low specificity of performance tests to measure endurance capacity, particularly in untrained subjects.

Endurance capacity was usually tested using exercise intensities at >80% $VO_{2\ max}$, a level well above the anaerobic threshold of most subjects (Hinton et al. 2000). At this level of exertion, iron is not involved in energy production, so low tissue iron would not limit endurance capacity (Haas & Brownlie 2001). However, in the study by Peeling and colleagues (2007), where a lower exercise intensity test was used (70% $VO_{2\ max}$), no improvement in endurance capacity was reported.

10.13 Summary of performance effects of iron deficiency

In summary, IDA impairs aerobic capacity, which can be corrected by increasing hemoglobin. Iron depletion without anemia does not affect oxygen-carrying capacity ($VO_{2\ max}$) or limit the functional role of iron in the tissues to carry out oxidative metabolism, so aerobic capacity is not impaired. There is now limited although convincing evidence that tissue iron deficiency, represented by sTfR at levels greater than 8.0 mg/L, together with very low iron stores, affects the functional role of iron in energy metabolism, and can impair an athlete's capacity to undertake aerobic training, as well as decrease work rate and energy efficiency. More studies are needed to determine the level at which tissue iron deficiency might affect performance in highly trained athletes before definitive recommendations can be made.

10.14 Dilutional pseudo-anemia or 'sports anemia'

Shaskey and Green (2000) recommend that the term 'dilutional pseudo-anemia' be used as the preferred terminology for the transient condition often referred to as 'sports anemia', 'athlete's anemia', 'runner's anemia', 'post-exercise anemia' or 'swimmer's anemia'. These terms are misleading and confusing. Dilutional pseudo-anemia is not genuine iron depletion or deficiency, but the result of a dilution effect on hematological markers. Several studies have shown that periods of intense training are accompanied by an increase in plasma volume—a 'normal' adaptive response to training—and a corresponding reduction in iron status measures (Schumacher, Schmid, Grathwohl et al. 2002; Malczewska et al. 2004; Merkel et al. 2005). Training increases plasma volume at greater rate than the increase in the red cell mass (Chatard et al. 1999). Hence the red cell mass appears diluted.

Up to a 20% increase in plasma volume has been reported in the 48 hours after a race in marathon runners and can persist for as long as a week (Dill et al. 1974; Brotherhood et al. 1975; Schmidt et al. 1989). There are usually no symptoms and performance is unlikely to be affected, as iron is not limiting red blood cell production.

Dilutional pseudo-anemia does not respond to iron supplements (Hegenauer et al. 1983; Magnusson et al. 1984). In clinical practice, differentiating between dilutional pseudo-anemia and true iron depletion using the usual hematological indicators is often difficult.

Does iron depletion affect fatigue? 10.15

Symptoms of fatigue and lethargy, common complaints in IDA, are not usually reported in people without anemia. In one study of forty-one competitive athletes with persistent fatigue, iron depletion accounted for only 3% of unexplained fatigue (Reid et al. 2004). In this study, the most common conditions linked to persistent fatigue were immune deficiency (28%) and unresolved viral infections (27%). Overtraining is also implicated (Toit & Locke 2007). In another study of fifty elite athletes who presented with short-term fatigue and tiredness of around 1–3 weeks, the main contributing factors were training related (28%) or a combination of training effects and infection (30%) (Fallon 2006). In this study, iron depletion was a minor contributor, with only 1% of athletes presenting with low ferritin stores.

Nevertheless, individual athletes with low SF values often complain of fatigue in the absence of any obvious clinical or physiological cause. Such symptoms can affect concentration and performance and increase the risk of injury. In one randomized, double-blind, placebo-controlled trial of untrained women with low SF values (mean SF about 30 μg/L), a significant improvement in unexplained fatigue was reported in the iron-supplemented group compared to controls (Verdon et al. 2003). The improvement was greatest in women with baseline SF ≤50 μg/L after iron supplementation. One explanation for unexplained fatigue in relation to iron depletion is a depressed activity of iron-dependent enzymes, which can affect the metabolism of neurotransmitters (Beard & Connor 2003). In athletes with low iron stores, unexplained fatigue, especially during physical activity, may be linked to tissue iron deficiency, but has not been studied. Future studies on the effects of low tissue iron status on performance should include measures of fatigue at rest and during activity to clarify this association. In summary, the reasons for short-term and persistent fatigue in athletes may be related to iron depletion or deficiency, although the primary contributors are training related or infection related. In some situations, a blood test may be warranted to confirm a diagnosis.

Does iron depletion affect immune function? 10.16

Strenuous prolonged exertion and heavy training are linked with depressed immune function and increased rate of infection (see Commentary C, p. 501), although the incidence of upper respiratory tract infections in swimmers training at the Australian Institute of Sport was similar to population data (Fricker et al. 2000). A low iron status and inadequate intake of iron and other micronutrients including zinc and vitamins A, E, B6 and B12 are also associated with immune dysfunction and possible exercise-induced immunosuppression (Konig et al. 1998; Gleeson et al. 2001). However, deficiencies of these micronutrients are rare in athletes and the extent by which low iron status, in isolation, may compromise the immune system is unknown.

Dietary iron absorption 10.17

Iron absorption and bioavailability (the amount of dietary iron available for metabolic functions) is influenced by the iron status of the individual and the type of iron consumed (Hurrell 1997). Iron absorption and metabolism is regulated by the small peptide hormone hepcidin, which is produced by the liver (Ganz 2003). One effect of high levels of circulating hepcidin is the inhibition of intestinal iron absorption (Ganz & Nemeth 2005). In contrast, its inhibitory effect on iron absorption diminishes when hepcidin levels decrease and more dietary iron is absorbed.

When iron stores are saturated, iron absorption is around 5–15% (Hallberg et al. 2000). In people with depleted iron stores or with high physiological requirements (e.g. to support growth, pregnancy or lactation), iron absorption increases to around 14–16% (Hallberg & Hulthen 1996; Fairweather-Tait 1996).

The type of dietary iron also affects iron absorption. Iron exists in two forms: heme (also known as haem) and non-heme (or non-haem). Heme iron is iron bound to protein complexes—hemoglobin or myoglobin—while the non-heme form is found as an iron salt in the ferric form (Fe^{3+}). Heme iron is more readily absorbed than non-heme iron, which needs to be converted into a soluble form to be absorbed. Meat, liver, seafood and poultry contain both forms whereas plant sources, mainly cereal and grains, legumes, vegetables, fruits, eggs, iron-fortified commercial foods (such as breakfast cereal) and iron supplements contain only the non-heme form (see Table 10.2).

Meat contains 30–70% of its total iron as heme iron (MacPhail et al. 1985; Rangan et al. 1997). In Australian meat, 60–70% of the total iron in cooked lean rump steak, lamb, pork and chicken is heme iron, whereas beef sausage, liver and tuna contain around 20–35% heme iron (Rangan et al. 1997). The heme iron content of lamb and beef is particularly high compared to that in chicken and fish, which explains why red meat is an excellent iron source. Although the contribution of heme iron in a western-style diet is around 10–15% of total iron intake, it contributes around one-third of the total iron absorbed (Hallberg 1981). The rest of the iron comes from non-heme sources.

TABLE 10.2 COMPONENTS IN FOOD THAT AFFECT BIOAVAILABILITY OF IRON, MAINLY FROM NON-HEME FOOD SOURCES

IRON ENHANCERS	IRON INHIBITORS
Vitamin C-rich foods (ascorbic acid)[a,b,k] such as salad, lightly cooked green vegetables, some fruits and citrus fruit juices and vitamin C-fortified fruit juices	Phytate (inositol hexaphosphate)[f,h], for example in cereal grains, wheat bran, legumes, nuts, peanut butter, seeds, bran, soy products, soy protein and spinach
Some fermented foods with a low pH[e,f] such as sauerkraut, miso and some types of soy sauce	Polyphenolic compounds[a,d,f], for example in strong tea and coffee, herb tea, cocoa, red wine and some spices (e.g. oregano)
Peptides from partially digested muscle tissue, which enhance both heme and non-heme iron[k,j]; this is often called the 'meat enhancement factor' and is found in beef, lamb, chicken, pork and liver—and fish (although fish isn't commonly thought of as a 'meat')	Calcium, which inhibits both heme and non-heme iron[a,b,c], for example in milk and cheese
Alcohol and some organic acids[f], for example in very low pH foods containing citric acid or tartaric acid, such as citrus fruit	Peptides from partially digested plant proteins[g,d,i,l], such as soy protein isolates and soy products
Vitamin A and beta carotene[m]	

Sources: [a]Hallberg 1981; [b]Hallberg, Rossander-Hulthen et al. 1993; [c]Cook et al. 1991; [d]Hallberg & Rossander 1982a; [e]Baynes et al. 1990; [f]Gillooly et al. 1983; [g]Lynch et al. 1994; [h]Brune et al. 1992; [i]Hurrell 1997; [j]Layrisse et al. 1984; [k]Gillooly et al. 1984; [l]Hallberg & Rossander 1982b; [m]Garcia-Casal et al. 1998, 2003

Dietary factors affecting dietary iron absorption 10.18

A large proportion of dietary iron is unavailable for absorption and is removed in the feces. The presence of vitamin C, vitamin A and protein from meat, fish and poultry enhance iron absorption, whereas phytates (found in legumes and grains), calcium, and polyphenols and tannins (in tea and coffee) inhibit iron absorption (see Table 10.2). Because of the presence of these inhibitors and enhancers in food, iron bioavailability from the total diet can vary tenfold from different meals with similar iron content (Hallberg et al. 2000).

Heme iron is efficiently absorbed from single foods (15–35%), although absorption is mildly affected by the inhibitors and enhancers in foods (Hallberg et al. 1997; Hunt 2001). Iron-rich plant sources of non-heme iron, including cereals, nuts, seeds, legumes and spinach, contain substantial quantities of inhibiting components that reduce the solubility of iron and limit its absorption. This explains why the 2–15% non-heme iron absorption from single meals is much lower than heme iron absorption (Hallberg et al. 1997). Soy beans and soy bean products contain several different inhibiting compounds and so have low bioavailability.

Inhibitors of dietary iron absorption 10.19

Phytates are salts of inositol hexaphosphate, found in cereal grains, legumes, seeds, nuts, vegetables and fruit, and can inhibit non-heme iron absorption by 50–80% (Hallberg et al. 1989).

Phytates concentrate in the bran and germ of cereal grains and legumes and are added via soy protein isolates to manufactured foods (Hurrell 1997). Although fiber itself does not inhibit iron absorption (Brune et al. 1992), foods rich in fiber are rich in phytates. High-bran cereals can have more than 3000 mg phytates/100 g cereal compared to cornflakes, which have about 70 mg phytates/100 g cereal (Harland & Oberleas 1987). Vegetables and fruits are poor sources of phytates, but even small amounts of phytates can have an inhibitory effect (Hallberg et al. 1989). Phytates are degraded in bread during dough fermentation and in milling of flour and rice, thereby increasing the bioavailability of the remaining iron (Hallberg et al. 2000).

Polyphenolic compounds found in plants, including phenolic acid and flavonoids (e.g. tannin), substantially inhibit non-heme iron absorption. Polyphenols are highest in black tea compared with other types of tea, such as herbal or green teas, and are also found in coffee, cocoa, red wine and many vegetables, including spinach and several herbs and spices (e.g. rosemary and oregano). In a western-style breakfast (toast and tea), the absorption of non-heme iron from bread was reduced by 60% because of concurrent consumption with black tea (Rossander et al. 1979). Coffee reduced absorption of non-heme iron by 35% from a hamburger meal, while tea reduced absorption by 62% (Hallberg & Rossander 1982a).

The inhibition of iron absorption by polyphenols in tea and other beverages is strongly dose related. Even at low tannin concentrations of 5 mg, absorption of iron was inhibited by 30%; at concentrations of 25 mg by 67%, and at concentrations of 100 mg by 88% (Brune et al. 1989). One glass of red wine (high in polyphenolic compounds) reduced iron absorption from a bread-based meal by 75% (Cook et al. 1995). In one study of adult female runners, coffee/tea consumption was significantly associated with low iron stores (Pate et al. 1993). Drinking tea or coffee with main meals is an important contributor to the high prevalence of iron deficiency in developing countries where strong beverages are consumed with each meal (Hallberg et al. 2000).

Calcium inhibits both heme and non-heme iron absorption although the inhibitory effects appear weaker than for phytates and polyphenols (Hurrell 1997). Although strong inhibitory effects have been reported from single-meal studies on non-heme iron absorption (Cook et al. 1991) and on heme iron absorption (Hallberg et al. 1991; Hallberg, Rossander-Hulthen et al. 1993), the overall weak effect of calcium on iron absorption from the whole diet does not justify avoidance of milk or dairy foods with iron-rich food at each meal (such as milk with breakfast cereal) (Reddy & Cook 1997; Grinder-Pedersen et al. 2004). Inadequate intakes of calcium in female and adolescent athletes are already a concern and removal of milk with breakfast cereal would further decrease calcium intakes.

Peptides, from the partial digestion of proteins, can either inhibit or enhance non-heme iron absorption depending on their source (Hurrell 1997). As shown in Table 10.2, peptides derived from legume proteins are inhibitory and bind iron in the intestine, while peptides from animal protein appear to enhance iron absorption, with the exception of calcium peptides from dairy foods (MacFarlane et al. 1988; Hurrell 1997).

10.20 Enhancers of dietary iron absorption

Several dietary enhancers of iron absorption have been identified: ascorbic acid, vitamin A, alcohol, some acidic foods and possibly peptides found in meat, seafood and poultry. There must be sufficient amounts of these enhancers present at the time of consumption for an enhancement effect. Vitamin A, vitamin C and other organic acids form a complex with inorganic (non-heme) iron, which enhances bioavailability by chemically reducing ferric iron to the more soluble ferrous form (Hurrell 1997; García-Casal et al. 1998).

Ascorbic acid (or vitamin C) is the most potent iron enhancer. See Hallberg and colleagues (1986) for a review. One glass of orange juice containing 100 mg of ascorbic acid consumed with a hamburger meal increased absorption of non-heme iron by 85% (Hallberg & Rossander 1982a). Large amounts of ascorbic acid in doses up to 500 mg are needed to negate the inhibitory effects of meals high in phytates and polyphenols (Hallberg et al. 1986, 1989). However, the absorption-enhancing effects of vitamin C are less pronounced from the whole diet than from single meals (Cook & Reddy 2001). As a general guideline for enhancing iron absorption, Hallberg and colleagues (1989) suggest that foods containing about 50 mg of ascorbic acid should be included with each main meal. Table 10.3 provides examples of ascorbic acid-rich foods.

Muscle tissue (meat, seafood and poultry) exerts a promoting effect on the absorption of both heme and non-heme iron. The heme iron in meat is efficiently absorbed. Other enhancers present in meat (and fish) also increase iron absorption in a meal otherwise from non-heme sources, although the mechanism of this enhancing effect is unknown. This enhancement effect explains why meat eaters have higher SF levels than non-meat eaters. An increase in non-heme iron absorption by two- to fourfold occurs when meat (or any animal tissue) is added to a vegetarian meal. Even small amounts of meat (around 50 g) can increase non-heme iron absorption from a high phytates (220 mg), low-ascorbic-acid meal, significantly reducing the inhibitory action of phytates (Baech et al. 2003).

10.21 Estimating iron bioavailability in meals or diets

Studies investigating the iron bioavailability from either single meals or the whole diet confirm the importance of combining foods as a means of maximizing iron absorption and minimizing the effects of inhibitors (Hulthen et al. 1995; Hallberg et al. 1997). Studies of

TABLE 10.3 EXAMPLES OF ASCORBIC ACID (VITAMIN C)-RICH FOODS

FOOD	SERVING SIZE	ASCORBIC ACID (VITAMIN C) (MG/SERVE)
FRUITS AND FRUIT JUICES		
Orange juice (commercial, with added vitamin C)	1 glass (200 mL)	109
Pawpaw	1 cup, diced (~150 g)	90
Apple juice (commercial, with added vitamin C)	1 glass (200 mL)	90
Blackcurrant juice	1 glass (200 mL)	86
Orange (navel), peeled	1 piece (160 g)	84
Fresh orange juice, home-squeezed	1 glass (200 mL)	70
Strawberry	1 cup (~150 g)	68
Kiwifruit	1 kiwifruit (50 g)	57
Rockmelon	1 cup, diced (165 g)	34
Fruit drink (such as orange and mango)	1 glass (200 mL)	27
VEGETABLES, INCLUDING SALAD VEGETABLES		
Capsicum (red/green) raw	½ cup, chopped (60 g)	102 (red)
		60 (green)
Brussels sprout (boiled, steamed, microwaved)	5 sprouts (85 g)	75
Cauliflower (boiled, steamed, microwaved)	4 flowerets (120 g)	61
Broccoli (boiled, steamed, microwaved)	4 flowerets (40 g)	34
Cabbage (boiled, steamed microwaved)	1 cup (135 g)	34
Tomato	1 medium (130 g)	30
Potato (boiled)	1 medium (145 g)	26

Sources: Food Standards Australia New Zealand: NUTTAB 2006; AUSNUT 2007

the bioavailability of iron from different diets designed for athletes or dietary intervention studies of athletes have not been conducted.

Several algorithms have been developed and validated to calculate the bioavailability of iron and allow estimations of iron absorption from whole diets, accounting for the effects of iron promoters and inhibitors (Hallberg & Hulthen 2000; Reddy et al. 2000). These can be used to predict iron absorption from various diets; to test the efficacy of iron intervention studies; and to evaluate the iron value/bioavailability of meals/diets when catering for any population, including athletes.

Causes of iron deficiency in athletes 10.22

Physiological, medical and dietary factors are responsible for iron deficiency in any population. In athletes, high iron requirements induced by athletic training, blood loss and growth, in combination with inadequate iron intake and low iron bioavailability, are potential causes. Roecker and colleagues (2005) suggest that chronically elevated hepcidin levels observed in athletes undertaking endurance exercise may lead to iron depletion. Table 10.4 summarizes physiological, medical and dietary factors linked with iron depletion that are specific to athletes.

10.23 Physiological causes

10.24 Athletic training and strenuous exercise

Athletic training can increase iron requirements, iron turnover in the tissue and iron losses, and potentially increase hepcidin levels. The greater the duration of training and intensity of workload, the greater the decline in iron stores, irrespective of sport (Telford & Cunningham 1991; Ashenden et al. 1998). In the absence of a dietary reason, no single physiological factor can explain the magnitude of the decline in iron status reported during an extended period of athletic training (Cook 1994), although the recent discovery of the iron regulatory hormone, hepcidin, may shed some light on this association (see section 10.38)

Athletes involved in high-intensity endurance training programs have the highest iron turnover and incidence of iron deficiency. In one large study of 747 trained athletes divided into three groups (power, endurance and mixed), the lowest iron stores were confirmed in the endurance athletes of both sexes, especially the runners (Schumacher, Schmid, Grathwohl et al. 2002). Significant decreases in iron status indicators have also been reported after 12 weeks resistance and weight training in young males and

TABLE 10.4 PHYSIOLOGICAL, MEDICAL AND DIETARY RISK FACTORS ASSOCIATED WITH IRON DEFICIENCY IN ATHLETES

RISK FACTORS	LINK WITH IRON DEFICIENCY
Athletic/strenuous training	Increases iron requirements by stimulating an increase in vascularity, red cell mass and hemoglobin, thereby decreasing iron stores
	Potentially causes high iron loss from sweating; from blood loss caused by injury or nose bleeds; from blood loss in the urine (hematuria) or from the gastrointestinal system; or from damage to red blood cells (hemolysis)
Growth and pregnancy	Increases iron requirements by stimulating an increase in vascularity, red cell mass and hemoglobin
Infection, parasites	Increases iron requirements
Chronic inflammatory diseases (e.g. inflammatory bowel disease and other non-infective inflammatory diseases)	Increases hepcidin, which inhibits iron absorption, resulting in depleted iron stores
Hereditary defects	Thalassaemia, sickle cell anemia as well as other nutritional deficiency, including folate and B12 deficiency
Other medical/physiological reasons for blood loss	Menstruation, ulcers, misuse of anti-inflammatory medications such as non-steroidal anti-inflammatories (NSAIDs) and aspirin, chronic use of antacids
Inadequate dietary iron intake/low dietary iron bioavailability	Poor food choices, unbalanced diets, low energy diets, high-CHO diets, avoidance of red meat/vegetarian or vegan diets, fad diets, low-heme iron intakes, avoidance of iron-fortified commercial foods

females (Deruisseau et al. 2004), in older men (Murray-Kolb et al. 2001) and in trained cyclists after 6 weeks of high-intensity interval training (Wilkinson et al. 2002). In these cyclists, SF had significantly decreased as early as week 5, although iron intake remained constant. Higher iron requirements in athletes are a consequence of increased vascularity accompanied by an increased red cell mass, hemoglobin and metabolic iron use, all of which are dependent on dietary iron.

Athletes involved in strenuous exercise also lose iron in several ways: through sweating (LaManca et al. 1988; Waller & Haymes 1996; Deruisseau et al. 2002), from gastrointestinal bleeding (Lampe et al. 1987; Natchtigall et al. 1996), by the breakdown of red blood cells caused by mechanical and capillary trauma (Miller et al. 1988), or from injury associated with blood loss.

Few studies have attempted to estimate accurately the extent of iron loss through sweat during prolonged exercise. Losses are relatively highest in distance runners and greater in female than male runners (LaManca et al. 1988). However, loss of iron via sweat is unlikely to be a major contributor to iron depletion. A study of male and female recreational cyclists found a decreased rate of sweat iron loss within 30–60 minutes of prolonged exercise, suggesting a possible iron conservation mechanism (Deruisseau et al. 2002). Gastrointestinal blood loss of large magnitude has been documented in male and female distance runners (McMahon et al. 1984; Lampe et al. 1987). It may be caused by desquamation of cells from the intestinal wall or ischemia of the stomach and intestinal lining. The presence of blood in the urine reported by athletes after strenuous physical activity (Siegal et al. 1979) may be caused by trauma to the bladder wall. Another source of iron loss called 'foot strike' hemolysis (destruction of red blood cells) has been associated with running on hard surfaces (Miller et al. 1988; Schumacher, Schmid, Grathwohl et al. 2002).

In summary, physiological factors associated with athletic training can cause iron depletion. A stimulation of hepcidin synthesis or chronically elevated hepcidin induced by very intensive training programs may further accelerate iron depletion if a physiological stress response is induced. In most highly trained athletes, an acute phase response to training is unlikely (Fallon et al. 2001), although to date, studies monitoring hepcidin levels in highly trained athletes have not been published. An athlete with low iron stores at the start of the training session, when recommencing training after an injury or in association with an increase in the duration and intensity of training, is at high risk of further iron depletion.

Moderate physical activity 10.25

Short- to long-term moderate physical activity or sports participation has no significant effect on iron status in studies of untrained or trained adults (Schumacher, Schmid, König et al. 2002) or in pubescent athletes and children. See Fogelholm (1999) for a review.

Growth, pregnancy and lactation, menstruation 10.26

Requirements for iron increase substantially in adolescents and children during a growth spurt, and for women in pregnancy and lactation, although a higher absorption of iron helps to compensate for this increase (Food & Nutrition Board 2000a). Iron loss from menstruation is not usually a major causal factor for iron deficiency in athletes, except in women with heavy menstrual losses. However, in one randomized, double-blind study of endurance athletes who had sufficient iron intakes, the principal cause of iron deficiency was attributed to menstrual blood loss (Malczewska et al. 2000). This is an unusual finding as a reduction in severity and frequency of menses with increased training loads is not uncommon. Nevertheless, a pregnant or lactating athlete has very high iron requirements and is unlikely to meet these from dietary sources.

These physiological states cannot be overlooked as contributors to iron depletion, particularly in adolescents, where reported iron intakes do not always meet increased requirements (Barr 1987; Risser & Risser 1990).

10.27 Blood loss and other medical causes

Blood loss from other causes—including injury, ulcers, misuse of anti-inflammatory medication (such as NSAIDs and aspirin), and the bacterium *Helicobacter pylori*—cannot be discounted as a possible cause of iron deficiency, nor can other pathological or hereditary factors.

Because non-heme iron absorption requires an acid environment, any condition or medication that decreases gastric acid secretion and is linked with gastrointestinal blood loss (e.g. *Helicobacter pylori* infection and chronic use of antacids) is associated with iron depletion and anemia (McColl et al. 1998; Sarker et al. 2004; Cardenas et al. 2006). Based on population data from the NHANES (1999–2000) study in the US, *Helicobacter pylori* infection accounted for 35% and 51% of cases of iron deficiency and IDA (Cardenas et al. 2006), so athletes with chronically low SF levels may need to be checked. The anemia that occurs with chronic infections, inflammation or malignant disorders differs from IDA but cannot be discounted in an athletic population as a reason for low iron stores (Handelman & Levin 2008).

10.28 Dietary causes

Habitual consumption of foods known to be low in total iron and heme iron, or that have a low iron bioavailability, are a major cause of iron deficiency, particularly in women. Western-style diets with high iron bioavailability can meet iron requirements for most women but as bioavailability decreases, meeting iron requirements becomes untenable from diet alone (Hallberg et al. 1998). Based on estimates of bioavailability from different diets, these authors estimate that 20–40% of women on diets with medium to low iron bioavailability cannot cover their iron requirements. These figures relate to non-athlete women and are likely to be even higher for athletes with increased requirements. Any athlete, irrespective of gender, will be at risk of iron depletion if they habitually follow the types of diets well known to be low in dietary iron or have low bioavailability of iron, such as those listed below.

10.29 Low-energy diets

Athletes on low-energy intakes are those most frequently reported as having diets that contain less-than-recommended intakes of iron (Barr 1987; Risser & Risser 1990; Haymes 1992).

10.30 Vegetarian diets and low heme iron intakes

Vegetarian diets have low iron bioavailability because they contain no or little heme iron, although they can provide as much or more total dietary iron than meat-based diets (American Dietetic Association 1997; Tetens et al. 2007) because of an increase in the variety of iron-fortified foods available in the food supply of western diets (Gerrior & Bente 2001).

Athletes following vegetarian-style diets or who eat little red meat (the highest heme iron source) have lower iron status than meat eaters, despite similar or higher iron intakes than meat eaters (Seiler et al. 1989; Snyder et al. 1989; Tetens et al. 2007). High-CHO diets recommended for athletes, if high in phytates and low in heme iron, have low bioavailability and increase risk of low iron stores. Several studies on athletes have confirmed an association between high CHO intakes and low iron stores (Telford et al. 1993; Pate et al. 1993), and low heme iron intake and low iron stores (Malczewska et al. 2001), although other physiological reasons were also linked.

Natural food eaters 10.31

Athletes who avoid commercial or packaged foods (such as breakfast cereals) are missing out on iron-fortified foods. For example, one serve of porridge contains about half the iron of most commercial breakfast cereals and is high in phytates, which strongly inhibit iron absorption. Contrary to popular belief, bread, breakfast cereals and other cereal-based products, not meat and meat products, provide the bulk of total iron in the Australian diet (McLennan & Podger 1998).

Fad diets and weight-control products 10.32

Some fad diets and weight-control products are marketed exclusively to athletes with claims of performance enhancement, weight gain or weight loss, but without adequate scientific substantiation for their claims. Weight reduction diets with fewer than 5000 kJ/d (1200 kcal/d) will not meet the energy, iron and other nutrient requirements of an athlete in training. Athletes who follow unusual eating regimens, consistently miss meals and have erratic eating patterns can also consume suboptimal intakes of iron. These types of dietary habits are not atypical of adolescents, a high-risk group for iron deficiency (Abrahams et al. 1988; Bothwell 1995).

Are athletes eating inadequate dietary iron intakes? 10.33

Dietary iron intakes of athletes are usually higher than or no different from non-athlete controls for both males and females and in prepubescent athletes and school children participating in sports (Resina et al. 1991; Fogelholm 1995, 1999), although athletes under-report dietary intakes in dietary surveys more than non-athlete controls (Haggarty et al. 1988).

Despite the potential bias from under-reporting in dietary surveys, female athletes are still likely to consume inadequate iron intakes. Male athletes tend to consume more dietary iron than females and easily meet or exceed iron intake recommendations (Fogelholm 1995).

Assessment of iron status of an athlete: clinical perspectives 10.34

Confirmation of a diagnosis of true iron depletion in athletes requires the use of a number of diagnostic criteria, including a comprehensive assessment of the physiological, medical, biochemical and dietary factors implicated in the etiology of iron deficiency. Blood tests alone do not always confirm a diagnosis of early iron depletion. The discovery of the small peptide hormone hepcidin, its identification as a regulator of iron metabolism and its measurement in plasma or urine, could be useful in the differential diagnosis of iron status in athletes (Ganz 2005).

10.35 Laboratory measures of iron status and their interpretation

The diagnosis of iron depletion and deficiency has been complicated by the absence of a clear and reliable reference method for detecting early iron depletion and the use of varying cut-offs for hematological markers at each stage. Several key hematological markers are used to assess iron status and define each stage in clinical practice: SF to measure depleted iron stores (stage 1), sTfR to measure functional iron deficiency (stage 2) and hemoglobin concentration to measure IDA (stage 3) (Skikne et al. 1990). The interpretation of these values and others commonly used in clinical practice are briefly described in sections 10.36–10.41.

Several hematological markers in the blood are used to fully assess iron status for research purposes, but only serum iron, SF, transferrin, transferrin saturation and hemoglobin are routinely measured in sports medicine practices, together with mean cell volume (MCV) and mean corpuscular hemoglobin concentration (MCHC). Early studies of athletes used either SF as a sole indicator of early iron depletion or a combination of these routine measures. More recent markers available include sTfR to measure the functional iron pool or sTfR/log SF index to determine the level of iron depletion and hepcidin.

Hematological markers of iron status collected on a single occasion do not always confirm iron deficiency. Repeated measures in combination with other diagnostic protocols, including clinical symptoms and dietary assessment, confirm the diagnosis (see Practice Tips). Even when clinical symptoms are evident, iron depletion or deficiency using hematological markers can easily be misdiagnosed in athletes. Reference ranges and cut-offs for evaluating iron status in athletes are based on population reference standards and, although these may be inappropriate for some athletes, they still serve as the benchmark for interpretation (see Table 10.5). Iron status measures below reference ranges could represent adequate iron status, especially in adolescents, and are closely associated with maturational age, body mass, sex, genetic factors and physical activity (Rossander-Hulten & Hallberg 1996).

The extent of iron depletion is determined by examining several markers found in the three main iron-containing compartments of the body: storage iron, transport iron and red blood cells.

10.36 Storage iron

Serum ferritin

Iron is stored within the reticuloendothelial system as molecular complexes called ferritin and hemosiderin, a partially degraded form of ferritin. Normally, small amounts of SF circulate in the blood in concentrations between 15 and 300 μg/L in adults (Worwood 1991). As storage iron increases, there is a corresponding increase in SF, which is why it is the best marker of iron stores in healthy people and athletes (Borch-Iohnsen 1995; Handelman & Levin 2008).

The mean SF in the NHANES II 1976–80 survey of US adults aged 20–65 years was 109 μg/L (range 66–285) in 649 men and 34 μg/L (range 12–94) in 409 women (Cook et al. 2003). In a survey of elite athletes aged 15–31 years training at the Australian Institute of Sport, the mean SF was 85 μg/L (range 16–288) in 105 males and 54 μg/L (range 8–205) in 166 females (Fallon 2004). The distribution of SF is skewed towards the lower end of the range in athletes and population surveys (Cook et al. 1974; Maes et al. 1997).

In athletes and non-athletes, SF varies with age, sex and physical activity, and is low in young children and in adolescents during the growth phase (Baynes 1996). Some male adolescent athletes have low SF, despite high dietary iron intakes and using iron supplements (Telford et al. 1993), which is probably physiologically 'normal' at this age. In population studies, a slow increase in SF and body iron occurs through adolescence followed by a substantial rise in males in late adolescence (Bothwell 1995; Bergstrom et al. 1996; Cook et al. 2003). Females do not show a late adolescent increase. Further increases in body iron stores occur in men with aging and in postmenopausal females, but not in younger women (Cook et al. 2003). SF has some day-to-day variability (Stupnicki et al. 2003) and can be distorted under different physiological conditions (see section 10.39).

In elite athletes, SF declines during the training season in both males and females. In 46 matched pairs of female Australian Institute of Sport athletes, SF decreased by around 25% during training seasons, with greater declines seen in weight-bearing sports (netball and basketball) than non-weight-bearing sports (swimming and rowing) (Ashenden et al. 1998).

Diagnostic cut-offs for serum ferritin to detect stage of iron depletion

There is no internationally accepted cut-off for diagnosing each stage of iron depletion. In untrained adults, SF below 30 μg/L suggests depleted iron stores (Crosby & O'Neill 1984) and 12 μg SF/L denotes exhaustion of iron stores (Cook et al. 1974). In one large study of 422 hospital patients with disease-specific anemia, the cut-off for diagnosing functional iron deficiency was 20.8 μg SF/L in combination with several other hematological markers) (Thomas & Thomas 2002). In another study, functional iron deficiency (stage 2) was detected at levels ≤15 μg SF/L, based on the absence of stainable iron in the bone marrow and other low-iron status markers in both male and female adolescents and women (Hallberg, Hulthen et al. 1993; Hallberg, Bengtsson et al. 1993). Cut-offs vary considerably in studies of iron depletion in athletes, so interpretation of low SF values needs to be cautious.

Diagnostic cut-offs for iron status indicators for adults cannot be applied reliably to adolescents because of the large variation reported during maturation (Bergstrom et al. 1996). Different reference ranges for male and female adults are recommended (see Table 10.5). Population reference ranges for children and adolescents are available in most biochemistry or hematology textbooks.

Transport iron 10.37

Hematological markers involved in transferring iron in the circulation are transferrin, serum iron and haptoglobin. Serum iron and serum transferrin in isolation are of limited value in determining iron status. Instead, total serum iron-binding capacity is usually estimated at the same time so that the percentage saturation of transferrin can be calculated. The combination of transferrin saturation and sTfR and possibly the sTfR/log SF index may be more useful to determine early-stage iron depletion than serum iron and serum transferrin (Cook et al. 2003).

TABLE 10.5 CLINICAL LABORATORY VALUES FOR MEASURING IRON DEFICIENCY ANEMIA IN A NON-ATHLETE POPULATION

IRON STATUS MEASURE	DIAGNOSTIC RANGE FOR IRON DEFICIENCY ANEMIA	REFERENCE RANGES FOR ADULTS (SI UNITS)	SI UNITS	CONVERSION FACTOR TO BRITISH* UNITS	REFERENCE RANGE TO BRITISH UNITS	BRITISH UNITS
Hemoglobin						
Females	<12.0	120–160	g/L	0.1	12.0–16.0	g/dL
Males	<13.0	140–180			14.0–17.5	
Hematocrit						
Females		0.33–0.43	Ratio	0.01	33–43	Ratio converted to %
Males		0.39–0.49			39–49	
MCV[a]	<80	76–100	fL	1	76–100	μm^3
Reticulocyte count[a]	NA	10–75	10^9/L	100	10000–75000	mm^3
SF	<22* (Stage 1) 22* (Stage 2) <12 (Stage 3)	*Males* 30–300 *Females* 10–160	μg/L	1	15–300	ng/mL
Serum iron						
Females	17.9	10–29	μmol/L	5.5	60–160	μg/dL
Males	17.9	14–32			80–180	
Serum transferrin[a]	< reference range	1.7–3.7	g/L	100	170–370	mg/dL
Total iron binding capacity (TIBC)[a]	< reference range	45–82	μmol/L	5.5	250–460	μg/dL

Transferrin saturation serum Fe/TIBC[a]	< reference range	20–40	%	1.00	20–40	%
Serum transferrin receptor[a]	≤2.75* (Stage 1) >2.75* (Stage 2) >2.8* (Stage 3)	1.15–2.75*	mg/L	NA	3–9	mg/L
Free transferrin receptor to ferritin index (Tfr-F index)[a]	≤1.8* (Stage 1) >3.6* (Stage 3) >2.2* (Stage 2)	0.63–1.8*	–	–	–	–

[a] No data available on male and female reference intervals for some measures. For these measures, reference intervals can be satisfactorily applied to both sexes.

NA = not available, stage 1 = depleted iron stores, stage 2 = functional iron deficiency, stage 3 = iron deficiency anemia, SI = Systeme International d'Unites, British units = Imperial units, L = liters, MCV = mean cell volume, SF = serum ferritin

– = no units used for a ratio

Sources: Expert Scientific Working Group 1985; INACG 1985; Ferguson et al. 1992; Food & Nutrition Board 2000a; *Suominen et al. 1998 using IDeA™ sTfR immunoenzymometric assay (IEMA) by Orion Diagnostics

Serum iron

Serum iron is unbound iron. It is generally lower in females than males, and appears unaffected by the menstrual cycle, but shows a large diurnal variation of around 20% (Beaton et al. 1989). The highest values occur in the morning and the lowest in the later part of the day (Jacobs 1974). Population reference ranges for serum iron are 14–32 µmol/L for males and 10–29 µmol/L for females (see Table 10.5). There is a true sex difference in values for serum iron similar to serum hemoglobin, irrespective of physical activity. However, the mean serum iron concentration is reported to be higher in untrained people than in athletes (Brotherhood et al. 1975).

Serum transferrin and transferrin saturation

Serum transferrin, the major plasma transport protein, binds iron (Fe^{3+} only) and carries it from the storage sites to the bone marrow (Handelman & Levin 2008). Transferrin saturation is the ratio of serum iron to iron-binding capacity and is considered an accurate indicator of iron supply to the bone marrow (Australian Iron Status Advisory Board 2005). In a non-athlete population, transferrin saturation is usually 20–40% saturated (see Table 10.5). Transferrin saturation, similar to serum iron, shows a wide diurnal variation and low specificity. A critical level of <16% transferrin saturation has been established for an adult as a level at which erythropoiesis is compromised (Bothwell et al. 1979; Finch & Cook 1984). Transferrin saturation levels >60% at the first blood test are suspect of hemochromatosis (see section 10.51). With depleted iron stores, transferrin saturation increases towards the upper end of the reference range, and then decreases when erythropoiesis is compromised.

Serum (soluble) transferrin receptor

Transferrin receptors (TfR), located on the surface of erythroblasts, control the uptake of iron delivered to the cell by transferrin. The remnant product of degradation of the receptor is released into the circulation in a soluble form and is called either serum or soluble transferrin receptor (sTfR). sTfR, which reflects the recruitment of receptors, provides a quantitative evaluation of mild tissue iron deficiency or functional iron depletion (Skikne et al. 1990; Ervasti et al. 2004), although the sensitivity of sTfR in isolation in detecting early and immediate stages of iron deficiency is low (Choi 2005). It is also used for detecting the use of erythropoietin, a banned performance-enhancing substance that increases erythropoiesis (Parisotto & Ashenden 2002).

sTfR levels *increase* as SF decreases and can be three to four times the 'normal' reference range in IDA (Huebers et al. 1990). In one study, sTfR levels were elevated at SF cut-off of 22 µg/L in healthy (non-athlete) adults (Suominen et al. 1998).

sTfR is not as sensitive as SF to changes in plasma volume induced by strenuous activity (Schumacher, Schmid, König et al. 2002) or growth spurts and is unaffected by any active acute phase response (e.g. inflammation or infection) compared to SF (Baynes 1996; Hulthen et al. 1998). However, it is unreliable in people with anemia, people with chronic diseases associated with hyperdestruction or hypoproliferation of red blood cells, or people with disorders in erythropoiesis (Beguin et al. 1993).

A longitudinal study of Swedish adolescents aged 15–21 years showed that, in both sexes, sTfR increased from age 15–17 years, then decreased from age 17–21 years (Samuelson et al. 2003), suggesting a skewed distribution in this age range. A decrease at 17–21 years in the females suggests that tissue iron needs were met although iron stores remained low. sTfR was found to be higher in boys aged 10–12 years than in men

(Virtanen et al. 1999). The distribution and kinetics of sTfR in elite athletes have not been investigated.

The use of sTfR in clinical practice added to the conventional iron status indicators to assess the stage of iron depletion did not, however, provide additional information compared to SF tests in a study on hospital outpatients and medical students (Mast et al. 1998) and in study on elite athletes (Pitsis et al. 2002), so is currently not supported for screening for iron depletion. The reagents used for the sTfR test are not yet standardized so different commercial testing kits give different values, further complicating interpretation. At the Australian Institute of Sport, sTfR is used only as an adjunct to other routine measures of iron status in cases of inflammation or persistent low ferritin levels after iron supplementation.

In performance effects of iron depletion in athletes, sTfR has been mainly used, in combination with other iron status markers, to recruit subjects with functional iron deficiency and as a benchmark to assess the effects of iron supplements or injections on performance (Brutsaert et al. 2003; Nikolaidis et al. 2003; Peeling et al. 2007; Hinton & Sinclair 2007). Diagnostic cut-offs for sTfR for each stage of iron depletion in healthy, non-athlete adults, based on recommendations by Suominen and colleagues (1998) are found in Table 10.5. Diagnostic cut-offs for children aged 5–15 years are also available (Zimmerman et al. 2005) and could be used in this age group until specific cut-offs for athletes become available.

Transferrin receptor-ferritin ratio (sTfR-F index)

As SF goes down, sTfR goes up in a linear manner (Skikne et al. 1990). The ratio of sTfR to log SF, called the sTfR/log SF index, is considered a more reliable determinant of iron status than either indicator used alone, especially in borderline cases (Cook et al. 2003; Punnonen et al. 1997; Suominen et al. 1998). A ratio of >1.8 for stage 1 (depleted iron stores) and ≥ 2.2 for stage 2 (functional iron deficiency or iron-deficient erythropoiesis) in 65 Finnish adults was the cut-off for differentiating between the stages (Suominen et al. 1998). These cut-offs have been used as benchmarks in two studies of athletes (Malczewska et al. 2001; Pitsis et al. 2002), but are mostly limited to research rather than clinical practice.

The advantages of these measures are that capillary rather than venous blood samples can be used (Cook et al. 2003), which could be useful for monitoring iron status in field studies. Conversion of the index into body iron stores (into mg/kg of body mass) allows a quantitative estimation of early iron depletion for an individual and avoids the problem of using arbitrary cut-offs for SF that are population based (see Cook et al. 2003 for the conversion equation).

The sTfR-F index has demonstrated excellent validity in estimating body iron stores in non-athletes (Cook et al. 2003), but it cannot be used widely because of the lack of standardization of sTfR assays (Brugnara 2003). Moreover, Stupnicki and colleagues (2003) challenged the validity of the sTfR-F index in athletes and found the within-subject day-to-day error of the ratio to be 50% higher in female athletes than in controls. This error was attributed mainly to fluctuations in SF in response to exercise-induced changes in plasma volume. Despite the significant daily fluctuations in SF reported in this study and others (Malczewska et al. 2001), the index remained stable over 10 days of training. These authors suggest that if the index is used to monitor iron status in elite athletes, reference values based on untrained people will need to be adjusted. Further studies are needed to test the index and justify this recommendation. At present this index is used in research rather than in clinical practice.

10.38 Red blood cell and other measures (full blood count, morphology and reticulocytes, hepcidin)

Full red blood cell count

Red blood cells undergo changes in number, size, hemoglobin concentration and composition in individuals developing iron deficiency. As iron depletes, red blood cell numbers eventually decrease if iron is limiting erythropoiesis, and low hemoglobin and abnormal red cell morphology occurs. Changes in red blood cell parameters of individual athletes who are developing iron deficiency are listed in Table 10.6. The technology needed to perform all tests listed in this table may not be readily available to sports medicine practices.

TABLE 10.6 CHANGES IN RED BLOOD CELL CHARACTERISTICS IN INDIVIDUALS DEVELOPING IRON DEFICIENCY
The cellular hemoglobin content of reticulocytes is reduced
% hypochromic and % microcytic cells are increased
The hemoglobin content of RBC is reduced (MCH)
RBC MCV is reduced
MCHC is reduced
Microcytic, hypochromic RBC may start to appear as the severity of iron depletion progresses

RBC = red blood count, MCV = mean cell volume, MCHC = mean corpuscular hemoglobin concentration
Source: Adapted from Pyne et al. 1997

Hemoglobin and hematocrit

Hemoglobin and hematocrit values decrease only when severe iron depletion is present (Bothwell et al. 1979) (see Table 10.5). These measures are subject to wide diurnal variations and individual variability in physiologically 'normal' levels (Beaton et al. 1989).

Hemoglobin and hematocrit values are similar for boys and girls until puberty, when they are higher in boys than girls and similar to adult values. However, in the absence of anemia, hemoglobin and hematocrit values are usually higher in adolescent athletes of both sexes (Nikolaidis et al. 2003b) and in adult athletes than in non-athletes (Brotherhood et al. 1975), higher in men than women (Sanborn & Jankowski 1994) and positively associated with a high body mass index (BMI) in athletes (Telford & Cunningham 1991).

Red cell morphology

With increasing severity of iron depletion, the number of red blood cells progressively decreases and the cells become microcytic and hypochromic. Occasional rod-shaped cells and target cells are also observed. Blood films are often examined directly to discriminate between different types of anemia and disorders of iron metabolism that affect red blood cells (e.g. IDA and thalassaemia, which is an inherited disorder of hemoglobin synthesis).

Reticulocytes and hemoglobin content in the reticulocytes

Reticulocytes are red blood cells recently released from the bone marrow. Determination of the reticulocyte hemoglobin content (CHr) provides an early and reliable measure of functional iron deficiency and bone marrow iron stores, but is unreliable in subjects with elevated MCV and thalassaemia (Mast et al. 2002). Low hemoglobin in reticulocytes, which circulate for only 1–2 days, results in low hemoglobin in mature red blood cells. Iron supplements may be beneficial at this point to boost iron stores and to prevent further iron depletion (Ashenden et al. 1998); however, this measure is not routinely used in clinical practice. Together with the sTfR-F index, CHr may allow for a more precise classification of iron depletion than other indicators (Brugnara 2003).

Hepcidin

Hepcidin is the hormone that regulates systemic iron metabolism. Measures in the urine and plasma may be useful to differentiate between the anemia of inflammation and other stages of iron deficiency and iron overload (Ganz 2005). High levels of circulating hepcidin inhibit intestinal iron absorption, activate release of iron from iron stores, and divert iron away from hemoglobin and red blood cell synthesis, resulting in decreased iron stores (Ganz 2005; Atanasiu et al. 2006). Hepcidin production and high circulating levels are induced by physiological stressors, including chronic infections, inflammation and—interestingly—chronic and acute high-intensity or endurance exercise. In one study, hepcidin was elevated four- to twenty-seven-fold compared to pre-race values in ten out of fourteen females on the day after a marathon (Roecker et al. 2005). Chronically elevated hepcidin in combination with inadequate dietary iron intake may explain the high prevalence of iron depletion reported in female endurance athletes.

In contrast, hepcidin production decreases when body iron requirements are high and erythropoiesis is active, as expected during growth and with low iron stores. Low levels have also been reported in athletes undertaking altitude training (Atanasiu et al. 2006), which stimulates erythropoesis. Presumably, in this study the altitude training was not at the level that induced a physiological stress response, otherwise hepcidin levels would be high. Currently, hepcidin levels in urine or plasma are not routinely measured in clinical practice or in athletes.

Errors in interpretation of laboratory measures of iron status 10.39

The use of hematological markers to diagnose iron status from a single or one-off blood test can be unreliable or misleading. Blood tests are susceptible to fluctuations from physiological and pathological conditions that confound interpretation, as indicated in Table 10.7. Hypohydration at the time of testing, for example, can cause hemoconcentration, resulting in an apparent increase in blood measures.

TABLE 10.7 FACTORS INFLUENCING INTERPRETATION OF LABORATORY MEASURES OF IRON STATUS AND METABOLISM

	HEMOGLOBIN (HB)
Hypohydration at the time of testing	↑
Chronic inflammation, malignancy	↓ or N
Infection (URTI, flu, virus)	N
After intense prolonged exercise (post-marathon)*	↓

N = normal, URTI = upper respiratory tract infection

Sources: Adapted from Smith & Roberts 1994 and Ganz 2005; *Fallon et al. 1999 and Roecker et al. 2005

In the absence of hypohydration, all hematological markers except SF and hepcidin and to a lesser extent sTfR decrease after acute short-term moderate to strenuous exercise; after prolonged aerobic exercise (such as cycling every day for 3–4 days) (Schumacher, Schmid, König et al. 2002); and after a marathon race (Lampe et al. 1986; Fallon et al. 1999; Roecker et al. 2005) because of exercise-induced plasma volume expansion resulting in hemodilution. As SF and hepcidin are acute phase reactants, infection, inflammation, liver disease, high alcohol consumption, reduced calorie intake and the physiological stress of strenuous exercise also falsely elevate these measures (Fallon et al. 1999; Hallberg & Hulthen 2003). At the levels of training undertaken by elite female netball and soccer teams at the Australian Institute of Sport, an acute phase response was not detected (Fallon et al. 2001).

Minor infections can induce an acute phase response. In one study of 1670 Swedish adolescents aged 15–16 years, 24.4% of those who had reported a mild common cold with fever during the preceding month had significant increases in SF, evidence of an acute phase response (Hulthen et al. 1998). In contrast, other indicators, such as hemoglobin, hematocrit, serum iron and transferrin, decrease with infection and inflammation (Finch & Huebers 1982). To avoid errors in SF, blood should be taken prior to any strenuous exercise.

10.40 Utility of screening iron status of athletes

The utility of routinely screening elite athletes, particularly female and endurance athletes, for a full blood count and SF has been questioned (Garza et al. 1997; Schnirring 2002; Fallon & Gerrard 2007). A recent prospective study of iron-status measures—ferritin and hemoglobin—at the Australian Institute of Sport suggests that routine screening for iron deficiency is recommended for athletes involved in an elite training program because of the high prevalence of low SF levels (Fallon & Gerrard 2007).

10.41 Summary of laboratory measures of iron status

Blood tests alone do not necessarily confirm a diagnosis of iron depletion, as iron status indicators that fall outside the diagnostic range may be 'normal' for some individuals. SF has been used routinely as a diagnostic measure in sports medicine practice and in research for initial assessment and prospective monitoring of stage 1 and stage 2 iron depletion in at-risk elite athletes, and remains, in combination with hemoglobin, the iron test of choice for early detection of iron depletion, despite its limitations. Routine screening of iron status may be warranted in athletes in an elite training program. More recently, sTfR, or the sTfR/log SF index, has been added to discriminate tissue or functional iron deficiency (stage 2), although more studies are needed in athletes to assess the utility of this index as a diagnostic tool. Hemoglobin and hematocrit without SF have limited use in early detection of iron depletion, as significant decreases in these markers are observed only in IDA. Serum iron and transferrin saturation show a wide diurnal variation, although high levels of transferrin saturation in association with low SF are an indication of early iron depletion. Measuring and monitoring changes in immature red blood cells (reticulocytes) is useful for evaluating relative changes in iron status in individual athletes, but not routinely used in clinical practice. Hepcidin levels are useful to differentiate between the anemia of inflammation and IDA. See Table 10.5 for population cut-offs and reference ranges, for most laboratory measures of iron status.

Clinical symptoms 10.42

IDA is associated with symptoms of weakness, breathlessness and impaired aerobic and endurance capacity. Even with depleted iron stores, some athletes look pale, may have a slightly elevated resting pulse rate, feel 'run-down' or 'washed out', and exhibit changes in mood state or have a diminished appetite. These types of symptoms are non-specific and may be indicative of overtraining, immune deficiency, psychosocial stress, unresolved viral infections, non-fasting hypoglycemia or sleep disorders; they may even be considered 'normal' in an athlete or adolescent. Conversely, athletes with low SF levels often have no symptoms. Despite an absence of clinical symptoms, one study reported that 100 intercollegiate female athletes considered their performance to be worse when iron depleted (Risser et al. 1988). Experienced elite athletes are often overly concerned about fatigue or SF levels, routinely request blood tests and self-supplement with iron when tired, despite normal SF levels (Fallon & Gerrard 2007). In anxious elite athletes with a history of iron depletion, any sign of fatigue or lethargy is often perceived as iron depletion.

Dietary assessment 10.43

Because iron is found in so many foods and its intake is highly variable, determining usual intakes with reliability requires many days of data collection, which is not possible in clinical practice. Dietary (and iron) intakes of individuals are assessed using several methods (such as diet records, food frequency questionnaires, diet histories and recalls) and are the main methods used by professionals in both research and clinical practice (see Chapter 2).

In clinical practice, dietary assessment of an individual usually involves a dietary and supplement history to estimate usual dietary intakes and to determine other dietary and lifestyle factors that influence food intake and iron absorption. Estimating the potential effects of physiological, training and medical factors on iron losses is a crucial component of the dietary interview. Techniques for assessing iron status are found in the Practice Tips.

A habitual low intake and low bioavailability of iron, in combination with clinical symptoms and several iron status measures that are below reference values, can usually confirm a diagnosis. However, any assessment of the usual diet and nutrient adequacy of an individual is imprecise, especially for iron, and must be interpreted cautiously because of the inherent problems in accurately assessing dietary intakes.

Dietary intervention for iron depletion and iron deficiency 10.44

Dietary intervention for the treatment of diagnosed iron depletion or deficiency usually requires iron supplements in combination with advice about increasing dietary iron intake to meet or exceed population recommendations and improve iron bioavailability.

Recommended dietary iron intakes for athletes 10.45

Average daily iron requirements or recommendations for athletes in different sports have not been established and are likely to be highly variable.

Daily iron losses in endurance runners have been estimated at 1.5–1.7 mg iron/d in men and 2.2–2.3 mg iron/d in women (Haymes & Lamanca 1989), although there is some debate about whether endurance athletes have truly low iron stores (Ashenden et al. 1998). Basal or obligatory iron losses in untrained adults are only 0.9–1.0 mg/d in men and 0.7–0.8 mg/d in women (excluding menstrual losses) (Bothwell 1996). To meet iron losses in distance runners, Haymes and Lamanca (1989) recommended iron intakes of 17.5 mg/d for men and around 23 mg/d in normally menstruating women, assuming iron absorption to be 10% of dietary iron from the total diet. Nutrient Reference Values (NRV) for iron are based on an average iron absorption of 18% from a mixed western diet (that includes animal foods) and 10% absorption from a vegetarian diet (Commonwealth Department of Health and Ageing et al. 2006).

The Australian NRV are based on the Dietary Reference Intakes (DRI) from the US and Canada, with some minor modifications in terminology. Multiple levels of nutrient reference values have been set: the Estimated Average Requirements (EAR), Adequate Intake (AI) and Upper Level of Intake (UL) or Upper Intake Level (UIL) in the US and Canada. These levels have different applications when used to assess and plan diets for individuals and groups, compared to previous usage (see Chapter 2). For assessment of an individual, the EAR is considered the best estimate of an individual's requirement (Food & Nutrition Board 2000b).

Although EAR may not be applicable for athletes without some adjustment, they can serve as a benchmark, in combination with the Recommended Dietary Intake, to examine the probability that usual intake is 'adequate' or 'inadequate' for an individual athlete (Food & Nutrition Board 2000b; Murphy et al. 2002). The Food and Nutrition Board (2000a) suggests that the EAR for iron should be 1.3–1.7 times higher than normal EAR values for athletes and 1.8 times higher for vegetarians (non-athletes) to account for low iron bioavailability. The EAR for female vegetarian athletes may be even higher than this because of increased requirements. Such high levels are unlikely to be met by dietary iron intake in this high-risk group without appropriate dietary planning.

10.46 Strategies to increase the total consumption of iron-rich food and enhance iron bioavailability

Iron-rich diets that have a high iron bioavailability are needed to prevent the development of iron depletion and to treat it. The Practice Tips provide practical dietary strategies to achieve these goals using different food combinations.

10.47 Medical intervention: iron supplements

Many athletes self-administer or are provided with iron supplements daily or intermittently as an ergogenic aid or as a preventive measure without being diagnosed with iron depletion. In a large cross-sectional survey of drug use in 658 Australian athletes, nearly 70% of the respondents in numerous team sports reported taking iron supplements regularly (Australian Sports Commission 1983). In another study, 30% of elite Australian swimmers (Baylis et al. 2001) and 89% of professional male cyclists riding on French teams (Deugnier et al. 2002) reported taking iron supplements. Whether the iron supplements were self-administered, provided to them or given under medical supervision was not assessed in these studies. This widespread and perhaps indiscriminate use of very high doses of iron supplements in athletes without iron deficiency is of concern for long-term safety, especially given the high prevalence of the genetic disorder hemochromatosis.

Iron supplements for clinical treatment of iron depletion 10.48

Nielsen and Natchtigall (1998) suggest that there are sufficient data from well-designed studies that support the use of iron supplements in therapeutic doses in athletes with low SF levels, although the level of SF at which supplementation should commence (from <12 to 35 µg/L) is still controversial (see section 10.36).

Decisions about using iron supplements are usually made on a case-by-case basis and are not necessarily based only on low SF levels but combine several iron markers. Full recovery from depleted or exhausted iron stores takes around 3 months using high doses of iron supplements (Nielsen & Natchtigall 1998) and is not possible using dietary intervention alone in this timeframe. Hallberg (1998) calculates that it takes about 2 to 3 years to attain around 80% of iron stores in men and women by dietary means alone, based on predictive equations. Therefore, iron supplements are important, at least for rapid recovery.

In most cases, supplements are discontinued when the measurement of SF or serum transferrin receptor returns to 'normal' for the individual athlete, and diet therapy is maintained. The importance of habitually consuming foods with a high bioavailability of iron is crucial to continued recovery.

Dosage and duration of oral iron supplementation 10.49

Iron supplements are available in two forms: ferrous and ferric. Ferrous salts—ferrous fumarate, ferrous sulphate and ferrous gluconate—are more readily absorbed than the ferric form (Hoffman et al. 2000). To replete exhausted iron stores, a dosage of around 100 mg elemental iron/d (the amount available for absorption) is necessary for more than 3 months (Nielsen & Natchtigall 1998), although doses of up to 300 mg/d have been used in severe cases (Balaban 1992). These doses are well above normal physiological levels.

Studies on non-athletes have found that iron supplements taken two to three times a week are just as effective in increasing SF and hemoglobin as supplements taken daily (Solomons 1997; Tee et al. 1999). In one study of 624 adolescent females in Malaysia with mild, moderate and borderline anemia, 120 mg of elemental iron taken once a week was found to be as effective in increasing hemoglobin and SF levels as 60 mg of elemental iron taken once a day (Tee et al. 1999). Research is needed to determine whether similar oral intakes are as effective in athletes. Hallberg (1998), however, is more in favor of daily iron supplementation, which increases depleted iron more rapidly than weekly doses. Current practice also favors daily supplement use in athletes to promote rapid recovery.

Side effects of iron supplementation 10.50

Some people do not tolerate iron supplements, especially in high doses; they complain of constipation, black stools, abdominal cramping and, to a lesser extent, diarrhea, nausea and vomiting. These adverse effects usually subside when iron is taken with food.

Iron supplements inhibit zinc and copper absorption, so there may be an increased risk of deficiency of these minerals in athletes who continually take supplements, although evidence for inducing an actual zinc or copper deficiency has not been substantiated.

10.51 Safety of long-term excess iron: risk of iron overload and hemochromatosis

Although iron is metabolically essential in small doses, it is also highly toxic if unbound and in excess in the blood, as is seen in iron overload and in the genetic disorder hemochromatosis. Free iron is toxic and acts as a pro-oxidant, accelerating the production of free oxygen radicals, which react with cell membrane lipids, resulting in organ damage and cell death (Ganz 2005). Excess iron in the blood is also linked to the pathogenesis of cardiovascular disease and cancer, to an alteration in immune defenses and to an increased risk of infection. For a review, see Reddy & Clarke (2004).

There is no evidence of a link between excessive dietary iron intake and iron overload in healthy subjects, including large intakes of red meat (Hallberg & Hulthen 2003; Heath & Fairweather-Tait 2003). However, there is some evidence of iron overload in people who regularly have iron injections and take iron supplements. In a survey of 1000 French male professional cyclists, 45% had SF levels >300 µg/L (Zotter et al. 2004), which is well above the diagnostic cut-off for iron overload. These high levels were largely attributed to repeated iron injections. High levels of SF from habitual iron supplement use were also reported in another study of professional cyclists (Deugnier et al. 2002). The long-term consequences of taking excessively high doses of iron supplements or iron injections in a healthy person are not known, but may mimic the effects of the genetic disorder hemochromatosis. Excess unabsorbed iron in the colon has been implicated in mucosal damage and possibly increases the risk of colorectal cancer (Reddy & Clarke 2004).

Hereditary hemochromatosis involves a group of genetic disorders associated with a deficiency of hepcidin, the hormone that regulates iron absorption and metabolism (Ganz 2005). As a consequence, iron is indiscriminately absorbed and slowly deposits in vital organs, resulting in irreversible damage. Only those homozygous for the gene express the condition, which occurs in around 0.3% of Caucasians (Bothwell 1995), although there is some evidence that carriers of the gene or its mutations—about 10–15% of Caucasians of northern European origin—are also at increased risk of health problems, particularly cardiovascular disease (Heath & Fairweather-Tait 2003). Clinical symptoms in the early stages of the condition are similar to those of iron deficiency and have been reported in patients as young as 20 years (Worwood 1998). In the last few years, we have picked up this condition in several young elite athletes from routine hematological screening or investigation of persistent fatigue. Indicators are high levels of SF (>150–200 µg/L) and other iron status indicators, particularly elevated transferrin saturation and serum iron; diagnosis is confirmed by genotyping. However, in one male athlete with a confirmed case of homozygous (C282Y) hemochromatosis, SF was in the normal range, although transferrin saturation and serum iron were substantially elevated (Fallon & Gerrard 2007).

The high prevalence of the gene in Caucasian populations and associated long-term health risks highlight the need for correct diagnosis of iron status in athletes and the importance of discouraging indiscriminate use of iron supplements, which are contraindicated in people carrying the gene for hemochromatosis.

Intramuscular iron therapy 10.52

There is no mechanism for getting rid of iron, so excess iron in the blood cannot be removed rapidly by normal physiological mechanisms. Problems with iron overload could be an outcome with injected iron. Although iron injection leads to a rapid increase in iron stores (Dawson et al. 2006; Peeling et al. 2007), it does carry a risk of anaphylactic shock, which can be fatal.

Summary 10.53

Although iron deficiency anemia is uncommon in athletes, iron depletion or deficiency remains a problem, particularly in female athletes, in athletes who follow vegetarian-style diets, and in runners and endurance athletes. Recent evidence using a relatively new marker of tissue iron status (or functional iron activity) called transferrin receptor suggests that iron depletion without anemia (i.e. iron deficiency) can reduce oxidative capacity and also impair endurance capacity in untrained people. When iron stores in both tissue and bone marrow become depleted, the capacity of muscle and other tissue to use oxygen and other iron-containing proteins for the oxidative production of energy can be compromised. More studies are needed on athletes to confirm these effects.

Treatment for iron depletion and deficiency (and iron deficiency anemia) requires a combination of iron supplements and dietary intervention. Dietary intervention with a high iron intake alone is unlikely to provide rapid recovery so supplements are essential. However, routine use of iron supplements as a preventive measure is not recommended because of the risk of iron overload and the high prevalence of the genetic disorder hemochromatosis, particularly in Caucasian populations. For those people with hemochromatosis, iron supplements are contraindicated and can cause irreversible damage to tissues and organs. For athletes without this disorder, an iron-rich diet with high bioavailability is the cornerstone to prevention and treatment of iron depletion and deficiency.

PRACTICE TIPS

VICKI DEAKIN

OVERVIEW

- Athletes involved in regular intensive training programs are at risk of depleting their iron stores, which can, if not detected and treated early, develop into the advanced condition of anemia. Athletes have higher iron requirements and potentially higher iron losses than non-athletes. Suboptimal intakes of iron are evident in athletes who follow low-energy diets, very high-CHO diets, fad diets and vegetarian diets, or who are natural food eaters. As athletes are encouraged to consume diets high in starchy CHO, there is a risk that inhibitors of iron absorption (found in cereal grains, nuts and legumes) will reduce iron bioavailability. Therefore, those athletes at risk of iron depletion need practical strategies for maintaining high CHO intakes without compromising iron status. Food combinations that enhance iron absorption are important to achieve this outcome.

BIOCHEMICAL DETECTION OF IRON DEFICIENCY

- Interpretation of biochemical indicators used to detect early iron depletion should be interpreted in a clinical context, as they can be affected by strenuous exercise just prior to testing, by chronic inflammation or infection, by hypohydration and even by mild infections. All low iron status measures in athletes should be treated as potential iron depletion.

MEDICAL OR PHYSIOLOGICAL CAUSES OF IRON DEFICIENCY

- Assessing the contribution of any medical or physiological factors implicated in the etiology of iron deficiency is important to target appropriate treatment or assign causation. These include:
  - increased iron requirement (such as recent pregnancy, growth spurt or sudden increase in the intensity or duration of training)
  - the habitual use of medications that decrease the acidity of the stomach, including the habitual use of antacids
  - potential blood loss (e.g. from frequent nose bleeds, menorrhagia, ulcers, chronic use of anti-inflammatory medications, being a blood donor)—signs of blood loss after competition or heavy training, including discolored urine or blood in stools
  - recent weight loss or illness
  - malabsorption of iron (e.g. inflammatory bowel disease, or bacterial infection such as *Helicobacter pylori*)

DIETARY ASSESSMENT OF IRON DEFICIENCY

- Diet-related risk factors that are linked to iron depletion include:
  - infrequent consumption of red meat, poultry or seafood
  - vegetarianism or very high CHO diets from mainly wholegrain cereals
  - irregular or erratic eating patterns
  - prolonged loss of appetite after physical activity

  - low intake of bread, breakfast cereal and iron-fortified foods
  - weight-reduction diets, some fad diets, inappropriate food combinations or limited variety of food choices
  - low intake of vitamin C- or vitamin A-rich foods with meals
  - regular consumption of strong tea or coffee with most meals
  - poor food knowledge, limited cooking skills, reliance on takeaway foods
- The EAR for iron is 6 mg/d for men (aged >19 years) and 8 mg/d for women (aged 19–50 years), and for adolescent males and females aged 14–18 years, 7.7 mg/d and 7.9 mg/d, respectively (Commonwealth Department of Health and Ageing et al. 2006). These values need to be adjusted for athletes and vegetarians, but can be used, in combination with the Recommended Dietary Intake/Recommended Dietary Allowance, as cut-offs to examine the probability that usual intake is inadequate or adequate for an individual.

DIETARY TREATMENT AND PREVENTION OF IRON DEFICIENCY

- Although dietary iron absorption increases in people with iron deficiency, the amount absorbed is not sufficient to allow quick recovery, especially in athletes with high requirements and losses. If depleted iron stores have progressed into an advanced condition of anemia, it could take up to 2 or 3 years for the full recovery of iron stores on diet alone (Hallberg et al. 1998). Nevertheless, an iron-rich diet, in combination with iron supplements and strategies to enhance iron absorption, is still the cornerstone of treatment of iron deficiency.

SOURCES OF DIETARY IRON

- The first strategy in treatment (and prevention) is to encourage athletes with iron depletion to increase total dietary iron intake and maintain high levels, especially after using supplements for treatment. Iron is found in a wide range of foods (see Table 10.8 overleaf). Red meat, including beef, veal and lamb, has a higher iron content than chicken and seafood. The color of meat is determined largely by its iron content; the 'redder' the meat, the higher the myoglobin (iron-containing pigment) content and hence iron content. Liver has the highest iron content because it stores iron. Iron-enriched breakfast cereal and bread are important iron sources, although iron from meat and other animal foods is better absorbed (i.e. these foods have a high iron bioavailability). Commercial breakfast cereals and cereal bars (especially wheat- and corn-based cereals) are excellent natural sources of iron, and many other foods (such as milk and fruit juice) are now iron-fortified in Australia. When eaten regularly, iron-fortified foods and, in particular, breakfast cereals provide a substantial amount of iron in the diet. One bowl of iron-enriched breakfast cereal has more than four times the iron content of a bowl of porridge.

PRACTICE TIPS

TABLE 10.8 IRON CONTENT OF AUSTRALIAN FOOD (MG/100 g)

	SERVING SIZE	AMOUNT OF TOTAL IRON PER SERVE (MG/SERVE)
ANIMAL SOURCES (GOOD SOURCES OF HEME AND NON-HEME IRON)		
Lean, cooked trim beef rump steak	1 small serve (100 g)	3.8
Lean, cooked trim lamb steak	1 small serve (100 g)	3.2
Egg	1 boiled egg (60 g)	1.7
Lean pork fillet, cooked; lean ham	1 small serve, ½ cup (100 g)	1.5
Tuna, dark flesh, cooked	½ cup (100g)	1.1
Lean grilled chicken, no skin	1 small breast (100 g)	0.8
Fish, white flesh, cooked	1 small fillet (~100 g)	0.4
PLANT SOURCES (GOOD SOURCES OF NON-HEME IRON)		
Commercial breakfast cereal (iron-fortified, such as Corn Flakes™)	average serve (60 g)	4.2–6.6
Muesli (untoasted, not iron-fortified)	1 cup (100 g)	6.1
Sustagen® Sport, Milo™	3 heaped teaspoons	6
Baked beans in tomato sauce	1 cup (275 g)	4.4
Bread (with added iron)	2 sandwich slices (60 g)	4
Bread (wholemeal or mixed grain, no added iron)	2 sandwich slices (60 g)	2.8
Cereal or breakfast bar (*e.g.* muesli bar)	1 bar (37 g)	2.2
Nuts (cashews, almonds)	50 g	1.6–3.8
Sweet corn	½ cup (120 g)	2.1
Porridge (cooked oats)	1 cup (260 g)	1.3
Green vegetables (*e.g.* broccoli, spinach, silverbeet, cabbage, Chinese green vegetables)	½ cup (120 g)	0.5–2
Pasta/noodles, cooked	1 cup	1.0
Rice, cooked	1 cup	0.7
Dried fruit (prunes, apricots)	5–6 (50 g)	0.6
Fruit (fresh)	1 average piece	0.3–0.5

Sources: Food Standards Australia New Zealand: NUTTAB 2006; AUSNUT 2007; manufacturers' food labels

- Wholemeal bread has nearly twice the iron content of white bread, although the higher phytate content in wholemeal flour reduces iron bio-availability. Legumes (such as lentils, baked beans, peanuts and soy beans) are good sources of iron, but high in inhibitory components (phytate and soy peptides). Dried fruit, sweet corn, green leafy vegetables (including broccoli, silverbeet and spinach) are also excellent sources of iron with a low phytate content and hence high bioavailability.
- The second strategy in treatment (and prevention) of iron depletion is to optimize iron absorption by improving food combinations in a meal.

LIMIT CONSUMPTION OF INHIBITORS OF IRON ABSORPTION WITH MEALS

- Only a small amount of iron consumed is actually absorbed. As foods high in phytate (see Table 10.9) and polyphenols (e.g. tea, coffee, cocoa and red wine) can strongly inhibit iron absorption from non-heme food sources and from iron supplements, advising athletes about food combinations that enhance and maximize iron absorption is important. Black tea and coffee contain almost twice as much polyphenol (expressed as tannin equivalents) as herb teas and green teas, which have similar amounts of tannin as red wine. Iron absorption is affected only when these beverages or inhibitors are consumed around the same time as iron-rich non-heme sources. White wine and other alcoholic beverages have only trace amounts of tannin and so have little effect on non-heme iron absorption.

TABLE 10.9 PHYTATE CONTENT IN FOODS

FOODS HIGH IN PHYTATE		FOODS LOW IN PHYTATE	
FOOD	MG PHYTATE/100 g EDIBLE PORTION*	FOOD	MG PHYTATE/100 g EDIBLE PORTION*
Wheat bran cereal (ready-to-eat) and wheat germ	~3200 (bran), 4000 (germ)	Most fruits and vegetables have a low phytate content	
Soy flour	~2300	Rye bread	~160
Cashew nuts (most nuts are high in phytate)	~1900	Rice cereal (such as Kelloggs Rice Bubbles™)	~140
Seeds (sesame, poppy—all high in phytate)	1616–2189	Oatmeal, porridge (cooked)	~100
Wheat cereal (ready-to-eat) (e.g. Wheaties™)	1500	Sweet corn	~130
Soy flour	~1400	Potato, boiled in skin	~100
Soy-based TVP, beef	~1270	Kelloggs Corn Flakes™	~ 70

(continued)

PRACTICE TIPS

TABLE 10.9 (continued)

FOODS HIGH IN PHYTATE		FOODS LOW IN PHYTATE	
FOOD	MG PHYTATE/100 g EDIBLE PORTION*	FOOD	MG PHYTATE/100 g EDIBLE PORTION*
Peanut and other nut butters/pastes	~1250	White bread (not fiber enriched)	~ 70
Oatmeal, uncooked (muesli)	~950	Apples (raw)	~65
Lentils (raw), chickpeas	~430–490	Green peas, boiled	~30
Wholemeal bread (wheat)	390	Broccoli	~20
Mixed grain breakfast cereal (i.e. Kelloggs Special K™)	270	Strawberries and other berries	~ 6

*All figures are rounded, TVP = textured vegetable protein, a soy product
Sources: Harland & Oberleas 1987; Hallberg & Hulthen 2000

INCLUDE FOODS THAT ENHANCE IRON ABSORPTION WITH MEALS OR NEGATE THE EFFECT OF INHIBITORS

- Inclusion of meat, poultry, seafood, vitamin C- or vitamin A-rich foods with meals (e.g. meat and salad on a sandwich, orange juice or fruit with breakfast cereal) enhances iron absorption substantially from non-heme foods. Vitamin C is a potent iron-enhancer and can override the inhibitory effects of phytates and tannins in a dose-dependent manner. Citrus fruit and juices are the richest natural sources of vitamin C, as indicated in Table 10.3. Many foods (including fruit juices) have added vitamin C, which enriches the food and also acts as an anti-oxidant to prevent vitamin C loss from oxidation. The presence of other organic acids in citrus fruits (e.g. grapefruit, orange, lemon and lime) also enhances iron absorption from non-heme foods.
- Table 10.10 shows two examples of food combinations with around the same amount of iron, but with different bioavailability. The high-bioavailability meals are lower in inhibitors (such as phytates and tannins) and provide more vitamin C-rich foods or meat with each meal, enhancing iron absorption and helping negate the effects of the inhibitors, while still maintaining a high CHO content.
- Table 10.11 provides practical strategies to increase iron density and improve iron bioavailability.

TABLE 10.10 EXAMPLES OF MEALS OF SIMILAR IRON CONTENT WITH HIGH AND LOW BIOAVAILABILITY OF IRON

HIGH BIOAVAILABILITY OF IRON			LOW BIOAVAILABILITY OF IRON		
FOOD ITEM	SERVE SIZE	IRON (MG/SERVE)	FOOD ITEM	SERVE SIZE	IRON (MG/SERVE)
Iron-fortified breakfast cereal (such as cornflakes)	1½ cups (60 g)	5.6	Muesli mixed with wheat germ and bran, unfortified	¾ cup (60 g)	3.0
Cow's milk	200 mL	trace	Soy milk, iron-fortified	200 mL	1.0
Fruit juice	1 glass (200 mL)	trace	Tea	1 cup	Trace
Ham and salad sandwich on white bread (30 g ham)	1 sandwich	1.4	Peanut butter sandwich on wholemeal bread	1 sandwich	3.0
Orange	1 medium (130 g)	0.5	Apple	1 medium (130 g)	0.1
Fruit juice, with vitamin C added	1 glass (200 mL)	trace	Soy milk, iron-fortified	1 glass (200 mL)	1.3
Pasta with lean ground beef (such as spaghetti bolognese)	2 cups (~500 g)	4.2	Pasta with tomato-based sauce	2 cups (~500 g)	2.6
Salad with lettuce, tomato, capsicum and carrot	1 cup (50 g)	1.0	Mixed lettuce	1 cup (50 g)	0.3
Fruit salad, fresh or canned, with yoghurt	½ cup (100 g)	0.3	Carton fruit yoghurt	200 g	0.2
			Dried fruit (no vitamin C) and mixed nuts	60 g	1.5
Total		13.0	Total		13.0

Source: Food Standards Australia New Zealand: NUTTAB 2006; AUSNUT 2007

TABLE 10.11 SUMMARY OF DIETARY STRATEGIES FOR ENHANCING IRON INTAKE AND BIOAVAILABILITY
• Eat lean red meat (beef, veal, lamb) in main meals at least three to four times a week. (This practice adds readily available iron to a meal and enhances absorption of iron from plant sources.) Add meat to high-CHO meals to enhance non-heme absorption (e.g. in a pasta sauce, in a stir-fry with rice or noodles or in meat and vegetable kabobs with rice).
• Use lean red meat, poultry or seafood on sandwiches, preferably daily.
• If vegetarian, ensure daily food choices are iron rich (e.g. choose iron-fortified cereal, baked beans, legumes, bread, fruits, green leafy vegetables—see Table 10.8). These are also excellent CHO sources.
• Combine plant foods with a high phytate content (such as cereal grains, breads, breakfast cereal and soy products) with vitamin C-rich foods. Good sources of vitamin C are citrus fruits, fruit juice, strawberries, broccoli, cabbage, cauliflower and capsicum.
• Eat iron-fortified breakfast cereal on most days and look for other foods that have been iron enriched. Porridge and some types of muesli, although excellent sources of CHO, are not iron fortified.
• If diagnosed with depleted iron stores or with iron deficiency, avoid or limit adding bran and wheat germ (rich in phytate) to meals and include a vitamin C-rich food to help negate the inhibitory effect of phytate (see Table 10.3 for vitamin C-rich foods and Table 10.9 for sources of phytate).
• If diagnosed with depleted iron stores or with iron deficiency, avoid drinking strong tea, coffee and red wine (all rich in polyphenols) with meals and substitute with a vitamin C-rich beverage to help negate the inhibitory effects of these beverages.

TREATMENT WITH IRON SUPPLEMENTS

- Where iron stores are exhausted, an iron-rich diet alone is insufficient to restore iron levels quickly. Iron supplements taken for at least 3 months in dosages of 80–100 mg elemental iron/day are necessary for full recovery of iron stores (see section 10.49). As most iron supplements have low iron bioavailability, consumption of vitamin C-rich food or a vitamin C supplement together with the iron supplement can enhance iron absorption. The ferrous form of iron supplement has a higher bioavailability than the ferric form and is often well tolerated. When iron supplements are taken on an empty stomach as indicated, further elimination of interference from inhibitors is possible, although the incidence of gastrointestinal side effects may increase. In our experience, adverse side effects are infrequently reported in athletes on short-term, prescribed iron dosages.

FOLLOW-UP

- Athletes should be discouraged from self-administering iron supplements, as iron supplements may induce deficiencies of copper and zinc and are contraindicated in hemochromatosis. Biochemical measures of iron status in elite athletes are usually reviewed at 12 weeks, and supplements are discontinued when iron status indicators are within the individual's usual levels or reference ranges.

FAILURE TO RESPOND TO INTERVENTION

- Reasons for failure to respond to dietary iron intervention and iron supplements may relate to:
  - poor compliance with the intervention
  - inadequate dosage of iron supplement: <50 mg elemental iron is associated with little improvement of hemoglobin and iron status (Haymes & Lamanca 1989)
  - inadequate iron density in the diet to meet individual requirements (iron intakes may need to be set at higher than previous levels)
  - poor food combinations that inhibit iron absorption from food or iron supplements
  - an underlying chronic medical condition (i.e. the anemia associated with inflammation or chronic disease) that does not respond to iron supplements (Handelman & Levin 2008) or parasite infection or *Helicobacter pylori* infection that was previously undetected
  - incorrect original diagnosis (consistently low biochemical measures of iron status), and the usual or normal levels for an individual athlete or hematological intakes were unreliable at the time of testing (see section 10.39)
- To provide a valid measure of usual or baseline levels for individual athletes, biochemical indicators need to be monitored over several months. Large fluctuations in these measures are usually indicative of dietary, physiological and training influences.

USEFUL WEBSITES

http://ods.od.nih.gov/factsheets/iron.asp
National Institutes of Health (US): Office of Dietary Supplements

http://www.sportsdietitians.com.au/content/506/IronDepletioninAthletes/
Sports Dietitians Australia: Iron fact sheet

REFERENCES

Abrahams SF, Mira M, Beaumont PJV, et al. Eating behaviours among young women. Med J Aust 1988;2:225–8.

American Dietetic Association. Position of the American Dietetic Association: vegetarian diets. J Am Diet Assoc 1997;97:1317–21.

Ashenden MJ, Martin DT, Dobson GP, et al. Serum ferritin and anaemia in trained female athletes. Int J Sport Nutr 1998;8:223–9.

Atanasiu V, Manolescu B, Stoian I. Hepcidin—central regulator of iron metabolism. Eur J Haem 2006;78:1–10.

Australian Iron Status Advisory Board. At http://www.ironpanel.org.au (accessed September 2005).

Australian Sports Commission. Survey of drug use in Australian sport. Canberra: Australian Sports Medicine Federation, 1983.

Baech SB, Hansen M, Bukhave K, et al. Nonheme-iron absorption from a phytate-rich meal is increased by the addition of small amounts of pork meat. Am J Clin Nutr 2003;77:173–9.

Balaban EP. Sports anaemia. Clin Sports Med 1992;10:313–25.

Barr SI. Women, nutrition and exercise: a review of athletes, intakes and a discussion of energy balance in active women. Prog Food Nutr Sc 1987;10:307–61.

Baylis A, Cameron-Smith D, Burke LM. Inadvertent doping through supplement use by athletes: assessment and management of the risk in Australia. Int J Sport Nutr & Exerc Metab 2001;10:365–83.

Baynes RD. Assessment of iron status. Clin Biochem 1996;29:209–15.

Baynes RD, Macfarlane BJ, Bothwell TH, et al. The promotive effect of soy sauce on iron absorption in human subjects. Eur J Clin Nutr 1990;44:419–24.

Beard JL. Iron biology in immune function, muscle metabolism and neural functioning. J Nutr 2001;131(Suppl):6568S–80S.

Beard JL, Connor JR. Iron status and neural functioning. Annu Rev Nutr 2003;23:41–58.

Beaton GH, Corey PN, Steele C. Conceptual and methodological issues regarding the epidemiology of iron deficiency and their implications for studies of the functional consequences of iron deficiency. Am J Clin Nutr 1989;50:575–88.

Beguin Y, Clemons GK, Pootrakul P, Fillet G. Quantitative assessment of erythropoiesis and functional characteristics of anemia based on measurements of serum transferrin receptor and erythropoietin. Blood 1993;81:1067–76.

Bergstrom E, Hernell O, Lonnerdal B, Persson LA. Sex differences in iron stores in adolescence. In: Hallberg L, Asp NG, eds. Iron nutrition in health and disease. London: John Libbey, 1996:157–63.

Borch-Iohnsen B. Determination of iron status: brief review of physiological effects on iron measures. Analyst 1995;8:891–3.

Bothwell TH. Iron balance and the capacity of regulatory systems to prevent the development of iron deficiency and overload. In: Hallberg L, Asp NG, eds. Iron nutrition in health and disease. London: John Libbey, 1996:3–16.

Bothwell TH. Iron deficiency in teenagers: new directions in management. Canberra: Australian Iron Status Advisory Panel, Symposium, November, 1995.

Bothwell TH, Charlton RW, Cook JD, Finch CA. Iron metabolism in man. London, Oxford: Blackwell Scientific Publications, 1979:88–104.

Brotherhood J, Brozovic B, Pugh LGC. Haematological status of middle- and long-distance runners. Clin Sci Molecular Med1975;48:139–45.

Brownlie TI, Utermohlen V, Hinton PS, et al. Marginal iron deficiency without anemia impairs aerobic adaptation among previously untrained women. Am J Clin Nutr 2002;75:734–42.

Brownlie TI, Utermohlen V, Hinton PS, Haas JD. Tissue iron deficiency without anemia impairs adaptation in endurance capacity after aerobic training in previously untrained women. Am J Clin Nutr 2004;79:437–43.

Brugnara C. Iron deficiency and erythropoiesis: new diagnostic approaches. Clin Chem 2003;49:1573–8.

Brune M, Rossander L, Hallberg L. Iron absorption and phenolic compounds: the importance of different phenolic structures. Eur J Clin Nutr 1989;43:547–8.

Brune M, Rossander-Hultén L, Hallberg L, et al. Iron absorption from bread in humans: inhibiting effects of cereal fiber, phytate and inositol phosphates with different numbers of phosphate groups. J Nutr 1992;122:442–9.

Brutsaert TD, Hernandez-Cordero S, Rivera J, et al. Iron supplementation improves progressive fatigue resistance during dynamic knee extensor exercise in iron-depleted, nonanemic women. Amer J Clin Nutr 2003;77:441–8.

Cardenas VM, Mulla ZD, Ortiz M, Graham DY. Iron deficiency and *Helicobacter pylori* infection in the United States. Am J Epidemiol 2006;163:127–34.

Celsing F, Blomstrand E, Werner B, et al. Effects of iron deficiency on endurance and muscle enzyme activity. Med Sci Sports Exerc 1986;18:156–61.

Chatard J, Mujika I, Guy C, Lacour J. Anaemia and iron deficiency in athletes. Practical recommendations for treatment. Sports Med 1999;27:229–40.

Choi J. Sensitivity, specificity, and predictive value of serum soluble transferrin receptor at different stages of iron deficiency. Ann Clin Lab Sci 2005;35:435–9.

Commonwealth Department of Health and Ageing, Ministry of Health, National Health and Medical Research Council. Nutrient reference values for Australia and New Zealand. Canberra: NHMRC, 2006.

Constantini NW, Eliakim A, Zigel L, Yaaron M, Falk B. Iron status of highly active adolescents: evidence of depleted iron stores in gymnasts. Int J Sport Nutr 2000;10:62–70.

Cook JD. The effect of endurance training on iron metabolism. Sem Hemat 1994;3:146–54.

Cook JD, Dassenko SA, Whittaker P. Calcium supplementation: effect on iron absorption. Am J Clin Nutr 1991;53:106–10.

Cook JD, Flowers CH, Skikne BS. The quantitative assessment of body iron. Blood 2003;101:3359–64.

Cook JD, Lipschitz DA, Laughton EM, Finch CA. Serum ferritin as a measure of iron stores in normal subjects. Am J Clin Nutr 1974;27:681–7.

Cook JD, Reddy MB. Effect of ascorbic acid intake on nonheme-iron absorption from a complete diet. Am J Clin Nutr 2001;73:93–8.

Cook JD, Reddy MB, Hurrell RF. The effect of red and white wine on non-heme iron absorption in humans. Am J Clin Nutr 1995;61:800–4.

Crosby WH, O'Neill MA. A small dose iron tolerance test as an indicator of mild iron deficiency. J Am Med Assoc 1984;251:1986–7.

Cusick SE, Mei ZG, Freedman DS, et al. Unexplained decline in the prevalence of anemia among US children and women between 1988–1994 and 1999–2002. Am J Clin Nutr 2008;88:1611–7.

Dawson B, Goodman C, Blee T, et al. Iron supplementation: oral tablets versus intramuscular injection. Int J Sport Nutr Exerc Metab 2006;16:180–6.

Deruisseau KC, Cheuvront SN, Haymes EM, Sharp RG. Sweat iron and zinc losses during prolonged exercise. Int J Sports Exerc Metab 2002:428–37.

Deruisseau KC, Roberts LM, Kushnick MR, et al. Iron status of young males and females performing weight-training exercise. Med Sci Sports Exerc 2004;36:241–8.

Deugnier Y, Loréal O, Carré F, et al. Increased body stores in elite road cyclists. Med Sci Sports Exerc 2002;34:878–80.

Dill DB, Braithwaite K, Adams WC. Blood volume of middle-distance runners: effect of 2,300 m altitude and comparison with non-athletes. Med Sc Sports Exerc 1974;6:1–7.

Dubnov G, Constantini NW. Prevalence of iron depletion and anemia in top-level basketball players. Int J Sport Nutr Exerc Metab 2004;14:30–7.

Dufaux B, Hoegerath A, Streitberger W, et al. Serum ferritin, transferrin, haptoglobin and iron in middle-distance and long-distance runners, elite rowers, and professional racing cyclists. Int J Sports Med 1981;2:43–6.

Ervasti M, Kotisaari S, Romppanen J, Punnonen K. In patients who have stainable iron in the bone marrow an elevated plasma transferrin receptor value may reflect functional iron deficiency. Clin Lab Haematology 2004;26:205–9.

Expert Scientific Working Group. Summary of a report on assessment of iron nutritional status of the United States population. Am J Clin Nutr 1985;42:1318–30.

Fairweather-Tait SJ. Iron requirements and prevalence of iron deficiency in adolescents: an overview. In: Hallberg L, Asp NG, eds. Iron nutrition in health and disease. London: John Libbey, 1996:137–48.

Fallon K. Utility of hematological and iron-related screening in elite athletes. Clin J Sports Med 2004;14:145–52.

Fallon KE. Clinical utility of blood tests in elite athletes with short term fatigue. Br J Sports Med 2006;40:541–4.

Fallon KE. The clinical utility of screening of biochemical parameters in elite athletes: analysis of 100 cases. Br J Sports Med 2008;42:334–7.

Fallon KE, Fallon SK, Boston T. The acute phase response and exercise: court and field sports. Br J Sports Med 2001;35:170–3.

Fallon KE, Gerrard DF. Blood tests in tired elite athletes: expectations of athletes, coaches and sport science/sports medicine staff. Commentary. Br J Sports Med 2007;41:41–4.

Fallon KE, Sivyer G, Sivyer K, Dare A. Changes in the haematological parameters and iron metabolism associated with a 1600 kilometre ultramarathon. Br J Sports Med 1999;33:27– 32.

Ferguson NJ, Skikne BS, Simpson KM, et al. Serum transferrin receptor distinguishes the anemia of chronic disease from iron deficiency anemia. J Lab Clin Med 1992;109:386– 90.

Finch CA, Cook JD. Iron deficiency. Am J Clin Nutr 1984;39:471–7.

Finch CA, Huebers H. Perspectives in iron metabolism. N Eng J Med 1982;306:1520–8.

Fogelholm M. Indicators of vitamin and mineral status in athletes' blood: a review. Int J Sports Nutr 1995;5:267–84.

Fogelholm M. Micronutrients; interaction between physical activity, intakes and requirements. Public Health Nutr 1999;2:349–56.

Fogelholm M, Jaakkola L, Lammpisjaervi T. Effect of iron supplementation in female athletes with low serum ferritin concentration. Int J Sports Med 1992;13:158–62.

Food and Nutrition Board, Institute of Medicine. Dietary reference intakes for vitamin A, vitamin K, arsenic, boron, chromium, copper, iodine, iron, manganese, molybdenum, nickel, silicon, vanadium and zinc. Washington DC: National Academy Press, 2000a.

Food and Nutrition Board, Institute of Medicine. Dietary reference intakes: Applications in dietary assessment. A report of the Subcommittee on Interpretation and Uses of Dietary Reference Intakes and the Standing Committee on the Scientific Evaluation of Dietary Reference Intakes, Washington DC: National Academy Press, 2000b.

Food Standards Australia New Zealand. AUSNUT 2007. At http://www.foodstandards.gov.au/monitoringandsurveillance/foodcompositionprogram/ausnut2007/index.cfm (accessed 24 April 2009).

Food Standards Australia New Zealand. NUTTAB 2006. At http://www.foodstandards.gov.au/monitoringandsurveillance/nuttab2006/onlineversionintroduction/onlineversion.cfm (accessed 23 April 2009).

Fricker PA, Gleeson M, Flanagan A, et al. A clinical snapshot: do elite swimmers experience more upper respiratory illness than non-athletes? Clin Exerc Physiol 2000;2:1508.

Friedmann B, Weller E, Mairbaeurl H, Baertsch P. Effects of iron repletion on blood volume and performance capacity in young athletes. Med Sci Sports Exerc 2001;33:741–6.

Ganz T. Hepcidin, a key regulator of iron metabolism and mediator of anemia of inflammation. Blood 2003;102:783–8.

Ganz T. Hepcidin—a regulator of intestinal iron absorption and iron recycling by macrophages. Best Pract Research Clin Haem 2005;18:171–82.

Ganz T, Nemeth E. Hepcidin and regulation of body iron metabolism. Am J Physiol Gastrointest Liver Physiol 2005:199–203.

García-Casal MN, Layrisse M, Peña-Rosas JP, et al. Iron absorption from elemental iron-fortified corn flakes in humans. Role of vitamins A and C. Nutr Res 2003;23:451–63.

García-Casal MN, Layrisse M, Solano L, et al. Vitamin A and beta-carotene can improve nonheme iron absorption from rice, wheat and corn by humans. J Nutr 1998;128:646–50.

Gardner GW, Edgertoe VR, Senewiratne B, et al. Physical work capacity and metabolic stress in subjects with iron deficiency. Am J Clin Nutr 1977:30:910–17.

Garza D, Shrier I, Kohl HW, et al. The clinical value of serum ferritin in endurance athletes. Clin J Sports Med 1997;7:46–53.

Gerrior S, Bente L. Nutrient content of the US food supply, 1909–1997. US Department of Agriculture, Center for Nutrition Policy and Promotion, Home Economics Research Report No. 54, Washington, DC: USDA, 2001.

Gillooly M, Bothwell TH, Torrance JD, et al. The effects of organic acids, phytates and polyphenols on the absorption of iron from vegetables. Br J Nutr 1983;49:331–42.

Gillooly M, Torrance JD, Bothwell TH, et al. The relative effect of ascorbic acid on iron absorption from soy-based and milk-based infant formulas. Am J Clin Nutr 1984;40:522–7.

Gleeson M, Lancaster G, Bishop N. Nutritional strategies to minimise exercise-induced immunosuppression in athletes. Can J Appl Physiol 2001;26(Suppl):23S–35S.

Grinder-Pedersen L, Bukhave K, Jensen M, et al. Calcium from milk or calcium-fortified foods does not inhibit nonheme-iron absorption from a whole diet consumed over a 4-day period. Am J Clin Nutr 2004;80:404–9.

Haas JD, Brownlie T. Iron deficiency and reduced work capacity: A critical review of the research to determine a causal relationship. J Nutr 2001;131(Suppl):676S–90S.

Haggarty P, McGraw BA, Maughan RJ, Fenn C. Energy expenditure of elite female athletes measured by the doubly-labeled water method. Proc Nutr Soc 1988;47:35A.

Hallberg L. Bioavailability of dietary iron in man. Annu Rev Nutr 1981;1:123–47.

Hallberg L. Combating iron deficiency: daily administration of iron is far superior to weekly administration. Am J Clin Nutr 1998;68:213–17.

Hallberg L, Brune M, Erlandsson E, et al. Calcium: effect of different amounts of nonheme- and heme-iron absorption in man. Am J Clin Nutr 1991;53:102–19.

Hallberg L, Brune M, Rossander L. Effect of ascorbic acid on iron absorption from different types of meals: studies with ascorbate rich foods and synthetic ascorbic acid given in different amounts with different meals. Hum Nutr: Appl Nutr 1986;40:97–103.

Hallberg L, Brune M, Rossander L. Iron absorption in man: ascorbic acid and dose-dependent inhibition by phytate. Am J Clin Nutr 1989;49:140–4.

Hallberg L, Hulthen L. Iron requirements, iron balance and iron deficiency in menstruating and pregnant women. In: Hallberg L, Asp NG, eds. Iron nutrition in health and disease. London: John Libbey, 1996:165–81.

Hallberg L, Hulthén L. Prediction of dietary iron absorption: an algorithm for calculating absorption and bioavailability of dietary iron. Am J Clin Nutr 2000;71:1147–60.

Hallberg L, Hulthen L. High serum ferritin is not identical to high iron stores. Amer J Clin Nutr 2003;78:122.

Hallberg L, Hulthén L, Garby L. Iron stores in man in relation to diet and iron requirements. Eur J Clin Nutr 1998;52:623–31.

Hallberg L, Hultén L, Gramatkovski E. Iron absorption from the whole diet in men: how effective is the regulation of iron absorption? Am J Clin Nutr 1997;66:347–56.

Hallberg L, Hulthén L, Linstedt G, et al. Prevalence of iron deficiency in Swedish adolescents. Paediatric Res 1993;34:680–7.

Hallberg L, Rossander, L. Effect of different drinks on the absorption of non-haem iron from composite meals. Hum Nutr Appl Nutr 1982a;36:116–23.

Hallberg L, Rossander L. Effect of soy protein on nonheme iron absorption in man. Am J Clin Nutr 1982b;36:514–20.

Hallberg L, Rossander Hulthen L, Brune M, Gleerup A. Inhibition of haem-iron absorption in man by calcium. Br J Nutr 1993;69:533–40.

Hallberg L, Sandstrom B, Ralph A, Arthur J. Iron, zinc and other trace elements. In: Garrow JS, James WPT, Ralph A, eds. Human nutrition and dietetics. Tenth edition. London: Churchill-Livingstone, 2000:177–210.

Handelman GJ, Levin NW. Iron and anemia in human biology: A review of mechanisms. Heart Fail Rev 2008;13:393–404.

Harland BF, Oberleas D. Phytate in food. Wld Rev Nutr Diet 1987;52:235–59.

Haymes EM, Lamanca JF. Iron loss in runners during exercise: implications and recommendations. Sports Med 1989;7:277–85.

Haymes EM. Nutrition and the physically active female. Women Sport Phys Act 1992;1:35– 47.

Heath ALM, Fairweather-Tait S. Health implications of iron overload: the role of diet and genotype. Nutr Rev 2003;61:45.

Hegenauer J, Strause L, Saltman P, et al. Transitory hematologic effects of moderate exercise are not influenced by iron supplements. Eur J Appl Physiol 1983;52:57–61.

Hinton P, Giordano C, Brownlie T, Haas JD. Iron supplementation improves endurance after training in iron-depleted, nonanemic women. J Appl Physiol 2000;88:1002–10.

Hinton P, Sinclair L. Iron supplementation maintains ventilatory threshold and improves energetic efficiency in iron-deficient nonanemic athletes. Eur J Clin Nutr 2007;61:30–9

Hoffman R, Benz E, Shattil S, et al. Disorders of iron metabolism: iron deficiency and overload. In: Hematology: basic principles and practice. NY: Churchill Livingstone, Harcourt Brace & Co, 2000.

Huebers HA, Begui Y, Pootrakul P, Einspar D, Finch CA. Intact transferrin receptors in human plasma and their relation to erythropoiesis. Blood 1990;1975:102–7.

Hulthen L, Gramatkovski E, Gleerup A, Hallberg L. Iron absorption from the whole diet: relation to meal composition, iron requirements and iron stores. Eur J Clin Nutr 1995;49:794–808.

Hulthen L, Lindstedt G, Lundberg PA, Hallberg L. Effect of a mild infection on serum ferritin concentration—clinical and epidemiological implications. Eur J Clin Nutr 1998;52:376–9.

Hunt JR. How important is dietary iron bioavailability? Am J Clin Nutr 2001;73:3–4.

Hurrell RF. Bioavailability of iron. Eur J Clin Nutr 1997;51(Suppl):4S–8S.

INACG (International Nutritional Anemia Consultative Group). Measurements of iron status. Washington DC: The Nutrition Foundation, 1985.

Israeli E, Merkel D, Constantini N, et al. Iron deficiency and the role of nutrition among female military recruits. Med Sci Sports Exerc 2008;40(11 Suppl):685S–90S.

Jacobs A. Erythropoiesis and iron deficiency anaemia. In: Jacobs A, Worwood M, eds. Iron in biochemistry and medicine. London and New York: Academic Press, 1974.

Klingshirn L, Pate R, Bourque S, et al. Effects of iron supplementation on endurance capacity in iron-depleted female runners. Med Sc Sports Exerc 1992;24:819–24.

Konig D, Weinstock C, Keul J, et al. Zinc, iron, and magnesium status in athletes—influence on the regulation of exercise-induced stress and immune function. Exerc Immunol Rev 1998;4:2–21.

LaManca JJ, Haymes EM. Effects of iron repletion on $VO_{2\,max}$, endurance and blood lactate in women. Med Sci Sports Exerc 1993;25:1386–92.

LaManca JJ, Haymes EM, Daly JA, et al. Sweat iron loss of male and female runners during exercise. Int J Sports Med 1988;9:52–5.

Lampe J, Ellefson M, Slavin J, et al. The effect of marathon running on gastrointestinal transit time and fecal blood loss in women runners. Med Sc Sport Exerc 1987;19(Suppl):21S.

Lampe JW, Slavin JL, Apple FS. Elevated serum ferritin concentrations in master runners after a marathon race. Int J Vit Nutr Res 1986;56:395–8.

Layrisse M, Martinez-Torres C, Leets I, et al. Effect of histidine, cysteine, glutathione or beef on iron absorption in humans. J Nutr 1984;104:217–23.

Looker A, Dallman P, Carroll M, Gunter E, Johnson C. Prevalence of iron deficiency in the United States. JAMA 1997;277:973–6.

Looker AC, Cogswell ME, Gunter EW. Iron deficiency, United States, 1999–2000. Morbidity and Mortality Weekly Report 2002;51:897–9.

Lynch SR, Dassenko SA, Cook JD, et al. Inhibitory effect of a soybean-protein related moiety on iron absorption in humans. Am J Clin Nutr 1994:60:567–72.

MacFarlane BJ, Baynes RD, Bothwell TH, et al. Effect of lupines, a protein-rich legume on iron absorption. Eur J Clin Nutr 1988;42:683–7.

MacPhail AP, Charlton R, Bothwell TH, Bezwoda WR. Experimental fortificants. In: Clydesdale FM, Weimer KL, eds. Iron fortification of foods. New York: Academic Press, 1985:55–75.

Maes M, Bosmans E, Sharpe S, et al. Components of biological variation in serum soluble transferrin receptor: relationships to serum iron, transferrin, and ferritin concentrations, and immune and haematological variables. Scan J Clin Lab Invest 1997;57;31–41.

Magnusson B, Hallberg L, Rossander L, Swolin B. Iron metabolism and sports anaemia: 10. A hematological comparison of elite runners and control subjects. Acta Med Scand 1984;216:157–64.

Malczewska J, Raczynski G, Stupnicki R. Iron status of female endurance athletes. Int J Sport Nutr Exerc Metab 2000;10:260–76.

Malczewska J, Stupnicki R, Blach W, Turek-Lepa E. The effects of physical exercise on the concentrations of ferritin and transferrin receptor in plasma of male judoists. Int J Sports Med 2004;25:516–21.

Malczewska J, Szczpanska B, Stupnicki R, Sendecki W. The assessment of frequency of iron deficiency in athletes from the transferrin receptor-ferritin index. Int J Sport Nutr Exerc Metab 2001;10:42–52.

Mast AE, Blinder M, Gronowski AM, et al. Clinical utility of the soluble transferrin receptor and comparison with serum ferritin in several populations. Clin Chem 1998;44:45–51.

Mast AE, Blinder MA, Lu Q, et al. Clinical utility of the reticulocyte hemoglobin content in the diagnosis of iron deficiency. Blood 2002;99:1489–91.

McColl KEL, El-Omar E, Gillen D. Interactions between *H. pylori* infection, gastric acid secretion and anti-secretory therapy. Br Med Bull 1998;54:121–38.

McLennan W, Podger A. National Nutrition Survey: nutrient intakes and physical measurements, Australia 1995. ABS Cat. No. 4805.0. Canberra: Australian Bureau of Statistics, 1998:80.

McMahon LF, Ryan MJ, Larson D, Fisher RL. Occult gastrointestinal blood loss in marathon runners. Ann Int Med 1984;100:846–7.

Merkel D, Huerta M, Grotto I, et al. Prevalence of iron deficiency and anemia among strenuously trained adolescents. J Adolescent Health 2005;37:220–3.

Miller BJ, Pate RR, Burgess W. Foot impact force and intravascular haemolysis during distance running. Int J Sports Med 1988;9:56–60.

Murphy S, Poos M. Dietary reference intakes: summary of applications in dietary assessment. Pub Health Nutr 2002;5:843–49.

Murray-Kolb L, Beard JL, Joseph LJ, et al. Resistance training affects iron status in older men and women. Int J Sports Nutr & Exerc Metab 2001;10:287–98.

Natchtigall DP, Nielsen P, Fischer R, et al. Iron deficiency in distance runners: a reinvestigation of 99 Fe-labeling and non invasive liver iron quantification. Int J Sports Med 1996;17:473–9.

Newhouse IJ, Clement DB. Iron status in athletes: an update. Sports Med 1988;5:337–52.

Newhouse IJ, Clement DB, Taunton JE, McKenzie DC. The effects of prelatent/latent iron deficiency on physical work capacity. Med Sc Sports Exerc 1989;21:263–8.

Nielsen P, Natchtigall D. Iron supplementation in athletes: current recommendations. Sports Med 1998;26:207–16.

Nikolaidis MG, Michailidis Y, Mougios V. Variation of soluble transferrin receptor and ferritin concentrations in human serum during recovery from exercise. Eur J Appl Physiol 2003;89:500–2.

Nikolaidis MG, Protosygellou MD, Petridou A, et al. Hematologic and biochemical profile of juvenile and adult athletes of both sexes: applications for clinical evaluation. Int J Sports Med 2003;24:506–11.

Parisotto R, Ashenden M. The development of a blood test for EPO abuse. Lab Hematol 2002;8:52–3.

Pate RR, Miller BJ, Davis JM, Slentz CA, Klingshirn LA. Iron status of female runners. Int J Sports Nutr 1993;3:222–31.

Peeling P, Blee T, Goodman C, et al. Effect of iron injections on aerobic-exercise performance of iron-depleted female athletes. Int J Sport Nutr Exerc Metabol 2007;17:221–31.

Pitsis G, Fallon KE, Fallon SK, Fazakerley R. Response of soluble transferrin receptor and iron-related parameters to iron supplementation in elite, iron-depleted nonanemic female athletes. Clin J Sports Med 2002;14:300–4.

Punnonen K, Irjala K, Rajamaki A. Serum transferrin receptor and its ratio to serum ferritin in the diagnosis of iron deficiency. Blood 1997;89:1052–7.

Pyne D, Parisotto, R, Ashenden M. Iron status in highly trained swimmers: guidelines for interpretation and supplementation. Aust Swim Coach 1997;13:45–50.

Rangan AM, Ho RWL, Blight GD, Binns CW. Haem iron content of Australian meats and fish. Food Aust 1997;49:508–10.

Reddy M. Clarke L. Iron, oxidative stress and disease risk. Nutr Rev 2004;62:120–4.

Reddy MB, Cook JD. Effect of calcium intake on nonheme-iron absorption from a complete diet. Am J Clin Nutr 1997;65:1820–5.

Reddy M, Hirrell RF, Cook JD. Estimation of non-heme iron bioavailability from meal composition. Amer J Clin Nutr 2000;71:937–43.

Reid VL, Gleeson M, Williams N, Clancy RL. Clinical investigation of athletes with persistent fatigue and/or recurrent infections. Br J Sports Med 2004;38:42–5.

Resina A, Gatteschi L, Giamberardino MA, et al. Hematological comparison of iron status in trained top-level soccer players and control subjects. Int J Sports Med 1991;12:453–6.

Risser WL, Lee EJ, Poindexter HBW, et al. Iron deficiency in female athletes: its prevalence and impact on performance. Med Sc Sports Exerc 1988;20:16–21.

Risser WL, Risser JMH. Iron deficiency in adolescents and young adults. Phys Sportsmed 1990;18:87–8, 91, 94, 96–8, 101.

Roecker L, Meir-Buttermilch R, Brechtel L, et al. Iron-regulatory protein hepcidin is increased in female athletes after a marathon. Eur J Appl Physiol 2005;95:569–71.

Rossander L, Hallberg L, Bjorn-Rasmussen E. Absorption of iron from breakfast meals. Am J Clin Nutr 1979;31:106–10.

Rossander-Hulten L, Hallberg L. Prevalence of iron deficiency in adolescents. In: Hallberg L, Asp NG, eds. Iron nutrition in health and disease. London: John Libbey, 1996:149–94.

Rowland TW, Deisroth MB, Green GM, Kelleher JF. The effect of iron therapy on the exercise capacity of nonanemic iron-deficient adolescent runners. Sports Med 1988;142:165–9.

Samuelson G, Lönnerdal B, Kempe B, et al. Serum ferritin and transferrin receptor concentrations during the transition from adolescence to adulthood in a healthy Swedish population. Acta Paediatrica 2003;92:5–10.

Sanborn CF, Jankowski CM. Physiologic considerations for women in sport. Clin Sports Med 1994;13:315–27.

Sarker SA, Davidsson L, Mahmud H, et al. *Helicobacter pylori* infection, iron absorption, and gastric acid secretion in Bangladeshi children. Am J Clin Nutr 2004;80:149–53.

Sauberlich HE. Laboratory tests for the assessment of nutritional status. Boca-Raton, Florida: CRC Press, 1999:343–70.

Schmidt W, Maassen N, Tegtbur U, Braumann KM. Changes in plasma volume and red cell formation after a marathon competition. Eur J Appl Physiol Occupat Physiol 1989;58:453–8.

Schnirring L. Screening athletes for low iron. Phys Sports Med 2002;30:5–6.

Schoene RB, Esciourrou P, Robertson HT, et al. Iron repletion decreases maximal exercise lactate concentration in female athletes with minimal iron-deficiency anaemia. J Lab Clin Med 1983; 102:306–12.

Schumacher YO, Schmid A, Grathwohl D, et al. Hematological indices and iron status in athletes of various sports and performances. Med Sci Sports Exer 2002;34:869–75.

Schumacher YO, Schmid A, König D, Berg A. Effects of exercise on soluble transferrin receptor and other variables of the iron status. Brit J Sports Med 2002;36:195–9.

Seiler D, Nager D, Franz H, et al. Effects of long-distance running on iron metabolism and hematological parameters. Int J Sports Med 1989;10:357–62.

Shaskey D, Green G. Sports haematology. Sports Med 2000;29:27–38.

Siegal AJ, Hennekens CH, Solomon HS, van Boeckel B. Exercise-related haematuria: findings in a group of marathon runners. J Am Med Ass 1979;241:391–2.

Skikne B, Flowers CH, Cook, JD. Serum transferrin receptor: a quantitative measure of tissue iron deficiency. Blood 1990;9:1870–6.

Smith DJ, Roberts D. Effects of high volume and/or intense exercise on selected blood chemistry parameters. 1994;27:435–40.

Snyder AC, Dvorak LL, Roepke JB. Influence of dietary iron source on measures of iron status among female runners. Med Sc Sports Exer 1989;21:7–10.

Solomons NW. Daily versus weekly iron: we still might not be asking the right questions. Nutr Rev 1997;55:141–2.

Stupnicki R, Malczewska J, Milde K, Hackney AC. Day to day variability in the transferrin receptor/ferritin index in female athletes. Br J Sports Med 2003;37:267–9.

Suominen P, Punnonen K, Rajamaki A, Irjala K. Serum transferrin receptor and transferrin receptor index identify health subjects with sub-clinical iron deficits. Blood 1998;92:2934–9.

Tee ES, Kandiah M, Awin N, et al. School-administered weekly iron-folate supplements improve haemoglobin and ferritin concentrations in Malaysian adolescent girls. Am J Clin Nutr 1999;69: 1249–56.

Telford RD, Bunney CJ, Catchpole EA, et al. Plasma ferritin concentration and physical work capacity in athletes. Int J Sport Nutr 1992;2:335–42.

Telford RD, Cunningham RB. Sex, sport and body-size dependency of hematology in highly trained athletes. Med Sc Sports Exerc 1991;23:778–94.

Telford RD, Cunningham RB, Deakin V, Kerr DA. Iron status and diet in athletes. Med Sc Sports Exerc 1993;25:796–800.

Tetens I, Bendtsen KM, Henriksen M, et al. The impact of a meat- versus a vegetable-based diet on iron status in women of childbearing age with small iron stores. Eur J Nutr 2007;46:439–45.

Thomas C, Thomas L. Biochemical markers and hematologic indices in the diagnosis of functional iron deficiency. Clin Chem 2002;48:1066–76.

Toit CD, Locke S. An audit of clinically relevant abnormal laboratory parameters investigating athletes with persistent symptoms of fatigue. J Sci Med Sport 2007;10:351–5.

Verdon F, Burnand B, Fallab Stubi CL, et al. Iron supplementation for unexplained fatigue in non-anaemic women: Double blind randomised placebo controlled trial. BMJ 2003;326:1014–18.

Virtanen M, Viinikka LU, Virtanen M, et al. Higher concentrations of serum transferrin receptor in children than in adults. Am J Clin Nutr 1999;69:256–60.

Waller MF, Haymes EM. The effects of heat and exercise on sweat iron loss. Med Sc Sports Exerc 1996;28:197–203.

Weight LM, Klein M, Noakes TD, Jacobs P. Sports anaemia—a real or apparent phenomenon in endurance trained athletes. Int J Sports Med 1992;13:344–7.

Wilkinson JG, Martin DT, Adams AA, Liebman M. Iron status in cyclists during high intensity interval training and recovery. Int J Sports Med 2002;23:544–8.

Worwood M. State of the art—ferritin. Blood Rev 1991;4:259–69.

Worwood M. Haemochromatosis. Clin Lab Haematol 1998;20:65–75.

Zhu YI, Haas JD. Altered metabolic response of iron-depleted nonanemic women during a 15-km time trial. J Appl Physiol 1998;84:1768–75.

Zimmerman MB, Molinari L, Staubli-Asobayire F, et al. Serum transferrin receptor and zinc protoporphyrin as indicators of iron status in African children. Am J Clin Nutr 2005;81:615–23.

Zotter H, Robinson N, Zorzoli M, et al. Abnormally high serum ferritin levels among professional road cyclists. Br J Sports Med 2004;38:704–8.

CHAPTER 11

Vitamin, mineral and anti-oxidant needs of athletes

MIKAEL FOGELHOLM

11.1 Introduction

Vitamins are organic compounds required in very small amounts (from a few micrograms to a few milligrams daily) to prevent clinical deficiency and deterioration in health, growth and reproduction. A distinct feature of vitamins is that the human body is not able to synthesize them. Classification of vitamins is based on their relative solubility: fat-soluble vitamins (A, D, E and K) are more soluble in organic solvents and water-soluble vitamins (B complex and C) in water.

Most vitamins participate in processes related to muscle contractions and energy expenditure (see Table 11.1). Vitamins of the B complex group (e.g. thiamin, riboflavin, vitamin B6, niacin, biotin and pantothenic acid) act as cofactors for enzymes regulating glycolysis, citric acid cycle, oxidative phosphorylation, b-oxidation (breakdown of fatty acids) and amino acid degradation. Folic acid and vitamin B12 are needed for heme synthesis. Ascorbic acid activates an enzyme regulating biosynthesis of carnitine, which is necessary for fatty acid transportation from cell cytosol into mitochondria. Finally, anti-oxidant vitamins (mainly vitamins C and E) participate in the buffer system against free radicals, which are produced by increased energy turnover.

Minerals are inorganic substances found naturally on the earth. Based on their daily requirements, minerals are usually classified as macrominerals (e.g. sodium, potassium, calcium, phosphorus and magnesium), or trace elements (e.g. iron, zinc, copper, chromium and selenium). The daily dietary allowance for macrominerals is more than 100 mg/d, whereas trace elements are needed in much smaller quantities (less than 20 mg/d).

Several minerals and trace elements, such as magnesium, iron, zinc and copper, act as enzyme activators in glycolysis, oxidative phosphorylation and in the system responsible for maintenance of acid-base equilibrium (Table 11.2). Iron is needed for heme synthesis. Minerals (electrolytes) also affect muscle contraction.

TABLE 11.1 SUMMARY OF THE MOST IMPORTANT EFFECTS OF VITAMINS ON BODY FUNCTIONS RELATED TO ATHLETIC TRAINING AND PERFORMANCE

	COFACTORS AND ACTIVATORS FOR ENERGY METABOLISM	NERVOUS FUNCTION, MUSCLE CONTRACTION	HEMO-GLOBIN SYNTHESIS	IMMUNE FUNCTION	ANTI-OXIDANT FUNCTION	BONE METABOLISM
WATER-SOLUBLE VITAMINS						
Thiamin	X	X				
Riboflavin	X	X				
Vitamin B6	X	X	X	X		
Folic acid	X	X				
Vitamin B12	X	X				
Niacin	X	X				
Pantothenic acid	X					
Biotin	X					
Vitamin C			X	X		
FAT-SOLUBLE VITAMINS						
Vitamin A				X	X	
Vitamin D						X
Vitamin E				X	X	

TABLE 11.2 SUMMARY OF THE MOST IMPORTANT EFFECTS OF MINERALS ON BODY FUNCTIONS RELATED TO ATHLETIC TRAINING AND PERFORMANCE

	COFACTORS AND ACTIVATORS FOR ENERGY METABOLISM	NERVOUS FUNCTION, MUSCLE CONTRACTION	HEMO-GLOBIN SYNTHESIS	IMMUNE FUNCTION	ANTI-OXIDANT FUNCTION	BONE METABOLISM
Sodium		X				
Potassium		X				
Calcium		X				X
Magnesium	X	X		X		X
Trace elements						
Iron	X		X		X	
Zinc	X			X	X	
Copper	X				X	
Chromium	X					
Selenium					X	

As evident from the introduction, micronutrients (vitamins and minerals) are essential for life. A well-balanced diet covers the needs for all micronutrients in healthy humans (NHMRC et al. 2006). Nevertheless, vitamin and mineral supplements—including vitamin C (especially), the B-complex vitamins, vitamin E and iron—are frequently used by athletes (Erdman et al. 2007; Tsitsimpikou et al. 2009). The common motivation for vitamin supplementation is to enhance recovery and improve sports performance.

The use of vitamin and mineral supplements at intakes below the Upper Intake Level (UIL) is only justified and necessary if a normal diet is unable to maintain an athlete's micronutrient status; if micronutrient supplements improve nutritional status and physiological functions of an athlete; and—most importantly—if supplements enhance athletic performance directly or indirectly (e.g. by enhancing recovery or by preventing infectious diseases).

This chapter aims to answer the following questions:

- Are micronutrient requirements increased in athletes?
- Are there any significant differences between indices of micronutrient status between athletes and untrained controls?
- If the supply of one or several micronutrients is marginal, would an athlete's functional capacity be less than optimal?
- If micronutrients are given in excess of daily dietary allowances, would this improve indices of micronutrient status, body functions and athletic performance?

Reviews on micronutrients and sports are addressed in chapters on measuring nutritional status of athletes (Chapter 2), calcium (Chapter 9) and iron (Chapter 10). Therefore, the above issues are not covered in the present chapter. Chapter 16 provides additional information on the supplementation practices of athletes.

11.2 Measuring vitamin and mineral status in athletes

11.3 What is nutritional status?

An organism has an adequate nutritional status if its cells, tissue, organs and anatomical systems, working together, can undertake all nutrient-dependent functions. The relationship between micronutrient supply and functional capacity is 'bell-shaped' (see Fig. 11.1) (Brubacher 1989). The core of the above relationship is that the output (functional capacity) is not improved after the 'minimal requirement for maximal output' is reached. In contrast, too high an intake may in some cases reduce the output below the maximal level.

Different body functions (single biochemical reactions, metabolic pathways, the function of anatomical systems and the function of the hosts themselves) reach their maximal output at different levels of supply. In other words, the supply (intake) needed for optimal function of an anatomical system (such as the muscle) may be quite different from the supply needed to maximize the activity of a single enzyme (Solomons & Allen 1983).

Short-term inadequacy of vitamin and mineral intake is characterized by the lowering of nutrient concentrations in different tissues and the lowering of certain enzyme activities (see Fig. 11.2). However, functional disturbances (such as decreased physical performance capacity) may appear later (Solomons & Allen 1983; Fogelholm 1995). In the opposite case, very large intakes increase the body pool and activity of some enzymes, but do not necessarily improve functional capacity (Fogelholm 1995).

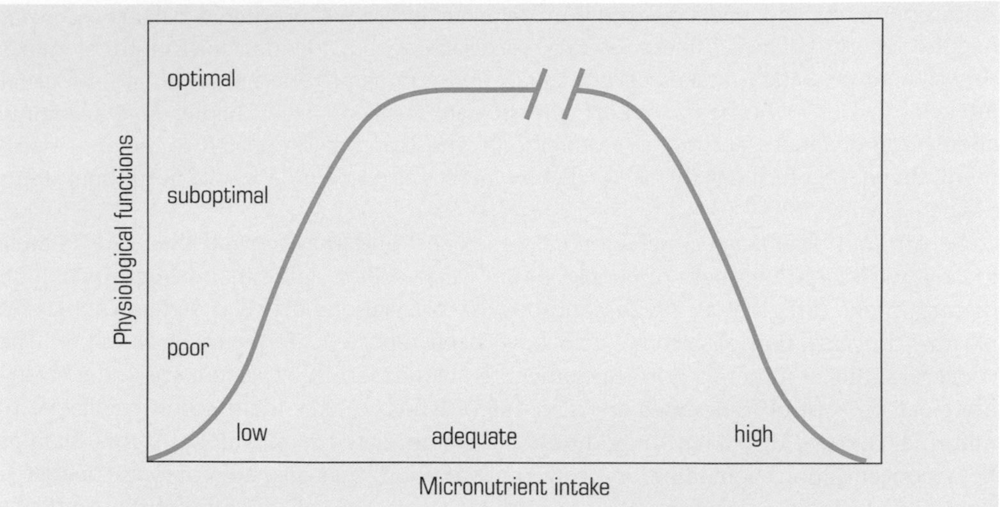

FIGURE 11.1 The relation between micronutrient supply and functional capacity (adapted from Brubacher 1989)

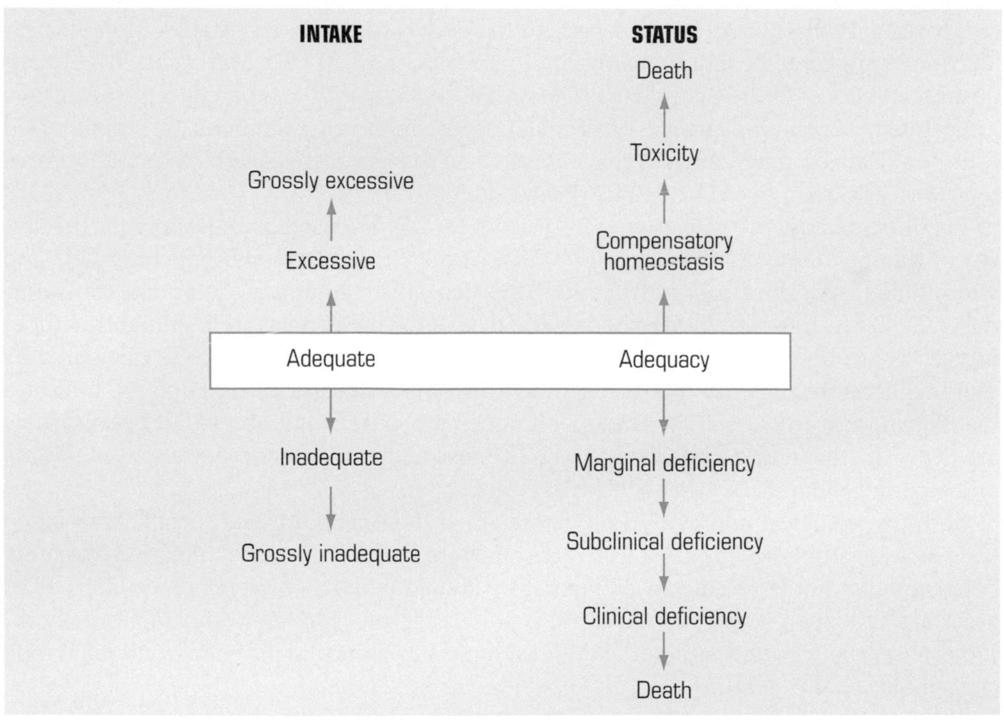

FIGURE 11.2 Dietary micronutrient intake and stages of micronutrient status

Assessment of nutritional status

11.4

Ideally, nutritional status should be assessed by combining the information obtained from different (clinical, anthropometric, dietary, biochemical) markers (see Chapter 2). Gross clinical deficiency of nutrients causes detectable changes in, for instance, the skin or eyes.

Anthropometric and body composition data are indicators of energy balance. Chronic negative energy balance is likely also to be associated with inadequate micronutrient intake. Assessment of dietary intakes of individuals and groups provide only estimates of 'usual' intakes of foods or nutrients and are not accurate measures (see Chapter 2). Uncertainty about an individual's nutritional requirements and inaccuracies related to dietary assessment, therefore, precludes the use of dietary intakes as a sole indicator of nutritional status (Aggett 1990).

Serum and plasma specimens are easy to collect and analyze, and therefore suitable for use with large numbers of people. Some water-soluble vitamins respond quickly to dietary intake (Singh et al. 1992b), and positive correlations between dietary intake and plasma concentration of ascorbic acid have been reported (Tur-Mari et al. 2006). The concentrations of minerals or trace elements in blood, serum or plasma are under strong homeostatic control (Solomons & Allen 1983), which makes them quite insensitive to marginal nutrient deficiency. In addition, factors unrelated to nutritional status, such as hemoconcentration, hemodilution or diurnal variation, may also affect blood chemistry. Therefore a single measurement of serum concentrations of micronutrients should be interpreted with great caution (Tur-Mari et al. 2006).

Because serum and plasma concentrations are rather insensitive to marginal micronutrient deficiency, substantial research has been undertaken to identify other body compartments that would better represent the body's micronutrient status. Mononuclear leucocytes appear to be more sensitive indicators of vitamin C (Tur-Mari et al. 2006), magnesium (Weller et al. 1998) and zinc (Dolev et al. 1995) status, compared to the respective indicators in serum or plasma. Unfortunately, these interesting methods are still not used routinely. Data on micronutrient concentrations in the leucocytes of athletes are too scarce to lead to any definitive conclusions (Peake 2003).

Erythrocyte enzyme activation co-efficients (E-AC) are used as indicators for the status of thiamin (enzyme: transketolase: TK), riboflavin (glutathione reductase: GR) and vitamin B6 (aspartate aminotransferase: AST, also called glutamate oxalacetate transaminase: GOT). In these methods, the activity of an enzyme is measured with and without in vitro cofactor (vitamin B) saturation. The activation co-efficient (AC) is calculated by dividing saturated activity by basal activity (Bayomi & Rosalki 1976). High AC indicates inadequate nutritional status. These techniques are extremely interesting, because they are truly functional rather than static, as is the case with nutrient concentrations in plasma and serum (Solomons & Allen 1983).

Both physiological and analytical factors affect the sensitivity and specificity of blood tests as indicators of vitamin status. These factors lead to a notable analytical variation between laboratories. Ideally, each laboratory should make its own reference interval, or ascertain that the chosen reference interval is made by precisely comparable methods. Otherwise, the reported number of athletes with 'sub-clinical deficiency' could be wrong (Fogelholm et al. 1993b).

The enzymes that are used for assessment of thiamin, riboflavin and vitamin B6 status represent one metabolic pathway in the erythrocytes. Therefore they do not necessarily indicate the function of other metabolic pathways in other tissues, for example glycolysis or the Kreb's cycle in the muscles. Moreover, when people follow a typical western mixed diet, erythrocyte concentrations of TK, GR and AST are not saturated in vivo by their cofactor. Consequently, after supplementation, their basal activity increases and activation co-efficient decreases (Guilland et al. 1989; Fogelholm et al. 1993b). However, these changes are not necessarily associated with improved physical performance (see section 11.11).

The relationships between exercise, free radicals and lipid peroxidation have raised considerable interest. Breath pentane, thiobarbituric acid reactive substances (TBARS) and malondialdehyde (MDA) are indicators of lipid peroxidation caused by free radicals in humans. Unfortunately, these markers indicate neither the source nor the timing of lipid peroxidation (Alessio 1993), nor do they permit quantitative correlation of peroxidation (Weber 1990). MDA and TBARS, for instance, may arise from other pathways besides lipid peroxidation (Weber 1990). Moreover, during sleep and light daily activities, products of lipid peroxidation may be produced and remain in regions where blood-flow is limited (Weber 1990). When blood-flow during exercise is increased and blood is redistributed to new regions, these products may then be 'washed out'.

Effects of exercise on vitamin and mineral requirements of athletes

11.5

Requirements of water-soluble vitamins and anti-oxidants

11.6

Physical activity increases energy expenditure. Van der Beek's review (1991) proposed that high metabolic activity might increase the turnover of several vitamins of the B-complex group. Indeed, some old data support the above view. For example, Sauberlich and colleagues (1979) found that thiamin requirements in male subjects were 30% higher when daily energy intake was 15.1 MJ (3600 kcal), compared with 11.7 MJ (2600 kcal). However, an energy-related requirement for thiamin has also been questioned (Caster & Mickelsen 1991). Vitamin losses through sweat are minimal, even in physically active people (Brotherhood 1984).

Energy production involves reduction of molecular oxygen (O_2) in the mitochondria. The reduction is not always complete, and about 2–5% of the molecular oxygen turns into a free radical (superoxide radical, O_2^-) (Sjödin et al. 1990). The free radicals are unstable, reactive and potentially harmful chemical substances with unpaired electrons in their outer orbitals (Sen 1995). An excessive production of free radicals, or an insufficient protection against them, has been linked to cell and mitochondria membrane damage, deterioration of the immune defense system, aging, cancer and atherosclerosis (Jacob & Burri 1996).

In humans, indirect evidence of lipid peroxidation during physical exertion includes increased pentane exhalation in the breath (Simon-Schnass & Pabst 1988; Dekkers et al. 1996; Leaf et al. 1997), elevated MDA in serum and erythrocytes (Dekkers et al. 1996; McBride et al. 1998; Nakhostin-Roohi et al. 2008), increased TBARS (Machefer et al. 2007) and increased levels of oxidized glutathione (Goldfarb et al. 2007). Not all studies show an exercise-induced increase in indices of lipid peroxidation (Laaksonen et al. 1995; Margaritis et al. 1997). It is, however, apparent that lipid peroxidation is increased if the preceding exercise is intense and strenuous enough (Leaf et al. 1997).

Scavenger enzymes and anti-oxidant vitamins (mainly vitamins C and E and β-carotene) build up a protection system against free radical attack. Mena and colleagues (1991) showed that highly trained athletes have higher activities of several scavenger enzymes, but the effects of moderate training are apparently much smaller (Tiidus et al. 1996). An increased need for endogenous defense against free radicals may, nevertheless, increase the requirement for anti-oxidant vitamins (Sen 1995; Dekkers et al. 1996; Jacob & Burri 1996). On the other hand, well-trained athletes may have a more developed endogenous anti-oxidant system than a sedentary individual, and hence the additional need for exogenous anti-oxidants (such as vitamins) may not be very high (Kanter 1998).

11.7 Requirements for minerals

The losses of magnesium and zinc through sweat may be important. The exercise-induced concentration of magnesium in sweat has varied between 3 and 36 mg/L in different studies (Beller et al. 1975; Costill et al. 1976, 1982; Verde et al. 1982; Wenk et al. 1989; Montain et al. 2007). Strenuous exercise increases magnesium requirements by 10–20% (Nielsen & Lukaski 2006). Similarly, the zinc concentration in sweat has varied between 0.6 and 1.5 mg/L (Beller et al. 1975; Aruoma et al. 1988; DeRuisseau et al. 2002; Montain et al. 2007), which would mean a 20–40% increase in the daily needs for each additional liter of sweat. Unfortunately, the interpretation of these data is difficult, because of several problems in sweat analyses. For instance, the composition of sweat varies with the collection site (Gutteridge et al. 1985; Aruoma et al. 1988). Moreover, it is uncertain whether a short sampling period represents long-term conditions. For instance, iron and zinc concentrations in sweat may decrease considerably after the first hour of exercise (DeRuisseau et al. 2002; Montain et al. 2007). The variation between different studies reflects the above-mentioned methodological problems.

In addition to sweating, micronutrients may be lost in urine or feces. On one day of physical exercise, Deuster and colleagues (1987) found elevated (22%) magnesium excretion. Similarly, higher excretion of magnesium (21–76%) (Singh et al. 1990a; Nuviala et al. 1999) and zinc (Lichton et al. 1988; Deuster et al. 1989) has been found in trained athletes compared with controls. Results are not without contradiction: Nuviala and colleagues (1999) reported similar urinary zinc excretion in female athletes and untrained controls, and Zorbas and colleagues (1999) found increased copper excretion in trained subjects only when their activity was markedly restricted. Moreover, Dressendorfer and colleagues (2002) did not find increased urinary excretion of magnesium, iron, zinc and copper during very high-intensity training in male cyclists. Finally, because of an increase in free radical formation during strenuous exercise, the requirements for zinc and copper (in Zn_2Cu_2-superoxide dismutase enzyme) and selenium (in glutathione peroxidase) may also be greater than normal in physically active people (Koury et al. 2004).

In summary, it is biologically plausible to assume that athletic training, especially if it leads to very high energy expenditure, increases the requirements for micronutrients (at least through losses in sweat and urine, and perhaps in feces) and through increased free radical production. Nevertheless, the data to date are insufficient to allow any quantification of micronutrient requirements in athletes. Because of a wide safety margin, the relevant cut-offs from the Dietary Reference Intakes (DRI)/ Nutrient Reference Values (NRV) for vitamins and minerals, with adjustments for iron, can still be used for assessing the probability of nutrient adequacy or inadequacy in athletes, although with caution. Guidelines for using the appropriate cut-off as benchmarks for assessing nutrient requirements of individuals and groups are found in section 2.24.

Biochemical indicators of vitamin and mineral status in athletes 11.8

Most biochemical measures that are indices of nutrient status in individuals are markers for risk and do not usually confirm a true diagnosis of nutrient overload or deficiency without other clinical and dietary assessment measures (see Chapter 2). One-off biochemical measures in individuals, although below the usual population measures, may be normal for those individuals. Biochemical measures of vitamins and minerals become diagnostic in individuals only in moderate to severe nutrient depletion states, which is unusual in an athlete population. Biochemical measures of vitamin and mineral status in athletes are useful in research to compare relative differences between athletes and non-athlete controls, and to allow an evaluation of nutrient requirements of groups of athletes involved in varying types of physical activity.

Biochemical indicators of water-soluble vitamin status 11.9

Vitamin B group 11.10

Cross-sectional studies comparing vitamin B status in athletes and untrained controls give inconclusive results. Guilland and colleagues (1989) found higher erythrocyte transketolase activation co-efficients (E-TKAC) in athletes than in untrained controls, whereas Fogelholm and colleagues (1992a, 1992b) found both lower and comparable E-TKAC in athletes. Keith and Alt (1991) found higher erythrocyte glutathione reductase activation co-efficients (E-GRAC) in female athletes, but Guilland and colleagues (1989) reported levels comparable to the controls. Only Guilland and colleagues (1989) have reported erythrocyte aspartate amino transferase activation co-efficient (E-ASTAC) values for both athletes and untrained controls; no difference was observed. All differences reported in the above studies were small, however, and most probably without any functional significance.

The effects of a 24-week fitness-type exercise program on micronutrient status in previously untrained female students have been studied (Fogelholm 1992). Indicators for thiamin and riboflavin status were unchanged throughout the study. E-ASTAC increased in exercise and decreased in control groups, which may indicate marginally impaired vitamin B6 status in the exercise group. However, the magnitude of the change (from 2.02 to 2.11) is not likely to affect functional capacity (Fogelholm et al. 1993a, 1993b).

The effects of varying the training volume on E-TKAC have also been studied in Finnish cross-country skiers (Fogelholm et al. 1992b). Despite very strenuous training in August and November, and clearly lighter training in February and in May, E-TKAC showed no seasonal variation.

Plasma total vitamin B6 concentration and/or pyridoxal-5′-phosphate concentration increase during short-term exercise, but decrease during very prolonged physical exertion (Crozier et al. 1994; Leonard & Leklem 2000). The physiological significance of these changes is not known.

Vitamin C 11.11

Reported data on vitamin C status in physically active people and untrained individuals are scarce. Serum ascorbic acid concentrations were the same (Guilland et al. 1989;

Fogelholm et al. 1992a; Rokitzki et al. 1994a) or higher (Fishbaine & Butterfield 1984) in athletes than in controls. The pooled mean concentrations for serum or plasma ascorbic acid in the above studies were 59 and 56 µmol/L for athletes ($n = 533$) and controls ($n = 193$), respectively. Moreover, studies have not shown any differences between athletes' and controls' urinary excretion of ascorbic acid (Peake 2003), which further suggests that athletic training does not have any special negative effects on vitamin C status that a slightly increased dietary intake could not counterbalance.

11.12 Biochemical indicators of fat-soluble vitamin status

11.13 Vitamin A

Serum concentration for β-carotene, the provitamin for retinol, is more responsive to marginal changes in status than retinol. Takatsuka and colleagues (1995) reported that hard physical activity was associated with lower β-carotene concentrations in Japanese men and women. The results in this cross-sectional study were adjusted for age, body mass index (BMI), diet, smoking, and serum cholesterol and serum triglycerides. Guilland and colleagues (1989) found comparable β-carotene concentrations in athletes and controls, whereas Watson and colleagues (2005) reported higher concentration in athletes.

11.14 Vitamin D

In a recent review, Willis and colleagues (2008) identified five studies with data on vitamin D intake in athletes. The intake was less than recommended in most of the studies and no different from controls. However, the subjects were selected from known high-risk groups where lean body mass and low energy intakes are commonly reported: ski jumpers, figure skaters, female soccer players, female cross-country skiers and runners. This introduces selection bias; therefore, although these data identify potential risk groups, they cannot be generalized to other disciplines and/or male athletes.

Biochemical indices of vitamin D-status in athletes have only been reported in a small number of studies of athletes. When serum 25(OH) vitamin D concentration was used as the indicator for vitamin D status, between 37% and 68% of the athletes studied showed deficient status (Willis et al. 2008). These figures are similar to the status in the general population, but nevertheless a clear concern. In one recent study in a high-risk group of female elite gymnasts, 15 out of 18 gymnasts had serum 25(OH) vitamin D below the cut-off concentration (Lovell 2008). Low vitamin D status is expected to be highest in those athletes who train inside and have little exposure to the sun but is certainly of concern to bone health in young athletes.

11.15 Vitamin E

Moderate physical activity has not been shown to have any negative effects on vitamin E (α-tocopherol) concentration in plasma (Kitamura et al. 1997; Thomas et al. 1998) or in the muscle (Tiidus et al. 1996). Only a few studies have compared plasma α-tocopherol levels between competitive athletes and controls, and the results are very contradictory. Watson and colleagues (2005) reported higher results in athletes, Guilland and colleagues (1989) reported similar results, and Karlsson and colleagues (1992) reported lower levels in athletes than in controls. Nevertheless, in this last study, the ratio between athletes' and controls' α-tocopherol concentration was precisely the same as the ratio between athletes' and controls' free cholesterol concentration in plasma. Because α-tocopherol is transported in lipoproteins together with cholesterol, dissimilar blood lipid profiles in athletes and controls might explain the difference found by Karlsson and colleagues (1992).

Biochemical indicators of mineral status 11.16

Iron 11.17

Biochemical indicators of iron status in athletes have been studied extensively and are reviewed in section 10.35.

Magnesium 11.18

The data on mineral status in athletes and controls, published between 1980 and 1994, have been pooled in an analytical review (Fogelholm 1995). The mean serum magnesium concentration in athletes (n = 516 in seven studies) was 0.84 mmol/L, and in controls (n = 251) was 0.85 mmol/L. Later studies reported that athletes had similar (Crespo et al. 1995; Nuviala et al. 1999) or even higher (Nuviala et al. 1999) serum magnesium concentration, as compared to sedentary controls. Lower (Casoni et al. 1990) or similar (Fogelholm et al. 1991) erythrocyte magnesium concentrations were found in athletes, compared with untrained controls. In a controlled intervention, a 24-week fitness-type exercise program did not affect serum or erythrocyte magnesium content in previously untrained young women (Fogelholm 1992).

Zinc 11.19

The mean serum zinc concentration, pooled from studies published between 1980 and 1994, was 13.5 μmol/L in athletes (n = 587 in 11 studies) and 13.7 μmol/L in controls (n = 244) (Fogelholm 1995). More recent studies have also found similar serum zinc levels in athletes and sedentary controls (Crespo et al. 1995; Nuviala et al. 1999). Following increased physical activity, three longitudinal studies found a negative time-trend for serum or plasma zinc (Miyamura et al. 1987; Lichton et al. 1988; Couzy et al. 1990). In contrast, serum zinc increased in competitive sailors during a 3-week transatlantic race (Fogelholm & Lahtinen 1991). Other studies have not found any associations between training volume and serum zinc concentration (Lukaski et al. 1990; Ohno et al. 1990; Fogelholm 1992; Fogelholm et al. 1992a; Dolev et al. 1995).

Data on zinc levels from other biomarkers are scarce, but the few findings are interesting. Several studies have reported a positive association between high or increased physical activity and erythrocyte zinc concentration (Ohno et al. 1990; Singh et al. 1990b; Fogelholm et al. 1991; Fogelholm 1992). Dolev and colleagues (1995) reported maintenance of zinc concentration in erythrocytes, but an increased concentration in mononuclear leucocytes, in male military recruits during an 11-week training program. The increase in erythrocyte and leukocyte zinc level might be related to increased amounts of intracellular zinc-dependent enzymes, such as superoxide dismutase.

Copper, chromium and selenium 11.20

In studies published between 1980 and 1994, the pooled mean results of plasma copper concentration tended to be higher for females and for athletes: 16.3 and 15.1 μmol/L for female athletes and controls, and 14.7 and 14.1 μmol/L for male athletes and controls, respectively (Fogelholm 1995). Similar serum copper and ceruloplasmin results for female collegiate athletes, compared with controls, were also reported more recently (Gropper et al. 2003). Data on other trace elements are even scarcer. Anderson and colleagues (1988) reported similar plasma chromium concentrations in athletes and untrained controls. A competitive sailing crew had lower serum selenium concentration than controls (Fogelholm & Lahtinen 1991). Nevertheless, even the sailing crew's results were clearly within the reference range for selenium.

In summary, the available indices of magnesium, zinc, copper, chromium and selenium do not suggest compromised status in physically active people. Because of the lack of sensitivity of these indices, this interpretation must be taken with caution.

11.21 Does marginal deficiency of vitamins and minerals affect physical performance?

Studies involving marginal deficiency of vitamins and minerals test the hypothesis that physical performance is impaired when the status of one or several micronutrients is indicative of marginal deficiency.

11.22 Vitamins

11.23 Thiamin

Earlier studies have shown that subclinical thiamin deficiency is associated with increased exercise-induced blood lactate concentrations, especially after a pre-exercise glucose load (Sauberlich 1967). The deterioration of physical capacity in marginal deficiency, however, is less evident. Despite a 5-week thiamin-depleted diet, Wood and colleagues (1980) did not find decreased working capacity in male students. E-TKAC decreased significantly, showing that the activity of this enzyme was affected faster than the activity of the enzymes of glycolysis and the citric acid cycle in working muscles.

11.24 Riboflavin

Significant changes in riboflavin supply affect both muscle metabolism and neuromuscular function. Data on the effects of marginal riboflavin supply are, however, scarce. In three studies (Belko et al. 1984, 1985; Trebler Winters et al. 1992), a 4- to 5-week marginal riboflavin intake lowered E-GRAC, but no relation between vitamin status and aerobic capacity was found. Similarly, Soares and colleagues (1993) did not find changes in muscular efficiency during moderate-intensity exercise after a 7-week period of riboflavin-restricted diet. Decreased urinary riboflavin excretion might be one mechanism to conserve riboflavin and prevent changes in riboflavin-dependent body functions during marginal depletion, which may explain the outcome of these studies.

11.25 Vitamin B6

In male wrestlers and judo athletes, a decrease in E-ASTAC indicated deteriorated vitamin B6 supply during a 3-week weight-loss regimen (Fogelholm et al. 1993a). Maximal anaerobic capacity, speed or strength was, however, not affected. Also, Coburn and colleagues (1991) showed that the muscle tissue was quite resistant to a 6-week vitamin B6 depletion.

Vitamin C 11.26

In one study (Van der Beek et al. 1990), a vitamin C-restricted diet reduced whole blood ascorbic acid concentration. Nevertheless, the marginal vitamin supply in the blood did not produce any significant effects on maximal aerobic capacity or lactate threshold in healthy volunteers. In contrast to the above study, Johnston and colleagues (1999) reported that a 3-week experimental vitamin C depletion was associated with reduced work efficiency during submaximal exercise and that work performance increased after repletion with vitamin C supplements (2 weeks, 500 mg/d).

Vitamin D 11.27

Although some studies have indicated marginal vitamin D deficiencies and intakes in athletes (Willis et al. 2008), there are no studies published that investigate the potential effects of marginal deficiency on athletic performance. Given the multiple roles of vitamin D in human metabolism, a prolonged inadequate intake and low biochemical status could increase the susceptibility for bone fracture. Another link between inadequate vitamin D status and performance could be through impaired immune function and increased susceptibility to upper respiratory tract infections (Laaksi et al. 2007). More research is needed to determine the effect (if any) of vitamin D supplementation on infection, illness and bone health in trained athletes.

Multivitamins 11.28

Finally, a combined depletion of thiamin, riboflavin, vitamin B6 and ascorbic acid has been found to affect both E-TKAC and aerobic working capacity (Van der Beek et al. 1988). Because of multiple depletion, the independent role of the single vitamins could not be demonstrated.

Minerals 11.29

Iron deficiency without anemia may have a negative impact on endurance performance (see Chapter 10). The effects of marginal status of other minerals on physical performance in healthy volunteers have been studied only rarely. Lukaski and Nielsen (2002) studied the effects of dietary magnesium restriction in postmenopausal women. In magnesium-depleted status, the energy cost during submaximal exercise was increased, compared with adequate magnesium intake. Unfortunately, there are no comparable data with athletes or physically fit young adults.

Van Loan and colleagues (1999) investigated the effects of induced zinc depletion on muscle function in eight male subjects who were fed a formula diet (<0.5 mg Zn/d for 33 or 41 days). The mean serum zinc concentration decreased from an initial 11.0 µmol/L to 3.4 µmol/L at the end of depletion. Muscle endurance (total work capacity in isokinetic exercise tests) declined, but peak force was not affected. The authors speculated that the effects observed could have been related to decreased activity of lactate dehydrogenase, a zinc-dependent enzyme, and a concomitant increase in blood lactate concentration. In a more recent study, marginal zinc deficiency, induced by a low zinc diet, lowered peak oxygen uptake and respiratory exchange ratio during a maximal exercise test in young adult men (Lukaski 2005).

11.30 Effects of supplementation on biochemical indices of micronutrient status and physical performance

It is assumed that the current recommended dietary allowances and dietary reference intakes are appropriate even for athletes (American College of Sports Medicine et al. 2000). Supplementation is warranted only if clear medical, nutritional and public health reasons are present (e.g. iron to treat iron deficiency anemia or folic acid to prevent birth defects). Although the available data suggest that micronutrient deficiencies in athletes are rare and no more common than in untrained subjects, depletion studies show that even marginal micronutrient deficiency conditions may impair physical performance. Even a small potential risk of marginal micronutrient deficiency may be a great concern for athletes and their coaches. Before making recommendations for or against micronutrient supplementation in athletes, two fundamental questions need to be reviewed:

1. Are the observed indicators of micronutrient status compatible with optimal athletic performance?
2. Would a nutrient intake beyond the daily dietary recommendations (supplementation) improve physical capacity?

11.31 Water-soluble vitamin supplementation

11.32 Thiamin

Thiamin supplementation (>7.5 mg/d) improves the activity of erythrocyte TK (Guilland et al. 1989; Fogelholm et al. 1993b). Nevertheless, despite improved indicators of thiamin status, several studies have shown that thiamin supplementation did not improve functional capacity in athletes who were not deficient (Telford et al. 1992a, 1992b; Webster 1998) or in young, moderately trained adults (Singh et al. 1992a, 1992b; Fogelholm et al. 1993b).

11.33 Riboflavin

Riboflavin supplementation improves the activity of erythrocyte GR (Weight et al. 1988b; Guilland et al. 1989; Fogelholm et al. 1993b) in athletes or trained students, even without indications of impaired vitamin status (Weight et al. 1988b). One early study suggested that supplementation and improved riboflavin status were related to improved neuromuscular function (Haralambie 1976). In contrast, later studies did not find any beneficial effects of riboflavin supplementation on maximal oxygen uptake (Weight et al. 1988a; Singh et al. 1992a, 1992b) or exercise-induced lactate appearance in the blood (Weight et al. 1988a; Fogelholm et al. 1993b).

11.34 Vitamin B6

Chronic supplementation of vitamin B6 increases the erythrocyte ASAT activity (Guilland et al. 1989; Fogelholm et al. 1993b) and plasma pyridoxal-5′-phosphate (PLP) concentration (Coburn et al. 1991) even in healthy subjects. Supplementation of vitamin B6, in combination with other B-complex vitamins, has improved shooting target performance (Bonke & Nickel 1989) in male athletes. In contrast, a number of other studies did not find any association between improved indicators of vitamin B6 status and maximal oxygen uptake (Weight et al. 1988a, 1988b), exercise-induced lactate appearance in blood (Manore & Leklem 1988; Weight et al. 1988a, 1988b; Fogelholm et al. 1993b) or other tests of physical performance (Telford et al. 1992a, 1992b; Virk et al. 1999). In fact, an increase in the biochemical indicators of vitamin B6 status is not necessarily associated with a change in intramuscular vitamin B6 content (Coburn et al. 1991).

It appears that vitamin B6, either as an infusion (Moretti et al. 1982) or given orally as a 20 mg/d supplement (Dunton et al. 1993), stimulates growth hormone production during exercise. The hypothetical mechanism behind this effect is that PLP acts as the coenzyme for dopa decarboxylase, and high concentrations might promote the conversion of L-dopa to dopamine (Manore 1994). The physiological significance of the above effect on muscle growth and strength is not known.

Folate and vitamin B12 11.35

There are only a few studies linking folic acid or vitamin B12 supply to sports-related functional capacity. Folate supplementation and increased serum folate concentration did not affect maximal oxygen uptake (Matter et al. 1987), anaerobic threshold (Matter et al. 1987) or other measures of physical performance (Telford et al. 1992a, 1992b). Together with thiamin and vitamin B6 supplementation, elevated intake of vitamin B12 was, however, associated with improved target shooting performance (Bonke & Nickel 1989).

Other B vitamins (such as thiamin and pantothenic acid) 11.36

Data on supplementation of other B vitamins and performance are even scarcer. Webster (1998) reported no effect of a combined thiamin and pantothenic acid supplementation on a 2000 m time trial by cycle ergometer.

Vitamin C 11.37

Athletes have been given vitamin C supplementation ranging from 85 to 1500 mg/d for a period from 1 day to 8 months (Peake 2003). About half of the studies reviewed by Peake (2003) showed no significant changes in plasma ascorbic acid concentration, whereas the remaining studies demonstrated significant increases. The non-responses may be explained by the fact that many athletes have a vitamin C intake that is close to the saturation of plasma concentration.

In an early review, Gerster (1989) concluded that a vast majority of studies have not shown any measurable effects of vitamin C supplementation on maximal oxygen uptake, lactate threshold or exercise-induced heart rate in well-nourished subjects. Recently, one study showed reduced levels of blood lactate concentration after a maximal exercise test after 90-day supplementation with vitamins C and E and β-carotene (Aguiló et al. 2007). However, one single study cannot be used for any recommendations.

An interesting aspect of interaction between vitamin C and physical activity is related to the proposed connection with upper respiratory tract infections (URTI). Strenuous physical activity seems to increase the risk for URTI during the first week or two after exercise (Nieman & Pedersen 1999). In a recent Cochrane analysis, Douglas and colleagues (2007) concluded that vitamin C supplementation does not affect the incidence or duration of common colds in the normal population. However, the data suggest that vitamin C supplementation could be justified as a preventive measure in people performing strenuous exercise, such as marathon or long-distance cross-country skiing. Nevertheless, the above data do not support the same effect for people taking supplementary vitamin C during moderate training. Moreover, it is not known whether the possible effect of vitamin C supplementation on the common cold in athletes undertaking strenuous exercise has any significant long-term effects on performance.

A potential mechanism for a reduced incidence of the common cold could be maintenance of neutrophil function during heavy exercise (Robson et al. 2003). However, recent studies have not confirmed that supplementation with vitamin C alone (Bryer & Goldfarb 2006; Davidson & Gleeson 2006, Nakhostin-Roohi et al. 2008) or in combination with other anti-oxidants (Mastaloudis et al. 2004; Traber 2006) has an effect on inflammatory markers, including neutrophil function.

Several recent studies have also shown that vitamin C supplementation for >2 weeks (Bryer & Goldfarb 2006; Nakhostin-Roohi et al. 2008) or a mixture of anti-oxidants, including vitamin C (Mastaloudis et al. 2004; Traber 2006; Goldfarb et al. 2007; Machefer et al. 2007), reduces indicators of exercise-induced lipid peroxidation. High doses of vitamin C (500–1500 mg/d for at least 1 week) also reduce exercise-induced increases in the levels of the stress hormone cortisol (Peake 2003). The practical significance of the above data is, however, not certain. Bryer and Goldfarb (2006) reported that vitamin C supplementation reduced post-exercise muscle soreness, but several other recent studies have not confirmed this effect (Connolly et al. 2006; Mastaloudis et al. 2006; Bloomer et al. 2007). Vitamin C might thus protect against reactive oxygen species during heavy exercise. The mechanisms are far from clear and it is not known whether vitamin C supplementation has any practical effects on muscle soreness or recovery in regularly training athletes.

A recent study by Gomez-Cabrera and colleagues (2008) presented interesting results that—if confirmed by others—could be used to warn against unnecessary vitamin C supplementation. The authors reported that vitamin C supplementation reduced endurance capacity by preventing some cellular adaptations to exercise. The adverse effects of vitamin C could result from its capacity to affect transcription factors involved in mitochondrial biogenesis. However, it is premature to draw any conclusions from this study.

11.38 Fat-soluble vitamin supplementation

There are no data on the effects of retinol, vitamin D or vitamin K supplementation on athletes' performances or other parameters. Based on several studies showing inadequate vitamin D status in female athletes, supplementation with around 10 or 20 μg vitamin D daily could be warranted at least for groups at risk of low dietary intake (Willis et al. 2008). However, further research is needed to show if this kind of a supplementation has an effect on immune function or injuries in athletes.

Many studies have shown that α-tocopherol supplementation (typical dose >100 mg/d) reduces breath pentane excretion (Simon-Schnass & Pabst 1988) and serum MDA concentration (determined as TBARs) (Simon-Schnass & Pabst 1988; Meydani et al. 1993; Rokitzki et al. 1994b) during exercise. Both breath pentane and serum MDA were used as indicators of lipid peroxidation. Unfortunately, many of these studies were poorly designed. In a critical review, Viitala and Newhouse (2004) concluded that studies with better design do not support the hypothesis that vitamin E alone attenuates lipid peroxidation during exercise. Moreover, studies have not supported the hypothesis that vitamin E attenuates exercise-induced muscle damage (Dekkers et al. 1996; Kaikkonen et al. 1998).

In one controlled trial (Simon-Schnass & Pabst 1988), vitamin E supplementation maintained aerobic working capacity at very high altitude (>5000 m). Later studies have not demonstrated that vitamin E intake exceeding daily recommendations would have any beneficial effects on athletic performance (Rokitzki et al. 1994b; Kanter & Williams 1998; Tiidus & Houston 1995; Buchman et al. 1999, Gaeini et al. 2006).

Mineral supplementation 11.39

Iron supplementation does not necessarily improve performance in athletes with low iron stores (i.e. low ferritin) (see section 10.11). However, the benefit of iron supplementation on performance in athletes with diagnosed iron deficiency anemia is well-established. Data on supplementation of minerals other than iron are scarce. Magnesium supplementation may improve performance in individuals with diagnosed magnesium deficiency (Nielsen & Lukaski 2006), but oral magnesium does not appear to have any beneficial effects in athletes with balanced magnesium status (Terblanche et al. 1992; Weller et al. 1998; Mooren et al. 2003). Similarly, in other studies (Singh et al. 1992b; Telford et al. 1992a), a supplement containing several minerals and trace elements failed to affect indicators of nutritional status and athletic performance.

Chromium supplementation, mainly as chromium picolinate, during training has been proposed to stimulate insulin function and to promote muscle growth and glycogen synthesis. In an earlier controlled trial, chromium (200 μg/d) or placebo was given to healthy, previously untrained students, during an 11-week weightlifting program (Hasten et al. 1992). Supplementation was associated with greater body-weight gain in women, but not in men. Strength was not affected. Despite this preliminary finding, more recent studies with athletes have not found any significant effects of chromium on weight, body composition, strength or glycogen synthesis (Clancy et al. 1994; Trent & Thieding-Cancel 1995; Lukaski et al. 1996; Walker et al. 1998; Volek et al. 2006). Hence, it seems that short-term (4–12 weeks) chromium supplementation with doses varying from 200 to 800 μg/d does not have any ergogenic effects in trained individuals (see also Chapter 16).

Potential risks of vitamin and mineral supplements 11.40

Risks related to high intake of water-soluble vitamins 11.41

Although the scientific data do not support the hypothesis that high vitamin and mineral intake enhance performance in well-nourished athletes, the use of supplements is very common (Erdman et al. 2007; Tsitsimpikou et al. 2009). Many athletes use supplements as a precaution,'just in case'. Nevertheless, very high, chronic intake of one or several micronutrients may involve risks. Therefore any precautionary use of supplements should remain within the safe recommended intake.

Thiamin, riboflavin and B6 11.42

Adverse reactions to chronic, elevated oral administration of thiamin are virtually unknown (Marks 1989; Meltzer et al. 2003). For chronic oral use, it is still safe at least 50–100 times the recommended daily intake: that is, above 100 mg daily. Riboflavin in large doses may cause a yellow discoloration of the urine, which might cause concern in people not aware of the source of the color (Alhadeff et al. 1984). However, there is no evidence of any harmful effects even with oral riboflavin doses exceeding 100 times the recommended daily intake (Marks 1989; Meltzer et al. 2003). In contrast to thiamin and riboflavin, megadoses of vitamin B6 may have toxic and possibly permanent effects. The most common disorder is sensory neuropathy (Bässler 1989). Long-term supplementation should not exceed 200 mg/d: that is, 100 times the recommended allowance (Marks 1989; Meltzer et al. 2003).

11.43 Folate and B12

The effects of high doses of folate have not been widely studied, but some results indicate a possible interference with zinc metabolism (Marks 1989; Reynolds 1994). The current estimate of the safety dose is between 50 and 100 times the daily recommended intake (Marks 1989). The safety margin for vitamin B12 appears to be much larger, because even doses as high as 30 mg/d (10 000 times the recommended intake) have been used without noticeable toxic effects (Marks 1989). However, a Nordic group recommended limiting vitamin B12 intake to levels corresponding to no more than 100 times the recommended level (Meltzer et al. 2003).

11.44 Other B vitamins (e.g. nicotinic acid, biotin and pantothenic acid)

Acute oral intake of at least 100 mg of nicotinic acid per day (at least five times the recommended daily allowance) causes vasodilatation and flushing, which is a rather harmless effect (Marks 1989). The safe chronic dose appears to be at least 50 times the recommended allowance or 1 g/d. There are no reported toxic effects of biotin and pantothenic acid intake up to 100 times the recommended allowance (Alhadeff et al. 1984; Marks 1989).

11.45 Vitamin C

Very high (>1 g/d), chronic doses of vitamin C may lead to the formation of oxalate stones, increased uric acid excretion, diarrhea, vitamin B12 destruction and iron overload (Alhadeff et al. 1984). However, excluding diarrhea, the risk for the above toxic effects is likely to be very low in healthy individuals, even with intake of several grams daily (Rivers 1989; Meltzer et al. 2003).

11.46 Risks related to high intake of fat-soluble vitamins

11.47 Vitamin A

Chronic toxic intake of pre-formed retinol (vitamin A) will cause joint or bone pain, hair loss, anorexia and liver damage. The safety level for chronic use is estimated to be 10 times the recommended allowance: that is, 10 g retinol daily (Marks 1989). Because of an increased risk of spontaneous abortion and birth defects, the safe level during pregnancy may be only 4 to 5 times the daily recommendation. β-carotene, a water-soluble form of vitamin A, in contrast to pre-formed retinol, is not toxic. This provitamin is stored under the skin and is converted to active retinol only when needed.

11.48 Vitamin D and vitamin E

Vitamin D is potentially toxic, causing hypercalcemia, hypercalciuria, soft-tissue calcification, anorexia and constipation, and eventually irreversible renal and cardiovascular damage

(Davies 1989). Intakes of 10 times the recommendation (75 μg/d) are safe, but the tolerable upper intake level may be at least 250 μg/d (Vieth 2007). High calcium intakes may enhance the toxicity of vitamin D. Vitamin E, in contrast to vitamins A and D, is apparently not toxic for healthy individuals (Machlin 1989). The safety factor for long-term administration is at least 100 times the recommended daily intake: that is, at least 1 g/d in oral use.

Risks related to high intake of minerals 11.49

The body pool of macrominerals, and especially of trace elements, is under strong homeostatic control. Therefore toxicity by dietary means or supplements is rare. If, however, toxic symptoms appear, they are severe and can even be fatal. Intakes needed for toxic effects are, luckily, extremely high. For instance, the first toxic symptoms (vomiting, diarrhea) of zinc overload are seen after a huge intake of at least 4 g (normal dietary intake is 10–15 mg/d). Extremely high intakes of copper can lead to liver cirrhosis or hepatic necrosis, and too much selenium causes changes in skin and hair, and neurological abnormalities. The threshold between the daily allowance and toxicity level of selenium is relatively small.

Although severe toxicity is very rare, high mineral intake may interfere with nutrient absorption at the intestinal mucosa (O'Dell 1985). Chronic zinc intake of 50 mg/d decreases both iron and copper bioavailability. Analogously, high intake of either iron or copper interferes with zinc absorption. Therefore, a surplus of one trace element may cause marginal deficiency of another trace element, especially when the intake of the latter is marginal. Because intestinal interactions are observed with rather low dosages, precautionary use of mineral supplements (not specifically to treat a diagnosed deficiency) that does not exceed five times the Recommended Dietary Intake (RDI)/Recommended Dietary Allowance (RDA) is warranted (Meltzer et al. 2003).

Summary 11.50

The daily requirement of at least some vitamins and minerals is increased beyond normal levels in highly physically active people. The potential reasons for this increased requirement are excretion through sweating and urine, and perhaps feces, and through increased free radical production. Unfortunately, it is not possible to quantify the micronutrient requirements of athletes. Measures on micronutrient status and supplementation trials are needed to evaluate whether or not normal dietary intakes in athletes are sufficient to cover the increased requirements.

Most studies have not revealed any significant differences between athletes' and controls' indices of micronutrient status. The results suggest that athletic training, of itself, does not lead to micronutrient deficiency. These data should, however, be interpreted very carefully. Because of the insensitivity of most indices to marginal deficiency, the results do not exclude the possibility of minor differences between the athletes and controls. In addition, the data do not exclude the possibility that some individual athletes (and controls) have inadequate status.

Physical performance can be affected even when micronutrient deficiency is only marginal. In depletion experiments, changes in one or more biochemical indices of micronutrient status were seen before or together with impairments in physical work capacity. Despite the associations between indices of micronutrient status and performance in depletion studies, the rationality of routine laboratory assessment of water-soluble vitamin, magnesium or trace element (excluding iron) status in athletes seems doubtful. Because the prevalence of even marginal deficiency is low, routine assessment would lead to numerous false-positive diagnoses.

Supplementation of water-soluble vitamins is associated with improved corresponding indicators in the blood. Moreover, supplementation of vitamin C may decrease the incidence of URTIs and attenuate stress response induced after very strenuous physical exercise. However, studies do not conclusively show that micronutrient supplementation would increase physical performance. Consequently, the levels of indicators of vitamin and mineral status seen in athletes are apparently compatible with optimal physical functions.

The evidence for benefits of vitamin and mineral supplements on athletic performance is extremely limited. In addition, high intake of single micronutrients may lead to physiological disturbances, especially if the diet is inadequate. Hence, an athlete should try to ensure adequate vitamin and mineral status mainly by a well-balanced diet. If, for any reason, an athlete wants to use micronutrient supplements as a precaution, a multivitamin–mineral supplement with amounts not exceeding two times the RDA is likely to be both safe and adequate for optimal sports performance.

PRACTICE TIPS

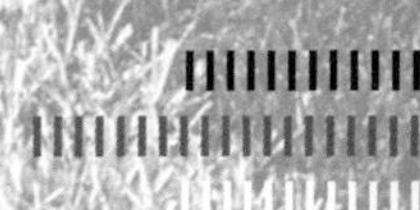

TRENT WATSON

DIETARY ASSESSMENT

- Population reference standards (NRV/DRI) for vitamins, minerals and anti-oxidants (micronutrients) are appropriate for use in athletes, because of a wide safety margin. However, some caution is needed for iron and calcium, where the requirements for athletes can be increased by special circumstances (see Chapters 9 and 10).
- Athletes who consume a variety of nutrient-rich foods and meet their energy requirements usually meet or exceed population reference levels (such as RDI/RDA) for most micronutrients. Those athletes who habitually restrict energy intake or have a limited variety of foods may be at risk of suboptimal micronutrient intakes.
- Determining the micronutrient status of an individual athlete is complex and involves a combination of dietary assessment, clinical history and biochemical and hematological measurements. Biochemical measures of micronutrient status do not necessarily reflect nutritional status and can be unreliable (see Chapters 2, 10 and 11). Food frequency questionnaires (FFQs) have multiple applications (see Chapter 2), including as a screening tool for checking nutrient or food intakes, and can also assist in educating athletes about food choice. FFQs targeting micronutrient intakes (e.g. β-carotene and retinol) (Ambrosini et al. 2001) or intakes of fruit and vegetables (Amanatidis et al. 2001) have been developed and validated for use in Australia and could be modified for use in athletes living in Australia or for athletes with similar food choices in other countries. The use of computer dietary analysis software can provide immediate objective evaluation of individual dietary intakes that can be used to determine micronutrient intakes, counsel an athlete and correct any deficiencies.

DIETARY STRATEGIES TO IMPROVE MICRONUTRIENT INTAKES

- Athletes' busy training schedules are often juggled with work, school and other family commitments, which can lead to missing meals or eating on the run and eating less than optimal energy and nutrient intakes. Therefore, it is not uncommon that the dietary intake that an athlete reports, and what they actually consume, differs. Most athletes accept that they need to physically train 'consistently' to achieve good results. Dietitians need to deliver strong messages and put it high on the agenda that 'athletes who require themselves to physically perform at consistently optimal levels need to consistently provide optimal fuel (nutrition) for this performance'.
- Creative menu planning assists athletes to broaden their food choices, which is particularly helpful for fussy eaters or those with limited food knowledge or imagination. For example, fortified soy products provide a calcium exchange for dairy products; berries and tropical fruits might provide a more inviting alternative for athletes who dislike fruit. For athletes who dislike vegetables, adding them to pizza, blended soups, casseroles and stir-fries or using vegetable juices are often acceptable substitutes.

PRACTICE TIPS

- Many athletes do not easily translate nutrient needs into food choices and are swayed by advertisements for vitamin and mineral supplements that claim our food is unable to supply us with our dietary requirements. The use of dietary analysis software at the time of consultation is visually effective as an intervention tool to identify micronutrient intakes and highlight food sources of micronutrients. Remind athletes that the combination of anti-oxidants and other phytochemicals found in food can provide greater benefits than isolated nutrients found in a supplement.

MICRONUTRIENT SUPPLEMENTATION: ADVANTAGES AND DISADVANTAGES

- Evaluate an athlete's supplementary practices at the initial interview. If an athlete takes micronutrient supplements, determine their beliefs, attitudes and reasons for the use.
- A supplement may be warranted where habitual dietary intake of micronutrients is unsatisfactory. For a multivitamin/mineral supplement (<2–3 times the RDI/RDA), a low dosage is recommended. Where a single micronutrient deficiency is diagnosed, a higher dosage supplement may be necessary for rapid recovery in the short term (e.g. a zinc or iron supplement); however, steps should also be taken to improve and maintain dietary intake to help prevent a relapse and avoid any potentially adverse effects of long-term supplement use.
- Even if advised not to continue with a supplement and the reasons for taking the supplement were unsubstantiated, an athlete may still take the supplement and possibly misuse it. It is important that the athlete is made aware of any potential disadvantages of this action, including cost, safety, poor quality control and risk of the product containing a banned substance.
- To date, there is some evidence to suggest that the consumption of additional vitamin, mineral and anti-oxidants above the known requirements of an athlete has protective effects against exercise-induced tissue damage; however, this has not translated into improved performance. It appears that these requirements can be best met via dietary intake. Thus the most prudent recommendation regarding optimal vitamin, mineral and anti-oxidant intakes for athletes should be to consume a diet containing a wide variety of nutrient-rich foods. Structured outlines of what to include in a training lunchbox (e.g. provide minimal requirements for each core food group), similar to the structured outlines for physical training sessions, work well. Guidelines for shopping, preparation of quick, easy meals and suitable snack ideas, and assistance with time management, ensure that an athlete's good eating habits are not disregarded in preference to training or other commitments.
- To remain abreast of current and increased availability of vitamin, mineral and anti-oxidant supplements on the market, it is worthwhile to meet regularly with sales representatives to obtain samples and to attend information sessions on supplements. However, be aware that your interest and attendance may be misinterpreted by multi-level marketing companies as a sign of endorsement of their product.

References

Aggett P. Scientific considerations in the formulation of RDI. Eur J Clin Nutr 1990;44:37–43.

Aguiló A, Tauler P, Sureda A, Cases N, Tur J, Pons A. Antioxidant diet supplementation enhances aerobic performance in amateur sportsmen. J Sports Sci. 2007;25:1203–10.

Alessio HM. Exercise-induced oxidative stress. Med Sci Sports Exerc 1993;25:218–24.

Alhadeff L, Gualtieri T, Lipton M. Toxic effects of water-soluble vitamins. Nutr Rev 1984;42:33–40.

Amanatidis S, Mackerras D, Simpson JM. Comparison of two food frequency questionnaires for quantifying fruit and vegetable intake. Pub Health Nutr 2001;4:233–9.

Ambrosini GL, de Klerk NH, Musk AW, Mackerras D. Agreement between a brief food frequency questionnaire and diet records using two statistical methods. Pub Health Nut 2001;4:255–64.

American College of Sports Medicine, American Dietetic Association, and Dieticians of Canada. Joint position statement: nutrition and athletic performance. Med Sci Sports Exerc 2000;32:2130–45.

Anderson RA, Bryden NA, Polansky MM, Deuster PA. Exercise effects on chromium excretion of trained and untrained men consuming a constant diet. J Appl Physiol 1988;64:249–52.

Aruoma OI, Reilly T, MacLaren D, Halliwell B. Iron, copper and zinc concentrations in human sweat and plasma: the effects of exercise. Clin Chem Acta 1988;177:81–8.

Bässler KH. Use and abuse of high dosages of vitamin B6. In: Walter P, Stähelin H, Brubacher G, eds. Elevated dosages of vitamins. Stuttgart: Hans Huber Publishers, 1989:120–6.

Bayomi RA, Rosalki SB. Evaluation of methods of coenzyme activation of erythrocyte enzymes for detection of deficiency of vitamins B1, B2, and B6. Clin Chem 1976;22:327–35.

Belko AZ, Meredith MP, Kalkwarf HJ, et al. Effects of exercise on riboflavin requirements: biological validation in weight reducing women. Am J Clin Nutr 1985;41:270–7.

Belko AZ, Obarzanec E, Roach R, et al. Effects of aerobic exercise and weight loss on riboflavin requirements of moderately obese, marginally deficient young women. Am J Clin Nutr 1984;40:553–61.

Beller GA, Maher JT, Hartley LH, Bass DE, Wacker WEC. Changes in serum and sweat magnesium levels during work in the heat. Aviat Space Environm Med 1975;46:709–12.

Bloomer RJ, Falvo MJ, Schilling BK, Smith WA. Prior exercise and antioxidant supplementation: effect on oxidative stress and muscle injury. J Int Soc Sports Nutr 2007;3:4–9.

Bonke D, Nickel B. Improvement of fine motoric movement control by elevated dosages of vitamin B1, B6, and B12 in target shooting. In: Walter P, Stähelin H, Brubacher G, eds. Elevated dosages of vitamins. Stuttgart: Hans Huber Publishers, 1989:198–204.

Brotherhood JR. Nutrition and sports performance. Sports Med 1984;1:350–89.

Brubacher GB. Scientific basis for the estimation of the daily requirements for vitamins. In: Walter P, Stähelin H, Brubacher G, eds. Elevated dosages of vitamins. Stuttgart: Hans Huber Publishers, 1989:3–11.

Bryer SC, Goldfarb AH. Effect of high dose vitamin C supplementation on muscle soreness, damage, function, and oxidative stress to eccentric exercise. Int J Sport Nutr Exerc Metab. 2006;16:270–80.

Buchman AL, Killip D, Ou CN, et al. Short-term vitamin E supplementation before marathon running: a placebo-controlled trial. Nutrition 1999;15:278–83.

Casoni I, Guglielmini C, Graziano L, et al. Changes of magnesium concentrations in endurance athletes. Int J Sports Med 1990;11:234–7.

Caster WO, Mickelsen O. Effect of diet and stress on the thiamin and pyramin excretion of normal young men maintained on controlled intakes of thiamin. Nutr Res 1991;11:549–58.

Clancy SP, Clarkson PM, DeCheke ME, et al. Effects of chromium picolinate supplementation on body composition, strength, and urinary chromium loss in football players. Int J Sport Nutr 1994;42:142–53.

Coburn SP, Ziegler PJ, Costill DL, et al. Response of vitamin B6 content of muscle to changes in vitamin B6 intake in men. Am J Clin Nutr 1991;53:1436–42.

Connolly DA, Lauzon C, Agnew J, Dunn M, Reed B. The effects of vitamin C supplementation on symptoms of delayed onset muscle soreness. J Sports Med Phys Fitness. 2006;46:462–7.

Costill DL, Cote R, Fink WJ. Dietary potassium and heavy exercise: effects on muscle water and electrolytes. Am J Clin Nutr 1982;36:266–75.

Costill DL, Cote R, Fink W. Muscle water and electrolytes following varied levels of dehydration in man. J Appl Physiol 1976;40:6–11.

Couzy F, Lafargue P, Guezennec CY. Zinc metabolism in the athlete: influence of training, nutrition and other factors. Int J Sports Med 1990;11:263–6.

Crespo R, Releca P, Lozano D, et al. Biochemical markers of nutrition in elite-marathon runners. J Sports Med Phys Fitness 1995;35:268–72.

Crozier PG, Cordain L, Sampson DA. Exercise-induced changes in plasma vitamin B-6 concentration do not vary with exercise intensity. Am J Clin Nutr 1994;60:552–8.

Davies M. High-dose vitamin D therapy: indications, benefits and hazards. In: Walter P, Stähelin H, Brubacher G, eds. Elevated dosages of vitamins. Stuttgart: Hans Huber Publishers, 1989:81–6.

Davison G, Gleeson M. The effect of 2 weeks vitamin C supplementation on immunoendocrine responses to 2.5 h cycling exercise in man. Eur J Appl Physiol 2006;97:454–61.

Dekkers JC, Van Doornen JP, Kemper HCG. The role of antioxidant vitamins and enzymes in the prevention of exercise-induced muscle damage. Sports Med 1996;21:213–38.

DeRuisseau KC, Chauvront SN, Haymes EM, Sharp RG. Sweat iron and zinc losses during prolonged exercise. Int J Sport Nutr Exerc Metab 2002;12:428–37.

Deuster PA, Dolev E, Kyle SB, Anderson RA, Schoomaker EB. Magnesium homeostasis during high-intensity aerobic exercise in men. J Appl Physiol 1987;62:545–50.

Deuster PA, Day BA, Singh A, Douglass L, Moser-Veillon PB. Zinc status of highly trained women runners and untrained women. Am J Clin Nutr 1989;49:1295–301.

Dolev E, Burstein R, Lubin F, et al. Interpretation of zinc status indicators in a strenuously exercising population. J Am Diet Assoc 1995;95:482–4.

Douglas RM, Hemilä H, Chalker E, Treacy B 2007. Vitamin C for preventing and treating the common cold. Cochrane Database of Systematic Reviews. Issue 18. Article No. CD000980.

Dressendorfer RH, Petersen SR, Lovshin SEM, Keen CL. Mineral metabolism in male cyclists during high-intensity endurance training. Int J Sports Nutr Exerc Metab 2002;12:63–72.

Dunton N, Virk R, Young J, Leklem J. The influence of vitamin B6 supplementation and exercise on vitamin B6 metabolism and growth hormone. FASEB Journal 1993;7:A727.

Erdman KA, Fung TS, Doyle-Baker PK, Verhoef MJ, Reimer RA. Dietary supplementation of high-performance Canadian athletes by age and gender. Clin J Sport Med 2007;17:458–64.

Fishbaine B, Butterfield G. Ascorbic acid status of running and sedentary men. Int J Vit Nutr Res 1984;54:273.

Fogelholm M. Micronutrient status in females during a 24-week fitness-type exercise program. Ann Nutr Metab 1992;36:209–18.

Fogelholm M. Indicators of vitamin and mineral status in athletes' blood: a review. Int J Sport Nutr 1995;5:267–86.

Fogelholm M, Laakso J, Lehto J, Ruokonen I. Dietary intake and indicators of magnesium and zinc status in male athletes. Nutr Res 1991a;11:1111–18.

Fogelholm M, Lahtinen P. Nutritional evaluation of a sailing crew during a transatlantic race. Scand J Med Sci Sports 1991b;1:99–103.

Fogelholm M, Himberg J-J, Alopaeus K, et al. Dietary and biochemical indices of nutritional status in male athletes and controls. J Am Coll Nutr 1992a;11:181–91.

Fogelholm M, Rehunen S, Gref CG, et al. Dietary intake and thiamin, iron and zinc status in elite Nordic skiers during different training periods. Int J Sport Nutr 1992b;2:351–65.

Fogelholm M, Koskinen R, Laakso J, Rankinen T, Ruokonen I. Gradual and rapid weight loss: effects on nutrition and performance in male athletes. Med Sci Sports Exerc 1993a;25:371–7.

Fogelholm M, Ruokonen I, Laakso J, Vuorimaa T, Himberg J-J. Lack of association between indices of vitamin B1, B2, and B6 status and exercise-induced blood lactate in young adults. Int J Sport Nutr 1993b;3:165–76.

Gaeini AA, Rahnama N, Hamedinia MR. Effects of vitamin E supplementation on oxidative stress at rest and after exercise to exhaustion in athletic students. J Sports Med Phys Fitness. 2006;46:458–61.

Gerster H. The role of vitamin C in athletic performance. J Am Coll Nutr 1989;8:636–43.

Goldfarb AH, McKenzie MJ, Bloomer RJ. Gender comparisons of exercise-induced oxidative stress: influence of antioxidant supplementation. Appl Physiol Nutr Metab. 2007;32:1124–31.

Gomez-Cabrera MC, Domenech E, Romagnoli M, Arduini A, Borras C, Pallardo FV, Sastre J, Vina J. Oral administration of vitamin C decreases muscle mitochondrial biogenesis and hampers training-induced adaptations in endurance performance. Am J Clin Nutr 2008;87:142–9.

Gropper SS, Sorrels LM, Blessing D. Copper status of collegiate female athletes involved in different sports. Int J Sports Nutr Exerc Metab 2003;13:343–57.

Guilland J-C, Penaranda T, Gallet C, et al. Vitamin status of young athletes including the effects of supplementation. Med Sci Sports Exerc 1989;21:441–4.

Gutteridge JMC, Rowley DA, Halliwell B, Cooper DF, Heeley DM. Copper and iron complexes catalytic for oxygen radical reactions in sweat from human athletes. Clin Chem Acta 1985;145:267–74.

Haralambie G. Vitamin B2 status in athletes and the influence of riboflavin administration on neuromuscular irritability. Nutr Metab 1976;20:1–8.

Hasten DL, Rome EP, Franks BD, Hegstedt M. Effects of chromium picolinate on beginning weight training students. Int J Sport Nutr 1992;2:343–50.

Jacob RA, Burri BJ. Oxidative damage and defence. Am J Clin Nutr 1996;63(Suppl):985S–90S.

Johnston CS, Swan PD, Corte C. Substrate utilization and work efficiency during submaximal exercise in vitamin C depleted-repleted adults. Int J Vitam Nutr Res 1999;69:41–4.

Kaikkonen J, Kosonen L, Nyyssönen K, et al. Effect of combined coenzyme Q10 and d-alpha-tocopheryl acetate supplementation on exercise-induced lipid peroxidation and muscular damage: a placebo-controlled double-blind study in marathon runners. Free Radic Res 1998;29:85–92.

Kanter M. Free radicals, exercise and antioxidant supplementation. Proceedings of the Nutrition Society 1998;57:9–13.

Kanter MM, Williams MH. Antioxidants, carnitine, and choline as putative ergogenic aids. Int J Sport Nutr 1998;5:S120–31.

Karlsson J, Diamant B, Edlund PO, et al. Plasma ubiquinone, alpha-tocopherol and cholesterol in man. Int J Vit Nutr Res 1992;62:160–4.

Keith RE, Alt LA. Riboflavin status of female athletes consuming normal diets. Nutr Res 1991;11:727–34.

Kitamura Y, Tanaka K, Kiyohara C, et al. Relationship of alcohol use, physical activity and dietary habits with serum carotenoids, retinol and alpha-tocopherol among male Japanese smokers. Int J Epidemiol 1997;26:307–14.

Koury JC, de Oliveira Jr AV, Portella ES, et al. Zinc and copper biochemical indices of antioxidant status in elite athletes of different modalities. Int J Sports Nutr Exerc Metab 2004;14:358–72.

Laaksi I, Ruohola JP, Tuohimaa P, Auvinen A, Haataja R, Pihlajamäki H, Ylikomi T. An association of serum vitamin D concentrations <40 nmol/L with acute respiratory tract infection in young Finnish men. Am J Clin Nutr 2007;86:714–7.

Laaksonen R, Fogelholm M, Himberg JJ, Laakso J, Salorinne Y. Ubiquinone supplementation and exercise capacity in trained young and older men. Eur J Appl Physiol 1995;72:95–100.

Leaf DA, Kleinman MT, Hamilton M, Barstow TJ. The effect of exercise intensity on lipid peroxidation. Med Sci Sports Exerc 1997;29:1036–9.

Leonard SW, Leklem JE. Plasma B-6 vitamin changes following a 50-km ultramarathon. Int J Sports Nutr Exerc Metab 2000;10:302–14.

Lichton IJ, Miyamura JB, McNutt SW. Nutritional evaluation of soldiers subsisting on meal, ready-to-eat operational rations for an extended period: body measurements, hydration, and blood nutrients. Am J Clin Nutr 1988;48:30–7.

Lovell G. Vitamin D status of females in an elite gymnastics program. Clin J Sport Med. 2008;18:159–61.

Lukaski HC. Low dietary zinc decreases erythrocyte carbonic anhydrase activities and impairs cardiorespiratory function in men during exercise. Am J Clin Nutr. 2005;81:1045–51.

Lukaski HC, Bolonchuk WW, Siders WA, Milne DB. Chromium supplementation and resistance training: effects on body composition, strength, and trace element status of men. Am J Clin Nutr 1996;63:954–65.

Lukaski HC, Hoverson BS, Gallagher SK, Bolonchuk WW. Physical training and copper, iron, and zinc status of swimmers. Am J Clin Nutr 1990;51:1093–9.

Lukaski HC, Nielsen FH. Dietary magnesium depletion affects metabolic responses during submaximal exercise in postmenopausal women. J Nutr 2002;132:930–5.

Machefer G, Groussard C, Vincent S, Zouhal H, Faure H, Cillard J, Radák Z, Gratas-Delamarche A. Multivitamin-mineral supplementation prevents lipid peroxidation during 'the Marathon des Sables'. J Am Coll Nutr 2007;26:111–20.

Machlin LJ. Use and safety of elevated dosages of vitamin E in adults. In: Walter P, Stähelin H, Brubacher G, eds. Elevated dosages of vitamins. Stuttgart: Hans Huber Publishers, 1989:56–68.

Manore M, Leklem JE. Effects of carbohydrate and vitamin B6 on fuel substrates during exercise in women. Med Sci Sports Exerc 1988;20:233–41.

Manore M. Vitamin B6 and exercise. Int J Sport Nutr 1994;4:89–103.

Margaritis I, Tessier F, Richard M-J, Marconnet P. No evidence of oxidative stress after a triathlon race in highly trained competitors. Int J Sports Med 1997;18:186–90.

Marks J. The safety of the vitamins: an overview. In: Walter P, Stähelin H, Brubacher G, eds. Elevated dosages of vitamins. Stuttgart: Hans Huber Publishers, 1989:12–20.

Mastaloudis A, Morrow JD, Hopkins DW, Devaraj S, Traber MG. Antioxidant supplementation prevents exercise-induced lipid peroxidation, but not inflammation, in ultramarathon runners. Free Radic Biol Med 2004;36:1329–41.

Mastaloudis A, Traber MG, Carstensen K, Widrick JJ. Antioxidants did not prevent muscle damage in response to an ultramarathon run. Med Sci Sports Exerc 2006;38:72–80.

Matter M, Stittfall T, Graves J, et al. The effect of iron and folate therapy on maximal exercise performance in female marathon runners with iron and folate deficiency. Clin Sci 1987;72:415–22.

McBride JF, Kraemer WJ, Triplett-McBride T, Sebastianelli W. Effect of resistance exercise on free radical production. Med Sci Sports Exerc 1998;30:67–72.

Meltzer HM, Aro A, Andersen NL, et al. Risk analysis applied to food fortification. Publ Health Nutr 2003;6:281–90.

Mena P, Maynar M, Gutierrez JM, et al. Erythrocyte free radical scavenger enzymes in bicycle professional racers: adaptation to training. Int J Sports Med 1991;12:563–6.

Meydani M, Evans WJ, Handelman G, et al. Protective effect of vitamin E on exercise-induced oxidative damage in young and older adults. Am J Physiol 1993;25:218–24.

Miyamura JB, McNutt SW, Lichton IJ, Wenkam NS. Altered zinc status of soldiers under field conditions. J Am Diet Assoc 1987;87:595–7.

Montain SJ, Cheuvront SN, Lukaski HC. Sweat mineral-element responses during 7 h of exercise-heat stress. Int J Sports Nutr Exerc Med 2007;17:574–82.

Mooren FC, Golf SW, Völker K. Effect of magnesium on granulocyte function and on the exercise induced inflammatory response. Magnes Res 2003;16:49–58.

Moretti C, Fabbri A, Gnessi L, et al. Pyridoxine (B6) suppresses the rise in prolactin and increases the rise in growth hormone induced by exercise. N Engl J Med 1982;307:444–5.

Nakhostin-Roohi B, Babaei P, Rahmani-Nia F, Bohlooli S. Effect of vitamin C supplementation on lipid peroxidation, muscle damage and inflammation after 30-min exercise at 75% VO_{2max}. J Sports Med Phys Fitness 2008;48:217–24.

National Health and Medical Research Council (NHMRC), Department of Health and Ageing & Ministry of Health. Nutrient reference values for Australia and New Zealand: executive summary. Canberra: NHMRC, 2006.

Nielsen FH, Lukaski HC. Update on the relationship between magnesium and exercise. Magnes Res 2006;19:180–9.

Nieman DC, Pedersen BK. Exercise and immune function: recent developments. Sports Med 1999; 27:73–80.

Nuviala RJ, Lapieza MG, Bernal E. Magnesium, zinc, and copper status in women involved in different sports. Int J Sport Nutr 1999;9:295–309.

O'Dell BL. Bioavailability of and interactions among trace elements. In: Chandra RK, ed. Trace elements in nutrition of children. New York: Nestlé Nutrition Vevey/Raven Press, 1985:41–59.

Ohno H, Sato Y, Ishikawa M, et al. Training effects on blood zinc levels in humans. J Sports Med Phys Fitness 1990;30:247–53.

Peake JM. Vitamin C: effects of exercise and requirements with training. Int J Sports Nutr Exerc Metab 2003;13:125–51.

Reynolds RD. Vitamin supplements: current controversies. J Am Coll Nutr 1994;13:118–26.

Rivers JM. Safety of high-level vitamin C ingestion. In: Walter P, Stähelin H, Brubacher G, eds. Elevated dosages of vitamins. Stuttgart: Hans Huber Publishers, 1989:95–102.

Robson PJ, Bouic JD, Myburgh KH. Antioxidant supplementation enhances neutrophil oxidative burst in trained runners following prolonged exercise. Int J Sports Nutr Exerc Metab 2003;13:369–81.

Rokitzki L, Hinkel S, Klemp C, Cufi D, Keul J. Dietary, serum and urine ascorbic acid status in male athletes. Int J Sports Med 1994a;5:435–40.

Rokitzki L, Logemann E, Huber G, Keck E, Keul J. α-tocopherol supplementation in racing cyclists during extreme endurance training. Int J Sports Nutr 1994b;4:253–64.

Sauberlich HE. Biochemical alterations in thiamin deficiency—their interpretation. Am J Clin Nutr 1967;20:528–42.

Sauberlich HE, Herman YF, Stevens CO, Herman RH. Thiamin requirement of the adult human. Am J Clin Nutr 1979;32:2237–48.

Sen CK. Oxidants and antioxidants in exercise. J Appl Physiol 1995;79:675–86.

Simon-Schnass I, Pabst H. Influence of vitamin E on physical performance. Int J Vit Nutr Res 1988;58:49–54.

Singh A, Deuster PA, Day BA, Moser-Veillon PB. Dietary intakes and biochemical markers of selected minerals: comparison of highly trained runners and untrained women. J Am Coll Nutr 1990a;9:65–75.

Singh A, Deuster PA, Moser PB. Zinc and copper status of women by physical activity and menstrual status. J Sports Med Phys Fitness 1990b;30:29–36.

Singh A, Moses FM, Deuster PA. Chronic multivitamin-mineral supplementation does not enhance physical performance. Med Sci Sports Exerc 1992a;24:726–32.

Singh A, Moses FM, Deuster PA. Vitamin and mineral status in physically active men: effects of high-potency supplement. Am J Clin Nutr 1992b;55:1–7.

Sjödin B, Hellsten Westing Y, Apple FS. Biochemical mechanisms for oxygen free radical formation during exercise. Sports Med 1990;10:236–54.

Soares MJ, Satyanarayana K, Bamji MS, et al. The effects of exercise on the riboflavin status of adult men. Br J Nutr 1993;69:541–51.

Solomons NW, Allen LH. The functional assessment of nutritional status: principles, practise and potential. Nutr Rev 1983;41:33–50.

Takatsuka N, Kawakami N, Ohwaki A, et al. Frequent hard physical activity lowered serum beta-carotene level in a population study of a rural city of Japan. Tohoku J Exp Med 1995;176:131–5.

Telford RD, Catchpole EA, Deakin V, Hahn AG, Plank AW. The effects of 7 to 8 months of vitamin/mineral supplementation on the vitamin and mineral status of athletes. Int J Sport Nutr 1992a;2:123–34.

Telford RD, Catchpole EA, Deakin V, Hahn AG, Plank AW. The effects of 7 to 8 months of vitamin/mineral supplementation on athletic performance. Int J Sport Nutr 1992b;2:35–53.

Terblanche S, Noakes TD, Dennis SC, Marais DW, Eckert M. Failure of magnesium supplementation to influence marathon running performance or recovery in magnesium-replete subjects. Int J Sport Nutr 1992;2:154–64.

Thomas TR, Ziogas G, Yan P, Schmitz D, LaFontaine T. Influence of activity level on vitamin E status in healthy men and women and cardiac patients. J Cardiopulm Rehabil 1998;18:52–9.

Tiidus PM, Houston ME. Vitamin E status and response to exercise training. Sports Med 1995;20:12–23.

Tiidus PM, Pushkarenko J, Houston ME. Lack of antioxidant adaptation to short-term aerobic training in human muscle. Am J Physiol 1996;271:R832–6.

Traber MG. Relationship of vitamin E metabolism and oxidation in exercising human subjects. Br J Nutr 2006;96(Suppl):34S–7S.

Trebler Winters LR, Yoon J-S, Kalkwarf HJ, et al. Riboflavin requirements and exercise adaptation in older women. Am J Clin Nutr 1992;56:526–32.

Trent LK, Thieding-Cancel D. Effects of chromium picolinate on body composition. J Sports Med Phys Fitness 1995;35:273–80.

Tsitsimpikou C, Tsiokanos A, Tsarouhas K, Schamasch P, Fitch KD, Valasiadis D, Jamurtas A. Medication use by athletes at the Athens 2004 Summer Olympic Games. Clin J Sport Med 2009;19:33–8.

Tur-Mari J, Sureda A, Pons A. Blood cells as functional markers of antioxidant vitamin status. Br J Nutr 2006;96(Suppl):38S–41S.

Van der Beek EJ. Vitamin supplementation and physical exercise performance. J Sports Sci 1991;9:77–89.

Van der Beek EJ, Van Dokkum W, Schrijver J, et al. Thiamin, riboflavin, and vitamins B6 and C: impact of combined restricted intake on functional performance in man. Am J Clin Nutr 1988;48:1451–62.

Van der Beek EJ, Van Dokkum W, Schriver J, et al. Controlled vitamin C restriction and physical performance in volunteers. J Am Coll Nutr 1990;9:332–9.

Van Loan MD, Sutherland B, Lowe NM, Turnlund JR, King JC. The effects of zinc depletion on peak force and total work of knee and shoulder extensor and flexor muscles. Int J Sport Nutr 1999;9:125–35.

Verde T, Shephard RJ, Corey P, Moore R. Sweat composition in exercise and in heat. J Appl Physiol 1982;53:1540–5.

Vieth R. Vitamin D toxicity, policy and science. J Bone Miner Res 2007;22(2 Suppl):V64–8.

Viitala P, Newhouse IJ. Vitamin E supplementation, exercise and lipid peroxidation in human participants. Eur J Appl Physiol 2004;93:108–15.

Virk RS, Dunton NJ, Young JC, Leklem JE. Effect of vitamin B6 supplementation on fuels, catecholamines, and amino acids during exercise in men. Med Sci Sports Exerc 1999;31:400–8.

Volek JS, Silvestre R, Kirwan JP, Sharman MJ, Judelson DA, Spiering BA, Vingren JL, Maresh CM, Vanheest JL, Kraemer WJ. Effects of chromium supplementation on glycogen synthesis after high-intensity exercise. Med Sci Sports Exerc. 2006;38:2102–9.

Walker LS, Bemben MG, Bemben DA, Knehans AW. Chromium picolinate effects on body composition and muscular performance in wrestlers. Med Sci Sports Exerc 1998;30:1730–7.

Watson TA, MacDonald-Wicks LK, Garg ML. Oxidative stress and antioxidants in athletes undertaking regular exercise training. Int J Sports Nutr Exerc Metab 2005;15:131–46.

Weber GF. The measurement of oxygen-derived free radicals and related substances in medicine. J Clin Chem Clin Biochem 1990;28:569–603.

Webster MJ. Physiological and performance responses to supplementation with thiamin and pantothenic acid derivatives. Eur J Appl Physiol 1998;77:486–91.

Weight LM, Myburgh KH, Noakes TD. Vitamin and mineral supplementation: effect on the running performance of trained athletes. Am J Clin Nutr 1988a;47:192–5.

Weight LM, Noakes TD, Labadarios D, et al. Vitamin and mineral status of trained athletes including the effects of supplementation. Am J Clin Nutr 1988b;47:186–91.

Weller E, Bachert P, Meinck H-M, et al. Lack of effect of oral Mg-supplementation on Mg in serum, blood cells, and calf muscle. Med Sci Sports Exerc 1998;30:1584–91.

Wenk C, Steiner G, Kunz P. Evaluation of the losses of water and minerals: description of the method with the example of a 10 000 m race. Int J Vit Nutr Res 1989;59:425.

Willis KS, Peterson NJ, Larson-Meyer DE. Should we be concerned about the vitamin D status of athletes? Int J Sport Nutr Exerc Metab 2008;18:204–24.

Wood B, Gijsbers A, Goode A, Davis S, Mulholland J, Breen K. A study of partial thiamin restriction in human volunteers. Am J Clin Nutr 1980;33:848–61.

Zorbas YG, Charapakin KP, Kakurin VJ. Daily copper supplement effects on copper balance in trained subjects during prolonged restriction of muscular activity. Biol Trace Elem Res 1999;69:81–98.

The science of anti-oxidants and exercise performance

TRENT WATSON

Introduction

Anti-oxidants protect the body from molecules known as reactive oxygen species (ROS). During exercise, the production of ROS increases. This could overwhelm the body's anti-oxidant defenses, damage cellular components (by increasing oxidative stress) and potentially reduce performance capacity. In animal studies, exercise capacity is significantly reduced when an anti-oxidant deficiency is induced; this highlights the vital role of anti-oxidants in exercise performance. Similar deficiency studies have not been undertaken in humans because of ethical constraints. Human studies have mostly focused on increasing anti-oxidant intakes above usual daily reference intakes by giving anti-oxidant supplements as a means to reduce oxidative stress and enhance exercise capacity. Results from these studies have been conflicting and inconsistent, so definitive conclusions or recommendations regarding anti-oxidant intake for athletes cannot be made.

Further controlled trials are needed to confirm the early evidence suggesting that athletes need higher anti-oxidant requirements than non-athletes, and to determine the level (or dosage) and combinations of anti-oxidants required, and the best form of delivery (whether via supplements or from food sources) before definitive recommendations can be made. Currently, the evidence from epidemiological studies and the limited number of studies conducted on athletes favors high intakes of anti-oxidants from food sources, rather than supplements.

Anti-oxidants

Anti-oxidants are defined as:

> Molecules that can be present in small concentrations compared to other oxidisable biologically-relevant molecules and prevent or reduce the extent of oxidative damage to other biologically-relevant molecules (Halliwell & Gutteridge 1989).

In other words, anti-oxidants neutralize or scavenge free radicals or, more specifically, ROS to relatively less toxic by-products and thus prevent oxidative damage to susceptible cells and cell components. Thus the extent of oxidative damage in an athlete is not only determined by the level of free radicals induced by exercise, but also by the capacity of anti-oxidant defenses to neutralize free radicals and prevent oxidative damage. However, if anti-oxidants are in excess (when taken in high doses as supplements, for example) they can become pro-oxidants and can themselves become free radicals (Bast & Haenen 2002; Vivekananthan et al. 2003).

Anti-oxidants are derived from both exogenous (dietary) and endogenous (body) sources. Endogenous anti-oxidants include uric acid, bilirubin, plasma proteins and the enzymes superoxide dismutase, glutathione peroxidase and catalase. Dietary anti-oxidants include vitamin C, vitamin E, carotenoids (mainly β-carotene), polyphenols (e.g. flavonoids), glutathione and coenzyme Q_{10}. They are found mainly in plant sources including dark-colored vegetables, and citrus fruits, legumes, nuts, grains, seeds and oils. Dietary anti-oxidants are added to many commercial foods to help prevent chemical deterioration (oxidation reactions from oxygen either naturally present in the food or from contact with the air). Some anti-oxidants (e.g. glutathione and coenzyme Q_{10}) can be produced both endogenously or consumed in the diet (Halliwell & Gutteridge 1989).

Free radicals, reactive oxygen species and oxidative stress

ROS are defined as reactive intermediates derived from the incomplete reduction of oxygen, and are generated as a normal part of our metabolism (McCord 2000). Most ROS are free radicals and are very reactive. Superoxide (O_2^-, hydrogen peroxide (H_2O_2) and the hydroxyl radical (HO^-) are commonly known ROS (McCord 2000). If the ROS generated are not mopped up by the body's anti-oxidant defenses they can react with surrounding cellular components including membrane lipids, cellular proteins and DNA. Around 2–5% of oxygen consumed by the body is reduced to form the superoxide radical, which can then go on to create the wider range of ROS (Sjodin et al. 1990). During exercise, whole body O_2 consumption can increase by ten- to fifteen-fold and the O_2 flux in active muscle has shown up to a 200-fold increase (Sen 1995). Thus if superoxide production increases in proportion to oxygen consumption during exercise, the potential for oxidative stress is substantially increased.

Oxidative stress is the term used to define the point at which the build-up of ROS exceeds the capacity of our anti-oxidant defense mechanisms, leaving ROS to react and damage cellular components (Jenkins 2000). Oxidative stress has been linked to the pathogenesis of chronic diseases (e.g. atherosclerosis, retinopathy, muscular dystrophy, some cancers, diabetes, rheumatoid arthritis, aging, ischemia-reperfusion injury, Alzheimer's disease) (Sen 1995; Schwemmer et al. 2000); fatigue (Powers & Hamilton 1999); muscle damage (Powers & Hamilton 1999); and reduced immune function (Bishop et al. 1999).

Exercise and oxidative stress

There is increasing evidence showing that acute exercise of varying intensities and duration increases the production of free radicals and oxidative stress in both animals (Alessio & Goldfarb 1988; Alessio et al. 1988; Bejma & Ji 1999; Davies et al. 1982; Jackson et al. 1985; Liu et al. 2000) and humans (Alessio et al. 1997; Ashton et al. 1998, 1999; Child et al. 1998, 2000; Kanter et al. 1993; Sen et al. 1994a; Laaksonen et al. 1996, 1999; Marzatico et al. 1997; Sacheck et al. 2003). Despite the potential for oxidative damage that occurs as a result of acute exercise, regular physical activity has well-known beneficial effects for health and performance outcomes. This apparently conflicting situation is often termed the exercise-oxidative stress (EXOS) paradox (Ashton et al. 1998). It is not known why the EXOS paradox exists, but it has been hypothesized that the capacity and adaptation of the body's anti-oxidant defenses may be part of the reason (Leeuwenburgh & Heinecke 2001).

Anti-oxidant adaptation to regular exercise

There is little doubt that anti-oxidant defenses eventually increase in response to athletic training, thereby improving the body's ability to defend against increased production of ROS induced during exercise. Three adaptive processes or mechanisms have been proposed to help attenuate the increased production and possible accumulation of ROS:

1. the up-regulation of endogenously produced anti-oxidant enzymes (Ji & Fu 1992; Ji 1993)
2. the increased de novo production of endogenous anti-oxidant molecules including glutathione (Ji 1999; Powers et al. 1999; Sen 1999; Sen & Packer 2000), urate (Westing et al. 1989; Liu et al. 1999; Svensson et al. 1999; Mastaloudis et al. 2001) and coenzyme Q_{10} (Beyer et al. 1984; Gohil et al. 1987)
3. the mobilization of anti-oxidant vitamins from tissue stores and their transfer through the plasma to sites undergoing oxidative stress (Gleeson et al. 1987; Pincemail et al. 1988; Bergholm et al. 1999).

To what extent these adaptive mechanisms improve the body's ability to defend against oxidative stress is unknown and the mechanisms behind these adaptive endogenous processes are not well understood.

Effects of dietary restriction of anti-oxidants on oxidative stress and exercise capacity

In animal studies, anti-oxidant deficiencies increase oxidative stress and reduce exercise capacity (Davies et al. 1982; Gohil et al. 1986; Sen et al. 1994b; Ji 1999). There is limited evidence from human studies to support these findings because in healthy, well fed subjects, particularly athletes, vitamin deficiencies are rare, difficult to create and unethical to induce.

The few human studies investigating the effects of short-term restriction of dietary intakes of anti-oxidants and oxidative stress or performance capacity have had varying results. These studies have predominantly restricted dietary intakes of a single anti-oxidant such as vitamin E or vitamin C over a short time. No differences in oxidative stress levels were observed between eleven female athletes who habitually consumed a diet low in fat and vitamin E compared to controls habitually consuming a higher-fat, higher-vitamin E diet prior to undertaking a 45-minute submaximal run (Sacheck et al. 2000). A difference in performance capacity between the groups was not reported in this study. In contrast, vitamin C restrictive diets (less than 10 mg/d) in six healthy men have been shown to reduce circulating vitamin C and lower other key anti-oxidant defenses (glutathione) (Van der Beek et al. 1990; Henning et al. 1991). Aerobic capacity was measured in one of these studies, but was unaffected (Van der Beek et al. 1990).

In a study of seventeen healthy male athletes oxidative stress was significantly increased during and following exercise when the athletes followed a restricted fruit and vegetable diet for only 2 weeks (and hence restricted a wider range of anti-oxidants than just a single anti-oxidant source), compared to the same athletes undertaking the same exercise test while consuming their habitually high anti-oxidant diet (Watson et al. 2005). Although exercise testing showed that time to exhaustion was not affected in the restricted diet group, subjects perceived that their levels of exertion had substantially increased. These findings indicate that anti-oxidant intakes were reduced threefold on a restricted anti-oxidant diet and the subjects' capacity to defend against the increased production of ROS during exercise was also potentially compromised. Although the level of anti-oxidant restriction did not induce measurable changes in exercise performance, it did increase the athletes' perception of effort. Further dietary anti-oxidant restriction beyond the levels used in this study may result in reduced exercise performance, but has not been tested. As suggested earlier, ethical concerns associated with inducing dietary deficiency in human subjects preclude further investigation.

Nevertheless, animal studies confirm that anti-oxidant deficiencies can increase oxidative stress and impair exercise capacity, providing strong biological plausibility. However, in human studies, short-term mild to moderate anti-oxidant restriction does not induce deficiency, which may explain why similar findings have not been confirmed in humans. The limited number of studies suggests that dietary anti-oxidants can provide some protection against the increased production of ROS during exercise, and so may be important to preventing further tissue damage and provide a more favorable oxidative environment for recovery and exercise performance.

Anti-oxidant supplements and exercise performance

Muscle-derived oxidants have been demonstrated to play a causal role in fatigue (Reid 2008), thus have the potential to effect exercise performance.

A number of animal studies have shown anti-oxidant supplementation to have positive effects on exercise performance (Shindoh et al. 1990; Novelli et al. 1990; Novelli et al. 1991; Leeuwenburgh & Ji 1998). Similar findings have not been observed in human studies—with one exception, a study conducted at high altitude. In this study, twelve mountain climbers were supplemented with 400 mg vitamin E daily (and a multivitamin and multimineral supplement) or a placebo during a 10-week expedition at high altitude (Simon-Schnass & Pabst 1988). During the course of the expedition, anaerobic threshold improved in the treatment group, whereas that of the placebo group decreased significantly. It was also found that the experimental group's pentane exhalation (an oxidative stress marker) showed no significant increase in the treatment group, compared to the control group, in which it was more than 100% higher. More research is needed to further explore whether the results of animal studies can be mimicked in humans.

Do athletes need higher dietary anti-oxidant intakes than non-athletes?

Manipulating dietary intakes of anti-oxidants could minimize the potential for free radicals to cause oxidative stress when adaptive endogenous anti-oxidant mechanisms can proceed no further, thereby providing a more favorable environment to enhance sporting performance. Only a few studies have reported the dietary intakes of anti-oxidants (Kanter et al. 1993; Alessio et al. 1997; Sacheck et al. 2000; Schroder et al. 2000; Watson et al. 2005) or considered the influence of food sources of anti-oxidants when testing the effects of exercise on oxidative stress (Balakrishnan & Anuradha 1998; Sacheck et al. 2000; Schroder et al. 2000; Watson et al. 2005). Consequently, the extent to which anti-oxidants from food defend against oxidative stress induced by exercise is largely unknown.

The available research suggests that athletes may require slightly higher amounts of anti-oxidants than the RDI/RDA to defend against exercise-induced oxidative stress. In athletes consuming a habitually high anti-oxidant diet (where vitamin C intakes were at least three times the RDI), oxidative stress was not elevated at completion of a submaximal and maximal test (Watson et al. 2005). This outcome suggests that these athletes were adequately protected against exercise-induced increases in oxidative stress. Interestingly, when the same athletes switched to a restrictive anti-oxidant diet for 2 weeks, oxidative stress levels observed at rest were no different from when they had been on the high anti-oxidant diet. This suggests that, even at rest, a restricted anti-oxidant diet was still adequate to protect against ROS. But after completing the same exercise test, significant increases in oxidative stress were observed during and following the exercise test in those athletes on the restricted diet. This response suggests that, for the subjects in this study, the 'low' level of dietary anti-oxidants consumed over 2 weeks (an intake that met the RDI for vitamin C and contained similar qualities of β-carotene to non-athletes) was not sufficient to defend against the acute increase in ROS production induced by submaximal and maximal exercise.

Moreover, decreases in anti-oxidant levels in the blood have been observed in elite basketball players during a season, despite maintaining high dietary intakes (Schroder et al. 2000). Other studies have confirmed lower circulating anti-oxidant concentrations at rest in athletes, compared with sedentary controls (Balakrishnan & Anuradha 1998). These differences suggest that the turnover of anti-oxidants is likely to be affected by athletic training and hence anti-oxidant intakes may need to be higher in elite athletes than sedentary people.

Are anti-oxidant supplements warranted?

Anti-oxidant supplements have been marketed to athletes to enhance training and recovery mainly for the purpose of reducing oxidative damage induced by exercise. In population studies, it is well accepted that diets rich in anti-oxidants are cardio-protective (Bazzano et al. 2003) and associated with lower risk of cancer (Block et al. 1992). Further, populations consuming diets rich in fruit, vegetables and wholegrains (and hence anti-oxidants) generally have higher plasma levels of anti-oxidants (e.g. vitamins C and E, carotenoids and certain flavonoids) than populations eating low intakes of these foods (Zino et al. 1997; Halliwell 1999). These findings led to the widespread promotion of anti-oxidant supplements to the general population as a preventive measure, although results from meta-analysis studies of intervention trials investigating the protective effects of single anti-oxidant supplements on health outcomes have not supported their widespread use. In contrast to earlier speculation of the protective effects of single anti-oxidant supplements, these meta-analyses actually revealed unfavorable health outcomes.

Authors of the first meta-analysis pooled clinical trials investigating the effect of vitamin E and β-carotene supplements on all-cause mortality and cardiovascular disease (Vivekananthan et al. 2003). β-carotene supplements were found to cause a small but significant increase in all-cause mortality and cardiovascular death, compared with controls, whereas vitamin E supplements did not provide any significant benefit or detriment. A second meta-analysis revealed an increase in all-cause mortality when vitamin E was supplemented at high doses (>400 IU/d for at least 1 year) (Miller et al. 2005). There appears to be a threshold effect with vitamin E supplements. In dose-response analyses, all-cause mortality progressively increased when vitamin E dosage exceeded 150 IU/d, but at dosages less than this mortality was decreased (Miller et al. 2005). A third meta-analysis (Bjelakovic et al.) also found that treatment with β-carotene, vitamin A, and vitamin E, singly or combined, significantly increased mortality, whereas, vitamin C and selenium had no significant effect on mortality.

Findings from two more recent studies have also shown that high-dose vitamin E supplementation (800 IU) had pro-oxidant effects during exercise of long duration, rather than the expected anti-oxidant effects (Nieman et al. 2004; McAnulty et al. 2005). Both studies used the reliable and sensitive oxidative stress marker, F_2-isoprostane. More recently, a combination of daily ingestion of vitamin C and vitamin E supplements (1000 mg/d and 400 IU/d, respectively) taken over 4 weeks actually blocked the beneficial effects of exercise on enhancing insulin sensitivity in both pre-trained and untrained male controls (Ristow et al. 2009). Prior to the results of these studies, high-dose anti-oxidant supplements were perceived at worst as innocuous. Despite these studies with negative effects, there is evidence to suggest that anti-oxidant supplements have favorable effects on oxidative stress markers during exercise (Sharman et al. 1976; Dillard et al. 1978; Sumida et al. 1989; Meydani 1992; Rokitzki et al. 1994; Mastaloudis et al. 2001). Clearly further research is required in at-risk groups.

In summary, the evidence suggests that the protective effect of diets rich in anti-oxidants is not simply attributed to anti-oxidants in isolation. Fruit, vegetables and wholegrains contain other compounds that have physiological functions that are protective (e.g. phyto-estrogens, polyphenols and flavonoids) (Halliwell 1999). Perhaps vitamin E and β-carotene are simply markers of fruit and vegetable intakes and may not be the primary protective compounds; or, more likely, anti-oxidants act in synergy with other anti-oxidants and nutrients in whole foods. It is not surprising that whole, unprocessed food appears to provide anti-oxidants in the right quantities and combinations to elicit health benefits. A diet that contains anti-oxidant nutrients in amounts that exceed RDIs as much as threefold is recommended (Watson et al. 2005). The levels or dosage and combination of anti-oxidant supplements that are needed to alter the anti-oxidant–pro-oxidant balance into one that is favorable for reducing oxidative stress induced by exercise is still unknown.

Conclusion

Current evidence supports a higher anti-oxidant requirement in athletes than non-athletes to help reduce oxidative damage induced by short-duration exercise. Population nutrient standards (e.g. RDI/RDA) are unlikely to match these higher requirements. Based on present evidence, dietary sources of anti-oxidants are preferable to single or even combined anti-oxidant supplements when consideration is given to the recent evidence from epidemiological studies demonstrating potential adverse health outcomes and pro-oxidant effects with prolonged use of high-dose anti-oxidant supplements. A diet that contains anti-oxidant nutrients in amounts that exceed the RDI as much as threefold is recommended. An anti-oxidant intake similar to the RDI appears less capable of protecting against exercise-induced oxidative stress.

The effects of anti-oxidant supplements on enhancing performance capacity in human studies are unclear, although strongly supportive based on results of animal studies. To date, there are not enough studies on the effects of anti-oxidant-rich diets rather than supplements on performance benefits to make any recommendations.

Until research suggests otherwise, the most prudent recommendation regarding anti-oxidant therapy to optimize the body's capacity to defend against increased ROS production during exercise is to consume a diet high enough in anti-oxidant-rich foods to exceed the RDIs for anti-oxidant nutrients, rather than use supplements. A low-dose anti-oxidant supplement containing several anti-oxidants together may be warranted in athletes who have difficulty meeting their higher anti-oxidant requirements. However, there is no clear evidence to suggest that an athlete will benefit from high dosages of anti-oxidant supplements, despite the theoretical basis. High dosages of anti-oxidant supplements may have pro-oxidant effects, which have the potential to cause more harm than good.

References

Alessio HM, Goldfarb AH. Lipid peroxidation and scavenger enzymes during exercise: adaptive response to training. J Appl Physiol 1988;64:1333–6.

Alessio HM, Goldfarb AH, Cao G. Exercise-induced oxidative stress before and after vitamin C supplementation. Int J Sport Nutr 1997;7:1–9.

Alessio HM, Goldfarb AH, Cutler RG. Content increases in fast- and slow-twitch skeletal muscle with intensity of exercise in a rat. Am J Physiol 1988;255:C874–7.

Ashton T, Rowlands CC, Jones E, et al. Electron spin resonance spectroscopic detection of oxygen-centred radicals in human serum following exhaustive exercise. Eur J Appl Physiol Occup Physiol 1998;77:498–502.

Ashton T, Young IS, Peters JR, et al. Electron spin resonance spectroscopy, exercise, and oxidative stress: an ascorbic acid intervention study. J Appl Physiol 1999;87:2032–6.

Balakrishnan SD, Anuradha CV. Exercise, depletion of antioxidants and antioxidant manipulation. Cell Biochem Funct 1998;16:269–75.

Bast A, Haenen GRMM. The toxicity of antioxidants and their metabolites. Environ Toxicol Pharmacol 2002;11:251–8.

Bazzano LA, Serdula MK, Liu S. Dietary intake of fruits and vegetables and risk of cardiovascular disease. Curr Atheroscler Rep 2003;5:492–9.

Bejma J, Ji LL. Aging and acute exercise enhance free radical generation in rat skeletal muscle. J Appl Physiol 1999;87:465–70.

Bergholm R, Makimattila S, Valkonen M, et al. Intense physical training decreases circulating antioxidants and endothelium-dependent vasodilatation in vivo. Atherosclerosis 1999;145:341–9.

Beyer RE, Morales-Corral PG, Ramp BJ, et al. Elevation of tissue coenzyme Q (ubiquinone) and cytochrome c concentrations by endurance exercise in the rat. Arch Biochem Biophys 1984;234:323–9.

Bishop NC, Blannin AK, Walsh NP, Robson PJ, Gleeson M. Nutritional aspects of immunosuppression in athletes. Sports Med 1999;28:151–76.

Bjelakovic G, Nikolova D, Gluud LL, et al. Mortality in randomised trials of antioxidant supplements for primary and secondary prevention. Systematic review and meta-analysis. JAMA 2007;297 (9):842–57.

Block G, Patterson B, Subar A. Fruit, vegetables, and cancer prevention: a review of the epidemiological evidence. Nutr Cancer 1992;18:1–29.

Child RB, Wilkinson DM, Fallowfield JL, Donnelly AE. Elevated serum antioxidant capacity and plasma malondialdehyde concentration in response to a simulated half-marathon run. Med Sci Sports Exerc 1998;30:1603–7.

Child RB, Wilkinson DM, Fallowfield JL. Effects of a training taper on tissue damage indices, serum antioxidant capacity and half-marathon running performance. Int J Sports Med 2000;21:325–31.

Davies KJ, Quintanilha AT, Brooks GA, Packer L. Free radicals and tissue damage produced by exercise. Biochem Biophys Res Commun 1982;107:1198–205.

Dillard CJ, Litov RE, Savin WM, Dumelin EE, Tappel AL. Effects of exercise, vitamin E, and ozone on pulmonary function and lipid peroxidation. J Appl Physiol 1978;45:927–32.

Gleeson M, Robertson JD, Maughan RJ. Influence of exercise on ascorbic acid status in man. Clin Sci (Lond) 1987;73:501–5.

Gohil K, Packer L, de Lumen B, Brooks GA, Terblanche SE. Vitamin E deficiency and vitamin C supplements: exercise and mitochondrial oxidation. J Appl Physiol 1986;60:1986–91.

Gohil K, Rothfuss L, Lang J, Packer L. Effect of exercise training on tissue vitamin E and ubiquinone content. J Appl Physiol 1987;63:1638–41.

Halliwell B. Establishing the significance and optimal intake of dietary antioxidants: the biomarker concept. Nutr Rev 1999;57:104–13.

Halliwell B, Gutteridge J. Free radicals in biology and medicine. Oxford: Clarendon Press; 1989.

Henning SM, Zhang JZ, McKee RW, Swendseid ME, Jacob RA. Glutathione blood levels and other oxidant defense indices in men fed diets low in vitamin C. J Nutr 1991;121:1969–75.

Jackson MJ, Edwards RH, Symons MC. Electron spin resonance studies of intact mammalian skeletal muscle. Biochim Biophys Acta 1985;847:185–90.

Jenkins RR. Exercise and oxidative stress methodology: a critique. Am J Clin Nutr 2000;72 (Suppl):670S–4S.

Ji LL. Antioxidant enzyme response to exercise and aging. Med Sci Sports Exerc 1993;25:225– 31.

Ji LL. Antioxidants and oxidative stress in exercise. Proc Soc Exp Biol Med 1999;222:283–92.

Ji LL, Fu R. Responses of glutathione system and antioxidant enzymes to exhaustive exercise and hydroperoxide. J Appl Physiol 1992;72:549–54.

Kanter MM, Nolte LA, Holloszy JO. Effects of an antioxidant vitamin mixture on lipid peroxidation at rest and postexercise. J Appl Physiol 1993;74:965–9.

Laaksonen DE, Atalay M, Niskanen L, Uusitupa M, Hanninen O, Sen CK. Increased resting and exercise-induced oxidative stress in young IDDM men. Diabetes Care 1996;19:569–74.

Laaksonen DE, Atalay M, Niskanen L, Uusitupa M, Hanninen O, Sen CK. Blood glutathione homeostasis as a determinant of resting and exercise-induced oxidative stress in young men. Redox Rep 1999;4:53–9.

Leeuwenburgh C, Heinecke JW. Oxidative stress and antioxidants in exercise. Curr Med Chem 2001;8:829–38.

Leeuwenburgh C, Ji LL. Glutathone and glutathione ethyl ester supplementation of mice alter glutathione homeostasis during exercise. J Nutr 1998;128:2420–6.

Liu J, Yeo HC, Overvik-Douki E, et al. Chronically and acutely exercised rats: biomarkers of oxidative stress and endogenous antioxidants. J Appl Physiol 2000;89:21–8.

Liu ML, Bergholm R, Makimattila S, et al. A marathon run increases the susceptibility of LDL to oxidation in vitro and modifies plasma antioxidants. Am J Physiol 1999;276:E1083–91.

Marzatico F, Pansarasa O, Bertorelli L, Somenzini L, Della Valle G. Blood free radical antioxidant enzymes and lipid peroxides following long-distance and lactacidemic performances in highly trained aerobic and sprint athletes. J Sports Med Phys Fitness 1997;37:235–9.

Mastaloudis A, Leonard SW, Traber MG. Oxidative stress in athletes during extreme endurance exercise. Free Radic Biol Med 2001;31:911–22.

McAnulty SR, McAnulty LS, Nieman DC, Morrow JD, Shooter LA, Holmes S, Heward C, Henson DA. Effect of alpha-tocopherol supplementation on plasma homocysteine and oxidative stree in highly trained althletes before and after exhaustive exercise. J Nut Bio 2005; 6:530–7.

McCord JM. The evolution of free radicals and oxidative stress. Am J Med 2000;108:652–9.

Meydani M. Vitamin E requirement in relation to dietary fish oil and oxidative stress in elderly. EXS 1992;62:411–18.

Miller 3rd ER, Pastor-Barriuso R, Dalal D, Riemersma RA, Appel LJ, Guallar E. Meta-analysis: high-dosage vitamin E supplementation may increase all-cause mortality. Ann Intern Med 2005;142:37–46.

Nieman DC, Henson DA, McAnulty SR, et al. Vitamin E and immunity after the Kona Triathlon World Championship. Med Sci Sports Exerc 2004;36:1328–35.

Novelli GP, Bracciotti G, Falsini S. Spin-trappers and vitamin E prolong endurance to muscle fatigue in mice. Free Radic Biol Med 1990;8:9–13.

Novelli GP, Falsini S, Bracciotti G. Exogenous glutathione increases endurance to muscle effort in mice. Pharmacol Res 1991;23:149–55.

Pincemail J, Deby C, Camus G, et al. Tocopherol mobilization during intensive exercise. Eur J Appl Physiol Occup Physiol 1988;57:189–91.

Powers SK, Hamilton K. Antioxidants and exercise. Clin Sports Med 1999;18:525–36.

Powers SK, Ji LL, Leeuwenburgh C. Exercise training-induced alterations in skeletal muscle antioxidant capacity: a brief review. Med & Sci Sports & Exerc 1999;31:987–97.

Ristow M, Zarse K, Oberbach A, et al. Antioxidants prevent health-promoting effects of physical exercise in humans. Proc National Acad Sci (Early Edition) 2009. At http://www.pnas.org/cgi/doi/10.1073/pnas.0903485106 (accessed 25 May 2009).

Reid MB. Free radical and muscle fatigue: of ROS, canaries, and the IOC. Free Rad Bio & Med 2008;44:169–79.

Rokitzki L, Logemann E, Huber G, Keck E, Keul J. Alpha-tocopherol supplementation in racing cyclists during extreme endurance training. Int J Sport Nutr 1994;4:253–64.

Sacheck JM, Decker EA, Clarkson PM. The effect of diet on vitamin E intake and oxidative stress in response to acute exercise in female athletes. Eur J Appl Physiol 2000;83:40–6.

Sacheck JM, Milbury PE, Cannon JG, Roubenoff R, Blumberg JB. Effect of vitamin E and eccentric exercise on selected biomarkers of oxidative stress in young and elderly men. Free Radic Biol Med 2003;34:1575–88.

Schroder H, Navarro E, Tramullas A, Mora J, Galiano D. Nutrition antioxidant status and oxidative stress in professional basketball players: effects of a three compound antioxidative supplement. Int J Sports Med 2000;21:146–50.

Schwemmer M, Fink B, Kockerbauer R, Bassenge E. How urine analysis reflects oxidative stress—nitrotyrosine as a potential marker. Clin Chim Acta 2000;297:207–16.

Sen CK. Oxidants and antioxidants in exercise. J Appl Physiol 1995;79:675–86.

Sen CK. Glutathione homeostasis in response to exercise training and nutritional supplements. Mol Cell Biochem 1999;196:31–42.

Sen CK, Rankinen T, Vaisanen S, Rauramaa R. Oxidative stress after human exercise: effect of N-acetylcysteine supplementation. J Appl Physiol 1994a;76:2570–7.

Sen CK, Atalay M, Hanninen O. Exercise-induced oxidative stress: glutathione supplementation and deficiency. J Appl Physiol 1994b;77:2177–87.

Sen CK, Packer L. Thiol homeostasis and supplements in physical exercise. Journal of Clinical Nutrition 2000;72(2 Suppl):653S–69S.

Sharman IM, Down MG, Norgan NG. The effects of vitamin E on physiological function and athletic performance of trained swimmers. J Sports Med Phys Fitness 1976;16:215–25.

Shindoh C, DiMarco A, Thomas A, Manubay P, Supinski G. Effect of N-acetylcysteine on diaphragm fatigue. J Appl Physiol 1990;68:2107–13.

Simon-Schnass I, Pabst H. Influence of vitamin E on physical performance. Int J Vitam Nutr Res 1988;58:49–54.

Sjodin B, Hellsten-Westing Y, Apple FS. Biochemical mechanisms for oxygen free radical formation during exercise. Sports Med 1990;10:236–54.

Sumida S, Tanaka K, Kitao H, Nakadomo F. Exercise-induced lipid peroxidation and leakage of enzymes before and after vitamin E supplementation. Int J Biochem 1989;21:835–8.

Svensson M, Malm C, Tonkonogi M, Ekblom B, Sjodin B, Sahlin K. Effect of Q10 supplementation on tissue Q10 levels and adenine nucleotide catabolism during high-intensity exercise. Int J Sport Nutr 1999;9:166–80.

Van der Beek EJ, Van Dokkum W, Schrijver J, Wesstra A, Kistemaker C, Hermus RJ. Controlled vitamin C restriction and physical performance in volunteers. J Am Coll Nutr 1990;9:332–9.

Vivekananthan DP, Penn MS, Sapp SK, Hsu A, Topol EJ. Use of antioxidant vitamins for the prevention of cardiovascular disease: meta-analysis of randomised trials. Lancet 2003;361:2017–23.

Watson TA, Callister R, Taylor RD, Sibbritt DW, MacDonald-Wicks LK, Garg ML. Antioxidant restriction and oxidative stress in short-duration exhaustive exercise. Med Sci Sports Exerc 2005;37:63–71.

Westing YH, Ekblom B, Sjodin B. The metabolic relation between hypoxanthine and uric acid in man following maximal short-distance running. Acta Physiol Scand 1989;137:341–5.

Zino S, Skeaff M, Williams S, Mann J. Randomised controlled trial of effect of fruit and vegetable consumption on plasma concentrations of lipids and antioxidants. BMJ 1997;314:1787–91.

CHAPTER 12

Preparation for competition

LOUISE BURKE

12.1 Introduction

The athlete's goal during competition is to perform to his or her optimum level. A range of factors can impair performance, including issues related to nutrition. 'Competition eating' is based on the principle of implementing nutrition strategies that can reduce or delay the onset of factors that cause fatigue or performance impairment. Of course, practical issues must also be considered, particularly in light of the frequency with which athletes are required to travel interstate or overseas to compete in their target events. Competition nutrition includes special eating strategies undertaken before, during and in the recovery from the event. In this chapter we will review the strategies undertaken in the hours or days prior to competition to prepare athletes to perform at their best.

12.2 Nutrition factors causing fatigue during performance

A variety of nutrition factors can reduce an athlete's ability to perform at their best during exercise (see Table 12.1). The risk and severity of an encounter during competition depends on issues including the:

- duration and intensity of the exercise involved
- environmental conditions, for example temperature and humidity
- training status of the athlete
- individual characteristics of the athlete
- success of nutrition strategies before and during the event

It is relatively easy to investigate the physiological factors limiting the performance of simple exercise tasks (such as running or cycling) undertaken in an exercise physiology laboratory. Furthermore, factors identified in laboratory simulations of simple competitive events such as these may well apply to the real-life performances of athletes. However,

TABLE 12.1 NUTRITION FACTORS ASSOCIATED WITH FATIGUE OR A DECLINE IN PERFORMANCE

• Depletion of glycogen stores in the active muscle
• Hypoglycemia
• Other mechanisms of 'central fatigue' involving neurotransmitters
• Dehydration
• Hyponatremia
• Gastrointestinal discomfort and upset

it is more complicated to measure or predict factors limiting the performance of complex sporting events, particularly ball games and racquet sports in which competition demands have a high degree of inter- and intra-athlete variability. Sports scientists try to pinpoint the likely risk that various factors will cause fatigue in a given sport or event, based on the available applied sports research, as well as accounts of the past competition experiences of the athletes involved. With this knowledge, athletes can then be guided to undertake specific competition nutrition strategies that will minimize or delay the onset of these problems.

Setting a competition nutrition plan to combat factors causing fatigue

12.3

Pre-competition nutrition strategies include dietary interventions that are implemented during the week prior to an event, as well as special tactics that are undertaken in the minutes or hours before the event begins. These nutrition strategies should target the specific physiological challenges that affect the performance of the athlete's sport. According to the characteristics of the event, strategies might aim to minimize fluid deficits, ensure fuel availability or prevent gastrointestinal discomfort. Ideally, an athlete should combat these challenges by undertaking a combination of nutrition strategies before, during and even in the recovery after an event. Although further systematic studies are needed to investigate the benefits of combining two or more strategies, it is logical that a multi-tasked approach would be superior to a single strategy. For example, it appears that the combination of carbohydrate (CHO) intake before, as well as during, an endurance event is superior to the performance benefits gained from undertaking each of these strategies in isolation (Wright et al. 1991; Burke et al. 1998; Chryssanthopoulous & Williams 1997). However, in practice, the athlete may not always be able to exploit each opportunity for a nutrition intervention. When one opportunity is missed or under-utilized, greater emphasis on tactics at another opportunity may help to compensate. For example, an athlete who has not been able to refuel muscle CHO stores before a prolonged event should place greater emphasis on consuming CHO during the event. Conversely, in events where opportunities to drink during exercise are limited and large fluid deficits occur, the athlete should pay extra attention to hydration before the event starts, and perhaps even experiment with hyperhydration (fluid overload). In any case, the athlete should set a complete plan for competition eating, using nutrition strategies that complement and enhance each other.

12.4 Pre-event fueling

The depletion of body CHO stores is a major cause of fatigue during exercise (see Chapter 1 for review). Optimizing CHO status in the muscle and liver is a primary goal of competition preparation. The key ingredients for glycogen storage are dietary CHO intake, and in the case of muscle stores, tapered exercise or rest (for review see Ivy 1991; Robergs 1991; Jentjens & Jeukendrup 2003a). The duration of pre-event fueling will depend on the balance between the anticipated fuel needs of the event and the preparation time that can be devoted to the event.

12.5 Muscle glycogen storage

Since the application of the biopsy technique to exercise metabolism in the 1960s, sports scientists have been able to directly measure the glycogen content in isolated muscle samples, and thus determine the factors that enhance or impair storage. More recently, indirect techniques of muscle glycogen measurement involving nuclear magnetic resonance spectroscopy (Roden & Shulman 1999) have increased the practical opportunities to study such factors.

Studies of glycogen synthesis (GS) describe a biphasic response, consisting of a rapid early phase for the first 24 hours (non-insulin-dependent) followed by a slow phase (insulin-dependent) lasting several days (Ivy & Kuo 1998). Early studies proposed that activity of the glycogen synthase enzyme plays a key role in determining the rates of GS in the muscle (Danforth 1965), although this relationship does not totally explain all observations of GS. For example, differences in post-exercise glycogen storage have been found in the absence of differences in GS activity (Ivy et al. 1988), and the increased GS activity observed immediately after glycogen-depleting exercise returns to normal in advance of the glycogen supercompensation that can be observed in trained muscle exposed to several days of high CHO intake (see Ivy & Kuo 1998). Insulin- or exercise-stimulated translocation of GLUT-4 protein transporter to the muscle membrane increases muscle glucose uptake and is also a determinant of glycogen resynthesis (McCoy et al. 1996). Factors affecting post-exercise resynthesis of glycogen exercise are discussed in greater detail in Chapter 14.

Investigators have reported that there are two separate glycogen pools within muscle, adding a new dimension to our understanding of GS and utilization. Research has identified a primer for GS, the protein glycogenin, which acts as both the core of the glycogen molecule and the enzyme stimulating self-glycosylation (Alonso et al. 1995). The initial accumulation of glucose units to glycogenin forms a glycogen type now known as proglycogen, which is of relatively smaller size. The storage of proglycogen is most prominent during the first phase of recovery and is sensitive to the provision of dietary CHO (Adamo et al. 1998). During the second phase of glycogen recovery, glycogen storage occurs mainly in the pool of macroglycogen, a glycogen molecule with greater amounts of glucose for each glycogenin core. It is an increase in the macroglycogen pool that appears to account for glycogen supercompensation in the muscle following 2–3 days of high CHO intake (Adamo et al. 1998).

Research indicates that the pools of proglycogen and macroglycogen are metabolically distinct. It is speculated that proglycogen is the small and dynamic intermediate form of glycogen, whereas macroglycogen is the larger storage form that increases on a relative basis as total glycogen increases (Adamo & Graham 1998). Adamo and Graham suggest that when the proglycogen pool has reached a critical limit in a favorable CHO environment, a portion is then synthesized into macroglycogen. Conversely, a study of a marathon race has shown that the pools of glycogen are utilized at separate rates (Asp et al. 1999). Future studies may allow us to exploit this information, and determine new factors and strategies that enhance the metabolic availability of glycogen pools or increase storage.

Fueling up for non-endurance events 12.6

In the absence of muscle damage, muscle glycogen stores can be normalized by 24 hours of rest and an adequate CHO intake: 7–10 g/kg body mass (BM) per day (Costill et al. 1981; Burke et al. 1995). Such stores appear adequate for the muscle fuel needs of events of less than 60–90 minutes in duration; at least, CHO loading to achieve supercompensated glycogen levels does not enhance the performance of these events (for review, see Hawley et al. 1997b).

Typically, the resting value for muscle glycogen in trained muscle is 100–120 mmol/kg wet weight (ww). Allowing for a typical rate of GS at ~5 mmol/kg ww/h, the athlete should set aside 24–36 hours following their last training session to normalize fuel stores prior to non-endurance events. For many athletes this might be as simple as scheduling a day of rest or light training before the event, while continuing to follow high-CHO eating patterns. However, not all athletes eat sufficient CHO in their typical or everyday diets to maximize glycogen storage, particularly females who restrict their total energy intake to control body fat levels (Burke 1995). These athletes may need education or encouragement to temporarily remove their energy restriction and prioritize refueling as the dietary goal on the day before competition. Similarly, some athletes may need to reorganize their training programs to allow a lighter training day or rest on the day prior to their event. At minimum, the athlete should avoid training sessions that cause significant muscle damage on the day before competition, since such damage interferes with glycogen storage (O'Reilly et al. 1987; Costill et al. 1990).

Carbohydrate loading for endurance events 12.7

CHO loading refers to practices that aim to maximize or supercompensate muscle glycogen stores prior to a competitive event that would otherwise deplete these fuel reserves. Such protocols may elevate muscle glycogen stores to ~150–250 mmol/kg ww. This will be an important strategy for events lasting more than 90 minutes, which would otherwise be limited by the depletion of muscle glycogen stores (for review, see Hawley et al. 1997b). The first CHO loading protocols were an outcome of studies undertaken in the late 1960s by Scandinavian sports scientists to examine muscle properties using biopsy techniques. In a series of studies (Bergstrom & Hultman 1966; Ahlborg et al. 1967; Bergstrom et al. 1967; Hermansen et al. 1967), these researchers found that endurance, or capacity for prolonged moderate intensity exercise, was determined by pre-exercise muscle glycogen stores. Several days of a low-CHO diet depleted the muscle glycogen stores and reduced cycling endurance compared with a normal-CHO diet. However, the subsequent high CHO intake over several days caused a supercompensation of glycogen stores and prolonged the cycling time to exhaustion. A clever research design involving one-legged cycling showed that glycogen supercompensation was localized to the muscle that had been previously depleted, and studies identified the activity of glycogen synthase enzyme as an important factor in GS. These pioneering studies produced the 'classical' 7-day model of CHO loading, involving a 3–4 day 'depletion' phase of hard training and low CHO intake, and finishing with a 3–4 day 'loading' phase of high CHO eating and exercise taper. Early field studies of prolonged running events showed that CHO loading might enhance sports performance, not by allowing the athlete to run faster, but by prolonging the time that race pace could be maintained (Karlsson & Saltin 1971).

Studies extended to trained subjects produced a 'modified' CHO loading strategy. Sherman and colleagues showed that well-trained athletes were able to supercompensate muscle glycogen stores without a depletion or 'glycogen stripping' phase (Sherman et al. 1981). The runners in this study elevated their muscle glycogen stores with 3 days of taper and high CHO intake, regardless of whether this was preceded by a depletion phase or a more typical diet and training preparation. For well-trained athletes at least, CHO loading may be seen as an extension of 'fueling up' (rest and high CHO intake) over 3–4 days. The modified CHO loading protocol offers a more practical strategy for competition preparation, by avoiding the fatigue and complexity of extreme diet and training requirements associated with the previous depletion phase.

The time course of glycogen storage was recently examined, investigating muscle glycogen concentrations after 1 and 3 days of rest and a high CHO intake (10 g/kg BM) in well-trained male athletes (Bussau et al. 2002). After 1 day, muscle glycogen content increased significantly from pre-loading levels of ~90 mmol/kg ww to values of ~180 mmol/kg ww, and thereafter remained stable despite another 2 days of rest and CHO intake. The authors concluded that this was an 'improved 1-day CHO loading protocol' and that a 24-hour period of physical inactivity and a high CHO intake was sufficient for trained athletes to maximize muscle glycogen levels. However, the rates of glycogen storage achieved in this study were not abnormally high compared to other literature values (90 mmol/kg ww in the 24-hour period of observation), and subjects started the 'loading' phase with high glycogen values since their last training session was undertaken on the day before the loading protocol officially started. In other words, the true loading phase was ~36 h. In essence, the study provides a midpoint to the glycogen storage observations of Sherman and colleagues (1981) and shows that the supercompensation is not linear and may not require a full 72-hour period in rested subjects. Therefore, rather than promoting a unique strategy for CHO loading, this study suggests that optimal refueling is probably achieved within 36–48 hours of the last exercise session, at least when the athlete rests and consumes adequate CHO intake. Of course, it is not always desirable for athletes to achieve total inactivity in the days prior to competition, since even in a taper some stimulus is required to maintain previously acquired training adaptations (Mujika & Padilla 2000).

More recently, an athlete's ability to repeat glycogen supercompensation protocols has been examined. Well-trained cyclists who undertook two consecutive periods of exercise depletion, followed by 48 hours of high CHO intake (12 g/kg/d) and rest, were found to elevate their glycogen stores above resting levels on the first occasion but not the next (McInerney et al. 2005). Further studies are needed to confirm this finding and determine why glycogen storage is attenuated with repeated CHO loading.

Although CHO loading is so well known that the term has entered everyday language, it seems difficult for athletes to master, even in its simplified form. At least one study has shown that in real life athletes may not have the knowledge to plan a suitable exercise taper; furthermore they fail to reach the daily CHO intake targets of 7–10 g/kg BM needed to maximize glycogen storage (Burke & Read 1987).

Carbohydrate loading and performance of endurance events

Theoretically, CHO loading could enhance the performance of exercise or sporting events that would otherwise be limited by glycogen depletion. An increase in pre-event glycogen stores can prolong the duration for which moderate intensity exercise can be undertaken before fatiguing. It may also enhance the performance of a set amount of work (a set distance) by preventing the decline in pace or work output that would otherwise occur as glycogen stores decline towards the end of the task. In a review of CHO loading studies, Hawley and colleagues (1997b) summarized the findings that supercompensation of glycogen stores is beneficial for the performance of exercise of greater than 90 minutes' duration, with the majority of studies investigating exercise protocols involving cycling or running. Typically, CHO loading will postpone fatigue and extend the duration of steady state exercise by ~20%, and improve performance over a set distance or workload by 2–3% (Hawley et al. 1997b). Such an intervention would provide a substantial improvement in most simple endurance events such as marathons, prolonged cycling and triathlon races, and cross-country skiing events. Shorter events of 45–90 minutes' duration do not show significant performance benefits from CHO loading (Sherman et al. 1981; Hawley et al. 1997a).

Some team and racquet sports extend for at least 60–90 minutes of playing time, although the work requirements of these activities are of a less predictable nature. The interaction of prolonged duration and intermittent high-intensity exercise, which is associated with an increased rate of glycogen utilization, might be expected to result in muscle glycogen depletion during the event. Theoretically, performance in such sports would be enhanced by supercompensation of muscle glycogen stores. In real life it is extremely difficult to undertake studies that measure the performance of complex and variable sports such as these. Sports that have been shown to benefit from pre-event enhancement of muscle glycogen stores include a soccer simulation (Bangsbo et al. 1992), an indoor soccer game (Balsom et al. 1999), and a real-life ice hockey game (Akermark et al. 1996). However, Abt and colleagues (1998) failed to show significant improvement in the performance of skill-based tasks in a simulation of a soccer match. Decisions about the benefits of CHO loading may be specific not only to the sport, but to the individual athlete, depending on the requirements of their position or style of play. Of course, the logistics of competition in many of these sports, where games may be played daily to twice a week, would prevent a full CHO loading preparation before each event. Nevertheless, athletes in these sports should fuel-up prior to each competition as much as is practical, and perhaps experiment with an extended preparation before the most important games, such as the final of the tournament.

It is of note that the majority of studies of CHO loading have failed to employ a placebo in their design: most studies have used a cross-over design in which subjects are fed a high-CHO preparation on one occasion, and a low–moderate-CHO diet as a control. Since the benefits of CHO loading are well known, it might be argued that the responses to the high-CHO preparation will be psychologically as well as physiologically driven. Indeed, it is interesting to note that the two studies that have employed a placebo design, masking the true diets, failed to find benefits from CHO loading (Hawley et al. 1997a;

do not appear detrimental to performance. One safeguard is to ensure that the amount of CHO in the pre-event meal is substantial rather than minor; thus, any increase in CHO utilization during exercise will be more than offset by the large increase in CHO availability.

In the field it is not always practical to consume a substantial CHO-rich meal or snack in the 4 hours before a sporting event. For example, it is unlikely that an athlete will want to sacrifice sleep to eat heartily before an early morning race start. Most will settle for a lighter meal or snack before the event, and consume CHO throughout the event to balance missed fueling opportunities. A smaller pre-event meal may also make sense for events or athletes predisposed to gastrointestinal discomfort. Foods with a low-fat, low-fiber and low–moderate protein content are the preferred choice for the pre-event menu since they are less prone to cause gastrointestinal upsets (Rehrer et al. 1992). Liquid meal supplements or CHO-containing drinks and bars are useful for athletes who suffer from pre-event nerves or an uncertain pre-event timetable. Above all, the individual athlete should choose a strategy that suits their situation and their past experiences, and can be fine-tuned with further experimentation.

12.11 Carbohydrate consumed in the hour before exercise

Not all studies of CHO intake before exercise have shown favorable outcomes. Foster and colleagues (1979) found that feeding 75 g of glucose 30 minutes prior to exercise impaired cycle time to exhaustion at 80% of $VO_{2\ max}$ compared to exercise in the fasted state. The pre-event feeding did not alter the length of time subjects were able to ride during more intense (100% of $VO_{2\ max}$) exercise. A rapid drop in blood glucose concentration was noted during the first 10 minutes of exercise after subjects had been fed CHO, but this response was transient and was not associated with fatigue. Although muscle glycogen content was not determined, the reduction in endurance following CHO feeding was attributed to an accelerated muscle glycogenolysis (Foster et al. 1979).

The results of this study have been so widely reported and publicized that warnings to avoid CHO intake during the hour prior to endurance exercise have become part of sports nutrition dogma (Inge & Brukner 1986; Wilmore & Costill 1994). However, reviews of the literature reveal that this is the *only* study to find a reduction in performance capacity after the ingestion of CHO in the hour before exercise (Coyle 1991; Hawley & Burke 1997). These reviews summarize that the findings of other investigations of pre-exercise CHO feeding range from no detrimental effect to improvements in performance in the order of 7–20% (Coyle 1991; Hawley & Burke 1997). In most cases, the decline in blood glucose observed during the first 20 minutes of exercise is self-corrected with no apparent effects on the athlete.

Nevertheless, there seems to be a small percentage of athletes who respond negatively to CHO feedings in the hour before exercise. These athletes experience an exaggerated CHO oxidation and decrease in blood glucose concentrations at the start of exercise, suffering a rapid onset of fatigue and symptoms of hypoglycemia. Why some athletes experience such an extreme reaction is not known. One study has suggested that risk factors include the intake of small amounts of CHO (<50 g), increased sensitivity to insulin, a lower sympathetic-induced counter-regulation, and exercise intensity of low–moderate workload (Kuipers et al. 1999). However, a series of related studies failed to find any differences in the mild decline in blood glucose during exercise or the prevalence of blood glucose concentrations defined as hypoglycemic (<3.5 mmol/L) with the systematic manipulation of the amount of CHO consumed 45 minutes before exercise (20–200 g) (Jentjens et al. 2003) or the intensity of exercise (55–90% $VO_{2\,max}$) (Achten & Jeukendrup 2003). Changing the timing of intake of 75 g CHO before exercise (15–75 minutes) caused differences in blood glucose concentrations at the beginning of exercise, with the later feeding times (45 and 75 minutes) being associated with a greater prevalence of hypoglycemic levels of blood glucose. Nevertheless, differences self-corrected within 10 minutes of cycling (Moseley et al. 2003). The intake of sugars with a lower glycemic index (GI) (such as trehalose or galactose) was associated with a reduced prevalence of hypoglycemic levels of blood glucose compared with glucose feedings (Jentjens & Jeukendrup 2003b). Finally, cyclists who developed hypoglycemic blood glucose levels did not differ in insulin sensitivity compared with subjects whose lowest blood glucose level remained above 3.5 mmol/L (Jentjens & Jeukendrup 2002).

Not all athletes who experience a major decline in blood glucose concentrations experience hypoglycemic symptoms; there is some evidence that sensitization to low glucose levels may adapt the athlete to an increased threshold before symptoms are reported (Kuipers et al. 1999). Nevertheless, these effects are so clear-cut that at-risk athletes will be identified easily. Preventive action for this group includes a number of options:

- Experiment to find the critical time before exercise that CHO intake should be avoided.
- Consume a substantial amount of CHO in the pre-event snack/meal (>1g/kg).
- Include low GI, CHO-rich choices in the pre-event menu; these have an attenuated and sustained blood glucose and insulin response.
- Include some high-intensity sprints during the warm-up to the event to stimulate hepatic glucose output.
- Consume CHO during the event.

Pre-exercise carbohydrate and the glycemic index 12.12

CHO-rich foods and drinks do not produce identical blood glucose and insulin responses; neither do athletes respond according to the dogma that 'simple' CHO types produce rapid and short-lived rises in blood glucose concentrations whereas 'complex' CHO-rich foods produce a flatter and sustained blood glucose rise. The GI offers a means to measure and utilize the individual blood glucose profiles achieved by consuming various CHO-rich foods and drinks. The GI provides a ranking of CHO foods based on the measured postprandial blood glucose response compared to that of a reference food (either glucose or white bread). It has been shown to provide a reliable and consistent measure of relative blood glucose response to CHO-rich foods and meals. Furthermore, GI values have been used to manipulate meals and diets to produce a desired metabolic or clinical outcome, which is useful for the treatment for diabetes, hyperlipidemias and, potentially, obesity (for reviews, see Wolever 1990; Brand Miller 1994).

Early studies of pre-exercise CHO feedings showed different outcomes according to the type of sugar ingested. Fructose, a low-GI saccharide, could be consumed before exercise without producing the metabolic impairments seen with glucose feedings (Hargreaves et al. 1985). Thomas and colleagues were the first to apply the GI of real foods to the arena of sports nutrition, by undertaking a manipulation of the glycemic response to pre-exercise CHO-rich meals (Thomas et al. 1991). A 1 g/kg CHO meal in the form of a low-GI food (lentils), eaten 1 hour prior to cycling at 67% of $VO_{2\,max}$, was found to prolong time to exhaustion compared with the ingestion of a high-GI food (potatoes). These results were attributed to lower glycemic and insulinemic responses to the low-GI trial compared with the high-GI meal, promoting more stable blood glucose levels during exercise, reduced rates of CHO oxidation and increased free fatty acid (FFA) concentrations. Although muscle glycogen was not measured, the authors suggested that glycogen sparing may have occurred with the low-GI CHO trial (Thomas et al. 1991). The results of the study have been publicized widely and are largely responsible for the general advice that athletes should choose pre-exercise meals based on low-GI, CHO-rich foods and drinks (Brand Miller et al. 1998). However, other studies have failed to find performance benefits following the intake of a low-GI pre-exercise meal. The literature pertaining to the GI of pre-exercise CHO feedings has been summarized in Table 12.2.

This literature shows that pre-exercise low-GI, CHO-rich meals generally achieve a lower post-prandial blood glucose response and a more sustained metabolic response throughout exercise compared to high-GI, CHO-rich foods (Sparks et al. 1998; DeMarco et al. 1999; Wee et al. 1999; Stevenson et al. 2006). These findings are not universal, however, with some studies finding that that glycemic differences prior to the onset of exercise are short-lived and of transient consequence to metabolism (Febbraio & Stewart 1996). While some studies show that the GI of the pre-exercise meal(s) has no effect on glycogen utilization during exercise (Febbraio & Stewart 1996; Stevenson et al. 2009), others show that glycogen utilization is reduced (Wee et al. 2005) or possibly lower (Febbraio et al. 2000) following low-GI meals or diets. Reduced availability of FFA during exercise in response to high-GI CHO feedings has also been associated with increased utilization of intramuscular triglyceride (Trennell et al. 2008; Stevenson et al. 2009). It has been suggested that these metabolic differences be further examined for outcomes related to loss of body fat and increased satiety in athletes (Stevenson et al. 2006).

Perhaps the greatest conflicts in the pre-event menu debate lie with the effect on exercise performance. As summarized in Table 12.2, some studies have reported that a low-GI meal before exercise enhances exercise capacity or performance compared with high-GI CHOs (Thomas et al. 1991; DeMarco et al. 1999; Wu & Williams 2006; Wong et al. 2008). However, other studies fail to find benefits from the consumption of a low-GI pre-event meal (Thomas et al. 1994; Febbraio & Stewart 1996; Sparks et al. 1998; Burke et al. 1998; Wee et al. 1999; Febbraio et al. 2000; Wong et al. 2009) even when metabolism has been altered throughout the exercise. An important factor in the interpretation of these studies, as with many areas of sports nutrition research, lies in the issue of defining and measuring 'performance'. It should be noted that three of the studies that report a beneficial exercise outcome following the lowering of the GI of the pre-event meal have measured time to exhaustion at a fixed work rate as their interpretation of performance (Thomas et al. 1991; DeMarco et al. 1999; Wu & Williams 2006). These findings are not readily applied to the world of competitive sport, where a successful performance is determined as being able to complete a set amount of work or set distance in the shortest possible time, and where the athlete is free to choose and vary their work rate. It is important if the results of studies are to be translated into practical advice for competitive athletes that the study design and variables should be chosen to mimic the situation of sport as closely as possible.

Finally, a central issue that is overlooked in the debate is the overall importance of pre-exercise feedings in determining CHO availability during prolonged exercise. In endurance exercise events, a typical and effective strategy used by athletes to promote CHO availability is to ingest CHO-rich drinks or foods during the event. Yet, in the

TABLE 12.2 STUDIES OF GI AND PRE-EXERCISE CHO INTAKE

STUDY	SUBJECTS	CHO FEEDINGS	EXERCISE PROTOCOL	ENHANCED PERFORMANCE	FINDINGS
STUDIES SHOWING BENEFIT OF LOW-GI MEALS OVER HIGH-GI, CHO-RICH MEALS					
Thomas et al. 1991	Trained cyclists (*n* = 8 M)	Water or 1 g/kg BM CHO high-GI (potatoes) low-GI (lentils) glucose 60 minutes pre-exercise	Cycling to exhaustion @ 67% $VO_{2\,max}$	Yes (low-GI versus high-GI foods) BUT No difference between low-GI and glucose	Compared with high-GI food, low-GI food reduced blood glucose changes (lower rise pre-exercise and smaller decline during exercise). Decrease in suppression of FFA also. CHO sparing/sustained CHO availability suggested as explanation for increased endurance (~20%) with low-GI compared with high-GI. No difference in performance time between low-GI and glucose trials.
DeMarco et al. 1999	Trained cyclists (*n* = 10 M + F)	Water or 1.5 g/kg CHO low-GI meal high-GI meal 30 minutes pre-exercise	Cycling for 120 minutes @ 70% $VO_{2\,max}$, followed by time to exhaustion @ 100% $VO_{2\,max}$	Yes	Low-GI meal maintained glucose during exercise and reduced CHO oxidation compared with high-GI meal. Time to exhaustion at maximal effort prolonged by 59%.
Wu & Williams 2006	Recreational runners (*n* = 8 M)	2 g/kg CHO low-GI meal high-GI meal 3 hours pre-exercise	Treadmill run at 70% $VO_{2\,max}$ until exhaustion	Yes	Time to exhaustion was longer ($p < 0.05$) in low-GI trial (108.8 min) versus high-GI trial (101.4 min). Fat oxidation was higher in low-GI trial.
Wong et al. 2008	Trained runners (*n* = 8 M)	1.5 g/kg CHO low-GI meal high-GI meal 2 hours pre-exercise	21 km run on treadmill: 5 km @ 70% $VO_{2\,max}$ + 16 km TT	Yes	21 km run time was faster with low-GI than high-GI trial (98.7 versus 101.5 min, $p < 0.01$). CHO increased and fat oxidation decreased in high-GI trial compared with low-GI trial.

(continued)

TABLE 12.2 *(continued)*

STUDY	SUBJECTS	CHO FEEDINGS	EXERCISE PROTOCOL	ENHANCED PERFORMANCE	FINDINGS
STUDIES SHOWING NO BENEFIT OF LOW-GI MEALS OVER HIGH-GI, CHO-RICH MEALS					
Thomas et al. 1994	Trained cyclists (*n* = 6 M)	1 g/kg CHO low-GI powdered food high-GI powdered food low-GI cereal high-GI cereal 60 minutes pre-exercise	Cycling to exhaustion @ 67% $VO_{2\,max}$	No	Inverse correlation between GI and decline in blood glucose, or suppression of FFA during exercise. No differences in performance times. No correlation between GI and endurance.
Febbraio & Stewart 1996	Well-trained cyclists (*n* = 6 M)	Placebo (low joule jelly) or 1 g/kg CHO high-GI (potatoes) low-GI (lentils) 45 minutes pre-exercise	120 minutes cycling @ 70% $VO_{2\,max}$ + 15 minutes TT	No	Low-GI food reduced pre-exercise rise in blood glucose compared with high-GI food. No differences during steady state exercise in blood glucose or insulin. No differences in total CHO oxidation between the two CHO treatments, and similar muscle glycogen utilization over 120 minutes. No differences in TT performance between three trials.
Sparks et al. 1998	Well-trained cyclists (*n* = 8 M)	Placebo (low-joule soft drink) or 1 g/kg CHO high-GI (potatoes) low-GI (lentils) 45 minutes pre-exercise	50 minutes cycling @ 67% $VO_{2\,max}$ + 15 minutes TT	No	Low-GI food reduced pre-exercise rise in blood glucose and decline during exercise compared with high-GI food. Higher CHO oxidation during exercise with high-GI trial. No differences in work completed in 15 minutes TT between trials.
Burke et al. 1998	Well-trained cyclists (*n* = 6 M)	Placebo (low-joule jelly) or 2 g/kg CHO low-GI (pasta) high-GI (potatoes) 120 minutes pre-exercise 10% CHO solution consumed during exercise to provide ~ 1g/kg CHO	120 minutes cycling @ 70% $VO_{2\,max}$ + 15 minutes TT	No	Low-GI food reduced rise in pre-exercise blood glucose compared with high-GI food. CHO fed during exercise minimized all differences in glucose, insulin, FFA during exercise. No difference in substrate oxidation or performance of TT between trials.

(continued)

STUDIES SHOWING NO BENEFIT OF LOW-GI MEALS OVER HIGH-GI, CHO-RICH MEALS					
Wee et al. 1999	Active subjects (n = 8 M + F)	2 g/kg CHO low-GI meal; high-GI meal 3 hours pre-exercise	Running to exhaustion @ 70% $VO_{2\,max}$	No	High-GI meal caused a decline in blood glucose at the onset of exercise. Low-GI meal attenuated this response and reduced CHO oxidation during first 80 minutes of exercise. No differences in endurance.
Febbraio et al. 2000	Endurance-trained cyclists (n = 8 M)	Placebo (low-joule jelly) or 1 g/kg CHO low-GI meal (muesli) high-GI meal (potatoes) 30 minutes pre-exercise	120 minutes cycling @ 70% $VO_{2\,max}$ + 30 minutes TT	No	High-GI meal caused self-correcting decline in blood glucose concentrations at onset of exercise compared with other trials, and suppression of FFA throughout steady state cycling. Increased CHO oxidation during high-GI trial due to increased glucose uptake and trend to increased muscle glycogenolysis. No differences in performance of TT between trials.
Wong et al. 2009	Trained runners (n = 9 M)	Placebo (low-joule jelly) or 1.5 g/kg CHO high-GI meal low-GI meal 120 min pre-exercise 6.6% CHO solution consumed during exercise to provide ~48 g/h	21 km run on treadmill: 5 km at @ 70% $VO_{2\,max}$ + 16 km TT	No	No difference in running times between trials (91.1, 91.8 and 92.9 for high-GI, low-GI and placebo, respectively, ns). Blood glucose concentrations, and rates of oxidation of fat and CHO were similar between trials.

TT = time trial, ns = not significant

typical pre-event meal study, athletes are expected to perform prolonged exercise while consuming water or with no intake at all. The final and practical message to the athlete can be considered only when the interaction of pre-exercise and during-exercise CHO intake has been studied. In one study, well-trained cyclists ate three different pre-event meals (high-GI, low-GI or placebo) on separate occasions before cycling for 120 minutes at 70% $VO_{2\,max}$, followed by a time trial to complete a set amount of work (Burke et al. 1998). During exercise, subjects ingested a 10% glucose solution, providing an intake of ~1 g CHO/kg/h. Despite pre-exercise differences in glucose, insulin and FFA concentrations between trials, there were no differences during exercise. Furthermore, there were no differences between any of the trials with regard to total CHO oxidation over the 120 minutes of steady-state exercise, or the oxidation of the CHO consumed from the glucose drink. There were no differences in the time to complete the performance ride.

A similarly designed study involving a running protocol provides further support for the importance of CHO intake during exercise (Wong et al. 2009). In that study, runners consumed a CHO-electrolyte drink providing ~0.8 g CHO/kg/h during a 21 km treadmill time trial that was preceded either by a placebo meal, or a meal providing 1.5 g/kg CHO from high- or low-GI sources. There were no differences in substrate utilization, blood glucose profiles and running performances between trials.

In summary, it appears likely that when CHO is consumed during exercise according to sports nutrition guidelines, any effects of pre-exercise CHO intake on either metabolism or performance are negligible or at least greatly diminished. Each athlete must judge the benefits and the practical issues associated with pre-exercise feedings in their particular situation. In cases where an athlete may not be able to consume CHO during a prolonged event or workout, they may find it useful to choose a menu based on low-GI CHO foods to promote a more sustained release of CHO throughout exercise. However, there is no evidence of universal benefits from such menu choices, particularly where the athlete is able to refuel during their session, or where their favored and familiar food choices happen to have a high GI. In the overall scheme, pre-event eating needs to balance a number of factors including the athlete's food likes, availability of choices and gastrointestinal comfort.

12.13 Pre-exercise hydration

Dehydration poses one of the most common nutrition problems occurring in sport. Chapter 13 details strategies to enhance fluid balance during training and competition sessions. Since on most occasions fluid intake during exercise will not match the rate of sweat loss, it is critical for the athlete to start the session well hydrated. Special attention is needed to ensure full restoration of fluid balance after previous exercise bouts, particularly if unusually large fluid losses have occurred. This can happen when athletes undertake deliberate dehydration to 'make weight' in weight-category sports (Chapter 7), or when athletes move to a hot environment and fail to adapt their fluid intake practices to cope with their new sweat losses. In the training scenario, at least, several studies employing measurements of urine specific gravity or osmolality show that some individuals begin the session in a hypohydrated state (Maughan et al. 2004; Godek et al. 2005; Shirreffs et al. 2005). Therefore, there is evidence that an education message promoting deliberate hydration strategies in the hours or days before exercise is warranted. However, the new awareness of the dangers of hyponatremia during prolonged exercise resulting from excessive fluid intake (see Chapter 13) provides a reminder that messages regarding fluid intake can be misinterpreted. Athletes need to be aware of fluid intake strategies that are commensurate with their fluid needs, and to undertake any overhydration strategies (section 12.14) under supervision. Chapter 14 deals with strategies to promote rapid restoration of fluid deficits.

Pre-exercise hydration and hyperhydration 12.14

Many athletes undertake events in which significant dehydration is inevitable and poses a challenge to both their health and their performance. Such dehydration can occur when an athlete's sweat rate is extremely high, when there is little opportunity to drink during the event, or when these factors are combined. Some athletes have experimented with hyperhydration or 'fluid overloading' in the hours prior to the event to attempt to reduce the total fluid deficit incurred. This practice has been shown to increase total body water, expand plasma volume and ultimately enhance performance in a subsequent exercise trial (Moroff & Bass 1980). However, there are some shortcomings and possible disadvantages to simple fluid overloading techniques. First, much of the fluid is excreted via urination, since the body has a well-developed system to regulate the volume and concentration of its fluid content both at rest and during exercise. Fluid overloading may have a detrimental effect on performance if it causes the significant interruption of having to urinate immediately before or in the early stages of the event. The discomfort of excess fluid in the gut has also been shown to impair the performance of moderate–high intensity exercise (Robinson et al. 1995). As previously mentioned, if taken to extreme levels and in susceptible individuals, excessive fluid intake may lead to hyponatremia. Clearly, fluid overloading just before an event is a strategy that needs to be researched before any more firm recommendations can be made to athletes.

In one study, heat-acclimatized subjects were required to double their usual fluid intake for a week, from a mean intake of 1980 mL/d to 4085 mL/d (Kristal-Boneh et al. 1995). This was found to reset normal fluid balance to retain an extra 600 mL of fluid. Several experimental trials in the heat found that superior hydration status increased heat tolerance and enhanced duration of work in the heat, allowed achievement of maximal aerobic workload at a lower heart rate and improved performance in a time trial. More work is needed to confirm these results, but they support the advice often given to athletes competing in a hot climate to increase their fluid intake over the days leading up to the event. Whether this advice merely ensures fluid balance, rather than promoting fluid overload, has not been tested adequately prior to this study.

Of course, the impact of any gain in BM as a result of increased fluid retention might need to be taken into account in sports that are weight-restricted (such as lightweight rowing) or weight-sensitive (such as running and uphill riding). In many sports an increase in BM may increase the energy cost of the activity, impede the speed of acceleration and change of direction, and decrease the 'power to weight' (BM) ratio. Whether this occurs and whether the small impairments in performance are more than offset by the improvement in fluid balance need to be individually studied.

Glycerol hyperhydration 12.15

A method of hyperhydration under current study involves the consumption of a small amount of glycerol (1–1.2 g/kg BM) along with a large fluid bolus (25–35 mL/kg) in the hours prior to exercise. Glycerol, a three-carbon alcohol, provides the backbone to triglyceride molecules and is released during lipolysis (see Chapter 16). Within the body it is evenly distributed throughout fluid compartments and exerts an osmotic pressure. When consumed orally, it is rapidly absorbed and distributed among body fluid compartments before being slowly metabolized via the liver and kidneys. When consumed in combination with a substantial fluid intake, the osmotic pressure will enhance the retention of this fluid and expansion of the various body fluid spaces. Typically, this allows a fluid expansion or retention of ~600 mL above a fluid bolus alone, by reducing urinary volume. Further information on glycerol as a hyperhydrating agent is found in Chapter 16 and in reviews by Robergs and Griffin (1998) and Nelson and Robergs (2007).

The effect of glycerol hyperhydration strategies on thermoregulation and exercise performance is at present unclear. Studies investigating the effects on sports performance have been summarized (see Chapter 16). This summary shows that at least some of the inconsistency in the literature is due to differences in study methodologies. However, the most promising scenario involves the use of glycerol to maximize the retention of fluid bolus just prior to an event in which a substantial fluid deficit cannot be prevented. In some, but not all, studies of this type, glycerol hyperhydration has been associated with performance benefits. Of particular interest are two studies undertaken with competitive athletes. In both studies, competitive cyclists were able to do more work in a time trial undertaken in the heat following hyperhydration with glycerol, compared with a trial using a fluid overload with a placebo drink (Hitchins et al. 1999; Anderson et al. 2001). Even if future studies confirm the beneficial effects of glycerol hyperhydration strategies, it may require careful research to determine the mechanisms behind the effect. At present the theoretical advantages of increased sweat losses and greater capacity for heat dissipation, and attenuation of cardiac and thermoregulatory challenges, are not consistently seen.

There are some concerns associated with glycerol hyperhydration strategies. As previously discussed, the cost of a gain in BM might need to be considered in some sports. Other side effects from the use of glycerol include nausea, gastrointestinal distress and headaches resulting from increased intracranial pressure. These problems have been reported among some, but not all, subjects in the current studies. Fine-tuning of protocols for individualized situations should always be undertaken, and may reduce the risk of these problems, but some individuals may remain at a greater risk than others.

The most important consideration with glycerol hyperhydration lies with its status within anti-doping codes. At the time of writing this review, the World Anti-Doping Agency (WADA) was in the process of adding oral glycerol to its List of Prohibited Substances in the class of plasma expanders. This would remove the opportunity for elite athletes who compete under the WADA Code from using glycerol hyperhydration (or rehydration) strategies. However, this ban may not be relevant to recreational athletes or those in active occupations such as the military and fire-fighters, who may need to perform in thermally stressful conditions.

12.16 Salt loading

Another protocol that has been shown to enhance fluid status prior to exercise is the consumption of a high sodium beverage. One strategy involves the intake of a moderate volume (10 mL/kg) of a high sodium beverage (~160 mmol/L) over a 60-minute period in the 2 hours prior to exercise. Studies involving trained males (Sims et al. 2007b) and females (Sims et al. 2007a) have shown that such a protocol increases plasma volume before exercise and is associated with less thermoregulatory and perceived strain during exercise and increased exercise capacity in warm conditions. Further studies are warranted.

Priming the stomach with a fluid bolus 12.17

Even if the athlete is not aiming to 'fluid overload', there can be good reasons to have a drink just before exercise. Effective rehydration during exercise depends on maximizing the rate of fluid delivery from the stomach to the intestine for absorption. One of the factors affecting gastric emptying is gastric distension due to the volume of stomach contents. According to Noakes and colleagues, optimal delivery of fluid from the stomach can be achieved by beginning exercise with a comfortable volume of fluid in the stomach, and adopting a pattern of periodic fluid intake during the exercise designed to top up gastric contents as it is partially emptied (Noakes et al. 1991). Obviously the athlete will need to experiment to determine what is a comfortable volume with which to prime gastric volume, and in particular how comfortable this feels once exercise has commenced. However, as a general rule of thumb, most athletes can tolerate a bolus of about 5 mL/kg BM (300–400 mL) of fluid immediately before the event starts. This may provide a useful start to fluid intake tactics during exercise (see Chapter 13).

Summary 12.18

The outcomes of pre-event nutrition strategies range from psychological wellbeing and confidence to optimal fluid and fuel status. The importance of these strategies will depend on the range and severity of physiological challenges that are likely to limit performance in the athlete's individual event. This may be determined by characteristics of the event itself, as well as the degree to which the athlete has been able to recover since their last workout or competition event. Nutrition strategies may include increased CHO intake during the day(s) prior to the event, as well as the extended fueling-up known as CHO loading, which has been shown to enhance endurance and the performance of prolonged exercise events. The pre-event meal also provides an opportunity to refuel muscle and liver glycogen stores. There is some concern that pre-exercise CHO feedings may increase CHO utilization during exercise, but the intake of substantial amounts of CHO can offset the increased rate of substrate use. The choice of low-GI, CHO-rich foods in the pre-event menu may also sustain the delivery of CHO during exercise, but this does not provide a guaranteed performance advantage, especially when additional CHO is consumed during the event. Pre-event preparation should also consider fluid balance, with strategies to rehydrate from previous dehydration associated with exercise or weight-making activities, as well as the potential for hyperhydration in preparation for events in which a large fluid deficit is unavoidable. A variety of eating practices can be chosen by the athlete to meet their competition preparation goals. These need to consider the practical aspects of nutrition such as gastrointestinal comfort, the athlete's likes and dislikes, and food availability. Above all, the athlete should experiment with their pre-event nutrition practices to find and fine-tune strategies that are successful. These may be individual to the athlete and their specific event. Pre-event nutrition practices should be undertaken as part of an integrated competition nutrition plan. Ideally, an athlete should combat these challenges of competition by undertaking a systematic plan of nutrition strategies before, during and even in the recovery after an event.

PRACTICE TIPS

LORNA GARDEN

FUELING UP FOR COMPETITION

- It is important for the sports dietitian to have an extensive understanding of the individual athlete's competition plan in order to advise on appropriate dietary preparation. Interview questions should help determine the usual pre-competition dietary habits of the athlete, the timing and place of competition, food and fluids available, support people, recovery time between events if appropriate, and the athlete's competition goals.
- The decision to CHO load needs to be made based on consideration of the physiological requirements of the athlete's event (see Table 12.3). The athlete needs to have a good comprehension of the rationale for loading, and the requirements, side effects and practical difficulties associated with achieving an exercise taper and high CHO intake.
- Where an athlete presents with medical problems such as diabetes or other endocrine disorders or gastrointestinal issues, it is important that the athlete, sports dietitian and physician work together in preparing the athlete for competition.
- It is useful for the athlete to know that CHO loading is likely to be associated with a BM gain of ~2 kg. This needs to be viewed as positive reinforcement that they have significantly increased glycogen stores. Encouraging the athlete to weigh in each morning, unclothed and after voiding, can help determine how the loading is progressing.
- For most athletes a CHO loading regimen will involve 3 days of a CHO intake between 8 and 12 g/kg BM/d, which may contribute 70–85% of energy. Since this may represent

TABLE 12.3 FACTORS AFFECTING THE DECISION TO CHO LOAD

CHO LOADING SHOULD BE CONSIDERED IF ...	CHO LOADING IS NOT NECESSARY IF ...
• the exercise is a high-intensity endurance activity (such as marathon, triathlon or cross-country skiing) where heavy demands are placed on glycogen stores	• the exercise is not an endurance activity and normal glycogen stores will be adequate to fuel the event
• the activity is likely to involve more than 90 minutes of continuous exercise	• the event will last less than 60–80 minutes
• the athlete's habitual diet provides less than 7–8 g CHO/kg BM/d and may not otherwise maximize glycogen stores	• the activity is high-intensity for a short duration and will be adversely affected by the weight gain associated with loading (such as sprint events and field events)
• the athlete is motivated to increase CHO intake for the specific purpose of fueling up for an important event	• the athlete is already eating sufficient CHO to allow glycogen stores to be replenished efficiently for their event (such as >8–9 g/kg BM/d)
• there are no medical reasons contraindicating a very high CHO diet for a 3–5-day period	• the athlete has unstable diabetes, or is hyperlipidemic, and a very high CHO diet is contraindicated

an unusual dietary pattern for many athletes, help will be needed to devise suitable food choices and meal plans. Useful resources for the athlete include CHO ready reckoners and an individualized CHO loading plan (see sample in Table 12.4).

- Some athletes will find it difficult to tolerate the higher fiber content of a high-CHO diet, particularly if wholegrain and wholemeal breads and cereals and large quantities of fruit are consumed. To avoid gastrointestinal symptoms such as flatulence, diarrhea and gut discomfort, the sports dietitian may need to advise on low fiber/residue alternatives such as white bread, plain cereals, tinned and peeled fruit and liquid forms of CHO.
- Athletes who struggle to meet higher CHO needs may need to include refined CHOs such as glucose confectionery, jelly, jam, honey and soft drinks to supplement more nutritious but bulkier forms of CHO. Liquid meal supplements and high-CHO supplements (e.g. polyjoule or polycose) are also useful as low-bulk, CHO-rich drinks.

TABLE 12.4 EXAMPLE OF A CHO LOADING MENU FOR ONE DAY

THIS PLAN FOR A 60 KG ATHLETE PROVIDES APPROXIMATELY 600 G CHO (74% E OR 10 G CHO/KG BM), 30 G FAT (8% E), 115 G PROTEIN (15% E, ~ G/KG BM) AND 13 MJ
BREAKFAST
2 cups plain breakfast cereal with low-fat milk
1 piece fresh fruit
2 slices wholemeal toast with jam
1 glass fruit juice
SNACK
1 muesli bar, low-fat
1 piece fresh fruit
LUNCH
2 rolls or bagels, 1 filled with meat and salad, 1 filled with sliced banana and honey
1 cup canned fruit
1 tub low-fat fruit yoghurt or light fromage frais
Water
SNACK
1 low-fat smoothie: blend ½ cup fruit salad with 1 cup low-fat milk and 2 scoops low-fat ice-cream
DINNER
2 cups Hokkein or egg noodles stir-fried with Asian vegetables and 1–2 tablespoons blackbean or sweet and sour sauce
200 g low-fat creamed rice with 1 diced mango or other seasonal fruit
1 can soft drink

PRACTICE TIPS

- Where training or competition schedules do not allow a 3-day CHO preparation, an athlete may be able to supercompensate their muscle glycogen stores with 36–48 hours of rest and a CHO intake of 10–12 g/kg/d. In this case, it may be useful to consider all techniques that maximize rates of GS. These are covered in Chapter 14 and include large amounts of CHO at frequent intervals during the 4 hours after the last training sessions, and emphasis on CHO foods with a high GI.
- Athletes should be encouraged to practice their CHO loading regimen well before important competitions to ensure they are familiar and comfortable with food choices and quantities. This may be appropriate before a long training session or a minor event.
- Athletes should be reassured that although their nutrition goals for some vitamins and minerals may not be met during CHO loading, this is not a problem as a balanced diet will be resumed after competition.

PRE-EVENT MEAL

- Athletes need an understanding of the role of the pre-event meal in topping up liver glycogen levels, and of the relative importance of a high-CHO diet in the days leading up to competition.
- The psychological role of the pre-event meal and the athlete's likes and dislikes need to be considered carefully when planning appropriate foods and fluids before competition. The psychological value of ingesting foods that are familiar and 'tried and true' should not be under-estimated.
- The pre-event meal should be based on high-CHO foods that are low in fat and protein to decrease the risk of gastrointestinal problems during the event (see Table 12.5). Athletes who are prone to gastric discomfort during competition may also benefit from reducing dietary fiber or choosing liquid meals prior to exercise.

TABLE 12.5 SUGGESTIONS FOR PRE-EVENT FOOD AND FLUID INTAKE
Plain breakfast cereal with low-fat milk and fruit
Porridge with low-fat milk and fruit juice
Pancakes/pikelets with maple syrup, honey or golden syrup
Toast, muffins, or crumpets with honey/jam/syrup
Baked beans on toast
Creamed rice (with low-fat milk) and tinned fruit
Spaghetti with low-fat, tomato-based sauce
Jacket potato with creamed corn
Low-fat breakfast bar or muesli bar and banana
Roll or sandwich with banana and honey
Fresh fruit salad with low-fat yoghurt or fromage frais
Smoothie based on low-fat milk or soy milk, low-fat yoghurt and mango/banana/berries

- Where an athlete is nervous pre-event and unable to eat or tolerate solid foods, the sports dietitian may need to advise on appropriate liquid meal supplements such as homemade smoothies or commercial beverages.
- Commercial liquid meal supplements may also be a useful pre-event meal when traveling for competition to countries where familiar foods are unlikely to be available.
- Athletes should be encouraged to experiment with pre-exercise eating before training sessions to find foods and drinks they are comfortable with. The timing of pre-event eating will be individual to the athlete and their event, but a general schedule of 2–4 hours before the event should be suitable for most athletes.
- Athletes involved in endurance events may wish to trial low-GI foods such as porridge, pasta, baked beans, multigrain bread, oranges and yoghurt in their pre-event meal. The evidence for performance benefits is unclear, but they are most likely to be useful before prolonged workouts, where a sustained release of fuel cannot be provided by intake during the session itself. When CHO can be consumed during exercise, it is likely to negate any metabolic differences arising from the GI of pre-event CHO meals.
- The response to eating high-GI foods immediately prior to exercise is likely to be individual and should be trialed and monitored during training, well before competition days. In most cases, where an athlete is eating 30–90 minutes before an event, practical issues such as convenience and tolerance will become more crucial than the GI in deciding the pre-event menu.
- Athletes who have dehydrated or are fluid-restricted to make weight will need an individualized plan to promote rapid rehydration between weighing in and commencing competition. If time is very limited, liquid meal supplements may be an option preferable to solid food prior to the event.
- Liquid meal supplements may also be useful as a pre-event meal for athletes who compete in sports where aesthetic requirements such as a 'flat stomach' are important (such as gymnastics, dancing and diving).

HYDRATION PRIOR TO THE EVENT

- Athletes should be encouraged to begin their events well hydrated. They should consume adequate fluids in the days leading up to competition to ensure that they hydrate after all training sessions and compensate for general sweat losses according to the environment.
- When the athlete has several events or races scheduled, a plan should be made to ensure that fluid losses are recovered after each exercise session. Monitoring of early morning urine levels can help the athlete to be aware of the success of their fluid intake plan (see Chapter 13).
- Hydration prior to competition should be carefully planned, especially before events carried out in hot and humid weather. Fluid intake before an event should include at least 300–600 mL fluid with the pre-event meal and then 300–450 mL in the 15–20 minutes before the event, leaving time for a toilet stop prior to the start of competition.

PRACTICE TIPS

- Effective rehydration during exercise can be enhanced by priming the stomach with a bolus of fluid prior to the event, to take advantage of the effect of gastric distension on gastric emptying. Athletes will need to experiment to determine the maximum volume that can be tolerated without stomach discomfort during the event. Most athletes will tolerate around 300–400 mL of fluid immediately before the event.
- All strategies to over-hydrate prior to competition should be undertaken under supervision, or with the awareness that excessive intake of fluid can lead to the dangerous condition of hyponatremia.
- Although water is adequate for hydration before shorter events, the use of CHO/ electrolyte beverages (sports drinks) prior to exercise can assist in meeting both fluid and CHO needs, particularly before endurance events. Beverages containing sodium, such as sports drinks, may also be useful in assisting with fluid retention prior to and during the event and can reduce the need for frequent urination.

REFERENCES

Abt G, Zhou S, Weatherby R. The effect of a high-carbohydrate diet on the skill performance of midfield soccer players after intermittent treadmill exercise. J Sci Med Sport 1998;1:203–12.

Achten J, Jeukendrup AE. Effects of pre-exercise ingestion of carbohydrate on glycaemic and insulinaemic responses during subsequent exercise at differing intensities. Eur J Appl Physiol 2003;88:466–71.

Adamo KB, Graham TE. Comparison of traditional measurements with macroglycogen and proglycogen analysis of muscle glycogen. J Appl Physiol 1998;84:908–13.

Adamo KB, Tarnopolsky MA, Graham TE. Dietary carbohydrate and postexercise synthesis of proglycogen and macroglycogen in human skeletal muscle. Am J Physiol 1998;275:E229–34.

Ahlborg B, Bergstrom J, Brohult J, et al. Human muscle glycogen content and capacity for prolonged exercise after different diets. Foersvarsmedicin 1967;85–99.

Akermark C, Jacobs I, Rasmusson M, Karlsson J. Diet and muscle glycogen concentration in relation to physical performance in Swedish elite ice hockey players. Int J Sport Nutr 1996;6:272–84.

Alonso MD, Lomako J, Lomako WM, Whelan WJ. A new look at the biogenesis of glycogen. FASEB J 1995;9:1126–37.

Anderson MJ, Cotter JD, Garnham AP, Casley DJ, Febbraio MA. Effect of glycerol-induced hyperhydration on thermoregulation and metabolism during exercise in the heat. Int J Sport Nutr Exerc Metab 2001;11:315–33.

Andrews JL, Sedlock DA, Flynn MG, Navalta JW, Ji H. Carbohydrate loading and supplementation in endurance trained women runners. J Appl Physiol 2003;95:584–90.

Asp S, Daugaard JR, Rohde T, Adamo KB, Graham T. Muscle glycogen accumulation after a marathon: roles of fiber type and pro- and macroglycogen. J Appl Physiol 1999;86:474–8.

Balsom PB, Wood K, Olsson P, Ekblom B. Carbohydrate intake and multiple sprint sports: with special reference to football (soccer). Int J Sports Med 1999;20:48–52.

Bangsbo J, Norregaard L, Thorsoe, F. The effect of carbohydrate diet on intermittent exercise performance. Int J Sports Med 1992;13:152–7.

Bergstrom J, Hermansen L, Hultman E, Saltin B. Diet, muscle glycogen and physical performance. Acta Physiol Scand 1967;71:140–50.

Bergstrom J, Hultman E. Muscle glycogen synthesis after exercise: an enhancing factor localised to the muscle cells in man. Nature 1966;210:309–10.

Brand Miller JC. Importance of glycemic index in diabetes. Am J Clin Nutr 1994;59(Suppl):747S– 52S.

Brand Miller J, Foster-Powell K, Colagiuri S, Leeds A. The GI factor. Second edition. Sydney: Hodder & Stoughton, 1998.

Burke LM. Nutrition for the female athlete. In: Krummel D, Kris-Etherton P, eds. Nutrition in women's health. Maryland: Aspen Publishers, 1995:263–98.

Burke LM, Claassen A, Hawley JA, Noakes TD. Carbohydrate intake during prolonged cycling minimizes effect of glycemic index of preexercise meal. J Appl Physiol 1998;85:2220–6.

Burke LM, Collier GR, Beasley SK, et al. Effect of coingestion of fat and protein with carbohydrate feedings on muscle glycogen storage. J Appl Physiol 1995;87:2187–92.

Burke LM, Hawley JA, Schabort EJ, St Clair Gibson A, Mujika I, Noakes TD. Carbohydrate loading failed to improve 100-km cycling performance in a placebo-controlled trial. J Appl Physiol 2000;80: 1284–90.

Burke LM, Read RSD. A study of carbohydrate loading techniques used by marathon runners. Can J Sports Sci 1987;12:6–10.

Bussau VA, Fairchild TJ, Rao A, Steele PD, Fournier PA. Carbohydrate loading in human muscle: an improved 1 day protocol. Eur J Appl Physiol 2002;87:290–5.

Chryssanthopoulos C, Williams C. Pre-exercise carbohydrate meal and endurance running capacity when carbohydrates are ingested during exercise. Int J Sports Med 1997;18:543–8.

Costill DL, Pascoe DD, Fink WJ, Robergs RA, Barr SI, Pearson D. Impaired muscle glycogen resynthesis after eccentric exercise. J Appl Physiol 1990;69:46–50.

Costill DL, Sherman WM, Fink WJ, Maresh C, Witten M, Miller JM. The role of dietary carbohydrates in muscle glycogen resynthesis after strenuous running. Am J Clin Nutr 1981;34:1831–6.

Coyle EF. Timing and method of increased carbohydrate intake to cope with heavy training, competition and recovery. J Sports Sci. 1991;9(Suppl):29S–52S.

Coyle EF, Coggan AR, Hemmert MK, Lowe RC, Walters TJ. Substrate usage during prolonged exercise following a preexercise meal. J Appl Physiol 1985;59:429–33.

Danforth W. Glycogen synthase activity in skeletal muscle. J Biol Chem 1965;240:588–93.

DeMarco HM, Sucher KP, Cisar CJ, Butterfield GE. Pre-exercise carbohydrate meals: application of glycemic index. Med Sci Sports Exercise 1999;31:164–70.

Febbraio MA, Keenan J, Angus DJ, Campbell SE, Garnham AP. Preexercise carbohydrate ingestion, glucose kinetics, and muscle glycogen use: effect of the glycemic index. J Appl Physiol 2000;89: 1845–51.

Febbraio MA, Stewart KL. CHO feeding before prolonged exercise: effect of glycemic index on muscle glycogenolysis and exercise performance. J Appl Physiol 1996;81:1115–20.

Foster C, Costill DL, Fink WJ. Effects of pre-exercise feedings on endurance performance. Med Sci Sports 1979;11:1–5.

Godek SF, Bartolozzi AR, Godek JJ. Sweat rate and fluid turnover in American football players compared with runners in a hot and humid environment. Br J Sports Med 2005;39:205–11.

Hackney AC. Effects of the menstrual cycle on resting muscle glycogen content. Horm Metab Res 1990;22:647.

Hargreaves M, Costill DL, Katz A, Fink WJ. Effects of fructose ingestion on muscle glycogen usage during exercise. Med Sci Sports Exerc 1985;17:360–3.

Hawley J, Burke L. Peak performance. Sydney: Allen & Unwin, 1998.

Hawley JA. Burke LM. Effect of meal frequency and timing on physical performance. Brit J Nutr 1997;77(Suppl):91S–103S.

Hawley JA, Palmer G, Noakes TD. Effects of 3 days of carbohydrate supplementation on muscle glycogen content and utilisation during a 1-h cycling. Eur J Appl Physiol 1997a;76:407–12.

Hawley JA, Schabort EJ, Noakes TD, Dennis SC. Carbohydrate-loading and exercise performance: an update. Sports Med 1997b;24:73–81.

Hermansen L, Hultman E, Saltin B. Muscle glycogen during prolonged severe exercise. Acta Physiol Scand 1967;129–39.

Hitchins S, Martin DT, Burke LM, et al. Glycerol hyperhydration improves cycle time trial performance in hot humid conditions. Eur J Appl Physiol 1999;80:494–501.

Inge K, Brukner P. Food for sport. Melbourne: William Heinemann Australia, 1986.

Ivy JL. Muscle glycogen synthesis before and after exercise. Sports Med 1991;11:6–19.

Ivy JL, Katz AL, Cutler CL, Sherman WM, Coyle EF. Muscle glycogen storage after exercise: effect of time of carbohydrate ingestion. J Appl Physiol 1988;65:1480–5.

Ivy JL, Kuo CH. Regulation of GLUT 4 protein and glycogen synthase during muscle glycogen synthesis after exercise. Acta Physiol Scand 1998;162:295–304.

James AP, Lorraine M, Cullen D, et al. Muscle glycogen supercompensation: absence of a gender-related difference. Eur J Appl Physiol 2001;85:533–8.

Jentjens RLPG, Jeukendrup AE. Prevalence of hypoglycemia following pre-exercise carbohydrate ingestion is not accompanied by higher insulin sensitivity. Int J Sport Nutr Exerc Metab 2002;12: 398–413.

Jentjens RLPG, Cale C, Gutch C, Jeukendrup AE. Effects of pre-exercise ingestion of differing amounts of carbohydrate on subsequent metabolism and cycling performance. Eur J Appl Physiol 2003a;88: 444–52.

Jentjens RLPG, Jeukendrup AE. Effects of pre-exercise ingestion of trehalose, galactose and glucose on subsequent metabolism and cycling performance. Eur J Appl Physiol 2003b;88:459–65.

Karlsson J, Saltin B. Diet, muscle glycogen, and endurance performance. J Appl Physiol 1971;31:203–6.

Kristal-Boneh E, Glusman JG, Shitrit R, Chaemovitz C, CassutoY. Physical performance and heat tolerance after chronic water loading and heat acclimation. Aviat Space Environ Med 1995;66:733–8.

Kuipers H, Fransen EJ, Keizer HA. Preexercise ingestion of carbohydrate and transient hypoglycemia during exercise. Int J Sports Med 1999;20:277–31.

Maughan RJ, Merson SJ, Broad NP, Shirreffs SM. Fluid and electrolyte intake and loss in elite soccer players during training. Int J Sport Nutr Exerc Metab 2004;14:333–46.

McCoy M, Proietto J, Hargreaves M. Skeletal muscle GLUT-4 and post-exercise muscle glycogen storage. J Appl Physiol 1996;80:411–16.

McInerney P, Lessord SJ, Burke LM, et al. Failure to repeatedly supercompensate muscle glycogen stores in highly trained men. Med Sci Sports Exerc 2005;37:404–11.

Moroff SV, Bass DE. Effects of over hydration on man's physiological responses to work in the heat. J Appl Physiol 1980;49:715–21.

Moseley L, Lancaster GI, Jeukendrup AE. Effects of timing of pre-exercise ingestion of carbohydrate on subsequent metabolism and cycling performance. Eur J Appl Physiol 2003;88:453–8.

Mujika I, Padilla S. Detraining: loss of training-induced physiological and performance adaptations. Part I: short term insufficient training stimulus. Sports Med 2000;30:79–87.

Nelson JL, Robergs RA. Exploring the potential ergogenic effects of glycerol hyperhydration. Sports Med 2007;37:981–1000.

Neufer PD, Costill DL, Flynn MG, Kirwan JP, Mitchell JB, Houmard J. Improvements in exercise performance: effects of carbohydrate feedings and diet. J Appl Physiol 1987;62:983–8.

Nicklas BJ, Hackney AC, Sharp RL. The menstrual cycle and exercise: performance, muscle glycogen, and substrate responses. Int J Sports Med 1989;10:264–9.

Noakes TD, Rehrer NJ, Maughan RJ. The importance of volume in regulating gastric emptying. Med Sci Sports Exerc 1991;23:307–13.

O'Reilly KP, Warhol MJ, Fielding RA, Frontera WR, Meredith CN, Evans WJ. Eccentric exercise-induced muscle damage impairs muscle glycogen repletion. J Appl Physiol 1987;63:252–7.

Paul DR, Mulroy SM, Horner JA, Jacobs KA, Lamb DR. Carbohydrate-loading during the follicular phase of the menstrual cycle: effects on muscle glycogen and exercise performance. Int J Sport Nutr Exerc Metab 2001;11:430–41.

Rauch LH, Rodger I, Wilson GR, et al. The effects of carbohydrate loading on muscle glycogen content and cycling performance. Int J Sports Nutr 1995;5:25–36.

Rehrer NJ, van Kemenade M, Meester W, Brouns F, Saris WHM. Gastrointestinal complaints in relation to dietary intake in triathletes. Int J Sport Nutr 1992;2:48–59.

Robergs RA. Nutrition and exercise determinants of postexercise glycogen synthesis. Int J Sport Nutr 1991;1:307–37.

Robergs RA, Griffin SE. Glycerol: biochemistry, pharmacokinetics and clinical and practical applications. Sports Med 1998;26:145–67.

Robinson TA, Hawley JA, Palmer GS, et al. Water ingestion does not improve 1-h cycling performance in moderate ambient temperatures. Eur J Appl Physiol 1995;14:153–60.

Roden M, Shulman GI. Applications of NMR spectroscopy to study muscle glycogen metabolism in man. Ann Rev Med 1999;50:277–90.

Sherman WM, Brodowicz G, Wright DA, Allen WK, Simonsen J, Dernbach A. Effects of 4 h preexercise carbohydrate feedings on cycling performance. Med Sci Sports Exerc 1989;21:598–604.

Sherman WM, Costill DL, Fink WJ, Miller JM. Effect of exercise-diet manipulation on muscle glycogen and its subsequent utilisation during performance. Int J Sports Med 1981;2:114–18.

Shirreffs SM, Aragon-Vargas LF, Chomorro M, et al. The sweating response of elite professional soccer players to training in the heat. Int J Sports Med 2005;26:90–5.

Sims ST, Rehrer NJ, Bell ML, Cotter JD. Preexercise sodium loading aids fluid balance and endurance for women exercising in the heat. J Appl Physiol 2007a;103:534–41.

Sims ST, van Vliet L, Cotter JD, Rehrer NJ. Sodium loading aids fluid balance and reduces physiological strain of trained men exercising in the heat. Med Sci Sports Exerc 2007b;39:123–30.

Sparks MJ, Selig SS, Febbraio MA. Pre-exercise carbohydrate ingestion: effect of the glycemic index on endurance exercise performance. Med Sci Sports Exerc 1998;30:844–9.

Stevenson EJ, Thelwall PE, Thomas K, Smith F, Brand-Miller J, Trenell MI. Dietary glycemic index influences lipid oxidation but not muscle or liver glycogen oxidation during exercise. Am J Physiol Endocrinol Metab 2009; 296:E1140–7.

Stevenson EJ, Williams C, Mass LE, Phillips B, Nute ML. Influence of high-carbohydrate mixed meals with different glycemic indexes on substrate utilization during subsequent exercise in women. Am J Clin Nutr 2006;84:354–60.

Tarnopolsky MA. Gender differences in metabolism. New York: CRC Press, 1999.

Tarnopolsky MA, Atkinson SA, Phillips SM, MacDougall JD. Carbohydrate loading and metabolism during exercise in men and women. J Appl Physiol 1995;75:2134–41.

Tarnopolsky MA, Zawada C, Richmond LB, et al. Gender differences in carbohydrate loading are related to energy intake. J Appl Physiol 2001;91:225–30.

Thomas DE, Brotherhood JE, Brand JC. Carbohydrate feeding before exercise: effect of glycemic index. Int J Sports Med 1991;12:180–6.

Thomas DE, Brotherhood JR, Brand Miller J. Plasma glucose levels after prolonged strenuous exercise correlate inversely with glycemic response to food consumed before exercise. Int J Sport Nutr 1994;4:361–73.

Trenell MI, Stevenson E, Stockmann K, Brand-Miller J. Effect of high and low glycaemic index recovery diets on intramuscular lipid oxidation during aerobic exercise. Br J Nutr 2008;99:326–32.

Walker JL, Heigenhauser GJF, Hultman E, Spriet LL. Dietary carbohydrate, muscle glycogen content and endurance performance in well trained women. J Appl Physiol 2000;88:2151–8.

Wee SL, Williams C, Gray S, Horabin J. Influence of high and low glycemic index meals on endurance running capacity. Med Sci Sports Exerc 1999;31:393–9.

Wee SL, Williams C, Tsintzas K, Boobis L. Ingestion of a high-glycemic index meal increases muscle glycogen storage at rest but augments its utilisation during subsequent exercise. J Appl Physiol 2005;99:707–14.

Widrick JJ, Costill DL, Fink WJ, Hickey MS, McConell GK, Tanaka H. Carbohydrate feedings and exercise performance: effect of initial muscle glycogen concentration. J Appl Physiol 1993;74:2998–3005.

Wilmore J, Costill DL. Physiology of sport and exercise. Champaign, Illinois: Human Kinetics, 1994.

Wolever TMS. The glycemic index. World Rev Nutr Diet 1990;62:120–85.

Wong SHS, Chan OW, Chen YJ, Hi HL, Lam CW, Chung PW. Effect of pre-exercise glycemic-index meal on running when CHO-electrolyte solution is consumed during exercise. Int J Sport Nutr Exerc Metab 2009;19: 222–42.

Wong SHS, Sui PM, Lok A, Chen YJ, Morris J, Lam CW. Effect of the glycaemic index of pre-exercise carbohydrate meals on running performance. Eur J Sports Sci 2008;8:23–33.

Wright DA, Sherman WM, Dernbach AR. Carbohydrate feedings before, during, or in combination improve cycling endurance performance. J Appl Physiol 1991;71:1082–8.

Wu CL, Williams C. A low glycemic index meal before exercise improves endurance running capacity in men. Int J Sport Nutr Exerc Metab 2006;16:510–27.

CHAPTER 13

Fluid and carbohydrate intake during exercise

RON MAUGHAN

13.1 Introduction

Athletes know that performance improvements can result from ingestion of drinks during exercise lasting more than about 40–60 minutes. Drinking water is generally better than drinking nothing, but carbohydrate (CHO)-electrolyte drinks are generally more effective than plain water. Although ingestion of CHO and fluids can improve performance, this is not necessarily true for all individuals in all situations. The choice of food and fluids to be consumed during exercise will be influenced by a variety of factors, including the nature and duration of the event, the climatic conditions, the pre-event nutritional status, and the physiological and biochemical characteristics of the individual. The circumstances of each athlete, each sport and each competition must therefore be considered when making choices of what or whether to drink. In a few situations, athletes can get it wrong, and performance can suffer if the type or amount of food and fluid ingested are inappropriate. In recent years, several recreational participants in endurance events have died due to excessive consumption of fluids, so drinking too much may be even more harmful than drinking too little (Hew-Butler et al. 2008).

Food and fluid consumed during competition are part of a specific, short-term nutritional strategy aimed at maximizing performance at that particular time. When choosing foods and fluids to be consumed during competition, there is no need to take account of long-term nutritional goals, except, perhaps—and even then to a limited extent—in extreme endurance events such as the Tour de France or in multi-day running events. In the Tour de France, prolonged exercise is performed on a daily basis over about 21 days and the food consumed during each day's competition may account for about half of the total daily intake (Saris et al. 1989). A balanced diet is therefore not necessary, and intake is targeted at minimizing the impact of those factors that are responsible for fatigue and impaired performance.

New information continues to emerge, and this sometimes changes our understanding of the needs of athletes and the advice that is given to them. These new insights, however, have not resulted in fundamental changes in our understanding, and the challenge is more to provide athletes with the available information in a useful format than to generate further confirmations of what we already know. The most recent fluid replacement guidelines from the American College of Sports Medicine (Sawka et al. 2007), for example, are different in many ways from its earlier guidelines. In particular, there is an increased awareness of the need to individualize recommendations and for any guidelines to be sufficiently flexible to meet the needs of athletes with very different physical characteristics exercising in a range of environmental conditions.

Fatigue during exercise 13.2

In the exercise physiology laboratory, fatigue and the nutritional interventions that influence the fatigue process are studied intensively. The subjects used in these studies are often relatively sedentary, and although club-level athletes may sometimes participate, it is seldom possible to recruit a population of elite athletes willing to take part in such investigations. The experimental models used in laboratory studies also differ from the competitive situation, usually involving exercise at a constant power output that has to be continued for as long as possible. Even where intermittent exercise or time trial models are used to simulate sporting events, subjects usually exercise alone in an artificial environment without many of the stresses that accompany competition. Advice given to athletes is therefore based on extrapolations from the available information, and it is not surprising that opinions differ on many of the key issues.

The role of CHO in muscle metabolism and in exercise performance is discussed in detail in Chapter 1. The extensive literature on the subject makes it clear that the availability of an adequate supply of CHO in the working muscles and in the bloodstream is central to the athlete's ability to sustain an intensive training load and to perform well in competition. In warm environments, however, fatigue occurs while substantial CHO stores remain (Parkin et al. 1999), and performance is limited more by factors associated with thermoregulatory function and hydration status. The mechanisms by which performance is affected by these factors are not entirely clear, but there are well recognized effects on the brain (Meeusen et al. 2006; Maughan et al. 2007a). The idea that fatigue is fundamentally a phenomenon of the central nervous system rather than the peripheral tissues dates back to the observations of physiologists during the latter part of the nineteenth century (Bainbridge 1919). These observations point clearly to some of the nutritional strategies that the athlete might adopt to improve performance.

Carbohydrate supplementation during exercise 13.3

The ingestion of CHO during exercise has a number of effects on metabolism and can provide a number of benefits for performance. These effects are well described in relation to prolonged bouts of moderate-intensity and intermittent-intensity exercise, but recent studies suggest that CHO ingestion may also be useful for the performance of high-intensity exercise of about 1 hour's duration. This section will discuss these various benefits.

13.4 Prevention of hypoglycemia

The blood glucose concentration is normally maintained within a narrow range by regulation of the addition of glucose to the circulation and its removal by peripheral tissues. Glucose can be added from the gastrointestinal tract after food intake or from the liver, which stores about 80–100 g of glycogen in the fully fed state and can also synthesize glucose from non-CHO sources. The primary hormones regulating the blood glucose concentration are insulin and glucagon, but it is increasingly recognized that a large number of other peptide hormones also play key roles in this process, either directly or by influencing the circulating insulin and glucagon levels. Important hormones in this respect are growth hormone, cortisol, somatostatin and the catecholamines. Because of the obvious difficulties in making the relevant measurements, there is a limited amount of data on the changes in liver glycogen content during prolonged exercise, but it is clear that a progressive fall occurs, with low levels being reached when subjects are exhausted (Hultman & Nilsson 1971).

It is important to maintain the circulating blood glucose concentration above about 2.5 mmol/L to provide a concentration gradient for transport into glucose-requiring cells. The cells of the central nervous system have an absolute requirement for glucose as a fuel, and when the blood glucose concentration falls below this level, the rate of uptake by the brain may not be sufficient to meet its metabolic needs. Hypoglycemia leads to a variety of symptoms, including dizziness, nausea and disorientation. Hypoglycemia was one of the earliest medical problems identified in marathon runners suffering from fatigue and collapse at the end of a race. Levine and colleagues (1924) obtained blood samples from runners at the end of the 1923 Boston marathon race and observed that three of the twelve runners studied finished the race in a very poor condition; these individuals had a blood glucose concentration of less than 2.8 mmol/L.

These same authors recognized that CHO feeding during the race could prevent the onset of hypoglycemic symptoms; this was shown to be the case in the following year's race, and an improvement in performance was also reported when CHO was consumed (Gordon et al. 1925). CHO ingested during exercise will enter the blood glucose pool at a rate that will be dictated by the rates of gastric emptying and absorption from the intestine; if this exogenous CHO can substitute for the body's limited endogenous glycogen stores, then exercise capacity should be increased in situations where liver or muscle glycogen availability limits endurance.

Several studies have shown that the ingestion of even modest amounts of glucose during prolonged exercise will maintain or raise the circulating glucose concentration (Costill et al. 1973; Pirnay et al. 1982; Erickson et al. 1987). Glucose can be replaced by a variety of other sugars, including sucrose, glucose polymers and mixtures of sugars, without markedly affecting this response. Ingestion of large amounts of fructose can also maintain or elevate the blood glucose concentration at the end of prolonged exhausting exercise (Maughan et al. 1989), although some studies have not reported a marked effect (Erickson et al. 1987). Fructose is absorbed relatively slowly in the intestine, and must be converted by the liver to glucose before it can be oxidized by muscle. Tracer studies show that the maximum rate of oxidation of orally ingested fructose is less than that for glucose, sucrose or oligosaccharides (Wagenmakers et al. 1993; Jeukendrup 2008). Perhaps for this reason, the ingestion of solutions containing only fructose is not generally effective in improving performance of prolonged exercise (Maughan et al. 1989; Murray et al. 1989). Jeukendrup and colleagues have recently shown that the maximum oxidation rate of exogenous CHO can be greatly increased by ingestion of drinks containing mixtures of different CHO sources (Jentjens et al. 2004; Jentjens & Jeukendrup 2005; Wallis et al. 2005). These observations may help to explain why fructose in combination with other sugars seems to be well tolerated, and can result in improved performance (Murray et al. 1987). There are also some suggestions that the addition of small amounts of caffeine to ingested CHO-electrolyte drinks can stimulate the intestinal absorption of glucose (Van Nieuwenhoven et al. 2000) and increase the contribution of exogenous CHO oxidation to energy supply during exercise (Yeo et al. 2005). Hulston and Jeukendrup (2008), however, have recently reported that co-ingestion of caffeine and CHO during exercise enhanced cycling time trial performance by 4.6% compared with CHO alone and 9.0% compared with water placebo, but that caffeine did not influence exogenous CHO oxidation or glucose kinetics during steady state exercise.

Although these studies have focused on attempts to maximize the provision of exogenous CHO for oxidation, there is good evidence that provision of even small amounts of glucose may improve performance (Maughan et al. 1996), and providing increased amounts of CHO does not necessarily provide further performance benefits (Davis et al. 1988). This apparent limitation may be overcome to some degree by the careful choice of both amount of CHO and combinations of different CHOs (Jeukendrup et al. 2008). Nonetheless, there remains a finite limit to the rate at which CHO consumed during exercise can be oxidized.

Additional fuel to the exercising muscle during prolonged exercise 13.5

The liver is a relatively small organ, with a limited capacity to store CHO. Although the glycogen concentration in muscle tissue is much less than in the liver, the total muscle glycogen store is large, amounting to about 300–400 g in the average 70 kg, well-fed, sedentary individual. The addition of those qualifications indicates the influence of body size, especially muscle mass, nutritional status and training status on muscle glycogen storage. The requirement for CHO to be available as a fuel to support muscle metabolism during intense exercise is well known. In trained marathoners running at racing pace, the rate of CHO oxidation can be about 3–4 g per minute, but if this was sustained, the available CHO stores would be depleted long before the finish line was reached. Certainly in cycling (Hermansen et al. 1967) and perhaps also in running (Williams 1998), the point of fatigue in prolonged exercise coincides closely with the depletion of glycogen in the exercising muscles. Increasing muscle glycogen stores prior to exercise can also improve performance in both cycling (Ahlborg et al. 1967) and running (Karlsson & Saltin 1971). The picture has not changed significantly in the 40 years or so since the first studies showing this.

Where performance is limited by the size of the body's endogenous liver or muscle glycogen stores, exercise capacity should be improved when CHO is consumed. This assumes, of course, that the ingestion of CHO does not stimulate an increase in the rate of utilization of endogenous CHO reserves, and the evidence indicates that this is indeed so. Several studies have shown that the ingestion of glucose during prolonged intense exercise will prevent the development of hypoglycemia by maintaining or raising the circulating glucose concentration (Costill et al. 1973; Pirnay et al. 1982; Erickson et al. 1987). In prolonged exercise, performance—which was measured in most of the early studies as the time for which a fixed power output could be sustained—is improved by the addition of an energy source in the form of CHO. More recent studies have used a variety of different experimental models and have confirmed that this improvement in performance seems to apply also to other exercise models. Beneficial effects of CHO ingestion are seen during constant effort cycling (Coggan & Coyle 1991) as well as during running (Tsintzsas et al. 1993). Jeukendrup and colleagues (2008) recently showed that ingestion of a 6% CHO-electrolyte drink did not improve performance in a cycling time trial that could be completed in about 25 minutes. Improvements in performance have also been reported in cycling time trials carried out in the laboratory, and in a variety of running models, including intermittent shuttle running tests. Williams (1989) and Williams and colleagues (1990) have used an experimental model in which the subject is able to adjust the treadmill speed while running; the subject can then be encouraged either to cover the maximum distance possible in a fixed time or to complete a fixed distance in the fastest time possible. They showed that ingestion of 1 liter of a glucose polymer-sucrose (50 g/L) solution did not increase the total distance covered in a 2-hour run, but that the running speed was greater over the last 30 minutes of exercise when CHO was given compared with a placebo trial (Williams 1989). They observed a similar effect when a CHO solution (50 g of glucose–glucose polymer, or 50 g of fructose–glucose polymer) or water was given in a 30-kilometer treadmill time trial (Williams et al. 1990). The running speed decreased over the last 10 kilometers of the water trial, but was maintained in the other two runs; there was no significant difference between the three trials in the time taken to cover the total distance. As with cycling exercise, the conclusion must be that ingestion of CHO-containing drinks is generally effective in improving performance in events lasting about an hour or more.

This ergogenic effect was initially attributed to a sparing of the body's limited muscle glycogen stores by the oxidation of the ingested CHO (Hargreaves et al. 1984; Erickson et al. 1987), but other studies have failed to show a glycogen-sparing effect of CHO ingested during prolonged exercise (Coyle 1991). The current consensus view seems to be that there is probably little or no sparing of muscle glycogen utilization, although liver glucose release is slowed (Bosch et al. 1994; McConnell et al. 1994). The primary benefit of ingested CHO is probably its role in supplementing the endogenous stores in the later stages of exercise (Coyle 1997).

13.6 Amount and timing of carbohydrate intake

It is clear from tracer studies that a substantial part of the CHO ingested during exercise is available for oxidation. Early studies suggested that there is an upper limit of about 1 g/min to the rate at which ingested CHO can be oxidized, even when much larger amounts are ingested (Wagenmakers et al. 1993). This has been used as an argument to suggest that CHO should not be ingested at rates of more than 1 g/min, but these high rates of oxidation will not be achieved if the amount ingested is not in excess of this. In prolonged exercise, ingested CHO can account for between about 10% and 30% of the total amount of CHO oxidized (Hawley et al. 1992). Gastric emptying and intestinal absorption rates should allow for a faster rate of CHO supply, and the fate of that fraction of the ingested CHO that is not oxidized is not clear at the present time (Rehrer et al. 1992). Based on the feeding protocols used in studies that show performance enhancements, it has been suggested that CHO should be ingested at a rate of about 30–60 g/h (Coyle 1991; American College of Sports Medicine 1996). Of course, this is meant as a general guideline that must be adapted to the needs of each sport and each athlete. In many sports these general guidelines appear adequate and can be met simultaneously with fluid needs by consuming commercial CHO-electrolyte drinks (see section 13.10).

More recent studies, however, have shown that much higher intakes of CHO—up to 1.8 g/min—are not only able to increase the contribution of exogenous CHO to oxidative metabolism (Jeukendrup 2008), but also lead to improvements in cycling time trial performance (Currell & Jeukendrup 2008). The success of such strategies, however, will depend on the type of CHO used as well as on the amount, as discussed below.

Tracer studies show that little of the ingested CHO is oxidized during the first 60 minutes of exercise (Hawley et al. 1992), but there are several studies that suggest that CHO intake should begin early in exercise, or at least well in advance of the onset of fatigue. For example, McConell and colleagues (1996) studied eight well-trained men who rode for 2 hours at 70% of $VO_{2\ max}$, followed immediately by a 15-minute time trial. Subjects ingested either 250 mL of a 7 g/100 mL CHO solution every 15 minutes throughout exercise, or a placebo for 90 minutes followed by a 21 g/100 mL CHO beverage at 90, 105 and 120 minutes. Although the protocol in which CHO was ingested late in exercise allowed subjects to start the time trial with significantly elevated plasma glucose concentrations, they completed a greater amount of work during the 15 minutes when they had been fed CHO *throughout* exercise. These results suggest that CHO ingestion improves performance through mechanisms other than, or in addition to, an increased CHO availability to the contracting muscles.

Of course, in most sports, practical considerations dictate the timing and frequency of CHO (and fluid) intake during the event. During many endurance events (e.g. running and cycling), energy replacement occurs while the athlete is literally 'on the run'. Saris and colleagues (1989) reported that about half of the daily energy intake of Tour de France cyclists was ingested during each day's cycling stage. Intake is generally much less in running events of comparable duration, as few runners are able to tolerate solid food, even when the exercise intensity is low. Intake during competition may be limited by consideration of the time lost in stopping or slowing down to consume food or fluid, or the impact of such ingestion on gastrointestinal discomfort. In other events, such as team sports, there are formal and informal pauses in play, and these may provide an opportunity to consume CHO/fluid. Athletes should be encouraged to make use of the opportunities provided in their sport to consume fluid and additional CHO. Experimentation and practice in training and in minor competitions will help to determine the best strategies for each situation.

13.7 Type of carbohydrate

In most of the early studies, CHO ingested during exercise was in the form of glucose, but glucose, sucrose and oligosaccharides have all been shown to be effective in maintaining the blood glucose concentration and in improving endurance capacity when ingested during prolonged exercise (Maughan 1994). There are theoretical advantages in the use of sugars other than glucose. Substitution of glucose polymers for glucose will allow an increased CHO content without an increased osmolality. If the osmolality of ingested drinks is too high, there will be a net flux of water into the intestinal lumen, leading to a reduction in plasma volume and increasing the risk of gastrointestinal distress (Evans et al. 2009). The use of glucose polymers may also have taste advantages as these are less sweet than glucose or sucrose, but the available evidence suggests that the use of glucose polymers rather than free glucose does not alter the blood glucose response or the effect on exercise performance (Ivy et al. 1979; Coyle et al. 1983, 1986; Maughan et al. 1987; Coggan & Coyle 1988; Hargreaves & Briggs 1988). Similar effects are seen with the feeding of sucrose (Sasaki et al. 1987) or mixtures of sugars (Murray et al. 1987; Mitchell et al. 1988; Carter & Gisolfi 1989). Mixtures of glucose and fructose in equal amounts seem to have some advantages: when ingested in combination there is an increased total exogenous CHO oxidation (Adopo et al. 1994). More recently, the rates of oxidation of various sugars when ingested singly or in combination have been systematically investigated by Jeukendrup and colleagues (Jentjens et al. 2004; Jentjens & Jeukendrup 2005; Jeukendrup 2008). These results seem to confirm speculation that intestinal transport is the rate-limiting step in the oxidation of CHO and that the ingestion of multiple CHOs that rely on different intestinal transporters may not only increase the rate of uptake and oxidation of ingested CHOs but also of water absorption (Shi et al. 1995). Fructose in high concentrations is generally best avoided on account of the risk of gastrointestinal upset. The argument advanced in favor of the ingestion of fructose during exercise, namely that it provides a readily available energy source but does not stimulate insulin release and consequent inhibition of fatty acid mobilization, is in any case not well founded: insulin secretion is suppressed during exercise. Some studies have suggested that long-chain glucose polymer solutions are more readily used by the muscles during exercise than are glucose or fructose solutions (Noakes 1990), but others have found no difference in the oxidation rates of ingested glucose or glucose polymer (Massicote et al. 1989; Rehrer 1990). Massicote and colleagues (1989) also found that ingested fructose was less readily oxidized than glucose or glucose polymers.

13.8 Effects on performance of other exercise events

Although most studies of the beneficial effects of CHO ingestion in exercise have concerned prolonged moderate-intensity or intermittent high-intensity exercise, recent studies have identified other situations of potential benefit. Studies in field situations, or in laboratory settings simulating competition, have shown that CHO ingestion during team and racquet games, sometimes (Vergauwen et al. 1998) but not always (Zeederberg et al. 1996) enhances measures of mental and physical skill by reducing the impairment seen with fatigue. Of considerable interest is the growing number of studies to report benefits of CHO ingestion during the performance of high-intensity exercise lasting about 1 hour (Below et al. 1995; Jeukendrup et al. 1997; Millard-Stafford et al. 1997). In these situations, the intake of a CHO drink was shown to enhance the performance of running and cycling time trials (~10 minutes) undertaken at the end of ~50 minutes of exercise, or cycling time trials lasting 1 hour. These studies have been reviewed by Coyle (2004). CHO availability to the muscle is not considered to be limiting in the performance of such exercise, and further research is needed to confirm and explain the effects. It is possible that benefits to 'central performance', involving the brain and nervous system, are involved. This hypothesis is given some support by the observation from a trial where a 6.4% maltodextrin solution (CHO) was rinsed around the mouth at intervals during a time trial lasting about 1 hour (Carter et al. 2004). Subjects were not allowed to swallow either the CHO solution or a water placebo, and each mouthful was spat out after a 5-second rinse. Performance time was significantly improved with CHO compared with the placebo (59.57 +/– 1.50 min versus 61.37 +/– 1.56 min, respectively, $p = 0.011$). There is some subsequent support for this finding (Rollo et al. 2008) but others have not been able to reproduce this performance benefit (Whitham & McKinney 2007), so further investigation is required.

Other effects of carbohydrate ingestion

13.9

Athletes in hard training are anxious to avoid any illness or injury that might interrupt training. These athletes may, however, be more susceptible than the sedentary individual to minor opportunistic infections, particularly those affecting the upper respiratory tract (Nieman & Pedersen 1999). While not serious in themselves, the disruption to training can have negative physical and psychological effects. Several reviews of the literature (Shephard 1997; Gleeson et al. 2004) suggest that exercise-induced increases in the release of catecholamines and glucocorticoids may be responsible for the reduced effectiveness of the immune system. Ingestion of CHO during exercise is effective in attenuating the rise in circulating catecholamine and cortisol concentrations that is normally observed during prolonged strenuous exercise, and has also been reported to reduce some of the immuno-suppressive effects of exercise (Nieman et al. 1997). In contrast to this finding, Bishop and colleagues (1999) reported that ingestion of a CHO drink before and during 90 minutes of an exercise session designed to simulate soccer match play had no effect on circulating cortisol concentration or on a number of markers of immune function. Notwithstanding the lack of an effect observed in this last study, it does seem that benefits may accrue to the athlete in hard training from the ingestion of CHO-containing drinks during each prolonged training session. The potential role of CHO ingestion during prolonged exercise as a strategy for staying well is covered in more detail in Commentary C, 'Nutrition for the athlete's immune system' (see page 501).

Another piece of evidence suggests that CHO ingestion during exercise may promote recovery of muscle glycogen stores in the post-exercise period (Kuo et al. 1999). In this study, rats performed two 3-hour swimming bouts, separated by 45 minutes of rest, to deplete muscle glycogen stores. A 50% glucose solution was administered by stomach tube at the end of each of the exercise bouts. CHO feeding resulted in glycogen super-compensation at 16 hours after exercise, an effect attributed to a stimulation of GLUT-4 protein expression in response to CHO. This suggests another reason for ingestion of CHO during exercise that is likely to result in substantial depletion of the muscle glycogen stores; this effect will be of particular significance when a second exercise bout—whether training or another competition—must follow after a short interval.

Effects of hyperthermia and dehydration on performance

13.10

It is a matter of common experience that the perception of effort is increased, and exercise capacity reduced, in hot climates. This was recognized by the early pedestrians: in a challenge race held in Curacao in August, 1808, the local man chose to start the race at the hottest time of day to gain an advantage over his European opponent, Lieutenant Fairman. Notwithstanding his disadvantage, Fairman won, but he declared the event to be much more stressful than any other event he participated in (Thom 1813). More recently, and under more controlled conditions, the effects of increasing ambient temperature were quantified when Galloway and Maughan (1997) showed that exercise capacity at a fixed power output was greatly reduced at 31°C (55 minutes) compared to the same exercise performed at 11°C (93 minutes). They also observed that the exercise time was already reduced (to 81 minutes) at the comparatively modest temperature of 21°C. Parkin and colleagues (1999) have shown similar effects and also showed that there remained a substantial amount of muscle glycogen at the point of fatigue when the ambient temperature was high (40°C).

When the ambient temperature is higher than skin temperature, the only mechanism by which heat can be lost from the body is evaporation of water from the skin and respiratory tract. Complete evaporation of 1 liter of water from the skin will remove 2.4 MJ (580 kcal) of heat from the body, and sweat losses are determined primarily by the intensity and duration of exercise and by the ambient temperature and humidity. Data for typical sweat losses in a range of sports activities have been compiled by Rehrer and Burke (1996). However, sweat rates vary greatly between individuals, even when the metabolic rate is apparently similar, and high sweat rates are sometimes necessary even at low ambient temperatures if an excessive rise in body temperature is to be prevented (Maughan 1985).

Water losses are derived in varying proportions from plasma, extracellular water, and intracellular water. Any decrease in plasma volume is likely to adversely affect thermal regulation and exercise capacity. When the metabolic rate is high, blood flow to the muscles must be maintained at a high level to supply oxygen and substrates, but a high blood flow to the skin is also necessary to convect heat to the body surface, where it can be dissipated (Nadel 1990). When the ambient temperature is high and blood volume has been decreased by sweat loss during prolonged exercise, there may be difficulty in meeting the requirement for a high blood flow to both these tissues. In this situation, skin blood flow is likely to be compromised, allowing body temperature to rise but preventing a catastrophic fall in central venous pressure (Rowell 1986). Muscle blood flow is also reduced, but oxygen extraction is increased to maintain oxidative energy metabolism (Gonzalez-Alonso et al. 1999).

Montain and Coyle have also investigated these factors and found that increases in core temperature and heart rate during prolonged exercise are graded according to the level of hypohydration achieved (Montain & Coyle 1992a). They also showed that the ingestion of fluid during exercise increases skin blood flow, and therefore thermoregulatory capacity, independent of increases in the circulating blood volume (Montain & Coyle 1992b). Plasma volume expansion using dextran/saline infusion was less effective in preventing a rise in core temperature than was the ingestion of sufficient volumes of a CHO-electrolyte drink to maintain plasma volume at a similar level. This suggests that oral intake achieves beneficial effects other than the maintenance of blood volume.

It is often reported that exercise performance is impaired when an individual is dehydrated by as little as 2% of body weight, and that losses in excess of 5% of body weight can decrease the capacity for work by about 30% (Saltin & Costill 1988). Although this observation has been broadly confirmed by later studies, the original data on which it is based are obscure. Dehydration can compromise performance in high-intensity exercise as well as endurance activities (Nielsen et al. 1982; Armstrong et al. 1985). Although sweat losses during brief exercise are small, prior dehydration (by as much as 10% of body mass) is common in weight-category sports where participants are often hypohydrated during competition (see Chapter 7). Nielsen and colleagues (1982) showed that prolonged exercise, which resulted in a loss of fluid corresponding to 2.5% of body weight, resulted in a 45% fall in the capacity to perform high-intensity exercise. It may be that even very small fluid deficits impair performance, but the methods used to measure performance are not sufficiently sensitive to detect small changes. Walsh and colleagues (1994) have reported that a fluid deficit of less than 2% of body mass results in impaired performance of a time-trial task.

The mechanisms responsible for the reduced exercise performance in the heat are not entirely clear, but Nielsen and colleagues (1993) have proposed that the high core temperature itself is involved. This proposition was based on the observation that a period of acclimatization was successful in delaying the point of fatigue, but that this occurred at the same core temperature. The primary effect of acclimatization was to lower the resting core temperature, and the rate of rise of temperature was the same on all trials. This observation is further supported by numerous studies that show that manipulation of the body heat content prior to exercise can alter exercise capacity: performance is extended by prior immersion in cold water and reduced by prior immersion in hot water (Gonzalez-Alonso et al. 1999).

Hypernatremia and hyponatremia

13.11

The sweat loss that accompanies prolonged exercise leads to a loss of electrolytes and water from the body. Although the volume loss is easily estimated from changes in body mass after correction for substrate oxidation and respiratory water loss, electrolyte loss is rather more difficult to quantify and the extent of these losses has been the subject of much debate. The values for sweat electrolyte content in Table 13.1 show the great inter-individual variability in the concentration of the major electrolytes.

Sodium, the most abundant cation of the extracellular space, is the major electrolyte in sweat; chloride, which is also mainly located in the extracellular space, is the major anion. This ensures that the greatest fraction of fluid loss is derived from the extracellular space, including the plasma. Although the composition of sweat is highly variable, sweat is always hypotonic with regard to body fluids, and the net effect of sweat loss is an increase in plasma osmolality. The plasma concentration of sodium and potassium also generally increases, suggesting that replacement of these electrolytes during exercise may not be necessary. There may, however, be a need to replace some of the sodium lost in sweat when these losses are high. Some indication of the extent of the individual variability in sweat electrolyte losses that can occur comes from reports of salt losses in football (soccer) players during training (Maughan et al. 2004; Shirreffs et al. 2005). Some players lost less than 2 g of salt (sodium chloride) in a 90-minute training session, while others incurred losses of close to 10 g. Substantial salt losses were also seen in some, but not all, players training in cold (5°C) conditions (Maughan et al. 2005).

Most participants in endurance events such as a marathon race or triathlon finish the event having lost more fluid than they consumed and are therefore relatively hypohydrated (Whiting et al. 1984). There have, however, been numerous publications in the scientific and medical literature over the last twenty years or so drawing attention to the fact that some participants in endurance events consume more fluid than they lose and therefore

TABLE 13.1 CONCENTRATION, IN MMOL/L, OF THE MAJOR ELECTROLYTES PRESENT IN SWEAT, PLASMA AND IN INTRACELLULAR (MUSCLE) WATER IN HUMANS

	PLASMA	SWEAT	INTRACELLULAR
Sodium	137–144	40–80	10
Potassium	3.5–4.9	4–8	148
Calcium	4.4–5.2	3–4	0–2
Magnesium	1.5–2.1	1–4	30–40
Chloride	100–108	30–70	2

Sources: The values are collated from a variety of sources: see Maughan 1994 for further details

complete the event in a hyperhydrated state (Noakes 2003). The main danger of excessive water intake is the development of hyponatremia; while often asymptomatic, this condition, if severe, can result in nausea, collapse, loss of consciousness, and even death. Early reports related almost exclusively to participants in ultra-endurance events where exercise intensity, and therefore sweat rate, was low and where opportunities for fluid intake were plentiful (Noakes et al. 1985, 1990; Hiller 1989). Noakes and colleagues (1985) reported four cases of exercise-induced hyponatremia; race times were between 7 and 10 hours, and post-race serum sodium concentrations were between 115 and 125 mmol/L. Estimated fluid intakes were between 6 and 12 liters, consisting of water or drinks containing low levels of electrolytes; estimated total sodium chloride intake during the race was 20–40 mmol. Frizell and colleagues (1986) reported even more astonishing fluid intakes of 20–24 L of fluids (an intake of almost 2.5 L/h sustained for a period of many hours, which is in excess of the maximum gastric emptying rate that has been reported) with a mean sodium content of only 5–10 mmol/L in two runners who collapsed after an ultramarathon run and who were found to be hyponatremic (serum sodium concentration 118–123 mmol/L).

A study of 488 participants in the 2002 Boston Marathon revealed that 13% had a serum sodium concentration equal to or less than 135 mmol/L, and were therefore diagnosed as being hyponatremic (Almond et al. 2005). Analysis of the results suggested that a substantial increase in body mass while running, a slow finishing time, and body-mass-index extremes were associated with hyponatremia; although female runners with low body mass had earlier been suggested to be at particular risk of this condition, the results did not support this. These results suggest that medical staff should be alert to the possibility of hyponatremia occurring in this situation, but this should not divert attention from the fact that most competitors will be both hypohydrated and hypernatremic. What is apparent is that participants in endurance events should not drink so much that they gain weight during the event (Sawka et al. 2007; Hew-Butler et al. 2008). Risk factors for the development of hyponatremia identified by Hew-Butler and colleagues (2008) are shown in Table 13.2.

TABLE 13.2 RISK FACTORS FOR THE DEVELOPMENT OF HYPONATREMIA
ATHLETE-RELATED
• Excessive drinking behavior
• Weight gain during exercise
• Low body weight
• Female sex
• Slow running or performance pace
• Event inexperience
• Non-steroidal anti-inflammatory agents
EVENT-RELATED
• High availability of drinking fluids
• >4 hours exercise duration
• Unusually hot conditions
• Extreme cold temperature

As outlined above, there are obvious benefits from the ingestion of fluids during exercise, and participants in endurance events should be encouraged to drink on a regular basis. There is, however, a need to apply common sense: slow runners on a cold day will lose little or no sweat and the primary need is for CHO intake. Drinking small amounts of concentrated CHO drinks will be an effective strategy. Fast runners in the heat may need to drink at a faster rate and are more likely to benefit from more dilute CHO-electrolyte drinks (Coyle 2004). It seems sensible to recommend that runners should drink enough to limit weight loss to not more than about 2% of body mass (Sawka et al. 2007) and perhaps even less than this on hot days. This recommendation puts some responsibility on the individual to experiment with different drinking strategies during training, but it cannot cater for the individual who enters a marathon to raise money for charity or for other reasons without having undertaken any preparation.

Fluid replacement and exercise performance

13.12

Most of the early studies carried out to investigate the effects of dehydration and rehydration on exercise in a military setting used very prolonged walking exercise as an experimental model and water as the fluid replacement. More recent studies have used a variety of exercise models more relevant to competitive sports situations, and most have investigated the effects of CHO-electrolyte drinks rather than of plain water. There have, however, been a few studies where the effects of plain water or of CHO-free electrolyte solutions have been investigated. In prolonged exercise at low intensity, water may be as effective as dilute saline solutions (Barr et al. 1991) or nutrient-electrolyte solutions (Levine et al. 1991) in maintaining cardiovascular and thermoregulatory function. Maughan and colleagues (1996) had twelve male subjects exercise to fatigue at about 70% of $VO_{2\,max}$ on four occasions after appropriate familiarization tests. When subjects ingested plain water (100 mL every 10 minutes) median exercise time was longer (93 minutes) than when no drink was given (81 minutes). Subjects also completed trials where dilute CHO-electrolyte drinks were given and these also resulted in extended exercise time compared to the no-drink trial. In a prolonged (90-minute) intermittent high-intensity shuttle running test designed to simulate the demands of competitive soccer, McGregor and colleagues (1999) found that ingestion of flavored water (5 mL/kg before the test and 2 mL/kg at 15-minute intervals) was effective in preventing a decline in performance of a soccer-specific skilled task. When no fluid was given, performance deteriorated.

It is clear that the addition of CHO has a number of potential benefits that may be important for performance (see sections 13.4–13.8). The separate effects of providing fluid and CHO were investigated by Below and colleagues (1995), who used an experimental model where subjects performed 50 minutes of exercise at about 80% of $VO_{2\,max}$ followed by a time trial where a set amount of work had to be completed as fast as possible. During the initial 50 minutes of exercise, subjects were given either a small volume (200 mL) of water, a small volume of water with added CHO (40% solution, 79 g maltodextrin), a large volume (1330 mL) of flavored water, or a large volume of water with the same amount of CHO as in the other CHO trial (as a 6% solution). They found water ingestion to be effective in improving performance; exercise time was 11.34 minutes on the placebo trial and 10.51 minutes on the water trial. Exercise time on the CHO trial was 10.55 minutes, indicating that CHO provision during exercise acted independently to improve performance, and the effects were found to be additive, with the shortest time (9.93 minutes) when the 6% CHO drink was given.

The results of these and other studies—see Maughan and Shirreffs (1998) for a review—suggest that fluid replacement is effective in improving exercise performance in a variety of different situations, and that an additional benefit is gained by the addition of CHO, and possibly also of electrolytes, to fluids ingested during exercise. The optimum formulation of drinks for use in different exercise situations has not, however, been clearly established at the present time.

13.13 Guidelines for replacing fluid and carbohydrate during exercise

The major components of the sports drink that can be manipulated to alter its functional properties are shown in Table 13.3. To some extent these factors can be manipulated independently, although addition of increasing amounts of CHO or electrolyte will generally be accompanied by an increase in osmolality, and alterations in the solute content will have an impact on taste characteristics, mouth feel and palatability.

As well as providing an energy substrate for the working muscles, the addition of CHO to ingested drinks will promote water absorption in the small intestine, provided the concentration is not too high. Because of the role of sugars and sodium in promoting water uptake in the small intestine, it is sometimes difficult to separate the effects of water replacement from those of substrate and electrolyte replacement when CHO-electrolyte solutions are ingested. Below and colleagues (1995) have shown that ingestion of CHO and water had separate and additive effects on exercise performance, and concluded that ingestion of dilute CHO solutions would optimize performance. Most reviews of the available literature have come to the same conclusion (Lamb & Brodowicz 1986; Murray 1987; Coyle & Hamilton 1990; Maughan & Shirreffs 1998).

13.14 Carbohydrate content

The amount of CHO and the types of CHO present in a drink will influence its efficacy when consumed during exercise. The optimum concentration of CHO to be added to a sports drink will depend on individual circumstances. High CHO concentrations will delay gastric emptying, thus reducing the amount of fluid that is available for absorption, but will increase the rate of CHO delivery. If the concentration is high enough to result in a markedly hypertonic solution, net secretion of water into the intestine will result, and this will

TABLE 13.3 VARIABLES THAT CAN BE MANIPULATED TO ALTER THE FUNCTIONAL CHARACTERISTICS OF A SPORTS DRINK

- CHO content: concentration and type
- Osmolality
- Electrolyte composition and concentration
- Flavoring components
- Other active ingredients

actually increase the danger of dehydration. High concentrations of sugars (>10%) may also result in gastrointestinal disturbances (Davis et al. 1988). Where the primary need is to supply an energy source during exercise, increasing the sugar content of drinks will increase the delivery of CHO to the site of absorption in the small intestine. Beyond a certain limit, however, simply increasing CHO intake will not continue to increase the rate of oxidation of exogenous CHO (Wagenmakers et al. 1993). Dilute glucose-electrolyte solutions may also be as effective, or even more effective, in improving performance as more concentrated solutions (Davis et al. 1988), and adding as little as 90 mmol/L (about 16 g/L or 1.6%) glucose may improve endurance performance (Maughan et al. 1996).

The consequences of severe dehydration and hyperthermia are potentially fatal, but the symptoms of CHO depletion are usually nothing more than severe fatigue. It seems sensible, therefore, to favor more dilute solutions, especially when training or competing in warm weather.

Osmolality

13.15

It has become common to refer to CHO-electrolyte sports drinks as isotonic drinks, as though the tonicity was their most important characteristic. The osmolality of ingested fluids is important as this can influence the rates of both gastric emptying and intestinal water flux; both of these processes together will determine the effectiveness of rehydration fluids at delivering water for rehydration and substrate for oxidation (Schedl et al. 1994). Ingestion of strongly hypertonic drinks will promote net secretion of water into the intestine and, although this effect is transient, it will result in a temporary exacerbation of the extent of dehydration. The composition of the drinks and the nature of the solutes is, however, of greater importance than the osmolality itself (Maughan 1994).

Osmolality is identified as an important factor influencing the rate of gastric emptying of liquid meals, but there seems to be rather little effect of variations in the concentration of electrolytes on the emptying rate, even when this substantially changes the test meal osmolality (Rehrer 1990). The effect of increasing osmolality seems to be important only when nutrient-containing solutions are examined, and energy density is undoubtedly the most significant factor influencing the rate of gastric emptying (Brener et al. 1983; Vist & Maughan 1994). There is some evidence that substitution of glucose polymers for free glucose, which will result in a decreased osmolality for the same CHO content, may be effective in increasing the volume of fluid and the amount of substrate delivered to the intestine. This is one reason for the inclusion of glucose polymers of varying chain length in the formulation of sports drinks. Vist and Maughan (1995) have shown that there is an acceleration of emptying when glucose polymer solutions are substituted for free glucose solutions with the same energy density. At low (about 40 g/L) concentrations, this effect is small, but it becomes appreciable at higher (180 g/L) concentrations; where the osmolality is the same (as in the 40 g/L glucose solution and 180 g/L polymer solution), the energy density is of far greater significance in determining the rate of gastric emptying. This effect may therefore be important when large amounts of energy must be replaced after exercise, but is unlikely to be a major factor during exercise where more dilute drinks are taken.

Water absorption occurs largely in the proximal segment of the small intestine and, although water movement is itself a passive process driven by local osmotic gradients, it is closely linked to the active transport of solute (Schedl et al. 1994). Net flux is determined largely by the osmotic gradient between the lumenal contents and intracellular fluid of the cells lining the intestine. Absorption of glucose is an active, energy-consuming process linked to the transport of sodium. The rate of glucose uptake is dependent on the lumenal concentrations of glucose and sodium, and dilute glucose-electrolyte solutions with an osmolality that is slightly hypotonic with respect to plasma will maximize the rate of water uptake (Wapnir & Lifshitz 1985). Solutions with a very high glucose concentration will not necessarily promote an increased glucose uptake relative to more dilute solutions, but, because of their high osmolality, will cause a net movement of fluid into the intestinal lumen (Gisolfi et al. 1990). This results in an effective loss of body water and will exacerbate any pre-existing dehydration. Other sugars, such as sucrose (Spiller et al. 1982) or glucose polymers (Jones et al. 1983, 1987), can be substituted for glucose without impairing glucose or water uptake, and may help by increasing the total transportable substrate without increasing osmolality. In contrast, iso-energetic solutions of fructose and glucose are isosmotic, and the absorption of fructose is not an active process in humans: it is absorbed less rapidly than glucose and promotes less water uptake (Fordtran 1975). The use of different sugars that are absorbed by different mechanisms and that might thus promote increased water uptake is supported by more recent evidence from an intestinal perfusion study (Shi et al. 1995).

Although most of the popular sports drinks are formulated to have an osmolality close to that of body fluids (Maughan 1994), and are promoted as isotonic drinks, there is good evidence that hypotonic solutions are more effective when rapid rehydration is desired (Wapnir & Lifshitz 1985). Although it is argued that a higher osmolality is inevitable when adequate amounts of CHO are to be included in sports drinks, the optimum amount of CHO necessary to improve exercise performance has not been clearly established.

13.16 Electrolyte composition and concentration

The available evidence indicates that the only electrolyte that should be added to drinks consumed during exercise is sodium, which is usually added in the form of sodium chloride (Maughan 1994). Sodium will stimulate sugar and water uptake in the small intestine and will help to maintain extracellular fluid volume. There is much debate as to the optimum sodium concentration, and it has been argued that equilibration occurs so rapidly in the upper part of the small intestine that addition of high concentrations of sodium is not necessary (Schedl et al. 1994). Although most soft drinks of the cola or lemonade variety contain virtually no sodium (1–2 mmol/L), sports drinks commonly contain about 10–30 mmol/L sodium and oral rehydration solutions intended for use in the treatment of diarrhea-induced dehydration, which may be fatal, have higher sodium concentrations, in the range 30–90 mmol/L. A high sodium content, although it may stimulate jejunal absorption of glucose and water, tends to make drinks unpalatable, and it is important that drinks intended for ingestion during or after exercise should have a pleasant taste in order to stimulate consumption. Specialist sports drinks are generally formulated to strike a balance between the twin aims of efficacy and palatability, although it must be admitted that not all achieve either of these aims.

13.17 Taste

Taste is an important factor influencing the consumption of fluids, and the choice of anion to accompany sodium may be important in this regard. The thirst mechanism is rather insensitive and will not stimulate drinking behavior until some degree of dehydration has been incurred (Hubbard et al. 1990). This absence of a drive to drink is reflected in the rather small volumes of fluid that are typically consumed during exercise. In endurance running events, voluntary intake seldom exceeds about 0.5 L/h (Noakes 1993), and seems to be largely unrelated to the sweating rate. Because the sweat losses normally exceed this, even in cool conditions, a fluid deficit is almost inevitable whenever prolonged exercise is performed. Anything that stimulates drinking behavior is therefore likely to be advantageous, and palatability is clearly important. Several factors will influence palatability, and the addition of a variety of flavors has been shown to increase fluid intake relative to that ingested when only plain water is available. Hubbard and colleagues (1984) and Szlyk and colleagues (1989) found that the addition of flavorings resulted in an increased consumption (by about 50%) of fluid during prolonged exercise. More recently, Bar-Or and Wilk (1996) have shown that the fluid intake during exercise of children presented with a variety of flavored drinks is very much influenced by taste preference; under the conditions of this study, sufficient fluid to offset sweat losses was ingested only when a grape-flavored beverage was available. In many of these studies, the addition of CHOs and/or electrolytes accompanied the flavoring agent, and the results must be interpreted with some degree of caution.

Given the need to add electrolytes to fluids intended to maximize the effectiveness of rehydration, there are clearly palatability issues that influence the formulation. Effective post-exercise rehydration requires replacement of electrolyte losses as well as the ingestion of a volume of fluid in excess of the volume of sweat loss (Shirreffs et al. 1996) (see section 13.10). When sweat electrolyte losses are high, replacement with drinks with a high sodium content can result in an unpalatable product. This can be alleviated to a large degree by substituting other anions for the chloride that is normally added. The addition of CHO has a major impact on taste and mouth feel, and a variety of different sugars with different taste characteristics can be added.

Temperature of ingested drinks 13.18

As well as affecting the taste and perceived pleasantness of drinks, the temperature at which they are ingested may have implications for exercise performance. When cold drinks are ingested, heat must be added to raise them to body temperature: if the volume of fluid ingested is large and the temperature differential is also large, a measurable fall in body temperature will occur. It is well recognized that performance of prolonged exercise in warm environments can be improved by prior immersion in cool water to lower body temperature (Gonzalez-Alonso et al. 1999), and there is emerging evidence that ingestion of cold drinks may have similar benefits. Wimer and colleagues (1997) found that, compared with the ingestion of approximately 1350 ml of water at 38°C, ingestion of the same volume of drinks at 0.5°C attenuated the rise in rectal temperature (T_{re}) during 2 hours of recumbent cycling at 51% $VO_{2\ peak}$ in a temperate environment (26°C, relative humidity 40%).

This observation was confirmed by Lee and Shirreffs (2007), who found that acute ingestion of 1 liter of drink at 10°C during 90 minutes of cycling at 53% $VO_{2\ peak}$ in a moderate environment (25°C, relative humidity 61%) was more effective in attenuating the rise in T_{re} than was ingestion of the same drink at 50°C. When drinks at 10°C and 50°C were consumed in four smaller aliquots of 400 ml each at intervals during 90 minutes of cycling at 50% $VO_{2\ peak}$ in a similar moderate environment (25°C, relative humidity 60%), the absolute rise in T_{re} at the end of exercise was similar. This can be explained by the initiation of appropriate thermoregulatory reflexes associated with ingestion of the cool and hot drinks (Lee et al. 2008a). Lee and colleagues (2008b) subsequently reported that time to fatigue in a cycling test at 66% of $VO_{2\,peak}$ in a hot (35°C), humid (relative humidity 60%) environment was improved when a drink ingested at intervals before and during exercise was given at a temperature of 4°C rather than 37°C.

13.19 Monitoring individual fluid needs

It is a matter of everyday observation that some people sweat more than others, even when the exercise and environmental conditions are the same. The crusted salt deposits that can be seen on the exercise clothing worn by some athletes also show them to be salty sweaters. From the information presented in the preceding section, it is also apparent that some athletes drink much more than others and that the match between what athletes choose to drink and their fluid needs is far from perfect. In addition, it must be remembered that most laboratory studies are conducted on subjects who are rested, fed and well hydrated prior to exercise; in the real world, many athletes may begin exercise while still recovering from an earlier exercise session and may be hypohydrated at the start of exercise.

Pre-exercise hydration status can be assessed in several different ways, but urine markers, especially color (Armstrong 2000) and osmolality (Shirreffs & Maughan 1998), are perhaps most reliable. Recent data suggest that many football players begin training with elevated urine osmolality, suggestive of significant hypohydration (Maughan et al. 2004; Shirreffs et al. 2005). A similar situation applies in the competitive environment, with as many as one-third of football players providing urine samples with an osmolality in excess of 900 mosmol/kg upon reporting for a competitive game (Maughan et al. 2007b).

It is often recommended that athletes should drink sufficient fluid during exercise to prevent any fall in body mass, as if this indicated a match between fluid intake and sweat losses. However, there is some loss of body mass during exercise due to substrate oxidation, and also some gain in body water due to the water of oxidation formed by oxidation of these fuels. It is also not apparent that there is an absolute need to replace all fluid losses. Two factors must be considered: the level of fluid deficit—or body mass loss—at which a decrement in performance occurs, and the potential benefit of the reduced body mass that follows from sweat loss in those sports where body mass must be supported. Body mass losses of up to 3% may be tolerable in cool environments without performance impairments, though smaller losses are tolerable in the heat (Coyle 2004). It might be more appropriate, therefore, to advise athletes to monitor their body mass losses during training or competition, and to drink sufficient to restrict body mass loss to not more than 1–2% of the initial value. This advice takes account of individual variations in sweating rate and in drinking behaviors, and also allows athletes to adjust drinking strategies to take account of the duration and intensity of an exercise session and of the climatic conditions. It does mean, though, that athletes must be willing to make these simple measures on themselves during training to allow anticipation of likely sweat losses in differing situations.

13.20 Summary

The intake of fluid and CHO offers benefits to the performance of a number of sports events and exercise activities. The effects of dehydration on performance are now well known, with the penalties ranging from subtle, but often important, decrements in performance at low levels of fluid deficit to the severe health risks associated with substantial fluid losses during exercise in the heat. Although evidence of the beneficial effects of CHO intake during exercise has existed for over 70 years, sports scientists are still to discover all the situations in which benefits occur and to explain the mechanisms involved. Optimal strategies for CHO and fluid intake during exercise will be determined by practical issues such as the opportunity to eat or drink during an event and gastrointestinal comfort. Variations in individual physiology and biochemistry will influence substrate use and sweat losses, so athletes must take responsibility for developing their personal plan based on individual circumstances.

PRACTICE TIPS

MICHELLE MINEHAN

NON-ENDURANCE SPORTS: EVENTS OF LESS THAN 30 MINUTES' DURATION

- The primary concern is minimal interference to competition.
- Recommendations:
  - Begin exercise in a well-hydrated condition.
  - Replace fluid losses between competition sessions.
- Athletes commonly approach competition in a hypohydrated condition as a result of failing to replace daily body fluid losses or as a result of deliberate dehydration strategies that are undertaken to 'make weight' in weight-limited sports (see Chapter 7). Exercising in a hypohydrated condition increases the risk of thermal injury and may reduce performance.
- Fluid ingested during exercise of less than 30 minutes' duration will not benefit performance, as it will not become available to the body within the timeframe of the competition. However, the ingestion of fluid may offer some advantages such as to alleviate dry mouth and improve perceived exertion. Athletes must weigh up any perceived benefits of drinking during exercise against potential disadvantages such as increased body mass and having to slow down to drink.
- Athletes competing in tournament situations or multiple events should aim to rehydrate between sessions to avoid a progressive dehydration over the competition.

EVENTS OF 30–60 MINUTES' DURATION

- The primary concerns are fluid intake with some support for CHO provision.
- Recommendations:
  - Begin exercise well hydrated.
  - Using a fluid intake plan that has been practiced in training, drink at a rate that is comfortable and practical to replace most of the fluid lost by sweating.
  - Use a beverage that is cool (15–20°C), palatable and provides CHO.
  - Ingest beverage regularly to maintain gastric volume and increase fluid availability.
  - Make the most of opportunities to drink within the confines and environment of the sport.
  - Replace fluid losses between competition sessions.
- Theoretically, athletes should aim to drink enough to offset most of their fluid losses. In practical terms, athletes should aim to drink as much as is comfortable and practical without exceeding the rate of their sweat losses so that they gain weight over the course of the event. Individuals vary enormously in their rates of gastric emptying, sweat loss and tolerance of fluid volume. Therefore each athlete must devise an individualized drinking schedule that is the best compromise between minimizing gastrointestinal discomfort and the time taken to drink, and minimizing the risk of dehydration. A guide to fluid requirements can be provided by weighing athletes before and after exercise

sessions to estimate fluid losses (see Fig. 13.1). A fluid replacement plan can then be developed, and practiced and refined during training. By experimenting and practicing, it is possible for athletes to train themselves to tolerate greater volumes and learn to drink at a rate that matches sweat losses as closely as possible. Hydration regimens should always be practiced in training before trying them in competitive situations.

- The volume of fluid ingested is more important than the timing, but drinking regularly will help to maintain a high rate of gastric emptying, as fluids leave the stomach faster when gastric volume is high. It also makes sense to begin drinking early in competition to minimize dehydration rather than trying to reverse a severe deficit later in competition.
- A supplementary source of CHO during exercise has been shown to improve performance of events of about 1 hour's duration, where fatigue would otherwise occur. A general recommendation of 30–60 g CHO per hour is suggested. Most sports drinks contain 60–80 g/L, making these rates of CHO ingestion easy to achieve. Gastric emptying slows as the energy density and osmolality of the fluid increase but solutions of up to 8% CHO can generally be tolerated, especially if a high gastric volume is maintained. Beverages that contain more than 8% CHO are more likely to cause gastrointestinal distress.
- Sodium chloride replacement is not necessary in short exercise periods, but the inclusion of sodium chloride in a sports drink may promote fluid retention in the extracellular compartment, help maintain the osmotic drive to drink and improve the palatability of the drink. Fluids will be consumed in greater amounts when they taste palatable during exercise, are kept cool (15–20°C), are served in a user-friendly container and are readily accessible.

1. Weigh athletes before and after training in minimal clothing and after towel-drying.
2. Monitor volume of fluid consumed during training.
3. Determine change in body mass (BM) before and after any toilet stops.

sweat loss (mL) = change in BM (g) + fluid intake (mL) − urine losses (g)

Note that these calculations do not take into account the changes in BM that occur during prolonged exercise as a result of factors other than sweat loss. This includes weight changes due to oxidation of metabolic fuels, and the formation of water during such reactions. In prolonged bouts of intense exercise, these factors become substantial (e.g. 1–2% BM) and monitoring changes in BM without correcting for these factors will cause an overestimation of the true fluid deficit.

FIGURE 13.1 Quick method for estimating sweat loss

PRACTICE TIPS

- Combinations of sucrose, glucose, fructose and maltodextrins are all acceptable forms of CHO for ingestion, provided that fructose does not predominate.
- The rules and conditions of some sports place restrictions on the opportunity to drink. Each athlete needs to identify opportunities to drink and practice strategies to utilize each opportunity. Sports such as netball, basketball and soccer restrict fluid intake to breaks in play, and drinks can only be taken from the sidelines. Players need to practice getting to the sidelines and distributing water bottles quickly. Other codes of football allow additional fluid to be provided by trainers on the field. Trainers need to monitor players and ensure fluids are distributed to all players. Players must make the effort to look for trainers and communicate their fluid needs. Opportunities for fluid intake in team sports are reviewed by Burke and Hawley (1997). Athletes competing in individual sports need to practice skills such as drinking on the run, grabbing drinks from drink stations, and so on.

ENDURANCE SPORTS: EVENTS OF 1–3 HOURS' DURATION

- The primary concerns are fluid replacement plus CHO provision.
- Recommendations:
  - Begin exercise well hydrated.
  - Use a fluid intake plan that has been practiced in training, and drink at a rate that is comfortable and practical to replace most of the fluid lost by sweating.
  - Use a beverage that is cool (15–20°C), palatable and provides CHO.
  - Begin ingesting fluid early in the exercise and continue to ingest beverage regularly to maintain gastric volume and increase fluid availability.
  - Plan to consume 30–60 g CHO per hour of exercise.
- Sports drinks are intended to cater for the masses and suit the average sports event. For some individuals in some situations it may be desirable to vary the standard sports drink formula. On occasions when CHO needs take priority over fluid needs (e.g. in prolonged events carried out in cold conditions), a more concentrated solution might be useful. Alternatively, a more dilute preparation (e.g. 4%) might be appropriate for exercise in extremely hot conditions when fluid needs are of greatest priority. The intake of larger volumes of the sports drink in warm conditions will automatically increase the total amount of CHO consumed.
- Athletes use a variety of foods, fluids and gels during competition. Some provide a more concentrated source of CHO and will slow gastric emptying. However, solids can be desirable during prolonged competition as they increase the flavor options available, provide different textures and help to relieve hunger. Solids and gels also have the advantage of being a compact form of CHO, reducing the amount of sports drink an athlete must carry to enable refueling. This is particularly useful for training sessions and for events conducted without the support of handlers or an intricate network of aid stations. Table 13.4 describes various food and fluids that may be used in competition.

TABLE 13.4 FOOD AND FLUID CHOICES FOR ENDURANCE EVENTS

DESCRIPTION	AMOUNT TO PROVIDE 50 G CHO	COMMENTS
Water		Does not assist with fuel needs, but may be drunk in addition to sports drinks or solid food to make up total fluid needs.
Sports drinks 4–8% CHO + electrolytes	600–1000 mL	Best option for meeting fluid and CHO requirements simultaneously. Has a good taste profile to encourage voluntary intake. Provides small amounts of electrolytes.
Soft drink 11% CHO	500 mL	May be more slowly absorbed due to CHO content. Negligible source of electrolytes. Provides alternative flavor during long events. Cola drinks provide a small amount of caffeine.
Fruit juices 8–12% CHO	500 mL	May be more slowly absorbed due to CHO content. Negligible source of electrolytes. Possible risk of gastrointestinal upset if juice is high in fructose.
Sports gel 60–70% CHO	1½–2 gels	Concentrated CHO source. Suitable for large fuel boost. Experiment to avoid gastrointestinal discomfort. Fluid requirements will need separate attention.
Banana	2–3 medium	Solid foods may cause gastrointestinal concerns in some individuals, but may help to relieve hunger during long events. Several portions are needed to provide substantial amounts of CHO. Fluid requirements will need separate attention.
Jelly beans	50 g	Compact CHO source. Large amounts may cause diarrhea. Fluid requirements will need separate attention.
Jam sandwich	2 thick slices + 4 teaspoons jam	Avoid adding fat sources (peanut butter, margarine). See comments for bananas.
Chocolate bar	1½ bars	High in fat, so may be more slowly absorbed. May help relieve hunger. Fluid requirements will need separate attention.
Muesli bar/cereal bar	1½–2 bars	Fat content varies from low to moderate. See comments for bananas.
Sports bars	1–1½ bars	Compact source of CHO. Varying levels of fat. May have various herbal additives of unknown function.

EVENTS OF GREATER THAN 3 HOURS' DURATION

- The primary concerns are fluid plus CHO plus sodium provision.
- Recommendations:
  - Begin exercise well hydrated.
  - Using a fluid intake plan that has been practiced in training, drink at a rate that is comfortable and practical to replace most of the fluid lost by sweating.

PRACTICE TIPS

- Use a beverage that is cool (15–20°C), palatable and provides CHO and sodium.
- Begin ingesting fluid early in the exercise and continue to ingest beverage regularly to maintain gastric volume and increase fluid availability.
- Plan to consume 30–60 g CHO per hour of exercise.
- Plan to replace sodium via sports drinks and foods.

- Hyponatremia is a possibility in ultra-endurance events. A beverage (or foods) containing sodium chloride should be consumed, and will help to replace some of the sodium lost in sweat. However, the chief cause of hyponatremia is excessive fluid consumption—drinking at a rate that exceeds the rate of sweat loss. Athletes should not drink in volumes that cause them to gain weight during an event. In fact, a loss of 1–2% body mass during prolonged events is likely to occur from factors unrelated to sweat losses and is acceptable.

SKILL-BASED SPORTS

- The primary concerns are fluid plus CHO provision.
- Recommendations:
  - Begin exercise well hydrated.
  - Using a fluid intake plan that has been practiced in training, drink at a rate that is comfortable and practical to replace most of the fluid lost by sweating.
  - Use a beverage that is cool (15–20°C) and palatable.
  - Plan to consume CHO in amounts similar to usual daily intake.
- Sports such as archery, shooting and bowling can involve long periods of competition, but the aerobic requirements of the sport are quite low. Drinking a fluid that is cool and palatable will encourage fluid intake. CHO from a variety of forms should be well tolerated as the aerobic demand is low. Athletes need to plan fluid and fuel replacement strategies that suit competition schedules.

REFERENCES

Adopo E, Perronet F, Massicote D, Brisson G, Hilaire-Marcel C. Respective oxidation of exogenous glucose and fructose given in the same drink during exercise. J Appl Physiol 1994;76:1014–19.

Ahlborg B, Bergstrom J, Brohult J, Ekelund L-G, Hultman E, Maschio G. Human muscle glycogen content and capacity for prolonged exercise after different diets. Forsvarsmedicin 1967;3:85–99.

Almond CS, Shin AY, Fortescue EB, Mannix RC, Wypij D, Binstadt BA, Duncan CN, Olson DP, Salerno AE, Newburger JW, Greenes DS. Hyponatremia among runners in the Boston marathon. N Engl J Med 2005;352:1550–6.

American College of Sports Medicine. Position stand: exercise and fluid replacement. Med Sci Sports Exerc 1996;28:i–vii.

Armstrong LE. Performing in extreme environments. Champaign: Human Kinetics, 2000.

Armstrong LE, Costill DL, Fink WJ. Influence of diuretic-induced dehydration on competitive running performance. Med Sci Sports Exerc 1985;17:456–61.

Bainbridge FA. The physiology of muscular exercise. London: Longmans, Green & Co, 1919.

Bar-Or O, Wilk B. Water and electrolyte replenishment in the exercising child. Int J Sport Nutr 1996;6:93–9.

Barr SI, Costill DL, Fink WJ. Fluid replacement during prolonged exercise: effects of water, saline or no fluid. Med Sci Sports Exerc 1991;23:811–17.

Below P, Mora-Rodriguez R, Gonzalez-Alonso J, Coyle EF. Fluid and carbohydrate ingestion independently improve performance during 1 h of intense cycling. Med Sci Sports Exerc 1995;27:200–10.

Bishop NC, Blannin AK, Robson PJ, Walsh NP, Gleeson M. The effects of carbohydrate supplementation on immune responses to a soccer-specific exercise protocol. J Sports Sci 1999;17:787–96.

Bosch AN, Dennis SC, Noakes TD. Influence of carbohydrate ingestion on fuel substrate turnover and oxidation during prolonged exercise. J Appl Physiol 1994;76:2364–72.

Brener W, Hendrix TR, McHugh PR. Regulation of the gastric emptying of glucose. Gastroenterol 1983;85:76–82.

Burke LM, Hawley JA, Fluid balance in team sports. Guidelines for optimal practices. Sports Med 1997;24:38–54.

Carter JE, Gisolfi CV. Fluid replacement during and after exercise in the heat. Med Sci Sports Exerc 1989;21:532–9.

Carter JM, Jeukendrup AE, Jones DA. The effect of carbohydrate mouth rinse on 1-h cycle time trial performance. Med Sci Sports Exerc 2004;36:2107–11.

Coggan AR, Coyle EF. Effect of carbohydrate feedings during high-intensity exercise. J Appl Physiol 1988;65:1703–9.

Coggan AR, Coyle EF. Carbohydrate ingestion during prolonged exercise: effects on metabolism and performance. Ex Sport Sci Rev 1991;19:1–40.

Costill DL, Bennett A, Branam G, Eddy D. Glucose ingestion at rest and during prolonged exercise. J Appl Physiol 1973;34:764–9.

Coyle EF. Timing and method of increased carbohydrate intake to cope with heavy training, competition and recovery. J Sports Sci 1991;9(Suppl):1S–40S.

Coyle EF. Fuels for sport performance. In: Lamb DR, Murray R, eds. Perspectives in exercise science and sports medicine. Vol 10: Optimising sport performance. Carmel: Benchmark Press, 1997:95–138.

Coyle EF. Fluid and fuel intake during exercise. J Sports Sci 2004;22:39–55.

Coyle EF, Coggan AR, Hemmert MK, Ivy JL. Muscle glycogen utilization during strenuous exercise when fed carbohydrate. J Appl Physiol 1986;61:165–72.

Coyle EF, Hagberg JM, Hurley BF, Martin WH, Ehsani AH, Holloszy JO. Carbohydrate feeding during prolonged strenuous exercise can delay fatigue. J Appl Physiol 1983;55:230–5.

Coyle EF, Hamilton M. Fluid replacement during exercise: effects on physiological homeostasis and performance. In: Gisolfi CV, Lamb DR, eds. Perspectives in exercise science and sports medicine. Vol 3: Fluid homeostasis during exercise. Carmel: Benchmark Press, 1990:281–308.

Currell K, Jeukendrup AE. Superior endurance performance with ingestion of multiple transportable carbohydrates. Med Sci Sports Exerc 2008;40:275–81.

Davis JM, Burgess WA, Slentz CA, Bartoli WA, Pate RR. Effects of ingesting 6% and 12% glucose/electrolyte beverages during prolonged intermittent cycling in the heat. Eur J Appl Physiol 1988;57:563–9.

Erickson MA, Schwartzkopf RJ, McKenzie RD. Effects of caffeine, fructose, and glucose ingestion on muscle glycogen utilisation during exercise. Med Sci Sports Exerc 1987;19:579–83.

Evans GH, Shirreffs SM, Maughan RJ. Acute effects of ingesting glucose solutions on blood and plasma volume. Br J Nutr 2009;101:1503–8.

Fordtran JS. Stimulation of active and passive sodium absorption by sugars in the human jejunum. J Clin Invest 1975;55:728–37.

Frizell RT, Lang GH, Lowance DC, Lathan SR. Hyponatraemia and ultramarathon running. JAMA 1986;255:772–4.

Galloway SD, Maughan RJ. Effects of ambient temperature on the capacity to perform cycle exercise in man. Med Sci Sports Exerc 1997:29:1240–9.

Gisolfi CV, Summers RW, Schedl HP. Intestinal absorption of fluids during rest and exercise. In CV Gisolfi, Lamb DR, eds. Perspectives in exercise science and sports medicine. Volume 3: Fluid homeostasis during exercise. Carmel: Benchmark Press, 1990:129–80.

Gleeson M, Nieman DC, Pedersen BK. Exercise, nutrition and immune function. J Sports Sci 2004;22:215–25.

Gonzalez-Alonso J, Teller C, Andersen CL, Jensen FB, Hyldig T, Nielsen B. Influence of body temperature on the development of fatigue during prolonged exercise in the heat. J Appl Physiol 1999;86;1032–9.

Gordon B, Cohn LA, Levine SA, Matton M, Scriver WDM, Whiting WB. Sugar content of the blood in runners following a marathon race. JAMA 1925;185:508–9.

Hargreaves M, Briggs CA. Effect of carbohydrate ingestion on exercise metabolism. J Appl Physiol 1988;65:1553–5.

Hargreaves M, Costill DL, Coggan A, Fink WJ, Nishibata I. Effect of carbohydrate feedings on muscle glycogen utilisation and exercise performance. Med Sci Sports Exerc 1984;16:219–22.

Hawley JA, Dennis SC, Noakes TD. Oxidation of carbohydrate ingested during prolonged endurance exercise. Sports Med 1992;14:27–42.

Hermansen L, Hultman E, Saltin B. Muscle glycogen during prolonged severe exercise. Acta Physiol Scand 1967;71:129–39.

Hew-Butler T, Ayus JC, Kipps C, Maughan RJ, Mettler S, Meeuwisse WH, Page AJ, Reid SA, Rehrer NJ, Roberts WO, Rogers IR, Rosner MH, Siegel AJ, Speedy DB, Stuempfle KJ, Verbalis JG, Weschler LB, Wharam P. Consensus Statement of the 2nd International Exercise-Associated Hyponatremia Consensus Development Conference. Clin J Sports Med 2008;18:111–21.

Hiller WDB. Dehydration and hyponatraemia during triathlons. Med Sci Sports Exerc 1989;21(Suppl): 219S–21S.

Hubbard RW, Sandick BL, Matthew WT, et al. Voluntary dehydration and alliesthesia for water. J Appl Physiol 1984;57:868–75.

Hubbard RW, Szlyk PC, Armstrong LE. Influence of thirst and fluid palatability on fluid ingestion during exercise. In: Gisolfi CV, Lamb DR, eds. Perspectives in exercise science and sports medicine. Vol 3: Fluid homeostasis during exercise. Carmel: Benchmark Press, 1990:39–95.

Hulston CJ, Jeukendrup AE. Substrate metabolism and exercise performance with caffeine and carbohydrate intake. Med Sci Sports Exerc 2008;40:2096–104.

Hultman E, Nilsson LH. Liver glycogen in man. Effect of different diets and muscular exercise. Adv Exp Biol Med 1971;11:143–51.

Ivy J, Costill DL, Fink WJ, Lower RW. Influence of caffeine and carbohydrate feedings on endurance performance. Med Sci Sports Exerc 1979;11:6–11.

Jentjens RL, Achten J, Jeulendrup AE. High oxidation rates from combined carbohydrates ingested during exercise. Med Sci Sports Exerc 2004;36:1551–8.

Jentjens RL, Jeukendrup AE. High rates of exogenous carbohydrate oxidation from a mixture of glucose and fructose ingested during prolonged cycling exercise. Br J Nutr 2005;93:485–92.

Jeukendrup A, Brouns F, Wagenmakers AJM, Saris WHM. Carbohydrate-electrolyte feedings improve 1 h time trial performance. Int J Sports Med 1997;18:125–9.

Jeukendrup AE. Carbohydrate feeding during exercise. Eur J Sport Sci 2008;8:77–86.

Jeukendrup AE, Hopkins S, Aragon-Vargas LF, Hulston C. No effect of carbohydrate feeding on 16 km cycling time trial performance. Eur J Appl Physiol 2008;104:831–7.

Jones BJM, Brown BE, Loran JS, Edgerton D, Kennedy JF. Glucose absorption from starch hydrolysates in the human jejunum. Gut 1983;24:1152–60.

Jones BJM, Higgins BE, Silk DBA. Glucose absorption from maltotriose and glucose oligomers in the human jejunum. Clin Sci 1987;72:409–14.

Karlsson J, Saltin B. Diet, muscle glycogen and endurance performance. J Appl Physiol 1971;31:203–6.

Kuo C-K, Hunt DG, Ding Z, Ivy JL. Effect of carbohydrate supplementation on post-exercise GLUT-4 protein expression in skeletal muscle. J Appl Physiol 1999;87:2290–6.

Lamb DR, Brodowicz GR. Optimal use of fluids of varying formulations to minimize exercise-induced disturbances in homeostasis. Sports Med 1986;3:247–74.

Lee JKW, Shirreffs SM. The influence of drink temperature on thermoregulatory responses during prolonged exercise in a moderate environment. J Sport Sci 2007;25:975–85.

Lee JKW, Shirreffs SM, Maughan RJ. The influence of serial feeding of drinks at different temperatures on thermoregulatory responses during prolonged exercise. J Sport Sci 2008a;26:583–90.

Lee JKW, Shirreffs SM, Maughan RJ. Cold drink ingestion improves exercise endurance capacity in the heat. Med Sci Sport Exerc 2008b;40:1637–44.

Levine SA, Gordon B, Derick CL. Some changes in the chemical constituents of the blood following a marathon race. JAMA 1924;82:1778–9.

Levine L, Rose MS, Francesconi RP, Neufer PD, Sawka MN. Fluid replacement during sustained activity: nutrient solution vs. water. Aviat Space Env Med 1991;62:559–64.

Massicotte D, Péronnet F, Brisson G, Bakkouch K, Hilaire-Marcel C. Oxidation of a glucose polymer during exercise: comparison with glucose and fructose. J Appl Physiol 1989;66:179–83.

Maughan RJ. Thermoregulation and fluid balance in marathon competition at low ambient temperature. Int J Sports Med 1985;6:15–19.

Maughan RJ. Fluid and electrolyte loss and replacement in exercise. In: Harries M, Williams C, Stanish WD, Micheli LL, eds. Oxford textbook of sports medicine. Oxford: Oxford University Press, 1994:82–93.

Maughan RJ, Bethell L, Leiper JB. Effects of ingested fluids on homeostasis and exercise performance in man. Exp Physiol 1996;81:847–59.

Maughan RJ, Fenn CE, Gleeson M, Leiper JB. Metabolic and circulatory responses to the ingestion of glucose polymer and glucose/electrolyte solutions during exercise in man. Eur J Appl Physiol 1987;56:356–2.

Maughan RJ, Fenn CE, Leiper JB. Effects of fluid, electrolyte and substrate ingestion on endurance capacity. Eur J Appl Physiol 1989;58:481–6.

Maughan RJ, Merson SJ, Broad NP, Shirreffs SM. Fluid and electrolyte intake and loss in elite soccer players during training. Int J Sport Nutr Ex Metab 2004;14:327–40.

Maughan RJ, Shirreffs SM. Fluid and electrolyte loss and replacement in exercise. In: Harries M, Williams C, Stanish WD, Micheli LL, eds. Oxford textbook of sports medicine. Second edition. New York: Oxford University Press, 1998:97–113.

Maughan RJ, Shirreffs SM, Merson SJ, Horswill CA. Fluid and electrolyte balance in elite male football (soccer) players training in a cool environment. J Sports Sci 2005;23:73–9.

Maughan RJ, Shirreffs SM, Watson P. Exercise, heat, hydration and the brain. J Am Coll Nutr 2007a; 26(Suppl):604S–12S.

Maughan RJ, P Watson, GH Evans, N Broad, SM Shirreffs. Water balance and salt losses in competitive football. Int J Sport Nutr Ex Metab 2007b;17:583–94

McConnell G, Fabris S, Proietto J, Hargreaves M. Effect of carbohydrate ingestion on glucose kinetics during exercise. J Appl Physiol 1994;77:1537–41.

McConell G, Kloot K, Hargreaves M. Effect of timing of carbohydrate ingestion on endurance exercise performance. Med Sci Sports Exerc 1996;28:1300–4.

McGregor SJ, Nicholas CW, Lakomy HKA, Williams C. The influence of intermittent high-intensity shuttle running and fluid ingestion on the performance of a soccer skill. J Sports Sci 1999;17:895–903.

Meeusen R, Watson P, Dvorak J. The brain and fatigue: new opportunities for nutritional interventions? J Sports Sci 2006;24:773–82.

Millard-Stafford M, Rosskopf LB, Snow TK, Hinson BT. Water versus carbohydrate-electrolyte ingestion before and during a 15-km run in the heat. Int J Sport Nutr 1997;7:26–38.

Mitchell JB, Costill DL, Houmard JA, Flynn MG, Fink WJ, Beltz JD. Effects of carbohydrate ingestion on gastric emptying and exercise performance. Med Sci Sports Exerc 1988;20:110–15.

Montain SJ, Coyle EF. Influence of graded dehydration on hyperthermia and cardiovascular drift during exercise. J Appl Physiol 1992a;73:1340–50.

Montain SJ, Coyle EF. Fluid ingestion during exercise increases skin blood flow independent of increases in blood volume. J Appl Physiol 1992b;73:903–10.

Murray R. The effects of consuming carbohydrate-electrolyte beverages on gastric emptying and fluid absorption during and following exercise. Sports Med 1987;4:322–51.

Murray R, Eddy DE, Murray TW, Seifert JG, Paul GL, Halaby GA. The effect of fluid and carbohydrate feedings during intermittent cycling exercise. Med Sci Sports Exerc 1987;19:597–604.

Murray R, Seifert JG, Eddy DE, Halaby GA. Carbohydrate feeding and exercise: effect of beverage carbohydrate content. Eur J Appl Physiol 1989;59:152–8.

Nadel ER, Mack GW, Nose H. Influence of fluid replacement beverages on body fluid homeostasis during exercise and recovery. In: Gisolfi CV, Lamb DR, eds. Perspectives in exercise science and sports medicine. Vol. 3: Fluid homeostasis during exercise. Carmel: Benchmark Press, 1990: 181–205.

Nielsen B, Hales JRS, Strange S, Christensen NJ, Warberg J, Saltin B. Human circulatory and thermoregulatory adaptations with heat acclimation and exercise in a hot, dry environment. J Physiol 1993;460:467–86.

Nielsen B, Kubica R, Bonnesen A, Rasmussen IB, Stoklosa J, Wilk B. Physical work capacity after dehydration and hyperthermia. Scand J Sports Sc 1982;3:2–10.

Nieman DC, Henson DA, Garner EB, et al. Carbohydrate affects natural killer cell redistribution but not function after running. Med Sci Sports Exerc 1997;29:1318–24.

Nieman DC, Pedersen BK. Exercise and immune function: recent developments. Sports Med 1999:27;73–80.

Noakes T. Fluid replacement during marathon running. Clin J Sports Med 2003;13:309–18.

Noakes TD. The dehydration myth and carbohydrate replacement during prolonged exercise. Cycling Science 1990;1:23–9.

Noakes TD. Fluid replacement during exercise. In: Holloszy JO, ed. Exercise and sports science reviews. Baltimore: Williams & Wilkins. Vol 21, 1993:297–330.

Noakes TD, Goodwin N, Rayner BL, Branken T, Taylor RKN. Water intoxication: a possible complication during endurance exercise. Med Sci Sports Exerc 1985;17:370–5.

Noakes TD, Norman RJ, Buck RH, Godlonton J, Stevenson K, Pittaway D. The incidence of hyponatremia during prolonged ultraendurance exercise. Med Sci Sports Exerc 1990;22:165–70.

Parkin JM, Carey MF, Zhao S, Febbraio MA. Effect of ambient temperature on human skeletal muscle metabolism during fatiguing submaximal exercise. J Appl Physiol 1999;86:902–8.

Pirnay F, Crielaard JM, Pallikarakis N, et al. Fate of exogenous glucose during exercise of different intensities in humans. J Appl Physiol 1982;53:1620–4.

Rehrer NJ. Limits to fluid availability during exercise. Haarlem, The Netherlands: De Vriesebosch, 1990.

Rehrer NJ, Burke LM. Sweat losses during various sports. Aust J Nutr Diet 1996;53(Suppl):13S–16S.

Rehrer NJ, Wagenmakers AJM, Beckers EJ, et al. Limits to liquid carbohydrate supplementation during exercise: gastric emptying, intestinal absorption and oxidation. J Appl Physiol 1992;72:468–75.

Rollo I, Williams C, Gant N, Nute M. The influence of carbohydrate mouth rinse on self-selected speeds during a 30-min treadmill run. Int J Sport Nutr Exerc Metab 2008;18:585–600.

Rowell LB. Human circulation. New York: Oxford University Press, 1986.

Saltin B, Costill DL. Fluid and electrolyte balance during prolonged exercise. In: Horton ES, Terjung RL, eds. Exercise, nutrition, and metabolism. New York: Macmillan, 1988:150–8.

Saris WHM, van Erp-Baart MA, Brouns F, Westerterp KR, ten Hoor F. Study on food intake and energy expenditure during extreme sustained exercise: the Tour de France. Int J Sports Med 1989;10(Suppl):26S–31S.

Sasaki H, Maeda J, Usui S, Ishiko T. Effect of sucrose and caffeine ingestion on performance of prolonged strenuous running. Int J Sports Med 1987;8:261–5.

Sawka MN, Burke LM, Eichner ER, Maughan RJ, Montain SJ, Stachenfeld NS. Exercise and fluid replacement. Med Sci Sports Exerc 2007;39:377–90.

Schedl HP, Maughan RJ, Gisolfi CV. Intestinal absorption during rest and exercise: implications for formulating oral rehydration beverages. Med Sci Sports Exerc 1994;26:267–80.

Shephard RJ. Physical activity, training, and the immune response. Carmel: Cooper Publishing, 1997.

Shi X, Summers RW, Schedl HP. Effect of carbohydrate type and concentration and solution osmolality on water absorption. J Appl Physiol 1995;27:1607–15.

Shirreffs SM, Aragon-Vargas LF, Chamorro M, Maughan RJ, Serratosa L, Zachwieja JJ. The sweating response of elite professional soccer players to training in the heat. Int J Sports Med 2005;26:90–5.

Shirreffs SM, Maughan, RJ. Urine osmolality and conductivity as markers of hydration status. Med Sci Sports Ex 1998;30:1598–602.

Shirreffs SM, Taylor AJ, Leiper JB, Maughan RJ. Post-exercise rehydration in man: effects of volume consumed and sodium content of ingested fluids. Med Sci Sports Exerc 1996;28:1260–71.

Spiller RC, Jones BJM, Brown BE, Silk DBA. Enhancement of carbohydrate absorption by the addition of sucrose to enteric diets. J Parent Ent Nut 1982;6:321.

Szlyk PC, Sils IV, Francesconi RP, Hubbard RW, Armstrong LE. Effects of water temperature and flavoring on voluntary dehydration in men. Physiol Behav 1989;45:639–47.

Thom W. Pedestrianism, or an account of the performance of celebrated pedestrians. Aberdeen: Chalmers, 1813.

Tsintzsas OK, Liu R, Williams C, Campbell I, Gaitanos G. The effect of carbohydrate ingestion on performance during a 30-km race. Int J Sport Nutr 1993;3:127–39.

Van Nieuwenhoven MA, Brummer RM, Brouns F. Gastrointestinal function during exercise: comparison of water, sports drink, and sports drink with caffeine. J Appl Physiol 2000;89:1079–85.

Vergauwen L, Brouns F, Hespel P. Carbohydrate supplementation improves stroke performance in tennis. Med Sci Sports Exerc 1998;30:1289–95.

Vist GE, Maughan RJ. The effect of increasing glucose concentration on the rate of gastric emptying in man. Med Sci Sports Exerc 1994;26:1269–73.

Vist GE, Maughan RJ. The effect of osmolality and carbohydrate content on the rate of gastric emptying of liquids in man. J Physiol 1995;486:523–31.

Wagenmakers AJM, Brouns F, Saris WH, Halliday D. Oxidation rates of orally ingested carbohydrates during prolonged exercise in men. J Appl Physiol 1993;75:274–80.

Wallis GA, Rowlands DS, Shaw C, Jentjens RL, Jeukendrup AE. Oxidation of combined ingestion of maltodextrins and fructose during exercise. Med Sci Sports Exerc 2005;37:426–32.

Walsh RM, Noakes TD, Hawley JA, Dennis SC. Impaired high-intensity cycling performance time at low levels of dehydration. Int J Sports Med 1994;15:392–8.

Wapnir RA, Lifshitz F. Osmolality and solute concentration—their relationship with oral rehydration solution effectiveness: an experimental assessment. Ped Res 1985;19:894–8.

Whitham M, McKinney J. Effect of a carbohydrate mouthwash on running time-trial performance. J Sports Sci 2007;25:1385–92.

Whiting PH, Maughan RJ, Miller JDB. Dehydration and serum biochemical changes in marathon runners. Eur J Appl Physiol 1984;52:183–7.

Williams C. Diet and endurance fitness. Am J Clin Nutr 1989;49:1077–83.

Williams C. Diet and sports performance. In: Harries M, Williams C, Stanish WD, Micheli LL, eds. Oxford textbook of sports medicine. Second edition. New York: Oxford University Press 1998:77–97.

Williams C, Nute MG, Broadbank L, Vinall S. Influence of fluid intake on endurance running performance: a comparison between water, glucose and fructose solutions. Eur J Appl Physiol 1990;60:112–19.

Wimer GS, Lamb DR, Sherman WM, Swanson SC. Temperature of ingested water and thermoregulation during moderate-intensity exercise. Can J Appl Physiol 1997;22:479–93.

Yeo SE, Jentjens RLGP, Wallis GA, Jeukendrup AE. Caffeine increases exogenous carbohydrate oxidation during exercise. J Appl Physiol 2005;99:844–50.

Zeederberg C, Leach L, Lambert EV, Noakes TD, Dennis SC, Hawley JA. The effect of carbohydrate ingestion on the motor skill of soccer players. Int J Sport Nutr 1996;6:348–55.

CHAPTER 14

Nutrition for recovery after training and competition

LOUISE BURKE

14.1 Introduction

Recovery after exercise poses an important challenge to the modern athlete. Athletes commonly undertake strenuous training programs involving one or more prolonged high-intensity exercise sessions each day, typically allowing 6–24 hours for recovery between workouts. In some sports, competition is conducted as a series of events or stages. In sports such as swimming or track and field, athletes are scheduled to compete in a number of brief races, or in a series involving heats, semi-finals and finals, often performing more than once each day. In tennis and team sport tournaments, or cycle stage races, competitors may be required to undertake one or more lengthy events each day, with the competition extending for 1–3 weeks. Even where athletes compete in a weekly fixture, optimal recovery is desired to allow the athlete to train between matches or races.

Recovery involves a complex array of desirable processes of adaptation to physiological stress. In the training situation, with correct planning of the workload and the recovery time, adaptation allows the body to become fitter, stronger or faster. In the competition scenario, however, there may be less control over the work:recovery ratio. A simpler but more realistic goal for the athlete may be to face the next opponent, or the next round or stage in a competition, as well prepared as possible.

Recovery encompasses a complex range of nutrition-related issues including:

- restoration of muscle and liver glycogen stores
- replacement of fluid and electrolytes lost in sweat
- regeneration, repair and adaptation processes following the catabolic stress and damage caused by the exercise

This last issue involves many processes described in other sections of this textbook, ranging from protein synthesis (see Chapter 4) to the activities of the immune and anti-oxidant defense systems (see Commentaries B and C, pages 295 and 501). The present chapter focuses on the well-defined and well-studied issues of restoration of fluid balance and glycogen stores, summarizing the current guidelines on strategies for post-exercise fluid and food intake to enhance these processes. Although this review and the resulting guidelines focus on fluid and carbohydrate (CHO) goals, some attention should be paid

TABLE 14.1 PRACTICAL FACTORS INTERFERING WITH POST-EXERCISE FLUID AND FOOD INTAKE

- Fatigue—interfering with ability/interest to obtain or eat food
- Loss of appetite following high-intensity exercise
- Limited access to (suitable) foods at exercise venue
- Other post-exercise commitments and priorities (such as coach meetings, drug tests, equipment maintenance and warm-down activities)
- Traditional post-competition activities (such as excessive alcohol intake)

to the simultaneous intake of other nutrients. While emerging research points to the importance of the quantity and timing of intake of protein for post-exercise recovery, it is possible that future studies may reveal the role of various micronutrients in promoting optimal function of the repair and adaptation processes.

In many situations, optimal recovery after training or competition will occur only with a specially organized nutrition plan. After all, thirst and voluntary fluid intake are unlikely to keep pace with large sweat losses. In addition, typical western eating patterns are unlikely to provide CHO intakes that reach the threshold of daily glycogen storage. These plans must be made in recognition of the practical factors that interfere with an athlete's post-exercise fluid and food intake plans (see Table 14.1). This is particularly important for the traveling athlete, who may be challenged by an inaccessible and foreign food supply. Special recognition of the needs of the traveling athlete is found in greater detail in Chapter 23.

Issues in post-exercise refueling 14.2

The depletion of muscle glycogen provides a strong drive for its own resynthesis (Zachwieja et al. 1991). Muscle glycogen resynthesis takes precedence over restoration of liver glycogen, and even in the absence of a dietary supply of CHO after exercise it occurs at a low rate—1–2 mmol/kg wet weight (ww) of muscle per hour—with some of the substrate being provided through gluconeogenesis (Maehlum & Hermansen 1978). High-intensity exercise that results in high post-exercise levels of lactate appears to be associated with rapid recovery of glycogen stores in the absence of additional CHO feeding (Hermansen & Vaage 1977). After moderate-intensity exercise, muscle glycogen synthesis is dependent on the provision of exogenous CHO. The rate of glycogen storage is affected by factors regulating glucose transport into the cell, such as the insulin- or exercise-stimulated translocation of GLUT-4 protein transporter to the muscle membrane (McCoy et al. 1996). It is also determined by factors regulating glucose disposal, such as the activity of glycogen synthase enzyme (Danforth 1965; McCoy et al. 1996). Changes in these factors are responsible for a bi-phasic muscle glycogen storage pattern, or a decline in glycogen storage rate over time (Ivy & Kuo 1998). Glycogen storage is impaired by damage to the muscle fiber, such as that caused by eccentric exercise or direct contact injury (Costill et al. 1988b, 1991).

Liver glycogen stores are more labile than muscle glycogen stores, and may be depleted by an overnight fast as well as by a prolonged bout of exercise. Strategies to enhance the restoration of liver glycogen stores have been less well studied due to practical problems in obtaining liver biopsy samples. Nevertheless it is considered that liver glycogen is restored by a single CHO-rich meal, and that fructose ingestion may cause a greater rate of liver glycogen synthesis than glucose intake (Blom et al. 1987).

The maximal rates of post-exercise muscle glycogen storage reported during the first 12 hours of recovery are within the range of 5–10 mmol/kg ww/h (Blom et al. 1987; Ivy et al. 1988a; Reed et al. 1989). Coyle (1991) has commented that with a mean glycogen storage rate of 5–6 mmol/kg ww/h, 20–24 hours of recovery are required for normalization of muscle glycogen levels following exercise depletion. In real life, the training and competition schedules of many athletes often provide considerably less time than this. Since performance in subsequent exercise sessions may depend on the success of muscle CHO restoration strategies, many athletes may compromise subsequent performance by beginning with inadequate muscle fuel stores. Several of the dietary factors that enhance or impair the rate of muscle glycogen storage are discussed in this chapter. Particular interest is focused on changes that have occurred in our knowledge over the past few years, and the resultant updates in guidelines for athletes.

14.3 Amount of carbohydrate intake

The most important dietary factor affecting muscle glycogen storage is the amount of CHO consumed. According to a summary of studies that have monitored muscle glycogen storage following 24 hours of recovery from glycogen-depleting exercise, there is a direct and positive relationship between the quantity of dietary CHO and post-exercise glycogen storage, at least until the muscle storage capacity or threshold has been reached (Burke et al. 2004). Only two studies have directly investigated this relationship by feeding different amounts of CHO to trained subjects over a 24-hour recovery period; the results of these studies show an increase in glycogen storage with increasing CHO intake and a glycogen storage threshold at a daily CHO intake of ~7–10 g/kg body mass (BM) (Costill et al. 1981; Burke et al. 1995).

Although these figures have evolved into the recommended CHO intakes for optimal muscle glycogen recovery, it is worth noting that they are derived from studies of glycogen storage during a passive recovery period (Burke et al. 2004). As a result, requirements for total daily CHO intake may be lower for athletes whose training programs do not challenge daily glycogen stores. However, they may be higher when the fuel requirements of continued heavy training are added to glycogen restoration needs. For example, well-trained cyclists undertaking 2 hours of training each day were found to have higher muscle glycogen stores after a week of a daily CHO intake of 12 g/kg BM than when consuming the 'recommended' CHO intake of 10 g/kg/d (Coyle et al. 2001). Furthermore, Tour de France cyclists riding at least 6 hours each day voluntarily consume CHO intakes of 12–13 g/kg/d (Saris et al. 1989), and the ingestion of substantial amounts of CHO during low- to moderate-intensity exercise has been reported to increase net glycogen storage during the session, particularly within non-active muscle fibers that have been previously depleted (Kuipers et al. 1987). Increased CHO intake may also be useful in the case of muscle damage (such as that following eccentric exercise), which typically impairs the rate of post-exercise glycogen resynthesis. Costill and colleagues (1991) reported that low rates of glycogen restoration in damaged muscles might be partially overcome by increased amounts of CHO intake during the first 24 hours of recovery.

Separate guidelines have been proposed to cover the CHO needs of the early phase (0–4 hours) of recovery. The 1991 consensus statement on nutrition for athletes by the

International Olympic Committee (IOC) recommended that athletes should consume 50 g (~1 g/kg BM) of CHO every 2 hours until meal patterns are resumed (Coyle 1991). These guidelines were based on studies that failed to find differences in post-exercise glycogen storage following CHO intakes of 0.7 and 1.4 g/kg BM (Blom et al. 1987), or between 1.5 and 3.0 g/kg BM (Ivy et al. 1988b), fed at 2-hourly intervals. However, newer studies of early post-exercise recovery (Doyle et al. 1993; Piehl Aulin et al. 2000; Van Hall et al. 2000) achieved glycogen synthesis rates of up to 10–11 mmol/kg ww/h, or about 30% higher than previous literature values. Features of these more recent studies include larger CHO intakes (e.g. 1–1.8 g/kg/h) and repeated small feedings (e.g. an intake every 15–60 minutes) rather than single or several large meals. Unfortunately, because these studies have not directly compared glycogen storage with different amounts of CHO and different feeding schedules, it is difficult to draw final conclusions about optimal CHO intake in the early recovery phase. Nevertheless, other studies (Van Loon et al. 2000; Jentjens et al. 2001) suggest that the threshold for early glycogen recovery is reached by a CHO feeding schedule providing 1.2 kg/h based on the failure to increase muscle glycogen storage when extra energy (protein) was consumed. These new recommendations were incorporated into the 2003 IOC consensus guidelines (Burke et al. 2004).

Timing of carbohydrate intake

14.4

The highest rates of muscle glycogen storage occur during the first hour after exercise (Ivy et al. 1988a), due to activation of glycogen synthase by glycogen depletion (Prats et al. 2009), exercise-induced increases in insulin sensitivity (Richter et al. 1989) and permeability of the muscle cell membrane to glucose. CHO feeding during these early stages appears to accentuate these effects by increasing blood glucose and insulin concentrations. Ivy and colleagues (1988a) reported that the immediate intake of CHO after prolonged exercise resulted in higher rates of glycogen storage (7.7 mmol/kg ww/h) during the first 2 hours of recovery, slowing thereafter to the more typical rates of storage (4.3 mmol/kg ww/h). Although this study has been interpreted to highlight the significantly higher rates of glycogen synthesis in early recovery, it is unlikely that these differences (7.7 compared to 4.3 mmol/kg ww/h) are of physiological importance. The most important finding of this study is that failure to consume CHO in the immediate phase of post-exercise recovery leads to very low rates of glycogen restoration until feeding occurs. Thus the importance of early intake of CHO following strenuous exercise is to avoid delaying the provision of substrate to the muscle cell, more than to take advantage of a period of moderately enhanced glycogen synthesis. This strategy is most important when there are only 4–8 hours of recovery between exercise sessions, but may be of less impact when there is a longer recovery time (12 hours or more). For example, Parkin and colleagues (1997) investigated glycogen storage over 8 hours and 24 hours of recovery when high glycemic index (GI) CHO meals were begun immediately after exercise, or delayed for 2 hours. They found no difference in glycogen restoration at either of these time points as a result of delaying the first CHO meal (Parkin et al. 1997).

Overall it appears that when the interval between exercise sessions is short, the athlete should maximize the effective recovery time by beginning CHO intake as soon as possible. However, when longer recovery periods are available, the athlete can choose their preferred meal schedule as long as total CHO intake goals are achieved. It is not always practical or enjoyable to consume substantial meals or snacks immediately after the finish of a strenuous workout.

Whether CHO is best consumed in large meals or as a series of snacks has also been studied. Studies investigating 24-hour recovery have found that restoration of muscle glycogen is the same whether a given amount of CHO is fed as two or seven meals (Costill et al. 1981) or as four large meals or sixteen hourly snacks (Burke et al. 1996). In the latter study, similar muscle glycogen storage was achieved despite marked differences in blood glucose and insulin profiles over 24 hours (Burke et al. 1996). In contrast, very high rates of glycogen synthesis during the first 4–6 hours of recovery have been reported when large amounts of CHO were fed at 15- to 30-minute intervals (Doyle et al. 1993; Van Hall et al. 2000; Van Loon et al. 2000; Jentjens et al. 2001) and attributed to the higher sustained insulin and glucose profiles achieved by such a feeding protocol. However, as previously noted, these outcomes were compared with other literature values of post-exercise glycogen restoration rather than directly tested against a control amount of CHO taken in less-frequent meals. One way to reconcile these apparently conflicting data is to propose that the effects of enhanced insulin and glucose concentrations on glycogen storage are most important during the first hours of recovery or when total CHO intake is below the threshold of maximum glycogen storage. However, during longer periods of recovery or when total CHO intake is above this threshold, manipulations of plasma substrates and hormones within physiological ranges do not add further benefit.

The practical implications of these studies are that meeting total CHO requirements is more important than the pattern of intake and, at least for long-term recovery, the athlete is advised to choose a food schedule that is practical and comfortable. A more frequent intake of smaller snacks may be useful in overcoming the gastric discomfort often associated with eating large amounts of bulky high-CHO foods, but may also provide direct benefits to glycogen storage during the early recovery phase.

14.5 Type of carbohydrate intake

Since glycogen storage is influenced by both insulin and a rapid supply of glucose substrate, it appears logical that CHO sources with a moderate to high GI would enhance post-exercise refueling. This hypothesis has been confirmed in the case of single nutrient feedings of mono- and disaccharides; intake of glucose and sucrose after prolonged exercise both produce higher rates of muscle glycogen recovery than the low-GI sugar, fructose (Blom et al. 1987). The results of early investigations of real foods (Costill et al. 1981; Roberts et al. 1988) were confusing, since they used the structural classification of 'simple' and 'complex or starchy' CHOs to construct recovery diets; the conflicting findings are probably due to the failure to achieve a real or consistent difference in the GI of the diets.

The first comparison of foods based on published GI values reported greater glycogen storage during 24 hours of post-exercise recovery with a CHO-rich diet based on high-GI foods compared with an identical amount of CHO eaten in the form of low-GI foods (Burke et al. 1993). However, the magnitude of increase in glycogen storage (~30%) was substantially greater than the difference in 24-hour blood glucose and insulin profiles. Researchers found that the meal consumed immediately after exercise produced a large glycemic and insulinemic response, independent of the GI of the CHO consumed, and overshadowed the differences in response to the rest of the diet. Other studies have confirmed an exaggerated glycemic response to CHO consumed immediately after exercise compared with the same feeding consumed at rest (Rose et al. 2001). This has been explained as a result of greater gut glucose output and greater hepatic glucose escape, favoring an increase in muscle glucose uptake and glycogen storage. Therefore, while it appears that high-GI CHO foods achieve superior post-exercise glycogen storage, this cannot be totally explained in terms of an enhanced glucose and insulin response.

An additional or alternative mechanism to explain less efficient glycogen storage with low-GI CHO-rich foods is that a considerable amount of the CHO in these foods may be malabsorbed (Wolever et al. 1986; Jenkins et al. 1987). Indeed, the poor digestibility of a high amylose starch mixture (low GI) was proposed as an explanation for lower muscle glycogen storage observed during 13 hours of post-exercise recovery compared with intake of high-GI CHOs, glucose, maltodextrins and a high amylopectin starch (Joszi et al. 1996). This study concluded that indigestible forms of CHO provide a poor substrate for muscle glycogen resynthesis and overestimate the available CHO consumed by subjects. This issue needs to be further studied in relation to real foods. Nevertheless, a study of chronic exposure to a lower GI diet in recreationally active people found that muscle glycogen storage declined over 30 days compared with pretrial values and was lower in comparison with the values on a high-GI trial (Kiens & Richter 1996).

In summary, when speedy restoration of glycogen is the goal, it seems prudent for low-GI foods to play a minor role in post-exercise meals. Typically, this does not need specific attention, since western eating patterns are generally based on high-GI CHO choices. However, the possible effect of the GI of recovery meals on metabolism during subsequent exercise requires further investigation (see Chapter 12) and may need to be taken into account.

Form of carbohydrate feeding

14.6

Both solid and liquid forms of CHO appear to be equally efficient in providing substrate for muscle glycogen synthesis (Keizer et al. 1986; Reed et al. 1989). Practical issues such as compactness and appetite appeal may be important in choosing CHO foods and fluids to meet the athlete's total CHO intake goals. Liquid forms of CHO or CHO foods with a high fluid content may be particularly appealing when athletes are fatigued and appetite-suppressed.

Infusion of carbohydrate

14.7

Intravenous (IV) delivery of CHO might be a practical way to ensure intake of recovery substrates when an athlete has impaired gastrointestinal function and/or limited time between workouts during which sleep and other activities compete with eating time. Such a situation can be found in events such as the Tour de France, where competitors need to recover overnight to tackle stages lasting 5–8 hours, and may finish each stage in a state of extreme fatigue and substantial dehydration. Certainly the expense and risks involved with CHO infusion mean that it might be considered only in extreme circumstances. Nevertheless the mystique of IV feeding has led to ideas that it might provide a superior method of restoration, promoting faster and higher levels of glycogen storage compared with the oral intake of similar amounts of CHO. Several studies argue against this idea. First, when oral CHO intake was compared with the infusion of matched amounts of CHO (infusion adjusted to match blood glucose concentrations achieved by eating CHO), the IV feeding route produced significantly lower insulin concentrations. Despite this, rates of glycogen storage were similar between treatments (Blom 1989).

More recently, Hansen and colleagues studied the effects of supra-physiological levels of blood glucose and insulin, achieved by infusions of both glucose and insulin (Hansen et al. 1999). IV delivery of glucose was undertaken to maintain glucose concentrations at ~20 mmol/L, while insulin infusion kept this hormone at its maximal effective concentration. After 8 hours, muscle glycogen had risen to the levels normally associated with glycogen supercompensation. Therefore it was concluded that infusion techniques can achieve glycogen storage at a faster rate. However, the IV feedings did not increase glycogen above levels that could be achieved by dietary means, albeit over a longer time period. Most importantly, the study was terminated for ethical reasons after the participation of only two subjects. Both became ill at the end of the study period, complaining of nausea and vomiting (Hansen et al. 1999).

In summary, maximal provision of glucose and insulin via infusion can increase the rate of glycogen storage over a period of 8 hours. However, similar total recovery can be achieved by dietary means given sufficient time, and with far less cost in terms of side effects, risks and expense.

14.8 Co-ingestion of other nutrients and total dietary energy intake

There is evidence that the relationship between CHO intake and glycogen storage is underpinned by consideration of total energy intake. In a study of CHO loading, female subjects showed a substantial enhancement of muscle glycogen storage associated with increased dietary CHO intake only after total energy intake was also increased (Tarnopolsky et al. 2001). The simplest way to consider this relationship is that dietary intake must provide for the body's immediate fuel requirements as well as storage opportunities. Greater proportions of available CHO substrates (such as dietary CHO) are likely to be oxidized to meet immediate energy needs during energy restriction, whereas CHO consumed during a period of energy balance or surplus may be available for storage within the muscle and liver.

It is possible that the co-ingestion of other macronutrients, either present in CHO-rich foods or consumed at the same meal, may directly influence muscle glycogen restoration as well as adding to energy intake. Although this hypothesis has not been systematically tested, factors that might directly or indirectly affect glycogen storage include the provision of gluconeogenic substrates, as well as effects on digestion, insulin secretion or the satiety of meals. The effects of protein have received most attention, but have become a source of debate, with some studies reporting an increase in post-exercise glycogen storage when protein is added to a CHO feeding (Zawadzki et al. 1992; Van Loon et al. 2000; Ivy et al. 2002) and others finding no effect (Tarnopolsky et al. 1995; Roy & Tarnopolsky 1998; Carrithers et al. 2000; Van Hall et al. 2000).

Some of the apparent conflict in these results, however, can be explained by differences in experimental design, including differences in the frequency of supplementation and in the amounts of CHO and protein provided. For example, studies that found an increase in muscle glycogen storage following the addition of protein to a CHO supplement generally used feeding intervals of 2 hours (Ivy et al. 2002; Zawadzki et al. 1992). By contrast, studies that did not demonstrate a beneficial effect of protein used 15- to 30-minute feeding intervals (Tarnopolsky et al. 1995; Carrithers et al. 2000; Van Hall et al. 2000; Jentjens et al. 2001). In addition, they generally consumed a high total amount of CHO

(Van Hall et al. 2000; Jentjens et al. 2001) and in some studies a low amount of protein (Tarnopolsky et al. 1995; Carrithers et al. 2000). Across these studies it appears that a high amount of CHO at frequent intervals negates the benefits of added protein. However, the co-ingestion of protein with CHO is likely to increase the efficiency of muscle glycogen storage when the amount of CHO ingested is below the threshold for maximal glycogen synthesis or when feeding intervals are greater than 1 hour (Zawadzki et al. 1992; Van Loon et al. 2000; Ivy et al. 2002). The benefits of protein in enhancing muscle glycogen storage may be limited to the very early phase (the first hour) of post-exercise recovery feedings. Ivy and colleagues (2002) found that glycogen storage was twice as fast for the first 40 minutes following a CHO-protein drink compared to an energy-matched CHO feeding, but differences were small at later phases of recovery. It is unclear whether any enhanced rates of glycogen storage due to co-ingestion of protein and CHO are achieved via the increased insulin response from protein per se, or as a result of the increase in energy intake. However, on the available evidence it seems that the presence of other macronutrients with CHO feedings does not substantially alter muscle glycogen synthesis when total CHO intake is at the level of the glycogen storage threshold. However, when the athlete's energy intake or food availability does not allow sufficient CHO to be consumed, the presence of protein in post-exercise meals and snacks may enhance overall glycogen recovery. Of course, protein plays an important role in recovery meals to enhance net protein balance, tissue repair and adaptations involving synthesis of new proteins (see Chapter 4). However, athletes are discouraged from consuming excessively large amounts of protein and fat if they displace CHO foods from the athletes' energy budget or eating comfort, thereby indirectly interfering with glycogen storage by preventing adequate CHO intake.

Excessive intake of alcohol

14.9

Since there is evidence that some athletes, particularly in team sports, consume alcohol in large amounts in the post-exercise period (Burke et al. 2003), it is important to consider the effect on recovery. With regard to muscle glycogen storage, rat studies have shown that intragastric administration of alcohol interferes with glycogen storage during 30 minutes of recovery from high-intensity exercise in oxidative but not non-oxidative fibers (Peters et al. 1996). Separate studies were undertaken in well-trained cyclists to monitor the effects of drinking a large amount of alcohol (~120 g or twelve standard drinks) after glycogen-depleting exercise on 8 hours and 24 hours of recovery (Burke et al. 2003). Muscle glycogen storage was impaired during both recovery periods when alcohol displaced an energy-matched amount of CHO from a standard recovery diet. This is a realistic comparison, since athletes typically forget about recovery programs, and forgo well-planned meals, during an alcohol binge and the pursuant hangover. Evidence for a direct effect of elevated blood alcohol concentrations on muscle glycogen synthesis was unclear, but it appeared that if an immediate impairment of glycogen synthesis existed, it might be compensated by adequate CHO intake and longer recovery time. It is likely that the most important effects of alcohol intake on glycogen resynthesis are indirect—by interfering with the athlete's ability, or interest, to achieve the recommended amounts of CHO required for optimal glycogen restoration. Athletes are therefore encouraged to follow the guidelines for sensible use of alcohol in sport (Burke & Maughan 2000) in conjunction with the well-supported recommendations for recovery eating.

14.10 Carbohydrate intake guidelines for training and recovery

The 2003 IOC Consensus on Nutrition for Athletes provided an opportunity to review the guidelines for CHO intake for training and competition, and to address issues regarding the communication of these guidelines. A summary of the updated guidelines produced by this meeting is provided in Table 14.2, and includes changes to recommendations for the type and timing of CHO intake during early recovery, as well as a comment on the general benefits of including protein in recovery meals. These issues were discussed in the previous

TABLE 14.2 UPDATED GUIDELINES FROM THE IOC CONSENSUS ON NUTRITION FOR ATHLETES FOR THE INTAKE OF CHO IN THE EVERYDAY OR TRAINING DIETS OF ATHLETES

RECOMMENDATIONS FOR
• Athletes should aim to achieve CHO intakes to meet the fuel requirements of their training program and to optimize restoration of muscle glycogen stores between workouts. General recommendations can be provided, but should be fine-tuned with individual consideration of total energy needs, specific training needs and feedback from training performance.
• Immediate recovery after exercise (0–4 h): 1–1.2 g/kg/h consumed at frequent intervals.
• Daily recovery: moderate duration/low-intensity training: 5–7 g/kg/d.
• Daily recovery: moderate to heavy endurance training: 7–12 g/kg/d.
• Daily recovery: extreme exercise program (4–6 h+ per day): 10–12 g/kg/d.
• It is valuable to choose nutrient-rich CHO foods and to add other foods to recovery meals and snacks to provide a good source of protein and other nutrients. These nutrients may assist in other recovery processes and, in the case of protein, may promote additional glycogen recovery when CHO intake is suboptimal or when frequent snacking is not possible.
• When the period between exercise sessions is <8 hours, the athlete should begin CHO intake as soon as practical after the first workout, to maximize the effective recovery time between sessions. There may be some advantages in meeting CHO intake targets as a series of snacks during the early recovery phase.
• During longer recovery periods (24 hours), the athlete should organize the pattern and timing of CHO-rich meals and snacks according to what is practical and comfortable for their individual situation. There is no difference in glycogen synthesis when liquid or solid forms of CHO are consumed.
• CHO-rich foods with a moderate to high GI provide a readily available source of CHO for muscle glycogen synthesis, and should be the major CHO choices in recovery meals.
• Adequate energy intake is also important for optimal glycogen recovery; the restrained eating practices of some athletes, particularly females, make it difficult to meet CHO intake targets and to optimize glycogen storage from this intake.
RECOMMENDATIONS AGAINST
• Guidelines for CHO (or other macronutrients) should not be provided in terms of percentage contributions to total dietary energy intake. Such recommendations are neither user-friendly nor strongly related to the muscle's absolute needs for fuel.
• The athlete should not consume excessive amounts of alcohol during the recovery period, since it is likely to interfere with their ability or interest to follow guidelines for post-exercise eating. The athlete should follow sensible drinking practices at all times, but particularly in the period after exercise.

Source: Burke et al. 2004

sections. Another issue meriting special comment was the recommendation to change the terminology in which CHO intake guidelines are given.

Terminology for carbohydrate intake recommendations

Previous dietary guidelines for athletes followed the tradition of community nutrition education messages in describing ideal CHO intake in terms of its contribution to total dietary energy intake. For example, athletes were advised to consume diets providing '60–65% of energy from CHO' by the American and Canadian Dietetic Associations (1995), 60–70% of dietary energy in the first consensus statement of the IOC (Devlin & Williams 1991) or 'at least 55% of energy from CHO' according to the 1994 position statement prepared for Fédération Internationale de Football Association (FIFA), the international governing body of soccer (Ekblom & Williams 1994). In the case of 'endurance' athletes, who undertake prolonged daily exercise session with increased fuel requirements, CHO intake recommendations have been set variously at '>60% of energy' in the 1995 position statement prepared for International Association of Athletics Federations (IAAF), the international governing body of athletics (Maughan & Horton 1995) or '65–70% of dietary energy' (American Dietetic Association & Dietitians of Canada 1995). Studies have typically reported that few individuals or groups of athletes achieve such CHO intake targets. A review of the dietary surveys of serious athletes published from 1970 to 2000 found that the mean values for the reported daily CHO intake of athletes was ~50–55% of total energy intake (Burke et al. 2001). Reported intakes of CHO as a percentage of energy were similar between male and female athletes, higher in endurance athletes compared with those involved in non-endurance sports, and appeared to have undergone a small increase during the 1990s when the previous guidelines existed.

The apparent failure of athletes to achieve such CHO-rich diets in training has caused some sports scientists to challenge the soundness of the advice (Noakes 1997), with the rationale that if it were advantageous to training adaptations and performance, we would expect athletes to follow the practice. While this is an interesting point, it fails to acknowledge that we have almost no knowledge of the dietary patterns of the world's best athletes; the available studies generally involve recreational to sub-elite performers. Furthermore, the 'mismatch' between sports nutrition guidelines and the real-life dietary patterns of these athletes can be largely explained as a result of the percentage energy terminology (Burke et al. 2001).

The new guidelines for CHO needs are derived from direct information regarding the fuel requirements of exercise or glycogen resynthesis, and are related to the athlete's body size/muscle mass as well as their exercise load (Burke et al. 2004). Even then, they should still be considered as 'ballpark' ranges that can be fine-tuned for the individual athlete, given more specific knowledge of their actual training program, their past and present response to training and their total energy budget. The dietary surveys of athletes published over the 1990s show mean values of reported daily CHO intake (g/kg BM) to be 7.6 and 5.8 for male endurance and non-endurance athletes, and 5.7 and 4.6 for their female counterparts (Burke et al. 2001).

Notwithstanding the limitations of self-reported information on dietary intakes, our assessment of athlete dietary surveys from the 1990s was that male athletes typically meet the notional guidelines for CHO intakes while female athletes have lower intakes, primarily due to lower energy intakes. These data also provided another interesting finding: a poor relationship between the percentage energy provided by CHO and the amount of CHO (g/kg) in the diets of athletes (see Fig. 14.1). In other words, percentage energy intakes provide a poor indicator of fuel intake in relation of the requirements of training. Because of the impractical nature and potentially misleading information provided by the use of percentage energy terminology, it has been removed and actively discouraged by the most recent sports nutrition guidelines for athletes (Burke et al. 2004; American Dietetic Association et al. 2009).

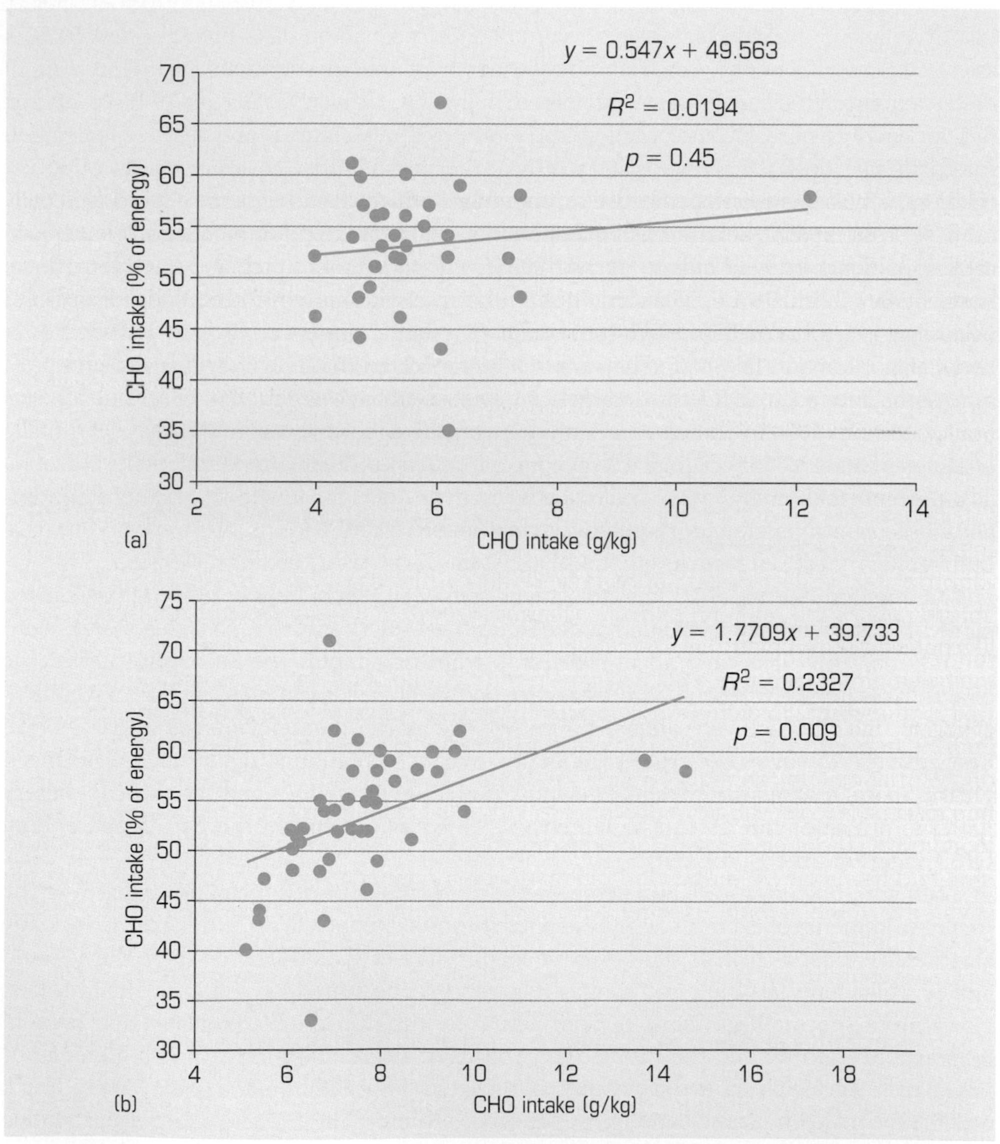

FIGURE 14.1 Relationship between dietary CHO intake (g/kg) and percentage of energy derived from CHO intake in training diets reported by serious male (b) and female (a) endurance athletes. Each data point represents the mean value from a dietary surveys published between 1970 and 1999. From Burke et al. 2001

Success of carbohydrate guidelines in promoting better performance through better recovery

It is relatively easy to find research literature that supports the acute benefits of a high-CHO diet in promoting recovery between exercise sessions. Numerous studies show that strategies to enhance glycogen stores between or before a prolonged exercise bout result in enhanced endurance and performance (for review see Chapter 12 and Hargreaves 1999). More specifically, Fallowfield and Williams (1993) reported that a high-CHO diet restored endurance capacity within 22.5 hours of recovery between running sessions, whereas an isocaloric diet of lower CHO content was associated with decreased endurance. Glycogen stores were not measured in this study, but the high-CHO recovery diet was presumed to promote greater resynthesis of glycogen in preparation for the second exercise trial (Fallowfield & Williams 1993).

Although a high CHO intake has been shown to benefit acute recovery and performance, it has been difficult to demonstrate clear benefits to repeated exercise performance over 7–28 days (Sherman & Wimer 1990; Burke et al. 2004). Theoretically, inadequate CHO intake during repeated days of exercise will lead to gradual depletion of muscle glycogen stores and subsequent impairment of exercise endurance. This hypothesis, based on observations of reduced muscle glycogen levels following successive days of running, was represented in a schematic in an early review paper by Costill and Miller (1980). Although this figure (see Fig. 14.2) has become perhaps the best known diagram in sports nutrition, and is often used to illustrate the relationship between high CHO intake and recovery, the results for the high-CHO diet are hypothetically derived rather than experimentally determined. In fact, a number of training studies have failed to find that a high-CHO diet (8–10 g CHO/kg BM/d) clearly enhances training adaptation or performance compared with a moderate CHO intake (5–7 g/kg BM/d), despite reports of local muscular fatigue or 'staleness' in the moderate-CHO group (Costill et al. 1988a; Lamb et al. 1990; Sherman et al. 1993). Although there is clear evidence of superior recovery of muscle glycogen with a higher CHO intake, a minority of the available studies shows enhancement of training outcomes (Simonsen et al. 1991; Achten et al. 2004).

It is curious that benefits from high-CHO eating have not been a universal outcome from training studies. Several methodological issues are important, including the overlap between what is considered a 'moderate' and 'high' CHO intake in various studies. Other important issues are whether sufficient time was allowed for differences in the training responses of athletes to lead to significant differences in the study performance outcome, and whether the protocol used to measure performance was sufficiently reliable to detect small but real improvements that would be of significance to a competitive athlete (Hopkins et al. 1999).

One possible conclusion from the available studies of chronic dietary patterns and exercise performance is that athletes can adapt to the lower muscle glycogen stores resulting from moderate CHO intakes such that it does not impair training or competition outcomes. This will be further considered below. However, no study shows that moderate CHO intakes promote superior training adaptations and performance compared with higher-CHO diets. Clearly, further research needs to be undertaken, using specialized and rigorous protocols, to better examine the issue of chronic CHO intake in heavily training athletes. Since such studies require painstaking control over a long duration, it is not surprising that there are few in the literature. In the meantime, although the lack

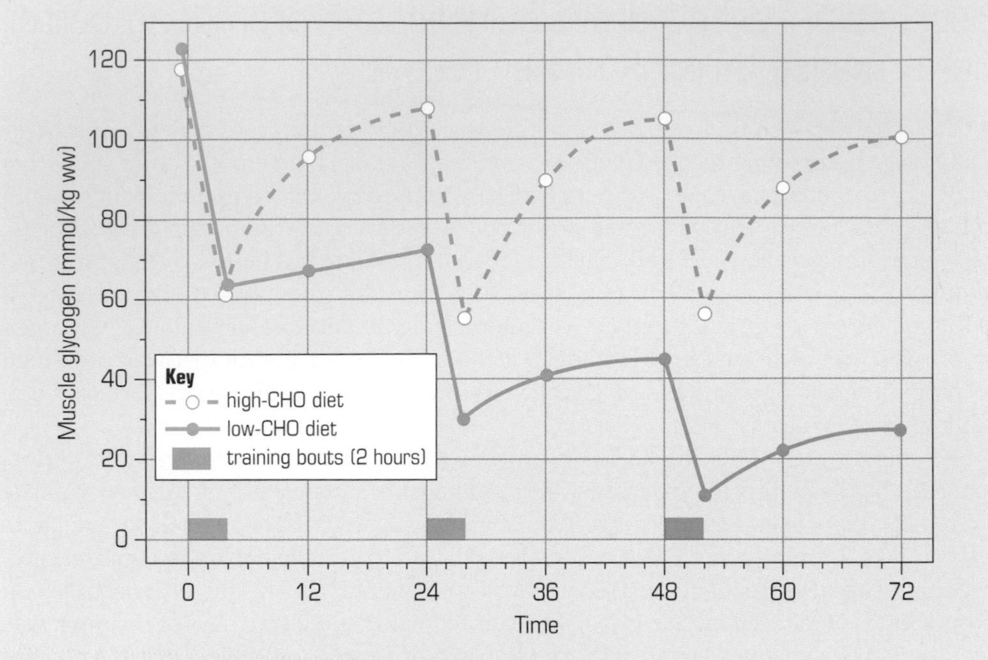

FIGURE 14.2 Graph prepared by Costill and Miller (1980), depicting the effect of moderate and high CHO intakes on restoration of muscle glycogen between daily training sessions. Although this figure has become famous as support for the benefits of high-CHO training diets, some of the data in this graph are extrapolated rather than taken from actual studies. Reprinted with permission Int J Sports Med 1980;1:2–14

of clear literature support is curious, the evidence from studies of acute CHO intake and exercise performance remains our best estimate of the chronic CHO needs of athletes.

14.13 Train low, compete high

New techniques that can examine molecular signaling within the muscle cell have allowed scientists to identify a range of pathways underpinning adaptations to training and form new hypotheses about the best strategies to promote these adaptations. Some studies have found that exercising with low muscle glycogen stores amplifies the activation of signaling proteins such as AMP-activated protein kinase (AMPK) and p38 mitogen-activated protein kinase (MAPK), which control the expression and activity of several transcription factors involved in mitochondrial biogenesis and other training adaptation (Hawley et al. 2006; Baar & McGee 2008). Exercise in a fasted state also promotes different cellular signaling responses to exercise undertaken with CHO intake prior to and during the session (Civitarese et al. 2005). These findings explain the recently described 'train low, compete high' protocol—training with low glycogen/CHO availability to enhance the training response, but competing with high fuel availability to promote performance. It is important to recognize that there are a number of potential ways to reduce CHO availability for the training environment, and these do not always promote a low-CHO diet per se nor restrict CHO availability for all training sessions (Burke 2009).

Our current interest in the concept of 'train low, compete high' was kick-started by a clever study from Danish researchers (Hansen et al. 2005) in which untrained males undertook a 10-week program of 'kicking' exercise while consuming a CHO-rich diet (~8 g/kg/d). Each leg did the same training program (5 x 1-hour sessions per week), but followed a different timetable. One leg was trained daily (refueling between sessions) while the other leg did two sessions back-to-back every second day, with a rest day in between (the second session on a training day was commenced with low glycogen stores). Compared to the leg that trained with normal glycogen reserves, the leg that commenced half of its training sessions with low muscle glycogen levels had a more pronounced increase in resting glycogen content and citrate synthase activity. Although the increase in maximal power was similar in each leg, the 'train low' leg had an almost twofold greater increase in time to fatigue compared to other leg.

Can the results of this study be applied to real-life athletes, especially elite competitors? Problems in translation include the potential differences between untrained and well-trained individuals, and the one-legged kicking exercise which bears little relationship to whole-body sporting activities. Importantly, the training sessions in the study were 'clamped' at a fixed submaximal intensity for the duration of the training program: athletes typically periodize their programs to incorporate a 'hard–easy' pattern to the overall organization of training, as well as progressive overload. Our group (Yeo et al. 2008) tried to address these issues in a recent study. Two groups of well-trained cyclists consumed a CHO-rich diet (~8 g/kg/d) over three weeks of training: with each week consisting of three steady state sessions (100 minutes at 70% $VO_{2\,peak}$) and three sessions of high-intensity intervals (8 x 5 minutes at maximal sustained power, with 1 minute's recovery). One group alternated between these sessions (High group), while another seven subjects trained every second day, with the steady state session followed an hour later by the interval session (Low group). Training intensity was measured as the self-selected power outputs achieved in the interval session, while performance was measured before and after the training block via a 1-hour time trial completed after an hour of steady state cycling. We found that resting muscle glycogen concentrations, rates of whole-body fat oxidation during steady-state cycling and muscle activities of enzymes citrate synthase and β-hydroxyacyl-CoA-dehydrogenase (HAD) were increased only in the group that undertook the interval sessions with low glycogen. However, total work completed in the interval sessions was reduced in the Low group compared with the High training group. Nevertheless, 1-hour cycling performance improved similarly (~10%) in both groups (Yeo et al. 2008).

Morton and colleagues (2009) studied three groups of recreationally active men who undertook four sessions of fixed-intensity 'interval' running over a 6-week period with either 'high' CHO availability (single day training), 'train low' (two training sessions, twice a week) or 'train low plus glucose' (as before, but with glucose intake before and during the second session). All groups recorded a similar improvement in $VO_{2\,max}$ (~10%) and distance run during an intermittent running test (~18%), although the group who trained with low availability of exogenous and endogenous CHO sources showed greater metabolic advantages, such as increased activity of the enzyme succinate dehydrogenase. The story of enhanced metabolic adaptations in the muscle, but similar gains in exercise capacity, has also been noted in studies comparing training in a fasted state versus training with a CHO drink in untrained or moderately trained groups (De Bock et al. 2008; Akerstrom et al. 2009).

The hypothesized benefits of 'train low' strategies include enhanced metabolic adaptations to a given training stimulus, increased ability to utilize fat as an exercise fuel and a reduced reliance on CHO. While there is support for such benefits, there is currently no clear evidence that this translates into a performance advantage. Other claimed benefits of 'train low' strategies are to enhance loss of body fat and reduce the need for CHO intake during competition (reducing the potential for gastrointestinal side effects by reducing the amount of food or sports drink an athlete might need to consume). These issues have not been studied, although work from our own group (Cox et al. unpublished observations) has shown that training with CHO intake increases oxidation rates of exogenous CHO, with the adaptation presumably occurring at the level of gut uptake.

Why don't the muscle and metabolic enhancements achieved with 'train low' strategies translate into clear performance benefits? The explanation for this apparent disconnect include the brevity of the study period, the possibility that performance is not reliant or quantitatively linked to the markers that have been measured, our failure to measure other counterproductive outcomes and our focus on the muscular contribution to performance while ignoring the brain and central nervous system. And, of course, we are ultimately limited by our ability to measure performance in a reliable and valid way.

Meanwhile, the potential for side effects arising from 'train low' strategies should also be considered (Burke 2009). There is already evidence that 'training low' reduces the ability to train—increasing the perception of effort and reducing power outputs. Most athletes and coaches fiercely guard the ability to generate high power outputs and work rates in training as a preparation for competition. Indeed, in our extensive work on fat adaptation (see Chapter 15), we have found evidence that adaptations that up-regulate fat utilization also down-regulate CHO utilization, leading to a reduction in ability to perform high-intensity exercise (Havemann et al. 2005). Finally, the effect of repeated training with low CHO status on the risk of illness, injury and overtraining needs to be considered (see Commentary C, page 501).

Practitioners who work with elite athletes appreciate that just as they periodize their training programs, they probably already periodize their fuel preparation for sessions. Many athletes may undertake some of their workouts in a fuel-restricted manner, either by accident (doing morning sessions in a fasted state because it is impractical to refuel before or during the session) or design (restricting CHO in an energy-restricted diet). Equally, these athletes will ensure that other sessions are done with better fuel support. The intricate mix and match of such sessions may be an art as well as a topic for further science.

14.14 Issues in post-exercise rehydration

As discussed in Chapter 12, hypohydration has a deleterious effect on exercise performance, with impairment of prolonged aerobic exercise and thermoregulation, particularly when exercise is performed in a hot environment (Sawka & Pandolf 1990), gastric emptying and comfort (Rehrer et al. 1991) and cognitive functioning (Gopinathan et al. 1988). Performance impairments can be detected when fluid deficits are as low as 1.8% of BM (Walsh et al. 1994); however, the effects are progressive throughout all levels of hypohydration (Montain & Coyle 1992). It is therefore undesirable to begin an exercise session with a pre-existing fluid deficit as a result of failure to rehydrate after previous exercise sessions, or as a result of dehydration protocols undertaken to make weight in a weight division event (see Chapter 7). In normal healthy people, the daily replacement of fluid losses and maintenance of fluid balance are well regulated by thirst and urine losses. However, under conditions of stress (e.g. exercise, environmental heat and cold, and altitude) thirst may not be a sufficient stimulus for maintaining euhydration (Greenleaf 1992). Furthermore, there may be a considerable lag of 4–24 hours before body fluid levels are restored following moderate to severe hypohydration.

Studies of voluntary fluid intake patterns across a range of sports show that athletes typically replace only 30–70% of the sweat losses incurred during exercise (Noakes et al. 1988; Broad et al. 1996). As a result, most athletes can expect to finish training or competition sessions with a mild to moderate level of hypohydration. After exercise, people fail to drink sufficient volumes of fluid to restore fluid balance, even when drinks are made freely available. Therefore, the fluid deficit can remain for prolonged periods. Rothstein and colleagues first described the failure to fully replace fluid losses as 'voluntary dehydration' and noted that it was exacerbated by factors that reduced the availability or palatability of fluids (Rothstein et al. 1947). However, this phenomenon has been more recently renamed 'involuntary dehydration' to recognize that the dehydrated individual has no volition to rehydrate even when fluids and the opportunity are available (Nadel et al. 1990). The factors affecting self-chosen drinking patterns are multi-faceted, and include behavioral issues such as social customs of drinking, as well as a genetic predisposition to be a reluctant or heavy drinker (Greenleaf 1992).

An additional challenge to post-exercise rehydration is that the athlete may continue to lose fluid during this phase, partly due to continued sweat losses, but principally due to urination. The success of post-exercise rehydration ultimately depends on the balance between fluid intake and urine losses. Ideally, an athlete should aim to fully restore fluid losses between exercise sessions so that the new event or workout can be commenced in a euhydrated state. This is difficult in situations where moderate to high levels of hypohydration have been incurred (deficits of 2–5% BM or greater) and the interval between sessions is less than 6–8 hours. Optimal rehydration requires a scheduled plan of fluid intake, to overcome physiological challenges such as inadequate thirst as well as practical problems such as poor access to fluids. A number of factors affecting post-exercise rehydration have been identified and will now be discussed.

Palatability of fluids 14.15

Numerous studies have reported that the palatability of fluids affects ad libitum (at any time) intake, with quality, flavor and temperature being identified as important variables (for review, see Hubbard et al. 1990). Since many of these studies have investigated rehydration during exercise, it is uncertain whether the findings apply directly to post-exercise recovery (when the athlete is at rest). Perceptions may change with environmental conditions and with the degree of dehydration; interestingly, there is some evidence that perception of palatability or pleasure may not always correlate with total intake of a rehydration fluid. Hubbard and colleagues (1990) reviewed studies and concluded that while very cold water (0°C) may be regarded as the most pleasurable, cool water (15°C) may be consumed in larger quantities.

Flavoring of drinks has also been considered to contribute to voluntary fluid intake, with studies reporting greater fluid intake during post-exercise recovery with sweetened drinks than with plain water. For example, Carter and Gisolfi (1989) investigated fluid intake during recovery after subjects had undertaken prolonged cycling to produce a fluid deficit of 2% BM. They found that subjects consumed significantly greater amounts of fluid when presented with a glucose-electrolyte drink than when plain water was provided. Water intake resulted in replacement of 63% of sweat losses, while the sweetened drink resulted in replacement of 79% ($p < 0.05$) of fluid losses. In both cases, ad libitum intake of fluid failed to meet total fluid losses, and the rate of intake decreased with time despite the continued fluid deficit. Whether subjects are responding to a sweet flavor or to energy replacement has not been systematically studied. There is some evidence that extreme sweetness and high CHO concentrations reduce voluntary intake, and that initial preferences for CHO-containing beverages may decrease after several hours (see Hubbard et al. 1990).

The addition of sodium to a beverage may also increase voluntary fluid intake, although there may be a concentration above which fluid intake is discouraged. Wemple and colleagues (1997) compared the volume of fluid consumed after dehydrating exercise when a flavored water beverage was provided with 0, 25 or 50 mmol/L concentrations of sodium. Subjects replaced a mean level of 123%, 163% and 133% of the volume of their sweat losses respectively. Sodium concentration is not only important in influencing the volume of a fluid that is consumed voluntarily, but also the amount that is then retained. This is discussed in the section below.

14.16 Replacement of electrolytes

Sodium is the principal electrolyte lost in sweat, and during prolonged bouts of heavy sweating, particularly in individuals with high-sodium sweat content, a substantial loss of body sodium can occur in each session of exercise. For example, in several studies of team sport players undertaking training sessions in hot weather, individuals recorded losses in excess of 7 g of salt (sodium chloride) in a single session (Maughan et al. 2004; Shirreffs et al. 2005). Although western dietary patterns are generally considered to be excessive in salt intake, athletes who lose such large amounts of sodium during exercise may need to undertake special strategies to actively replace sodium losses during and after exercise (Bergeron 2003). Even if the loss of sodium during an exercise session is not substantial and will be replaced eventually by dietary means, there are good reasons for including sodium in recovery fluids and snacks.

When water is ingested following exercise-induced dehydration, there is a dilution of plasma osmolality and sodium content, which results in an increased diuresis and reduced thirst. Nose and colleagues (1988) compared rehydration with water plus sodium capsules with water plus a placebo capsule in subjects who had been dehydrated by approximately 2.5% BM. They found that intake of sodium (equivalent to a solution of approximately 80 mmol/L) achieved more rapid restoration of plasma volume than the water trial, due to a greater voluntary intake of fluid and lower urine output.

Maughan and Leiper (1995) dehydrated subjects by 2% BM via exercise in a hot environment, then observed them for 6 hours of recovery after they had consumed 150% of their fluid losses with test drinks providing varying levels of sodium. Fluid was consumed over a 30-minute period, beginning 30 minutes after the end of the exercise bout. After 90 minutes of recovery there was a significant treatment effect, with greater urine losses being observed with 2 mmol/L (no sodium) and 26 mmol/L sodium (low sodium) drinks than with the 52 and 100 mmol/L sodium solutions (see Fig. 14.3). After 6 hours the difference in mean urine output between the no-sodium and 100 mmol/L sodium drinks was in the order of 800 mL.

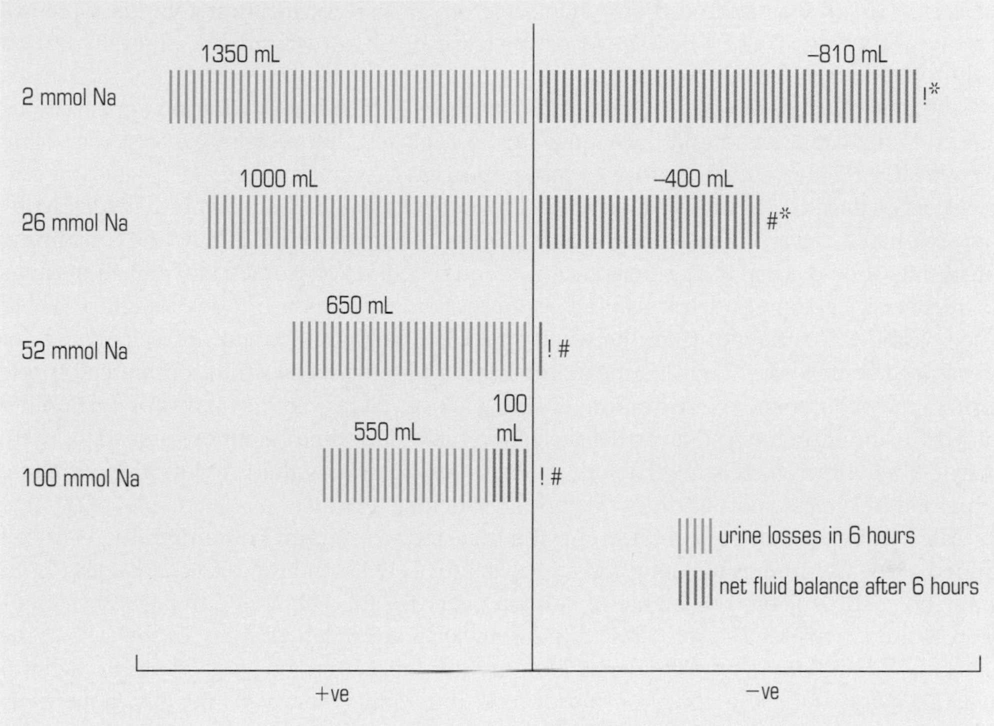

FIGURE 14.3 Effect of sodium content of fluid on urine losses and restoration of fluid balance following intake of volumes of fluid representing 150% of fluid deficit incurred by exercising in the heat. Fluids contain sodium content of 2 mmol/L, 26 mmol/L, 52 mmol/L and 100 mmol/L.
* significantly different to pre-exercise, # significantly different to 2 mmol/L, ! significantly different to 26 mmol/L. Data redrawn from Maughan & Leiper 1995

Subjects were in fluid balance by the end of the recovery period when they consumed the two higher-sodium beverages, but were still in net negative fluid balance on the no- and low-sodium trials, despite the intake of a volume of fluid that was 1.5 times their estimated sweat losses. Retention of the ingested fluid was related to the sodium content, but there was no difference in net fluid balance between the 52 and 100 mmol/L sodium trials.

There is some argument about the optimal sodium level for a post-exercise rehydration fluid. The World Health Organization recommends a sodium level of 90 mmol/L for oral rehydration solutions used in the treatment of diarrhea-induced dehydration (Walker-Smith 1992). However, this is based on the need to replace the sodium lost through diarrhea as well as optimize intestinal absorption of fluid and retention of ingested fluid. Sodium losses in sweat vary markedly, with typical sweat sodium levels believed to be in the range of 20–80 mmol/L (Verde et al. 1982; Armstrong et al. 1987). Therefore a post-exercise recovery drink with sodium levels of ~50 mmol/L may well be justified. Nevertheless, to be palatable and to have commercial appeal across a wide market, sports drinks have gravitated to a more moderate sodium content (10–25 mmol/L). When fluids are freely chosen, the interaction between the palatability of a drink (voluntary intake) and its sodium content (retention of fluid) are important. In one study, subjects chose to drink greater volumes (~2.5 L) when an orange juice/lemonade or sports drink was offered than when water or an oral rehydration solution were the recovery beverages (~1.7 L). However, urine losses were lowest with the oral rehydration solution (Maughan & Leiper 1993).

The effectiveness of such moderate sodium levels in restoring hydration appears to be slight. Gonzalez-Alonso and colleagues (1992) reported that a commercial sports drink (6% CHO, 20 mmol/L sodium) was more effective than plain water in promoting restoration of fluid levels after exercise-induced dehydration. Subjects were dehydrated by approximately 2.5% BM and were studied during 2 hours of rehydration while consuming a volume of fluid equal to this deficit, as two equal boluses consumed at 0 and 45 minutes of recovery. The sports drink trial achieved greater restoration of body weight (73% of the volume was retained) than the water trial (65% volume retained), principally due to decreased urine losses. Thus it appears from this and other studies that commercial sports drinks may confer some rehydration advantages over plain water, in terms of palatability as well as fluid retention. Nevertheless, where maximum fluid retention is desired, there may be benefits in increasing the sodium levels of rehydration fluids to levels above those provided in typical sports drinks (Maughan & Leiper 1995).

Alternatively, additional sodium may be ingested via sodium-containing foods or salt added to meals. Studies by Maughan and colleagues (1996) and Ray and colleagues (1998) have both shown that the intake of salt via everyday food choices enhances the retention of fluid consumed to rehydrate after exercise-induced dehydration. In the case of the study by Maughan and colleagues (1996), greater fluid retention (less urine production) was seen following the consumption of food plus fluid, than a drink only, potentially because of the greater electrolyte content. In this study, subjects were dehydrated by 2% BM by exercising in the heat. Over 60 minutes (beginning 30 minutes into the recovery period), they consumed fluid equal to 150% of sweat losses, either in the form of a sports drink (20 mmol/L sodium) or as a meal plus a low sodium drink (the water content of the meal was included to match the total fluid intake of the other trial). At the end of 6 hours of recovery, total urine production was lower following the meal plus drink and subjects were in a euhydrated state. The sports drink trial resulted in a net negative fluid balance of approximately 350 mL over the same period.

The addition of potassium (25 mmol/L) to a rehydration beverage is also effective in retaining fluids ingested during recovery from exercise-induced dehydration (Maughan et al. 1994). However, there is no additive effect of including both potassium and sodium, and the replacement of sodium would appear to be a priority, since sweat losses of sodium can be significant. According to the review of Shirreffs and colleagues (2004) for the 2003 IOC Consensus on Nutrition for Athletes, there is no convincing justification for the addition of other electrolytes such as magnesium in recovery fluids. Although some magnesium is lost in sweat, the reduction in plasma magnesium concentration that accompanies exercise is likely to be due to a redistribution of compartmental fluids rather than large magnesium losses.

14.17 Volume and pattern of drinking

As sweating and obligatory urine losses continue during the rehydration phase, fluids must be consumed in volumes greater than the post-exercise fluid deficit (exercise sweat loss) to restore fluid balance. A general finding of the previously reviewed studies is that replacement of fluid in volumes equal to sweat losses results in 50–70% rehydration over 2–4 hours of recovery (based on body weight restoration). Several studies have reported on the effect of the volume of rehydration fluids on restoration of body water deficit. Mitchell and colleagues (1994) dehydrated subjects by 2.5% BM by exercising them in a hot environment, then rehydrated them using a dilute electrolyte solution (15 mmol/L sodium) in volumes equivalent to 100% or 150% of their body weight deficit. Thirty percent of the total volume was consumed as a priming dose, with the remainder of the fluid being consumed in five equal volumes at 30-minute intervals. Gastric emptying was measured, and fluid restoration was determined as body weight gain corrected for fluid remaining in the stomach. During the 3-hour rehydration period, the 150% rehydration protocol resulted in greater rates and amounts of fluid emptied from the stomach, and a greater net fluid restoration (68% restoration of BM losses versus 48% restoration). The rate of gastric emptying and regain of body weight decreased over time. Interestingly, there was no further restoration of fluid balance achieved through hours 2–3 of recovery with either protocol, due to an increase in urine production. Even the 150% rehydration protocol achieved restoration of only 68% of loss of BM, although this figure may be lower than results calculated from other studies due to the correction for gastric contents. Thus these authors conclude that even forced rehydration with a low-electrolyte beverage does not achieve restoration of fluid balance, and while ingestion of large volumes of fluid is more effective than an equal replacement of the lost fluid, the possible gastrointestinal fullness and discomfort that follow must be taken into account. This may be a practical consideration if a subsequent bout of exercise is scheduled within 2–4 hours post-recovery.

Similar conclusions were reported by Shirreffs and colleagues (1996) regarding the volume of fluid required to restore hydration after exercise. They studied subjects who exercised to dehydrate by 2% BM, then consumed volumes, equivalent to 50%, 100%, 150% and 200% of BM loss, of solutions containing sodium concentrations of 23 mmol/L or 61 mmol/L. Fluids were consumed in four equal volumes at 15-minute intervals, and fluid balance was monitored over 6 hours of recovery. They found that urine production was related to the volume of fluid consumed. In the case of the high-sodium fluids, consumption of 150% and 200% of fluid losses resulted in euhydration and hyperhydration, respectively, after 6 hours of recovery. All other trials resulted in residual hypohydration. These results show that a drink volume greater than the sweat loss during exercise must be ingested to restore fluid balance, but unless the sodium content of the beverage is sufficiently high this will result merely in an increased urinary output.

Whether the pattern of fluid intake influences rehydration has been investigated, comparing intakes of larger amounts of fluid in the immediate post-exercise period with the same total volume of fluid being spread equally over 5–6 hours of recovery (Kovacs et al. 2002). Early replacement of large volumes of fluid was associated with better restoration of fluid balance during the first hours of recovery despite an increase in urinary output; however, differences in fluid restoration between hydration patterns disappeared by 5–6 hours of recovery. In another study, spacing fluid intake over several hours of recovery after exercise was more effective in restoring fluid balance, via reduction in urine losses, than consuming it as a large bolus immediately after the exercise (Archer & Shirreffs 2001). Of course, factors such as gastric comfort need to be considered when undertaking forced post-exercise rehydration practices, especially if the athlete needs to perform another exercise session within the next hours.

Finally, the consumption of a meal may be a useful adjunct to rehydration. Hubbard and colleagues (1990) note that food consumption may provide a social or psychological stimulus to increase voluntary fluid intake. Furthermore, the sodium content of the meal will enhance fluid retention (Maughan et al 1996; Ray et al. 1998).

14.18 Caffeine and alcohol: potential diuretics

Diuresis may be stimulated by several factors commonly found in beverages consumed by dehydrated athletes. Gonzalez-Alonso and colleagues (1992) reported that consumption of a diet cola drink containing caffeine resulted in less effective regain of body fluid losses than their water or sports drink trials (see section 14.17). Ingestion of diet cola in a volume equal to sweat losses resulted in restoration of 54% of BM losses; urine losses were significantly increased compared to the other trials and there was a small but significantly greater loss of fluid through continued sweating and respiratory losses (Gonzalez-Alonso et al. 1992). This finding fits with the common advice that caffeine-containing fluids are not ideal rehydration beverages and should be avoided in relation to exercise or other situations of dehydration (such as air travel). However, a large review of caffeine and hydration status found that there is a lack of rigorously collected data to show that caffeine intake impairs fluid status (Armstrong 2002). It concluded that the effect of caffeine on diuresis is overstated, and may be minimal in people who are habitual caffeine users. Indeed, a more recent study observed hydration status and urine losses in subjects who were first habituated to a daily caffeine intake of 3 mg/kg, then changed to 5 days of caffeine doses of 0, 3 or 6 mg/kg/d (Armstrong et al. 2005). There were no differences in BM, urine losses or serum osmolality as a result of the different intakes of caffeine, questioning the theory that caffeine consumption acts chronically as a diuretic. In addition, any small increase in fluid losses from caffeine-containing drinks may be more than offset by the increased voluntary intake of fluids that are enjoyed by the athlete, or part of social rituals and eating behaviors. If the athlete is suddenly asked to remove such beverages from their diet or post-exercise meals, they may not compensate by drinking an equal volume of other less familiar or well-liked fluids.

Alcohol consumption has also been shown to increase urinary losses during post-exercise recovery. Subjects consuming drinks containing 4% alcohol reported greater urinary losses than when drinks containing 0, 1 or 2% alcohol were consumed (Shirreffs & Maughan 1995). Subjects exercised in the heat to dehydrate by 2% BM and rehydrated over a 60-minute period by consuming drinks equivalent to 150% of their fluid deficit of varying alcohol content. The total volume of urine produced over the 6-hour recovery period was related to the alcohol content of the fluid; however, only the 4% alcohol drink trial approached significance with a net retention of 40% of ingested fluid compared to 59% in the no-alcohol trial.

14.19 Intravenous rehydration

In the situation of severe dehydration, especially when fluid intake is compromised by gastrointestinal dysfunction and/or the collapse of the subject, rapid rehydration may be attempted via IV delivery of saline solutions. It has become fashionable in some sports for athletes to receive IV rehydration at the end of their event to aid recovery. This is understandable in events such as the Tour de France and tennis tournaments, where moderate to severe fluid deficits are usual, the period between stages or games is brief, and the athlete has to juggle time to allow adequate sleep as well as recovery nutrition. However, it has recently become more common across a range of sports in which athletes incur moderate fluid deficits and have no gastrointestinal impediments to oral rehydration. Many athletes and coaches believe that IV rehydration has advantages of itself in enhancing recovery and the performance of subsequent exercise. This idea needs to be considered, and balanced against the expense and slight medical risk involved with IV procedures (especially when carried out in the field).

A series of studies compared the effects of oral and IV rehydration on restoration of fluid balance, and thermoregulation, metabolism and performance in subsequent exercise trials (Castellani et al. 1997; Riebe et al. 1997; Casa et al. 2000a, 2000b; Maresh et al. 2001). Protocols involved exercise-induced dehydration, followed by no rehydration, or matched replacement of fluid via oral or IV delivery. After a period of recovery, subjects undertook a second bout of exercise in hot conditions. These studies showed that fluid replacement protocols achieved equal improvement in plasma volume and thermoregulation during subsequent exercise, compared with the no-rehydration trial (Castellani et al. 1997). However, oral rehydration was superior to IV rehydration in relation to reducing thirst and lowering the perception of effort in the second exercise trial (Riebe et al. 1997). In this study, exercise tolerance was better following oral rehydration compared with IV fluid replacement, apparently because of the reduced perception of workload. In the other series, oral and IV rehydration were equally effective in improving exercise performance compared with no rehydration, although it seemed that oral rehydration was associated with better return of physiological parameters (Casa et al. 2000a, 2000b; Maresh et al. 2001). Therefore, there is evidence that oral rehydration is at least as effective as IV therapy in treating moderate and uncomplicated situations of dehydration. The psychological sensation of drinking appears to provide an important component of recovery, enabling the athlete to feel better when tackling the next event or workout. On the other hand, IV hydration attenuated the loss of thirst that accompanies oral intake of fluid, even before fluid restoration is achieved. On this basis, it could be argued that a combination of the strategies might provide the best hydration technique. However, the medical and financial aspects of IV feeding protocols must be considered.

Alcohol and recovery

14.20

Although it is difficult to gain reliable data on people's alcohol intake practices, there is at least preliminary evidence and testimonials of binge drinking behavior by some athletes, particularly during the post-competition period. This appears to be most prevalent in team sports where the culture may promote, or at least fail to discourage, post-game alcohol binges (see Burke & Maughan 2000). Unfortunately, the post-exercise intake of alcohol is subject to many rationalizations and justifications by athletes, including 'everyone is doing it', 'I only drink once a week' and 'I can run/sauna it off the next morning'.

Heavy intake of alcohol may interfere with post-exercise recovery in a number of ways. The most important effects of alcohol are the impairment of judgment and reduced inhibition; heavy drinking has a major impact on the behavior of athletes during the post-exercise recovery period, increasing high-risk behaviors that may lead to a poor image, accidents and injury and, sometimes, death.

Alcohol consumption is highly correlated with accidents of drowning, spinal injury and other problems in recreational water activities (see O'Brien 1993), and is a major factor in road accidents. The intoxicated athlete is likely to be distracted from sound recovery strategies related to nutrition, injury treatment and sleep. There is some evidence that alcohol may directly affect physiological processes such as rehydration and glycogen storage (see above). Many sporting activities are associated with muscle damage and soft tissue injuries, as a direct consequence of the exercise, as a result of accidents, or due to the tackling and collisions involved in contact sports. Standard medical practice is to treat soft tissue injuries with vasoconstrictive techniques (such as rest, ice, compression and elevation). Since alcohol is a potent vasodilator of cutaneous blood vessels it has been suggested that the intake of large amounts of alcohol might cause or increase undesirable swelling around damaged sites, and might impede repair processes. Although this effect has not been systematically studied, there are case histories that report these findings. Overall, heavy alcohol intake after exercise is likely to directly and indirectly prevent the athlete from achieving optimal recovery.

Alcohol is strongly linked with modern sport. The alcohol intakes and drinking patterns of athletes merit further study and a well-considered plan of education, particularly to target the binge drinking practices often associated with post-competition socializing. In addition to being targeted for education about sensible drinking practices, athletes might be used as spokespeople for community education messages. Athletes are admired in the community and may be effective educators in this area. Alcohol is consumed by many adults and merits education messages about how it might be used to enhance lifestyle rather than detract from health and performance.

14.21 Summary

Recovery after exercise poses an important challenge to the modern athlete. Important nutrition goals include restoration of liver and muscle glycogen stores, and the replacement of fluid and electrolytes lost in sweat. Although future research may identify occasions in which an athlete may enhance training adaptations through deliberate restriction of fuel status, enhanced performance of key training sessions and competitive events merit attention to fuel needs. Rapid resynthesis of muscle glycogen stores over the first 4 hours of recovery is aided by the immediate intake of CHO (1 g/kg BM every hour), particularly of CHO-rich foods of high GI, and perhaps consumed as a series of small snacks every 15–20 minutes. Such rapid refueling during the first hours may be important for the athlete who has less than 8 hours between lengthy exercise sessions. To ensure maximal glycogen synthesis over longer term (24-hour) recovery, the athlete should achieve a total CHO intake of 7–12 g/kg BM, depending on factors such as the presence of muscle damage and continued exercise during this period. In situations where daily training does not heavily deplete muscle glycogen stores, dietary CHO needs are lower, for example 3–5 g/kg/d. Provided adequate CHO is consumed, it appears that the frequency of intake, the form (liquid versus solid) and the presence of other macronutrients do not appear to affect the rate of glycogen storage. Practical considerations, such as the availability and appetite appeal of foods or drinks, and gastrointestinal comfort, may determine ideal CHO choices and intake patterns.

Rehydration requires a special fluid intake plan since thirst and voluntary intake will not provide for full restoration of sweat losses in the acute phase (0–6 hours) of recovery. When the fluid deficit following exercise exceeds ~2% of BM, it may be necessary to consume volumes equivalent to 150% of fluid losses over the hours following exercise to allow for complete fluid restoration. Steps should be taken to ensure that a supply of palatable drinks is available after exercise. Sweetened drinks are generally preferred and can contribute towards achieving CHO intake goals. Replacement of sodium lost in sweat is important for maximizing the retention of ingested fluids. A sodium content of 50–90 mmol/L may be necessary for optimal rehydration; however, commercial sports drinks are formulated with a more moderate sodium content (10–25 mmol/L) to allow a greater overall use and palatability. Of course, sodium replacement can occur via salt added or eaten within meals and snacks. Excessive intake of alcohol is not recommended during the recovery period, because it is associated with high-risk behaviors while distracting the athlete from undertaking ideal recovery strategies. Alcohol intake may also provide a direct impairment of rehydration, glycogen synthesis and other recovery processes. Although concerns have been raised about the diuresis associated with caffeine-associated drinks, it appears that the overall effects on urine losses and hydration status are minimal, at least in habitual consumers of caffeine. Since athletes often compete in a foreign environment, the practical issues of food availability and food preparation facilities must be considered when making recommendations for post-exercise nutrition.

PRACTICE TIPS

LOUISE BURKE

Practice tips have been taken from Burke and Maughan (2000) and Burke (2007).

REFUELING AFTER EXERCISE

- Effective refueling begins only after a substantial amount of CHO has been consumed. When there are less than 8 hours between workouts or events that deplete glycogen stores, the athlete should maximize effective recovery time by consuming a high-CHO meal or snack within 30 minutes of completing each session. This will mean being organized to have suitable food and drinks available—at the exercise venue if necessary.
- The athlete should aim to consume 1 g of CHO per kilogram of their BM immediately after exercise, and repeat after an hour or until normal meal patterns are resumed (see Table 14.3). Recovery snacks and meals should contribute towards a daily CHO intake of 7–12 g/kg BM. Total CHO requirements need to be individualized to each athlete's exercise program and energy budget, and athletes are advised to seek expert advice from a sports dietitian, especially when they are trying to restrict total energy intake.

TABLE 14.3 IDEAS FOR RECOVERY SNACKS
CHO-RICH SNACKS (50 G CHO SERVES) PROVIDING AT LEAST 10 G OF PROTEIN
250–350 mL of liquid meal supplement
250–350 mL of milk-shake or fruit smoothie
500 mL flavored low-fat milk
Many sports bars (check labels for protein and CHO content)
60 g (1½–2 cups) breakfast cereal with ½ cup milk
1 round of sandwiches including cheese/meat/chicken filling, and 1 large piece of fruit or 300 mL sports drink
1 cup of fruit salad with 200 g carton fruit-flavored yoghurt or custard
200 g carton fruit-flavored yoghurt or 300 mL flavored milk and 30–35 g cereal bar
2 crumpets or English muffins with thick spread of peanut butter or 2 slices of cheese
200 g (cup or small tin) of baked beans on 2 slices of toast
250 g (large) baked potato with cottage cheese or grated cheese filling
150 g thick crust pizza with meat/chicken/seafood topping
50 G CHO SNACKS
800–1000 mL of sports drink
800 mL of cordial
500 mL of fruit juice, soft drink or flavored mineral water
60–70 g packet of jelly beans or jube sweets
2 sports gels

TABLE 14.3 *(continued)*
50 G CHO SNACKS *(continued)*
3 medium pieces of fruit or 2 bananas
1 round of thick-sliced sandwiches with jam or honey
2 large (35 g) or 3 small (25 g) cereal bars
1 large chocolate bar (70–80 g)

Note: The athlete should use this guide to consume snacks or light meals providing at least 1 g CHO per kilogram of their BM, to ensure speedy recovery of glycogen stores (post-exercise recovery) or to 'top up' fuel stores prior to a workout (pre-exercise snack). In the case of post-exercise recovery, this strategy should be repeated after an hour or until normal eating patterns have been resumed. The intake of protein (~20 g) in conjunction with CHO snacks will help to meet goals for enhanced net protein synthesis.
Source: Burke 2000

- The consumption of protein within recovery snacks and meals will enhance the synthesis of new proteins underpinning adaptations to the workout as well as contribute to any increase in protein requirements related to exercise (see Chapter 4). The intake of a high-quality protein source providing 10–25 g of protein will have a substantial to maximal effect on net protein synthesis. It is likely that such an intake will be exceeded in the meals provided within a well-chosen diet. Choices for snacks that provide a good source of CHO and protein include breakfast cereal and milk, flavored milk drinks and specially formulated sports bars and liquid meal supplements (see Table 14.3).
- When CHO needs are high, and appetite is suppressed or gastric discomfort is a problem, the athlete should focus on compact forms of CHO, including low-fiber choices of CHO-rich foods, sugar-rich foods and special sports supplements such as sports bars.
- CHO-containing fluids are also low in fiber and may be appealing to athletes who are fatigued and dehydrated. These include sports drinks, soft drinks and juices, commercial liquid meal supplements, milk-shakes and fruit smoothies.
- Low-GI CHO foods such as lentils and other legumes may be less suitable for speedy glycogen recovery and should not be the principal CHO source in recovery meals. This is generally not a problem as typical western diets are based on CHO-rich foods of moderate and high GI.
- Small, frequent meals may assist the athlete to achieve high CHO intakes without the discomfort of overeating. However, the athlete should organize their routine of meals and snacks to suit individual preferences, timetable and appetite/comfort. In long-term recovery (24 hours), as long as enough CHO is consumed, it does not appear to matter how intake is spaced throughout the day. There may be benefits in increasing the frequency of intake of CHO (such as snacks every 30–60 minutes) during the first hours of recovery.
- When stomach discomfort or total energy requirements limit total food intake, high-fat foods and excessive amounts of protein should not be consumed at the expense of CHO choices.

PRACTICE TIPS

- Nutritious CHO foods and drinks contain other nutrients including vitamins and minerals that may be important in other post-exercise recovery processes. These nutrients are also important in the overall diet. Future research may show that intake early after exercise could enhance other activities of repair and rebuilding, as well as the immune system.

SPECIAL COMMENTS FOR THE ATHLETE WITH A RESTRICTED ENERGY BUDGET

- Recovery snacks should not contribute additional energy to a restricted energy budget. Rather, when rapid recovery is desirable, the energy-restricted athlete should change the timing of their existing meal structure to allow for immediate intake after exercise sessions. One option is to reschedule training sessions or meals so that the athlete is able to eat their normal meal as soon as possible after the workout. Where this is not practical, the athlete may be able to take a small snack from within their usual meal plan to consume immediately after training or as a pre-resistance training snack (e.g. fruit and flavored yoghurt usually consumed as a dessert with dinner), then consume the remainder of their meal at the usual time.
- Since the athlete may have increased requirements for protein and micronutrients as a result of their exercise program, it is important that foods consumed as recovery snacks contribute to overall nutrient intake goals as well as immediate recovery needs. Nutrient-rich choices (e.g. fruit, flavored milk drinks and dairy foods, sandwiches with meat and salad fillings) are more valuable than lower nutrient choices (e.g. lollies or candies, soft drink, bread with jam or honey).
- The energy-restricted athlete should also make use of foods with a high-fiber content (e.g. fresh fruit rather than juice), high volume/low energy density (salad fillings added to sandwiches) or low-GI (rolled oat cereals rather than cornflakes) to maximize the satiety value of meals and snacks. The addition of protein to meals and snacks (e.g. yoghurt with fruit, meat or cheese in sandwich) also improves satiety. Guidelines for low-fat eating are also important.
- The energy-restricted athlete is unlikely to have a sufficient energy budget to cover the guidelines for optimal intakes of some macronutrients (e.g. CHO for optimal daily glycogen synthesis). Specialized dietary advice from a sports dietitian is valuable in ensuring that the athlete has reasonable goals related to their energy requirements and physique goals, and is able to organize meal plans to optimize their nutrient intake within this energy budget. It may be valuable to cycle between nutritional goals—restrict energy during periods suitable for loss of body fat, while liberalizing energy and CHO intake to promote better fueling and recovery for key sessions or competition.

RAPID REHYDRATION

- Dehydration will have a negative effect on subsequent exercise sessions if not fully corrected before the next workout. However, moderate to severe fluid deficits can also have an effect on recovery, since they are associated with an increased risk of gastrointestinal upset and discomfort, potentially limiting the athlete's ability to ingest substantial amounts of nutrients. Therefore, rehydration should be considered an immediate priority, especially where gastrointestinal function is compromised. Early recovery strategies may need to focus on rehydration goals (e.g. consuming dilute fluids) before the athlete is able to consume significant amounts of the macronutrients needed for refueling and protein recovery.

- The athlete should not rely on thirst or opportunity to dictate fluid intake to reverse a situation of dehydration. A 'hit and miss' approach may be acceptable when fluid deficits are 1 L or less, but when fluid losses are greater an organized schedule is required.
- The athlete should monitor changes in BM from pre- to post-exercise to evaluate the success of drinking strategies during exercise, and the residual fluid deficit that must now be replaced. A loss of 1 kg is equivalent to 1 L of fluid. Since fluid losses will continue during the recovery period via urine losses and ongoing sweating, the athlete will need to consume additional fluid to counter this. Typically, a volume equal to ~150% of the post-exercise fluid deficit should be consumed over the subsequent 2–4 hours to fully restore fluid balance.
- It is important to ensure that an adequate supply of palatable drinks is available. This may be difficult when the athlete is at a remote competition venue, or traveling in a country where bottled water must be consumed instead of the local water supply.
- In situations where fluid intake needs to be encouraged, the provision of flavored drinks is a useful strategy. Since most people prefer sweet-tasting drinks, they are likely to increase their voluntary intake of such fluids. Keeping drinks at a refreshing temperature is also known to encourage greater intake. Cool drinks (10–15°C) are preferred in most situations. Very cold fluids (0–5°C) may seem ideal when the environment or the athlete is hot, but it is often challenging to drink them quickly or in large volumes.
- CHO-containing drinks are also useful in assisting with refueling goals and allow the athlete to tackle a number of recovery goals simultaneously.
- In the situation of moderate to large fluid deficits (e.g. >2 L), sodium replacement will assist the retention of ingested fluids, by minimizing urine losses. Options include sports drinks, commercial oral rehydration solutions (such as Gastrolyte™), salty foods or salt added to post-exercise meals. A high sodium beverage such as an oral rehydration solution (50–90 mmol/L or 2–5 g of salt per liter), or salt added to post-exercise meals along with substantial fluid intake, should guarantee that sufficient fluid and sodium have been replaced.
- Athletes are often educated that the production of 'copious amounts of clear urine' is a desirable state and a sign of good hydration status. Measurements of urinary specific gravity or osmolality are sometimes undertaken to provide an indicator of euhydration and good hydration practices. Although this may be true in the long-term situation, the athlete is to be reminded that during the acute period of fluid replacement immediately following dehydration, mismatch of fluid and electrolyte

PRACTICE TIPS

replacement can lead to production of large amounts of dilute urine despite the continuing existence of substantial fluid deficits. Thus, in the case of significant fluid loss, the athlete should be aware of the need for electrolyte replacement, and should know that 'urine checks' over the first hours of fluid intake often provide false readings. Dietary strategies that minimize urine losses during the rehydration period not only enhance the speed of regaining fluid balance, but help the athlete to achieve better quality rest or sleep without frequent disturbances related to having to get up to urinate.

- Caffeine-containing fluids (e.g. cola drinks, tea, coffee and energy drinks) are generally not considered to be ideal rehydration beverages, since caffeine may increase urine losses. It is often suggested that alternative choices should be used for early post-exercise rehydration, and that once fluid balance has been substantially restored, the athlete may have greater freedom in making drink choices. It should be noted that a recent review of the caffeine literature concluded that the diuretic effect of caffeine is overstated in habitual caffeine drinkers. Furthermore, greater voluntary consumption of favorite beverages such as cola drinks may lead to a better hydration status even if they are associated with a slightly greater urine production.
- Alcohol also causes an increase in urine losses, and drinks containing significant amounts of alcohol (4% or more of volume) are not considered ideal rehydration beverages. Nevertheless, athletes are to be reminded that alcohol exerts its main effect on recovery through indirect means: the intoxicated athlete is unlikely to follow sound nutritional practices and is more likely to undertake high-risk behavior and suffer an increased risk of accidents.
- Where possible, the athlete should avoid post-exercise activities that exacerbate sweat losses—for example, long exposure to hot-spas, saunas or sun.

ALCOHOL INTAKE AND SPORT

- Alcohol is not an essential component of a diet. It is a personal choice of the athlete whether to consume alcohol at all. However, there is no evidence of impairments to health and performance when alcohol is used sensibly.
- The athlete should be guided by community guidelines, which suggest general intakes of alcohol that are 'safe and healthy'. This varies from country to country, but in general, it is suggested that mean daily alcohol intake should be less than 40–50 g (perhaps 20–30 g per day for females), and that 'binge' drinking is discouraged. Since individual tolerance to alcohol is variable, it is difficult to set a precise definition of 'heavy' intake or an alcohol 'binge'. However, intakes of about 80–100 g at a single sitting are likely to constitute a heavy intake for most people.
- Alcohol is a high-energy (and nutrient-poor) fluid and should be restricted when the athlete is attempting to reduce body fat.

- The athlete should avoid heavy intake of alcohol on the night before competition. It appears unlikely that the intake of 1–2 standard drinks will have negative effects in most people.
- The intake of alcohol immediately before or during exercise does not enhance performance and in fact may impair performance in many people. Psychomotor performance and judgment are most affected. Therefore, the athlete should not consume alcohol deliberately to aid performance, and should be wary of exercise that is conducted in conjunction with the social intake of alcohol.
- Heavy alcohol intake is likely to have a major impact on post-exercise recovery. It may have direct physiological effects on rehydration, glycogen recovery and repair of soft-tissue damage. More importantly, the athlete is unlikely to remember or undertake strategies for optimal recovery when intoxicated. Therefore, the athlete should attend to these strategies first before any alcohol is consumed. No alcohol should be consumed for 24 hours in the case of an athlete who has suffered a major soft-tissue injury.
- The athlete should rehydrate with appropriate fluids in volumes that are greater than their existing fluid deficit. Suitable fluid choices include sports drinks, fruit juices, soft drinks (all containing CHO) and water (when refueling is not a major issue). However, sodium replacement via sports drinks, oral rehydration solutions or salt-containing foods is also important to encourage the retention of these rehydration fluids. Low-alcohol beers and beer-soft drink mixes may be suitable and seem to encourage large volume intakes. However, drinks containing greater than 2% alcohol are not recommended as ideal rehydration drinks.
- Before consuming any alcohol after exercise, the athlete should consume a high-CHO meal or snack to aid muscle glycogen recovery. Food intake will also help to reduce the rate of alcohol absorption and thus reduce the rate of intoxication.
- Once post-exercise recovery priorities have been addressed, the athlete who chooses to drink is encouraged to do so 'in moderation'. Drink-driving education messages in various countries may provide a guide to sensible and well-paced drinking.
- Athletes who drink heavily after competition, or at other times, should take care to avoid driving and other hazardous activities.
- It appears likely that it will be difficult to change the attitudes and behaviors of athletes with regard to alcohol. However, coaches, managers and sports medicine staff can encourage guidelines such as these, and specifically target the 'old wives' tales' and rationalizations that support binge drinking practices. Importantly, they should reinforce these guidelines with an infrastructure that promotes sensible drinking practices. For example, alcohol might be banned from locker rooms, and fluids and foods appropriate to post-exercise recovery provided instead. In many cases, athletes drink in a peer-group situation and it may be easier to change the environment in which this occurs than the immediate attitudes of the athletes.

References

Achten J, Halson SH, Moseley L, et al. Higher dietary carbohydrate content during intensified running training results in better maintenance of performance and mood state. J Appl Physiol 2004;96: 1331–40.

Akerstrom TC, Fischer CP, Plomgaard P, Thomsen C, Van Hall G, Pedersen BK. Glucose ingestion during endurance training does not alter adaptation. J Appl Physiol 2009;106:1771–9.

American Dietetic Association, Canadian Dietetic Association. Position stand of the American Dietetic Association and Canadian Dietetic Association: nutrition for physical fitness and athletic performance for adults. J Am Diet Assoc 1995;93:691–6.

American Dietetic Association, Dietitians of Canada, American College of Sports Medicine, Rodriguez NR, Di Marco NM, Langley S. American College of Sports Medicine position stand: nutrition and athletic performance. Med Sci Sports Exerc 2009;41:709–31.

Archer DT, Shirreffs SM. Effect of fluid ingestion rate on post-exercise rehydration in man. Proc Nutr Soc 2001;60:200A.

Armstrong LE. Caffeine, body fluid-electrolyte balance, and exercise performance. Int J Sport Nutr Exerc Metab 2002;12:189–206.

Armstrong LE, Costill DL, Fink WJ. Changes in body water and electrolytes during heat acclimation: effects of dietary sodium. Aviat Space Environ Med 1987;58:143–8.

Armstrong LE, Pumerantz AC, Roti MW, et al. Fluid, electrolyte, and renal indices of hydration during 11 days of controlled caffeine consumption. Int J Sport Nutr Exerc Metab 2005;15: 252–65.

Baar K, McGee SL. Optimizing training adaptations by manipulating glycogen. Eur J Sport Sci 2008;8: 97–106.

Bergeron MF. Heat cramps: fluid and electrolyte challenges during tennis in the heat. J Sci Med Sport 2003;6:19–27.

Blom CS. Post-exercise glucose uptake and glycogen synthesis in human muscle during oral or IV glucose intake. Eur J Appl Physiol 1989;58:327–33.

Blom PSC, Hostmark AT, Vaage O, Kardel KR, Maehlum S. Effect of different post-exercise sugar diets on the rate of muscle glycogen synthesis. Med Sci Sports Exerc 1987;19:491–6.

Broad EM, Burke LM, Gox GR, Heeley P, Riley M. Body weight changes and voluntary fluid intakes during training and competition sessions in team sports. Int J Sport Nutr 1996;6:307–20.

Burke LM. Nutrition for the female athlete. In: Krummel D, Kris-Etherton P, eds. Nutrition in women's health. Maryland: Aspen Publishers, 1995:263–98.

Burke LM. Nutrition for post-exercise recovery. Aust J Sci Med Sports 1996;29(1):3–10.

Burke LM. Practical sports nutrition. Champaign: Illinois, Human Kinetics Publishers, 2007.

Burke LM. Fuelling strategies to optimise performance—train low or train high? Scand J Med Sci Sports 2009 (in press).

Burke LM, Collier GR, Beasley SK, et al. Effect of coingestion of fat and protein with carbohydrate feedings on muscle glycogen storage. J Appl Physiol 1995;78:2187–92.

Burke LM, Collier GR, Broad EM, et al. Effect of alcohol intake on muscle glycogen storage after prolonged exercise. J Appl Physiol 2003;95:983–90.

Burke LM, Collier GR, Davis PG, Fricker PA, Sanigorski AJ, Hargreaves M. Muscle glycogen storage following prolonged exercise: effect of the frequency of carbohydrate feedings. Am J Clin Nutr 1996;64:115–19.

Burke LM, Collier GR, Hargreaves M. Muscle glycogen storage following prolonged exercise: effect of the glycaemic index of carbohydrate feedings. J Appl Physiol 1993;75:1019–23.

Burke LM, Cox GR, Cummings N, Desbrow B. Guidelines for daily CHO intake: do athletes achieve them? Sports Med 2001;31:267–99.

Burke LM, Kiens B, Ivy JL. Carbohydrates and fat for training and recovery. J Sports Sci 2004;22:15–30.

Burke LM, Maughan RJ. Alcohol in sport. In: Maughan RJ, ed. Nutrition in sport. Oxford: Blackwell Science, 2000:405–14.

Carrithers JA, Williamson DL, Gallagher PM, et al. Effects of postexercise carbohydrate-protein feedings on muscle glycogen restoration. J Appl Physiol 2000;88:1976–82.

Carter JE, Gisolfi CV. Fluid replacement during and after exercise in the heat. Med Sci Sports Exerc 1989;21:532–9.

Casa DJ, Maresh CM, Armstrong LE, et al. Intravenous versus oral rehydration during a brief period: responses to subsequent exercise in the heat. Med Sci Sports Exerc 2000a;32:124–33.

Casa DJ, Maresh CM, Armstrong LE, et al. Intravenous versus oral rehydration during a brief period: stress hormone responses to subsequent exhaustive exercise in the heat. Int J Sport Nutr Exerc Metab 2000b;10:361–74.

Castellani JW, Maresh CM, Armstrong LE, et al. Intravenous vs. oral rehydration: effects on subsequent exercise-heat stress. J Appl Physiol 1997;82:799–806.

Civitarese AE, Hesselink MK, Russell AP, Ravussin E, Schrauwen P. Glucose ingestion during exercise blunts exercise-induced gene expression of skeletal muscle fat oxidative genes. Am J Physiol Endocrinol Metab 2005; 289:E1023–9.

Costill DL, Flynn MG, Kirwan JP, et al. Effects of repeated days of intensified training on muscle glycogen and swimming performance. Med Sci Sports Exerc 1988a;20:249–54.

Costill DL, Miller JM. Nutrition for endurance sport: carbohydrate and fluid balance. Int J Sports Med 1980;1:2–14.

Costill DL, Pascoe DD, Fink WJ, Robergs RA, Barr SI, Pearson D. Impaired muscle glycogen resynthesis after eccentric exercise. J Appl Physiol 1991;69:46–50.

Costill DL, Pearson DR, Fink WJ. Impaired muscle glycogen storage after muscle biopsy. J Appl Physiol 1988b;64:2245–8.

Costill DL, Sherman WM, Fink WJ, Maresh C, Witten M, Miller JM. The role of dietary carbohydrates in muscle glycogen resynthesis after strenuous running. Am J Clin Nutr 1981;34:1831–6.

Coyle EF. Timing and method of increased carbohydrate intake to cope with heavy training, competition and recovery. J Sports Sci 1991;9(special issue):29–52.

Coyle ET, Jeukendrup AE, Oseto MC, et al. Low-fat diet alters intramuscular substrates and reduces lipolysis and fat oxidation during exercise. Am J Physiol 2001;280:E391–8.

Danforth W. Glycogen synthase activity in skeletal muscle. J Biol Chem 1965;240:588–93.

De Bock K, Derave W, Eijnde BO, Hesselink MK, Koninckx E, Rose AJ, Schrauwen P, Bonen A, Richter EA, Hespel P. Effect of training in the fasted state on metabolic responses during exercise with carbohydrate intake. J Appl Physiol 2008;104:1045–55.

Devlin JT, Williams C, eds. Final consensus statement: foods, nutrition and sports performance. J Sports Sci 1991;9(Suppl):iiiS.

Doyle JA, Sherman WM, Strauss RL. Effects of eccentric and concentric exercise on muscle glycogen replenishment. J Appl Physiol 1993;74:1848–55.

Ekblom B, Williams C, eds. Final consensus statement: foods, nutrition and soccer performance. J Sports Sci 1994;12(Suppl):3S.

Fallowfield JL, Williams C. Carbohydrate intake and recovery from prolonged exercise. Int J Sport Nutr 1993;3:150–64.

Gonzalez-Alonso J, Heaps CL, Coyle EF. Rehydration after exercise with common beverages and water. Int J Sports Med 1992;13:399–406.

Gopinathan PM, Pichan G, Sharma VM. Role of dehydration in heat-stress induced variations in mental performance. Arch Environ Health. 1988;43:15–17.

Greenleaf JE. Problem: thirst, drinking behaviour, and involuntary dehydration. Med Sci Sports Exerc 1992;24:645–56.

Hansen AK, Fischer CP, Plomgaard P, Andersen JL, Saltin B, Pedersen BK. Skeletal muscle adaptation: training twice every second day vs. training once daily. J Appl Physiol 2005;98: 93–9.

Hansen BF, Asp S, Kiens B, Richter E. Glycogen concentration in human skeletal muscle: effect of prolonged insulin and glucose infusion. Scand J Med Sci Sports 1999;9:209–13.

Hargreaves M. Metabolic responses to carbohydrate ingestion: effect on exercise performance. In: Lamb DR, Murray, R, eds. Perspectives in exercise science and sports medicine. Volume 12. The metabolic basis of performance in exercise and sport. Carmel, Indiana: Cooper Publishing Company, 1999:93–124.

Havemann L, West SJ, Goedecke JH, Macdonald IA, St Clair Gibson A, Noakes TD, Lambert EV. Fat adaptation followed by carbohydrate loading compromises high-intensity sprint performance. J Appl Physiol 2006;100:194–202.

Hawley JA, Tipton KD, Millard-Stafford ML. Promoting training adaptations through nutritional interventions. J Sports Sci 2006;24:709–21.

Hermansen L, Vaage O. Lactate disappearance and glycogen synthesis in human muscles after maximal exercise. Am J Physiol 1977;233:E422–9.

Hopkins WG, Hawley JA, Burke LM. Design and analysis of research on sport performance enhancement. Med Sci Sports Exerc 1999;31:472–85.

Hubbard RW, Szlyk PC, Armstrong LE. Influence of thirst and fluid palatability on fluid ingestion during exercise. In: Gisolfi CV, Lamb DR, eds. Perspectives in exercise science and sports medicine. Volume 3. Fluid homeostasis during exercise. Carmel, Indiana: Benchmark Press, 1990:39–96.

Ivy JL, Goforth HW, Damon BD, et al. Early post-exercise muscle glycogen recovery is enhanced with a carbohydrate-protein supplement. J Appl Physiol 2002;93:1337–44.

Ivy JL, Katz AL, Cutler CL, Sherman WM, Coyle EF. Muscle glycogen synthesis after exercise: effect of time of carbohydrate ingestion. J Appl Physiol 1988a;64:1480–5.

Ivy JL, Kuo CH. Regulation of GLUT4 protein and glycogen synthase during muscle glycogen synthesis after exercise. Acta Physiol Scand 1998;162:295–304.

Ivy JL, Lee MC, Bronzinick JT, Reed MC. Muscle glycogen storage following different amounts of carbohydrate ingestion. J Appl Physiol 1988b;65:2018–23.

Jenkins DJA, Cuff D, Wolever TMS, et al. Digestibility of carbohydrate foods in an ileostomate: relationship to dietary fibre, in vitro digestibility, and glycemic response. Am J Gastroenterol 1987;82:709–17.

Jentjens RL, van Loon LJC, Mann CH, Wagenmakers AJM, Jeukendrup AE. Addition of protein and amino acids to carbohydrates does not enhance postexercise muscle glycogen synthesis. J Appl Physiol 2001;91:839–46.

Joszi AC, Trappe TA, Starling RD, et al. The influence of starch structure on glycogen resynthesis and subsequent cycling performance. Int J Sports Med 1996;17:373–8.

Keizer HA, Kuipers H, Van Kranenburg G, Guerten P. Influence of liquid and solid meals on muscle glycogen resynthesis, plasma fuel hormone response, and maximal physical work capacity. Int J Sports Med 1986;8:99–104.

Kiens B, Richter EA. Types of carbohydrate in an ordinary diet affect insulin action and muscle substrates in humans. Am J Clin Nutr 1996;63:47–53.

Kovacs EMR, Schmahl RM, Senden JMG, Brouns F. Effect of high and low rates of fluid intake on post-exercise rehydration. Int J Sport Nutr Exerc Metab 2002;12:14–23.

Kuipers H, Keizer HA, Brouns F, Saris WHM. Carbohydrate feeding and glycogen synthesis during exercise in man. Pflugers Arch 1987;410:652–6.

Lamb DR, Rinehardt KF, Bartels RL, Sherman WM, Snook JT. Dietary carbohydrate and intensity of interval swim training. Am J Clin Nutr 1990;52:1058–63.

Maehlum S, Hermansen L. Muscle glycogen concentration during recovery after prolonged severe exercise in fasting subjects. Scand J Clin Lab Invest 1978;38:447–60.

Maresh CM, Herrera-Soto JA, Armstrong LE, et al. Perceptual responses in the heat after brief intravenous versus oral rehydration. Med Sci Sports Exerc 2001;33:1039–45.

Maughan RJ, Horton ES, eds. Final consensus statement: current issues in nutrition in athletics. J Sports Sci 1995;13(Suppl):1S.

Maughan RJ, Leiper JB. Post-exercise rehydration in man: effects of voluntary intake of four different beverages (Abst). Med Sci Sports Exerc 1993;25(Suppl):2S.

Maughan RJ, Leiper JB. Sodium intake and post-exercise rehydration in man. European J Appl Phys 1995;71:311–19.

Maughan RJ, Leiper JB, Shirreffs SM. Restoration of fluid balance after exercise-induced dehydration: effects of food and fluid intake. Eur J Appl Physiol 1996;73:317–25.

Maughan RJ, Merson SJ, Broad NP, Shirreffs SM. Fluid and electrolyte intake and loss in elite soccer players during training. Int J Sport Nutr Exerc Metab 2004;14:333–46.

Maughan RJ, Owen JH, Shirreffs SM, Leiper JB. Post-exercise rehydration in man: effects of electrolyte addition to ingested fluids. Eur J Appl Physiol 1994;69:209–15.

McCoy M, Proietto J, Hargreaves M. Skeletal muscle GLUT-4 and postexercise muscle glycogen storage in humans. J Appl Physiol 1996;80:411–15.

Mitchell JB, Grandjean PW, Pizza FX, Starling RD, Holtz RW. The effect of volume ingested on rehydration and gastric emptying following exercise-induced dehydration. Med Sci Sports Exerc 1994;26:1135–43.

Montain SJ, Coyle EF. Influence of graded dehydration on hyperthermia and cardiovascular drift during exercise. J Appl Physiol 1992;73:1340–50.

Morton JP, Croft L, Bartlett JD, Maclaren DP, Reilly T, Evans L, McArdle A, Drust B. Reduced carbohydrate availability does not modulate training-induced heat shock protein adaptations but does upregulate oxidative enzyme activity in human skeletal muscle. J Appl Physiol 2009;106:1513–21.

Nadel ER, Mack GW, Nose HN. Influence of fluid replacement beverages on body fluid homeostasis during exercise and recovery. In: Gisolfi CV, Lamb DR, eds. Perspectives in exercise science and sports medicine. Volume 3. Fluid homeostasis during exercise. Carmel, Indiana: Benchmark Press, 1990:181–205.

Noakes TD. Challenging beliefs: ex Africa semper aliquid novi. Med Sci Sports Exerc 1997;29:571–90.

Noakes TD, Adams BA, Myburgh KH, Greff C, Lotz T, Nathan M. The danger of inadequate water intake during prolonged exercise. Eur J Appl Physiol 1988;57:210–19.

Nose H, Mack GW, Shi X, Nadel ER. Role of osmolality and plasma volume during rehydration in humans. J Appl Physiol 1988;65:325–31.

O'Brien CP. Alcohol and sport: impact of social drinking on recreational and competitive sports performance. Sports Med 1993;15:71–7.

Parkin JAM, Carey MF, Martin IK, Stojanovska L, Febbraio MA. Muscle glycogen storage following prolonged exercise: effect of timing of ingestion of high glycemic index food. Med Sci Sports Exerc 1997;29:220–4.

Peters TJ, Nikolovski S, Raja GK, Palmer N, Fournier PA. Ethanol acutely impairs glycogen repletion in skeletal muscle following high intensity short duration exercise in the rat. Addiction Biology 1996;1:289–95.

Piehl Aulin K, Soderlund K, Hultman E. Muscle glycogen resynthesis in humans after supplementation of drinks containing carbohydrates with low and high molecular masses. Eur J Appl Physiol 2000;81:346–51.

Prats C, Helge JW, Nordby P, Qvortrup K, Ploug T, Dela F, Wojtaszewski JF. Dual regulation of muscle glycogen synthase during exercise by activation and compartmentalization. J Biol Chem 2009;284:15692–700.

Ray ML, Bryan MW, Ruden TM, Baier SM, Sharp RL, King DS. Effect of sodium in a rehydration beverage when consumed as a fluid or meal. J Appl Physiol 1998;85:1329–36.

Reed MJ, Brozinick JT, Lee MC, Ivy JL. Muscle glycogen storage postexercise: effect of mode of carbohydrate administration. J Appl Physiol 1989;66:720–6.

Rehrer NJ, Beckers EJ, Brouns F, ten Hoor F, Saris WHM. Effects of dehydration on gastric emptying and gastrointestinal distress while running. Med Sci Sports Exerc 1991;22:790–5.

Richter EA, Mikines KJ, Galbo H, Kiens B. Effects of exercise on insulin action in human skeletal muscle. J Appl Physiol 1989;66:876–85.

Riebe D, Maresh C, Armstrong, LE, et al. Effects of oral and intravenous rehydration on ratings of perceived exertion and thirst. Med Sci Sports Exerc 1997;29:117–24.

Roberts KM, Noble EG, Hayden DB, Taylor AW. Simple and complex carbohydrate-rich diets and muscle glycogen content of marathon runners. Eur J Appl Physiol 1988;57:70–4.

Rose AJ, Howlett K, King DS, Hargreaves M. Effect of prior exercise on glucose metabolism in trained men. Am J Physiol Endocrinol Metab 2001;281:E766–71.

Rothstein A, Adolph EF and Wills JH. Voluntary dehydration. In: Adolph EF, et al. Physiology of man in the desert. Interscience, New York, 1947:254–70.

Roy BD, Tarnopolsky MA. Influence of differing macronutrient intakes on muscle glycogen resynthesis after resistance exercise. J Appl Physiol 1998;84:890–6.

Saris WHM, van Erp-Baart MA, Brouns F, Westerterp KR, ten Hoor F. Study on food intake and energy expenditure during extreme sustained exercise: the Tour de France. Int J Sports Med 1989;10(1 Suppl):26S–31S.

Sawka MN, Pandolf KB. Effects of body water loss on physiological function and exercise performance. In: Gisolfi CV & Lamb DR, eds. Perspectives in exercise science and sports medicine, Vol 3. Fluid homeostasis during exercise. Carmel, Indiana: Benchmark Press, 1990:3–38.

Sherman WM, Wimer GS. Insufficient dietary carbohydrate during training: does it impair athletic performance? Int J Sport Nutr 1990;1:28–44.

Sherman WM, Doyle JA, Lamb DR, Strauss RH. Dietary carbohydrate, muscle glycogen, and exercise performance during 7 d of training. Am J Clin Nutr 1993;57:27–31.

Shirreffs SM, Aragon-Vargas LF, Chamorro M, et al. The sweating response of elite professional soccer players to training in the heat. Int J Sports Med 2005;26:90–5.

Shirreffs SM, Armstrong LE, Cheuvront SN. Fluid and electrolyte needs for preparation and recovery from training and competition. J Sports Sci 2004;22:57–63.

Shirreffs SM, Maughan RJ. The effect of alcohol consumption on fluid retention following exercise-induced dehydration in man. J Physiol 1995;489:33P–4P.

Shirreffs SM, Taylor AJ, Leiper JB, Maughan RJ. Post-exercise rehydration in man: effects of volume consumed and sodium content of ingested fluids. Med Sci Sports Exerc 1996;28:1260–71.

Simonsen JC, Sherman WM, Lamb DR, et al. Dietary carbohydrate, muscle glycogen, and power output during rowing training. J Appl Physiol 1991;70:1500–5.

Tarnopolsky MA, Atkinson SA, Phillips SM, MacDougall JD. Carbohydrate loading and metabolism during exercise in men and women. J Appl Physiol 1995;78:1360–8.

Tarnopolsky MA, Zawada C, Richmond LB, et al. Gender differences in carbohydrate loading are related to energy intake. J Appl Physiol 2001;91:225–30.

Van Hall G, Shirreffs SM, Calbert JAL. Muscle glycogen resynthesis during recovery from cycle exercise: no effect of additional protein ingestion. J Appl Physiol 2000;88:1631–6.

Van Loon LJC, Saris WHM, Kruijshoop M, Wagenmakers AJM. Maximizing postexercise muscle glycogen synthesis: carbohydrate supplementation and the application of amino acid or protein hydrolysate mixtures. Am J Clin Nutr 2000;72:106–11.

Verde T, Shepherd RJ, Corey P, Moore R. Sweat composition in exercise and in heat. J Appl Physiol 1982;53:1540–5.

Walker-Smith JA. Recommendations for composition of oral rehydration solutions for children in Europe. J Pediat Gastro 1992;14:113–15.

Walsh RM, Noakes TD, Hawley JA, Dennis SC. Impaired high-intensity cycling performance time at low levels of dehydration. Int J Sports Med 1994;15:392–8.

Wemple RD, Morocco TS, Mack GW. Influence of sodium replacement on fluid ingestion following exercise-induced dehydration. Int J Sport Nutr 1997;7:104–16.

Wolever TMS, Cohen Z, Thompson LU, et al. Ileal loss of available carbohydrate in man: comparison of a breath hydrogen method with direct measurement using a human ileostomy model. Am J Gastroenterol 1986;81:115–22.

Yeo WK, Paton CD, Garnham AP, Burke LM, Carey AL, Hawley JA. Skeletal muscle adaptation and performance responses to once a day versus twice every second day endurance training regimens. J Appl Physiol 2008;105:1462–70.

Zachwieja JJ, Costill DL, Pascoe DD, Robergs RA, Fink WJ. Influence of muscle glycogen depletion on the rate of resynthesis. Med Sci Sports Exerc 1991;23:44–8.

Zawadzki KM, Yaspelkis BB, Ivy JL. Carbohydrate-protein complex increases the rate of muscle glycogen storage after exercise. J Appl Physiol 1992;72:1854–9.

CHAPTER 15

Nutritional strategies to enhance fat oxidation during aerobic exercise

LOUISE BURKE AND JOHN HAWLEY

Introduction

15.1

Compared with the finite stores of carbohydrate (CHO), endogenous fat depots in humans are large, and represent a potentially unlimited source of fuel for skeletal muscle metabolism during aerobic exercise. However, fatty acid (FA) oxidation by muscle is limited, especially during the high power outputs and intensities sustained by athletes in training and compctition. In the never-ending search for strategies to improve athletic performance, there has been considerable interest in several nutritional interventions that might, theoretically, promote FA oxidation, attenuate the rate of muscle glycogen utilization and improve exercise performance. This chapter presents an overview of the role of endogenous fat as an energy substrate for skeletal muscle during exercise, discusses the methods for quantifying fat oxidation during exercise, examines the effect of exercise intensity on the regulation of fat metabolism, and provides a synopsis of some of the processes that could limit FA during exercise. Given this theoretical background, some of the nutritional procedures that may enhance fat utilization and improve aerobic exercise performance in humans are reviewed, and practical recommendations on their use provided for the practitioner.

Triacylglycerol as an energy source during exercise

15.2

Lipids provide the largest nutrient store of chemical energy that can be used to power biological work (see Fig. 15.1). As an energy source, triacylglycerol (TG) has several advantages over CHO: the energy density of lipid is higher (37.5 kJ/g for stearic acid versus 16.9 kJ/g for glucose), while the relative weight as stored energy is lower. TG also provides more adenosine triphosphate (ATP) per molecule than glucose (147 versus 38 ATP), although the complete oxidation of FA requires more oxygen than the oxidation

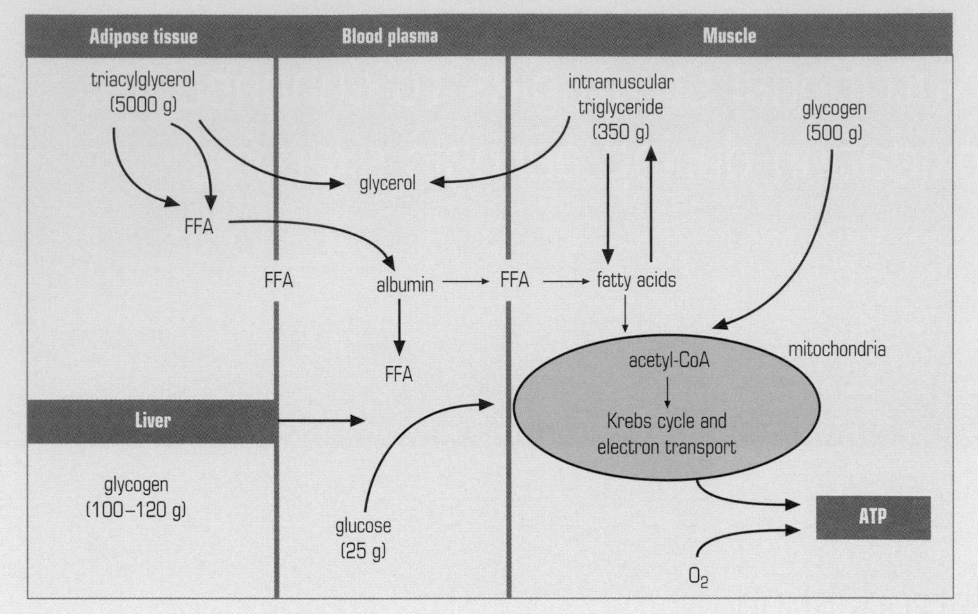

FIGURE 15.1 A schema of the major endogenous storage sites of carbohydrate and fat. Reprinted with permission from Coyle 1997

of CHO (6 versus 26 mol of oxygen per mole of substrate for glucose and stearic acid oxidation, respectively). Adipose tissue TG constitutes by far the largest energy store in the body (see Fig. 15.1), sufficient to sustain skeletal muscle contraction for ~120 hours at marathon running pace! On the other hand, if only CHO were utilized as a fuel, it would deliver energy for only ~90 minutes of running. As the men's world record for the marathon is ~125 minutes, this highlights the importance of fuel integration during prolonged exercise. The size of the adipose tissue TG pool is difficult to estimate and obviously depends on the fat mass of each individual, but is likely to range from 50 000 to 100 000 kcal (200–400 MJ) in men and women with 10–30% body fat (see Fig. 15.1). In order for this TG to be used as a substrate for oxidative metabolism, it has to be exported from adipose tissue and transported by the blood to the active tissues where it will be utilized.

Another important physiological store of TG can be found within the skeletal muscle (IMTG), mostly adjacent to the mitochondria: the total active muscle mass may contain up to 300 g of TG within the myocyte as small lipid droplets, although this amount can vary substantially due to individual differences in fiber type (type I fibers contain a greater concentration of IMTG than type II fibers), endurance training status (Kiens et al. 1993; Martin et al. 1993) and diet (Starling et al. 1997).

Finally, FA can also be derived from circulating TG (chylomicrons) and very low density lipoproteins (VLDL) formed from dietary fat in the post-absorptive state. Evidence suggests that if all the circulating VLDL-TG were taken up and oxidized, VLDL-TG degradation could contribute up to 50% of the lipid oxidized during submaximal exercise (Kiens 1998).

Intramuscular triacylglycerol and insulin resistance: the metabolic paradox 15.3

Elevated IMTG stores have been associated with reduced muscle insulin sensitivity in sedentary, obese and/or insulin-resistant individuals in some studies (Ebeling et al. 1998; Goodpaster et al. 2001) but not all studies (Bruce et al. 2003). In contrast, regular endurance training elicits an increase in IMTG concentration in healthy individuals (Kiens et al. 1993; Pruchnic et al. 2004) and is associated with increased insulin sensitivity (Staudacher et al. 2001). This greater storage of IMTG in the athlete represents an adaptive response to endurance training, allowing a greater contribution of the IMTG pool as a substrate for oxidative metabolism during exercise. In contrast, the elevated IMTG stores in the obese and/or type 2 diabetic patient seems to be secondary to a structural imbalance between FA availability, storage and oxidation (Kelley 2002). As such, the reported correlations between IMTG content and insulin resistance do not necessarily represent a functional relationship, as this association is strongly modulated by training status, habitual physical activity and muscle fiber composition. As 'fitness status' is better reflected through measures of skeletal muscle oxidative capacity rather than more traditional measures of whole body maximal aerobic power (Bruce et al. 2003), it has been suggested that IMTG content should be expressed relative to this muscle marker, rather than in isolation (Van Loon & Goodpaster 2006).

Processes that could limit fatty acid oxidation during exercise 15.4

Despite the vast stores of endogenous TG, the capacity for FA oxidation during exercise is limited. Unlike CHO oxidation, which is closely geared to the energy requirements of the working muscle, there are no mechanisms for matching the availability and utilization of FA to the rate of energy expenditure (Holloszy et al. 1998). There are many potential sites at which the ultimate control of FA oxidation may reside (see Fig. 15.2), with the relative importance of each site depending on a myriad of external factors, such as the aerobic training status of the individual, habitual dietary intake, ingestion of substrates (CHO and fat) before and during exercise, gender, and both the relative and absolute exercise intensity. A comprehensive analysis of the processes that potentially limit FA oxidation during exercise is beyond the scope of this chapter, and the reader is referred to several excellent reviews of the topic (Van der Vusse & Reneman 1996; Jeukendrup 1997; Holloszy et al. 1998; Wolfe 1998).

Mobilization of fatty acids from adipose triacylglycerol: lipolysis 15.5

Triacylglycerols cannot be oxidized by skeletal muscle directly; first they must be hydrolyzed into their components, non-esterified fatty acids (NEFA) and glycerol. This process, called lipolysis, is largely dependent on the activation of the enzyme hormone-sensitive TG lipase

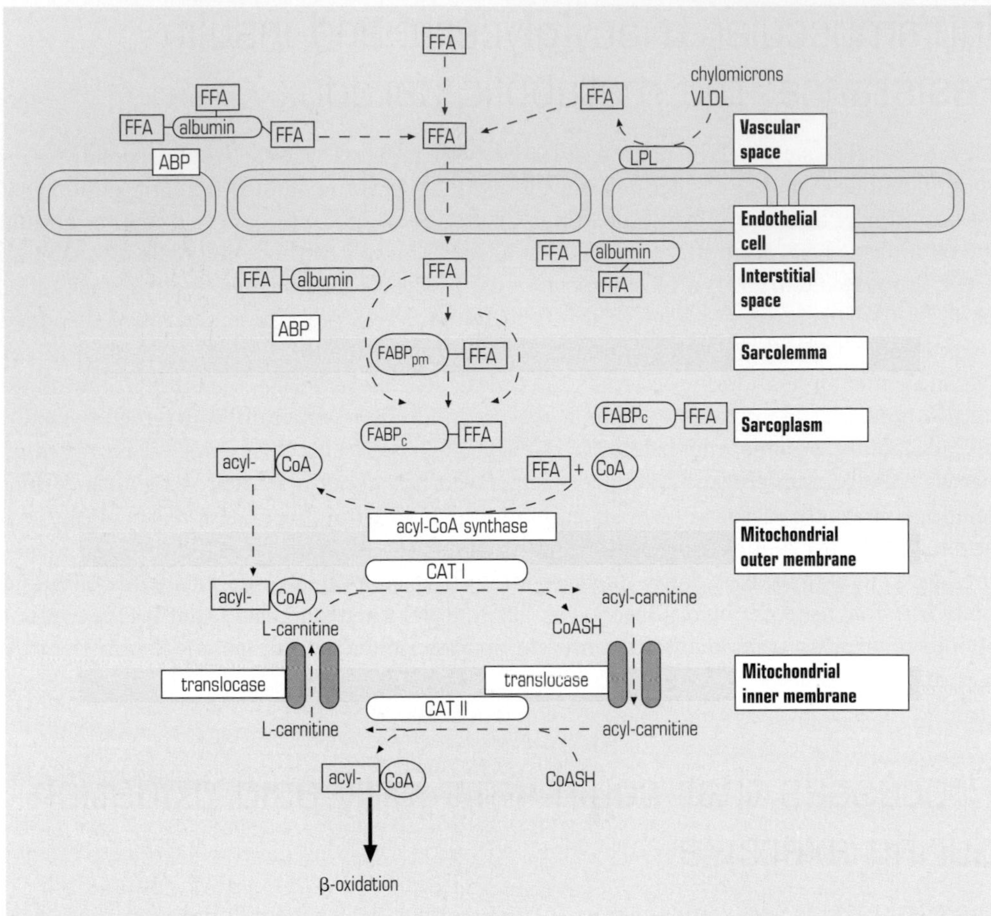

FIGURE 15.2 A schema of the transport of fatty acids from the vascular space to the inner mitochondria of the skeletal muscle where β-oxidation occurs. CAT I = carnitine acyl transferase I; CAT II = carnitine acyl transferase II; $FABP_c$ = fatty acid binding protein; $FABP_{pm}$ = plasma-membrane-bound fatty acid binding protein; FFA = free fatty acid; VLDL = very low density lipoprotein. The various processes are described in detail in the text. Reproduced with permission from Jeukendrup 1997

(HSL) in adipose tissue. Binding of hormone to plasma membrane receptors on adipocytes activates adenyl cyclase and initiates the lipolytic cascade (see Fig. 15.2). Epinephrine and glucagon activate HSL, while high levels of plasma glucose and insulin inhibit the activity of the lipase and reduce lipolysis. FA and glycerol derived from lipolysis in adipose tissue are released into the circulation: FA are bound by serum albumin and transported to tissues for oxidation and production of ATP (discussed subsequently), while glycerol returns to the liver and can be either phosphorylated to glycerol 3-phosphate and used to form TG, or converted to dihydroxyacetone and enter the glycolytic or gluconeogenic pathways. An isoform of the enzyme HSL is also present in skeletal muscle, where it acts to break down IMTG stores.

Transport of fatty acids across the sarcolemmal membrane into skeletal muscle

15.6

During transport of FA from blood to muscle there are several potential processes that limit eventual FA uptake. These are the membranes of the vascular endothelial cells, the interstitial space between endothelium and muscle cell, and finally the muscle cell membrane. Although FA transport across the sarcolemmal membrane into the muscle fiber was originally thought to occur exclusively by simple passive diffusion along a concentration gradient, there is now good evidence of a long-chain fatty acid (LCFA) transport system involving FA binding proteins (FABP), FA translocases (FAT) and FA transport proteins (FATP) (for review, see Glatz et al. 2001, 2002). Of interest is the finding that FABP content is higher in type I (slow twitch) than type II (fast twitch) muscle fibers, and is also increased with endurance training. This suggests a functional relationship between the FA binding capacity and the degree of oxidative metabolism in the muscle (Kiens 1998). Once FA enter the cytoplasm of muscle cell they can either be esterified and stored as IMTG, or the FA can be bound to FABP for transport to the site of oxidation and activated to a fatty acyl-CoA (co-enzyme-A) by the enzyme acyl-CoA synthase.

Oxidation of fatty acids

15.7

Whereas most fatty acyl-CoA is formed outside the mitochondria, the oxidative machinery is inside the inner membrane, which is impermeable to CoA. To overcome this problem, there exists a specific carnitine-dependent shuttle to carry acyl groups across the membrane (see Fig. 15.3).

Enzymes on both sides of the membrane transfer acyl groups between CoA and carnitine. On the outer mitochondrial membrane, the acyl group is transferred to carnitine catalyzed by carnitine palmityltransferase I (CPTI). Acylcarnitine then exchanges across the inner mitochondrial membrane with free carnitine by a carnitine-acylcarnitine antiporter translocase. Finally, the fatty acyl group is transferred back to CoA by carnitine palmityltransferase II (CPTII) located on the matrix side of the inner membrane. This mitochondrial transport of fatty acyl-CoA functions primarily with chain lengths of C12–C18. Medium- and short-chain fatty acid (MCFA and SCFA) can freely diffuse into the mitochondrial matrix and do not require a carnitine-dependent shuttle mechanism to allow transport across the mitochondrial inner membrane. There is some evidence to suggest that carnitine-dependent transport of LCFA into the mitochondria might be a rate-limiting step for FA oxidation (see below).

The process of β-oxidation, which occurs in the mitochondria, comprises four separate reactions in which the fatty acyl-CoA is sequentially degraded to acetyl-CoA and an acyl-CoA residue that has had 2C sequestered. The acetyl-CoA units enter the tricarboxylic acid (TCA) cycle and follow the same pathway as acetyl-CoA units from pyruvate. The rate at which FA are oxidized depends on the chain length and the degree of saturation: MCFA are oxidized more rapidly and more completely than LCFA.

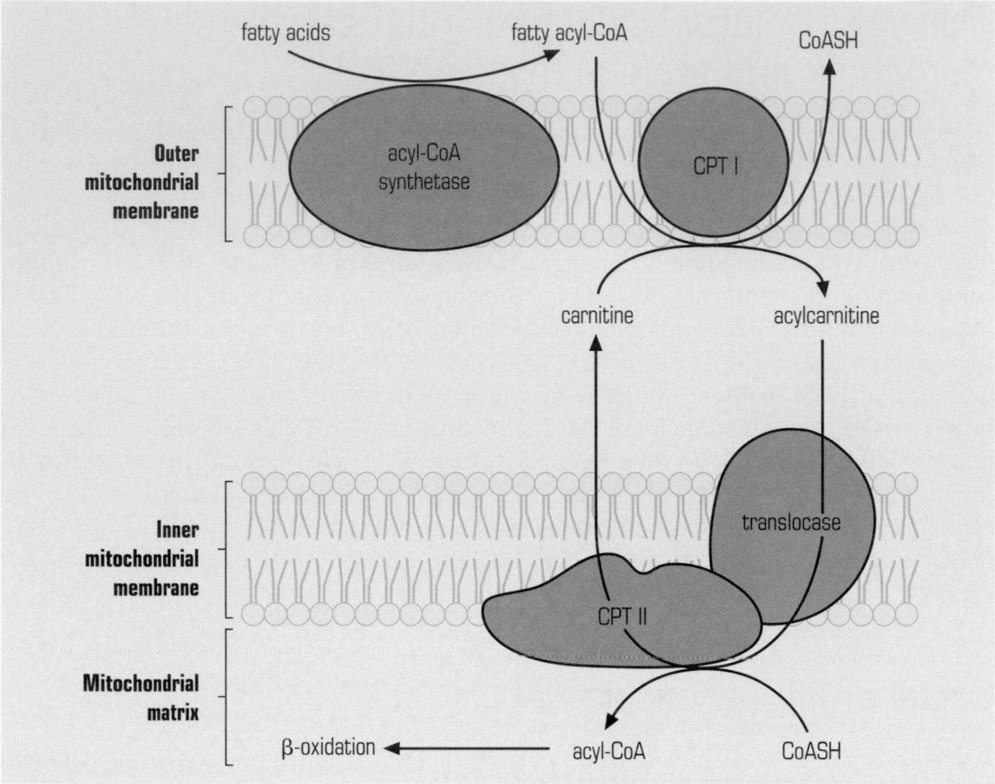

FIGURE 15.3 The transport of long-chain fatty acids from the cytosol through the inner mitochondrial membrane for oxidation is dependent on the carnitine palmityltransferase complex (see text for further details). Reproduced from TM Devlin, Textbook of biochemistry (fourth edition), Wiley-Liss, New York, 1997

15.8 Methods to quantify lipid metabolism during exercise

A background knowledge of some of the methods used to measure substrate metabolism during laboratory-based investigations is essential for the sports practitioner striving to comprehend and interpret the findings of such studies in a meaningful and practical manner to athletes and coaches. Our understanding of the regulation of fat metabolism has been advanced considerably by modern-day investigations that have used a combination of stable isotope techniques in association with conventional indirect calorimetry (Romijn et al. 1992, 1993). As the three most abundant FA are oxidized in proportion to their relative concentration in the plasma FA pool, total plasma FA kinetics can be estimated from stable isotope infusions of either oleate or palmitate. The rate of appearance (Ra) of an FA (palmitate) in the bloodstream gives an index of the release of FA into the plasma and represents the net balance between the rate of adipose tissue lipolysis and the rate of FA uptake and re-esterification. Glycerol, on the other hand, cannot be produced by the body other than from lipolysis. Furthermore, all glycerol released during lipolysis, whether from adipose tissue or skeletal muscle, appears in the plasma. Accordingly, the Ra of glycerol provides a useful indicator of the rate of whole body lipolysis. An estimation of total fuel utilization (fat and CHO) during steady state exercise can be obtained from the respiratory exchange ratio, the volume of carbon dioxide produced (VCO_2) divided by the oxygen consumed (VO_2):

$$\text{CHO oxidation (g/min)} = 4.585\ VCO_2 - 3.226\ VO_2$$
$$\text{fat oxidation (g/min)} = 1.695\ VO_2 - 1.701\ VCO_2$$

Rates of substrate oxidation are usually expressed relative to an individual's body mass (BM) (or sometimes their lean muscle mass or fat-free mass). Accordingly, the rate of CHO oxidation (μmol/kg/min) is determined by converting the g/min rate of CHO oxidation to its molar equivalent, assuming 6 mol of O_2 are consumed and 6 mol of CO_2 produced for each mole (180 g) oxidized. Rates of FA oxidation (μmol/kg/min) are determined by converting the g/min rate of TG oxidation to its molar equivalent, assuming the average molecular weight of TG to be 855.26 g/mole and multiplying the molar rate of TG oxidation by three, because each molecule contains 3 mmol of FA.

Given the tracer-derived rates of total lipolysis and total FA released into the plasma, it is possible to distinguish peripheral lipolysis from adipose TG and intramuscular lipolysis:

$$\underset{(\mu mol/kg/min)}{\text{IMTG FA oxidation}} = \underset{(\mu mol/kg/min)}{\text{total FA oxidation}} - \underset{(\mu mol/kg/min)}{\text{FA uptake (FARd)}}$$

For every three FA molecules released from the IMTG pool, one glycerol molecule will be released into the plasma. Consequently, the minimum rate of release of glycerol from the IMTG pool gives an estimation of IMTG lipolysis and can be estimated from the following equation (FFA stands for free fatty acids):

$$\text{intramuscular FA oxidation } (\mu mol/kg/min) \div (3\mu mol\ FFA \div \mu mol\ glycerol)$$

The rate of total glycerol release (Ra glycerol) equals the glycerol released from adipocyte TG and glycerol released from the IMTG pool. Accordingly it is possible to calculate the rate of adipose (peripheral) TG lipolysis from the following equation:

$$\underset{(\mu mol/kg/min)}{\text{adipose lipolysis}} = \underset{(\mu mol/kg/min)}{\text{total Ra glycerol}} - \underset{(\mu mol/kg/min)}{\text{IMTG lipolysis}}$$

Using a combination of these techniques, it has been possible to estimate the effect of exercise intensity and duration on fat metabolism (Romijn et al. 1993).

The effects of exercise intensity on lipid metabolism

15.9

In the post-absorptive state, FA oxidation provides a major portion of the energy requirements for skeletal muscle: at rest, the rate of total FA oxidation is ~4 μmol/kg/min, which represents about 50% of oxygen consumption. The rate of lipolysis at rest is usually in excess of that required to provide resting energy requirements such that, at the onset of low- to moderate-intensity exercise, a significant increase in FA oxidation could occur even if there were no instant increase in lipolysis. During low-intensity exercise (25% of $VO_{2\,max}$), an intensity comparable to walking, most of the energy requirements can be met from plasma FA oxidation, with a small contribution from the oxidation of plasma glucose. At exercise of low intensity the Ra of FA in plasma matches closely the rate of FA oxidation. Even when low-intensity exercise is sustained for 1–2 hours, the pattern of fuel utilization does not change considerably. Presumably this is because the muscle energy requirements can be met almost exclusively from the oxidation of the FA mobilized from the large adipose TG stores, and lipolysis is not limited by blood flow.

With an increase in exercise intensity from 25% to 65% of $VO_{2\,max}$ (the pace that could be sustained by a trained person for up to 8 hours), total fat oxidation reaches its peak, despite a slight decline in the Ra of plasma FA. The higher rate of total FA oxidation at 65% compared to 25% of $VO_{2\,max}$ reflects a substantial increase in the oxidation of IMTG. Of interest is that even when the absolute rate of FA oxidation is at a peak, fat only contributes about 50% to the total fuel requirements of exercise, with the remainder of the energy coming from CHO (see Fig. 15.4).

During high-intensity exercise at 85% of $VO_{2\,max}$ (race pace for endurance events lasting ~90 minutes) there is a decline in total FA oxidation compared to moderate-intensity exercise (see Fig. 15.4). This is largely due to a marked reduction in the Ra of plasma FA. It is likely the Ra for plasma FA decreases with increasing exercise intensity because of an insufficient blood flow and albumin delivery to transport FA from adipose tissue into the bloodstream. On the other hand, glycerol is water-soluble and so its appearance in the plasma is not blood-flow-dependent; consequently the Ra for glycerol is not affected. In addition, continuous high-intensity exercise is associated with high rates of glycogenolysis (see Fig. 15.4) and the concomitant production of lactic acid that accumulates in muscle and blood. This increased glycolytic flux also acts to inhibit FA oxidation by skeletal muscle (see below).

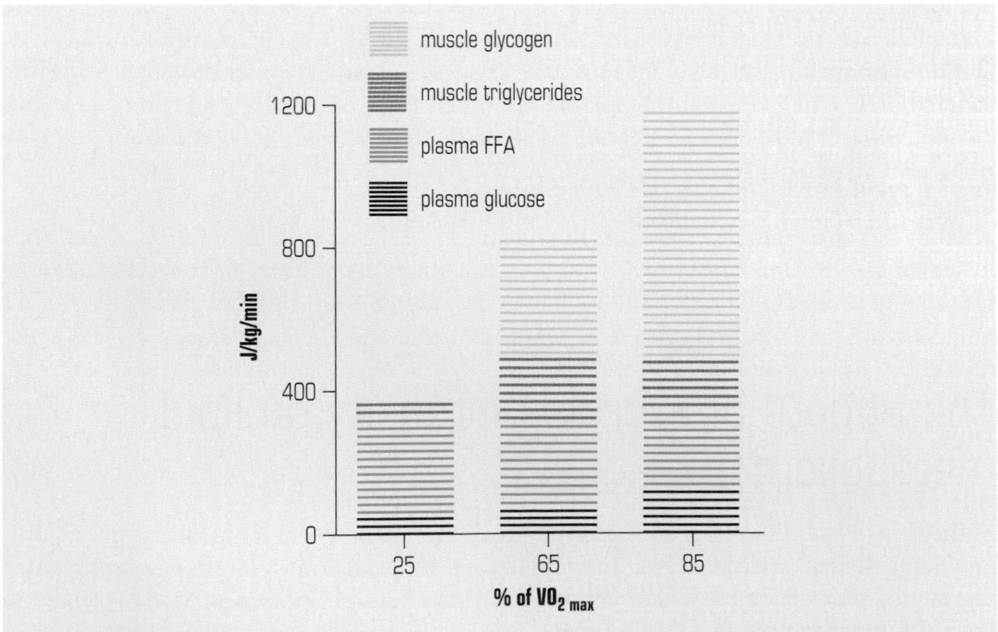

FIGURE 15.4 The effect of exercise intensity on the contribution from the four major substrates to energy expenditure. Redrawn from Romijn et al. 1993. Reproduced with permission from the American Physiological Society

Why can't fatty acid oxidation sustain intense exercise?

At rest, the Ra of plasma FA (lipolysis) normally exceeds the energy requirements of skeletal muscle. During low-intensity exercise, when lipolysis increases further, there is still a sufficient supply of FA to meet the muscles' energy demand. However, there is little further increase in lipolysis (the Ra FA) when exercise intensity increases to 65% of $VO_{2\,max}$; at such work rates Ra FA closely matches FA oxidation. During high-intensity exercise, lipolysis is markedly suppressed and the contribution of FA oxidation to the total energy requirement of exercise is diminished. These observations would support the notion that the reduced availability of FA (a reduction in lipolysis) may contribute to a part of the decline in FA oxidation during intense exercise.

To evaluate the extent to which decreased FA availability contributes to the lower rates of FA oxidation during intense exercise, Romijn and colleagues (1995) studied well-trained endurance subjects during 30 minutes of intense (85% of $VO_{2\,max}$) cycling, once during a 'control' trial when plasma FFA concentration was normal (0.3 mM), and again when plasma FFA concentration was elevated to ~2 mM by an infusion of lipid (Intralipid™) and heparin. Total FA oxidation was increased 27% (from 26.7 to 34.0 μmol/kg/min) with the lipid infusion compared to control. However, the elevation of plasma FFA concentration (increased availability) during intense exercise only resulted in a partial restoration of FA oxidation, as the rates of total fat oxidation at 85% of $VO_{2\,max}$ were still lower than those observed in normal conditions at 65% of $VO_{2\,max}$. These findings indicate that FA oxidation is impaired during intense exercise because of a failure of lipolysis to meet the energy demands of the muscle. Therefore, in theory, TG lipolysis establishes the upper limit to FA oxidation during high-intensity exercise.

However, even when lipid is infused well in excess of the muscle requirements during high-intensity exercise, less than half of the total energy requirement is met by FA oxidation. This is because the muscle is also a major site of control of the rate of FA oxidation during such exercise. Specifically, the increased rate of glycogenolysis during intense exercise appears to inhibit the entry of LCFA into the mitochondria. Sidossis and colleagues (1997) reported that during cycling at 80% of $VO_{2\,max}$, the accelerated glycolytic flux associated with the high work rates resulted in high rates of pyruvate and acetyl-CoA formation, which inhibited CPT-I activity and, in turn, FA entry into the mitochondria. Coyle and colleagues (1997) also showed that CHO metabolism (glycolytic flux) regulates FA oxidation during exercise. Their subjects ingested CHO before exercise (in order to produce high concentrations of plasma glucose and insulin) and the rates of oxidation of an LCFA (palmitate) and an MCFA (octanoate) were subsequently determined. Unlike palmitate, which requires CPT-I for transport into skeletal muscle mitochondria, octanoate is not limited by mitochondrial transport. The increased glycolytic flux from pre-exercise glucose ingestion significantly reduced palmitate oxidation, but had no effect on octanoate oxidation. Even when FA availability is maintained by an infusion of lipid, CHO ingestion still inhibits LCFA oxidation (Sidossis et al. 1996), presumably because of the anti-lipolytic effects of elevated insulin concentrations. Taken collectively, these findings suggest that although the rate of lipolysis is important, the primary site of control of FA oxidation during moderate to intense exercise resides at the muscle tissue level (Wolfe 1998). Furthermore, increased glycolytic flux resulting from either CHO ingestion

(Coyle et al. 1997; Horowitz et al. 1997, 1999) and the concomitant rise in plasma insulin, or an increase in exercise intensity (Romijn et al. 1995; Sidossis et al. 1997) directly inhibits LCFA oxidation.

15.11 Nutritional strategies to enhance fat oxidation during exercise

As endogenous CHO reserves are limited, and as muscle and liver glycogen depletion often coincide with fatigue during both endurance events and many team sports (McInerney et al. 2005), there has been a recent surge of interest among athletes, coaches and sports practitioners in several nutritional practices which, in theory at least, could promote FA oxidation, attenuate the normal rate of CHO utilization and improve exercise capacity. Many of these so-called 'ergogenic aids' have received scientific investigation (for review, see Brouns & Van der Vusse 1998; Hawley et al. 1998; Coyle & Hodgkinson 1999; Hawley et al. 2000b). They include ingestion of fat and caffeine before exercise; LCFA and MCFA feedings during exercise; chronic adaptation to high-fat diets; and 'train low' strategies, where exercise is specifically undertaken with low CHO availability (see Chapter 14) and L-carnitine supplementation. Although intravenous infusion of lipid (Intralipid™) accompanied by heparin is a potent lipolytic stimulant that increases FA oxidation and spares muscle glycogen stores during both moderate (Odland et al. 1996, 1998) and intense (Dyck et al. 1993, 1996) exercise, such a procedure is impractical in most sporting environments. Furthermore, intravenous infusions contravene the doping regulations of the World Anti-Doping Agency. As such, a critique of this technique has not been included in this chapter. The reader is referred to the excellent reviews of Spriet and Dyck (1996) and Spriet (1999) for further information on this topic.

15.12 Caffeine ingestion before exercise

Caffeine, a common drug used throughout the world, is a pharmacological agent used by many athletes as an ergogenic aid to improve both short-term high-intensity and prolonged moderate-intensity exercise performance (see Chapter 16). Caffeine has direct effects on the central nervous system, reducing an individual's perception of effort (Cole et al. 1996), and also on neuromuscular function (Kalmar & Cafarelli 1999). However, the early studies investigating the effects of caffeine ingestion on exercise capacity focused on changes in FFA availability and subsequent FA oxidation, the so-called 'metabolic theory' (Spriet 1997).

In a series of investigations conducted 30 years ago, Costill and colleagues were the first to report that the ingestion of moderate doses of caffeine (~5 mg/kg) ~1 hour before exercise stimulated lipolysis-enhanced rates of total FA oxidation (as estimated from RER measurements) and decreased the utilization of muscle glycogen (Costill et al. 1978; Ivy et al. 1979; Essig et al. 1980). Caffeine was proposed to mobilize FA from adipose tissue and/or IMTG stores by increasing plasma epinephrine concentrations and/or directly antagonizing adipocyte tissue adenosine receptors. The increased circulating FFA would then increase FA uptake and oxidation by muscle and spare endogenous CHO reserves. More recent evidence against the metabolic theory is provided by Graham and colleagues

(2000), who quantified muscle metabolism by a combination of direct arteriovenous balance methods and muscle biopsies after ingestion of 6 mg/kg caffeine during 1 hour of submaximal exercise. They found that, although caffeine ingestion stimulated the sympathetic nervous system, it did not alter leg FA uptake, net muscle glycogenolysis or rates of CHO and fat metabolism in the monitored leg. Another study from this group confirmed that intake of caffeine can prolong endurance during cycling at 80% $VO_{2\,max}$ without affecting muscle glycogen utilization (Greer et al. 2000). However, others have found individual variability in the metabolic response to caffeine: half of a group of subjects was shown to 'spare' glycogen during the first 15 minutes of exercise following caffeine intake (9 mg/kg) compared with a placebo treatment, while glycogen utilization was unaffected in the other half of the group following caffeine treatment (Chesley et al. 1998). Taken collectively, the results of these studies indicate that glycogen sparing following caffeine ingestion is a variable response, but seems most likely to occur with larger caffeine doses (>6 mg/kg) and power outputs eliciting ≥70% $VO_{2\,max}$.

Fat feeding before exercise 15.13

Several studies have investigated the effects of fat feeding before exercise on the subsequent rates of substrate oxidation and exercise performance. The results from these investigations are equivocal with regard to the effect of fat feeding on metabolism and also performance. Costill and colleagues (1977) first reported that fat feeding in combination with intravenous administration of heparin stimulated lipolysis, elevated plasma FFA concentrations and decreased the rate of muscle glycogen utilization by 40% compared to a control condition during 30 minutes of running at 70% of $VO_{2\,max}$. A more recent study from the same laboratory also reported muscle glycogen sparing with fat feeding and IV heparin compared to control during 60 minutes of cycling at 70% of $VO_{2\,max}$ (Vukovich et al. 1993).

On the other hand, Okano and colleagues (1996, 1998) reported only small differences in the rates of fat and CHO oxidation in response to high-fat or high-CHO meals ingested 4 hours before prolonged submaximal cycling (2 hours at 67% of $VO_{2\,max}$ followed by a ride to exhaustion at 78% of $VO_{2\,max}$). Furthermore, most of the differences in metabolism (a lower RER) after the fat feeding were evident only in the early stages of exercise, and did not result in an improved performance time. Whitley and colleagues (1998) also found that high-fat or high-CHO meals ingested 4 hours before exercise failed to substantially alter the pattern of fuel utilization during 90 minutes of moderate-intensity cycling, or affect a subsequent 10 km cycle time trial. Wee and colleagues (1999) fed six endurance-trained runners a random order of either a high-fat, a high-CHO or a high-fat–high-CHO meal 3 hours before a run to exhaustion at 71% of $VO_{2\,max}$. Despite the rate of fat oxidation being elevated after the high-fat compared to the high-CHO and high-fat–high-CHO meals (19% and 14%, respectively), endurance time was 14% less after the high-fat meal. These workers concluded that CHO, rather than fat availability before exercise, exerts a predominant control over substrate selection during subsequent exercise.

Only one study has compared the effect of fat feeding versus CHO feeding on metabolism and performance during intense (80% of $VO_{2\,max}$) exercise. Hawley and colleagues (2000a) reported that a high-fat feeding increased fat availability and elevated rates of FA oxidation during 20 minutes of exercise, but that the small reduction in CHO oxidation after such a regimen did not enhance intense exercise lasting ~30 minutes.

The only study to find an increase in exercise capacity with fat feeding was that of Pitsaladis and colleagues (1999). These workers found that cycling time to exhaustion was prolonged (from 118 to 128 minutes) when their trained subjects ingested a high-fat (90% of energy) versus a high-CHO (70% of energy) meal 4 hours prior to exercise. As no significant differences in total CHO oxidation were reported between trials (383 g versus 362 g for the CHO and fat meals respectively), it is difficult to explain the prolonged exercise time in that study.

15.14 Long- and medium-chain triglyceride ingestion during exercise

Nearly 30 years ago Ivy and colleagues (1980) were the first to compare the effects of MCFA and LCFA ingestion on FA oxidation during exercise. Lipids (~30 g) were ingested by ten well-trained subjects 1 hour before a bout of moderate-intensity exercise lasting 60 minutes. LCFA ingestion increased serum TG concentrations, but neither MCFA nor LCFA had any effects on the rates of FA oxidation. These workers did report that when more than 50 g of MCFA or LCFA were ingested, severe gastrointestinal problems were experienced by the majority of subjects, and recommended a maximum amount of 30 g that could be tolerated by most athletes (Ivy et al. 1980).

Satabin and colleagues (1987) also compared the effect of MCFA with LCFA on rates of fat and CHO oxidation and exercise time to exhaustion at 60% of $VO_{2\ max}$. These workers used stable isotope tracers ([1-^{13}C] octanoate, [1-^{13}C] palmitate) to track the fate of ingested substrates during exercise. The most striking effect of MCFA ingestion was a rise in blood ketone bodies. On the other hand, blood ketone concentrations were unchanged with LCFA ingestion. Not surprisingly, the ingested LCFA were oxidized to a lesser extent than the MCFA (9% versus 43% of the amount ingested), although exercise times to exhaustion were similar.

In contrast to LCFA, which slow the rate of gastric emptying and enter the systemic circulation as chylomicrons, MCFA are emptied very rapidly from the stomach and are absorbed into the bloodstream almost as fast as glucose (Beckers et al. 1992). As such, interest has focused on the potential ergogenic effect of ingesting MCFA solutions on endurance performance (Jeukendrup et al. 1995, 1996, 1998; Goedecke et al. 1999b; Angus et al. 2000). These studies are summarized in Chapter 16.

The first study to investigate the effects of MCFA, in the form of medium chain triglyceride (MCT) ingestion during exercise was undertaken by Massicotte and colleagues (1992). These researchers compared the oxidation of ingested MCFA to glucose during 2 hours of cycling at 65% of $VO_{2\ max}$. They found that the contribution of fat and CHO to total energy requirements during exercise was similar between the two interventions.

Jeukendrup and colleagues (1995) investigated the effects of a combination of CHO and MCFA ingested during 3 hours of moderate-intensity (57% $VO_{2\ max}$) exercise in well-trained cyclists. When 10 g of MCFA was co-ingested with CHO each hour, ~70% of the MCFA consumed was oxidized compared to only 33% when the MCFA was ingested alone. Towards the end of exercise the rate of ingested MCFA oxidation closely matched the rate of ingestion. Even so, the contribution of ingested MCFA to total energy expenditure was only 7%. In a separate study, Jeukendrup and colleagues (1996) examined the effects of MCFA ingestion on the rates of muscle glycogen utilization during 180 minutes of moderate-intensity cycling. MCFA ingested at a rate of ~10 g/h had no effect on the rates of total CHO oxidation, or the rates of muscle glycogen utilization. Even when subjects commence exercise with low muscle glycogen content, MCT ingestion has no effect on CHO utilization (Jeukendrup et al. 1996). More recently, Angus and colleagues (2000) compared the ingestion of CHO (60 g/h) with a CHO (60 g/h) plus MCFA solution (~24 g/h) on cycling time trial performance. Subjects completed a set amount of work equal to ~100 km as fast as possible. Compared to a placebo (178 ± 11 minutes), the time to complete the ride was reduced after the ingestion of both CHO (166 ± 7 minutes) and CHO plus MCFA (169 ± 7 minutes). However, the addition of the MCFA did not provide any further performance enhancement over CHO alone.

To date, only one study has reported a beneficial effect of MCFA ingestion on FA metabolism and performance. Van Zyl and colleagues (1996) reported that when large doses (~30 g/h) of MCFA were co-ingested with a 10% glucose beverage, serum FA concentrations were elevated, FA oxidation was increased, estimated muscle glycogen utilization reduced, and a 40-km cycle performance (which followed 2 hours of submaximal exercise at 60% of $VO_{2\ max}$) improved by 2.5% compared to when glucose was ingested alone. However, that study is the exception. Jeukendrup and colleagues (1998) fed well-trained subjects a similar MCFA–CHO solution to that given by Van Zyl and colleagues (1996) and found no difference in the performance of a work bout lasting ~15 minutes that was preceded by 2 hours at 60% of $VO_{2\ max}$. Interestingly, both these investigations reported that when MCFA was ingested alone, performance was reduced compared to CHO. Jeukendrup and colleagues (1998) also found that MCFA ingestion resulted in a worse performance than when subjects ingested a water placebo. On a practical note, the ingestion of large (>15 g/h) amounts of MCFA is likely to produce gastrointestinal problems in most athletes, which would be expected to be detrimental to performance.

Adaptation to high-fat, low-carbohydrate diets 15.15

It has long been known that modifying an individual's habitual diet can significantly alter the subsequent patterns of substrate utilization during aerobic exercise, and influence performance (Christensen & Hansen 1939). The consumption of a high-fat (>60% of energy intake), low-CHO (less than 20% of energy) diet for 1–3 days markedly reduces resting muscle glycogen content and increases FA oxidation during submaximal exercise (Jansson & Kaijser 1982). Such a shift in substrate utilization is commonly associated with impairment in exercise capacity (for review, see Hawley et al. 1998).

In contrast to the negative effects on exercise capacity that seem to result from short-term (1–3 days) exposure to high-fat diets, there is some evidence to suggest that longer periods of adaptation to high-fat diets may induce adaptive responses that are fundamentally different from the acute lowering of body CHO reserves. Such adaptations have been proposed to eventually induce a reversal of some of the mitochondrial adaptations that favor CHO oxidation and 'retool' the working muscle to increase its capacity for FA oxidation (Lambert et al. 1997).

The most frequently cited study to support the use of high-fat diets to improve athletic performance is that of Phinney and colleagues (1983), who examined the effects of 28 days of a high-fat diet (85% of energy) versus a eucaloric diet containing 66% of energy from CHO on submaximal cycle time to exhaustion. The high-fat diet reduced the average resting muscle glycogen content of their five trained subjects by 47% (143 versus 76 mmol/kg ww).

Consequently, when cycling at ~63% of $VO_{2\ max}$, the RER values were 0.72 (95% of energy from fat, 5% from CHO) and 0.83 (56% of energy from fat, 44% from CHO) for the high-fat and normal diets, respectively. Remarkably, the mean exercise time at this moderate work intensity was not statistically significantly different after the two dietary interventions (147 and 151 minutes for the eucaloric and high-fat diets, respectively). However, this 'performance' result needs to be interpreted with caution. First, it has previously been reported that trained subjects can ride for 3–4 hours at moderate intensities when fasted and fed CHO throughout exercise (Coyle et al. 1986). Second, the performance data are heavily skewed in favor of the fat diet, largely as a result of one individual who rode ~60% longer after the high-fat compared to the normal diet. Finally, competitive endurance athletes training and racing in events lasting less than 4 hours rarely exercise at such low intensities (Bergman & Brooks 1999).

Lambert and colleagues (1994) used a randomized crossover design to investigate the effects of 14 days of either a high-fat (67% MJ) or a high-CHO (74% MJ) diet in five trained cyclists. After dietary adaptation, subjects undertook a comprehensive battery of physical tests including a 30-second Wingate anaerobic test, a ride to exhaustion at ~90% of $VO_{2\ max}$, and, following a 30-minute rest, a further ride to volitional fatigue at 60% of $VO_{2\ max}$. Although the high-fat diet significantly reduced pre-exercise muscle glycogen content from 121 mmol/kg ww after the normal diet to 68 mmol/kg ww after the high-CHO diet, mean 30-second anaerobic power was similar between the two conditions (862 versus 804 Watts for the high-fat and CHO diet respectively). Neither was there an effect of dietary manipulation on the time subjects could ride at a work rate eliciting ~90% of $VO_{2\ max}$ (8.3 versus 12.5 minutes for the high-fat and CHO trials). However, although failing to attain statistical significance, a margin of 4.2 minutes at such a work rate would result in a huge difference in athletic performance (Hopkins et al. 1999). The only effect of the high-fat diet was to prolong submaximal endurance time during the third and final laboratory test (the ride to exhaustion at 60% of $VO_{2\ max}$) from 42 to 80 minutes, despite significantly lower starting muscle glycogen content (32 versus 73 mmol/kg ww). Such increases in endurance were associated with a marked decrease in the average rate of CHO oxidation (2.2 versus 1.4 g/min) and a significant increase in the rate of fat oxidation from 0.3 to 0.6 g/min. The results of this investigation are difficult to interpret because of the unorthodox study design, but they strongly suggest that submaximal exercise capacity can be preserved in spite of low pre-exercise muscle glycogen content when trained individuals are adapted to a high-fat diet.

Probably the longest exposure to a CHO-restricted diet was the investigation of Helge and colleagues (1996), who examined diet–training interactions in two groups of ten untrained subjects participating in a 7-week endurance-training program while consuming either a high-fat (62% MJ) or high-CHO (65% MJ) diet. Cycle time to exhaustion at 70% of $VO_{2\ max}$ increased by 191% after the high-CHO diet, but only by 68% in those subjects who consumed the high-fat diet. In order to determine if the impairment in endurance observed after the high-fat diet could be reversed, subjects then switched to a high-CHO diet during the eighth week of the study and the exercise task was repeated. Even after a week of ingesting CHO, the mean performance time only improved by 12 minutes, leading these workers to conclude that 'a combination of training and a fat-rich diet did not reveal an additive effect on physical performance'. A similar study from these same authors that investigated 4 weeks of training on a high-fat or high-CHO diet did not find any difference between the gains in endurance of the groups (Helge et al. 1998). This suggests that a long duration of exposure to high-fat eating may impair the response to training; such a finding needs to be investigated in well-trained athletes.

In summary, compared to a high-CHO diet, a period of adaptation to a high-fat diet will increase the relative contribution from FA oxidation by ~40% to the total energy requirements of exercise. However, adaptation to high-fat diets does not appear to alter the rate of muscle glycogen utilization or improve prolonged, moderate-intensity exercise (for review, see Kiens & Helge 2000). Although it has been suggested that as long as 20 weeks of exposure should be allowed if humans wish to adapt to high-fat diets (Kronfeld 1973), adherence to such an extreme diet for a long period is impractical and could also pose health problems for athletes. High-fat diets are associated with increased risk of a number of diseases (Sternfeld 1992; Sarna & Kaprio 1994) and although regular physical activity attenuates these risks, individuals should limit their long-term exposure to high-fat diets. Short-term exposure to high-fat diets is also associated with insulin resistance in the liver (Kraegen et al. 1991), resulting in a failure to suppress hepatic glucose output and an attenuation of liver glycogen synthesis.

Short-term 'adaptation' to high-fat diets followed by acute high-carbohydrate diets 15.16

It has been proposed that nutritional preparation for endurance and ultra-endurance events should encompass periods of 'nutritional periodization' (Hawley & Hopkins 1995). In such a scenario athletes might train for most of the year on a high-CHO diet, adapting to a high-fat diet for several days early in the week prior to a major event, then CHO-loading in the final 48 hours immediately prior to competition. Such nutritional periodization would still permit endurance athletes to train hard throughout the year and maximize their endogenous CHO stores before competition while, theoretically, allowing the working muscles to optimize their capacity for FA oxidation during a major endurance race. More to the point, a short (3–5 days) period of exposure to a high-fat diet represents a more manageable period for extreme dietary change while minimizing any potential health risks. The results of a study by Goedecke and colleagues suggest that most of the adaptive responses that facilitate an increased rate of FA oxidation are complete after as little as 5 days of a high-fat diet (Goedecke et al. 1999a); nutritional periodization would seem a prudent and perhaps optimal strategy for endurance and ultra-endurance athletes to follow.

In order to test this hypothesis, we and colleagues have undertaken a series of investigations designed to determine the effects of either a 5-day adaptation to a high-fat diet (4.0 g/kg of fat/d, 2.4 g/kg of CHO/d) followed by 1 day of CHO restoration, or an isoenergetic CHO diet (9.6 g/kg of CHO/d) on metabolism and performance of endurance and ultra-endurance cycling (Burke et al. 2000, 2002; Carey et al. 2001; Stellingwerff et al. 2006). Competitive cyclists or triathletes with a history of regular endurance training were recruited for these studies; such individuals would be expected to have the muscle adaptations that favor FA oxidation (Brooks & Mercier 1994). All investigations employed a protocol in which these subjects undertook supervised training while consuming either a high-fat or high-CHO diet for 5–6 days, then resting and eating a high-CHO intake for 1 day to restore muscle glycogen content.

In agreement with other investigations (Phinney et al. 1983; Lambert et al. 1994), following a high-fat diet while undertaking a substantial training program resulted in a drastic reduction in resting muscle glycogen concentration (451 to 255 mmol/kg dry mass) (Burke et al. 2000). However, 1 day of a high-CHO diet was sufficient to restore muscle glycogen concentration to an equally supercompensated level, irrespective of the previous diet (~550–600 mmol/kg dry mass). With this preparation, the athletes cycled for 2 hours at a steady state submaximal pace before undertaking a time trial lasting about 30 minutes. In our first study (Burke et al. 2000), this was undertaken after an overnight fast and with the intake of water during exercise. Total CHO utilization was substantially reduced after fat adaptation, with a 'sparing' of muscle glycogen use accounting for this reduction. Rates of FA oxidation were elevated by ~50% above the CHO trial following fat adaptation. Unfortunately, the techniques utilized in this study did not enable us to determine whether this was due to an increase in FFA release, uptake and oxidation, or an increased reliance on IMTG. However, despite the brevity of the adaptation period, the high-fat diet elicited large shifts in favor of FA oxidation, an impressive adaptation in light of the already enhanced capacity for FA oxidation in such highly trained subjects. Despite these metabolic shifts, there was no significant effect on performance. The time-trial outcome was similar on each dietary treatment, although there was some evidence of better preservation of blood glucose concentrations following fat adaptation, which helped to reduce the risk of hypoglycemia in susceptible subjects.

Because the conditions of the first trial are not commensurate with the nutritional practices of athletes, we undertook a follow-up investigation (Burke et al. 2002) in which subjects consumed a pre-trial CHO-rich breakfast and ingested CHO throughout the ride, as recommended by sports nutrition guidelines (American Dietetic Association et al. 2009). Since CHO ingestion effectively eliminates any rise in plasma FFA concentration, an effect that can persist for several hours after ingestion (Horowitz et al. 1997), it would be expected that FA oxidation would also be suppressed during exercise. Indeed, compared to the first experiment (Burke et al. 2000), the overall rate of FA oxidation was lower. However, total FA oxidation was maintained at higher levels throughout the bout of exercise with the fat-adaptation trial compared to the control (CHO) diet (see Fig. 15.5), indicating that our fat-adaptation treatment achieved metabolic 'retooling' that persists even when CHO availability during exercise is high. Again, however, the performance of the time trial was similar after the two dietary regimens.

A final study was undertaken to see whether the metabolic benefits of fat adaptation/CHO restoration required an ultra-endurance protocol before performance changes became apparent (Carey et al. 2001). In this study, the metabolic differences achieved by the fat adaptation were apparent throughout a 4-hour steady-state cycling protocol despite a pre-exercise CHO-rich breakfast and the intake of >1 g/kg of CHO during exercise. However, performances of the subsequent 1-hour time trial were similar between trials.

A variety of explanations has been offered to explain the apparent lack of transfer of the clear metabolic changes to performance outcomes (Burke & Hawley 2002). They include the failure of scientists to detect small changes in performance that might be worthwhile in real-life sport (Hopkins et al. 1999), and the existence of 'responders' and 'non-responders' to fat-adaptation strategies (Phinney et al. 1983; Burke et al. 2000) which are hidden within group statistics. Two more recent studies have lent weight to an alternative theory. Previous investigations have considered that metabolic changes occurring with fat-adaptation strategies represent an up-regulation of fat metabolism. Mechanisms have included increases in putative FA transporters as well as enzymes of fat metabolism (for review, see Kiens & Helge 2000; Burke & Hawley 2002). However,

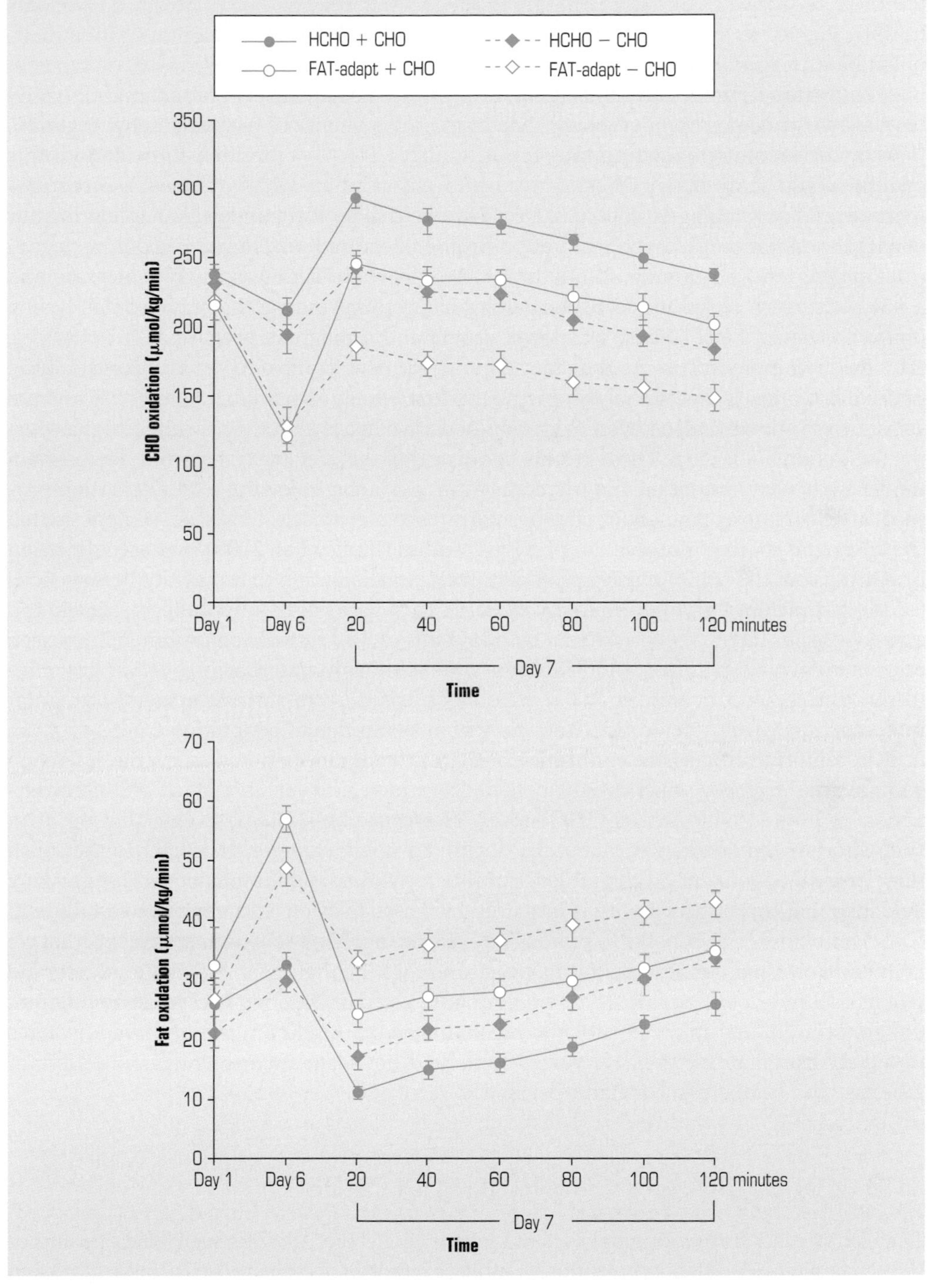

FIGURE 15.5 The effects of short-term (5 days) adaptation to high-fat diet and 1 day of CHO restoration (FAT-adapt) on rates of whole-body CHO (upper graph) and fat oxidation (lower graph) during continuous cycling at 70% of maximal aerobic power compared with control trial (HCHO). Values are mean ± SEM for eight subjects at day 1 (baseline), day 6 (after fat adaptation) and during 120 minutes of steady-state cycling on day 7 (after fat adaptation and glycogen restoration). Reproduced with permission from Medicine and Science in Sports and Exercise (Burke 2002)

the most recent work on fat-adaptation strategies has provided evidence that what was initially viewed as 'glycogen sparing' may be, in fact, a down-regulation of CHO metabolism or 'glycogen impairment'.

A study targeting the mechanisms underpinning the outcomes of fat-adaptation/CHO restoration strategies found a robust reduction in the activity of pyruvate dehydrogenase (PDH), the enzyme regulating the step in which CHO is committed to oxidation; this change would act to impair rates of glycogenolysis at a time when muscle CHO requirements are high (Stellingwerff et al. 2006). The exercise protocol undertaken following our usual fat-adaptation/glycogen restoration protocol featured a 20 minutes' bout of steady-state cycling and a 1-minute all-out sprint. As expected, there was a ~45% increase and a ~30% decrease in fat and CHO oxidation, respectively, during the submaximal cycling phase. However, PDH activity was lower at rest and throughout exercise at 70% $VO_{2\,peak}$, and the 1-minute sprint in the 'fat-adapt' treatment compared to the control trial. Estimates of muscle glycogenolysis during the first minute of submaximal exercise and the 1-minute sprint were also lower. Hormone-sensitive lipase activity was ~20% higher during submaximal exercise. These results confirm that the previously reported decreases in whole-body CHO oxidation and increases in fat oxidation following a fat-adaptation protocol are a function of metabolic changes within skeletal muscle. However, it suggests that the 'glycogen sparing' observed in previous studies (Burke et al. 2000) may actually be an impairment of the rate of muscle glycogenolysis, an adaptation that may not be beneficial for the performance of high-intensity exercise. In support of this hypothesis, Havemann and colleagues (2006) reported that a fat-adaptation/CHO restoration treatment increased rates of fat oxidation during a 100-km time trial. Although there was no overall difference to the time taken to complete 100 km between trials, 1-km sprints repeated at regular intervals during the 100 km ride were compromised in the fat-adaptation trial.

It is tempting to classify endurance and ultra-endurance sports as events involving submaximal exercise, which might benefit from increased fat utilization and a conservation of limited endogenous CHO stores. However, the strategic events that occur in such sports—the breakaway, the surge during an uphill stage or the sprint to the finish line—are all dependent on the athlete's ability to work at high intensities. With growing evidence that this critical ability is impaired by 'fat-adaptation' strategies, and a failure to find clear evidence of benefits to prolonged exercise involving self-pacing, it seems that we are near to closing the door on 'fat-loading' and high-fat diets as a genuine ergogenic aid (Kiens & Burke 2006). Scientists may remain interested in the body's response to different dietary stimuli, and may hunt for the mechanisms that underpin the observed changes in metabolism and function. However, there does not seem a worthwhile application for athletes who compete in conventional sports.

15.17 The 'Zone' diet and high-fat sports bars

The claims made in the original versions of the 'Zone' diet (the '40:30:30' diet) by author Barry Sears included the optimization of athletic performance (Sears 1995, 1997). However, as reviewed in Chapter 6, if an athlete's diet is constructed according to the instruction in these books, it would achieve an intake that restricts total energy and CHO to levels that could not sustain the daily training undertaken by most serious athletes. These instructions included pegging protein intake to levels that are consistent with recommended intakes for athletes, but pegging the rest of the diet so that protein now provides 30% of the new total energy intake. Essentially, this cuts typical energy intake in half. CHO and fat intake then fall into line at 40% and 30% of this new low energy intake. As a result, the 'Zone' diet would provide a 75 kg athlete with a total energy intake of ~2000 kcal (8.4 MJ) per day, of which the contribution from CHO would be only ~200 g, or less than 3 g of CHO/kg BM/d. Such a CHO intake is well below the self-reported daily intakes of athletes (for review, see Burke et al. 2001) and far less than currently recommended by sports nutrition guidelines (Burke et al. 2004). The rationale promoted for the 40:30:30 diet is that it will allow the athlete to 'tap into their body fat'. However, this effect should be true of all energy-restricted diets.

How the 'Zone' diet should be constructed for an athlete with a high energy expenditure and no desire to reduce their body fat levels is not clear from the earlier books. One option is to increase all dietary constituents within the 40:30:30 ratio to meet real energy needs. However, this would lead to absolute intakes of protein and CHO that are above the levels that Sears considers healthy or helpful. The other option is to leave protein and CHO at the Zone-stated levels and to increase fat intake to meet the high energy needs of training. Modeling of this approach, for typical athletes undertaking daily training sessions, shows that fat intakes are likely to be 60–70% of total energy intake (Burke 2007).

As summarized in this chapter, there is no clear evidence of benefits from such a dietary program, and some evidence of impaired performance (Havemann et al. 2006) and training adaptations (Helge et al. 1996). Despite the popularity of the 'Zone' diet books, websites and products, there have been only two studies involving the original 'Zone' philosophy and exercise or athletic performance; these do not report favorable effects (Jarvis et al. 2002; Bosse et al. 2004).

In addition to the diet itself, a variety of commercially available 'Zone-friendly' sports bars and other products have been promoted as 'fat burners' capable of reducing CHO metabolism. Like the diet, these bars contain a 40:30:30 mixture of CHO, fat and protein. To date, only one study has examined the effects of ingestion of such a sports bar on metabolism and ultra-endurance performance. Rauch and colleagues (1999) studied six highly trained endurance cyclists who rode for 5.5 hours at ~55% of $VO_{2\,max}$ before performing a time trial lasting ~25 minutes. During the 5.5-hour ride, subjects ingested 1.5 sports bars and 700 mL of water every hour, or 700 mL of a 10% glucose polymer solution, such that the total energy ingested during the two prolonged rides was similar. Although the rates of fat oxidation were significantly greater at the end of the submaximal ride when subjects ingested the bar compared to CHO (1.09 versus 0.73 g/min), two subjects were so fatigued that they failed to complete the time trial. Furthermore, the drop-off in time-trial performance following ingestion of the bar was directly related to the drop in the rate of CHO oxidation, suggesting that even when FA oxidation is increased, it is insufficient to meet the demands of intense exercise (see section 15.18).

The most recent evolution of the 'Zone' diet (http://www.zonediet.com) also includes athletes among its list of those who potentially would benefit. The 40:30:30 mantra promoted in the previous books does not appear to be so dominant in the new information: instead there is a focus on eating a diet based on 'healthy fats' and 'healthy' (low glycemic index) CHO, and supplementation with fish oils and polyphenol supplements (as well as other 'Zone' dietary products/supplements). The idea that the athletes should not follow sports nutrition messages to consume 'high-CHO diets' is still part of the 'Zone' philosophy; it appears that Dr Sears is not aware that sports nutrition guidelines for athletes now recommend that athletes consume a CHO-adequate diet based on the real fuel requirements of their exercise program rather than 'high CHO' per se (see Chapter 14). While there are many pieces of sound nutritional advice within the 'Zone' information, and it seems likely that the 'Zone' diet and sports nutrition guidelines have both moved towards middle ground, it is still difficult to access the real formula behind the 'Zone' diet for athletes. At best it may explore some of the 'train low, compete high' strategies that were covered in Chapter 14. At worst it may be a cover for selling Zone products or a hit-and-miss approach to training and competition needs.

15.18 L-carnitine supplementation

The carnitine pool in a healthy individual is about ~100 mmol, of which ~98% is found in skeletal and cardiac muscle, 1.6% in the liver and kidneys and 0.4% in the extracellular fluid. Over half of the daily requirements of carnitine are found in a balanced diet that includes meat, poultry, fish and some dairy products. The remainder is synthesized from methionine and lysine. Daily urine losses of carnitine are usually less than 2% of the total body carnitine store.

LCFA oxidation in all tissues is carnitine-dependent (see section 15.7). Therefore, hereditary and acquired conditions associated with carnitine deficiency result in TG accumulation in the skeletal muscles, insulin resistance, an impaired utilization of FA and reduced exercise capacity. These pathological changes can normally be reversed by carnitine supplementation. It has been hypothesized that increased availability of L-carnitine by supplementary ingestion might up-regulate the capacity to transport FA into the mitochondria and increase FA oxidation. If this were possible, then carnitine supplementation would be of significant benefit both to endurance athletes and to individuals wishing to increase their lean BM by reducing their levels of adipose tissue.

There have been many well-controlled studies examining the effects of carnitine supplementation on metabolism and athletic performance in both moderately trained individuals and well-trained athletes (see Chapter 16). The doses administered in these studies have varied between 2 and 6 g/d, with the length of administration from 5 days up to 4 weeks. The results of these and many other investigations convincingly demonstrate that carnitine supplementation has no effect on patterns of fuel utilization either at rest or during exercise. As lipid metabolism during exercise is unaltered after supplementation regimens, it is not surprising that there is no change in the rate of working muscle glycogen utilization (Vukovich et al. 1994). Even when CHO availability has been compromised before exercise by reducing muscle glycogen stores, carnitine supplementation still fails to alter substrate utilization (lipid metabolism) during submaximal exercise (Decombaz et al. 1993).

As carnitine has a physiological role in the metabolism of FA, it is not surprising that it has also been marketed as a potential fat-loss agent. In those sports in which making weight and body-fat loss are deemed important for successful performance (e.g. wrestling, rowing, gymnastics and bodybuilding), carnitine use has been vigorously promoted. However, there is no scientific evidence to suggest that carnitine enhances FA oxidation, helps reduce body fat, or aids an athlete to 'make weight'.

Finally, many studies have shown that there is little or no loss of carnitine from skeletal muscle during either low- or high-intensity exercise (see Heinonen 1996 for review). More to the point, in healthy athletes eating conventional diets, training does not appear to induce any physiologically substantial changes in muscle carnitine levels. Even massive doses of carnitine increase muscle carnitine levels by only 1–2%. Therefore there is little reason for carnitine supplementation in moderately active individuals or athletes in hard training.

Summary and recommendations for sports practitioners

15.19

Many nutritional strategies have been employed in an attempt to promote FA oxidation, attenuate the rate of utilization of endogenous CHO stores, and thereby enhance athletic performance. Some of these practices have not been subjected to *any* rigorous scientific testing (e.g. the 'Zone' diet) and are not recommended to athletes. Others (e.g. L-carnitine supplementation) have been well investigated and clearly have no effect on the rates of FA oxidation, muscle glycogen utilization or subsequent performance.

While the ingestion of small to moderate doses of caffeine (2–6 mg/kg BM) in most individuals has been shown to enhance endurance capacity even if it does not improve FA oxidation (Cox et al. 2002), the ingestion of small (10 g/h) amounts of MCFA has no major effects on fat metabolism, nor does it improve exercise performance. Although the ingestion of larger (30 g/h) quantities of MCFA *may* increase fat availability and rates of FA oxidation, such amounts are likely to produce gastrointestinal problems in most athletes, which would be expected to be detrimental to performance.

With regard to the ingestion of high-fat diets, the results of several studies show that both acute (2–3 days) and more prolonged (7 days to 4 weeks) exposure to such diets reduces resting muscle glycogen levels and increase the relative contribution from FA oxidation to the total energy requirements of submaximal exercise. However, such diets significantly impair subsequent endurance performance. While dietary periodization (high-fat diets followed by acute high-CHO diets) may be of benefit to a select group of ultra-endurance athletes, there is currently insufficient scientific evidence to recommend that athletes 'fat load' during training or before competition, and growing evidence to warn against the practice. The recent paradigm of commencing training with low muscle glycogen stores to enhance rates of fat oxidation and further drive the training adaptation (the so-called 'train low, compete high' model) is interesting (Hansen et al. 2005), but coaches and athletes should be careful not to draw practical consequences from the results of a single study (Hansen et al. 2005) with regard to current training regimens. In the real world, training with a high muscle glycogen content may allow the athlete to train for longer periods and thereby obtain better results.

Finally, even those agents that have been shown to have an ergogenic effect when tested under well-controlled conditions may be ergolytic in certain individuals; there are likely to be many scientific studies that, because of a lack of a positive finding, have never been published. Accordingly, it is important for sports practitioners to recognize that there is wide inter-individual variability in the response to many fat-enhancing/performance-enhancing substances. Any nutritional strategies should be undertaken under the supervision of qualified medical personnel, and fine-tuned during daily training to suit each individual's specific needs.

REFERENCES

American Dietetic Association, Dietitians of Canada, American College of Sports Medicine, Rodriguez NR, Di Marco NM, Langley S. American College of Sports Medicine position stand: nutrition and athletic performance. Med Sci Sports Exerc 2009;41:709–31.

Angus DJ, Hargreaves M, Dancey J, Febbraio MA. Effect of carbohydrate or carbohydrate plus medium chain triglyceride ingestion on cycling time trial performance. J Appl Physiol 2000;88:113–19.

Beckers EJ, Jeukendrup AE, Brouns F, Wagenmakers AJM, Saris WHM. Gastric emptying of carbohydrate-medium chain triglyceride suspensions at rest. Int J Sports Med 1992;13:581–4.

Bergman BC, Brooks GA. Respiratory gas-exchange ratios during graded exercise in fed and fasted trained and untrained men. J Appl Physiol 1999;86:479–87.

Bosse MC, Davis SC, Puhl SM, et al. Effects of Zone diet macronutrient proportions on blood lipids, blood glucose, body composition, and treadmill exercise performance. Nutr Res 2004;24:521–30.

Brooks GA, Mercier J. Balance of carbohydrate and lipid utilization during exercise: the 'crossover' concept. J Appl Physiol 1994;76:2253–61.

Brouns F, Van der Vusse GJ. Utilization of lipids during exercise in human subjects: metabolic and dietary constraints. Br J Nutr 1998;79:117–28.

Bruce CR, Anderson MJ, Carey AL, Newman DG, Bonen A, Kriketos AD, Cooney GJ, Hawley JA. Muscle oxidative capacity is a better predictor of insulin sensitivity than lipid status. J Clin Endocrinol Metab 2003;88:5444–51.

Burke LM. Practical sports nutrition. Champaign, Illinois: Human Kinetics, 2007.

Burke LM, Angus DJ, Cox GR, Cummings NK, Febbraio MA, Gawthorn K, Hawley JA, Minehan M, Martin DT, Hargreaves M. Effect of fat adaptation and carbohydrate restoration on metabolism and performance during prolonged cycling. J Appl Physiol. 2000;89:2413–21.

Burke LM, Cox GR, Cummings NK, Desbrow B. Guidelines for daily CHO intake: do athletes achieve them? Sports Med. 2001;31:267–99.

Burke LM, Hawley JA. Effects of short-term fat adaptation on metabolism and performance of prolonged exercise. Med Sci Sports Exerc 2002;34:1492–8.

Burke LM, Hawley JA, Angus DJ, Cox GR, Clark SA, Cummings NK, Desbrow B, Hargreaves M. Adaptations to short-term high-fat diet persist during exercise despite high carbohydrate availability. Med Sci Sports Exerc 2002;34:83–91.

Burke LM, Kiens B, Ivy JL. Carbohydrates and fat for training and recovery. J Sports Sci 2004;22:15–30.

Carey AL, Staudacher HM, Cummings NK, Stepto NK, Nikolopoulos V, Burke LM, Hawley JA. Effects of fat adaptation and carbohydrate restoration on prolonged endurance exercise. J Appl Physiol 2001;91:115–22.

Chesley A, Howlett RA, Heigenhauser GJF, Hultman E, Spriet LL. Regulation of muscle glycogenolytic flux during intense aerobic exercise after caffeine ingestion. Am J Physiol 1998;275:R596–603.

Christensen EH, Hansen O. Zur Methiodik der respiratorischem Quotientbestimmung in Ruhe und bei Arbeit. III: Arbeitsfahigkeit und Ernahrung. Scand Arch Physiol 1939;81:160–71.

Cole KJ, Costill DL, Starling RD, Goodpaster BH, Trappe SW, Fink WJ. Effect of caffeine ingestion on perception of effort and subsequent work production. Int J Sport Nutr 1996;6:14–23.

Costill DL, Coyle EF, Dalsky G, Evans W, Fink W, Hoopes D. Effects of elevated plasma FFA and insulin on muscle glycogen usage during exercise. J Appl Physiol 1977;43:695–9.

Costill DL, Dalsky GP, Fink WJ. Effects of caffeine ingestion on metabolism and exercise performance. Med Sci Sports 1978;10:155–8.

Cox GR, Desbrow B, Montgomery PG, Anderson ME, Bruce CR, Macrides TA, Martin DT, Moquin A, Roberts A, Hawley JA, Burke LM. Effect of different protocols of caffeine intake on metabolism and endurance performance. J Appl Physiol 2002;93:990–9.

Coyle EF. Fuels for sports performance. In: Lamb DR, Murray R, eds. Perspectives in exercise science and sports medicine. Volume 10. Optimising sport performance. Cooper Publishing Group, Indiana, 1997:95–129.

Coyle EF, Coggan AR, Hemmert MK, Ivy JL. Muscle glycogen utilization during prolonged strenuous exercise when fed carbohydrate. J Appl Physiol 1986;61:165–72.

Coyle EF, Hodgkinson BJ. Influence of dietary fat and carbohydrate on exercise metabolism and performance. In: Lamb DR, Murray R, eds. Perspectives in exercise science and sports medicine.

Volume 12. The metabolic basis of performance in exercise and sport. Cooper Publishing Group, Indiana, 1999;165–98.

Coyle EF, Jeukendrup AE, Wagenmakers AJM, Saris WHM. Fatty acid oxidation is directly regulated by carbohydrate metabolism during exercise. Am J Physiol 1997;273:E268–75.

Decombaz J, Deriaz O, Acheson K, Gmuender B, Jequier E. Effect of L-carnitine on submaximal exercise metabolism after depletion of muscle glycogen. Med Sci Sports Exerc 1993;25:733–40.

Dyck DJ, Peters SA, Wendling PS, Chesley A, Hultman E, Spriet LL. Regulation of muscle glycogen phosphorylase activity during intense aerobic cycling with elevated FFA. Am J Physiol 1996;265:E116–25.

Dyck DJ, Putman CT, Heigenhauser GJF, Hultman E, Spriet LL. Regulation of fat-carbohydrate interaction in skeletal muscle during intense aerobic cycling. Am J Physiol 1993;265:E852–9.

Ebeling P, Essen-Gustavsson B, Tuominen JA, Koivisto VA. Intramuscular triglyceride content is increased in IDMM. Diabetologica 1998;41:111–15.

Essig D, Costill DL, Van Handel PJ. Effects of caffeine ingestion on utilization of muscle glycogen and lipid during ergometer cycling. Int J Sports Med 1980;1:86–90.

Glatz JF, Bonen A, Luiken JJ. Exercise and insulin increase muscle fatty acid uptake by recruiting putative fatty acid transporters to the sarcolemma. Curr Opin Clin Nutr Metab Care 2002;5:365–70.

Glatz JF, Luiken JJ, Bonen A. Involvement of membrane-associated proteins in the acute regulation of cellular fatty acid uptake. J Mol Neurosci 2001;16:123–32.

Goedecke JH, Christie C, Wilson G, Dennis SC, Noakes TD, Hopkins WG, et al. Metabolic adaptations to a high-fat diet in endurance cyclists. Metabolism 1999a;48:1509–17.

Goedecke JH, Elmer-English R, Dennis SC, Schloss I, Noakes TD, Lambert EV. Effects of medium-chain triacylglycerol ingested with carbohydrate on metabolism and exercise performance. Int J Sport Nutr 1999b;9:35–47.

Graham TE, Helge JW, MacLean DA, Kiens B, Richter EA. Caffeine ingestion does not alter carbohydrate or fat metabolism in human skeletal muscle during exercise. J Physiol 2000;529:837–47.

Goodpaster BH, He J, Watkins S, Kelley DE. Skeletal muscle lipid content and insulin resistance: evidence for a paradox in endurance-trained athletes. J Clin Endocrinal Metab 2001;86:5755–61.

Greer F, Friars D, Graham TE. Comparison of caffeine and theophylline ingestion: exercise metabolism and endurance. J Appl Physiol 2000;89:1837–44.

Hansen AK, Fischer CP, Plomgaard P, Andersen JL, Saltin B, Pedersen BK. Skeletal muscle adaptation: training twice every second day vs. training once daily. J Appl Physiol 2005;98:93–9.

Havemann L, West SJ, Goedecke JH, Macdonald IA, St Clair Gibson A, Noakes TD, Lambert EV. Fat adaptation followed by carbohydrate-loading compromises high-intensity sprint performance. J Appl Physiol 2006;100:194–202.

Hawley JA, Brouns F, Jeukendrup AE. Strategies to enhance fat utilisation during exercise. Sports Med 1998;25;241–57.

Hawley JA, Burke LM, Angus DJ, Fallon KE, Martin DT, Febbraio MA. Effect of altering substrate availability on metabolism and performance during intense exercise. Br J Nutr 2000a;84:829–38.

Hawley JA, Hopkins WG. Aerobic glycolytic and aerobic lipolytic power systems. A new paradigm with implications for endurance and ultraendurance events. Sports Med 1995;19:240–50.

Hawley JA, Jeukendrup AE, Brouns F. Fat metabolism during exercise. In: Maughan RJ, ed. Nutrition in sport. Oxford: Blackwell Science, 2000b:192–7.

Heinonen OJ. Carnitine supplementation and physical exercise. Sports Med 1996;22:109–32.

Helge JW, Richter EA, Kiens B. Interaction of training and diet on metabolism and endurance during exercise in man. J Physiol 1996;492:293–306.

Helge JW, Wulff B, Kiens B. Impact of a fat-rich diet on endurance in man: role of the dietary period. Med Sci Sports Exerc 1998;30:456–61.

Holloszy JO, Kohrt WM, Hansen PA. The regulation of carbohydrate and fat metabolism during and after exercise. Front Biosci 1998;15;3:D1011–27.

Hopkins WG, Hawley JA, Burke LM. Design and analysis of research on sport performance. Med Sci Sports Exerc 1999;31:472–85.

Horowitz JF, Mora-Rodriguez R, Byerley LO, Coyle EF. Lipolytic suppression following carbohydrate ingestion limits fat oxidation during exercise. Am J Physiol 1997;273:E768–75.

Horowitz JF, Mora-Rodriguez R, Byerley LO, Coyle EF. Substrate metabolism when subjects are fed carbohydrate during exercise. Am J Physiol 1999;276:E828–35.

Ivy JL, Costill DL, Fink WJ. Contribution of medium and long chain triglyceride intake to energy metabolism during prolonged exercise. Int J Sports Med 1980;1:15–20.

Ivy JL, Costill DL, Fink WJ, Lower RW. Influence of caffeine and carbohydrate feedings on endurance performance. Med Sci Sports 1979;11:6–11.

Jansson E, Kaijser L. Effect of diet on the utilization of blood-borne and intramuscular substrates during exercise in man. Acta Physiol Scand 1982;115:19–30.

Jarvis M, McNaughton L, Seddon A, et al. The acute 1 week effects of the Zone diet on body composition, blood lipid levels, and performance in recreational endurance athletes. J Strength Cond Res 2002;16:50–7.

Jeukendrup AE. Aspects of carbohydrate and fat metabolism. Haarlem, The Netherlands: De Vrieseborch, 1997.

Jeukendrup AE, Saris WHM, Schrauwen P, Brouns F, Wagenmakers AJM. Metabolic availability of medium chain triglycerides co-ingested with carbohydrates during prolonged exercise. J Appl Physiol 1995;79:756–62.

Jeukendrup AE, Saris WH, Brouns F, Halliday D, Wagenmakers JM. Effects of carbohydrate (CHO) and fat supplementation on CHO metabolism during prolonged exercise. Metabolism 1996;45:915–21.

Jeukendrup AE, Thielen JJ, Wagenmakers AJM, Brouns F, Saris WHM. Effect of MCT and carbohydrate ingestion on substrate utilization and cycling performance. Am J Clin Nutr 1998;67:397–404.

Kalmar JM, Cafarelli E. Effects of caffeine on neuromuscular function. J Appl Physiol 1999;87:801–8.

Kelley DE. Skeletal muscle triglycerides: an aspect of regional adiposity and insulin resistance. Ann NY Acad Sci 2002;967:135–45.

Kiens B. Training and fatty acid metabolism. In: Richter EA, Kiens B, Galbo H, Saltin B, eds. Advances in experimental medicine and biology. Volume 441. Skeletal muscle metabolism in exercise and diabetes. New York: Plenum Press, 1998:229–38.

Kiens B, Burke LM. 'Fat adaptation' for athletic performance—the nail in the coffin? J Appl Physiol 2006;100:7–8.

Kiens B, Essen-Gustavsson B, Christensen NJ, Saltin B. Skeletal muscle substrate utilization during submaximal exercise in man: effect of endurance training. J Physiol 1993;469:459–78.

Kiens B, Helge JW. Adaptations to a high fat diet. In: Maughan RJ, ed. Nutrition in sport. Oxford: Blackwell Science, 2000:192–202.

Kraegen EW, Clark PW, Jenkins AB, Daley EA, Chisholm DJ, Storlien LH. Development of muscle insulin resistance after liver insulin resistance in high-fat fed rats. Diabetes 1991;40:1397–403.

Kronfeld DS. Diet and the performance of racing sled dogs. J Am Vet Med Assoc 1973;162:470–3.

Lambert EV, Hawley JA, Goedecke J, Noakes TD, Dennis SC. Nutritional strategies for promoting fat utilization and delaying the onset of fatigue during prolonged exercise. J Sports Sci 1997; 15:315–24.

Lambert EV, Speechly DP, Dennis SC, Noakes TD. Enhanced endurance in trained cyclists during moderate intensity exercise following 2 weeks adaptation to a high fat diet. Eur J Appl Physiol 1994;69:287–93.

Martin WH, Dalsky GP, Hurley BF, Matthews DE, Bier DM, Hagberg JM, et al. Effect of endurance training on plasma free fatty acid turnover and oxidation during exercise. Am J Phsyiol 1993;265:E708–14.

Massicotte D, Peronnet F, Brisson GR, Hillaire-Marcel C. Oxidation of exogenous medium-chain free fatty acids during prolonged exercise—comparison with glucose. J Appl Physiol 1992;73:1334–9.

McInerney P, Lessard SJ, Burke LM, Coffey VG, Lo Giudice SL, Southgate RJ, Hawley JA. Failure to repeatedly supercompensate muscle glycogen stores in highly trained men. Med Sci Sports Exerc 2005;37:404–11.

Odland LM, Heigenhauser GJ, Lopaschuk GD, Spriet LL. Human skeletal muscle malonyl-CoA at rest and during prolonged submaximal exercise. Am J Physiol 1996;270:E541–4.

Odland LM, Heigenhauser GJ, Wong D, Hollidge-Horvat MG, Spriet LL. Effects of increased fat availability on fat-carbohydrate interaction during prolonged aerobic exercise in humans. Am J Physiol 1998;274:R894–902.

Okano G, Sato Y, Murata Y. Effect of elevated blood FFA levels on endurance performance after a single fat meal ingestion. Med Sci Sports Exerc 1998;30:763–8.

Okano G, Sato Y, Takumi Y, Sugawara M. Effect of 4-h pre-exercise high carbohydrate and high fat meal ingestion on endurance performance and metabolism. Int J Sports Med 1996;17:530–4.

Phinney SD, Bistrian BR, Evans WF. The human metabolic response to chronic ketosis without caloric restriction: preservation of submaximal exercise capacity with reduced carbohydrate oxidation. Metabolism 1983;32:769–76.

Pitsiladis YP, Smith I, Maughan RJ. Increased fat availability enhances the capacity of trained individuals to perform prolonged exercise. Med Sci Sports Exerc 1999;31:1570–9.

Pruchnic R, Katsiaras A, He J, Kelley DE, Winters C, Goodpaster BH. Exercise training increases intramyocellular lipid and oxidative capacity in older adults. Am J Physiol Endocrinol Metab 2004;287:E857–62.

Rauch LGH, Hawley JA, Woodey M, Dennis SC, Noakes TD. Effects of ingesting a sports bar versus glucose polymer on substrate utilization and ultra-endurance performance. Int J Sports Med 1999;20:252–7.

Romijn JA, Coyle EF, Hibbert J, Wolfe RR. Comparison of indirect calorimetry and a new breath: $^{13}C/^{12}C$ ratio method during strenuous exercise. Am J Physiol 1992;263:E64–71.

Romijn JA, Coyle EF, Sidossis LS, Gastaldelli A, Horowitz JF, Endert E, et al. Regulation of endogenous fat and carbohydrate in relation to exercise intensity. Am J Physiol 1993;E380–91.

Romijn JA, Coyle EF, Sidossis LS, Zhang XJ, Wolfe RR. Relationship between fatty acid delivery and fatty acid oxidation during strenuous exercise. J Appl Physiol 1995;79:1939–45.

Sarna S, Kaprio J. Life expectancy of former athletes. Sports Med 1994;17:149–51.

Satabin P, Portero P, Defer G, Bricout J, Guezennec CY. Metabolic and hormonal responses to lipid and carbohydrate diets during exercise in man. Med Sci Sports Exerc 1987;19:218–23.

Sears B. The Zone diet: a dietary road map. New York: Regan Books, 1995.

Sears B. Mastering the Zone: the next step in achieving superhealth and permanent fat loss. New York: Regan Books, 1997.

Sidossis LS, Gastaldelli A, Klein S, Wolfe RR. Regulation of plasma fatty acid oxidation during low- and high-intensity exercise. Am J Physiol 1997;272:E1065–70.

Sidossis LS, Stuart CA, Schulman GI, Lopaschuk GD, Wolfe RR. Glucose plus insulin regulate fat oxidation by controlling the rate of fatty acid entry into the mitochondria. J Clin Invest 1996;98:2244–50.

Spriet LL. Ergogenic aids: recent advances and retreats. In: Lamb DR, Murray R, eds. Perspectives in exercise science and sports medicine. Volume 10. Optimizing sports performance. Carmel, Indiana: Cooper Publishing Company, 1997:185–234.

Spriet LL. Biochemical regulation of carbohydrate-lipid interaction in skeletal muscle during low and moderate intensity exercise. In: Hargreaves M, Thompson M, eds. Biochemistry of exercise X. Champaign, Illinois: Human Kinetics, 1999:241–61.

Spriet LL, Dyck DJ. The glucose-fatty acid cycle in skeletal muscle at rest and during exercise. In: Maughan RJ, Shirreffs SM, eds. Biochemistry of exercise IX. Champaign, Illinois: Human Kinetics, 1996:127–55.

Starling RD, Trappe TA, Parcell AC, Kerr CG, Fink WJ, Costill DL. Effects of diet on muscle triglyceride and endurance performance. J Appl Physiol 1997;82:1185–9.

Staudacher HM, Carey AL, Cummings NK, Hawley JA, Burke LM. Short-term high-fat diet alters substrate utilization during exercise but not glucose tolerance in highly trained athletes. Int J Sport Nutr Exerc Metab 2001;11:273–86.

Stellingwerff T, Spriet LL, Watt MJ, Kimber NE, Hargreaves M, Hawley JA, Burke LM. Decreased PDH activation and glycogenesis during exercise following fat adaptation with carbohydrate restoration. Am J Physiol 2006: 290:E380–8.

Sternfeld B. Cancer and the protective effect of physical activity: the epidemiological evidence. Med Sci Sports Exerc 1992;4:1195–209.

Van der Vusse D, Reneman RS. Lipid metabolism in muscle. In: Rowell LB, Shepherd JT, eds. Handbook of physiology. Exercise: Regulation and integration of multiple systems. Chapter 21. New York: American Physiological Society, Oxford Press, 1996:952–94.

Van Loon LJ, Goodpaster BH. Increased intramuscular lipid storage in the insulin-resistant and endurance-trained state. Pflugers Arch 2006;451:606–16.

Van Zyl CG, Lambert EV, Hawley JA, Noakes TD, Dennis SC. Effects of medium-chain triglyceride ingestion on carbohydrate metabolism and cycling performance. J Appl Physiol 1996;80:2217–25.

Vukovich MD, Costill DL, Fink WJ. Carnitine supplementation: effect on muscle carnitine and glycogen content during exercise. Med Sci Sports Exerc 1994;26:1122–9.

Vukovich MD, Costill DL, Hickey MS, Trappe SW, Cole KJ, Fink WJ. Effect of fat emulsion, infusion and fat feeding on muscle glycogen utilization during cycle exercise. J Appl Physiol 1993;75:1513–18.

Wee SL, Williams C, Garcia-Roves P. Carbohydrate availability determines endurance running capacity in fasted subjects. Med Sci Sports Exerc 1999;31(Suppl):91S.

Whitley HA, Humphreys SM, Campbell IT, Keegan MA, Jayanetti TD, Sperry DA, et al. Metabolic and performance responses during endurance exercise after high-fat and high-carbohydrate meals. J Appl Physiol 1998;85:418–24.

Wolfe RR. Fat metabolism in exercise. In: Richter EA, Kiens B, Galbo H, Saltin B, eds. Advances in experimental medicine and biology. Vol. 441. Skeletal muscle metabolism in exercise and diabetes. New York: Plenum Press, 1998:147–56.

CHAPTER 16

Supplements and sports foods

LOUISE BURKE, ELIZABETH BROAD, GREG COX, BEN DESBROW, CHRISTINE DZIEDZIC, STEPHEN GURR, BENITA LALOR, GREG SHAW, NIKKI SHAW, GARY SLATER

Introduction 16.1

Supplement use is a widespread and accepted practice among athletes, with a high prevalence of use and a large range of different types and brands of products. Such observations are illustrated by the results of a study of seventy-seven elite Australian swimmers (Baylis et al. 2001), which found that 94% of the group reported the use of supplements in pill and powder form. When the use of specialized sports foods such as sports drinks was also taken into account, 99% of swimmers reported supplement use and a total of 207 different products was identified. According to other studies, supplement use is also widespread among athletes at high school and collegiate levels (Massad et al. 1995; Krumbach et al. 1999; Froiland et al. 2004).

Overview of supplements and sports foods 16.2

'Dietary supplements', 'nutritional ergogenic aids', 'sports supplements', 'sports foods' and 'therapeutic nutritional supplements'—these are some of the terms used to describe the range of products that collectively form the sports supplement industry. Just as there is a variety of names for these products, there is a variety of definitions or classification systems. Characteristics that can be used to categorize supplements include:

- function (e.g. muscle building, immune boosting, fuel providing)
- form (e.g. pills, powders, foods or drinks)
- availability (e.g. over-the-counter, mail order, Internet, multi-level marketing)
- scientific merit for claims (e.g. well-supported, unsupported, undecided)

This last approach has been adopted recently by the Australian Institute of Sport (AIS) to guide the use of supplements by the athletes within its programs. The goal of this approach is to provide objective information to athletes, coaches and sports administrators regarding the likely efficacy of these products so that individuals can make informed decisions about their intended use. The specific details of the AIS Sports Supplement Program will be addressed later in this chapter.

For the purposes of this chapter we will discuss supplements and sports foods that meet one or more of the following definitions:

- They provide a convenient and practical means of meeting a known nutrient requirement to optimize daily training or competition performance (e.g. a liquid meal supplement, sports drink, carbohydrate gel, sports bar).
- They contain nutrients in large quantities in order to treat a known nutritional deficiency (e.g. an iron supplement).
- They contain nutrients or other components in amounts that directly enhance sports performance or maintain/restore health and immune function—scientifically supported or otherwise (e.g. caffeine, creatine, glycerol, ginseng).

There is an ever-increasing range of supplements and sports foods readily accessible to athletes and coaches. It is of primary importance for the sports nutrition professional to have a thorough working knowledge of the various sports foods and supplements in order to provide sound advice about appropriate situations of use, possible benefits, potential side effects and risks associated with use.

16.3 Regulation of supplements and sports foods

The regulation of supplements and sports foods is a contentious area and encompasses issues of manufacture, labeling and marketing. In addition to the concerns of efficacy and safety faced by the general consumer, athletes are faced with the problem of contamination with prohibited substances, leading to a positive doping offence. There is no universal system of regulation of sports foods and supplements. Countries differ in their approach and practice of the regulation of sports foods and supplements, with some involving a single government body (such as the Food and Drug Administration—FDA—in the US), while others fall under several government agencies (e.g. Food Standards Australia New Zealand for food-based products and the Therapeutic Goods Administration for pill-based products in Australia).

Athletes need to have a global understanding of the regulation of dietary supplements, since regular travel and modern conveniences such as mail order and the Internet provide them with easy access to products that fall outside the scrutiny of their own country's system. Although it is outside the scope of this chapter to review the various regulatory issues in different countries, the important changes that can be attributed to the *Dietary Supplement Health and Education Act 1994* in the US are worthy of special mention. This Act reduced the regulation of supplements and broadened the category to include new ingredients, such as herbal and botanical products, and constituents or metabolites of other dietary supplements. As a result, a new group of products flooded the US and international market: the 'pro-hormones' or compounds including androstenedione, DHEA, 19-norandrostenedione and other metabolites found in the steroid pathways that can be converted in the body to testosterone or the anabolic steroid nandrolone (Blue & Lombardo 1999). These products will be discussed later in the context of doping and inadvertent doping outcomes. The other important outcome of the *Dietary Supplement Health and Education Act 1994* was to shift responsibility from the supplement manufacturer to the FDA to enforce safety and claim guidelines. Since the passing of the Act, good manufacturing practice has not been enforced within the supplement industry, leaving non-compliant products or manufacturers to flourish unless there is specific intervention by the FDA.

Athletes and coaches often fail to understand that, in the absence or minimization of rigorous government evaluation, the quality control of supplement manufacture is trusted to supplement companies. Large companies that produce conventional supplements such as vitamins and minerals, particularly to manufacturing standards used in the preparation of pharmaceutical products, are likely to achieve good quality control. This includes precision with ingredient levels and labeling, and avoidance of undeclared ingredients or contaminants. However, this does not appear to be true for all supplement types or manufacturers, with many examples of poor compliance with labeling laws (Gurley et al. 1998; Parasrampuria et al. 1998; Hahm et al. 1999) and the presence of contaminants and undeclared ingredients (see sections 16.8 and 16.9).

Although manufacturers are not meant to make unsupported claims about health or performance benefits elicited by supplements, product advertisements and testimonials show ample evidence that this aspect of supplement marketing is unregulated and exploited. For example, a survey of five issues of bodybuilding magazines found 800 individual performance claims for 624 different products within advertisements (Grunewald & Bailey 1993). It is easy to see how enthusiastic and emotive claims provide a false sense of confidence about the products. Most consumers are unaware that the regulation of such advertising is generally not enforced. Therefore, athletes are likely to believe that claims about supplements are medically and scientifically supported, simply because they believe that untrue claims would not be allowed to exist.

16.4 The pros and cons of using supplements and sports foods

The decision by an athlete to use a supplement or sports food should be made after careful consideration of several issues. Figure 16.1 overleaf provides an overview of important questions that should be answered regarding the safety, efficacy and legality of any product. It also characterizes the balance between the arguments for and against the use of the product. The potential for both positive and negative outcomes will now be discussed in greater detail.

16.5 Pros—true performance benefits

Some supplements and sports foods offer real advantages to athletic performance. Some products 'work' by producing a direct performance-enhancing (ergogenic) effect. Other products can be used by athletes to meet their nutrition goals and, as an indirect outcome, allow the athlete to achieve optimal performance. In some cases these effects are so well known and easily demonstrated that beneficial uses of sports foods or supplements are clear-cut. For example, there are many studies that support the benefits of consuming sports drinks to supply carbohydrate (CHO) and fluid during exercise (see Coombes & Hamilton 2000). But even when indirect nutritional benefits or true ergogenic outcomes from supplement use are small, they are often worthwhile in the competitive world of sport (Hopkins et al. 1999). Of course, athletes need to be aware that it is the use of the product

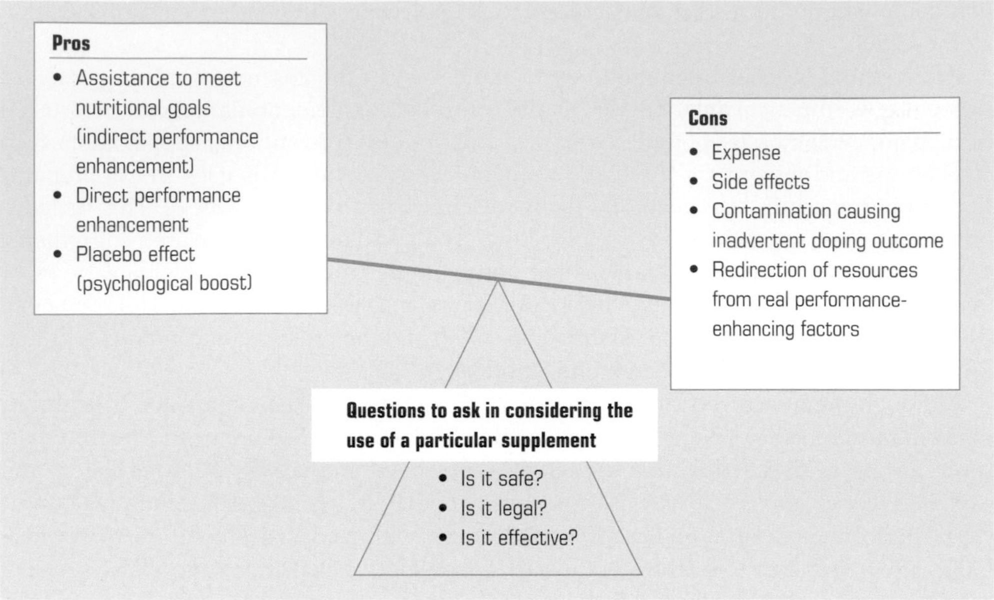

Pros

- Assistance to meet nutritional goals (indirect performance enhancement)
- Direct performance enhancement
- Placebo effect (psychological boost)

Cons

- Expense
- Side effects
- Contamination causing inadvertent doping outcome
- Redirection of resources from real performance-enhancing factors

Questions to ask in considering the use of a particular supplement

- Is it safe?
- Is it legal?
- Is it effective?

FIGURE 16.1 Issues to consider in the decision to take a supplement

as much as the product itself that leads to the beneficial outcome. Therefore education about specific situations and strategies for the use of supplements and sports foods is just as important as the formulation of the product.

16.6 Pros—the placebo effect

Even where a sports food does not produce a true physiological or ergogenic benefit, an athlete might attain some performance benefit because of a psychological boost or 'placebo' effect. The placebo effect describes a favorable outcome arising simply from an individual's belief that they have received a beneficial treatment. In a clinical environment, a placebo is often given in the form of a harmless but inactive substance or treatment that satisfies the patient's symbolic need to receive a 'therapy'. In a sports setting, an athlete who receives enthusiastic marketing material about a new supplement or hears glowing testimonials from other athletes who have used it is more likely to report a positive experience. Despite our belief that the placebo effect is real and potentially substantial, only a few studies have tried to document this effect in relation to sport. In one investigation, weightlifters who received saline injections that they believed to be anabolic steroids increased their gains in lean body mass (BM) (Ariel & Saville 1972). Another investigation in which athletes were given either a sports drink or a sweetened placebo during a 1-hour cycling time trial found that performance was affected by the information provided to the subjects (Clark et al. 2000). The placebo effect caused by thinking they were receiving a CHO drink allowed the subjects to achieve a small but worthwhile increase in performance of 4%. Being unsure of which treatment was being received increased the variability of performance, illustrating that the greatest benefits from supplement use occur when athletes are confident they are receiving a useful product.

Additional well-controlled studies are needed to better describe the potential size and duration of the placebo effect and whether it applies equally to all athletes and across all types of performance. In the meantime we can accept that the placebo effect exists and may explain, at least partially, why athletes report performance benefits after trying a new supplement or dietary treatment.

Cons—expense

16.7

An obvious issue with supplement use is the expense, which in extreme cases can equal or exceed the athlete's weekly food budget. Such extremes include the small number of athletes identified in many surveys (Baylis et al. 2001) who report a 'polypharmacy' approach to supplements, identifying long lists of products that often overlap in ingredients and claimed functions. However, even a targeted interest in a small number of supplements can be expensive: the cost of some individual products, such as ribose or colostrum, can exceed A$50 per week to achieve the manufacturer's recommended dose or the amounts found to have a true ergogenic outcome in scientific studies. The issue of expense is compounded for teams and sports programs that have to supply the needs of a group of athletes.

Expense must be carefully considered when there is little scientific evidence to support a product's claims of direct or indirect benefits to athletic performance. But even where benefits do exist, cost is an issue that athletes must acknowledge and prioritize appropriately within their total budget. Supplements or sports food generally provide nutrients or food constituents at a price that is considerably higher than that of everyday foods. At times, the expense of a supplement or sports food may be deemed money well spent, particularly when the product provides the most practical and palatable way to achieve a nutrition goal, or when the ergogenic benefits have been well documented. On other occasions, the athlete may choose to limit the use of expensive products to the most important events or training periods. There are often lower-cost alternatives to some supplements and sports foods that the budget-conscious athlete can use on less critical occasions; for example, a fruit smoothie fortified with milk powder or a commercial liquid meal replacement product is a less expensive choice to supplement energy and protein intake than most protein-rich 'bodybuilder' products.

Cons—side effects

16.8

Since most supplements are considered by regulatory bodies to be relatively safe, in many countries there are no official or mandatory accounting processes to document adverse side effects arising from the use of these products. Nevertheless, information from medical registers (Perharic et al. 1994; Kozyrskyj 1997; Shaw et al. 1997) shows that while the overall risk to public health from the use of supplements and herbal and traditional remedies is low, cases of toxicity and side effects include allergic reactions to some products (e.g. royal jelly), overexposure as a result of self-medication and poisoning due to contaminants. During the 1980s, deaths and medical problems resulted from the use of tryptophan supplements (Roufs 1992); products containing ephedra and caffeine are a more recent source of medical problems, sometimes causing deaths in susceptible individuals. Many reports call for better regulation and surveillance of supplements and herbal products, and increased awareness of potential hazards (Perharic et al. 1994; Kozyrskyj 1997; Shaw et al. 1997).

16.9 Cons—doping outcomes

A number of ingredients that may be found in supplements are considered prohibited substances by the codes of the World Anti-Doping Agency (WADA) and other sports bodies. These include pro-hormones (steroid-related compounds such as androstenedione, DHEA and 19-norandrostenedione) and stimulants such as ephedrine or related substances. Although the group of pro-hormone substances is not available for sale in Australia, they can be bought as over-the-counter products in countries such as the US. Drug education programs highlight the need for athletes to read the labels of supplements and sports foods carefully to ensure that they do not contain such banned substances. This is a responsibility that athletes must master to prevent inadvertent doping outcomes.

However, even when athletes take such precautions, inadvertent intake of banned substances from supplement products can still occur. This is because some supplements contain banned products without declaring them as ingredients; this is a result of contamination or poor labeling within lax manufacturing processes. The pro-hormone substances seem to provide the greatest risk of inadvertent consumption via supplement use, with a positive test for the steroid nandrolone being one of the possible outcomes. The most striking evidence of these problems was uncovered by a study carried out by a laboratory accredited by the International Olympic Committee (Geyer et al. 2004). This study analyzed 634 supplements from 215 suppliers in thirteen countries, with products being sourced from retail outlets (91%), the Internet (8%) and telephone sales. None of these supplements declared pro-hormones as ingredients, and came from manufacturers who produced other supplements containing pro-hormones as well as companies who did not sell these products. Ninety-four of the supplements (15% of the sample) were found to contain hormones or pro-hormones that were not stated on the product label. A further 10% of samples provided technical difficulties in analysis such that the absence of hormones could not be guaranteed. Of the 'positive' supplements, 68% contained pro-hormones of testosterone, 7% contained pro-hormones of nandrolone, and 25% contained compounds related to both. Forty-nine of the supplements contained only one steroid, but forty-five contained more than one, with eight products containing five or more different steroid products. According to the labels on the products, the countries of *manufacture* of all supplements containing steroids were the US, The Netherlands, the UK, Italy and Germany; however, these products were *purchased* in other countries. In fact, 10–20% of products purchased in Spain and Austria were found to be contaminated. Just over 20% of the products made by companies selling pro-hormones were positive for undeclared pro-hormones, but 10% of products from companies that did not sell steroid-containing supplements were also positive. The brand names of the 'positive' products were not provided in the study, but included amino acid supplements, protein powders, and products containing creatine, carnitine, ribose, guarana, zinc, pyruvate, HMB, *Tribulus terrestris*, herbal extracts and vitamins/minerals. It was noted that a positive urinary test for nandrolone metabolites occurs in the hours following uptake of as little of 1 μg of nandrolone pro-hormones. The positive supplements contained steroid concentrations ranging from 0.01 to 190 μg per gram of product.

This is a major area of concern for serious athletes who compete in competitions that apply anti-doping codes, since many of these codes place liability with the athlete for ingestion of banned substances, regardless of the circumstances and the source of ingestion. As such, full penalties can be expected for a positive doping test arising from the ingestion of a banned substance that is a contaminant or undeclared ingredient of a supplement. Further information on contamination of supplements can be found in reviews by Maughan (2005) and Geyer and colleagues (2008). Athletes should make enquiries at the anti-doping agencies within their countries for advice on the specific risks identified with supplement use, and any initiatives to reduce this risk.

Cons—displacement of real priorities 16.10

A more subtle outcome of reliance on supplements is the displacement of the athlete's real priorities. Successful sports performance is the product of superior genetics, long-term training, optimal nutrition, adequate sleep and recovery, state-of-the-art equipment and a committed attitude. These factors cannot be replaced by the use of supplements, but often appear less exciting or more demanding than the enthusiastic and emotive claims made for many supplements and sports foods. Athletes can sometimes be sidetracked from the true elements of success in search of short-cuts from bottles and packets. Most sports dietitians are familiar with individual athletes who are reliant on supplements while failing to address some of the basic elements of good training and lifestyle.

Special issues for the young athletes and supplement use 16.11

Success in sports involves obtaining an 'edge' over the competition, and children and adolescents may be uniquely vulnerable to the lure of supplements. The pressure to 'win at all costs', extensive coverage in lay publications, and hype from manufacturers with exciting and emotive claims all play a role in the use of supplements by young athletes. The knowledge that famous athletes and other role models use or promote supplements and sports foods adds to the allure.

An array of ethical issues arises in the consideration of supplement use by young athletes, including all the factors previously outlined in this section. Displaced priorities and the failure to build a foundation of sound training, diet and recovery strategies are particularly important since a long-term career in sport is underpinned by such an investment. The lack of information about the long-term safety of ingesting various compounds on a growing or developing body is a special concern.

Various expert groups have made strong statements against the use of supplements by young athletes. The American Academy of Pediatrics policy statement on the use of performance-enhancing substances (2005) condemns the use of ergogenic aids, including various dietary supplements, by children and adolescents. The American College of Sports Medicine recommends that creatine not be used by people under 18 years of age (American College of Sports Medicine 2000). These policies are based on the unknown but potentially adverse health consequences of some supplements and the implications of supplement use on the morals of a young athlete. Many people consider supplements to be an 'entry point' to the decision to take more serious compounds, including prohibited drugs.

16.12 Finding proof of the efficacy of supplements and sports foods

The process of substantiating the performance benefits or outcomes from supplement use is difficult. To various audiences, 'proof' comes in different forms, including testimonials from 'satisfied customers' and scientific theories that predict the outcome from the use of a product. On evaluation, however, these methods are flawed in their ability to provide definite support for the actions of a supplement. The scientific trial remains the best option for measuring the potential benefits of the use of a product. Nevertheless, the limitations of scientific studies need to be understood before a full interpretation of the results can be applied to real-life sport.

16.13 Scientific theories

The current focus of the sports supplement industry is on compounds and nutrients that act as cofactors, intermediary metabolites or stimulants of key reactions in exercise metabolism. The rationale behind supplementation is that if the system is 'supercharged' with additional amounts of these compounds, metabolic processes will proceed faster or for longer time, thus enhancing sports performance. The marketing of many contemporary supplements is accompanied by sophisticated descriptions of metabolic pathways and biochemical reactions, with claims that enhancement of these will lead to athletic success. In some cases, these descriptions are supplemented with data from studies on patients with an inherited deficiency of these compounds—these patients respond when supplementation is able to correct their deficiency.

To the scientist, a theory that links an increased level of a compound with performance enhancement may be a hypothesis that is worthy of testing, but it does not constitute proof for the idea. To the public, however, a hypothesis can be made to sound like a fait accompli, and athletes can be induced to buy products on the strength of a 'scientific breakthrough' that exists only on paper. In an era when sports scientists feel challenged by the apparent sophistication of the scientific theories presented by supplement companies, it is unlikely that athletes will possess sufficient scientific knowledge to be critical of these proposals.

While a 'supercharging' hypothesis may appear plausible at first glance, there are many reasons why it may not occur. Other issues to be considered include:

- Will oral ingestion of the compound increase concentrations at the sites that are critical?
- Does the present level of compound fall below the critical level for optimal metabolism?
- Is this reaction the rate-limiting step in metabolism or are other reactions setting the pace?

A scientific theory or hypothesis should be developed and fine-tuned before setting up a supplementation study. Since studies are expensive in time, money and resources, it is important that ideas that make it to trial are based on sound logic. But while a scientific theory should be developed in preparation for a study (or to explain the data collected in a study), it cannot be accepted as proof of the efficacy of a supplement until verified by actual research.

Anecdotal support

16.14

Testimonials provide a powerful force in the advertising and marketing of sports supplements, particularly in the case of products that target the bodybuilding or resistance-training industry. This is also true of supplements sold through multi-level marketing schemes, where individual distributors are encouraged to have a 'personal story' of how the product has enhanced their life. Testimonials for supplements and sports foods highlight the successful health or performance outcomes that people have achieved, allegedly as a result of their use of a supplement product. Often famous athletes or media stars supply these testimonials, but sometimes they also feature the exploits of 'everyday' people. Although people sometimes receive payment for their testimonials, in other cases the endorsement for a supplement is provided by hearsay, observation or direct recommendation from a 'satisfied customer'. Successful athletes and teams are perpetually being asked to nominate the secrets of their success by peers, fans or the media. In the following reviews of well-known ergogenic aids, there are many examples where public interest in a product can be traced back to the recommendation or testimonial of a winning sportsperson.

It is hard for athletes to understand that success in sport results from a complicated and multifactorial recipe, and that even the most successful athletes may not fully appreciate the factors behind their prowess. In many cases, it is likely that the athlete has succeeded without the effects of the supplements they are taking—and in some cases, perhaps, in spite of them! Unsupported beliefs and superstition are key reasons behind many decisions to use supplements. The idea that 'everyone is doing it' provides a powerful motivation to the athlete contemplating a new product. Sometimes, this manifests as a fear that 'others may have a winning edge that I don't have'. The ad hoc and undiscriminating patterns of supplement use reported by some athletes are testament to the power of 'word of mouth'.

Of course, the anecdotal experiences of athletes may be useful when considering the scientific investigation of a supplement. These experiences may support the case for expending resources on a study, or help in deciding on protocols for using a supplement or for measuring the outcomes. However, by itself, a self-reported experience provides very weak support for the benefits of a supplement. Many of the benefits perceived by athletes who try a new supplement result from the psychological boost or placebo effect that accompanies a new experience or special treatment.

The scientific trial

16.15

The scientific trial remains the 'gold standard' for investigating the effects of dietary supplements and nutritional ergogenic aids on sports performance. Scientists undertaking scientific trials should test the effects of the supplement in a context that simulates sports

TABLE 16.1 FACTORS IN CONDUCTING RESEARCH ON SUPPLEMENTS AND SPORTS FOODS

FACTORS TO CONSIDER IN DESIGNING A RESEARCH PROTOCOL TO SELECT INDEPENDENT AND DEPENDENT VARIABLES OF IMPORTANCE
• Subject variables—age, gender, level of training, nutritional status
• Measurement variables—validity and reproducibility of techniques, costs, availability of equipment, subjective versus objective measures, application to the hypothesis being tested
• Study design—acute versus chronic supplementation, lab versus field, 'blinding' of subjects and researchers, crossover versus parallel group design, placebo control
• Supplementation protocols—timing and quantity of doses, duration of the supplementation period
STRATEGIES TO UNDERTAKE TO ELIMINATE OR STANDARDIZE THE VARIABLES THAT MIGHT OTHERWISE CONFOUND THE RESULTS OF A SUPPLEMENT STUDY
• Recruit well-trained athletes, as the subject's level of training may alter the effect of the supplement and will affect the precision of measurement of performance.
• Incorporate the use of a placebo treatment to overcome the psychological effect of supplementation.
• Use repeated measures or crossover design to increase statistical power; each subject acts as their own control by undertaking both treatment and placebo.
• Allow a suitable wash-out period between treatments.
• Randomly assign subjects to treatment and placebo groups and counterbalance the order of treatment.
• Employ a double-blind allocation of treatments to remove the subjective bias of both researcher and subjects.
• Standardize the pre-trial training and dietary status of subjects.
• Design the parallel conditions to mimic real-life practices of athletes.
• Choose measurement variables that are sufficiently reliable to allow changes due to the supplement to be detected, and that are applicable to the hypothesis being tested.
• Choose a performance test that is highly reliable and applicable to the real-life performances of athletes.
• Choose a supplementation protocol that maximizes the likelihood of a positive outcome.
• Interpret the results in light of what is important to sports performance.

performance as closely as possible. Additional studies might be needed to elucidate the mechanisms by which these effects occur, but, overall, sports science research must be able to deliver answers to questions related to real-life sport.

It is beyond the scope of this chapter to fully explore the characteristics of good research design. However, there are many variables that interfere with the outcomes of research and that need to be considered. Table 16.1 summarizes the issues that need to be addressed to control for these variables, along with other issues to consider in designing trials to test the effects of supplements on sports performance. Several factors that are important to consider in the interpretation of results will now be discussed.

16.16 Are we testing the athlete's definition of improvement?

In the world of sport, the difference between winning and losing can be measured in hundredths of seconds and in millimeters. To the athlete or coach, that hundredth of a second or millimeter seems a meaningful improvement in performance. This helps to explain why supplements that promise a performance boost are greeted with such enthusiasm—the chance of the tiniest improvement seems worth the investment. Unfortunately, the traditional framework of sports science research works on a different basis. The scientist aims to detect (i.e. declare statistically significant) an effect, with acceptably low rates for detection of non-existent effects (5%) and failed detection of a real effect (20%). Most scientific investigations of supplements are biased towards rejecting the hypothesis that the product enhances performance, due to small sample sizes and performance-testing protocols with low reliability. In effect, most intervention studies are able to detect only large differences in performance outcomes. Changes that are smaller than this large effect are declared to be 'not statistically significant' and are dismissed.

Hopkins and colleagues attempted to find some middle ground between what scientists and athletes consider significant (Hopkins et al. 1999). First, they established that an athlete's required improvement is *not* the tiny margin between the place-getters in a race (also known as between-athlete variation). Each athlete has their own day-to-day or event-to-event variability in performance, known as the within-athlete variation or coefficient of variation (CV) of performance. This variation would influence the outcome of an event if it were to be rerun without any intervention. By modeling the results of various sporting events in track and field, Hopkins suggested that 'worthwhile' changes to the outcome of most events require a performance change equal to ~0.4–0.7 times the CV of performance for that event. Note that this 'worthwhile' change does not *guarantee* that an athlete would win an event, but would make a reasonable change to an athlete's likelihood of winning—for example, improve the probability of winning, for an athlete who has a true probability of winning the race 20% of the time, to 30%. Across a range of track and field events, Hopkins noted that the CV of performance of top athletes was within the range of 0.5–5%, thus making performance changes of up to 3% important to detect (Hopkins et al. 1999).

Even though 'worthwhile' performance differences are larger than the tiny margins considered important by athletes, these changes are still outside the realms of detection for many of the studies commonly published in scientific journals. As discussed by Hopkins and colleagues (1999), a change of 0.7 of the CV in a parameter requires a sample size of about 32 for detection in a crossover study in which every athlete receives an experimental and placebo treatment. For a parallel group designed study, 128 subjects would be needed. Such sample sizes are beyond the patience and resources of most sport scientists!

To bridge the gap between science and the athlete on the issue of a significant performance change, Hopkins proposed a new approach to reporting and interpreting the results of intervention studies (Hopkins et al. 1999). He suggested that outcomes should be as a percent change in a measure of athletic performance—for example, a study may find a 1% enhancement in time, caused by a 0.8% improvement in mean power, as a result of the use of a supplement. The reporting of the 95% or 90% confidence limits for the outcome will provide the likely range of the true effect of the treatment on the typical subject. For example, in our study, the 95% confident interval (CI) for the change in time might be –1% to +3%. This can then be interpreted in terms of the likely effect on athletes in an event. For example, the outcome in this study includes the possibility of a small decrement in performance as well as a substantial improvement in performance. Both possibilities could change the outcome of an event, and the athlete needs to consider the small risk of a negative outcome as well as the more likely chance of a noticeable improvement in finishing order. It is hoped that sports scientists will undertake such interpretations of the results of their studies.

16.17 Individual responses

Notwithstanding the general variability in performance, there is evidence that some treatments cause a range of different responses in individual athletes. In some cases, the same intervention can produce favorable responses in some individuals, neutral responses in others and, sometimes, detrimental outcomes to another group. For example, research has identified that some athletes are 'non-responders' to caffeine or creatine supplementation (Graham & Spriet 1991; Greenhaff et al. 1994). It is useful to have metabolic or other mechanistic data to substantiate real differences in response, and to differentiate these from the general variability of performance. For example, it has been shown that subjects whose muscle creatine levels did not increase by at least 20% as a result of creatine supplementation did not show the functional changes and performance enhancements seen by the rest of the experimental group (Greenhaff et al. 1994).

Studies employing simple group analysis and small sample sizes are not appropriate for situations in which there is true variability in the size and direction of the response to an intervention. Such studies will fail to detect a difference in performance, even though this is a real outcome for some subjects in the group. Ideally, studies employing large sample sizes and co-variate analysis should be used; this approach will allow real changes to be detected and may also identify the characteristics of individuals that predict 'response' and 'non-response'. At present, such studies are rare.

16.18 AIS Sports Supplement Program

In some cases, sporting organizations or institutions make policies or programs for supplement use on behalf of athletes within their care. This may range from a single sporting team to an entire sports program, such as that of the National Collegiate Athletics Association (Burke 2001). Since 2000, the AIS has implemented a supplement program for athletes within its funding program with the stated goals of:

- allowing its athletes to focus on the sound use of supplements and special sports foods as part of their special nutrition plans
- ensuring that supplements and sports foods are used correctly and appropriately to deliver maximum benefits to the immune system, recovery and performance
- giving its athletes the confidence that they receive 'cutting edge' advice and achieve 'state-of-the-art' nutrition practices
- ensuring that supplement use does not lead to an inadvertent doping offense

A key part of the AIS program is a ranking system for supplements and sports foods, based on a risk:benefit analysis of each product by a panel of experts in sports nutrition, medicine and science. This ranking system has four tiers, each of which has a prescribed level of use by AIS-funded athletes. Although the hierarchy of categories was developed for long-term use, there is a regular assessment of supplements and sports foods to ensure that they are placed in the category that best fits the available scientific evidence. The hierarchical system allows the program to avoid the 'black and white' assessment that any particular product works or fails to live up to claims. Rather, the available science is reviewed to place supplements into categories ranked from what is most likely to provide a benefit for little risk, to what provides least benefit and a definite risk. Table 16.2 provides a summary of the AIS Sports Supplement Program at the time of publication. The remainder of this chapter provides a summary of the current scientific support for a range of products within the various supplement categories.

TABLE 16.2 AIS SPORTS SUPPLEMENT PROGRAM 2009 (see http://www.ausport.gov.au/ais/nutrition/supplements)

SUPPLEMENT CATEGORY AND EXPLANATION OF USE WITHIN THE AIS SPORTS SUPPLEMENT PROGRAM	PRODUCTS INCLUDED IN CATEGORY[a]
Group A: Approved supplements • Provide a useful and timely source of energy and nutrients in the athlete's diet, or • Have been shown in scientific trials to provide a performance benefit, when used according to a specific protocol in a specific situation in sport. *AIS Sports Supplement Panel position* We know that athletes and coaches are interested in using supplements to achieve optimal performance. Our supplement program aims to focus this interest on products and protocols that have documented benefits, by: • making these supplements available and accessible to the AIS athletes who will benefit from their appropriate use. In particular, to provide these supplements at no cost to AIS sports programs, through systems managed by appropriate sports science/medicine departments. Strategies to provide products range from individual 'prescription' of supplements requiring careful use (e.g. creatine) to creative programs that make valuable sports foods and everyday foods accessible to athletes in situations of nutritional need (e.g. post-exercise recovery bars) • providing education to athletes and coaches about the beneficial uses of these supplements/sports foods and their appropriate use, with the emphasis on state-of-the-art sports nutrition • ensuring that supplements/sports foods used by AIS athletes carry a minimal risk of doping safety problems • providing immediate access to research opportunities	• Sports drinks • Liquid meal supplements • Sports gels • Sports bars • Caffeine[b] • Creatine • Bicarbonate and citrate • Anti-oxidants: vitamin C, vitamin E • Electrolyte replacement • Multivitamin/mineral supplement • Iron supplement • Calcium supplement • Vitamin D • Probiotics (for gastrointestinal health)
Group B: Supplements under consideration Supplements may be classified as belonging to Group B if they have no substantial proof of health or performance benefits, but: • remain of interest to AIS coaches or athletes • are too new to have received adequate scientific attention • have preliminary data that hint at possible benefits *AIS Sports Supplement Panel position* These supplements can be used at the AIS under the auspices of a controlled scientific trial or a supervised therapeutic program. Inadvertent doping risk from the use of these products is carefully considered.	• B-alanine • Glutamine • Hydroxymethylbutyrate (HMB) • Colostrum • Probiotics (for boost to immune system) • Ribose • Glucosamine[b] • Melatonin[b]
Group C: Supplements that have no clear proof of beneficial effects This category contains the majority of supplements and sports products promoted to athletes. Supplements not specifically listed within this system probably belong here. These supplements, despite enjoying a cyclical pattern of popularity and widespread use, have not been proven to provide a worthwhile enhancement of sports performance. Although we can't categorically state that they don't 'work', current scientific evidence shows that either the likelihood of benefits is very	• Amino acids (these can be provided by everyday foods or sports foods in Group A) • Carnitine • Chromium picolinate • *Cordyceps* • Co-enzyme Q10 • Gamma-oryzanol and ferulic acid • Ginseng

(continued)

TABLE 16.2 (continued)

SUPPLEMENT CATEGORY AND EXPLANATION OF USE WITHIN THE AIS SPORTS SUPPLEMENT PROGRAM	PRODUCTS INCLUDED IN CATEGORY[a]
small or that any benefits that occur are too small to be useful. In fact, in some cases these supplements have been shown to impair sports performance or health, with a clear mechanism to explain these results. *AIS Sports Supplement Panel position* In the absence of proof of benefits, these supplements should not be provided to AIS athletes from AIS program budgets. If an individual athlete or coach wishes to use a supplement from this category, they may do so providing: • they are responsible for payment for this supplement • any sponsorship arrangements are within guidelines of AIS marketing • the supplement brand has been assessed for doping safety and is considered 'low risk', and • the use is reported to an AIS sports dietitian or physician	• Inosine • Lact-Away™ • Medium-chain triglycerides • Nitric oxide stimulators • Oxygenated waters • Pyruvate • *Rhodiola rosea* • Vitamins when used in situations other than described in Group A • ZMA (zinc monomethionine aspartate and magnesium aspartate) • Most other supplements not listed probably belong here
Group D: Banned supplements These supplements are either directly banned by the WADA anti-doping code or provide a high risk of producing a positive doping outcome. *AIS Sports Supplement Panel position* These supplements should not be used by AIS athletes.	• Glycerol[c] • Androstenedione • DHEA (dehydroepiandrosterone) • 19 norandrostenedione and 19-norandrostenediol • *Tribulus terrestris* and other herbal testosterone supplements • Ephedra • Strychnine

[a]Note that the AIS does not support the use of products provided by Network Marketing Supplements.
[b]These supplements are not made available to athletes under the AIS Sports Supplement Program.
[c]At the time of publication, glycerol was being considered for placement on the 2010 List of Prohibited Substances of the WADA.

16.19 Supplements in Group A of the AIS Sports Supplement Program

According to the judgments of the expert panel of the AIS Sports Supplement Program, products listed in Group A have scientific support to show that they can be used within an athlete's nutritional plan to provide direct or indirect benefits to performance.

16.20 Sports foods and dietary supplements that achieve nutritional goals

Sports foods that provide a practical way to meet goals of sports nutrition are among the most valuable special products available to athletes. Table 16.3 summarizes the major classes of sports foods, together with the situations or goals of sports nutrition that they can be used to address. Substantiation for many of these nutrition goals is well accepted and often includes situations where a measurable enhancement of performance can be detected as a result of the correct use of the sports food. More detail about the uses of these products can be found in various chapters throughout this text (see Table 16.3 for cross-referencing).

TABLE 16.3 SPORTS FOODS AND DIETARY SUPPLEMENTS USED TO MEET NUTRITIONAL GOALS

SUPPLEMENT	FORM	COMPOSITION	SPORTS-RELATED USE	CHAPTER
Sports drink	Powder or liquid	5–8% CHO 10–35 mmol/L sodium 3–5 mmol/L potassium	Optimum delivery of fluid + CHO during exercise	13
			Post-exercise rehydration	14
			Post-exercise refueling	14
Sports gel	Gel 30–40 g sachets or larger tubes	60–70% CHO (~25 g CHO per sachet)	Supplement high-CHO training diet	14
		Some contain caffeine or electrolytes	CHO loading	12
			Post-exercise CHO recovery	14
			May be used during exercise when CHO needs exceed fluid requirements	13
Electrolyte replacement supplements	Powder sachets or tablets	≤2% CHO 50–60 mmol/L sodium 10–20 mmol/L potassium	Rapid and effective rehydration following dehydration undertaken for weight-making	7
			Replacement of large sodium losses during ultra-endurance activities	13
			Rapid and effective rehydration following moderate to large fluid and sodium deficits (e.g. post-exercise)	14
Liquid meal supplement	Powder (mix with water or milk) or liquid	1–1.5 kcal/mL 15–20% protein 50–70% CHO low to moderate fat vitamins/minerals: 500–1000 mL supplies RDI/RDAs	Supplement high-energy/ CHO/nutrient diet (especially during heavy training/competition or weight gain)	14
			Low-bulk meal replacement (especially pre-event meal)	12
			Post-exercise recovery—provides CHO, pro- and micronutrients	4, 14
			Portable nutrition for traveling athlete	23
Sports bar	Bar (50–60 g)	40–50 g CHO 5–10 g protein Usually low in fat and fiber	CHO source during exercise	13
			Post-exercise recovery—provides CHO, protein and micronutrients	5, 14
		Vitamins/minerals: 50–100% of RDA/RDIs	Supplements high-energy/ CHO/nutrient diet	14
		May contain creatine, amino acids	Portable nutrition (traveling)	23

(continued)

TABLE 16.3 (continued)

SUPPLEMENT	FORM	COMPOSITION	SPORTS-RELATED USE	CHAPTER
Vitamin/mineral supplement	Capsule/tablet	Broad range 1–4 × RDI/RDAs of vitamins and minerals	Micronutrient support for low-energy or weight-loss diet	6
			Micronutrient support for restricted variety diets (e.g. vegetarian)	20
			Micronutrient support for unreliable food supply (e.g. traveling athlete)	23
			Heavy competition schedule where normal eating patterns may be disrupted	
Iron supplement	Capsule/tablet	Ferrous sulfate/gluconate/fumarate	Supervised management of iron deficiency (including treatment and prevention)	10
Calcium supplement	Tablet	Calcium carbonate/phosphate/lactate	Calcium supplementation in low-energy or low dairy food diet	9
			Treatment/prevention of osteopenia	9

CHO = carbohydrate, RDA = Recommended Dietary Allowance, RDI = Recommended Dietary Intake

Although most sports foods have specialized uses in sport, some products (e.g. sports drinks) have crossed successfully into the general market. As long as consumers are prepared to pay the premium price for a niche product and sports nutrition messages are left intact, most sports nutrition experts are not unduly concerned by this outcome. In fact, there is some support for the use of products such as sports drinks by 'weekend warriors' and recreational exercisers, since the benefits of fluid intake and CHO replacement during a workout are determined by the physiology of exercise rather than the caliber of the person who is exercising. In fact, most studies of sports drinks have been undertaken on moderately trained to well-trained performers rather than elite athletes; therefore, where evidence of a performance benefit does exist, it is directly relevant to these sub-elite populations.

Vitamin and mineral supplements that are used to correct or prevent a suboptimal nutrient status can also be considered as supplements that help an athlete achieve their nutritional goals. These include multivitamin, iron and calcium supplements used in specific situations or individuals (see Table 16.3).

16.21 Caffeine

Caffeine is a drug that enjoys social acceptance and widespread use around the world. This acceptance now includes its use in competitive sport following the removal of caffeine from the WADA list of prohibited substances in January 2004. Caffeine is the best known member of the methylxanthines, a family of naturally occurring stimulants found in the leaves, nuts and seeds of a number of plants. Major dietary sources of caffeine—such as tea, coffee, chocolate, cola and energy drinks—typically provide 30–200 mg of caffeine per serve, whereas some non-prescriptive medications contain 100–200 mg of caffeine per tablet. The recent introduction of caffeine (or guarana) to 'energy drinks', confectionery and sports foods/supplements has increased the opportunities for athletes to consume caffeine, either as part of their everyday diet or for specific use as an ergogenic aid.

The complex range of actions of caffeine on the human body has been extensively researched (Tarnopolsky 1994; Spriet 1997; Fredholm et al. 1999; Graham 2001a, 2001b). Briefly, caffeine has several effects on skeletal muscle, involving calcium handling, sodium–potassium pump activity, elevation of cyclic-AMP and direct action on enzymes such as glycogen phosphorylase (see Chapter 1). Increased catecholamine action, and the direct effect of caffeine on cyclic-AMP, may both act to increase lipolysis in adipose and muscle tissue, causing an increase in plasma free fatty acid concentrations and increased availability of intramuscular triglyceride. It has been proposed that an increased potential for fat oxidation during moderate-intensity exercise promotes glycogen sparing. However, studies have found this effect to be short-lived or confined to certain individuals, and are unable to explain the ergogenic effects seen with caffeine supplementation (for review, see section 15.12). Caffeine may also influence athletic performance via central nervous system effects, such as a reduced perception of effort or an enhanced recruitment of motor units. Breakdown products of caffeine such as paraxanthine and theophylline may also have actions within the body. Caffeine supplementation is a complex issue to investigate due to the difficulty in isolating individual effects of caffeine, and the potential for variability between subjects.

The effect of caffeine on exercise has received extensive scientific attention for a century (Rivers 1907), with excellent reviews by Spriet (1997), Graham (2001a, 2001b) and Doherty and Smith (2004, 2005) covering a large range of studies. Burke (2008) concentrates on the literature that is most relevant to sports performance rather than exercise capacity per se, reviewing studies involving trained individuals and defined tasks rather than exercise to fatigue protocols. Due to the large volume and turnover of such research we will present our summary of the available peer-reviewed literature as a continually updated online publication at the website: http://www.ausport.gov.au/ais/nutrition/supplements. This resource includes a tabulation of the results of studies of caffeine supplementation and sports performance, divided according to the type of exercise task and the method of administration of caffeine administration. Some of the key information from this resource will now be presented to summarize our current knowledge of the effects of the quantity, timing and source of caffeine on exercise performance.

Caffeine dose

An obvious interest of athletes is to find the dose of caffeine that elicits the greatest benefit to their specific performance for the minimum level of risk or side effect. Unfortunately, it is difficult to conduct this analysis across all of the available literature due to the mixture of studies providing caffeine in absolute doses (e.g. 250 mg caffeine) and relative doses (e.g. 3 mg/kg BM of caffeine) across populations of differing body sizes. Studies that have investigated a dose–response relationship with caffeine supplementation, by examining the performance outcomes following the intake of different doses of caffeine by the same subjects, deserve specific comment. These include a number of brief high-intensity performances (<20 minutes) in relatively untrained (Perkins & Williams 1975; Dodd et al. 1991) and trained subjects (Anderson et al. 2000; Bruce et al. 2000). In untrained subjects, the data show that caffeine supplementation in any dose fails to provide a detectable change in exercise capacity. However, in the studies undertaken by trained subjects who were familiarized to the performance protocol (Anderson et al. 2000; Bruce et al. 2000), 6 and 9 mg/kg of caffeine had similarly positive effects on a time trial performance.

In events of slightly longer duration (~1 hour) the effects of caffeine supplementation appear more consistent. Similar benefits to endurance or performance were identified at caffeine doses of 5, 9 and 13 mg/kg (Pasman et al. 1995) and at 3 and 6 mg/kg (Graham & Spriet 1995). Kovacs and colleagues (1998) demonstrated a threshold of the performance benefits to a cycling time trial at a caffeine dose of 3.2 mg/kg dose (that is, no further benefit with 4.5 mg/kg). Whereas caffeine did not have a detectable benefit to the performance of a half-marathon in the heat at intakes of 5 or 7 mg/kg (Cohen et al. 1996), Cox and colleagues (2002) found that intakes of as little as 1–2 mg/kg caffeine enhanced the performance of a time trial at the end of 2 hours of cycling to the same degree as an intake of 6 mg/kg. In some trials (Graham & Spriet 1995), large amounts of caffeine (9 mg/kg) reduced endurance compared to smaller doses.

Overall, it appears that, for the performance of events lasting 1 hour or longer, benefits are seen at low doses of caffeine (1–3 mg/kg), and there do not seem to be further benefits at doses higher than this. Further research of this type is warranted so that athletes can identify the *smallest* dose of caffeine that produces a worthwhile benefit to their performance.

Timing of intake of caffeine

Caffeine is rapidly absorbed, reaching peak concentrations in the blood within 1 hour after ingestion (for a review of caffeine pharmacokinetics see Fredholm et al. 1999). This explains why the traditional approach to caffeine supplementation has been to consume the caffeine dose 1 hour prior to exercise. In the case of prolonged exercise (>60 minutes), this protocol of intake is often associated with a benefit to endurance or performance, whereas the effect on shorter-term high-intensity exercise is less consistent (see the tables on caffeine supplementation at http://www.ausport.gov.au/ais/nutrition/supplements). Whether this relates to the real outcome, the reliability of the exercise in allowing changes to performance to be detected, or the timing of the intake of caffeine is unknown.

Caffeine is slowly catabolized (half-life 4–6 hours) with peak concentrations being maintained for 3–4 hours (Graham 2001a, 2001b). Studies have reported that the ergogenic benefits of caffeine may be sustained for up to 6 hours post-ingestion (Bell & McLellan 2002), even after a prior bout of exhaustive exercise (Bell & McLellan 2003).

Although early studies (Ivy et al. 1979) demonstrated the potential benefits of consuming caffeine both before and throughout an exercise task, it is only recently that there has been a renewed interest in investigating the effects of divided or progressive doses of caffeine during exercise (Kovacs et al. 1998; Cox et al. 2002; Hunter et al. 2002; Conway et al. 2003). Conway and colleagues (2003) investigated the performance of a time trial following 90 minutes of submaximal cycling with supplementation of 6 mg/kg caffeine, either 1 hour pre-trial or 3 mg/kg pre-trial and 3 mg/kg at 45 minutes of exercise (= 3 + 3 mg/kg). There was a large reduction (that is, an improvement) in the mean time to complete the task (28.3, 24.2 and 23.4 minutes for placebo, 6 mg/kg and 3 + 3 mg/kg, respectively); however, differences between trials were not found to be statistically significant (see section 16.16).

We showed that similar performance benefits of a 3% improvement in time trial performance were achieved when six doses of caffeine of 1 mg/kg were spread throughout a 2-hour submaximal cycling bout prior to the time trial, when 6 mg/kg of caffeine was consumed 1 hour prior to the cycling bout, or when small amounts of caffeine (~1.5 mg/kg) were consumed over the last third of the protocol (Cox et al. 2002). It may be that subjects become more sensitive to small amounts of caffeine as they become fatigued. Further investigations are required to confirm this and the potential for strategic timing of intake of caffeine in various sporting and exercise activities.

Source of caffeine

A number of studies have investigated the effects of caffeine on exercise, using coffee as the source of caffeine (i.e. providing subjects with decaffeinated coffee ± added caffeine) (Costill et al. 1978; Wiles et al. 1992; Trice & Haymes 1995; Graham et al. 1998; Vanakoski et al. 1998; McLellan & Bell 2004). The results of these studies have shown that coffee intake can both enhance performance (Costill et al. 1978; Wiles et al. 1992; Trice & Haymes 1995; McLellan & Bell 2004) and fail to have a detectable effect (Graham et al. 1998; Vanakoski et al. 1998). Only two of these studies (Graham et al. 1998; McLellan & Bell 2004) included trials in which the performance responses to caffeinated coffee were compared to responses to pure caffeine. Graham and colleagues found that runners increased their treadmill running time to exhaustion following the intake of pure caffeine compared to their endurance following the intake of the same amount of caffeine consumed in coffee. The differences in performance occurred despite similar appearance rates of caffeine and other caffeine metabolites; it has been suggested that other components within coffee might antagonize the responses to the caffeine or counteract its ergogenic effects by directly impairing performances. However, McLellan and Bell (2004) demonstrated that the consumption of one cup of coffee (either decaffeinated or caffeinated) prior to the consumption of pure caffeine failed to dampen the ergogenic effect gained from the larger caffeine doses. Further research is needed on this issue, since in the 'real world', athletes often consume coffee before competing or training, either as part of their normal social and dietary patterns, or as an intentional source of caffeine as an ergogenic aid.

Food tables generally provide a range for the typical caffeine content of coffee, to account for the variable quantities of caffeine in the coffee bean and differences in the way that coffee drinks are prepared for consumption by individuals—even among the same 'type' of drink prepared under seemingly standard conditions. For example, we have recently demonstrated larger than anticipated variations in the caffeine content of an individual serve of retail preparations using ground coffee. We found that the caffeine content of a single espresso purchased from a large number of separate outlets varied from 25 to 214 mg/serve (Desbrow et al. 2007). This unexpectedly large, and otherwise unknown, variation in the caffeine content of coffee and the potential interaction between the caffeine and other active ingredients in coffee (e.g. derivates of the chlogogenic acids) suggest that coffee should not be the preferred source of caffeine for athletes.

Only one study (Cox et al. 2002) has investigated the effect of the use of cola-containing beverages on the performance of endurance cycling, to mimic the patterns practiced in real life, where athletes consume a sports (CHO-electrolyte) drink for the first two-thirds of their event before switching to de-fizzed cola drinks. We found that the consumption of ~750 mL of Coca-cola™ towards the end of our cycling protocol enhanced the performance of a time trial to a similar extent as larger amounts of caffeine. A separate study was then conducted to test whether this effect was achieved by the presence of the caffeine (~1–2 mg/kg BM) or the increase in CHO concentration between the cola and sports drink. The second study confirmed the finding of a 3% enhancement of performance of the time trial with the intake of Coca-cola™ towards the end of the trial, finding that the majority of this effect (2%, $p < 0.05$) could be explained by the caffeine content (Cox et al. 2002).

Similarly, a single study has been published on the effects of caffeine on exercise when ingested in the form of an 'energy drink' (Alford et al. 2001). This study reported that the consumption of Red Bull Energy Drink™ (a CHO-containing drink with the additional ingredients of caffeine, taurine and glucuronolactone) enhanced performance in a battery of tests, including measures of aerobic and anaerobic performance, and psychomotor traits. Unfortunately, this study did not distinguish the contribution of caffeine, and the authors concluded that the results reflected the effects of the combination of ingredients.

Summary of caffeine and exercise

- There is sound evidence that caffeine enhances endurance and provides a small but worthwhile enhancement of performance over a range of exercise protocols. There is still no consensus on the mechanism to explain this performance improvement, but it is unlikely to result from the so-called 'metabolic theory' (increase in fat oxidation and 'sparing' of glycogen utilization during exercise). Instead, altered perception of fatigue and effort, or direct effects on the muscle, may underpin performance changes. Most studies of caffeine and performance have been undertaken in laboratories; studies that investigate performance effects in elite athletes under field conditions or during real-life sports events are scarce. Caffeine may enhance competition performance, but is also likely to be a useful training aid, allowing the athlete to undertake better and more consistent training.
- There is evidence, particularly from recent studies, that beneficial effects from caffeine occur at very modest levels of intake (1–3 mg/kg BM or ~70–150 mg caffeine), when it is taken before and/or during exercise. Furthermore, there is little evidence of a dose–response relationship to caffeine—that is, performance benefits do *not* appear to increase with increases in the caffeine dose. This information is an advance on the traditional caffeine supplementation protocols, which provided intakes of 6–9 mg/kg BM (e.g. 400–600 mg) 1 hour prior to the exercise. Further research is needed to define the range of caffeine intake protocols that provide performance enhancements across various sports or exercise activities.
- The effects of caffeine supplementation differ between individuals. Some people are non-responders and others experience negative side effects such as tremors, increased heart rate, headaches and impaired sleep. Such side effects are more common at higher doses—for example, exceeding 6–9 mg/kg BM—and may cause a direct impairment of performance. They may also indirectly impair exercise outcomes—for example, disturbing the sleep patterns of athletes who compete in a multi-day sport and need to recover between days of competition.
- Coffee is not an ideal vehicle for caffeine supplementation by athletes, because of the variability of caffeine content and the possible presence of chemicals that impair exercise performance. Furthermore, there is a lack of investigations of the effects of available caffeine sources, such as cola drinks, energy drinks and caffeinated sports products, compared to those of pure caffeine. Therefore many athletes may find it difficult to apply the results of caffeine studies to their 'real world' scenarios.

Creatine

When the first edition of this book was written in 1994, creatine was the latest 'hot supplement', with testimonials from gold medal winners at the 1992 Barcelona Olympic Games. However, unlike many supplements that draw the attention of athletes, creatine enjoyed some scientific support, with the 1992 publication of a study that showed that muscle creatine stores could be increased by the intake of large doses of an oral source of creatine (Harris et al. 1992). Since then, creatine supplements have become a phenomenon in sports nutrition—an ergogenic aid that records huge annual sales and has been the topic of over 200 investigations, book chapters and reviews. It is not often that scientists and athletes are excited by the same product. The coincidental rise of the Internet has assisted the rapid spread of scientific and testimonial information.

Although some lay publications and manufacturers have labeled creatine as a 'legal steroid', this is an incorrect and unfair comparison. In fact, creatine is a muscle fuel, and the ability of creatine supplementation to increase muscle creatine stores makes it similar to CHO loading. Creatine (methylguanidine-acetic acid) is a compound derived from amino acids and is stored primarily in skeletal muscle at typical concentrations of 100–150 mmol/kg/dry weight (dw) of muscle. About 60–65% of this creatine is phosphorylated. Creatine phosphate (CrP) provides a rapid but brief source of phosphate for the resynthesis of adenosine triphosphate (ATP) during maximal exercise, and is therefore an important fuel source in maximal sprints of 5–10 seconds. Other functions of creatine phosphate metabolism are the buffering of hydrogen ions produced during anaerobic glycolysis and the transport of ATP, generated by aerobic metabolism, from the muscle cell mitochondria to the cytoplasm, where it can be utilized for muscle contraction. Creatine metabolism is covered in more detail in Chapter 1 and in reviews of creatine metabolism and supplementation (Spriet 1997; Greenhaff 2000, 2001; Hespel et al. 2001).

The daily turnover of creatine, eliminated as creatinine, is approximately 1– 2 g/d. This can be partially replaced from dietary creatine intake, found in animal muscle products such as meat and eggs, and typically consumed in amounts of ~1–2 g/d in an omnivorous diet. Additional creatine needs are endogenously synthesized from arginine, glycine and methionine, principally in the liver, and transported to the muscle for uptake. Creatine is transported into the muscle against a high concentration gradient, via saturable transport processes that are stimulated by insulin (Green et al. 1996a, 1996b). High dietary intakes temporarily suppress endogenous creatine production. Vegetarians who do not consume a dietary source of creatine are believed to have a reduced body creatine store, suggesting that they do not totally compensate for the lack of dietary intake (Green et al. 1997). The reason for the variability of muscle creatine concentrations between individuals is uncertain. There are some suggestions that females typically have higher muscle creatine concentrations (Forsberg et al. 1991) and it appears that creatine stores decline with aging. The effect of training on creatine concentrations also requires further study.

Protocols for creatine supplementation

The watershed study by Harris and colleagues showed that muscle creatine levels were increased as a result of supplementation with repeated doses of creatine, large enough to sustain plasma creatine levels above the threshold for maximal creatine transport into the muscle cell (Harris et al. 1992). The protocol provided four to six doses of 5 g creatine (monohydrate) for 5 days to increase total muscle creatine concentrations by 20%, and reach an apparent muscle threshold of ~150–160 mmol/kg dw. About 20% of the increased muscle creatine content was stored as CrP and saturation occurred after 2–3 days. Increases in muscle creatine stores were greatest in those who had the lowest pre-supplementation concentrations and when coupled with intensive daily exercise.

Although this discovery appears to be recent, in fact, studies showing that oral creatine doses are largely retained in the body were available 80 years ago (Chanutin 1926). However, it is only now that muscle biopsy procedures and imaging techniques are available to enable scientists to monitor muscle stores of creatine and investigate the success of creatine loading protocols. Over the past decade a number of studies have refined our knowledge of supplementation protocols. Rapid loading is achieved by consuming a daily creatine dose of 20–25 g, in split doses, for 5 days. Alternatively, a daily dose of 3 g/d will achieve a slow loading over 28 days (Hultman et al. 1996). Elevated muscle creatine stores are maintained by continued daily supplementation of 2–3 g (Hultman et al. 1996). Across studies there is evidence that the creatine loading response varies between individuals, with ~30% of individuals being 'non-responders' or failing to significantly increase muscle creatine stores (Spriet 1997; Greenhaff 2000). Co-ingestion of substantial amounts of CHO (75–100 g) with creatine doses has been shown to enhance creatine accumulation (Green et al. 1996a, 1996b) and to assist individuals to reach the muscle creatine threshold of 160 mmol/kg dw. Creatine appears to be trapped in the muscle; in the absence of continued supplementation, it takes ~4–5 weeks to return to resting creatine concentrations (Hultman et al. 1996). Many studies have reported an acute gain in BM of ~1 kg during rapid creatine loading. This is likely to be primarily a gain in body water, and is mirrored by a reduction in urine output during the loading days (Hultman et al. 1996).

Effects of creatine supplementation on performance

Many studies have investigated the effect of creatine supplementation on muscle function exercise and performance. Studies vary according to the characteristics of subjects (e.g. gender, age, and training status), the mode of exercise, and whether supplementation involved an acute loading intervention or a chronic effect on training adaptations. It is beyond the scope of this chapter to summarize the large and growing body of literature on creatine supplementation and performance effects—even those that are carried out in trained individuals with relevance to sports activities. We will provide this information via an updated online resource (http://www.ausport.gov.au/ais/nutrition/supplements). However, we offer the following summary of this literature, and of reviews (Juhn & Tarnopolsky 1998a, 1998b; Kraemer & Volek 1999; Branch 2003; Rawson & Volek 2003; Bemben & Lamont 2005):

- The major benefit of creatine supplementation appears to be an increase in the rate of creatine phosphate resynthesis during the recovery between bouts of high-intensity exercise, producing higher creatine phosphate levels at the start of the subsequent exercise bout. Creatine supplementation can enhance the performance of repeated 6–30-second bouts of maximal exercise, interspersed with short recovery intervals (20 seconds to 5 minutes), where it can attenuate the normal decrease in force or power production that occurs over the course of the session.
- Oral creatine supplementation cannot be considered ergogenic for single-bout or first-bout sprints because the likely benefit is too small to be consistently detected.
- The exercise situations that have been most consistently demonstrated to benefit from creatine supplementation are laboratory protocols of repeated high-intensity intervals, involving isolated muscular efforts or weight-supported activities such as cycling.
- In theory, acute creatine supplementation might be beneficial for a single competitive event in sports involving repeated high-intensity intervals with brief recovery periods.

This description includes team games and racquet sports. Similarly, chronic creatine supplementation may allow the athlete to train harder at exercise programs based on repeated high-intensity exercise, and make greater performance gains. These benefits may apply to the across-season performance of athletes in team and racquet sports, as well as the preparation of athletes who undertake interval training and resistance training (e.g. swimmers and sprinters).

- For many specific sports, the benefits of creatine are theoretical, since few studies have been undertaken with elite athletes or as 'field studies'. Performance enhancements may not always occur in complex games and sports; even if changes in strength or speed are achieved by creatine-assisted training, these may not translate into improvements in game outcomes (for instance, goals scored).
- Evidence that creatine supplementation is of benefit to endurance exercise is absent or inconsistent, although it may enhance muscle glycogen storage.
- Acute creatine loading is associated with an increase in BM of ~0.6–1.0 kg. Performance enhancements will occur in weight-bearing and weight-sensitive sports (such as lightweight rowing and rock climbing) only if gains in muscular output compensate for increases in BM.
- There is variability in the performance response to creatine supplementation within and between studies. This may reflect the difficulty of detecting small changes in performance, individual responses to treatment or a combination of both factors.
- Whether the long-term gains in muscle mass reported in studies of resistance training are caused by direct stimulation of increased myofibrillar protein synthesis by creatine, enhanced ability to undertake resistance training, or a combination of both factors remains to be determined.

Concerns with creatine use

Whether there are side effects from long-term use of creatine, particularly with the large doses associated with rapid loading, remains to be determined. To date, there are anecdotal reports of nausea, gastrointestinal upset, headaches and muscle cramping/strains linked to some creatine supplementation protocols. Some of these adverse effects are plausible, particularly in light of increased water retention within skeletal muscle (and perhaps brain) cells. At this time, however, studies have failed to find evidence of an increased prevalence or risk of these problems among creatine users (Greenwood et al. 2003, 2004; Kreider et al. 2003b). Some concern is directed to long-term creatine users, particularly those who self-medicate with doses far in excess of the recommended creatine usage protocols in this chapter. Although it is commonly suggested that creatine supplementation may cause renal impairments, these are limited to case reports in a few patients with pre-existing renal dysfunction. Longitudinal studies have reported that creatine intake had no detrimental effects on renal responses in various athletic populations (Poortmans et al. 1997; Mayhew et al. 2002). Nevertheless, until long-term and large population studies can be undertaken, bodies such as the American College of Sports Medicine have taken a cautious view on the benefits and side effects of creatine supplementation (American College of Sports Medicine 2000). However, a suggestion from a French food safety agency that creatine supplementation is carcinogenic has been discredited (see Hespel et al. 2001). Creatine supplementation should be limited to well-developed athletes. Young athletes are able to make substantial gains in performance through maturation in age and training, without the need to expose themselves to the expense or small potential for long-term consequences of creatine use.

16.23 Bicarbonate and citrate

Anaerobic glycolysis provides the primary fuel source for exercise of near-maximal intensity lasting longer than approximately 20–30 seconds. The total capacity of this system is limited by the progressive increase in the acidity of the intracellular environment, caused by the accumulation of lactate and hydrogen ions (see Chapter 1). When intracellular buffering capacity is exceeded, lactate and hydrogen ions diffuse into the extracellular space, perhaps aided by a positive pH gradient. Since the 1930s it has been recognized that dietary strategies that decrease blood pH (e.g. intake of acid salts) impair high-intensity exercise, while alkalotic therapies improve such performance (Dennig et al. 1931; Dill et al. 1932). In theory, an increase in extracellular buffering capacity should delay the onset of muscular fatigue during prolonged anaerobic metabolism by increasing the muscle's ability to dispose of excess hydrogen ions.

Protocols for supplementation with bicarbonate and citrate

The two most popular buffering agents are sodium bicarbonate and sodium citrate. Athletes have practiced 'soda loading' or 'bicarbonate loading' for over 70 years, with sodium bicarbonate being ingested in the form of the household product 'bicarb soda' or as pharmaceutical urinary alkalinizers such as Ural™. The general protocol for bicarbonate loading is to ingest 0.3 g of sodium bicarbonate/kg BM 1–2 hours prior to exercise; this equates to 4–5 teaspoons of bicarbonate powder. Bicarbonate loading is not considered to pose any major health risk, although some individuals suffer gastrointestinal distress such as cramping or diarrhea. Consuming sodium bicarbonate with plenty of water (e.g. a liter or more) may help to prevent hyperosmotic diarrhea. Sodium citrate is also usually ingested in doses of 0.3–0.5 g/kg BM. Bicarbonate or citrate loading is not considered a banned practice for human performance, although it is not permitted in dog or horse racing. It is difficult to detect the use of bicarbonate- or citrate-loading strategies by athletes, since urinary pH varies according to dietary practices such as vegetarianism and high CHO intake (Heigenhauser & Jones 1991).

Some athletes need to compete in heats, semis and finals to decide the outcome of their event. Swimmers, rowers and track athletes may compete several times over a series of days, and sometimes more than once on the same day. Whether buffering protocols can be repeated on each occasion and how such protocols are best undertaken are questions that require investigation. Issues for study include the determination of the lowest effective dose of bicarbonate or citrate, in order to minimize side effects such as gastrointestinal discomfort or disturbances to post-race recovery. After all, although an acute supplementation protocol may enhance the performance of the immediate race, side effects in the post-race period could jeopardize the outcomes of the following events. It is also important to investigate whether subsequent doses are still effective and without side effects at this level. It is possible that a lower dose may be effective in a repeated supplementation protocol, especially if the first dose has not been completely washed out. It is also possible that a subsequent dose may have a reduced or absent effect. In this case the athlete might need to decide if the priority is to enhance performance to make the final, or to trust that they will make the final without aid and save any supplementation protocols for the most important race.

In the case of bicarbonate, a 'chronic' loading protocol has been investigated as an alternative to the repetition of acute protocols. McNaughton and colleagues studied the effect of 5–6 days of bicarbonate supplementation with a total of 500 mg/kg/d, spread into four doses over the day (McNaughton et al. 1999a; McNaughton & Thompson 2001). This protocol was found to achieve an increase in plasma base excess, which was sustained over the days of bicarbonate intake. Further, it enhanced the performance of a prolonged sprint undertaken on the 1–2 days *after* the bicarbonate supplementation ceased compared to the pre-trial performance (McNaughton & Thompson 2001). The persistence of the ergogenic outcome may be a desirable feature for sports involving a series of competition events. Alternatively, it may allow the athlete to finish their intake of bicarbonate (and the risk of gastrointestinal side effects) on the day prior to their competition, while maintaining the benefit to performance. Further study of such buffering strategies is needed over a wider range of exercise protocols.

Effect of buffering protocols on performance

Bicarbonate or citrate loading strategies are 'purpose-built' for strategies that might otherwise be limited by disturbances to acid-base balance. It is beyond the scope of this chapter to review individually the fifty or more studies of the effects of bicarbonate or citrate loading on exercise capacity in humans (for reviews see Heigenhauser & Jones 1991; Linderman & Fahey 1991; McNaughton 2000). Instead, we will focus our interest to studies involving trained subjects or protocols with relevance to sport or athletic events (see Table 16.4). There is evidence that strategies to increase extracellular buffering can benefit events that are conducted at near-maximum intensity for the duration of 1–7 minutes (e.g. 400–1500 m running, 100–400 m swimming, kayaking, rowing and canoeing events) and, perhaps, sports that are dependent on repeated anaerobic bursts, such as team games. There is some evidence of benefits to the performance of prolonged high-intensity events conducted at intensities around the so-called anaerobic threshold.

In addition to looking at the results of individual studies, the results of a meta-analysis of the general literature on bicarbonate supplementation (Matson & Tran 1993) provide some interesting insights. This analysis included twenty-nine randomized double-blind crossover investigations of bicarbonate loading and physical performance, examining thirty-five effect sizes from a total pool of 285 subjects (mainly healthy male college students). There was some variation in the protocols of bicarbonate loading, with different doses and times of ingestion being employed. While cycling was the most frequently used mode of exercise, there were a variety of exercise protocols (single efforts of 30 seconds to 5–7 minutes of near-maximal intensity, or repeated intervals of 1 minute with short rest times between) and a variety of performance outcomes (changes in power over a given time period, total work performed in a specified time, or time to exhaustion at a specific exercise intensity).

Overall, this meta-analysis concluded that the ingestion of sodium bicarbonate has a moderate positive effect on exercise performance, with a weighted effect size of 0.44—that is, the mean performance of the bicarbonate trial was, on average, 0.44 standard deviations better than the placebo trial. Overall, there was only a weak relationship reported between the increased blood alkalinity (increase in pH and bicarbonate) attained in the bicarbonate trial and the performance outcome. However, ergogenic effects were related to the level of metabolic acidosis achieved during the exercise, suggesting the importance of attaining a threshold pH gradient across the cell membrane from the combination of the accumulation of intracellular H^+ and the extracellular alkalosis. Significant variability within studies suggests that bicarbonate ingestion has an individual effect on different subjects.

TABLE 16.4 STUDIES OF BICARBONATE OR CITRATE LOADING WITH RELEVANCE TO SPORTS PERFORMANCE; FOR UPDATES SEE http://www.ausport.gov.au/ais/nutrition/supplements

REFERENCE	SUBJECTS	DOSE	EXERCISE PROTOCOL	PERFORMANCE ENHANCEMENT	SUMMARY
SUPPLEMENTATION AS SUPPORT FOR TRAINING OUTCOMES					
Edge et al. 2006	16 moderately trained females (team sports and rowing) Parallel group design	400 mg/kg sodium bicarbonate for 8 weeks, spread at 90 and 30 minutes before training (3/wk interval training with 6–12 reps × 2 minutes high-intensity + 1 minute rest)	Team sport relevance Cycling • $VO_{2\,peak}$ • TTE @ 100% pre-training $VO_{2\,peak}$	Yes	Both placebo and bicarbonate groups increased $VO_{2\,peak}$, lactate threshold and TTE after training. The bicarbonate group had significantly greater improvements in lactate threshold (26 versus 15%) and TTE (164 versus 123%) than the placebo group.
CHRONIC SUPPLEMENTATION PROTOCOL BEFORE AN EXERCISE TEST					
Douroudos et al. 2006	24 untrained males Parallel group design	0, 300 or 500 mg/kg sodium bicarbonate in two divided doses per day for 5 days	Cycling • Wingate anaerobic cycling test	Yes, in dose-dependent manner	Performance increased with bicarbonate supplementation; larger increase in higher bicarbonate group (7.7 W/kg vs. 7.3 W/kg and 6.7 W/kg for 500, 300 and 0 mg/kg, respectively), in line with adjustments in resting blood bicarbonate concentration.
McNaughton & Thompson 2001	8 recreationally active males Unblinded crossover design	500 mg/kg sodium bicarbonate days in four divided doses per day for 6 days (chronic) or 500 mg/kg sodium bicarbonate 90 minutes pre-trial (acute)	Cycling • 90-second TT Tests conducted on day of intake, plus following day	Yes, for both acute and chronic ingestion	Similar improvement in performance with acute and chronic bicarbonate supplementation on the first day of testing. However, performance improvement was maintained only in the chronic trial on the day after ceasing last bicarbonate dose. Increase in blood bicarbonate and pH following 1 day of supplementation that was maintained throughout study in the chronic group.
McNaughton et al. 1999b	8 recreationally active males Unblinded single group design with order effect	500 mg/kg sodium bicarbonate in four divided doses per day for 5 days	Cycling • 60-second TT Tests conducted pre-trial, post-supplementation and 1 month later (control trial)	Yes	Greater PPO and total work at end of chronic bicarbonate supplementation period compared to pre-trial and control test 1 month after supplementation. Increase in blood bicarbonate and pH following 1 day of supplementation that was maintained throughout study.

ACUTE SUPPLEMENTATION BEFORE AN EXERCISE TEST					
Pruscino et al. 2008	6 elite male swimmers Crossover design	300 mg/kg sodium bicarbonate 120–30 minutes pre-trial 6 mg/kg caffeine 45 minutes pre-trial	Swimming • 2 × 200 m TT on 30-minute recovery	No, for a one-off 200 m time-trial Yes, for repeat 200 m time-trials	Bicarbonate enhanced performance, with and without caffeine on repeat performance. Effect was less evident for a single effort. Majority of athletes recorded fastest TT for single and repeat performance from the combination of bicarbonate and caffeine.
Lindh et al. 2008	9 elite male swimmers Crossover design	300 mg/kg sodium bicarbonate 90–60 minutes pre-trial	Swimming • 1 × 200 m TT	Yes	Swimming TT with bicarbonate trial was 1.6% faster than placebo trial in internationally competitive swimmers.
Artioli et al. 2007	9 national level judo athletes Crossover design 14 national level judo athletes Crossover design	300 mg/kg sodium bicarbonate 120 minutes pre-trial 300 mg/kg sodium bicarbonate 120 minutes pre-trial	Judo • Three judo-specific throwing fitness tests on 5 minutes recovery • Four Wingate anaerobic upper body tests on 3 minutes recovery	Yes Yes	Bicarbonate supplementation increased total throws completed, primarily in bouts two and three. Greater mean power with bicarbonate supplementation in bouts three and four and greater PPO in bout four.
Bishop & Claudius 2005	7 female team sports players Crossover design	2 × 200 mg/kg bicarbonate @ 90 minutes and 20 minutes pre-exercise	Team sport simulation • Intermittent cycling protocol of 2 × 36-minute 'halves' involving repeated 2-minute blocks (all-out 4-second sprint, 100-second active recovery at 35% $VO_{2\,peak}$, and 20 seconds of rest)	Yes	Bicarbonate supplementation failed to produce any effect on performance in first half, but caused trend towards improved total work in the second half ($p = 0.08$). In particular, subjects completed significantly more work in 7 of 18 4-second sprints in second half in the bicarbonate trial.

(continued)

TABLE 16.4 *(continued)*

REFERENCE	SUBJECTS	DOSE	EXERCISE PROTOCOL	PERFORMANCE ENHANCEMENT	SUMMARY
Montfoort et al. 2004	15 competitive male distance runners Crossover design	300 mg/kg sodium bicarbonate or 525 mg/kg sodium citrate 90–180 minutes pre-race	Running • Treadmill run to exhaustion at speed designed to last 1–2 minutes	Yes for bicarbonate Perhaps for citrate	Analysis estimated likelihood of treatments increasing endurance compared to placebo by at least 0.5% (considered to be the smallest worthwhile improvement). Bicarbonate produced 2.7% enhancement of endurance (96% chance of improvement); citrate enhanced endurance by 0.5% (50% chance). Overall, authors concluded that bicarbonate is most effective, and citrate is possibly not as effective. No difference in gastrointestinal symptoms.
Bishop et al. 2004	10 recreational team sports players (F) Parallel group design	0.3 g/kg sodium bicarbonate, 90 minutes before exercise	Cycling • 5 × 6-second maximal sprints, every 30 seconds	Yes	Compared to the control group there was a significant increase in total work for five sprints and peak power output in sprints 3–5.
Mero et al. 2004	8 male + 8 female national level swimmers Crossover design (30-day washout)	300 mg/kg bicarbonate or gelatin placebo, 2 hours pre-exercise (6 days @ 20 g/d creatine also taken prior to bicarbonate trial)	Swimming • 2 × 100 m swims with 10 m passive recovery	Yes (?)	Faster time for second swim with creatine/bicarbonate trial than with placebo: 1-second reduction in performance from first swim in placebo compared with 0.1 s drop-off in supplement trial ($p < 0.05$). Study unable to indicate individual effect of bicarbonate.
Price et al. 2003	8 active male runners Crossover design	300 mg/kg sodium bicarbonate 1 hour pre-exercise	Team sport simulation: • Intermittent cycling protocol of 30 minutes involving repeated 3-minute blocks (90 seconds at 40%, 60 seconds at 60% $VO_{2\,max}$ and 14 seconds at maximal sprint)	Yes	Significant main effect with greater PPO achieved in 14-second sprints across protocol in bicarbonate trial, whereas placebo trial showed gradual decline in PPO across time. Blood lactate levels elevated to 10–12 mmol/L by 10 minutes and remained elevated across rest of protocol. Such values are higher than is generally reported in team sports; thus movement patterns may not reflect the true workloads or physiological limitations of team sports.

Oopik et al. 2003	17 male collegiate distance runners Crossover design	500 mg/kg sodium citrate 2 hours pre-exercise	Running • 5000 m treadmill run	Yes	Performance significantly faster ($p < 0.05$) for citrate trial (1153 seconds) compared with placebo trial (1183 seconds). High risk of gastrointestinal distress. Blood lactate concentration higher after race with citrate trial. No change in RPE.
Stephens et al. 2002	6 well-trained male cyclists/triathletes and 1 cross-country skier Crossover design	300 mg/kg sodium bicarbonate 2 hours pre-exercise	Cycling • 30 minutes at 77% $VO_{2\,max}$ + TT (~30 minutes)	No	Increase in blood lactate but no difference in TT performance time, muscle glycogen utilization or lactate.
Shave et al. 2001	7 elite male + 2 elite female athletes Crossover design	500 mg/kg sodium citrate 1.5 hours pre-race	Running • 3000 m	Yes	Performance time significantly faster ($p < 0.05$) for citrate trial (610.9 seconds) compared with placebo trial (621.6 seconds). High risk of gastrointestinal distress.
Schabort et al. 2000	8 endurance-trained male cyclists and triathletes Crossover design	200 mg/kg, 400 mg/kg and 600 mg/kg sodium citrate 1 hour pre-exercise	Cycling • 40 km TT including 500 m, 1 km and 2 km sprints	No	Increasing citrate dose increased blood pH but no effect on sprint performances or overall 40 km TT performance (58:46, 60:24, 61:47 and 60:02 minutes for citrate (200, 400 and 600 mg/kg doses) and placebo.
McNaughton et al. 1999b	10 well-trained male cyclists Crossover design	300 mg/kg sodium bicarbonate 90 minutes pre-exercise	Cycling • 60-minute TT	Yes	14% more work completed with bicarbonate
Potteiger et al. 1996a	8 trained male cyclists Crossover design	500 mg/kg sodium citrate 90 minutes pre-exercise	Cycling • 30 km TT	Yes	Reduction in TT time (57:36 minutes versus 59:22). Sodium citrate raised pH values from 10 km onwards and improved power output in the initial 25 minutes.
Potteiger et al. 1996b	7 well-trained male runners Crossover design	300 mg/kg sodium bicarbonate and 500 mg/kg sodium citrate 2 hours pre-exercise	Running • 30 minutes at LT + TTE at 110% LT	No	Both citrate and bicarbonate supplementation increased blood pH during steady state run. No differences in run to exhaustion: 287 seconds, 172.8 seconds, 222.3 seconds for bicarbonate, citrate and placebo respectively.

(continued)

TABLE 16.4 ***(continued)***

REFERENCE	SUBJECTS	DOSE	EXERCISE PROTOCOL	PERFORMANCE ENHANCEMENT	SUMMARY
Tiryaki & Atterbom 1995	11 collegiate female runners + 4 trained non-athletes Crossover design	300 mg/kg sodium citrate or sodium bicarbonate 2.5 hours pre-exercise	Running • 600 m	No	No performance effect despite significant changes to acid–base status.
Bird et al. 1995	10 trained middle-distance runners Crossover design	300 mg/kg sodium bicarbonate (half at 120 and half at 90 minutes pre-exercise)	Running • 1500 m	Yes	Performance in bicarbonate trial improved compared with placebo trial (253.9 versus 256.8 seconds, $p < 0.05$).
Pierce et al. 1992	7 male collegiate swimmers Crossover design	200 mg/kg bicarbonate, sodium chloride placebo or control, 1 hour pre-exercise	Swimming • 100 yards freestyle • 2 × 200 yards swims 20-minute recovery between each race (simulation of competition program)	No No	No difference in swim times between trials.
McNaughton & Cedaro 1991	5 highly trained male rowers Crossover design	300 mg/kg sodium bicarbonate 95 minutes pre-exercise	Rowing • 6-minute maximum effort on ergometer	Yes	Increased work and distance rowed in bicarbonate trial (1861 m versus 1813 m). Increased lactate levels.
Goldfinch et al. 1988	6 trained male runners Crossover design	400 mg/kg sodium bicarbonate 60 minutes pre-exercise	Running • 400 m	Yes	Improved running time (56.94 seconds versus 58.63 for placebo and 58.46 for control). Elevated post-exercise values for pH and base excess.
Gao et al. 1988	10 male collegiate swimmers Crossover design	250 mg/kg sodium bicarbonate 1 hour pre-exercise	Swimming • 5 × 100 yard swim with 2 minutes rest (simulation of training program)	Yes	Faster times in fourth and fifth swim ($p < 0.05$). Supplementation also associated with higher post-race blood lactate concentrations.
Wilkes et al. 1983	6 varsity track male athletes Crossover design	300 mg/kg sodium bicarbonate 2.5 hours pre-exercise	Running • 800 m	Yes	Improved running time (2:02.9 minutes versus 2:05.1 for placebo and 2:05.8 for control). Elevated post-exercise values for pH, lactate and blood bicarbonate.

LT = lactate threshold, PO = power output, PPO = peak power output, RPE = rating of perceived exertion, TT = time trial, TTE = time to exhaustion, W/kg = watts per kilogram

Popular theories about bicarbonate and citrate loading include the likelihood that anaerobically trained athletes should show less response to protocols because their intrinsic buffering capacity is already better, and the risk that performance of *prolonged* high-intensity exercise will be impaired if bicarbonate/citrate supplementation leads to increased rates of glycogen utilization. However, studies that have examined bicarbonate or citrate loading using sports-specific protocols and well-trained subjects (see Table 16.4) fail to support these theories. Some, but not all, studies of well-trained athletes have found performance improvements following bicarbonate/lactate loading prior to brief (1–10 minutes) or prolonged (30–60 minutes) events involving high-intensity exercise (see Table 16.4).

Until further research can clarify the range of exercise activities that might benefit from bicarbonate or citrate enhancement, individual athletes are advised to experiment in training and minor competitions to judge their own case. It is important that experimentation is conducted in a competition-simulated environment, including the need to undertake multiple loading strategies for heats and finals of an event; the athlete needs to discover not only the potential for performance improvement but also the likelihood of unwanted side effects.

Finally, there is some preliminary evidence that bicarbonate loading may be used to enhance training outcomes. Edge and colleagues (2006) monitored moderately trained female team athletes over an 8-week program that included three interval training sessions per week: one group undertook an acute bicarbonate loading protocol prior to each of these sessions, while a matched group took a placebo. While the groups increased their maximal aerobic capacity equally, the bicarbonate loading group recorded a larger increase in lactate threshold and the ability to exercise at the pre-training level of $VO_{2\,peak}$ for a longer duration than the placebo group. Further work is warranted.

Supplements in Group B of the AIS Sports Supplement Program 16.24

According to the AIS Sports Supplement Program, some supplements enjoy preliminary data that are supportive of performance benefits or hypotheses that strongly suggest such benefits. However, this information is not sufficient to be sure of a positive outcome, or to define the situations and protocols that would achieve an optimal result. Because these supplements are of interest to athletes and coaches, they should be prioritized for additional research to either confirm their value to athletes or downgrade the interest.

Beta-alanine 16.25

Carnosine is a dipeptide, formed from the amino acids β-alanine and histidine found in large amounts in the brain and muscle, especially fast twitch muscle. The availability of β-alanine, the only amino acid that occurs naturally in a beta-form, is believed to be the limiting factor in carnosine production. Dietary sources of carnosine and β-alanine include meats, especially 'white' (fast twitch) meat such as the breast meat of poultry and birds and of sea animals that are exposed to hypoxia, such as whale. Vegetarians have lower resting muscle carnosine concentrations than meat eaters (Harris et al. 2007). Carnosine has an anti-oxidant role and accounts for about 10% of the muscle's ability to buffer the acidity (H^+ ions) produced by high-intensity exercise.

Recent studies have shown that supplementation with 5-6 g/d (~65 mg/kg) β-alanine can increase muscle carnosine content by ~60% after 4 weeks and ~80% after 10 weeks of supplementation (Harris et al. 2006). The present literature is unclear on how long supplementation needs to continue to maximize muscle carnosine concentrations, or how long muscle carnosine remains elevated if supplementation is stopped. However, it appears that the rise and fall of muscle carnosine may take several months to occur. To date, the major side effect that has been described is paresthesia—a prickling or 'pins and needles' sensation—occurring for ~60 minutes about 15–20 minutes following a dose of β-alanine. This is apparently related to the rate in the rise of plasma β-alanine concentrations and is frequently reported with doses greater than 10 mg/kg. There are anecdotal reports that symptoms disappear over a period of weeks of continued supplementation but are increased by exercise prior to a dose of the supplement. It may be beneficial to take β-alanine in split doses over the day and to consume it with CHO-rich foods. The benefits may include an enhanced muscle uptake as well as a reduction in side effects. Alternatively, a 'controlled-release' supplement (CarnoSyn™) has been reported to provide an equivalent 'area under the curve' increase in plasma β-alanine concentrations compared with a standard β-alanine, without any evidence of the associated side effects (Harris et al. 2008).

Increasing muscle carnosine levels may offer an alternative to bicarbonate/citrate loading for sustained or intermittent high-intensity exercise that is limited by the build-up of H^+ ion through anaerobic glycolysis (see section 16.23). It may also offer an additional strategy, since muscle carnosine is an intracellular buffer, while bicarbonate/citrate loading provides extracellular buffering. The present literature of β-alanine supplementation and exercise capacity or performance is limited (see Table 16.5), especially with relevance to well-trained individuals. However, there is some evidence of benefits to training adaptations and the performance of a single exercise protocol that warrants further investigation.

16.26 Colostrum

Colostrum is a protein-rich substance secreted in breast milk in the first few days after a mother has given birth. It is high in immunoglobulins and insulin-like growth factors (IGFs). Unlike the adult gut, the gut of a baby has 'leaky' junctions that allow it to absorb whole proteins, including immunoglobulins, thus developing the immuno-competence needed to survive outside the uterus.

A number of companies have developed supplements rich in bovine colostrum (colostrum derived from cows) for use by humans. In 1997, attention was focused on these products after a study reported that sprinters and jumpers who consumed a colostrum supplement (Bioenervie™) for 8 days while undertaking resistance and speed training experienced an increase in plasma IGF-1 levels (Mero et al. 1997). Although supplementation failed to improve vertical jump performance in these athletes, the study raised several intriguing issues. First, it appeared to show that humans could absorb intact proteins from a supplement and, second, it appeared to show that colostrum could provide a dietary source of IGF, an anabolic hormone, the intentional intake of which is banned by WADA. Subsequent discussion of this paper suggested that the increase in IGF concentrations was spurious, caused by inaccurate techniques for measuring these growth factors. However, a follow-up study by this group (Mero et al. 2002) reported an increase in plasma IGF-1 following supplementation with another colostrum product (Dynamic™). In this follow-up study, gel electrophoresis techniques showed that there was little direct absorption of

TABLE 16.5 STUDIES OF β-ALANINE SUPPLEMENTATION ON EXERCISE CAPACITY OR PERFORMANCE; FOR UPDATES SEE http://www.ausport.gov.au/ais/nutrition/supplements

STUDY	SUBJECTS	β-ALANINE DOSE	EXERCISE PROTOCOL	ENHANCED PERFORMANCE	COMMENTS
Van Thienen et al. 2009	Moderate–well-trained male cyclists Parallel group design	2–4 g/d for 8 weeks	Testing at baseline and 8 weeks: • 10-minute TT • 30-second sprint after 110 minutes submaximal cycling on ergometer	 No Yes	Mean power output during the time trial (~300 W) was similar between placebo and β-alanine group at baseline and 8 weeks testing. However, compared with placebo, during the final sprint after the time trial, the β-alanine group increased peak power output by 11.4% (7.8–14.9%, $p = 0.0001$), whereas mean power output increased by 5.0% (2.0– 8.1%, $p = 0.005$). Blood lactate and pH values were similar between groups at any time.
Smith et al. 2009a	46 recreationally active men Parallel group design	6 g/d for 3 weeks + 3 g/d for 3 weeks High-intensity interval training 3/wk	Testing at baseline, 3 and 6 weeks: • $VO_{2\,peak}$ • TTE at 110% $VO_{2\,peak}$ • total work done in TTE	 Perhaps Perhaps Perhaps	Both groups improved after 3 weeks in all tests (e.g. 50% increase in Total Work Done during TTE), but only the β-alanine group made further significant improvements over the subsequent 3-week period in $VO_{2\,peak}$ and TTE at at110% $VO_{2\,peak}$. Trend to greater improvement in total work done in second period (32% versus 18%). Trend to greater training volume in β-alanine group plus significant increase in LBM with training only in β-alanine group. A companion paper (Smith et al. 2009b) failed to find differences between groups in the improvements in the fatigue threshold determined by muscle electromyography (EMG) tests.
Hoffman et al. 2008a	8 resistance-trained men Crossover design with 4-week washout	4.8 g/d sustained release β-alanine or placebo for 30 days (dose gradually built up from 2.4 g/d over first 8 days) Resistance training undertaken 4/wk	Testing at baseline and 4 weeks of each treatment: • 1 RM squat • training workout of 6 × 12 × 70% 1 RM	 No Yes	Authors acknowledged that 4-week washout may not be sufficient for return to baseline of muscle carnosine content. 4 weeks of β-alanine treatment resulted in greater increase in volume of training and number of repetitions than placebo treatment. However, no difference in gains in strength or BM at end of treatment. No difference in acute hormonal response to a resistance-training workout.

(continued)

TABLE 16.5 *(continued)*

STUDY	SUBJECTS	β-ALANINE DOSE	EXERCISE PROTOCOL	ENHANCED PERFORMANCE	COMMENTS
Hoffman et al. 2008b	Collegiate football players Parallel group design	4.5 g/d for 30 days (3-week + 9-day training camp)	Testing at day 1 of training camp • 60-second Wingate test • 3 line drills (200-yard runs with 2 minutes rest)	 No No	Authors claim trend to lower fatigue rate in Wingate test in β-alanine group on day 1 of camp than placebo group. Higher training volume and reduced self-reported ratings of soreness during camp.
Kendrick et al. 2008	26 untrained males Parallel group design	6.4 g/d β-alanine or placebo for 10 weeks Resistance training program 4/wk	Testing at baseline and 10 weeks: • whole body strength (1 RM box squat + bench press + deadlift) • isokinetic knee force • upper arm curl test	 No No No	No change in muscle carnosine with training alone, but β-alanine group showed 60% increase. Both groups gained LBM and increased whole body strength, knee isokinetic force and muscle endurance of arm curl, but no difference between groups. Structure of resistance program may not have stressed muscle acidity limits.
Stout et al. 2007	22 young females Training status unreported Parallel group design	6.4 g/d (~86 mg/kg/d) sustained release β-alanine or placebo for 4 weeks 'Normal exercise program' unreported	Incremental cycling test at baseline and 4 weeks: • PWC at fatigue threshold • ventilatory threshold • $VO_{2\,max}$ • time to exhaustion	 Yes Yes No Yes	The β-alanine group showed a ~13% increase in PWC at fatigue threshold and ventilatory thresholds at post-supplementation testing compared with pre-supplementation testing, and a 2.5% increase in time to exhaustion in the graded incremental cycling test. The placebo group showed no differences between pre- and post-supplementation test results.
Derave et al. 2007	15 sprint-trained track and field athletes (400 m time < 53 seconds) Parallel group design	4.8 g/d sustained release β-alanine or placebo for 4–5 weeks (dose gradually built up from 2.4 g/d over first 8 days) Track training undertaken ~ 6/wk	Testing at baseline and 4 weeks: • average peak torque during 5 × 30 knee extensions on dynamometer • endurance at isometric contraction at 45% mean voluntary contraction • 400 m run (indoor track)	 Yes No No	Non-invasive measurement of muscle carnosine (proton magnetic resonance spectroscopy) found average increase of ~40% in calf muscles resulting from supplementation. Response was not related to initial carnosine concentration and did not appear to reach maximal threshold as a result of supplementation. β-alanine supplementation associated with attenuation of fatigue with repeated dynamic contractions. Failure to see clear enhancement of 400 m performance perhaps related to under-powering of study design, failure of sufficient increase in muscle carnosine/muscle buffering or failure of H^+ ion accumulation to limit 400 m performance. No relationship between change in 400 m performance, change in muscle carnosine or post-race lactate concentration.

Zoeller et al. 2007	55 males Training status unreported Parallel group design	6.4 g/d sustained-release β-alanine for 6 days then 3.2 g/d for 22 days OR 21 g creatine + CHO for 6 days then 10 g/d for 22 days OR creatine + β-alanine combined 'Normal exercise program' unreported	Testing at baseline and 4 weeks: • graded incremental cycling test to exhaustion	 No	No between group differences for time to exhaustion, $VO_{2\,max}$ in test.
Hill et al. 2007	25 physically active males Parallel group design	6.4 g/d sustained release β-alanine or placebo for 4 or 10 weeks (dose gradually built up over first 4 weeks) No committed training undertaken before or during treatment	Testing at baseline, 4 weeks, 10 weeks • cycling to exhaustion at 110% maximal power output	 Yes	Increase in total work done in cycling test at 4 weeks and 10 weeks in β-alanine group but no difference in placebo group.
Hoffman et al. 2006	33 resistance-trained male collegiate football players Parallel group design	10 weeks of 10.5 g/d creatine + 3.2 g β-alanine OR 10.5 g/d creatine alone Resistance training program 4/wk	Testing at baseline and 10 weeks: • 1 RM squat • 1 RM bench press • 2 × 30-second cycling Wingate • 20 × vertical jump	Difference between β-alanine and β-alanine + Cr No No No No	No differences in cycling and jump over the training period in any group. Improvement in strength with creatine but no further improvement with creatine + β-alanine. Addition of β-alanine appeared to enhance training volume, and appeared to enhance DXA-determined loss of body fat and gain of lean BM.
Stout et al. 2006	51 males Training status unreported Parallel group design	6.4 g/d β-alanine for 6 days then 3.2 g/d for 22 days OR 21 g creatine + CHO for 6 days then 10 g/d for 22 days OR creatine + β-alanine combined 'Normal exercise program' unreported	Incremental cycling test at baseline and 4 weeks: • PWC at fatigue threshold	 Yes for β-alanine	β-alanine and β-alanine + creatine group showed ~14% increase in PWC. Creatine alone or in combination did not provide a benefit.

DXA = dual energy X-ray absorptiometry, LBM = lean body mass, PWC = physical work capacity, RM = repetition maximum TT = time trial, TTE = time to exhaustion

IGF-1 from the oral supplement. This suggests that the intake of colostrum stimulated endogenous production of growth factors. Nevertheless, other studies have failed to demonstrate any change in IGF-1 levels in response to colostrum supplementation (Buckley et al. 2002; Kuipers et al. 2002). There are also inconsistencies in effect of colostrum supplementation on immune parameters, with various studies showing either an increase (Mero et al. 2002) or no change (Mero et al. 1997) in salivary immunoglobulin A (IgA). One study reported a reduction in the self-reported symptoms of upper respiratory tract infections following colostrum supplementation in a large group of subjects (Brinkworth & Buckley 2003); this finding warrants further investigation.

A number of studies have investigated the chronic effects of supplementation with colostrum products, particularly an Australian product (Intact™), on the outcome of training programs undertaken by both trained and previously untrained subjects. The results of these studies are summarized in Table 16.6. Buckley and colleagues studied the effects of 8 weeks of running training (3 × 45 minutes/wk) in combination with 60 g/d of colostrum powder or a whey placebo in two groups of previously untrained men (Buckley et al. 2002). The test set, consisting of two incremental treadmill runs to exhaustion, with a 20-minute recovery interval, was undertaken at 0, 4 and 8 weeks. The study found that after 8 weeks the treatment group completed more work and ran further in the second of two treadmill runs than subjects in the placebo group. However, no differences were seen at 4 weeks, and no measurements were taken to explain the performance improvements seen in the second run at 8 weeks. Another study involving trained cyclists (Coombes et al. 2002) also used a protocol involving two incremental tests to exhaustion separated by 20 minutes. In contrast to the results of the previous study, neither the colostrum nor the placebo groups improved their cycling 'max test' performance in either of the two tests after 4 or 8 weeks of supplementation with colostrum. However, another measure of performance was undertaken by these cyclists on a separate day, in the form of a submaximal ride followed by a time trial. In this protocol, cyclists who had received colostrum recorded a greater improvement in the performance of the time trial at week 8 compared with those who had received a placebo. Again, there were no mechanisms to explain this enhancement of performance.

In several other studies, there have been reports of an enhancement of the performance of the treatment group compared with the group taking a placebo product. However, there is inconsistency in the literature, with one study reporting an improvement in vertical jump in previously untrained subjects who undertook plyometric and resistance training (Buckley et al. 2003) and others finding no enhancement in vertical jump in highly trained team sport players (Hofman et al. 2002) or track and field athletes (Mero et al. 1997). Similarly, colostrum supplementation has been reported to enhance the improvement in sprint performance in one study of previously untrained men (Buckley et al. 2003), while failing to alter this outcome in trained team sport athletes (Hofman et al. 2002). Reports of the changes in body composition have also showed inconsistencies. While one study has reported an increase in lean body mass (LBM) following a period of colostrum supplementation (Antonio et al. 2001), other studies have found no changes in BM or body composition (Hofman et al. 2002). The finding that a colostrum-supplemented group showed an increase in subcutaneous fat and skin thickness in their arms following resistance training is curious (Brinkworth et al. 2004). The only consistent findings from the present studies of colostrum supplementation are that there are no apparent benefits to the outcomes of resistance training (Antonio et al. 2001; Buckley et al. 2003; Brinkworth

TABLE 16.6 STUDIES OF COLOSTRUM SUPPLEMENTATION ON EXERCISE CAPACITY/PERFORMANCE OR ILLNESS; FOR UPDATES SEE http://www.ausport.gov.au/ais/nutrition/supplements

REFERENCE	SUBJECTS	COLOSTRUM DOSE AND TRAINING	EXERCISE PROTOCOL	PERFORMANCE ENHANCEMENT	COMMENTS
COLOSTRUM AND EXERCISE/SPORTS PERFORMANCE					
Shing et al. 2006	29 highly trained male cyclists Parallel group design	8 weeks @ 10 g/d colostrum or placebo (whey protein) 5 weeks normal training (cycling) + 5 days HIT + return to normal training	Cycling • $VO_{2\,max}$ test • Time to fatigue @ 110% ventilatory threshold • 40 km TT • baseline, after normal training, after HIT and after return to normal training	No—after normal training Yes—after HIT	The effect of colostrum after normal training was unclear however after 5 days' HIT there was a likely benefit (~2% enhancement) to TT performance compared to placebo. This difference disappeared when normal training recommenced.
Brinkworth et al. 2004	34 active male subjects Parallel group design	8 weeks @ 60 g/d colostrum or placebo (whey protein) 4/wk one-armed resistance training	Tests @ baseline and 8 weeks: • 1 RM biceps curl	No	Increase in biceps curl 1 RM in trained arm, but no difference between placebo and colostrum group. Increase in circumference and MRI-determined cross-sectional area of trained arm of colostrum group compared with placebo group ($p < 0.05$), principally due to increase in subcutaneous fat and skin.
Buckley et al. 2003	51 active males (colostrum = 26; placebo = 25) Parallel group design	8 wk @ 60 g/d Resistance and plyometric training, 6/wk	Tests at baseline, 4 weeks and 8 weeks • 3 × vertical jump • 3 × 10-second cycle sprints • 1 RM of a number of resistance movements	 Yes—only @ 8 weeks Yes—only @ 8 weeks No	At week 4, no differences in peak cycling power, anaerobic work capacity or peak vertical jump power between groups. At week 8, peak vertical jump power and peak cycle power higher in colostrum group, but no differences in anaerobic work capacity. No difference in strength over eight different movements. No changes in IGF-1 in either group.

(continued)

TABLE 16.6 *(continued)*

COLOSTRUM AND EXERCISE/SPORTS PERFORMANCE					
REFERENCE	**SUBJECTS**	**COLOSTRUM DOSE AND TRAINING**	**EXERCISE PROTOCOL**	**PERFORMANCE ENHANCEMENT**	**COMMENTS**
Buckley et al. 2002	30 active males (colostrum = 17; placebo = 13) Parallel group design	8 weeks @ 60 g/d colostrum or placebo (whey protein) 45 minutes running @ 3/wk	Tests at baseline, 4 and 8 weeks • 2 × ~30 min incremental running tests to exhaustion separated by 20 minutes	4 week—no for either run 8 week—no for first run, yes for second run	Training improved peak running speed in both runs in both groups at week 8. No differences between groups in either run at week 4 although trend to lower peak speed in second run with colostrum group. At week 8, no difference in peak speed in first run, but greater speed in second run in colostrum group ($p < 0.05$), suggesting better recovery between runs.
Brinkworth et al. 2002	13 elite female rowers (colostrum = 6; placebo = 7) Parallel group design	9 weeks @ 60 g/d of colostrum or placebo (whey protein) 18 hr/wk rowing + 3/wk resistance training	Tests @ baseline and 9 weeks • 2 × incremental rowing tests with 15-minute recovery interval (each = 3 × 4 min submaximal workloads + 4 min maximal effort)	No	Rowing performance increased by week 9 in both groups. No difference between groups at week 9 for either maximal rowing performance. Higher value for index of blood buffering capacity at week 9 in colostrum group.
Coombes et al. 2002	28 trained male cyclists (high-dose colostrum = 10; low-dose colostrum = 9; placebo = 9) Parallel group design	8 week @ 60 g/d colostrum or 20 g/d colostrum + 40g/d whey or placebo (40 g/d whey protein) 1.5 hr/d cycling	Tests @ baseline and 8 week on separate days • 2 × $VO_{2\,max}$ tests separated by 20 minutes • 2 hours @ 65% $VO_{2\,max}$ + ~12-minute TT	No Yes	No difference between groups or between weeks for performance of either $VO_{2\,max}$ test. Greater improvement at week 8 in TT following 2-hour submaximal ride in both colostrum groups (4%; 19%; 16% $p < 0.05$ for placebo, low dose and high dose).
Hofman et al. 2002	17 female and 18 male highly trained hockey players Parallel group design	8 weeks @ 60 g/d of colostrum or placebo (whey protein) 3/wk training + game 1/wk	Tests at baseline and 8 weeks • 5 × 10 m sprint • vertical jump • shuttle run • 'suicide' agility test	Yes No No No	No improvements in shuttle run, jump or agility run over 8 weeks in either group. Significant improvement in sprint performance for both groups with larger improvement in colostrum group (0.64 seconds versus 0.33 seconds, $p < 0.05$). Similar increases in LBM in both groups.

Antonio et al. 2001	Active male + females Parallel group design	8 week @ 20 g/d of colostrum or placebo (whey protein) 3/wk aerobic and resistance training	Tests @ baseline and 8 weeks • treadmill run to exhaustion • bench press: 1 RM • submaximal repetitions to exhaustion	 No No No	Colostrum group experienced significant increase in LBM (1.5 kg), while placebo group showed increase in BM (2 kg) as measured by DXA.
Mero et al. 1997	9 male sprinters and jumpers Crossover design with 13-day wash-out	8 d @ 25 mL/d colostrum or 125 mL/d or placebo (milk whey) 6 sessions speed and resistance training	Tests @ day 6 of each program • counter-movement jump	 No	Serum IGF-1 increased over time with colostrum supplementation (although still within physiological ranges) compared with placebo. No change in serum or saliva immunoglobulins between treatments.

COLOSTRUM AND ILLNESS

REFERENCE	SUBJECTS	COLOSTRUM DOSE AND TRAINING	TEST PROTOCOL	CHANGES IN ILLNESS	COMMENTS
Shing et al. 2007	29 highly trained male cyclists Parallel group design	8 weeks @ 10 g/d colostrum or placebo (whey protein) 5 weeks normal training (cycling) + 5 days HIT + return to normal training	Tests @ baseline, after 5 weeks normal training, after HIT and after return to normal training • illness log • salivary IgA • serum immunoglobulin • serum cytokines	No changes in URTI symptoms	No significant changes were seen in symptoms of URTI. Although no changes in actual illness frequency or severity were seen changes in immune markers were seen.
Crooks et al. 2006	35 recreational distance runners (aged 35–58 years) (15 female, 20 male) Parallel group design	12 weeks @ 26 g commercially available colostrum powder or skim milk placebo	Tests @ baseline, 4 8,12 and 14 weeks • salivary IgA • training log • wellness log	No—for upper respiratory symptoms	Salivary IgAs increased significantly in the colostrum group but this had no effect on upper respiratory symptoms.
Brinkworth et al. 2003	174 physically active males (aged 18–35 years) (colostrum = 93; whey protein placebo = 81) Parallel group design	8 weeks @ 60 g/d^{-1} commercial colostrum powder or whey protein placebo	Illness logs kept daily	Yes—for URTI symptoms during supplementation period. No—for reduction in duration of URTI	The number of subjects reporting symptoms of URTI was less in the colostrum group compared to placebo group for the period of supplementation. Duration of symptoms did not differ between groups.

BM = body mass, DXA = dual energy X-ray absorptiometry, HIT = high-intensity training, LBM = lean body mass, RM = repetition maximum, TT = time trial, URTI = upper respiratory tract infection

et al. 2004), and that when benefits are detected, they are apparent only after more than 4 weeks of treatment (Buckley et al. 2002, 2003).

The results of the current literature have been aggressively marketed by the manufacturers of colostrum supplements. Claims include enhanced recovery, superior muscle buffering capacity and increased growth of muscle contractile proteins. Furthermore, the benefits have been transferred from athletes to other groups, including manual workers and sufferers of chronic fatigue. Although the observations of enhanced training or performance outcomes are of real interest to athletes and coaches, there are several explanations for the reluctance of most sports scientists to consider colostrum as a proven ergogenic aid. The inconsistency of the literature is problematic, even when the difficulties of detecting small changes in performance are taken into account. The lack of a plausible hypothesis to explain how colostrum might enhance the response to exercise is also an important absence. Not only is there a lack of support for the current observations, but, without a possible mechanism to explore or exploit, there are difficulties in identifying the type of athletes or situations of exercise that might benefit from colostrum supplementation. Whether all colostrum supplements are of equal quality or efficacy is also a concern.

Finally, colostrum is an expensive supplement. The typical dose provided to subjects in the current studies is 60 g per day, which would cost about A$70 per week at retail rates. In light of this expense, and the suggestion that it may take up to 8 weeks to provide a detectable outcome, greater levels of support for colostrum are needed before it can pass a cost–benefit analysis.

16.27 Ribose

Ribose is a pentose (5-carbon) sugar that provides part of the structure of a variety of important chemicals in the body (including DNA and RNA) and the adenine nucleotides adenosine triphosphate (ATP), adenosine monophosphate (AMP) and adenosine diphosphate (ADP). Ribose is found naturally in the diet but purified forms have also been released onto the market, finding their way into sports supplements. Oral ribose is quickly absorbed and tolerated even at intakes of 100 g, but, at A$700 per kg, ribose powders represent an expensive form of CHO.

In the body, the pentose phosphate pathway is a rate-limiting pathway for the interconversion of glucose and ribose-5-phosphate. The ribose-5-phosphate can be converted to phosphoribosyl pyrophosphate (PRPP), which is then involved in the synthesis or salvaging of the adenine nucleotide pool. It has been suggested that suboptimal amounts of PRPP may limit these processes, and ribose infusion has been shown to enhance ATP recovery and exercise function in animal models of myocardial ischemia (see Op 't Eijnde et al. 2001). High-intensity exercise has been shown to cause a reduction in the muscle ATP content and the total adenine nucleotide pool, possibly because the rate of nucleotide salvaging and synthesis falls behind the massive rates of nucleotide degradation.

It has been suggested that oral intake of ribose might increase the rate of nucleotide salvaging/synthesis and achieve quicker recovery of exercise-mediated reductions in the muscle total adenine nucleotide pool. Sports supplements containing ribose typically provide doses of 3–5 g of this sugar, often in combination with creatine. Marketing claims for such products include 'dramatic reductions in recovery from 72 hours to 12 hours' and 'the most sophisticated energy support systems'. Several early studies that appeared in abstract form from conference presentations reported favorable results following ribose supplementation in heavily training athletes. However, the brief form of these reports does not provide sufficient information to judge the quality of the study and the interpretation of results.

To date, only six studies have been published in full in peer-reviewed journals (see Table 16.7). These studies have investigated daily doses of 2–40 g ribose in conjunction with programs of intermittent high-intensity exercise such as weight training or interval training. Two studies have tracked the muscle content of adenine nucleotides in response to fatiguing protocols of intermittent exercise and ribose supplementation (Op 't Eijnde et al. 2001; Hellsten et al. 2004). In one study, muscle ATP content and power/force characteristics were compared after two intermittent training sessions 24 hours apart on two occasions; the first occasion was a baseline measure on active subjects, whereas the second test set followed a 7-day training program involving two bouts of intermittent exercise each day while taking ribose (four doses of 4 g/d) or placebo. The first exercise bout in each testing occasion caused a decrease in muscle total adenine nucleotide, with muscle ATP content being reduced by 20% at the time of the second bout. However, ribose supplementation did not alter the loss or recovery of ATP resulting from this exercise protocol, nor did it change muscle force or power characteristics during maximal testing (Op 't Eijnde et al. 2001). The authors suggested that plasma ribose concentrations achieved by the supplementation were too low to achieve a significant change in nucleotide synthesis/salvage. However, the doses used in the study were already higher than that recommended by most supplement manufacturers.

In the other study, daily ribose supplementation of 600 mg/kg BM (~42 g for a 70 kg subject) was provided after a 7-day training program involving twice-daily bouts of sprint training (Hellsten et al. 2004). Muscle ATP content was reduced by ~25% immediately after the last training bout, and remained low at 24 hours, in both the supplementation and placebo trials. By 72 hours, however, ribose supplementation elevated muscle ATP above that seen in the placebo trial and restored it to pre-training levels. This was not accompanied by superior performance of the intermittent sprint protocol. The authors concluded that even though the availability of ribose in the muscle may be a limiting factor for the rate of resynthesis of ATP, the reduction in muscle ATP observed after intense training is not limiting for the performance of intermittent high-intensity exercise.

Overall, the published evidence for benefits from ribose supplementation is not promising. Only one of the published studies has reported an enhancement of performance following ribose use; recreational bodybuilders who consumed 10 g/d over a four-week period of resistance training achieved larger gains in strength and muscular endurance than a group receiving a placebo (Van Gammeren et al. 2002). Five other studies failed to detect any performance benefits from the use of ribose. Several of the authors have noted that their ribose treatments were well in excess of the doses recommended by manufacturer and, given the expense of this supplement, there are questions about its cost-effectiveness (Berardi & Ziegenfuss 2003).

HMB 16.28

β-hydroxy-β-methylbutyrate (HMB), a metabolite of the amino acid leucine, is claimed to increase the gains in strength and LBM associated with resistance training and enhance recovery from exercise (see Slater & Jenkins 2000). HMB is claimed to act as an anti-catabolic agent, minimizing protein breakdown and the cellular damage that occurs with high-intensity exercise. The hypothesis underpinning these claims is that the anti-catabolic effects that are sometimes associated with leucine feeding during times of stress are mediated by HMB. Interest in HMB supplementation stemmed from animal studies, with some but not all investigations finding that HMB supplementation increased gains in carcass weight or feed efficiency, defined as weight gain per unit feed, during periods of growth (for review, see Slater & Jenkins 2000). HMB supplements were first introduced to the sports

TABLE 16.7 PLACEBO-CONTROLLED STUDIES OF RIBOSE SUPPLEMENTATION AND EXERCISE PERFORMANCE; FOR UPDATES SEE http://www.ausport.gov.au/ais/nutrition/supplements

STUDY	SUBJECTS	RIBOSE DOSE AND TRAINING	EXERCISE PROTOCOL	PERFORMANCE ENHANCEMENT	COMMENTS
Hellsten et al. 2004	8 active males Crossover design 5-day washout	3 days @ 3 × 200 mg/kg ribose following 7 days of 2/d repetition of sprint training (15 × 10-second all-out sprints)	Cycling sprints • 15 × 10-second all-out sprints, separated by a 50-second rest period, undertaken 72 hours after last training session and following supplementation	No	7-day training program caused reduction in muscle ATP by ~25% immediately after last bout. ATP remained lower at 5- and 24-hour supplementation. After 72 hours, muscle ATP had returned to pre-training in ribose trial but was still lower in placebo trial. However, mean and peak power outputs during the test performed at 72 hours were similar in both trials.
Kreider et al. 2003a	19 resistance-trained males Parallel group design	10 g/d D-ribose (2 × 5 g daily) for 5 days	Cycling sprints • two 30-second Wingate anaerobic sprint tests separated by 3 minutes of rest recovery	No	Test protocol achieved a decrease in power output across 30 s of sprinting, and a lower work output in sprint 2 compared with sprint 1. No difference between pre- and post-supplementation values for peak power, average power, fatigue index or time to peak power for either group. Ribose group showed a higher total work for second sprint during post-supplementation trial than placebo group, due to deterioration in placebo group. No difference in blood lactate and ammonia profiles between groups.
Berardi & Ziegenfuss 2003	8 recreationally active males Crossover design	32 g powdered ribose spread over 3 days (4 × 8 g doses)	Cycling sprints • 6 × 10-second cycling sprints with 60-second recovery Test protocol undertaken day 1 × 2 (a.m. and p.m.) and day 3 × 1 (p.m.)	No	Ribose supplementation caused a marginal and inconsistent increase in power characteristics of the sprint protocol on day 3 compared with placebo trial. It was concluded from this study that ribose supplementation does not have a consistent or substantial effect on anaerobic cycle sprinting.
Falk et al. 2003	28 resistance-trained males Parallel group design	2 g/d for 8 weeks (as part of an effervescent supplement also containing CHO, creatine and glutamine) Resistance training	Resistance training • 1 RM bench press • repetitions 80% RM bench press to fatigue	No No	Both groups increased LBM, muscle strength and strength endurance over 8 weeks of training, but no differences between groups. Did not utilize a protocol likely to disturb adenine levels, thus may not have allowed the proposed mechanism of ribose supplementation to take effect.

Van Gammeren et al. 2002	19 male recreational bodybuilders Crossover design	10 g/d for 4 weeks (2/d, 30–60 minutes pre- and post-training) Resistance training	Resistance training • 1 RM bench press (muscular strength test) • 10 sets @ bench press at 100% BM to exhaustion with 1 minute recovery (muscular endurance test)	 Yes Yes	Both groups increased muscle strength and endurance over 4 weeks of training. However, only in the case of the ribose group did these training effects reach statistical significance, e.g. 20% versus 12% increase in 1 RM for bench press for ribose and placebo groups, respectively. Ribose-supplemented group experienced a significant increase in muscular strength and endurance. This improvement may be related to the role that ribose might play in the phosphagen system. However, ribose-supplemented group seemed to be less trained than placebo group.
Op 't Eijnde et al. 2001	19 recreationally active males involved in sprint and resistance activities Parallel group design	16 g/d for 6 day (4 × 4 g/d) 2/d training: bout of 15 × 12 knee extensions with 15 seconds' recovery	Isolated leg extensions • Two exercise bouts separated by 60 minutes Each bout = 15 × 12 maximal intermittent knee extensions with the right leg with 15 seconds' rest	No	Oral ribose supplementation at 16 g/day did not enhance the restoration of the fall in ATP concentrations following each exercise bout. The 6-day exercise protocol achieved training effect; mean power output in post-trial testing was 10% higher than pre-trial testing. However, no differences between ribose and placebo group. Authors suggested that the ribose dose was too low to increase plasma levels enough to increase muscle uptake, although dose was higher than recommended by most manufacturers.

RM = repetition maximum

market in the mid-1990s and by 1998 were achieving annual sales of US$30–50 million in the US alone (Slater & Jenkins 2000).

A number of scientific investigations of HMB supplementation and resistance training have been undertaken with a focus on changes in body composition and strength. The results of investigations that have been published in full in peer-reviewed journals are summarized in Table 16.8. This table shows there is mixed support for the hypothesis that HMB can enhance the response to resistance training as a result of reducing exercise-induced protein breakdown or damage. While some studies have reported a benefit of HMB supplementation (Nissen et al. 1996; Panton et al. 2000; Jowko et al. 2001; Thomson 2004), others have failed to detect any enhancement of the training response (Kreider et al. 1999; Slater et al. 2001; O'Connor & Crowe 2003; Ransone et al. 2003; Hoffman et al. 2004). Other studies that have simply monitored indices of muscle damage following eccentric exercise have found that HMB supplementation either reduced (Knitter et al. 2000) or failed to change the normal responses (Paddon-Jones et al. 2001). A meta-analysis of the studies published up until 2001 reported that HMB supplementation significantly increased net lean mass and strength gains above resistance training alone. However, the effect sizes of these improvements were trivial to small; effect sizes for gain in muscle mass = 0.15 and strength = 0.19 (Nissen & Sharp 2003). In addition, this meta-analysis has received criticism on the basis that the studies emanate from only three different laboratories, and may show experimental bias because of interdependence (Decombaz et al. 2003).

It is difficult to find a common thread to the findings of the present HMB research. One theory is that HMB supplementation might be most valuable in the early phases of a new training program, or when previously untrained subjects undertake resistance training, where it is able to reduce the large catabolic response or damage produced by unaccustomed exercise. However, once adaptation to training occurs, reducing the residual catabolism/damage response, HMB supplementation no longer provides a detectable benefit. If this were the case, it would explain why HMB tends to produce favorable results in novice resistance trainers rather than well-trained subjects, and why positive results are reported in shorter studies (2–4 weeks) but not at the end of longer studies (8 weeks). Further well-controlled studies are required to clarify if, and under what circumstances, HMB is a useful training aid. Short-term supplementation with HMB does not appear to cause any adverse effects on indices of health (Gallagher et al. 2000; Crowe et al. 2003). Athletes are warned that although HMB itself is not banned by anti-doping codes and does not lead to a positive doping finding (Slater et al. 2000), supplements that are popularly promoted as 'bodybuilding' or 'legal alternatives to steroids' are often at risk of contamination with banned substances such as pro-hormones.

16.29 Glutamine

Glutamine is the most abundant free amino acid in human muscle and plasma. Likely roles of glutamine within the body including transfer of nitrogen between organs, the maintenance of the acid–base balance during acidosis, regulation of protein synthesis and degradation, provision of a nitrogen precursor for synthesis of nucleotides and, finally, a fuel source for gut mucosal cells and cells of the immune system (for review, see Rowbottom et al. 1996). Numerous studies have been conducted to investigate the effects of glutamine supplementation on the immunosuppression that occurs after strenuous exercise; the consensus from this literature will be discussed in the commentary on nutrition for the immune system (see Commentary C at the end of this chapter). This section will focus only on the studies that have directly investigated the effects of acute or long-term glutamine supplementation on exercise performance. These studies are summarized in Table 16.9.

TABLE 16.8 STUDIES OF HMB SUPPLEMENTATION ON EXERCISE CAPACITY OR PERFORMANCE; FOR UPDATES SEE http://www.ausport.gov.au/ais/nutrition/supplements

STUDY	SUBJECTS	HMB DOSE AND TRAINING	EXERCISE PROTOCOL	PERFORMANCE ENHANCEMENT	COMMENTS
O'Connor & Crowe 2007	30 elite male rugby league players Parallel group design	3 g/d HMB or 3 g/d HMB-creatine for 6 weeks, no placebo Sports-related training	Tests @ baseline and 6 weeks • 3 RM strength testing • Upper body muscular endurance • 10-second max cycling test • surface anthropometry	 No No No No	No significant differences in muscular strength and endurance, leg power or anthropometric parameters among control, HMB or HMB-creatine groups.
Lamboley et al. 2007	16 (8 male, 8 female) active university students Parallel group design	3 g/d HMB or placebo for 5 weeks Treadmill interval training 3 d/wk	Tests @ baseline and 5 weeks • $VO_{2\,peak}$ • time to exhaustion at maximal aerobic speed • body composition	 Yes Yes No	Significantly greater increase in maximal aerobic capacity. Body composition did not change throughout the study, nor differ between groups.
Hoffman et al. 2004	26 male collegiate football players Parallel group design	3 g/d HMB for 10 days Sports-related training 2/d	Tests @ baseline and @ 10 days • Wingate anaerobic power test, 30-second sprint @ maximum speed	 No	No difference in anaerobic power was seen between groups. Plasma concentrations of cortisol decreased and CK increased over the 10-day training in both groups.
Thomson 2004	34 resistance-trained males Parallel group design	3 g/d HMB for 9 weeks Resistance training	Tests @ baseline and @ 9 weeks • 1 RM strength testing	 Yes	Significant increase in leg extension strength following HMB supplementation. No effect of HMB supplementation on body composition.
O'Connor & Crowe 2003	27 elite male rugby league players Parallel group design	3 g/d HMB or 3 g/d HMB-creatine for 6 weeks, no placebo Sports-related training	Tests @ baseline and 6 weeks • multi-stage fitness test • 60-second max cycling test	 No No	No differences in aerobic power from multi-stage fitness test or anaerobic capacity (peak power, total work and peak lactate levels) between groups at end of trial.

(continued)

TABLE 16.8 *(continued)*

STUDY	SUBJECTS	HMB DOSE AND TRAINING	EXERCISE PROTOCOL	PERFORMANCE ENHANCEMENT	COMMENTS
Ransone et al. 2003	35 male collegiate football players Crossover design	3 g/d HMB for 4 weeks Sports-specific fitness and strength training (20 hr/wk)	Tests @ baseline and 4 weeks supplementation • bench press • squats • power cleans	 No No No	No significant changes in muscular strength or in BM or body fat levels due to supplementation.
Slater et al. 2001	27 elite male rowers and male water polo players Parallel group design	3 g/d conventional or time-release HMB for 6 weeks Sports-related training including 3/wk resistance training Provided with nutritional advice + CHO/protein supplement	Tests @ baseline, 3 and 6 weeks • bench press • leg press • chin-ups	 No No No	All groups increased strength and LBM with no differences in response between groups. No differences in urinary 3-MH or plasma CK—crude markers of muscle breakdown and damage between groups.
Jowko et al. 2001	40 untrained males Parallel group design	3 g/d HMB, 3 g/d HMB-creatine, or creatine for 3 weeks Resistance training 3/wk	Tests @ baseline and 3 weeks • strength in various resistance exercises	Yes	Creatine caused greater increase in LBM and strength than placebo group. Greater strength and trend to greater increase in LBM with HMB than placebo. Effects were additive. HMB reduced plasma CK levels and urea, suggesting nitrogen sparing.
Vukovich & Dreifort 2001	8 trained male cyclists Crossover study (2-week washout)	3 g/d leucine or 3 g/d HMB for 2 weeks Cycling training	Tests @ baseline and 2 weeks supplementation • $VO_{2\,peak}$	Yes	Significant increase in $VO_{2\,peak}$, time to reach $VO_{2\,peak}$ and time to reach peak lactate threshold following HMB supplementation but not other supplementation periods.
Panton et al. 2000	39 males and 36 females of varying training status Parallel group design	3 g/d HMB for 4 weeks Resistance training 3/wk	Tests @ baseline and 4 weeks • strength in various resistance exercises	Yes	Data pooled across training status and gender. HMB group showed greater increase in upper body strength and a trend to greater gains in LBM, and loss of body fat than placebo, regardless of gender or training status.

Gallagher et al. 2000	37 untrained males Parallel group design	3 g/d or 6 g/d HMB for 8 weeks Resistance training 3/wk	Tests @ baseline and 8 weeks • muscle strength • peak isokinetic or isometric torque	 No No	No differences in strength gains between treatments. 3 g/d HMB supplementation increased gains in some measures of isokinetic or isometric torque and LBM, and decreased the rise in plasma CK.
Kreider et al. 1999	40 resistance-trained males Parallel group design	3 or 6 g/d HMB for 4 weeks Resistance training 7 hr/wk	Tests @ baseline and 4 weeks • bench press • leg press	 No No	No difference in improvements in strength between groups, or changes in LBM or body fat levels. No differences between plasma CK level and LDH levels (another marker of catabolism).
Nissen et al. 1996	41 untrained males Parallel group design	1.5 g/d or 3 g/d for 3 weeks Resistance training 1.5 hours 3/wk Groups further divided into 117 or 175 g/d protein	Tests at baseline and 3 weeks • weight lifted in training session	 Yes	HMB associated with decrease in urinary 3-MH and plasma CK. Trend to increased gain in LBM with HMB. Dose-responsive increase in weight lifted during training session with HMB compared with placebo.
Nissen et al. 1996	32 resistance-trained males Parallel group design	3 g/d for 7 weeks Resistance training 2–3 hr/d, 6/wk	Tests @ baseline and 7 weeks • bench press • squat • clean	 Yes No No	Control group was stronger at baseline in upper body strength; gains made by HMB group simply caused groups to be equal in upper and lower body strength at end of study. Greater increase in LBM during early part of study in HMB group was absent by 7 weeks. Effects of HMB diminish over time. Diet not controlled.

CHO = carbohydrate, CK = creatine kinase, LBM = lean body mass, RM = repetition maximum

TABLE 16.9 STUDIES OF GLUTAMINE SUPPLEMENTATION ON EXERCISE CAPACITY OR PERFORMANCE; FOR UPDATES SEE http://www.ausport.gov.au/ais/nutrition/supplements

STUDY	SUBJECTS	GLUTAMINE DOSE AND TRAINING	EXERCISE PROTOCOL	PERFORMANCE ENHANCEMENT	COMMENTS
ACUTE SUPPLEMENTATION					
Antonio et al. 2002	6 resistance-trained male subjects Crossover design	0.3 g/kg BM glutamine or 0.3 g/kg BM glycine ingested 60 minutes prior to test protocol	Resistance training: sets of exercise to fatigue • 2 × leg press @ 200% BM • 2 × bench press @ 100% BM	 No No	No difference in performance of resistance sets between trials. Plasma lactate and pH not measured to test out the hypothesis that acute glutamine supplementation would enhance buffering capacity.
Haub et al. 1998	10 active male subjects Crossover design	0.03 g/kg BM glutamine, ingested 90 minutes prior to test protocol	Cycling • 4 × 60-second bouts @ 100% of maximal PO followed by a TTE effort	No	Although researchers speculated that glutamine ingestion would increase buffering capacity, no differences were observed in plasma bicarbonate concentration at any time point.
CHRONIC SUPPLEMENTATION					
Falk et al. 2003	28 resistance-trained male subjects Parallel group design	3 g/d glutamine for 8 weeks (as part of effervescent supplement with creatine + ribose) Resistance training	• 1 RM bench press • repetitions 80% RM bench press to fatigue	No No	Both groups increased LBM, muscle strength and strength endurance over 8 weeks of training, but no differences between groups.
Lehmkuhl et al. 2003	19 male and female collegiate track and field athletes Parallel group design	4 g/d glutamine in addition to creatine for 8 weeks (glutamine + creatine versus creatine alone) Supervised event-specific resistance training program	• 5 × 5-second cycling sprints with 50-second recovery • static jump • counter-movement jump	No No No	Creatine supplementation in conjunction with training was associated with an increase in cycling power and increase in LBM. However, the addition of glutamine did not further enhance these gains.
Candow et al. 2001	31 untrained male and female subjects Parallel group design	0.9 g/kg lean tissue mass/ day for 6 weeks (consumed after training and prior to bed) Resistance training	• 1 RM bench press • 1 RM squat • peak knee extensor torque	No No No	Both groups increased in strength, knee extensor torque, LBM and index of muscle protein degradation (urinary 3-methyl histidine) in response to training. No differences seen between groups.

BM = body mass, LBM = lean body mass, PO = power output, RM = repetition maximum, TTE = time to exhaustion

Although the acute intake of glutamine prior to exercise has been hypothesized to enhance blood buffering capacity, the available studies fail to support this theory or any beneficial outcome on the performance of exercise (Haub et al. 1998; Antonio et al. 2002). Similarly, chronic protocols of supplementation with glutamine have not been associated with any enhancement of the adaptations to training (Candow et al. 2001; Falk et al. 2003; Lehmkuhl et al. 2003).

Supplements in Group C of the AIS Sports Supplement Program 16.30

The claims made for the majority of supplements available to athletes are not supported by sound scientific research. This is because the products have not been studied, or because the available literature has failed to provide evidence of a detectable benefit to training or competition performance.

Herbal products 16.31

Ginseng

Ginseng, extracted from the roots of ginseng plants, has enjoyed popularity as a health supplement for many centuries. The chemical composition of commercial ginseng supplements is highly variable due to differences in the genetic nature of the plant source, variation in active ingredients according to the season and to cultivation methods, and differences in the methods of production into supplements. Several species of ginseng are known to exist: American, Chinese, Korean and Japanese (Bahrke & Morgan 1994). These belong to the genus *Panax* and are related. However, Russian or Siberian ginseng is extracted from a different plant (*Eleutherococcus senticosus*) and often goes by the name of ciwujia.

A number of chemically similar steroid glycosides or saponin chemicals, known as ginsenosides, have been identified as active ingredients in ginsengs. Unfortunately for the process of scientific study, there is a great variability in the active ingredients within and between products. The bioavailability of supplements can also vary according to the method of administration (e.g. chewing gum, pill, capsule, tablet or liquid). Some ginseng preparations also provide additional agents such as vitamins, minerals or other herbal compounds.

Ginseng has been used widely in the herbal medicines of oriental cultures to cure fatigue, relieve pain and headaches, and improve mental function and vigor. It is also claimed to increase non-specific resistance to various stressors, described by Russian and Eastern European scientists as an adaptogenic response. An adaptogen is a substance purported to normalize physiology after exposure to a variety of stresses. It exhibits a lack of specificity in its actions and can both reduce and increase a response that has been altered by a stressor. This theory represents a philosophy of physiology or medicine different from the traditional western understanding.

Despite the history of use in eastern or traditional medicine, ginseng has only relatively recently emerged as a purported ergogenic aid for exercise performance. In athletes, ginseng is claimed to reduce fatigue and improve aerobic conditioning, strength, mental alertness and recovery. However, several reviews of the literature on supplementation with ginsengs on exercise have noted that there is a lack of well-controlled research to support these claims (Bahrke & Morgan 1994; Dowling et al. 1996; Bahrke & Morgan 2000; Goulet 2005). In many cases, the studies that appear to show benefits to athletic performance are either flawed in design (e.g. failure to include a control or placebo group) or lacking in detail due to their publication in a foreign language journal. Our review of the literature on ginseng supplement and exercise outcomes (see Table 16.10) has not included these studies. Studies that have appeared in abstract form, and have not been published in a peer-reviewed forum, have also been omitted. Finally, we have included only studies that have involved a measurement of exercise capacity or performance.

On the whole, the studies included in Table 16.10 fail to provide clear support for any benefits to performance following ginseng supplementation. Although a few studies have reported enhancement of physical exercise capacity or performance following chronic ginseng use (McNaughton et al. 1989; Liang et al. 2005), the majority have failed to detect an enhanced outcome (Dowling et al. 1996; Morris et al. 1996; Engels et al. 2001, 2003; Hsu et al. 2005). There are claims that ginseng supplementation may be valuable for athletic training in producing an enhancement of immune function, reduction in muscle damage or improved levels of psychomotor performance and wellbeing. Indeed there is some support for some of these claims (Ziemba et al. 1999; Hsu et al. 2005). However, other studies found a failure of supplementation with ginseng to enhance immune system parameters in athletes (Gaffney et al. 2001) or untrained subjects undertaking exercise (Engels et al. 2003), or to improve psychological function or wellbeing (Cardinal & Engels 2001).

A noticeable feature of the summary provided in Table 16.10 is that there are few studies of supplementation with ginseng in trained subjects. Therefore it is fair to say that the effect of ginseng supplementation on athletic performance has not been adequately researched. However, the range in the types of ginseng and the variability in the content of commercial ginseng supplements creates a difficulty in undertaking a thorough investigation in any population. Furthermore, these factors would also create caution in applying the results of a particular study to general education for athletes. For example, Chong and Oberholzer (1998) assayed fifty commercial ginseng preparations and noted that forty-four products ranged in ginsenoside concentration from 1.9–9.0%, with the other six preparations failing to produce a detectable level of ginsenosides. Thus, even if well-controlled studies were to report beneficial outcomes from ginseng use, athletes could not be certain of receiving the appropriate dose and type of active ingredients from all preparations in the commercially available range. Furthermore, one product that was included in this assay contained large amounts of ephedrine (Chong & Oberholzer 1988); this would be a cause of an inadvertent doping outcome. The conclusion that must be made about ginseng at the current time is that there is no substantial evidence to support claims that this supplement is of benefit to performance or recovery.

Cordyceps sinensis and *Rhodiola rosea*

Several other herbal compounds with a history of medical use or as tonics in other cultures have recently become available in supplements promoted to athletes. These include *Cordyceps sinensis*, a Chinese herb extracted from a mushroom, and *Rhodiola rosea*, popular in Asian and Eastern European medicine. Whereas *Cordyceps* is claimed to increase vasodilation and facilitate the delivery of oxygen to the working tissue, *Rhodiola* is said to stimulate the nervous system (De Bock et al. 2004; Earnest et al. 2004; Parcell et al. 2004). The small amount of literature on supplementation with these products on exercise capacity or performance is summarized in Table 16.11 (page 471). To date, there is little evidence to support any of

TABLE 16.10 PLACEBO-CONTROLLED STUDIES OF GINSENG SUPPLEMENTATION AND PERFORMANCE; FOR UPDATES SEE http://www.ausport.gov.au/ais/nutrition/supplements

STUDY	SUBJECTS	GINSENG DOSE	EXERCISE PROTOCOL	PERFORMANCE ENHANCEMENT	COMMENTS
Liang et al. 2005	29 active males and females Parallel group design	Chinese ginseng *Panax notoginseng* 1350 mg/d for 30 days	Cycling • Incremental test to exhaustion	Yes	Ginseng group improved endurance by 7 minutes ($p < 0.05$) over treatment while no change seen in placebo group. Ginseng treatment also associated with a reduction in blood pressure and VO_2 during exercise.
Engels et al. 2003	27 active males and females Parallel group design	G115 Chinese/Korean ginseng (*Panax ginseng* CA Meyer) 400 mg/d for 8 weeks	Cycling • 3 consecutive 30-second Wingate tests with 3-minute recovery periods	No	Comparison of post-test to pre-test scores showed no difference between groups in power during cycling or heart rate response. No difference in salivary IgA response to exercise due to ginseng.
Engels et al. 2001	19 active females Parallel group design	G115 Chinese/Korean ginseng (*Panax ginseng* CA Meyer) 400 mg/d for 8 weeks	Cycling • 30-second Wingate test	No	Comparison of post-test to pre-test scores showed no difference between groups in power during cycling or heart rate response.
Ziemba et al. 1999	15 male soccer players Parallel group design	Unspecified *Panax* sp. ginseng 350 mg/d for 6 weeks	Cycling • Incremental test to exhaustion • Reaction time measured at each stage	No Yes	No change in lactate threshold or $VO_{2\,max}$. However, enhanced reaction time at submaximal workloads.
Allen et al. 1998	28 active males and females Parallel group design	Chinese/Korean ginseng (*Panax ginseng* CA Meyer) 200 mg/d for 3 weeks	Cycling • Incremental test to exhaustion	No	No enhancement of total workload, RPE and lactate at submaximal loads or $VO_{2\,max}$ due to ginseng supplementation.
Morris et al. 1996	8 active males and females Crossover design	Unspecified ginseng 8 mg/kg/d or 16 mg/kg/d for 1 week	Cycling • Time to exhaustion @ 75% $VO_{2\,max}$	No	No change in time to exhaustion or metabolic parameters. No change in RPE.

(continued)

TABLE 16.10 (continued)

STUDY	SUBJECTS	GINSENG DOSE	EXERCISE PROTOCOL	PERFORMANCE ENHANCEMENT	COMMENTS
Hsu et al. 2005	13 active males Crossover design	American ginseng 400 mg/d for 4 weeks	Running • 80% $VO_{2\,max}$ to fatigue	No	No difference in endurance with ginseng supplementation; however, plasma CK levels were lower during exercise and for 2 hours post-exercise in ginseng trial, indicating lower levels of muscle damage.
Dowling et al. 1996	20 highly trained male and female runners Parallel group design	Siberian ginseng (*Eleutherococcus senticosus*) 60 drops/d (maximum recommended dose) for 6 weeks	Running • 10-minute treadmill test at 10 km race pace • Maximal treadmill test	No No	No change in metabolic characteristics at race pace or performance of treadmill max. and RPE. Low statistical power may prevent small changes from being detected.
Pieralisi et al. 1991	Active male subjects Crossover design	Ginsana 115 2 capsules/d for 6 weeks (ginseng, vitamins, bitartrate + minerals)	Running • Incremental treadmill test to exhaustion	Yes	Increased $VO_{2\,max}$ and reduced O_2 consumption at submaximal workloads.
McNaughton et al. 1989	30 active males and females Crossover design	Chinese ginseng (*Panax ginseng* CA Meyer) or Siberian ginseng (*Eleutherococcus senticosus*) 1 g/d for 6 weeks	Physical testing • $VO_{2\,max}$, grip • pectoral strength • quadriceps strength	Yes Yes Yes	Significantly greater increase in $VO_{2\,max}$ and pectoral and grip strength with Chinese ginseng. Trends for enhancement with Siberian ginseng.

CK = creatine kinase, RPE = ratings of perceived exertion

TABLE 16.11 PLACEBO-CONTROLLED STUDIES OF SUPPLEMENTATION WITH *CORDYCEPS SINENSIS* OR *RHODIOLA ROSEA* ON PERFORMANCE; FOR UPDATES SEE http://www.ausport.gov.au/ais/nutrition/supplements

STUDY	SUBJECTS	SUPPLEMENT DOSE	EXERCISE PROTOCOL	PERFORMANCE ENHANCEMENT	COMMENTS
ACUTE SUPPLEMENTATION					
De Bock et al. 2004	24 active males Crossover design	200 mg *Rhodiola rosea* 1 hour pre-exercise	Battery of tests • incremental cycling to fatigue • isokinetic knee torque • speed of limb movement • reaction time • sustained attention	 Yes No No No No	Compared with placebo, supplementation with *Rhodiola rosea* produced increased time to exhaustion in cycling protocol. No effect seen on muscle strength, or measures of reaction time and responsiveness to stimuli.
CHRONIC SUPPLEMENTATION					
Parcell et al. 2004	22 well-trained male cyclists Parallel group design	3.15 g/d *Cordyceps sinensis* (CordyMax Cs-4™) for 5 weeks Normal training	Cycling • $VO_{2\,peak}$ + • TT lasting ~1 hour	 No No	No change in aerobic capacity ($VO_{2\,peak}$) over time in either group. No change in time to complete cycling time trial over time or between groups.
Earnest et al. 2004	17 endurance-trained male cyclists Parallel group design	1 g/d *Cordyceps sinensis* + 300 mg *Rhodiola rosea* for 2 weeks (+ chromium, pyruvate, phosphate, ribose, adenosine) Optygen	Cycling • Incremental cycling time to exhaustion to assess peak power output, $VO_{2\,peak}$	 No	No change in cycling endurance or aerobic capacity in either group over time.
De Bock et al. 2004	23 active males Parallel group design	200 mg *Rhodiola rosea* for 4 weeks	Battery of tests: • incremental cycling to fatigue • isokinetic knee torque • speed of limb movement • reaction time • sustained attention	 No No No No No	Neither treatment nor placebo group showed any changes in response to test battery. Previously seen benefits of acute intake of *Rhodiola rosea* on exercise capacity not apparent after chronic supplementation.

the claims made for these compounds. There has been insufficient research on the effects of these supplements on exercise or athletic performance to allow further discussion.

16.32 Carnitine

The first reports on carnitine in the early 1900s described it as a vitamin (an essential component of the diet). Following the discovery that carnitine can be manufactured in the liver and kidney from amino acid precursors (lysine and methionine), it is now considered to be a non-essential nutrient. Most animal foods provide a dietary source of carnitine, but due to losses in the cooking and preparation of foods there are few data on the total content of the diet. Carnitine ingested or synthesized by humans is in the *l*-isoform and is carried via the blood for storage, predominantly in the heart and skeletal muscle. Within these tissues, carnitine plays a number of roles related to fat and CHO metabolism.

Carnitine is a component of the enzymes carnitine palmityltransferase I (CPTI), carnitine palmityltransferase II (CPTII) and carnitine acylcarnitine translocase (CAT). These enzymes are involved in the transportation of long-chain fatty acids (LCFAs) across the mitochondrial membrane to the site of their oxidation (see Chapter 15). Because of this function, it has been suggested that carnitine supplementation might enhance fatty acid transport and oxidation. As a result, carnitine is a popular component of supplements claimed to enhance the loss of body fat, and has been embraced by bodybuilders wanting to 'cut up' and by other populations interested in weight loss. An increase in fatty acid oxidation during exercise could be of advantage to endurance athletes if it resulted in a sparing of glycogen during events in which CHO stores are otherwise limiting.

During exercise, carnitine also plays the role of a 'sink' for acetyl-CoA production. By converting this to acetyl-carnitine and CoA, carnitine helps to maintain CoA availability and to decrease the ratio of acetyl-CoA:CoA. If carnitine supplementation could increase this function it might enhance flux through the citric acid cycle. Furthermore, it could enhance the activity of the enzyme pyruvate dehydrogenase, which is otherwise inhibited by high levels of acetyl-CoA, thus increasing oxidative metabolism of glucose. If this results in lower lactate production, it might enhance exercise performance in situations that might otherwise be limited by excess lactate and hydrogen ion accumulation. Extensive reviews of carnitine function are available (Cerretelli & Marconi 1990; Wagenmakers 1991; Clarkson 1992; Heinonen 1996).

When muscle carnitine activity is inadequate, as in the case of inborn errors of metabolism or certain disease states (such as in hemodialysis), individuals demonstrate lipid abnormalities and reduced exercise capacity. Carnitine supplementation is an established medical therapy for these conditions and helps to attenuate such symptoms. However, whether additional oral carnitine intake in healthy individuals enhances metabolism and exercise performance is a different issue. A positive outcome would require one or more of the following scenarios: heavy training causing suboptimal levels of muscle carnitine; carnitine supplementation increasing muscle carnitine content; carnitine being a limiting factor in fatty acid transport; or carnitine being a limiting factor in pyruvate dehydrogenase activity or citric acid cycle flux. However, thorough reviews cast doubt on the potential for enhanced metabolic function via enhanced carnitine status (Wagenmakers 1991; Heinonen 1996). These reviews summarize that normal muscle carnitine levels appear to be adequate for maximal function of CPTI and CPTII, and that there is no proof that fatty acid transport is the rate-limiting step in fat oxidation. Furthermore, pyruvate dehydrogenase is believed to be fully active within seconds of high-intensity exercise, and additional carnitine is unlikely to stimulate this activity further.

Optimal muscle carnitine content in athletes is probably the most important issue to address. Exercise is known to increase carnitine excretion and it is possible that muscle carnitine content may decrease during intense training. However, a series of reviews conclude that although most human studies find an increase in *plasma* carnitine levels following carnitine supplementation of 1–6 g/d, there is no compelling evidence that *muscle* carnitine levels are enhanced as a result of oral carnitine supplementation (Cerretelli & Marconi 1990; Wagenmakers 1991; Heinonen 1996) unless plasma insulin concentrations are at relatively high levels (>90 mU/L-1; Stephens et al. 2006a) or substantial CHO (>94 g) is consumed with each dose of carnitine (Stephens et al. 2006b).

While one study has reported an increase in lipid utilization during exercise following chronic carnitine supplementation in trained men (Gorostiaga et al. 1989), the majority of studies have not reported any changes in substrate utilization during exercise as a result of carnitine use per se (Broad et al. 2008), even under conditions in which fat availability was increased (Vukovich et al. 1994) or muscle glycogen stores were depleted (Decombaz et al. 1993). Studies that have investigated the effects of carnitine supplementation on exercise performance are summarized in Table 16.12 overleaf. On balance, there is little credible evidence of increased performance during submaximal or high-intensity exercise resulting from carnitine supplementation. Despite the popularity of carnitine in fat-loss supplements and the marketing claims associated with these products, the effect of carnitine supplementation on body-fat levels has not been studied in athletes.

Coenzyme Q10 16.33

Coenzyme Q10, or ubiquinone, is a non-essential, lipid-soluble nutrient found predominantly in animal foods and in low levels in plant foods. It is located in the body primarily in skeletal and cardiac muscle, inside the mitochondria. Coenzyme Q10 is part of the mitochondrial anti-oxidant defense system, preventing damage to DNA and cell membranes, and provides a link in the electron transport chain producing ATP. Some cardiac and neuromuscular dysfunction is believed to result from coenzyme Q10 deficiency. Indeed, patients with ischemic heart disease are often seen to have lower plasma coenzyme Q10 concentrations and improve their exercise capacity following coenzyme Q10 supplementation. The marketing campaigns for coenzyme Q10 supplement promote increased vigor and youthfulness as a benefit of their use. For athletes, there are claims of enhanced energy production and reduced oxidative damage from exercise.

Peer-reviewed studies of coenzyme Q10 supplementation on exercise metabolism, oxidative damage caused by exercise and performance are summarized in Table 16.13. There are few data that support an ergogenic benefit of coenzyme Q10 on exercise performance. In contrast, several studies have shown that coenzyme Q10 has an *ergolytic,* or negative, effect on high-intensity performance and training adaptations (Laaksonen et al. 1995; Malm et al. 1996, 1997; Svensson et al. 1999). A series of studies found that coenzyme Q10 supplementation had no effect on indices of lipid oxidation (indicated by plasma malondialdehyde concentrations) or catabolism of adenine nucleotides (indicated by plasma uric acid and hypoxanthine concentrations) when previously untrained men undertook twice daily sessions of repeated sprints (Svensson et al. 1999). In fact, supplementation with coenzyme Q10 may have increased oxidative damage, as indicated by higher plasma creatine kinase levels in response to exercise compared with the placebo trial (Malm et al. 1996). In these circumstances, coenzyme Q10 was believed to act as a pro-oxidant rather than an anti-oxidant. Training adaptations were impaired by coenzyme Q10, with the placebo group outperforming the coenzyme Q10 group either during training or at the

TABLE 16.12 STUDIES OF CARNITINE SUPPLEMENTATION ON EXERCISE CAPACITY OR PERFORMANCE

STUDY	SUBJECTS	CARNITINE DOSE	EXERCISE PROTOCOL	PERFORMANCE ENHANCEMENT	COMMENTS
ACUTE SUPPLEMENTATION STUDIES					
Siliprandi et al. 1990	10 moderately trained males Crossover design	Acute administration 2 g @ 1 hour before exercise	Cycling • Cycle to exhaustion	Yes	Increased time to exhaustion. Carnitine reduced the increase in plasma lactate and pyruvate after maximal progressive work. However, dose and timeframe for uptake into muscle seem unrealistic.
Vecchiet et al. 1990	10 moderately trained males Crossover design	Acute administration 2 g @ 1 hour before exercise	Cycling • Incremental cycling to exhaustion	Yes	Increase in time (and work) until exhaustion. Decrease in lactate production and oxygen consumption at same workload. However, dose and timeframe for uptake into muscle seem unrealistic.
CHRONIC SUPPLEMENTATION STUDIES					
Broad et al. 2008	20 male cyclists Double blind, placebo-controlled, pair-matched parallel design	2 g/d for 2 weeks	90 minutes cycling	No difference in CHO or fat metabolism during exercise	Suppressed ammonia accumulation during exercise with L-carnitine.
Colombani et al. 1996	7 endurance-trained male athletes Crossover design	2 g @ 2 hours before run and at 20 km mark	Running • Marathon run + submaximal performance test day after marathon	No	No change in exercise metabolism or marathon running time. No change in recovery and submaximal test performance on following day.

Trappe et al. 1994	20 highly trained male collegiate swimmers Parallel group design	4 g/d for 7 days	Swimming • 5 × 91.4 m swims (100 y)	No	No difference in performance times between trials or between groups.
Greig et al. 1987	9 untrained males and females + 10 untrained males and females Crossover design	2 g/d for 2 weeks 2 g for 4 weeks	Cycling • Progressive test to exhaustion	No	No significant physiological changes. Changes in performance were small and inconsistent.
Marconi et al. 1985	6 national class walkers Crossover design	4 g/d for 2 weeks	Running • supramaximal work (jumps) • treadmill $VO_{2\,max}$	 No Yes?	Increase in $VO_{2\,max}$ by 6%. However, no effects on oxygen utilization and RER at submaximal loads, or change in lactate accumulation with jumps. Results appear inconsistent.

RER = respiratory exchange ratio

TABLE 16.13 STUDIES OF COENZYME Q10 SUPPLEMENTATION AND EXERCISE PERFORMANCE; FOR UPDATES SEE http://www.ausport.gov.au/ais/nutrition/supplements

STUDY	SUBJECTS	COENZYME Q10 DOSE	EXERCISE PROTOCOL	PERFORMANCE ENHANCEMENT	COMMENTS
Bonetti et al. 2000	28 recreational cyclists Parallel group design	100 mg/d for 8 weeks	Cycling • Incremental test with increase of 50 W/minutes until exhaustion	No	Supplementation did increase plasma coenzyme Q10 levels, but did not improve aerobic power.
Nielsen et al. 1999	7 well-trained male triathletes Crossover design	100 mg/d for 6 weeks (+ vitamin E + vitamin C)	Cycling • Incremental $VO_{2\,max}$ test to exhaustion	No	No effect on maximal oxygen uptake or muscle energy metabolism (determined by nuclear magnetic resonance spectroscopy).
Malm et al. 1997	18 males Parallel group design	120 mg/d for 22 days Days 2–9: usual activity Days 11–14: 2/d anaerobic training Days 15–22: recovery	Cycling anaerobic test (days 1, 11, 15 and 20) • 30-second Wingate cycle + 5-minute recovery + 10 × 10-second sprints Aerobic test (pre-trial and day 18) • Cycling $VO_{2\,max}$ Aerobic test (pre-trial and day 22) • Running $VO_{2\,max}$	No—in fact, impairment No No	Placebo and Q10 group both improved performance of repeated sprint test after training, however, only placebo group maintained this improvement during recovery to day 20. Placebo group achieved higher average power, and greater improvement in latter intervals during anaerobic training sessions. No change in $VO_{2\,max}$ outcomes in either group over time or in oxygen use during submaximal cycling.
Weston et al. 1997	18 trained male cyclists and triathletes Parallel group design	1 mg/kg/d for 28 days	Cycling • Incremental test to exhaustion	No	Test undertaken pre- and post 28 days of training; coenzyme Q10 did not enhance performance compared with placebo group.
Ylikoski et al. 1997	25 national-level cross-country skiers Parallel group design	90 mg/d for 6 weeks	Cross-country skiing • Treadmill pole-walking to exhaustion	Yes	Improved $VO_{2\,max}$ with coenzyme Q10 supplementation. Increase in aerobic and anaerobic thresholds. No control of exercise during supplementation periods.

Malm et al. 1996	15 active males Parallel group design	120 mg/d for 20 days Days 2–10: usual activity Days 11–15: 2/d anaerobic training Days 16–20: recovery	Cycling • Days 1, 11, 15 and 20 • 30-second Wingate cycle + 5-minute recovery + 10 × 10-second sprints	No—in fact, impairment	Placebo group improved anaerobic work capacity at day 15 or 20—training effect. However, Q10 group did achieve this training effect. CK levels maintained during placebo trial but were increased at various time points in Q10 group.
Laaksonen et al. 1995	11 young and 8 older trained males Crossover design	120 mg/d for 6 weeks	Cycling • Prolonged endurance test to exhaustion	No—in fact, performance impairment	No change in muscle coenzyme Q10 concentrations or plasma malondialdehyde as a result of coenzyme Q10 supplementation. Negative effect on time to exhaustion (placebo had greater endurance).
Snider et al. 1992	11 highly trained triathletes Crossover design	100 mg/d for 4 weeks (+ vitamin E, inosine, cytochrome c)	Cycling and running • 90 minutes on treadmill @ 70% VO_{2max} + cycling @ 70% VO_2 max to exhaustion	No	No difference in time to exhaustion between trials. No differences in blood metabolites or RPE.
Braun et al. 1991	10 male cyclists Parallel group design	100 mg/d for 8 weeks	Cycling • Incremental test to exhaustion	No	Performance increased equally in both groups from pre- to post-supplementation. Coenzyme Q10 had no effect on cycling performance or any measured parameters. Malondialdehyde concentrations reduced in both groups after training.

CK = creatine kinase, RPE = rating of perceived exertion, W = watts

end of the supplementation phase (Malm et al. 1996, 1997). Similarly, a crossover study found that trained subjects had greater endurance during a cycling test at the end of the placebo trial compared with the period of coenzyme Q10 supplementation. An increase in plasma Q10 concentrations in response to supplementation is not associated with an increase in Q10 concentrations in skeletal muscle or isolated skeletal muscle mitochondria (Svensson et al. 1999).

Further work is required to investigate the effects of coenzyme Q10 supplementation on exercise performance and training. However, at present there is no clear evidence to recommend coenzyme Q10 supplementation to athletes undertaking high-intensity training.

16.34 Inosine

Inosine is a nucleic acid derivative that occurs naturally in brewer's yeast, and in liver and other glandular organ meats. It is a non-essential nutrient, since our bodies can make all nucleic acids from their amino acid and sugar precursors provided in protein and CHO foods. Specifically, inosine is a purine nucleoside and a precursor of the nucleotide, inosine monophosphate (IMP). This is, in turn, an intermediary in the degradation and salvage of the adenine nucleotides ATP, AMP and ADP. Thus, it has been hypothesized that inosine supplementation could increase the muscle content of ATP. Other mechanisms by which inosine supplementation is claimed to enhance exercise performance include an increase in 2,3-diphosphoglycerate in red blood cells, which theoretically shifts the oxyhemoglobin curve to increase the release of oxygen into the muscle. Inosine is also believed to have vasodilatory effects and anti-oxidant properties. However, these are only hypothetical situations that have not been supported by research. Further information on inosine can be found in Williams and colleagues (1990) and Starling and colleagues (1996).

The main support for inosine supplementation is testimonial, with reports from athletes, especially from Russian and ex-Eastern-bloc countries, and muscle-building magazines. One popular magazine, *Muscle and Fitness*, published an article describing a 6-week study of inosine supplementation on four trained athletes (Colgan 1988). The report claimed the study was undertaken using a double-blind crossover design and found strength gains as a result of the supplementation. This study has not appeared in a peer-reviewed publication or in adequate detail to judge the validity of these claims. The athletes reported irritability and fatigue while taking the inosine supplements.

Table 16.14 summarizes the results of the only three well-controlled studies of inosine supplementation that have been published in the peer-reviewed literature. Inosine was also an ingredient in a multi-compound ergogenic aid (CAPS) that failed to enhance performance of triathletes in a study by Snider and colleagues (1992); this study has been reviewed in Table 16.13. The three studies of isolated inosine supplementation all failed to find either favorable metabolic changes or performance benefits following inosine supplementation in well-trained subjects (Williams et al. 1990; Starling et al. 1996; McNaughton et al. 1999c). There were no data to support any of the theoretical actions of inosine supplementation. Although muscle substrates were not directly measured in these studies, purported changes to ATP concentrations are unlikely to enhance exercise performance, since ATP is not depleted by exercise, even at the point of fatigue (see Chapter 1).

TABLE 16.14 STUDIES OF INOSINE SUPPLEMENTATION AND EXERCISE PERFORMANCE; FOR UPDATES SEE http://www.ausport.gov.au/ais/nutrition/supplements

STUDY	SUBJECTS	INOSINE 10 000 DOSE	EXERCISE PROTOCOL	ENHANCED PERFORMANCE	COMMENTS
Williams et al. 1990	9 highly trained male and female endurance runners Crossover design	6000 mg/d for 2 days (maximum recommended dose)	Running • Submaximal warm-up run • 3-mile treadmill TT • maximal treadmill run	No—in fact, performance impairment	No effect on 3-mile run time, $VO_{2\ peak}$ or other variables. Negative effect on maximal run.
Starling et al. 1996	10 competitive male cyclists Crossover design	5000 mg/d for 5 days	Cycling • Wingate 30-second test • 30-minute TT • supramaximal sprint to fatigue	No—in fact, performance impairment	No difference in Wingate performance or 30-minute cycle. Negative effect on time to fatigue. Increase in plasma uric acid concentration.
McNaughton et al. 1999c	7 well-trained males Crossover design	10 000 mg for 5 and 10 days	Cycling • 5 × 6-second sprints • 30-second sprint • 20-minute TT	No	No improvements in sprint times or TT performance. Increase in plasma uric acid concentrations.

TT = time trial

Of note, two studies reported that subjects showed better performance of high-intensity tasks while on the placebo treatment than on the inosine trial, suggesting that inosine supplementation might actually impair the performance of high-intensity exercise (Williams et al. 1990; Starling et al. 1996). Potential mechanisms for exercise impairment include an increased formation of IMP in the muscle, either at rest or during exercise. High IMP concentrations have been found at the point of fatigue in many exercise studies; furthermore, IMP has been shown to inhibit ATPase activity (Sahlin 1992). It is possible that increased resting concentrations of muscle IMP reduced the duration of high-intensity exercise before critically high levels were reached, causing premature fatigue. Such a theory can only be investigated by direct measurements of muscle nucleosides. Another possible mechanism of performance impairment is an increase in levels of uric acid, a product of inosine degradation. In the present studies, 2 days of inosine supplementation did not change uric acid levels; however, 5 days and 10 days of intake doubled blood concentrations to levels above the normal range (Williams et al. 1990; Starling et al. 1996; McNaughton et al. 1999c). Thus, chronic inosine supplementation may pose a health risk, since high uric acid levels are implicated as a cause of gout. In summary, since there is a lack of evidence of performance benefits, and the possibility of performance decrements and side effects, there is little to recommend the use of inosine supplements by athletes.

16.34 Chromium picolinate

Chromium is an essential trace mineral. Good sources of dietary chromium include liver, eggs, poultry and wholegrain cereals; however, absorption of chromium from food is poor. Insufficient data exist to establish a recommended dietary intake for chromium. Adequate intakes, determined from estimates of nutrient intake by healthy people, are within the range of 25–35 μg per day. The lack of reliable food composition data on the chromium content of foods often causes an underestimation of chromium intake.

Chromium plays many roles in maintaining proper metabolism, including roles in glucose, lipid and amino acid metabolism (see Stoecker 1996). Glucose tolerance factor (GTF), found in brewer's yeast, may be the most biologically active and absorbable form of chromium. GTF potentiates insulin activity and is responsible for normal insulin function related to uptake of glucose and amino acids into the cell. Optimal chromium intake appears to decrease the amount of insulin required to maintain normal blood glucose levels. Chromium deficiency is rare, but it is suggested that marginal chromium intakes may contribute to the development of conditions such as insulin resistance and poor growth. People with chromium deficiencies often show improvements in growth or glucose tolerance in response to chromium supplementation (Stoecker 1996). However, research is yet to show convincing proof that chromium supplementation improves glucose metabolism in people with type 2 diabetes. Since exercise has been shown to increase the urinary excretion of chromium, it has been suggested that athletes are at risk of becoming chromium deficient and that supplementation would be beneficial. Further research is required to determine if the body adapts to increased excretion of chromium by increasing the absorption of chromium. As is the case for many micronutrients, athletes with restricted energy intakes are most at risk of low chromium intakes.

Chromium supplements are available in the form of chromium nicotinate, chloride and picolinate. Chromium picolinate is claimed to be the most biologically active form, and the claims for the efficacy of chromium picolinate have caused an interesting public debate between the patent holders and other trace element/mineral experts (Levafi et al. 1992; Evans 1993; Levafi 1993). A concern with chromium supplementation is that chromium potentially competes with trivalent iron for binding to transferrin, thus predisposing those with chronically high intakes of chromium to iron deficiency (Lukaski et al. 1996). Some (Lukaski et al. 1996), but not all (Campbell et al. 1997), studies have reported a reduction in iron status as a result of chromium picolinate supplementation.

The main claims for chromium supplements are that they will enhance handling of glucose, amino acids and fatty acids, allow dramatic gains in muscle mass and strength, and reduce body fat. Initial studies reported increases in muscle mass and a reduction in body fat following supplementation with chromium picolinate in subjects undertaking aerobic exercise classes (Evans 1993) and weight training (Evans 1989). These studies have been criticized for methodological flaws, such as lack of a control group, inadequate control of diet or training status, and the reliance on unreliable and insensitive methods of assessing body composition (Levafi et al. 1992; Levafi 1993). We have not included such investigations in our summary of the literature (Table 16.15 overleaf). This summary shows that studies that use 'gold standard' techniques for measuring body composition (underwater weighing, dual X-ray absorptiometry and magnetic resonance imaging) have found no change in LBM or loss of body fat above the effects achieved by training alone. A study in which chromium picolinate was added to a sports drink consumed during exercise found that there were no additional benefits to exercise performance above that achieved by the CHO in the drink (Davis et al. 2000). Therefore, chromium picolinate supplementation does not appear to provide any acute benefits to CHO metabolism.

In summary, there is certainly no support for the dramatic claims made in some advertisements that position chromium picolinate is a 'legal anabolic' agent. The only situation in which chromium supplementation is likely to be useful is in treating individuals whose dietary intake is inadequate.

Medium chain triglycerides 16.36

Medium-chain triglycerides (MCTs) are fats composed of medium-chain fatty acids (MCFA) with a chain length of six to ten carbon molecules. They are digested and metabolized differently from the long-chain fatty acids that make up most of our dietary fat intake. Specifically, MCTs can be digested within the intestinal lumen with less need for bile and pancreatic juices than long-chain triglycerides, with MCFAs being absorbed via the portal circulation. MCFAs can be taken up into the mitochondria without the need for carnitine-assisted transport (see Chapter 15 for more details on fat metabolism). In clinical nutrition, MCT supplements derived from palm kernel and coconut oil are used as energy supplements for patients who have various digestive or lipid metabolism disorders. In the sports world, MCTs have been positioned as easily absorbed and oxidized fuel sources, and have been marketed to bodybuilders as fat sources that are less likely to deposit as body fat. However, the role of MCTs in the general diet of athletes has not been studied.

Another role for MCTs in sport is to provide a fuel source during endurance and ultra-endurance events that could potentially spare glycogen, and prolong the availability of important CHO stores. Jeukendrup and colleagues (1995) reported that the co-ingestion of MCT with CHO during prolonged exercise increased the rate of MCT oxidation, possibly by increasing its rate of absorption; the maximum rate of MCT oxidation was achieved at around 120–180 minutes of exercise, with values of 0.12 g/min. Table 16.16 (page 484) summarizes the findings of studies that have examined the effect of the co-ingestion of MCT and CHO on ultra-endurance performance; the results are inconsistent and appear to depend on the amount of MCT that can be ingested and the prevailing hormonal conditions. Studies in which the intake of large amounts of MCT raised plasma free fatty

TABLE 16.15 STUDIES OF CHROMIUM PICOLINATE SUPPLEMENTATION AND BODY COMPOSITION AND PERFORMANCE; FOR UPDATES SEE http://www.ausport.gov.au/ais/nutrition/supplements

STUDY	SUBJECTS	CHROMIUM DOSE AND FORM	EXERCISE PROTOCOL	ENHANCED PERFORMANCE	COMMENTS
ACUTE SUPPLEMENTATION STUDIES					
Davis et al. 2000	8 active males Crossover design	400 μg/d Cr-Pic (400)	Intermittent high-intensity exercise • shuttle running and fatigue test	 No	Cr added to a CHO-electrolyte sports drink did not enhance performance beyond the benefit of ingesting CHO during exercise.
CHRONIC SUPPLEMENTATION STUDIES					
Livolsi et al. 2001	15 female collegiate softball players Parallel group design	500 μg/d Cr-Pic for 6 weeks Resistance training program	Testing at baseline and 6 weeks strength • IRM for variety of lifts • body composition (hydrostatic weighing)	 No No	Muscle strength increased with training but no difference between groups. No significant differences in body fat or LBM. Urinary Cr excretion increased in treatment group.
Walker et al. 1998	20 male collegiate wrestlers Parallel group design	200 μg/d Cr-Pic for 14 weeks Resistance and conditioning training program	Testing at baseline and 14 weeks • strength • peak power • body composition • Wingate test • $VO_{2\,max}$ on run treadmill	 No No No No No	No enhancement of body composition or performance variables beyond improvements seen with training alone.
Hallmark et al. 1996	16 untrained males Parallel group design	200 μg/d Cr-Pic for 12 weeks Resistance training program	Testing at baseline and 12 weeks: • strength • body composition	 No No	No differences in body composition with training or supplement. Strength increases independent of supplement.

Lukaski et al. 1996	36 untrained males Parallel group design	3–4 μmol/d (~200 μg/d) Cr-Pic or Cr-chloride for 8 weeks Resistance training program	Testing at baseline and 8 weeks: • strength • body composition • iron status	 No No No	No beneficial effects on LBM, body fat or strength above training effect. No difference between chromium preparations. Trend for ↓ iron status (↓ transferrin status) with chromium picolinate.
Clancy et al. 1994	36 male collegiate football (gridiron) players Parallel group design	200 μg/d Cr-Pic for 9 weeks Pre-season resistance and conditioning training	Testing at baseline, mid and 9 weeks: • strength • body composition	 No No	No enhancement of BM, body composition or strength above placebo group.
Hasten et al. 1992	59 male and female college students Parallel group design	200 μg/d Cr-Pic for 12 weeks Resistance training program	Testing at baseline and 12 weeks • strength • body composition	 No No—males Yes—females	Both groups gained BM and reduced body fat. Greater ↑ in BM in females with chromium but no difference with males. No differences in strength changes due to chromium picolinate.

BM = body mass, LBM = lean body mass

TABLE 16.16 STUDIES OF MEDIUM-CHAIN TRIGLYCERIDES + CHO SUPPLEMENTATION AND ULTRA-ENDURANCE PERFORMANCE; FOR UPDATES SEE http://www.ausport.gov.au/ais/nutrition/supplements

STUDY	SUBJECTS	MCT DOSE	EXERCISE PROTOCOL	ENHANCED PERFORMANCE	COMMENTS
Goedecke et al. 2005	8 male endurance-trained cyclists Crossover design	1 hour pre-exercise 75 g CHO or 32 g MCT During exercise 600 mL/h of 10% CHO or 10% CHO + 4.2% MCT Total intake of MCT = 148 g over 6 hours	Cycling • 4.5 hours @ 50% PPO + 200 kJ TT (~15 minutes)	No—in fact impaired	No difference in substrate utilization (RER) during submaximal exercise. Half the subjects experienced gastrointestinal side effects with MCT. Overall, TT performance compromised in MCT trial (12.36 versus 14.30 minutes)
Vistisen et al. 2003	Well-trained cyclists (7 males) Crossover design	2.4 g/kg CHO or 2.4 g/kg CHO + 1.5 g/kg MCT/LCFA mixture over 4 hours Total intake of MCT mixture = 93–128 g over 4 hours	Cycling • 3 h @ 55% $\dot{V}O_{2\,max}$ + 800 kJ TT (~50 minutes)	No	No difference in TT performance between CHO and CHO + MCT mixture (50.8 ± 3.6 versus 50.0 ± 1.8 minutes, NS). Significantly lower RER (greater fat use) during first hour of ride, but not significantly different thereafter, indicating only minor differences in substrate utilization as a result of the treatment. No major gastrointestinal side effects during trial, but problems experienced next day with CHO + MCT mixture trial.
Angus et al. 2000	8 endurance-trained male cyclists/ triathletes Crossover design	1 L per hour of 6% CHO + 4% MCT (versus 6% CHO or placebo) Total intake of MCT = 42 g/h or ~120 g	Cycling • 100 km TT (~3 hours)	No	CHO enhanced performance over placebo, but addition of MCT did not provide further benefits. 4 subjects experienced gastrointestinal problems with MCT. No differences in fat oxidation, plasma FFA between MCT and CHO + MCT. Suppression of fat oxidation may be due to high exercise intensity or pre-trial CHO meal causing high insulin concentrations.

Goedecke et al. 1999	9 endurance-trained male cyclists Crossover design	1.6 L of 10% CHO or 10% CHO + 1.7% MCT or 10% CHO + 3.4% MCT Total intake of MCT = 26 or 52 g	Cycling • 2 hours @ 63% $VO_{2\,max}$ + 40 km TT (~70 minutes)	No	No differences in TT performance. 2 subjects experienced gastrointestinal distress with higher MCT intake. Higher FFA with MCT but no change in CHO oxidation.
Jeukendrup et al. 1998	9 endurance-trained male cyclists/ triathletes Crossover design	20 mL/kg of 10% CHO or 10% CHO + 5% MCT or 5% MCT or placebo Total intake of MCT = 86 g	Cycling • 2 hours @ 60% $VO_{2\,max}$ + TT (~15 minutes)	No	No difference between CHO, CHO + MCT or placebo (~14 minutes) but MCT alone impaired performance (17.3 minutes). MCT + CHO showed slightly higher fat oxidation than CHO alone. No glycogen sparing.
Van Zyl et al. 1996	6 endurance-trained cyclists Crossover design	2 L of 4.3% MCT or 10% CHO or 10% CHO + 4.3% MCT Total intake of MCT = 86 g	Cycling • 2 hours @ 60% $VO_{2\,max}$ + 40 km TT (~70 minutes)	Yes	MCT + CHO enhanced TT performance times (65.1 minutes) compared with CHO (66.8 minutes) and MCT (72.1 minutes). Increase in FFA and glycogen sparing with MCT + CHO.

acid (FFA) concentrations and allowed glycogen sparing reported a performance benefit at the end of prolonged exercise (Van Zyl et al. 1996). However, these metabolic (and performance) benefits may be compromised when exercise is commenced with higher insulin levels, as is the case following a CHO-rich pre-exercise meal (Goedecke et al. 1999; Angus et al. 2000). Critical to the whole issue is the ability of subjects to tolerate the substantial amount of MCT oils required to have a metabolic impact. Jeukendrup and colleagues found that the gastrointestinal tolerance of MCT is limited to a total intake of about 30 g, which would limit its fuel contribution to 3–7% of the total energy expenditure during typical ultra-endurance events (Jeukendrup et al. 1995). At greater intakes, subjects report gastrointestinal reactions that range in severity from insignificant (Van Zyl et al. 1996) to performance-limiting (Jeukendrup et al. 1998; Goedecke et al. 2005). Differences in gastrointestinal tolerance between studies or within studies may reflect differences in the mean chain length of MCTs found in the supplements, or increased tolerance in some athletes due to constant exposure to MCTs. The intensity and mode of exercise may also affect gastrointestinal symptoms.

In summary, although some CHO gels are marketed with the addition of MCTs, there is little evidence to support an ergogenic effect from these special products. In fact, Goedecke and colleagues (2005) reported a performance decrement in an ultra-endurance protocol following the intake of MCTs before and during cycling. This appeared to have causes other than the gastrointestinal disturbances, since all subjects experienced an impairment of time trial performance, while only half the group reported gastrointestinal problems.

16.37

Supplements in Group D of the AIS Sports Supplement Program

While we do not typically consider supplements that are prohibited for use under anti-doping codes, the case of glycerol for hyperhydration is still of interest. At the time of publication of this edition, it was proposed that glycerol be added to the WADA List of Prohibited Substances and Methods as a plasma expander. Since this decision is still pending, and because glycerol hyperhydration may have some value for non-elite athletes and others whose occupational activities expose them to situations in which moderate–severe fluid deficits occur (e.g. firefighters), we will consider the potential value of hyperhydration prior to exercise in hot conditions.

16.32

Glycerol

Glycerol, a three-carbon alcohol, provides the backbone to the triglyceride molecule. It is released during lipolysis and slowly metabolized via the liver and kidneys. Athletes are interested in glycerol not for its energy potential but, rather, its role as a hyperhydration agent. Oral intake of glycerol, via glycerine or special hyperhydration supplements, achieves a rapid absorption and distribution of glycerol around all body fluid compartments, adding to osmotic pressure. When a substantial volume of fluid is consumed simultaneously with glycerol, there is an expansion of fluid spaces and retention of this fluid. Effective protocols for glycerol hyperhydration are 1–1.5 g/kg glycerol with an intake of 25–35 mL/kg of fluid. Typically, such a protocol achieves a fluid expansion or retention of about 600 mL above a fluid bolus alone via a reduction in urinary volume (see review by Robergs & Griffin 1998).

Glycerol hyperhydration may be useful in the preparation for events that challenge fluid status and thermoregulation, for example for exercise at high intensity and/or in hot and humid environments, where sweat losses are high and opportunities to replace fluid are substantially less than the rates of fluid loss. It may also be useful to enhance the recovery of a moderate-to-large fluid deficit, for example in brief recovery periods between events or important training sessions, or between the weigh-in and competition following 'weight making' strategies in weight-division sports. Scientific investigations have focused on its potential for hyperhydrating prior to an endurance event (see Table 16.17 overleaf).

Some of the apparent inconsistency in the results of these investigations occurs because of differences in study methodologies. For example, some studies have investigated the effect of glycerol in assisting the body to retain larger amounts of a fluid bolus consumed in the hours before exercise, whereas others have used protocols in which glycerol is consumed with only a modest fluid intake (Inder et al. 1998). At present, the best-supported scenario involves the use of glycerol to maximize the retention of fluid bolus just prior to an event in which a substantial fluid deficit cannot be prevented. In some, but not all, studies of this type, glycerol hyperhydration has been associated with performance benefits, particularly in well-trained athletes (Hitchins et al. 1999; Anderson et al. 2001; Coutts et al. 2002). However, the mechanism for this effect is not clear, since the theoretical advantages of increased sweat losses and greater capacity for heat dissipation, and attenuation of cardiac and thermoregulatory challenges, are not consistently seen. Further investigation is needed to replicate and explain performance benefits.

Side effects reported by some subjects following glycerol use include nausea, gastrointestinal distress and headaches resulting from increased intracranial pressure. Fine-tuning of protocols may reduce the risk of these problems, yet some individuals may remain at a greater risk than others. Even when it is permissible to use glycerol hyperhydration strategies during sport or occupational activities in hot conditions, it should remain an activity that is used only after adequate experimentation and fine-tuning have occurred.

Summary 16.39

Sports dietitians frequently observe a chaotic pattern of use of supplements and sports foods by athletes and coaches, and the appearance on the market of an almost never-ending range of products that are claimed to achieve benefits needed to enhance sports performance. The poor regulation of supplements and sports foods in many countries allows athletes and coaches to be the target of marketing campaigns based on exaggerated claims and hype rather than documented benefits. However, scientific study has identified a number of products that offer true benefits to performance or the achievement of nutritional goals.

A systematic approach to educating athletes and coaches about supplements and sports foods, and managing their provision to athletes and teams, can allow sportspeople to include the successful use of these products with the activities that underpin optimal performance.

TABLE 16.17 PLACEBO-CONTROLLED CROSSOVER DESIGNED STUDIES OF GLYCEROL HYPERHYDRATION AND PERFORMANCE; FOR UPDATES SEE http://www.ausport.gov.au/ais/nutrition/supplements

STUDY	SUBJECTS	GLYCEROL DOSE	EXERCISE PROTOCOL	ENHANCED PERFORMANCE	COMMENTS
Coutts et al. 2002	7 male + 3 female well-trained triathletes Crossover design Difference in conditions: • hot day (30°C) • warm day (25°C)	1.2 g/kg BM + 25 mL/kg sports drink, 2 hours pre-exercise (compared with sports drink placebo)	Olympic distance triathlon (field conditions) Hot conditions 25–30°C	Yes	Decrease in triathlon performance (especially run time) between warm and hot conditions was greater in placebo group (11:40 minutes) than glycerol group (1:47 minutes). Greatest difference in times between placebo and glycerol group was found on hot day. Hyperhydration increased fluid retention of drink and reduced diuresis.
Anderson et al. 2001	6 well-trained male cyclists Crossover design	1 g/kg with 20 mL/kg low-joule cordial (compared with low-joule cordial overload)	Cycling • 90 minutes @ 98% LT + 15 minutes TT hot environment (35°C)	Yes	Glycerol allowed retention of additional 400 mL of fluid above hyperhydration with cordial alone. 5% improvement in work done in 15 minutes TT. No change in muscle metabolism. Reduced rectal temperature at 90 minutes with glycerol trial.
Hitchins et al. 1999	8 well-trained male cyclists Crossover design	1 g/kg with 22 mL/kg dilute sports drink, 2.5 hours pre-exercise (compared with sports drink overload)	Cycling • 30 minutes @ fixed power + 30 minutes TT. Hot environment (32°C)	Yes	Glycerol treatment expanded body water by 600 mL and increased (5%) work achieved in TT. This was achieved largely by preventing the drop in power seen at the start of placebo TT. No difference in power profile at end of TTs. No difference in cardiovascular, thermoregulatory, RPE between trials despite differences in power output.

Inder et al. 1998	8 highly trained male triathletes Crossover design	1 g/kg with 500 mL water, 4 hours pre-exercise (compared with 500 mL water)	Cycling • 60 minutes @ 70% $VO_{2\,max}$ + incremental ride to exhaustion	No	Glycerol was consumed with a modest fluid load. No increase in pre-exercise hydration status, sweat losses or urine production during exercise. No difference in time to exhaustion or workload reached. Three subjects experienced gastrointestinal problems with glycerol.
Latzka et al. 1998	8 heat-acclimatized athletes Crossover design	1.2 g/kg LBM + 29 mL/kg water, 1 hour pre-exercise (compared with water hyperhydration or control)	Running • Treadmill running at 55% $VO_{2\,max}$ until exhaustion or high rectal temperature. Hot environment (35°C) without further fluid intake	Yes (better than control but equal to water hyperhydration)	Both hyperhydration trials increased body fluid by ~1400 mL. Time to exhaustion longer in both trials compared with control. Performance changes not explained by differences in sweat losses, cardiac output or temperature control. Some gastrointestinal and headache symptoms with glycerol.
Montner et al. 1996	11 active male and female cyclists, 7 active male and female cyclists Crossover design	1.2 g/kg with 26 mL/kg water, 1 hour pre-exercise, same pre-treatment + sports drink during exercise	Cycling • Cycling @ 60% Wmax until exhaustion	Yes	Reduced heart rate and increased time to exhaustion with pre-exercise glycerol treatment by ~20%.

RPE = rating of perceived exertion, TT = time trial

REFERENCES

Alford C, Cox H, Wescott R. The effects of Red Bull Energy Drink on human performance and mood. Amino Acids 2001;21:139–50.

Allen JD, McLung J, Nelson AG, Welsch M. Ginseng supplementation does not enhance healthy young adults' peak aerobic exercise performance. J Am Coll Nutr 1998;17:462–6.

American Academy of Pediatrics Committee on Sports Medicine and Fitness. Position on use of performance-enhancing substances. Pediatrics 2005;115:1103–6.

American College of Sports Medicine. Roundtable: The physiological and health effects of oral creatine supplementation. Med Sci Sports Exerc 2000;32:706–17.

Anderson ME, Bruce CR, Fraser SF, Stepto NK, Klein R, Hopkins WG, Hawley JA. Improved 2000-metre rowing performance in competitive oarswomen after caffeine ingestion. Int J Sport Nutr Exerc Metab 2000;10:436–47.

Anderson MJ, Cotter JD, Garnham AP, Casley DJ, Febbraio MA. Effect of glycerol-induced hyperhydration on thermoregulation and metabolism in the heat. Int J Sport Nutr Exerc Metab 2001;11:315–33.

Angus DJ, Hargreaves M, Dancey J, Febbraio MA. Effect of carbohydrate or carbohydrate plus medium-chain triglyceride ingestion on cycling time trial performance. J Appl Physiol 2000;88:113–19.

Antonio J, Sanders MS, Kalman D, Woodgate D, Street C. The effects of high-dose glutamine ingestion on weightlifting performance. J Strength Cond Res 2002;16:157–60.

Antonio J, Sanders MS, Van Gammeren D. The effects of bovine colostrum supplementation on body composition and exercise performance in active men and women. Nutrition 2001;17:243–7.

Ariel G, Saville W. Anabolic steroids: the physiological effects of placebos. Med Sci Sports Exerc 1972;4:124–6.

Artioli GG, Gualano B, Coelho DF, Benatti FB, Gailey AW, Lancha AH, Jr. Does sodium-bicarbonate ingestion improve simulated judo performance? Int J Sport Nutr Exerc Metab 2007;17:206–17.

Bahrke MS, Morgan WP. Evaluation of the ergogenic properties of ginseng. Sports Med 1994;18:229–48.

Bahrke MS, Morgan WR. Evaluation of the ergogenic properties of ginseng: an update. Sports Med 2000;29:113–33.

Baylis A, Cameron-Smith D, Burke LM. Inadvertent doping though supplement use by athletes: assessment and management of the risk in Australia. Int J Sport Nutr Exerc Metab 2001;11: 365–83.

Bell DG, McLellan TM. Exercise endurance 1, 3, and 6 h after caffeine ingestion in caffeine users and nonusers. J Appl Physiol 2002;93:1227–34.

Bell DG, McLellan TM. Effect of repeated caffeine ingestion on repeated exhaustive exercise endurance. Med Sci Sports Exerc 2003;35:1348–54.

Bemben MG, Lamont HS. Creatine supplementation and exercise performance. Recent findings. Sports Med 2005;35:107–25.

Berardi JM, Ziegenfuss TN. Effects of ribose supplementation on repeated sprint performance in men. Int J Sport Nutr Exerc Metab 2003;17:47–52.

Bird SR, Wiles J, Robbins J. The effect of sodium bicarbonate ingestion on 1500-m racing time. J Sports Sci 1995;13:399–403.

Bishop D, Edge J, Davis C, Goodman C. Induced metabolic alkalosis affects muscle metabolism and repeated-sprint ability. Med Sci Sports Exerc 2004;36:807–13.

Bishop D, Claudius B. Effects of induced metabolic alkalosis on prolonged intermittent-sprint performance. Med Sci Sports Exerc 2005;37:759–67.

Blue JG, Lombardo JA. Steroids and steroid-like compounds. Clin Sports Med 1999;18:667–89.

Bonetti A, Solito F, Carmosino G, Bargossi AM, Fiorella PL. Effect of ubidecarenone oral treatment on aerobic power in middle-aged trained subjects. J Sports Med Phys Fitness 2000;40:51–7.

Branch JD. Effect of creatine supplementation on body composition and performance: a meta-analysis. Int J Sport Nutr Exerc Metab 2003;13:198–226.

Braun B, Clarkson PM, Freedson PS, Kohl RL. Effects of coenzyme Q10 supplementation and exercise performance, $VO_{2\ max}$, and lipid perodixation in trained subjects. Int J Sport Nutr 1991;1:353–65.

Brinkworth GD, Buckley JD. Concentrated bovine colostrum protein supplementation reduces the incidence of self-reported symptoms of upper respiratory tract infection in adult males. Eur J Nutr 2003;42:228–32.

Brinkworth GD, Buckley JD, Bourdon PC, Gulbin JP, David AZ. Oral bovine colostrum supplementation enhances buffer capacity but not rowing performance in elite female rowers. Int J Sport Nutr Exerc Metab 2002;12:349–63.

Brinkworth GD, Buckley JD, Slavotinek JP, Kurmis AP. Effect of bovine colostrum supplementation on the composition of resistance trained and untrained limbs in healthy young men. Eur J Appl Physiol 2004;91:53–60.

Broad EM, Maughan RJ, Galloway SD. Carbohydrate, protein, and fat metabolism during exercise after oral carnitine supplementation in humans. Int J Sport Nutr Exerc Metab 2008;18: 567–84.

Bruce CR, Anderson ME, Fraser SF, Stepto NK, Klein R, Hopkins WG, Hawley JA. Enhancement of 2000-m rowing performance after caffeine ingestion. Med Sci Sports Exerc 2000;32:1958–63.

Buckley JD, Abbott MJ, Brinkworth GD, Whyte PBD. Bovine colostrum supplementation during endurance running training improves recovery, but not performance. J Sci Med Sport 2002;5: 65–79.

Buckley JD, Brinkworth GD, Abbott MJ. Effect of bovine colostrum on anaerobic exercise performance and plasma insulin-like growth factor. J Sports Sci 2003;21:577–88.

Burke LM. An interview with Dr Gary Green about supplements and doping problems from an NCAA perspective. Int J Sport Nutr Exerc Metab 2001;11:397–400.

Burke LM. Caffeine and sports performance. Appl Physiol Nutr Metab 2008;33:1319–34.

Campbell WW, Beard JL, Joseph LJ, Davey SL, Evans WJ. Chromium picolinate supplementation and resistive training by older men: effects on iron-status and hematologic indexes. Am J Clin Nutr 1997;66:944–9.

Candow DG, Chilibeck PD, Burke DG, Davison KS, Smith-Palmer T. Effect of glutamine supplementation combined with resistance training in young adults. Eur J Appl Physiol 2001;86:142–9.

Cardinal BJ, Engels HJ. Ginseng does not enhance psychological well-being in healthy, young adults: results of a double blind, placebo-controlled, randomized clinical trial. J Am Diet Assoc 2001;101:655–60.

Cerretelli P, Marconi C. L-carnitine supplementation in humans. The effects on physical performance. Int J Sports Med 1990;11:1–14.

Chanutin A. The fate of creatine when administered to man. J Biol Chem 1926;67:29–37.

Chong SKF, Oberholzer VGP. Ginseng—is there a clinical use in medicine? Postgrad Med 1988;65:841–6.

Clancy SP, Clarkson PM, DeCheke ME, Nosaka K, Freedson PS, Cunningham JJ, Valentine B. Effects of chromium picolinate supplementation on body composition, strength, and urinary chromium loss in football players. Int J Sport Nutr 1994;4:142–53.

Clark VR, Hopkins WG, Hawley JA, Burke LM. Placebo effect of carbohydrate feedings during a 40-km cycling time trial. Med Sci Sports Exerc 2000;32:1642–7.

Clarkson PM. Nutritional ergogenic aids: carnitine. Int J Sport Nutr 1992;2:185–90.

Cohen BS, Nelson AG, Prevost MC, Thompson GD, Marx BD, Morris GS. Effects of caffeine ingestion on endurance racing in heat and humidity. Eur J Appl Physiol 1996;73:358–63.

Colgan M. Inosine. Muscle and Fitness 1988;49:94–6, 204, 206, 210.

Colombani P, Wenk C, Kunz I, Krahenbuhl S, Kuhnt M, Arnold M, Frey-Rindova P, Frey W, Langhans W. Effects of L-carnitine supplementation on physical performance and energy metabolism of endurance-trained athletes: a double-blind crossover field study. Eur J App Phys 1996;73:434–9.

Conway KJ, Orr R, Stannard SR. Effect of a divided dose of endurance cycling performance, postexercise urinary caffeine concentration and plasma paraxanthine. J Appl Physiol 2003;94:1557–62.

Coombes JS, Conacher M, Austen SK, Marshall PA. Dose effects of oral bovine colostrum on physical work capacity in cyclists. Med Sci Sports Exerc 2002;34:1184–8.

Coombes JS, Hamilton KL. The effectiveness of commercially available sports drinks. Sports Med 2000;29:181–209.

Costill DL, Dalsky GP, Fink WJ. Effects of caffeine ingestion on metabolism and exercise performance. Med Sci Sports Exerc 1978;10:155–8.

Coutts A, Reaburn P, Mummery K, Holmes M. The effect of glycerol hyperhydration on Olympic distance triathlon performance in high ambient temperatures. Int J Sport Nutr Exerc Metab 2002;12:105–19.

Cox GR, Desbrow B, Montgomery PG, Anderson ME, Bruce CR, Macrides TA, Martin DT, Moquin A, Roberts A, Hawley JA, Burke LM. Effect of different protocols of caffeine intake on metabolism and endurance performance. J Appl Physiol 2002;93:990–9.

Crooks CV, Wall CR, Cross ML, Rutherfurd-Markwick KJ. The effect of bovine colostrum supplementation on salivary IgA in distance runners. Int J Sport Nutr Exerc Metab 2006;16:47–64.

Crowe MJ, O'Connor DM, Lukins JE. The effects of B-hydroxy-B-methylbutyrate (HMB) and HMB/creatine supplementation on indices of health in highly trained athletes. Int J Sport Nutr Exerc Metab 2003;13:184–97.

Davis JM, Welsh RS, Alderson NA. Effects of carbohydrate and chromium ingestion during intermittent high-intensity exercise to fatigue. Int J Sport Nutr Exerc Metab 2000;10:476–85.

De Bock K, Eijnde BO, Ramaekers M, Hespel P. Acute *Rhodiola rosea* intake can improve endurance exercise performance. Int J Sport Nutr Exerc Metab 2004;14:298–307.

Decombaz J, Bury A, Hager C. HMB meta-analysis and the clustering of data sources (letter to editor). J Appl Physiol 2003;95:2180–2.

Decombaz J, Deriaz O, Acheson K, Gmuender B, Jequier E. Effect of L-carnitine on submaximal exercise metabolism after depletion of muscle glycogen. Med Sci Sports Exerc 1993;25:733–40.

Dennig H, Talbot JH, Edwards HT, Dill B. Effects of acidosis and alkalosis upon the capacity for work. J Clin Invest 1931;9:601–13.

Derave W, Ozdemir MS, Harris RC, Pottier A, Reyngoudt H, Koppo K, Wise JA, Achten E. Beta-alanine supplementation augments muscle carnosine content and attenuates fatigue during repeated isokinetic contraction bouts in trained sprinters. J Appl Physiol 2007;103:1736–43.

Desbrow B, Hughes R, Leveritt M, Scheelings P. An examination of consumer exposure to caffeine from retail coffee outlets. Food Chem Toxicol 2007;45:1588–92.

Dill DB, Edwards HT, Talbot JH. Alkalosis and the capacity for work. J Biol Chem 1932;97:58–9.

Dodd SL, Brooks E, Powers SK, Tulley R. The effects of caffeine on graded exercise performance in caffeine naive versus habituated subjects. Eur J Appl Physiol 1991;62:424–9.

Doherty M, Smith PM. Effects of caffeine ingestion on exercise testing. Int J Sport Nutr Exerc Metab 2004;14:626–46.

Doherty M, Smith PM. Effects of caffeine ingestion on rating of perceived exertion during and after exercise: a meta-analysis. Scand J Med Sci Sports 2005;15:69–78.

Douroudos II, Fatouros IG, Gourgoulis V, Jamurtas AZ, Tsitsios T, Hatzinikolaou A, Margonis K, Mavromatidis K, Taxildaris K. Dose-related effects of prolonged $NaHCO_3$ ingestion during high-intensity exercise. Med Sci Sports Exerc 2006; 38:1746–53.

Dowling EA, Redondo DR, Branch JD, Jones SGM, Williams MH. Effect of *Eleutherococcus senticosus* on submaximal and maximal exercise performance. Med Sci Sports Exerc 1996;28:482–9.

Earnest CP, Morss GM, Wyatt F, Jordan AN, Colson S, Church TS, Fitzgerald Y, Autrey L, Jurca R, Lucia A. Effects of a commercial herbal-based formula on exercise performance in cyclists. Med Sci Sports Exerc 2004;36:504–9.

Edge J, Bishop D, Goodman C. Effects of chronic $NaHCO_3$ ingestion during interval training on changes to muscle buffer capacity, metabolism, and short-term endurance performance. J Appl Physiol 2006;101:918–25.

Engels HJ, Fahlman MM, Wirth JC. Effects of ginseng on secretory IgA, performance, and recovery from interval exercise. Med Sci Sports Exerc 2003;35:690–6.

Engels HJ, Kolokouri I, Cieslak TJ, Wirth JC. Effects of ginseng supplementation on supramaximal exercise performance and short-term recovery. J Strength Cond Res 2001;15:290–5.

Evans GW. The effect of chromium picolinate on insulin controlled parameters in humans. Int J Bio Med Res 1989;11:163–80.

Evans GW. Chromium picolinate is an efficacious and safe supplement (letter). Int J Sport Nutr 1993;3:117–22.

Falk DJ, Heelan KA, Thyfault JP, Koch AJ. Effects of effervescent creatine, ribose, and glutamine supplementation on muscular strength, muscular endurance, and body composition. J Strength Cond Res 2003;17:810–16.

Forsberg AM, Nilsson E, Werneman J, Bergstrom J, Hultman E. Muscle composition in relation to age and sex. Clin Sci 1991;81:249–56.

Fredholm B, Battig K, Holmen J, Nehlig A, Zvartau E. Actions of caffeine in the brain with special reference to factors that contribute to its widespread use. Pharmacol Rev 1999;51:83–133.

Froiland K, Koszewski W, Hingst J, Kopecky L. Nutritional supplement use among college athletes and their sources of information. Int J Sport Nutr Exerc Metab 2004;14:104–20.

Gaffney BT, Hugel HM, Rich PA. The effects of *Eleutherococcus senticosus* and *Panax ginseng* on steroidal hormone indices of stress and lymphocyte subset numbers in endurance athletes. Life Sci 2001;70:431–42.

Gallagher PM, Carrithers JA, Godard MP, Schulze KE, Trappe SW. Beta-hydroxy-beta-methyl-butyrate ingestion, Part I: effects on strength and fat free mass. Med Sci Sports Exerc 2000;32:2109–15.

Gao J, Costill DL, Horswill CA, Park SH. Sodium bicarbonate ingestion improves performance in interval swimming. Eur J App Phys 1988;58:171–4.

Geyer H, Parr MK, Koehler K, Mareck U, Schänzer W, Thevis M. Nutritional supplements cross-contaminated and faked with doping substances. J Mass Spectrom 2008;43:892–902.

Geyer H, Parr MK, Mareck U, Reinhart U, Schrader Y, Schanzer W. Analysis of non-hormonal nutritional supplements for anabolic-androgenic steroids—results of an international study. Int J Sports Med 2004;25:124–9.

Goedecke JH, Clark VR, Noakes TD, Lambert EV. The effects of medium-chain triacylglycerol and carbohydrate ingestion on ultra-endurance exercise performance. Int J Sport Nutr Exerc Metab 2005;15:15–28.

Goedecke JH, Elmer-English R, Dennis SC, Schloss I, Noakes TD, Lambert EV. Effects of medium-chain triacylglycerol ingested with carbohydrate on metabolism and exercise performance. Int J Sport Nutr 1999;9:35–47.

Goldfinch J, McNaughton L, Davies P. Induced metabolic alkalosis and its effects on 400-m racing time. Eur J App Phys 1988;57:45–8.

Gorostiaga EM, Maurer CA, Eclache JP. Decrease in respiratory quotient during exercise following L-carnitine supplementation. Int J Sports Med 1989;10:169–74.

Goulet EDB. Assessment of the effects of *Eleutherococcus senticosus* on endurance performance. Int J Sport Nutr Exerc Metab 2005;15:75–83.

Graham TE. Caffeine and exercise: metabolism, endurance and performance. Sports Med 2001a;31: 765–807.

Graham TE. Caffeine, coffee and ephedrine: impact on exercise performance and metabolism. Can J Appl Physiol 2001b;26(Suppl):103S–9S.

Graham TE, Hibbert E, Sathasivam P. Metabolic and exercise endurance effects of coffee and caffeine ingestion. J Appl Physiol 1998;85:883–9.

Graham TE, Spriet LL. Performance and metabolic responses to a high caffeine dose during prolonged exercise. J Appl Physiol 1991;71:2292–8.

Graham TE, Spriet LL. Metabolic, catecholamine, and exercise performance responses to various doses of caffeine. J Appl Physiol 1995;78:867–74.

Green AL, Hultman E, Macdonald IA, Sewell DA, Greenhaff PL. Carbohydrate ingestion augments skeletal muscle creatine accumulation during supplementation in man. Am J Physiol Endocrinol Metab 1996a;271:E812–26.

Green AL, MacDonald IA, Greenhaff PL. The effects of creatine and carbohydrate on whole body creatine retention in vegetarians. Proc Nutr Soc 1997;56:81A.

Green AL, Simpson EJ, Littlewood JJ, MacDonald IA, Greenhaff PL. Carbohydrate ingestion augments creatine retention during creatine feeding in humans. Acta Physiol Scand 1996b;158:195–202.

Greenhaff PL. Creatine. In: Maughan RJ, ed. Nutrition in sport. Oxford: Blackwell Science, 2000:367–78.

Greenhaff PL. The creatine-phosphocreatine system: there's more than one song in its repertoire. J Physiol (Lond) 2001;537:657.

Greenhaff PL, Bodin K, Soderlund K, Hultman E. Effect of oral creatine supplementation on skeletal phosphocreatine resynthesis. Am J Phys Endocrin Metab 1994;266:E725–30.

Greenwood M, Kreider RB, Greenwood L, Byars A. Cramping and injury incidence in collegiate football players are reduced by creatine supplementation. J Ath Train 2004;38:216–19.

Greenwood M, Kreider RB, Melton C, Rasmussen C, Lancaster S, Cantler E, Milnor P, Almada A. Creatine supplementation during college football training does not increase the incidence of cramping or injury. Mol and Cell Biochem 2003;244:83–8.

Greig C, Finch KM, Jones DA, Cooper M, Sargeant AJ, Forte CA. The effect of oral supplementation with L-carnitine on maximum and submaximum exercise capacity. Eur J App Phys 1987;56: 457–60.

Grunewald KK, Bailey RS. Commercially marketed supplements for bodybuilding athletes. Sports Med 1993;15:90–103.

Gurley BJ, Wang P, Gardner SF. Ephedrine-type alkaloid content of nutritional supplements containing *Ephedra sinica* (Ma Huang) as determined by high performance liquid chromatography. J Pharm Sc 1998;87:1547–53.

Hahm H, Kujawa J, Ausberger L. Comparison of melatonin products against USP's nutritional supplements standards and other criteria. J Am Pharm Assoc (Wash) 1999;39:27–31.

Hallmark MA, Reynolds TH, deSouza CA, Dotson CO, Anderson RA, Rogers MA. Effects of chromium and resistive training on muscle strength and body composition. Med Sci Sports Exerc 1996;28: 139–44.

Harris RC, Jones G, Hill CA, Kendrick IP, Boobis L, Kim C, Kim H, DangVH, Edge J, Wise JA. The carnosine content of V Lateralis in vegetarians and omnivores (abst). FASEB Journal 2007; 21:769.20

Harris RC, Jones G, Wise JA. The plasma concentration-time profile of beta-alanine using a controlled release formulation (Carnosyn) (abst). FASEB Journal 2008; 22: 701.9

Harris RC, Soderlund K, Hultman E. Elevation of creatine in resting and exercised muscle of normal subjects by creatine supplementation. Clin Sci 1992;83:367–74.

Harris RC, Tallon MJ, Dunnett M, Boobis L, Coakley J, Kim HJ, Fallowfield JL, Hill CA, Sale C, Wise JA. The absorption of orally supplied beta-alanine and its effect on muscle carnosine synthesis in human vastus lateralis. Amino Acids 2006;30:279–89.

Hasten DL, Rome EP, Franks BD, Hegsted M. Effects of chromium picolinate on beginning weight training students. Int J Sport Nutr 1992;2:343–50.

Haub MD, Potteiger JA, Nau KL, Webster MJ, Zebas CJ. Acute L-glutamine ingestion does not improve maximal effort exercise. J Sports Med Phys Fitness 1998;38:240–4.

Heigenhauser GJF, Jones NL. Bicarbonate loading. In: Lamb DR and Williams MH, eds. Perspectives in exercise science and sports medicine. Dubuque, IN: Brown & Benchmark, 1991:183–212.

Heinonen OJ. Carnitine and physical exercise. Sports Med 1996;22:109–32.

Hellsten Y, Skadhauge L, Bangsbo J. Effect of ribose supplementation on resynthesis of adenine nucleotides after intense training in humans. Am J Physiol Reg 2004;286:R182–8.

Hespel P, Op 't Eijnde B, Derave W, Richter EA. Creatine supplementation: exploring the role of the creatine kinase/phosphocreatine system in the human muscle. Can J Appl Physiol 2001; 26(Suppl):79S–102S.

Hill CA, Harris RC, Kim HJ, Harris BD, Sale C, Boobis LH, Kim CK, Wise JA. Influence of beta-alanine supplementation on skeletal muscle carnosine concentrations and high intensity cycling capacity. Amino Acids 2007;32:225–33.

Hitchins S, Martin DT, Burke L, Yates K, Fallon K, Hahn A, Dobson GP. Glycerol hyperhydration improves cycle time trial performance in hot humid conditions. Eur J App Phys 1999;80: 494–501.

Hoffman JR, Cooper J, Wendell M, Im J, Kang J. Effects of beta-hydroxy-beta-methylbutyrate on power performance and indices of muscle damage and stress during high-intensity training. J Strength Cond Res 2004;18:747–52.

Hoffman J, Ratamess N, Kang J, Mangine G, Faigenbaum A, Stout J. Effect of creatine and beta-alanine supplementation on performance and endocrine responses in strength/power athletes. Int J Sport Nutr Exerc Metab 2006;16:430–46.

Hoffman J, Ratamess NA, Ross R, Kang J, Magrelli J, Neese K, Faigenbaum AD, Wise JA. Beta-alanine and the hormonal response to exercise. Int J Sports Med 2008a;29:952–8.

Hoffman JR, Ratamess NA, Faigenbaum AD, Ross R, Kang J, Stout JR, Wise JA. Short-duration beta-alanine supplementation increases training volume and reduces subjective feelings of fatigue in college football players. Nutr Res 2008b;28:31–5

Hofman Z, Smeets R, Verlaan G, Van der Lugt R, Verstappen PA. The effect of bovine colostrum supplementation on exercise performance in elite field hockey players. Int J Sport Nutr Exerc Metab 2002;12:461–9.

Hopkins WG, Hawley JA, Burke LM. Design and analysis of research on sport performance enhancement. Med Sci Sports Exerc 1999;31:472–85.

Hsu CC, Ho MC, Lin LC, Su B, Hsu MC. American ginseng supplementation attenuates creatine kinase level induced by submaximal exercise in human beings. World J Gastroenterol 2005;11:5327–31.

Hultman E, Soderlund K, Timmons JA, Cederblad G, Greenhaff PL. Muscle creatine loading in men. J Appl Physiol 1996;81:232–7.

Hunter AM, St Clair Gibson A, Collins M, Lambert M, Noakes TD. Caffeine ingestion does not alter performance during a 100-km cycling time-trial performance. Int J Sport Nutr Exerc Metab 2002;12:438–52.

Inder WJ, Swanney MP, Donald RA, Prickett TCR, Hellemans J. The effect of glycerol and desmopressin on exercise performance and hydration in triathletes. Med Sci Sports Exerc 1998;30:1263–9.

Ivy JL, Costill DL, Fink WJ, Lower RW. Influence of caffeine and carbohydrate feedings on endurance performance. Med Sci Sports Exerc 1979;11:6–11.

Jeukendrup AE, Saris WHM, Schrauwen P, Brouns F, Wagenmakers AJM. Metabolic availability of medium-chain triglycerides coingested with carbohydrates during prolonged exercise. J Appl Physiol 1995;79:756–62.

Jeukendrup AE, Thielen JJHC, Wagenmakers AJM, Brouns F, Saris WHM. Effect of medium-chain triacylglycerol and carbohydrate ingestion during exercise on substrate utilization and subsequent cycling performance. Am J Clin Nutr 1998;67:397–404.

Jowko E, Ostaszewski P, Jank M, Sacharuk J, Zieniewicz A, Wilczak J, Nissen S. Creatine and beta-hydroxy-beta-methylbutyrate (HMB) additively increase lean body mass and muscle strength during a weight-training program. Nutrition 2001;17:558–66.

Juhn MS, Tarnopolsky M. Potential side-effects of oral creatine supplementation: a critical review. Clin J Sport Med 1998a;8:298–304.

Juhn MS, Tarnopolsky M. Oral creatine supplementation and athletic performance: a critical review. Clin J Sport Med 1998b;8:286–97.

Kendrick IP, Harris RC, Kim HJ, Kim CK, Dang VH, Lam TQ, Bui TT, Smith M, Wise JA. The effects of 10 weeks of resistance training combined with beta-alanine supplementation on whole body strength, force production, muscular endurance and body composition. Amino Acids 2008;34:547–54.

Knitter AE, Panton L, Rathmacher JA, Petersen A, Sharp R. Effects of beta-hydroxy-beta-methylbutyrate on muscle damage after a prolonged run. J Appl Physiol 2000;89:1340–4.

Kovacs EMR, Stegen JHCH, Brouns F. Effect of caffeinated drinks on substrate metabolism, caffeine excretion, and performance. J Appl Physiol 1998;85:709–15.

Kozyrskyj A. Herbal products in Canada. How safe are they? Can Fam Physician 1997;43:697–702.

Kraemer WJ, Volek JS. Creatine supplementation: its role in human performance. Clin Sports Med 1999;18:651–66.

Kreider RB, Ferreira M, Wilson M, Almada AL. Effects of calcium β-hydroxy-β-methylbutyrate (HMB) supplementation during resistance-training on markers of catabolism, body composition and strength. Int J Sports Med 1999;20:503–9.

Kreider RB, Melton C, Greenwood M, Rasmussen CJ, Lundberg J, Earnest C, Almada AL. Effects of oral D-ribose supplementation on anaerobic capacity and selected metabolic markers in healthy males. Int J Sport Nutr Exerc Metab 2003a;13:76–86.

Kreider RB, Melton C, Rasmussen CJ, Greenwood M, Lancaster S, Cantler EC, Milnor P, Almada AL. Long-term creatine supplementation does not significantly affect clinical markers of health in athletes. Mol and Cell Biochem 2003b;244:95–104.

Krumbach CJ, Ellis DR, Driskell JA. A report of vitamin and mineral supplement use among university athletes in a Division I institution. Int J Sport Nutr 1999;9:416–25.

Kuipers H, Van Breda E, Verlaan G, Smeets R. Effects of oral bovine colostrum supplementation on serum insulin-like growth factor 1 levels. Nutrition 2002;18:566–7.

Laaksonen R, Fogelholm M, Himberg JJ, Laakso J, Salorinne Y. Ubiquinone supplementation and exercise capacity in trained young and older men. Eur J App Phys 1995;72:95–100.

Lamboley CR, Royer D, Dionne IJ. Effects of beta-hydroxy-beta-methylbutyrate on aerobic-performance components and body composition in college students. Int J Sport Nutr Exerc Metab 2007;17: 56–69.

Latzka WA, Sawka MN, Montain SJ, Skrinar GS, Fielding RA, Matott RP, Pandolf KB. Hyperhydration: tolerance and cardiovascular effects during uncompensable exercise-heat stress. J Appl Physiol 1998;84:1858–64.

Lehmkuhl MJ, Malone M, Justice B, Trone G, Pistilli EE, Vinci D, Haff EE, Kilgore JL, Haff GG. The effects of 8 weeks of creatine monohydrate and glutamine supplementation on body composition and performance measures. J Strength Cond Res 2003;17:425–38.

Levafi RG. Response to GW Evans. Int J Sport Nutr 1993;3:120–1.

Levafi RG, Anderson RA, Keith RE, Wilson GD, McMillan JL, Stone MH. Efficacy of chromium supplementation in athletes: emphasis on anabolism. Int J Sport Nutr 1992;2:111–22.

Liang MT, Podolka TD, Chuang WJ. *Panax notoginseng* supplementation enhances physical performance during endurance exercise. J Strength Cond Res 2005;19:108–14.

Linderman J, Fahey TD. Sodium bicarbonate ingestion and exercise performance. Sports Med 1991;11:71–7.

Lindh AM, Peyrebrune MC, Ingham SA, Bailey DM, Folland JP. Sodium bicarbonate improves swimming performance. Int J Sports Med 2008;29:519–23.

Livolsi JM, Adams GM, Laguna PL. The effect of chromium picolinate on muscular strength and body composition in women athletes. J Strength Cond Res 2001;15:161–6.

Lukaski HC, Bolonchuk WW, Siders WA, Milne DB. Chromium supplementation and resistance training: effects on body composition, strength, and trace element status of men. Am J Clin Nutr 1996;63:954–63.

Malm C, Svensson M, Ekblom B, Sjodin B. Effects of ubiquinone-10 supplementation and high intensity training on physical performance in humans. Acta Physiol Scand 1997;161:379–84.

Malm C, Svensson M, Sjoberg B, Ekblom B, Sjodin B. Supplementation with ubiquinone-10 causes cellular damage during intense exercise. Acta Physiol Scand 1996;157:511–12.

Marconi C, Sassi G, Carpinelli A, Cerretelli P. Effects of L-carnitine loading on the aerobic and anaerobic performance of endurance athletes. Eur J App Phys 1985;54:131–5.

Massad SJ, Shier NW, Koceja DM, Ellis NT. High school athletes and nutritional supplements: a study of knowledge and use. Int J Sport Nutr 1995;5:232–45.

Matson LG, Tran ZT. Effects of sodium bicarbonate ingestion on anaerobic performance: a meta-analytic review. Int J Sport Nutr 1993;3:2–28.

Maughan RJ. Contamination of dietary supplements and positive drug tests in sport. J Sports Sci 2005:23;883–9.

Mayhew DL, Mayhew JL, Ware JS. Effects of long-term creatine supplementation on liver and kidney functions in American college football players. Int J Sport Nutr Exerc Metab 2002;12:453–60.

McLellan TM, Bell DG. The impact of prior coffee consumption on the subsequent ergogenic effect of anhydrous caffeine. Int J Sport Nutr Exerc Metab 2004;14:698–708.

McNaughton L, Backx K, Palmer G, Strange N. Effects of chronic bicarbonate ingestion on the performance of high-intensity work. Eur J App Phys 1999a;80:333–6.

McNaughton L, Dalton B, Palmer G. Sodium bicarbonate can be used as an ergogenic aid in high-intensity, competitive cycle ergometry of 1 h duration. Eur J App Phys 1999b;80:64–9.

McNaughton L, Dalton B, Tarr J. Inosine supplementation has no effect on aerobic or anaerobic cycling performance. Int J Sport Nutr 1999c;9:333–44.

McNaughton L, Egan G, Caelli G. A comparison of Chinese and Russian ginseng as ergogenic aids to improve various facets of physical fitness. Int Clin Nutr Rev 1989;9:32–5.

McNaughton L, Thompson D. Acute versus chronic sodium bicarbonate ingestion and anaerobic work and power output. J Sports Med Phys Fitness 2001;41:456–62.

McNaughton LR, Cedaro R. The effect of sodium bicarbonate on rowing ergometer performance in elite rowers. Aust J Sci Med Sport 1991;23:66–9.

McNaughton LR. Bicarbonate and citrate. In: Maughan RJ, ed. Nutrition in sport. Oxford: Blackwell Science, 2000:393–404.

Mero A, Kahkonen J, Nykanen T, Parviainen T, Jokinen I, Takala T, Nikula T, Rasi S, Leppaluoto J. IGF-I, IgA, and IgG responses to bovine colostrum supplementation during training. J Appl Physiol 2002;93:732–9.

Mero AA, Keskinen KL, Malvela MT, Sallinen JM. Combined creatine and sodium bicarbonate supplementation enhances interval swimming. J Strength Cond Res 2004;18:306–10.

Mero A, Mikkulainen H, Riski J, Pakkanen R, Aalto J, Takala T. Effects of bovine colostrum supplement on serum IGF-1, IgG, hormone and saliva IgA during training. J Appl Physiol 1997;83:1144–51.

Montfoort MCE, Van Dieren L, Hopkins WG, Shearman JP. Effects of ingestion of bicarbonate, citrate, lactate, and chloride on sprint running. Med Sci Sports Exerc 2004;36:1239–43.

Montner P, Stark DM, Riedesel ML, Murata G, Robergs R, Timms M, Chick TW. Pre-exercise glycerol hydration improves cycling endurance time. Int J Sports Med 1996;17:27–33.

Morris AC, Jacobs I, McLellan TM, Klugerman A, Wang LCH, Zamecnik J. No ergogenic effects of ginseng ingestion. Int J Sport Nutr 1996;6:263–71.

Nielsen AN, Mizuno M, Ratkevicius A, Mohr T, Rohde M, Mortensen SA, Quistorff B. No effect of antioxidant supplementation in triathletes on maximal oxygen uptake, 31P-NMRS detected muscle energy metabolism and muscle fatigue. Int J Sports Med 1999;20:154–8.

Nissen S, Sharp R, Ray M, Rathmacher JA, Rice D, Fuller JC, Connelly AS, Abumrad N. Effect of leucine metabolite β-hydroxy-β-methylbutyrate on muscle metabolism during resistance-exercise training. J Appl Physiol 1996;81:2095–104.

Nissen SL, Sharp RL. Effect of dietary supplements on lean mass and strength gains with resistance exercise: a meta-analysis. J Appl Physiol 2003;94:651–9.

O'Connor DM, Crowe MJ. Effects of beta-hydroxy-beta-methylbutyrate and creatine monohydrate on aerobic and anaerobic capacity of highly trained athletes. J Sports Med Phys Fitness 2003;41:64–8.

Oopik V, Saaremets I, Medijainen L, Karelson K, Janson T, Timpmann S. Effects of sodium citrate ingestion before exercise on endurance performance in well-trained runners. Br J Sports Med 2003;37:485–9.

Op 't Eijnde B, van Leemputte M, Brouns F, Van Der Vusse GJ, Larbarque V, Ramaekers M, van Schuylenberg R, Verbessem P, Wijnen H, Hespel P. No effects of oral ribose supplementation on repeated maximal exercise and ATP resynthesis. J Appl Physiol 2001;91:2274–81.

Paddon-Jones D, Keech A, Jenkins D. Short-term B-hydroxy-B-methylbutyrate supplementation does not reduce symptoms of eccentric muscle damage. Int J Sport Nutr Exerc Metab 2001;11:442–50.

Panton LB, Rathmacher JA, Baier S, Nissen S. Nutritional supplementation of the leucine metabolite beta-hydroxy-beta-methylbutyrate (HMB) during resistance training. Nutrition 2000;16:734–9.

Parasrampuria J, Schwartz K, Petesch R. Quality control of dehydroepiandrosterone dietary supplement products. J Am Med Assoc 1998;280:1565.

Parcell AC, Smith JM, Schulthies SS, Myrer JW, Fellingham G. *Cordyceps sinensis* (CordyMax Cs-4) supplementation does not improve endurance exercise performance. Int J Sport Nutr Exerc Metab 2004;14:236–42.

Pasman WJ, van Baak MA, Jeukendrup AE, de Haan A. The effect of different dosages of caffeine on endurance performance time. Int J Sports Med 1995;16:225–30.

Perharic L, Shaw D, Collbridge M, House I, Leon C, Murray V. Toxicological problems resulting from exposure to traditional remedies and food supplements. Drug Saf 1994;11:284–94.

Perkins R, Williams MH. Effect of caffeine upon maximal muscular endurance of females. Med Sci Sports Exerc 1975;7:221–4.

Pieralisi G, Ripari P, Vecchiet L. Effects of standardised ginseng extract combined with dimethylaminoethanol bitartrate, vitamins, minerals and trace elements on physical performance during exercise. Clin Therapeut 1991;12:373–82.

Pierce EF, Eastman NW, Hammer WH, Lynn TD. Effect of induced alkalosis on swimming time trials. J Sports Sci 1992:255–9.

Poortmans JR, Auquier H, Renaut V, Durussel A, Saugy M, Brisson GR. Effect of short-term creatine supplementation on renal responses in men. Eur J App Phys 1997;76:566–7.

Potteiger JA, Nickel GL, Webster MJ, Haub MD, Palmer RJ. Sodium citrate ingestion enhances 30 km cycling performance. Int J Sports Med 1996a;17:7–11.

Potteiger JA, Webster MJ, Nickel GK, Haub MD, Palmer RJ. The effects of buffer ingestion on metabolic factors related to distance running performance. Eur J App Phys 1996b;72:365–71.

Price M, Moss P, Rance S. Effects of sodium bicarbonate ingestion on prolonged intermittent exercise. Med Sci Sports Exerc 2003;38:1303–8.

Pruscino CL, Ross ML, Gregory JR, Savage B, Flanagan TR. Effects of sodium bicarbonate, caffeine, and their combination on repeated 200-m freestyle performance. Int J Sport Nutr Exerc Metab 2008;18:116–130.

Ransone J, Neighbours K, Lefavi R, Chromiak J. The effect of B-hydroxy-B-methylbutyrate on muscular strength and body composition in collegiate football players. J Strength Cond Res 2003;17:34–9.

Rawson ES, Volek JS. Effects of creatine supplementation and resistance training on muscle strength and weightlifting performance. J Strength Cond Res 2003;17:822–31.

Rivers W, Webber H. The action of caffeine on the capacity for muscular work. J Physiol 1907; 36:33–47.

Robergs RA, Griffin SE. Glycerol: biochemistry, pharmacokinetics and clinical and practical applications. Sports Med 1998;26:145–67.

Roufs JB. Review of L-tryptophan and eosinophilia-myalgia syndrome. J Am Diet Assoc 1992;92: 844–50.

Rowbottom DG, Keast D, Morton AR. The emerging role of glutamine as an indicator of exercise stress and overtraining. Sports Med 1996;21:80–97.

Sahlin K. Metabolic factors in fatigue. Sports Med 1992;13:99–107.

Schabort EJ, Wilson G, Noakes TD. Dose-related elevations in venous pH with citrate ingestion do not alter 40-km cycling time-trial performance. Eur J App Phys 2000;83:320–7.

Shave R, Whyte G, Siemann A, Doggart L. The effects of sodium citrate ingestion on 3,000-metre time-trial performance. J Strength Cond Res 2001;15:230–4.

Shaw D, Leon C, Kolev S, Murray V. Traditional remedies and food supplements. A 5-year toxicological study (1991–1995). Drug Saf 1997;17:342–56.

Shing CM, Jenkins DG, Stevenson L, Coombes JS. The influence of bovine colostrum supplementation on exercise performance in highly trained cyclists. Br J Sports Med 2006;40:797–801.

Shing CM, Peake J, Suzuki K, Okutsu M, Pereira R, Stevenson L, Jenkins DG, Coombes JS. Effects of bovine colostrum supplementation on immune variables in highly trained cyclists. J Appl Physiol 2007;102:1113–22.

Siliprandi N, Di Lisa F, Pieralisi G, Ripari P, Maccari F, Menabo R, Giamberardino MA, Vecchiet L. Metabolic changes induced by maximal exercise in human subjects following L-carnitine administration. Biochim Biophys Acta 1990;1034:17–21.

Slater G, Jenkins D, Logan P, Lee H, Vukovich M, Rathmacher JA, Hahn AG. B-hydroxy-B-methylbutyrate (HMB) supplementation does not affect changes in strength or body composition during resistance training in trained men. Int J Sport Nutr Exerc Metab 2001;11:384–96.

Slater GJ, Jenkins D. B-hydroxy-B-methylbutyrate (HMB) supplementation and the promotion of muscle growth and strength. Sports Med 2000;30:105–16.

Smith AE, Moon JR, Kendall KL, Graef JL, Lockwood CM, Walter AA, Beck TW, Cramer JT, Stout JR. The effects of beta-alanine supplementation and high-intensity interval training on neuromuscular fatigue and muscle function. Eur J Appl Physiol 2009a;105:357–63.

Smith AE, Walter AA, Graef JL, Kendall KL, Moon JR, Lockwood CM, Fukuda DH, Beck TW, Cramer JT, Stout JR. Effects of beta-alanine supplementation and high-intensity interval training on endurance performance and body composition in men; a double-blind trial. J Int Soc Sports Nutr 2009b;11:6:5

Snider IP, Bazzarre TL, Murdoch SD, Goldfarb A. Effects of coenzyme athletic performance system as an ergogenic aid on endurance performance to exhaustion. Int J Sport Nutr 1992;2: 272–86.

Spriet LL. Ergogenic aids: recent advances and retreats. In: Lamb DR, Murray R, eds. Perspectives in exercise science and sports medicine. Carmel, IN: Cooper, 1997:185–238.

Starling RD, Trappe TA, Short KR, Sheffield-Moore M, Joszi AC, Fink WJ, Costill DL. Effect of inosine supplementation on aerobic and anaerobic cycling performance. Med Sci Sports Exerc 1996;28:1193–8.

Stephens FB, Constantin-Teodosiu D, Laithwaite D, Simpson EJ, Greenhaff PL. Insulin stimulates L-carnitine accumulation in human skeletal muscle. FASEB J 2006a 20:377–9.

Stephens FB, Constantin-Teodosiu D, Laithwaite D, Simpson EJ, Greenhaff PL. An acute increase in skeletal muscle carnitine content alters fuel metabolism in resting human skeletal muscle. J Clin Endocrinol Metab 2006b;91:5013–8.

Stephens TJ, McKenna MJ, Canny BJ, Snow RJ, McConell GK. Effect of sodium bicarbonate on muscle metabolism during intense endurance cycling. Med Sci Sports Exerc 2002;34:614–21.

Stoecker BJ. Chromium. In: Ziegler EE, Filer LJ, eds. Present knowledge in nutrition. Seventh edition. Washington: ILSI Press, 1996:344–52.

Stout JR, Cramer JT, Mielke M, O'Kroy J, Torok DJ, Zoeller RF. Effects of twenty-eight days of beta-alanine and creatine monohydrate supplementation on the physical working capacity at neuromuscular fatigue threshold. J Strength Cond Res 2006;20:928–31.

Stout JR, Cramer JT, Zoeller RF, Torok D, Costa P, Hoffman JR, Harris RC, O'Kroy J. Effects of beta-alanine supplementation on the onset of neuromuscular fatigue and ventilatory threshold in women. Amino Acids 2007;32:381–6.

Svensson M, Malm C, Tonkonogi M, Ekblom B, Sjodin B, Sahlin K. Effect of Q10 supplementation on tissue Q10 levels and adenine nucleotide catabolism during high-intensity exercise. Int J Sport Nutr 1999;9:166–80.

Tarnopolsky MA. Caffeine and endurance performance. Sports Med 1994;18:109–25.

Thomson JS. Beta-hydroxy-beta-methylbutyrate (HMB) supplementation of resistance trained men. Asia Pac J Clin Nutr 2004;13(Suppl):59S.

Tiryaki GR, Atterbom HA. The effects of sodium bicarbonate and sodium citrate on 600 m running time of trained females. J Sports Med Phys Fitness 1995;35:194–8.

Trappe SW, Costill DL, Goodpaster B, Vukovich MD, Fink WJ. The effects of L-carnitine supplementation on performance during interval swimming. Int J Sports Med 1994;15:181–5.

Trice I, Haymes EM. Effects of caffeine ingestion on exercise-induced changes during high-intensity intermittent exercise. Int J Sport Nutr 1995;5:37–44.

Van Gammeren D, Falk D, Antonio J. The effects of four weeks of ribose supplementation on body composition and exercise performance in healthy, young, male recreational body builders: a double-blind, placebo-controlled trial. Cur Therapeut Res 2002;63:486–95.

Van Thienen R, Van Proeyen K, Vanden Eynde B, Puype J, Lefere T, Hespel P. Beta-alanine improves sprint performance in endurance cycling. Med Sci Sports Exerc 2009;41:898–903.

Van Zyl CG, Lambert EV, Hawley JA, Noakes TD, Dennis SC. The effect of medium-chain triglyceride ingestion on fuel metabolism and cycling performance. J Appl Physiol 1996; 80:2217–25.

Vanakoski J, Kosunen V, Merirrine E, Seppala T. Creatine and caffeine in anaerobic and aerobic exercise: effects of physical performance and pharmacokinetic considerations. Int J Clin Pharmac Therapeut 1998;36:258–63.

Vecchiet L, Di Lisa F, Pieralisi G, Ripari P, Menabo R, Giamberardino MA, Siliprandi N. Influence of L-carnitine administration on maximal physical exercise. Eur J App Phys 1990;61:486–90.

Vistisen B, Nybo L, Xuebing X, Hoy CE, Kiens B. Minor amounts of plasma medium-chain fatty acids and no improved time trial performance after consuming lipids. J Appl Physiol 2003; 95:2434–43.

Vukovich MD, Costill DL, Fink WJ. Carnitine supplementation: effect on muscle carnitine and glycogen content during exercise. Med Sci Sports Exerc 1994;26:1122–9.

Vukovich MD, Dreifort GD. Effect of B-hydroxy-B-methylbutyrate on the onset of blood lactate accumulation and $VO_{2\ peak}$ in endurance-trained cyclists. J Strength Cond Res 2001;15:491–7.

Wagenmakers AJM. L-carnitine supplementation and performance in man. In: Brouns F, ed. Advances in nutrition and top sport. Basel: Karger, 1991:110–27.

Walker LS, Bemben MG, Bemben DA, Knehans AW. Chromium picolinate effects on body composition and muscular performance in wrestlers. Med Sci Sports Exerc 1998;30:1730–7.

Weston SB, Zhou S, Weatherby RP, Robson SJ. Does exogenous coenzyme Q10 affect aerobic capacity in endurance athletes? Int J Sport Nutr 1997;7:197–206.

Wiles JD, Bird SR, Hopkins J, Riley M. Effect of caffeinated coffee on running speed, respiratory factors, blood lactate and perceived exertion during 1500-m treadmill running. Br J Sports Med 1992;26:116–20.

Wilkes D, Geldhill N, Smyth R. Effect of acute induced metabolic alkalosis on 800-m racing time. Med Sci Sports Exerc 1983;15:277–80.

Williams MH, Kreider RB, Hunter DW, Somma CT, Shall LM, Woodhouse ML, Rokitzki L. Effect of inosine supplementation on 3-mile treadmill run performance and $VO_{2\ peak}$. Med Sci Sports Exerc 1990;22:517–22.

Ylikoski T, Piirainen J, Hanninen O, Penttinen J. The effect of coenzyme Q10 on the exercise performance of cross-country skiers. Mol Aspects Med 1997;18(Suppl):283S–90S.

Ziemba AW, Chmura J, Kaciuba-Uscilko H, Nazar K, Wisnik P, Gawronski W. Ginseng treatment improves psychomotor performance at rest and during graded exercise in young athletes. Int J Sport Nutr 1999;9:371–7.

Zoeller RF, Stout JR, O'kroy JA, Torok DJ, Mielke M. Effects of 28 days of beta-alanine and creatine monohydrate supplementation on aerobic power, ventilatory and lactate thresholds, and time to exhaustion. Amino Acids 2007;33:505–10.

Nutrition for the athlete's immune system: eating to stay well during training and competition

DAVID PYNE

Introduction

The links between nutrition, supplements and immunity in athletes undertaking high-level training generate considerable discussion in sporting circles. The diets of most athletes have sufficient energy, macro- and micronutrients to maintain health and immune function. In most circumstances, resistance to illness and infection is unlikely to be compromised in otherwise healthy athletes. However, there are two groups of athletes who may be more at risk of nutrition-related immune system disturbance: those athletes who voluntarily restrict energy and nutrient intake to make weight limits or for aesthetic and performance reasons (more commonly female athletes), and athletes who consume large amounts of energy and nutritional supplements in the expectation of performance improvements and/or muscle bulking (more commonly male athletes). Experimental evidence indicates that immune responses can be impaired by both inadequate and excessive intake of certain nutrients. Many athletes falsely assume that higher intake of nutrient supplements automatically elicits beneficial effects on health, immunity and performance.

A key consideration for clinicians is the combination of poor nutritional practices and the cumulative stress of intensive training on immune function. The stress of high-level athletic training is influenced by the intensity and duration of exercise, the fitness level of the athlete, and the balance between training loads and recovery practices. Just as poor nutrition can impair immune function, the clinical effects of infection can adversely affect nutritional status by suppressing appetite and nutrient absorption, and increasing nutrient losses and requirements (Calder & Jackson 2000). These observations lend support for the notion of a two-way interaction between nutrition and infective processes.

The immune system

The human immune system is comprised of physical, cellular and soluble elements that work in concert to defend the body's tissues against pathogenic agents, and promote repair and healing of tissues damaged by injury or trauma. The physical elements include the skin, epithelial cells, mucosal secretions and hair-like cilia that line the upper respiratory tract. The cellular (white blood cells such as neutrophils, lymphocytes and natural killer cells) and soluble (various proteins including immunoglobulins, complement, lactoferrin and lysozyme) elements work collectively to provide specific (acquired) and non-specific (innate) immunity. The immune system is linked integrally with the nervous and hormonal systems. Stress hormones such as adrenaline, noradrenaline and cortisol can exert potent immunomodulatory effects. There is intricate control of the immune system involving feed-forward and feed-back regulation, underpinned in part by a large group of cytokines or regulatory proteins that up- or down-regulate responses to pathogens or tissue damage (Malm 2002). The immune system is also characterized by redundancy and counter-regulation such that deficiencies or abnormalities in one aspect are usually compensated by other immune responses so that good health is maintained.

Immune function is influenced by a range of factors, including the presence of injury-related tissue damage and/or inflammation, physical stress of acute exercise or prolonged periods of training, psychological stress, environmental factors such as ambient temperature, the degree of pathogen exposure, and nutrition (Pyne et al. 2000). Immune cells require water, glucose, proteins and electrolytes to maintain normal functioning. The extent of relationships between conditions such as protein energy malnutrition and inadequate intake of carbohydrate, fat and micronutrients are well established (Chandra 1991, 1999). The emergence of exercise immunology and sports nutrition as legitimate scientific disciplines has facilitated ongoing interest in exercise, nutrition and immune function. Several reviews of exercise, nutrition and immune function in the sports science literature have been published (Bishop et al. 1999; Nieman 2001; Venkatraman & Pendergast 2002; Gleeson et al. 2004).

Athletes in periods of heavy training, or in the final preparations for competition, can show signs of perturbations in immune function. Several prospective and cross-sectional studies in a variety of sports have reported exercise or training-induced immunosuppression in some individuals. Typically, the immunosuppression is mild and transient in nature and without the long-term clinical consequences associated with clinically diagnosed immunosuppression associated with various diseases. Moreover, not all athletes with evidence of exercise- or training-induced immunosuppression will experience illness unless the magnitude of the immunosuppression is greater than the typical homeostatic limits of immune function (Smith 1995). A large 11-year retrospective study of the medical records of athletes resident at the Australian Institute of Sport (AIS) showed that approximately 10% did not report illness, while ~15% or 1 in 7 experienced four or more episodes of illness in a given scholarship year (Fricker et al. 2000). Athletes can be reassured that they can train hard without necessarily fearing the negative consequences of illness and impaired performance.

The importance of maintaining good health and adequate immune protection is highlighted by evidence that some athletes presenting with symptoms of illness have a higher risk of a substantial impairment in performance. However, given there is substantial between-subject variation in the likelihood that athletes with symptoms will suffer impairment, maintenance or even improvement in performance (Pyne et al. 2005), the onset of illness does not necessarily mean a poor performance will ensue. Athletes, coaches and support staff should employ a range of practical strategies, including nutritional practices, to maintain or improve immune function, and limit the risk of illness compromising training and competitive performance (Gleeson 2000; Pyne et al. 2000).

Clinical approach to maintaining immune function

Clinical advice for athletes trying to maintain or improve immune function in the context of nutrition and training centers on three key areas: long-term nutritional strategies during training and preparations for competition; short-term strategies to maintain immune function before, during and after acute bouts of exercise, training or competition; and nutritional strategies during periods of illness or infection. Athletes presenting with persistent or recurrent illness are typically seen by a physician for medical review. The review process can also include the sports dietitian, psychologist, team or individual coach, strength and conditioning coach, and sports physiologist. The review process should be broad-based and address issues such as medical history, training background and lifestyle. Practical issues—such as the typical home and normal training environment, and travel when the athletes are eating 'on the road' for domestic or international tournaments or competitions—should also be considered.

Long-term nutritional recommendations during training

The macronutrients CHO, fat and protein all play critical roles in maintaining immunocompetence. Unless dietary intake is extremely low or high, and excessive volumes of training are undertaken, immune function is unlikely to be substantially compromised. Athletes undertaking large volumes of training may consume less energy than expended, potentially compromising inflammatory and anti-oxidant mechanisms (Venkatraman & Pendergast 2002). Inadequate intake of protein can impair immune function, leading to an increased incidence of opportunistic infections (Chandra 1999). Inadequate protein can impair cell replication and protein synthesis necessary for the production of key immune cells and soluble factors such as immunoglobulins, acute phase proteins and cytokines. However, prolonged or extreme deficiencies of protein are unlikely in athletes undertaking high-level training or competition schedules. Even highly trained vegetarian athletes with low protein intakes appear to have normal immune function. Athletes who are overtrained or fatigued might benefit from a higher protein diet over a 2- or 3-week period (Venkatraman & Pendergast 2002). Two specific proteins, glutamine and colostrum, appear to boost immunity (Cynober 2001), but further research is required before definitive guidelines and recommendations for athletes and coaches can be established. There is also theoretical support for supplementation with lactoferrin, given its important role in antiviral and antibacterial defense (Lönnerdal 2009). Bovine lactoferrin, isolated by dairy technology, as well as recombinant human lactoferrin, are commercially available and can be added to foods and clinical products. Protein intakes of ~15% of total energy intake should be sufficient for most athletes (see Chapter 4).

Dietary CHO is a critical fuel source for both muscle and immune cells. The requirement for CHO by immune cells is greatly amplified during an immune response when cell proliferation is up-regulated. Glucose has both direct and indirect effects on immune function. Exercise or training-induced reduction in blood glucose has been linked to increased release of cortisol and decreased release of growth hormone in various athletic settings (Gleeson & Bishop 2000; Bishop et al. 2001, 2002). Greater perturbations in leucocyte and lymphocyte numbers, lymphocyte proliferative responses and cytokine production have been linked with exercise undertaken in a CHO-depleted state. Particular attention should be placed on the daily CHO intake during training and acute exercise (Tarnopolsky 2008). The recommendations for daily intakes of CHO scaled to the training load (see Chapter 14) should be a high priority.

In contrast to protein and CHO, there is relatively little information on the importance of fat intake in maintaining immune function in highly trained athletes. Immune function is influenced by the type of dietary fat and its utilization as a fuel during prolonged exercise. Low intakes of fat may compromise intramuscular energy stores and provide insufficient levels of essential micronutrients. One strategy that has attracted interest from researchers is whether manipulations of fat intake modulate the balance of pro- and anti-inflammatory cytokines. Some studies have examined whether high intakes of polyunsaturated fatty acids impair inflammation and immune function in athletes (Konig et al. 1997). It appears that increased intake of dietary fat can improve extended endurance performance without adverse effects on plasma levels of cortisol.

However, fatty acid supplementation during strenuous exercise in one study did not substantially influence pro- and anti-inflammatory cytokine balance (Toft et al. 2000).

An adequate intake of the minerals iron and zinc, and vitamins A, E, B6 and B12, is important for maintaining immune function. In most mixed western diets there is sufficient intake of vitamins and minerals to maintain immune function, and deficiencies are rare in athletic populations. Some researchers have suggested that supplementation with anti-oxidant vitamins and trace minerals such as vitamins E and C and β-carotene may be beneficial (Bishop et al. 1999). Athletes are also advised to consume foods rich in zinc, and supplementation may be useful for those individuals on low-calorie or vegetarian diets. However, megadoses of vitamins may have deleterious consequences for immune function, and in some circumstances elicit toxic effects. Iron plays an important role in immune function, although the clinical consequences of long-term supplementation are unclear. Vitamin E dosages in the range of 300–600 mg are known to impair lymphocyte proliferation (Prasad 1980) and increase oxidative and inflammatory cytokine responses during a triathlon (Nieman et al. 2004). Megadoses of vitamin A can impair inflammatory responses and complement formation (Bishop et al. 1999). Clearly, athletes should be educated to adopt prudent vitamin supplementation practices.

The health benefits of vitamin C supplementation have been debated widely in the general and medical communities for over 40 years. Vitamin C is thought to play important roles in various immune functions, including lymphocyte proliferation, neutrophil activity and viral replication (Peters 1997). Early studies by Peters and colleagues showed that daily 600 mg supplementation of vitamin C reduced the incidence of illness in runners undertaking an ultramarathon of 90 km (Peters et al. 1993). However, subsequent double-blind placebo-controlled studies using doses of vitamin C up to 1000 mg for 8 days (Himmelstein et al. 1998) or 2 months (Nieman et al. 1997) in runners have not been able to replicate the initial findings. Vitamin C supplementation by athletes may not have a consistent effect on markers of oxidative stress or muscle damage, and any linkage to immune perturbations remains speculative (Nieman et al. 2002).

Probiotics or yoghurt preparations contain so-called 'good' gut bacteria that are purported to enhance gut health and immunity. Although studies with athletes are lacking there is evidence in studies of healthy volunteers that probiotic administration can enhance discrete aspects of immune function (Kopp-Hoolihan 2001). The mechanisms by which probiotics exert their effects are largely unknown, but are thought to include modification of gut pH, production of antimicrobial compounds, and stimulation of immunomodulatory cells (Kopp-Hoolihan 2001). Marathon runners taking the probiotic *Lactobacillus rhamnosus* daily for 12 weeks had a similar rate of gastrointestinal illness to control subjects, but episodes were substantially shorter in duration (Kekkonen et al. 2007). Further studies on the clinical effects of probiotics are required before specific guidelines can be issued for clinicians, coaches and athletes.

In summary, few supplements have been shown to reduce substantially the risk of common respiratory and gut illness in athletes in randomized controlled trials (Akerström & Pedersen 2007). Further research is required on both macro- and micronutrient intake, supplementation, and health and performance outcomes in highly trained athletes.

Nutrition to maintain immune function during exercise

It is important to implement appropriate nutritional strategies before, during and after single events such as individual training sessions, a competitive game in the context of team sports, or single events or races for individual athletes. Longer endurance events, such as a marathon, triathlon or road cycling race, provide opportunities for athletes to ingest sports drinks, gels or foods for maintenance of fluid and energy levels. Given the importance of CHO in the energy supply during exercise, and its likely depletion after prolonged high-intensity exercise, the primary nutritional strategy during prolonged exercise is to replace glycogen and glucose. Current recommendations suggest that 30–60 g per hour of CHO in drinks or gels should attenuate various aspects of immunosuppression during prolonged exercise (Gleeson et al. 2004). The influence of this practice on clinical outcomes has not been evaluated. The post-event period is also a critical time for nutrient replenishment, particularly as it coincides with the so-called window of opportunity for infections to become established (Nieman 1993). The immune system can experience transient suppression in the first few hours after intense and/or prolonged exercise. Co-ingestion of CHO and protein should replenish critical sources of glucose and glutamine, and whole-body net protein balance (Howarth et al. 2009). Although plasma glutamine levels decrease during exercise, it is unclear whether immediate post-exercise supplementation of glutamine has a substantial effect on immune function (Gleeson & Bishop 2000). Another interesting question relates to the direct effect of fluid intake on immune function. A controlled trial comparing 2 hours of cycling at 65% of maximal oxygen uptake with and without fluid ingestion showed no substantial differences in neutrophil responses (Bishop et al. 2004). However, fluid replacement is still an important strategy during prolonged or intensive exercise, to maintain hydration levels and performance.

Nutritional intervention during illness

Despite the best of intentions, and careful self-management practices, most athletes will occasionally experience illness of varying type, severity and duration. Most of these illnesses in otherwise healthy athletes are usually mild and self-limiting in nature, with symptoms generally resolving in a few days. The general advice for athletes is to reduce the overall load (frequency, volume and intensity) of their training program. Where signs and/or symptoms of moderate to severe illness persist for several days, a medical opinion should be sought. The need for additional fluids during periods of illness is well established in clinical practice and home remedies. A series of studies with marathon and ultramarathon runners suggests that vitamin C supplementation can be effective in reducing the incidence of illness. There is some evidence that therapeutic ingestion of vitamin C and zinc at the onset of upper respiratory tract illness may be helpful in alleviating symptoms (Swain & Kaplan 1998) although other research on this practice is contradictory (Gleeson et al. 2004). There is ongoing interest in the use of phytosupplements (herbal preparations) such as *Echinacea*, which is purported to have important clinical effects (Barrett 2003). However, a placebo-controlled intervention trial involving the administration of *Echinacea* in 148 young adults presenting with symptoms of the common cold did not show any substantial health benefits (Barrett et al. 2002). Further research is needed to confirm the effectiveness of phytosupplements in boosting immune function and reducing signs and symptoms of illness in athletes.

Summary

Clinical and laboratory studies provide compelling evidence of a two-way interaction between nutrition and immune function. The combination of poor nutrition and heavy training loads in some athletes can exert measurable effects on immune function. A well-chosen diet meeting the underlying energy demands should provide sufficient macro- and micronutrients to maintain adequate immune function. Athletes on energy-restricted diets or undertaking very high training loads may benefit from supplements and specific nutritional strategies. Regular CHO ingestion during training and acute exercise can attenuate fluctuations in key hormones and immune parameters. The immunological and clinical benefits of megadoses of vitamins and minerals, particularly the anti-oxidant supplements of vitamin C and E, remain unclear. Further studies on glutamine and probiotics are required before specific clinical guidelines on these supplements can be developed.

References

Akerström TC, Pedersen BK. Strategies to enhance immune function for marathon runners: what can be done? Sports Med 2007;37:416–19.

Barrett BP, Brown RL, Locken K, et al. Treatment of the common cold with unrefined *Echinacea*: a randomized double-blind, placebo-controlled trial. Annals Int Med 2002;137:939–46.

Barrett B. Medicinal properties of *Echinacea*: critical review. Phytomed 2003;10:66–86.

Bishop NC, Blannin AK, Walsh NP, Gleeson M. Carbohydrate beverage ingestion and neutrophil degranulation responses following cycling to fatigue at 75% $VO_{2\ max}$. Int J Sports Med 2001;22:226–31.

Bishop NC, Blannin AK, Walsh NP, Robson PJ. Nutritional aspects of immunosuppression in athletes. Sports Med 1999;28:151–76.

Bishop NC, Gleeson M, Nicholas CW, Ali A. Influence of carbohydrate supplementation on plasma cytokine and neutrophil degranulation responses to high intensity intermittent exercise. Int J Sport Nutr Exer Metab 2002;12:145–56.

Bishop NC, Scanlon GA, Walsh NP, McCallum LJ, Walker GJ. No effect of fluid intake on neutrophil responses to prolonged cycling. J Sports Sci 2004;22:1091–8.

Calder PC, Jackson AA. Undernutrition, infection and immune function. Nutr Res Rev 2000;13:3–29.

Chandra RK. 1990 McCollum Award Lecture: nutrition and immunity—lessons from the past and new insights into the future. Am J Clin Nutr 1991;53:1087–101.

Chandra RK. Nutrition and immunology: from the clinic to cellular biology and back again. PNS 1999;58:681–3.

Cynober L. Do we have unrealistic expectations of the potential of immuno-nutrition? Can J Appl Physiol 2001;26(Suppl):36S–44S.

Fricker PA, Gleeson M, Flanagan A, et al. A clinical snapshot: do elite swimmers experience more upper respiratory illness than non-athletes? J Clin Exer Physiol 2000;2:155–8.

Gleeson M. The scientific basis of practical strategies to maintain immunocompetence in elite athletes. Exer Immunol Rev 2000;6:75–101.

Gleeson M, Bishop NC. Modification of immune responses to exercise by carbohydrate, glutamine and anti-oxidant supplements. Immune Cell Biol 2000;78:554–61.

Gleeson M, Nieman DC, Pedersen BK. Exercise, nutrition and immune function. J Sports Sci 2004;22: 115–25.

Howarth KR, Moreau NA, Phillips SM, Gibala MJ. Co-ingestion of protein with carbohydrate during recovery from endurance exercise stimulates skeletal muscle protein synthesis in humans. J Appl Physiol 2009;106: 1934–402.

Himmelstein SA, Robergs RA, Koehler KM, Lewis SL, Qualls CR. Vitamin C supplementation and upper respiratory tract infections in marathon runners. J Ex Phys 1998;1:1–17.

Kekkonen RA, Vasankari TJ, Vuorimaa T, Haahtela T, Julkunen I, Korpela R. The effect of probiotics on respiratory infections and gastrointestinal symptoms during training in marathon runners. Int J Sport Nutr Exer Metab 2007;17:352–63.

Konig D, Berg A, Weinstock C, Keul J, Northoff H. Essential fatty acids, immune function and exercise. Exer Immunol Rev 1997;3:1–31.

Kopp-Hoolihan L. Prophylactic and therapeutic uses of probiotics: a review. J Am Diet Assoc 2001;101: 229–41.

Lönnerdal B. Nutritional roles of lactoferrin. Review. Curr Opin Clin Nutr Metab Care 2009;12:393–7.

Malm C. Exercise immunology: a skeletal muscle perspective. Exer Immunol Rev 2002;8:116–67.

Nieman DC. Exercise and upper respiratory tract infection. Sports Med Tr Rehab 1993;4:1–14.

Nieman DC. Exercise immunology: nutritional countermeasures. Can J Appl Physiol 2001;26(Suppl):45S–55S.

Nieman DC, Henson DA, Butterworth DE, et al. Vitamin C supplementation does not alter the immune response to 2.5 hours of running. Int J Sport Nutr Exer Metab 1997;7:173–84.

Nieman DC, Henson DA, McAnulty SR, et al. Influence of vitamin C supplementation on oxidative and immune changes after an ultramarathon. J Appl Physiol 2002;92:1970–7.

Nieman DC, Henson DA, McAnulty SR, et al. Vitamin E and immunity after the Kona triathlon World Championship. Med Sci Sports Exer 2004;36:1328–35.

Peters EM. Exercise, immunology and upper respiratory tract infections. Int J Sports Med 1997;18(Suppl): 69S–77S.

Peters EM, Goetzsche JM, Grobbelaar B, Noakes TD. Vitamin C supplementation reduces the incidence of postrace symptoms of upper-respiratory-tract infection in ultramarathon runners. Am J Clin Nutr 1993;57:170–4.

Prasad JS. Effect of vitamin E supplementation on leucocyte function. Am J Clin Nutr 1980;33:606–8.

Pyne DB, Gleeson M, McDonald WA, et al. Training strategies to maintain immunocompetence in athletes. Int J Sports Med 2000;21(Suppl):51S–60S.

Pyne DB, Gleeson M, Batterham A, Hopkins WG, Fricker PA. Individual response to illness in elite swimmers. Brit J Sports Med 2005;39:752–6.

Smith JA. Guidelines, standards, and perspectives in exercise immunology. Med Sci Sports Exer 1995;27: 497–506.

Swain RA, Kaplan B. Upper respiratory infections: treatment selection for active patients. Phys and Sports 1998;26:85–96.

Tarnopolsky MA. Nutritional consideration in the aging athlete. Clin J Sports Med 2008;18:531–538.

Toft AD, Ostrowski K, Asp S, et al. The effects of n-3 PUFA on the cytokine response to strenuous exercise. J Appl Physiol 2000;89:2401–5.

Venkatraman JT, Pendergast DR. Effect of dietary intake on immune function in athletes. Sports Med 2002;32:323–37.

CHAPTER 17

Nutrition for special populations: children and young athletes

SHONA BASS AND KAREN INGE

17.1 Introduction

Physical activity during childhood and adolescence is widely recommended for short- and long-term physiological, sociological and psychological benefits. There are concerns, however, about the possible negative effects of intense training on growth and maturation, and, in particular, the combination of intense training with suboptimal energy and nutrient intakes.

Understanding growth, development and maturation is clinically important because exposure to risk or protective factors may result in site-specific effects depending on the timing and duration of exposure. Sections 17.2–17.20 describe the different temporal patterns of skeletal growth and maturation, how maturation is clinically assessed, and how diet and intense exercise may affect skeletal growth and maturation. Sections 17.21–17.41 consider the nutritional requirements of children and adolescents participating in sport at an elite level, and the chapter concludes with lifestyle issues, food habits and counseling strategies for sports dietitians who are working with this special population.

17.2 Skeletal growth and maturation in young elite athletes

Growth and maturation refer to two distinct biological processes—growth refers to an increase in the total body size, and/or the size attained by specific parts of the body, whereas maturation refers to the tempo and timing of progress towards the mature biological state. Growth focuses on size, and maturation focuses on the progress of attaining size (Malina & Bouchard 1991). Understanding skeletal development—growth in size and bone mineral accrual—becomes clinically important when exposure to risk and protective factors (such as disease, poor nutrition and exercise) affect the attainment of final stature and peak bone mass.

Skeletal growth

17.3

Skeletal growth can be viewed as two distinct but interrelated processes: an increase in bone length and an increase in bone mass (bone mineral accrual). There are different temporal patterns of growth in bone length and bone mineral accrual (Bass et al. 1999). These different patterns are characterized by the stage of maturation, the gender and the skeletal region (axial or appendicular). The clinical importance of understanding this heterogeneity in skeletal development lies in the site-specific (e.g. hip or spine) surfeits or deficits that may occur due to exposure to risk or protective factors at different stages of development.

Skeletal growth is categorized by unique biological phases that are linked to hormonal regulation. The entire growth process is divided into three additive and partly superimposed components: infancy, childhood and puberty (Karlberg 1989a, 1989b, 1990). Growth during infancy is thought to be a continuation of post-natal 'fetal growth' and is predominantly regulated by insulin and insulin-like growth factors I and II (IGF-I and IGF-II) (Gluckman 1989, 1996; Wollmann & Ranke 1996). It is independent of growth hormone (GH) and probably thyroid function. GH and IGF-I are responsible for growth during childhood, provided thyroid function is normal, while growth during puberty is related to GH and sex steroids (Karlberg 1989a, 1989b; Wollmann & Ranke 1996). The three phases of growth are also distinguished by the different temporal patterns of growth in stature. There is rapid fetal growth with a peak intra-uterine growth velocity at 4 months gestational age. From this point there is a marked deceleration of linear growth that continues after birth until 6 to 12 months. Childhood growth is characterized by a growth spurt occurring early, and then a gradually decelerating velocity through childhood. Puberty is characterized by acceleration of growth velocity (growth spurt).

Growth in bone length

17.4

During infancy

Body size at birth is primarily dependent on intra-uterine conditions (nutrition and oxygen). After birth, most infants make growth adjustments (increased or decreased velocity) in their first 2 years to reach their genetically determined growth potential (Karlberg 1989b; Rogol 1995). As a result of this, infants are known to 'shift centiles' during the first 12–18 months of life. The second year of life seems to be an important period of growth of bone length because environment and/or diseases may delay the onset of the GH-dependent growth spurt (Karlberg 1989b). Further, the position on the growth curve at 2 years of age is generally tracked for the remaining growth period (Smith et al. 1976; Karlberg 1989b; Cooper et al. 1995). Growth is more stable during the third year of life, when the infancy component of growth has virtually disappeared and growth is predominated by the GH-dependent childhood component.

During childhood

The onset of the GH-dependent childhood component is characterized by a growth spurt between the ages of 6 and 12 months. There is an obvious and abrupt increase in growth rate, which results in a slowing of the rapid deceleration in growth velocity. The peak velocity during this growth spurt is approximately 17 cm/yr (Karlberg 1989a, 1989b, 1990; Wollmann & Ranke 1996). Of particular interest is that this growth spurt is characterized by an acceleration of growth of the legs; growth velocity of the trunk remains constant.

The childhood component, often referred to as prepubertal growth, is nearly identical in girls and boys, as shown in Figure 17.1. During this phase, there is an initial rapid decrease in velocity, and then a slow, consistent decline in velocity to reach a minimal prepubertal height velocity of about 5 cm/yr in both sexes (Karlberg 1989a, 1989b; Prader 1992). A mid-childhood growth spurt at 7 to 8 years has been observed in two-thirds of healthy children. This transient acceleration in height is thought to be due to adrenal androgens, involves growth in all dimensions, and is similar for both genders. The subsequent decline in growth immediately before puberty often highlights this mid-childhood spurt (Karlberg 1989a, 1989b; Prader 1992).

The childhood patterns of long-bone growth are very stable and orderly compared to those of infancy and puberty. Changes in percentile levels with increasing age are minimal (Maresh 1955; Karlberg 1989b). Growth in the childhood component is dominated by growth of the legs compared to trunk growth (Karlberg 1989b). At 12 years of age, the gain in height for both sexes due to childhood growth is about equal (Karlberg 1989b).

During puberty

Growth during puberty is more complex than in the childhood years (when growth rate is relatively constant). Similar to the infancy phase of growth, there is also a growth spurt during puberty. In contrast to the infancy component, however, the growth spurt during puberty is dominated by an acceleration in trunk length; growth of the legs proceeds with constant velocity. Approximately 15% of the final stature is achieved during the pubertal growth spurt and 97% of final stature has been attained by the time of menarche (Faulkner et al. 1993; Bass et al. 1999). Pubertal growth is often considered to be a growth-promoting event and the final height-limiting process. This is because although height velocity is

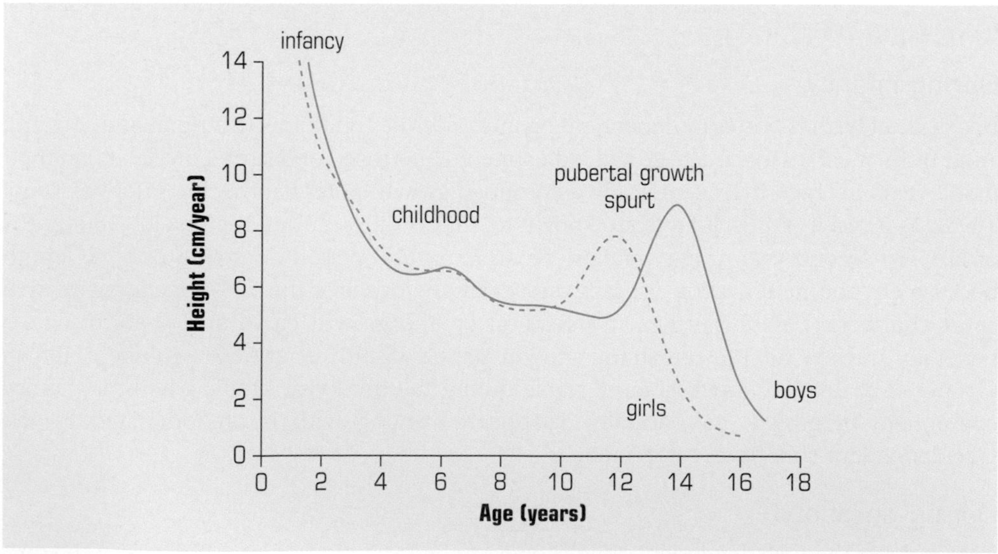

FIGURE 17.1 Skeletal growth velocity. The childhood component, often referred to as prepubertal growth, is nearly identical in girls and boys. During this phase, there is an initial rapid decrease in velocity, and then a slow consistent decline in velocity. The pubertal component is characterized by a growth spurt. Girls generally start their growth spurt and attain their peak height velocity (PHV) approximately 2 years earlier than boys. Adapted from Preece & Ratcliffe 1992

markedly increased, the rate of skeletal maturation is also increased, which eventually leads to fusion of the epiphyseal cartilage (Bourguignon 1988). This pubertal growth spurt is directly related to hormonal changes that accompany sexual development, and is characterized by three phases (Cara 1993):

1. minimal height velocity just before the spurt (prepubertal growth lag)
2. maximal growth—peak height velocity (PHV)
3. decreasing height velocity (epiphyses fuse and final height is achieved)

Girls generally start their growth spurt and attain their PHV 2 years earlier than boys (see Fig. 17.1). Early in puberty, girls tend to be taller than boys because they begin their spurt earlier, and grow faster in the early phases of the growth spurt (Preece 1982; Buckler 1990; Preece & Ratcliffe 1992).

17.5 Bone mineral accrual

During skeletal growth there is an increase in bone length and a corresponding increase in bone size and bone mass. At birth, the newborn skeleton contains approximately 30 g of calcium, and in the next 20 years of life approximately 1500 g of calcium is accrued in the skeleton. This increase is more than three times the calcium that is lost during 40 years of ageing. During childhood, bone mass is accrued at a constant rate, similar to the pattern of longitudinal bone growth; there are minimal differences in bone size or mass at most skeletal sites between prepubertal girls and boys (Faulkner et al. 1993). The pubertal growth spurt contributes proportionally more to peak bone mass than to final stature. The majority (80–90%) of peak bone mass has been accrued by the end of puberty; less than half of this is achieved during the 10 to 12 years of prepubertal growth and is non-sex-hormone-dependent. In both boys and girls (depending on the site), 50–80% of bone mineral is accrued very rapidly during 2–4 years of pubertal growth (Faulkner et al. 1993; Bass et al. 1999; Bradney et al. 2000). These results highlight the important contribution of bone mineral accrual during puberty for the attainment of peak bone mass in young women (Bachrach et al. 1991).

The pubertal growth spurt is also characterized by different temporal patterns of growth in bone length and bone mineral accrual (Bass et al. 1999; Bradney et al. 2000) (see Fig. 17.2 overleaf). For instance, the age of PHV occurs approximately 1 year earlier than the peak rate of bone mineral accrual. It is thought that bone fragility increases at this time because there is a rapid increase in bone length, without a corresponding increase in bone mass. Interestingly, this time of temporal dissociation between length and mass corresponds to the time when there is an increase in the number of childhood fractures. Increased physical activity or an increase in the number of falls does not account for this increased number of fractures (Bailey et al. 1989; Blimkie et al. 1993).

17.6 Maturation

Maturation refers to progress (timing and tempo) towards the biological mature state. Timing refers to when specific maturational events occur, and tempo refers to the rate at which maturation progresses. Individuals vary in the timing and tempo of maturation; this may affect the ability of some children to train and compete against other children who are the same chronological age, but at a different stage of maturation. Techniques for estimating maturity vary depending on the biological system being assessed. Commonly used systems include skeletal maturation, sexual maturation and somatic (physical) maturation. Dental maturation also can be used as a maturity indicator.

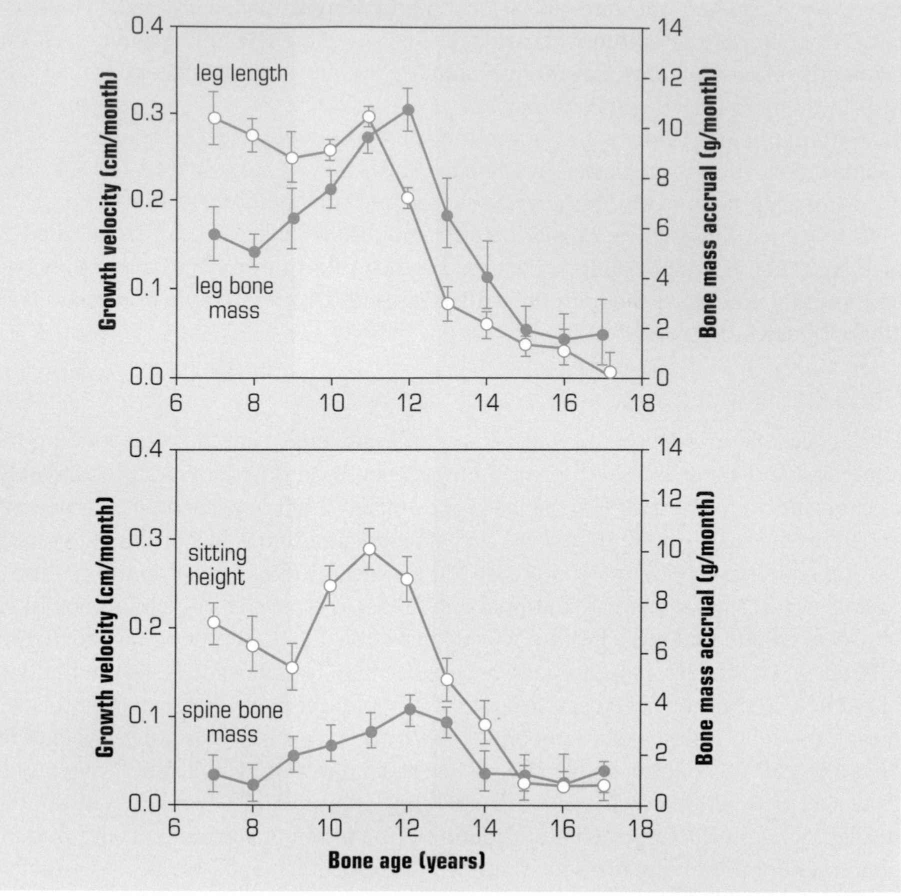

FIGURE 17.2 Growth velocity and mineral accrual during childhood and adolescence. The pubertal growth spurt is characterized by different temporal patterns of growth in bone length (centimeters/month) and bone mass (grams/month accrual). The age of PHV occurs approximately 1 year earlier than the peak rate of bone mineral accrual. The shaded region represents the pubertal years (Tanner stage 2 to menarche). Adapted from Bass et al. 1999

17.7 Skeletal age

The skeleton develops from cartilage in the prenatal period to fully developed bone in early adulthood. Skeletal age (or bone age) is based on the maturation of the skeleton—it reflects the development of calcified or ossified areas of bone and the external contour changes that result from bone growth and ossification (Malina & Bouchard 1991). As the epiphyseal growth plate matures, its shape and width change in a predictable fashion, with eventual fusion of the epiphysis and elimination of the radiological visible 'gap' between the epiphysis and its corresponding metaphysis (Gertner 1999). Therefore a mature skeleton will have more bone development and less cartilage compared to a less mature skeleton.

X-rays are used to determine the amount of bone development and how close the shape and contours of the bones are to adult status. The left hand (wrist area) is the site most often used, as there are many bones in the area to assess, it is reasonably typical of the skeleton as a whole, and the gonads are not exposed to radiation. Bone age is assigned by averaging the developmental stage of the bones in the wrist (Tanner et al. 1975; Grimston et al. 1990). Figure 17.3 shows the different stages of skeletal maturation in the wrist bones of two individuals.

Bone age gives a better assessment of skeletal and biological maturity than chronological age (years since birth). Skeletal maturation is also thought to be the best method for assessing biological age or maturity status as it is the only method that spans the entire growth period—from birth to adulthood (Malina & Bouchard 1991). Three methods used to evaluate skeletal development are the Greulich-Pyle, Tanner-Whitehouse and Fels methods (Greulich & Pyle 1959; Tanner et al. 1975, 1983; Roche et al. 1988). The systems are complex and require extensive experience to be used accurately and reliably.

Sexual maturation

17.8

The principal physical events of puberty include the growth spurt, and the development of reproductive organs and secondary sexual characteristics. Changes also occur in body composition and in the cardiorespiratory system. While skeletal age is the only maturational indicator that can be applied over the entire growth period, it does not predict pubertal events. Assessing sexual maturation is useful because sexual maturation is highly related to the overall process of physiological maturation (Tanner 1962).

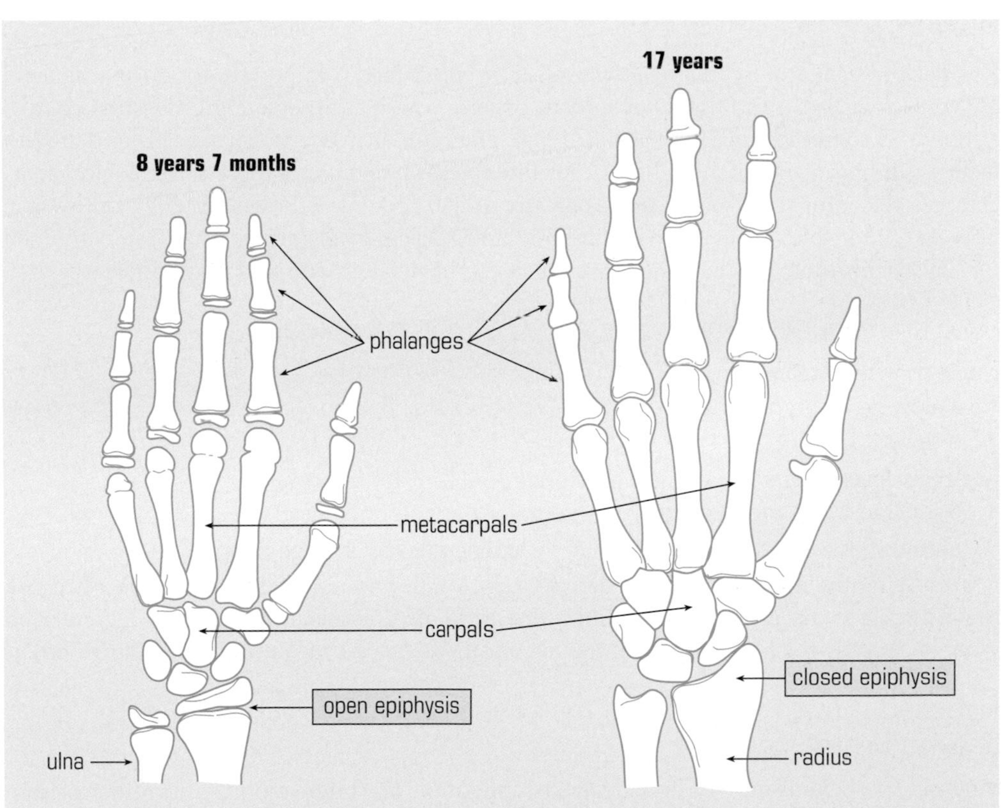

FIGURE 17.3 The different stages of skeletal maturation in the wrist bones of two individuals

Sexual maturation is assessed by the stage of development of secondary sex characteristics, including breast development and age of menarche in girls, genital development in boys, and pubic hair development in both sexes. Tanner (1962) devised categories based on specific secondary sex characteristics consisting of five stages of maturation from Stage 1 (prepubertal children) to Stage 5 (full maturation). Other maturity indicators include the development of axillary (armpit) hair in boys and girls, and facial hair and voice changes in boys.

The assessment of skeletal age reflects the development of calcified or ossified areas of bone and changes in shape that result from bone growth and ossification. The epiphyses are open in the younger child and closed in the adolescent.

Gender differences in maturation are most apparent during puberty. While the overall sequence of maturation is similar in girls and boys, there are considerable differences in the timing of onset of pubertal events. Thus the growth spurt of boys tends to be 2 years after that of girls, because boys enter puberty 1 year later and the relative placement of the growth spurt and PHV in male puberty is also 1 year later (compared with female puberty) (Preece & Ratcliffe 1992). The time between the start and the end of the pubertal development of the male genitalia is very short, only about 2.5 years. This short time reflects the powerful effect of testosterone on development of the male genitalia (Prader 1992).

17.9 Factors influencing the temporal patterns of skeletal growth and maturation

Regular physical activity in a healthy, well-nourished child is important for normal skeletal and muscle growth, and the development of cardiovascular fitness, neuromuscular coordination and cognitive function (Malina 1994). The rapid increase in sex steroids and growth factors during puberty is thought to accelerate the development of these physiological characteristics, leading to increased trainability for athletic potential (Rowland 1997). In contrast, however, intense training during childhood and adolescence, particularly when combined with poor nutrition, can have negative effects on skeletal growth and maturation.

17.10 How are reduced growth and delayed maturation detected?

Compromised skeletal growth is characterized by:

- a slowing of prepubertal growth to a velocity close to zero, and
- reduced or no PHV

whereas delayed maturation is characterized by:

- bone age being more than 2 years younger than chronological age, and
- failure to have the first menstrual cycle (menarche) by the age of 16 years

Assessing the effect of physical activity on growth and maturation is complex because it is difficult to discern the contribution due to familial associations (genetic factors) and what is causally related to environmental conditions (such as training and/or nutrition).

17.11 Reduced growth and delayed maturation in elite athletes: inherited or environmental factors?

Slowing of skeletal growth and delayed maturation are often reported in athletes from sports where there is emphasis on leanness (10–20% below desired weight) or in aesthetic sports where there is a focus on a petite build or small body mass (BM) (such as gymnastics, long distance running, skiing, figure skating and ballet) (Warren 1980; Frisch et al. 1981; Warren 1983; Neinstein 1985; Brooks-Gunn et al. 1987; Warren & Stiehl 1999). Proponents of the position that gymnastics training has no apparent effect on growth and maturation typically build their case on evidence that claims elite or high-level gymnasts were relatively small before they began training and that gymnasts who persist with their sport tend to be smaller and lighter than those who drop out (Baxter-Jones et al. 2003). There is no question that gymnasts are short and often have delayed maturation; the strict selection criteria of this sport identify individuals with familial short stature, constitutionally delayed growth or idiopathic delayed puberty. However, the question to be addressed is not whether gymnasts have short stature or late maturation, but, rather, does gymnastics training itself alter the tempo and rate of growth and maturation? That is, are some gymnasts growing and maturing differently than they would have had they not undertaken training and participated in competitive gymnastics?

Several research groups have documented growth and maturation in elite gymnasts from 2 years (Theintz et al. 1993; Bass et al. 2000) to 5 years (Lindholm et al. 1994; Zonderland et al. 1997). Findings of these studies indicated that gymnasts grew more slowly than controls, their growth spurt was either absent or delayed, and the delay in skeletal maturation increased with longer duration of training.

There is also evidence that intense exercise may be associated with delayed maturation. Bass and colleagues (2000) reported that skeletal maturation in twenty-one gymnasts (aged 11 years) was delayed by 1.8 years and became more delayed by an additional 0.5 years after 2 years of training. Similar findings have been reported in rhythmic gymnasts aged 11–23 years (Georgopoulos et al. 1999). Their skeletal maturation was delayed by 1.3 years, and their mean age of menarche was older than that of their mothers and sisters. In this study the delay in skeletal maturation and the age of menarche was positively correlated to the intensity of training, and negatively correlated to body fat. Furthermore, the prevalence of delayed menarche in ballet dancers varies from 5–40%, with an average delay of around 2 years (Warren & Brooks-Gunn 1989). Some dancers do not menstruate until their early 20s (Warren 1980, 1983; Warren & Stiehl 1999). Slowing of skeletal growth and delayed maturation associated with intense training has also been reported in case studies of young female and male athletes (Laron & Klinger 1989), monozygotic twins (Constantini et al. 1997) and triplets (Tveit-Milligan et al. 1993).

17.12 Not all elite athletes are at risk of reduced growth and delayed maturation

Methodological approaches also limit the ability to detect the occurrence of reduced growth and delayed maturation. For instance, the effect of gymnastics training on growth and maturation is often reported as averaged data, an approach that does not identify individual growth patterns (Daly et al. 2003, 2005). Large differences in growth and maturation have been observed between individual gymnasts involved in similar training regimens. In the study by Bass and colleagues (2000), some gymnasts had delayed skeletal maturation by up to 3.2 years and yet others of a similar age and training schedule were not delayed. Further, over the course of the study the delay in skeletal maturation improved in some, but became more delayed in others. Only thirteen of the twenty-two gymnasts followed by Lindholm and colleagues (1994) showed an attenuated growth curve. In the study by Theintz and colleagues (1993), the height standard deviation scores in some gymnasts were positive and remained positive over the course of the study; in others, the height standard deviation scores were reduced and worsened. These data support the notion that not all gymnasts involved in elite training programs are at risk of reduced growth and delayed maturation. Therefore it is important to identify gymnasts who are likely to be at risk (see section 17.19).

17.13 Do attenuated skeletal growth patterns occur uniformly in all bones?

Short stature in elite young athletes may be the result of attenuated growth at one skeletal site, but not others (Bass et al. 2000). For instance, Theintz and colleagues (1993) reported that the reduced growth of twenty-two gymnasts was related to a slower growth velocity of the legs, not the trunk. However, sampling bias may have affected these results, as the controls were swimmers who were taller than average, with greater-than-average growth velocities. In contrast, Bass and colleagues (2000) reported that reduced leg length in the gymnasts was present at baseline, but did not worsen with increasing duration of gymnastic training; the deficit in trunk length was only detectable after 2 years of training and worsened with increasing years of training. Therefore Bass and colleagues (2000) proposed that the reduced leg length of gymnasts may be due to selection bias, and the acquired component of the deficit in stature was the result of a progressive deficit in trunk length. Site-specific deficits in longitudinal growth have also been reported in ballet dancers—their trunk length was shorter relative to leg length as demonstrated by the decreased upper- to lower-body ratio compared to other female family members (Warren 1980).

17.14 Other factors that may influence skeletal growth and maturation

The mechanism for the attenuated growth and delayed maturation reported in athletes is unclear, but nutritional insufficiency may be a major contributing factor (see Chapter 9). Growth failure and impaired maturation have been reported in healthy, non-athletic children who regularly restricted kilojoules (Pugliese et al. 1983). Similar eating behavior is not uncommon in young athletes striving for a lean BM. For many young athletes, energy and nutrient intakes may be insufficient to support the nutritional needs for normal growth and maturation as well as intense exercise (Caine et al. 2003). Puberty, the period of accelerated growth, may be particularly influenced by poor nutrition (Largo 1993), and young athletes may be at increased risk if dietary energy intakes are restricted. Often diets designed for elite gymnasts are nutrient-dense and well-balanced, but may be too low in energy (Lindholm et al. 1995; Bass et al. 2000). In most instances, however, young athletes who are following very low-energy diets are unsupervised—hence it is likely that their diets are unbalanced and are both low in energy and suboptimal in nutrient density.

Unfortunately, little is known about the energy requirements of gymnastic training (Van Erp-Baart et al. 1985; Davies et al. 1997; Caine et al. 2001), so determining daily energy expenditures and energy balance in gymnastics is not possible. If young athletes are in negative energy balance, chronic mild under-nutrition may result, leading to compromised skeletal growth and delayed maturation (Malina 1994). Negative energy balance is known to reduce the levels of IGF-I, and the relationship between IGF-I and growth is well known (Smith et al. 1995). Low IGF-I values have been reported in young female gymnasts (Jahreis 1991; Bass et al. 1998). In a study of twenty-one gymnasts, energy intake was an independent predictor of growth velocity and correlated with the delay in skeletal maturation (Bass et al. 2000).

Environmental influences on growth and maturation 17.15

Other factors that may interact with intense exercise and negative energy balance to alter growth potential include:

- the psychological and emotional stress associated with maintaining BM when the natural course is to gain
- year-long training (including training programs with little time-out)
- frequent competitions
- altered social relationships with peers
- demanding parents and/or coaches (Malina 1994)

In addition, reduced skeletal growth may be due to repetitive stress and physical trauma damaging the epiphyses. Immature bones with open epiphyses are susceptible to stress injuries such as little-leaguer elbow, Osgood-Schlatter disease and iliac crest apophysitis. Stress changes, stress fractures and abnormal bone growth in the epiphysis of the radius have also been reported in gymnasts (Micheli 1983; Caine et al. 1989, 1992; Mandelbaum et al. 1989; Meeussen & Borms 1992). However, there has been little investigation into the effects of repetitive loading on an open epiphysis (Borms 1986; Maffulli & King 1992). Interestingly, there are limited animal-based data that show that repetitive load may inhibit the long bone growth, and that non-weight-bearing exercise (swimming) may facilitate long bone growth (Swissa-Sivan et al. 1989; Maffulli & King 1992).

Catch-up growth: can impaired growth and delayed maturation be reversed? 17.16

The most convincing evidence for an adverse effect of intense training on growth and maturation are the data on gymnasts who have retired or have time off due to injury. If participation in the sport has no effect on growth and maturation then it would follow that cessation of the sport would also have no effect on the tempo or rate of growth. However, this does not appear to be the case.

Catch-up growth is generally associated in a clinical sense when a temporary cause of growth retardation has been removed and the child returns to their normal growth channel. This occurs after any type of temporary growth disturbance (e.g. after malnutrition, corticoid therapy, renal acidosis, and after initiation of substitution in GH deficiency or hypothyroidism) (Boersma et al. 1995). Catch-up growth is characterized by accelerated and/or protracted skeletal growth. In some cases, prolonged catch-up growth continues until early adulthood, and in other cases growth velocity can be as high as four times the 'usual' rate (Largo 1993; Boersma et al. 1995).

Examples of catch-up growth in athletes 17.17

Bass and colleagues (2000) monitored the growth and maturation in thirteen elite gymnasts 12 months before and 12 months after retirement. Figure 17.4 overleaf shows that the gymnasts who were more than 10 years of age exhibited the well-documented pattern of catch-up growth characterized by an increase and maintenance of growth velocity well above that expected for their chronological age. This catch-up growth occurred and varied according to the age at retirement from the sport. Tonz and colleagues (1990) also reported a slowing of growth in gymnasts during the peripubertal years (relative to controls) and catch-up growth later in puberty. Lindholm and colleagues (1994) reported that catch-up growth was evident in gymnasts during times of reduced training schedules. It has also been reported that ballet dancers progressed very rapidly through pubertal development during periods of reduced training. While normal girls progress from Tanner Breast Stage 2 to 4 over an average of 2 years, dancers have been shown to make the same progression in as little as 4 months when they cease or reduce training (Warren 1980). Catch-up growth observed during reduced training schedules or following retirement is also reported in case studies of young female and male athletes (Laron & Klinger 1989), monozygotic twins (Constantini et al. 1997) and triplets (Tveit-Milligan et al. 1993).

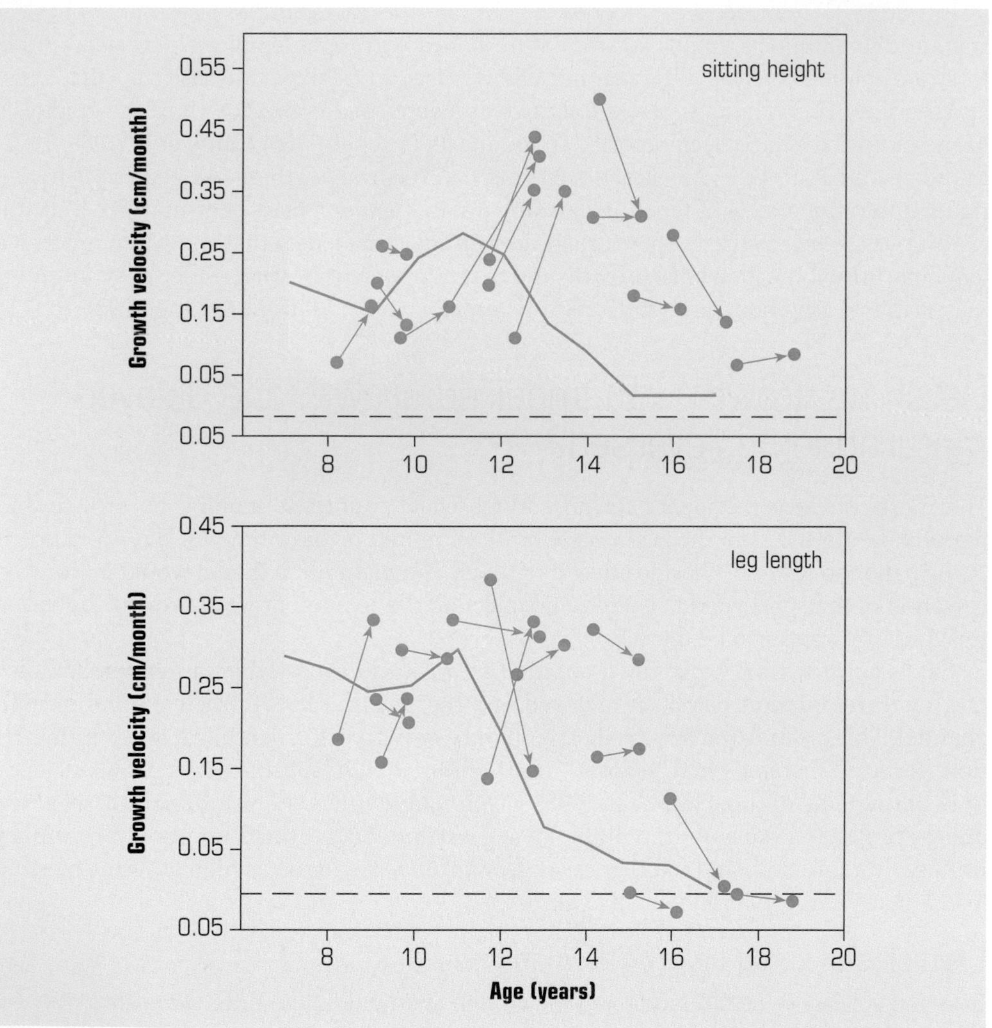

FIGURE 17.4 Catch-up growth in elite gymnasts. Growth velocity of thirteen elite gymnasts, 12 months before (tail of arrow), and 12 months after retirement (head of the arrow) from gymnastic training. Catch-up growth was evident in sitting height in the gymnasts who were more than 10 years of age. There was no evidence of catch-up growth in leg length at any age. The shaded area represents the growth velocity of young healthy non-athlete controls (mean ± 1 SD). Adapted from Bass et al. 2000

Is catch-up growth always complete? 17.18

Even if catch-up growth does occur, the evidence is inconclusive as to whether normal height is achieved (Mosier 1989; Largo 1993). Long-term cohort studies where final height is compared to predicted height provide evidence that final height may be compromised in some gymnasts (Caine et al. 2003). Usually when growth in length is retarded, so is bone maturation, but not always to the same extent. Theoretically, any imbalance could result in incomplete catch-up growth. However, catch-up of bone age may be slower than that of bone length; thus, in most cases the equilibrium of both parameters is re-established (Mosier 1986; Van den Brande 1986; Prader 1992). The timing and magnitude of the negative energy balance may also influence the ability of the child to achieve complete catch-up growth. Generally, the more severe the delay in skeletal maturation, the higher the risk of incomplete catch-up growth.

In healthy, non-athlete children, normal skeletal maturation is defined as bone age being within 1 year of chronological age. In late-maturing children, bone age is delayed between 1 and 2 years, and delayed maturation is defined as bone age being delayed by more than 2 years (Blethen et al. 1984; Mosier 1986; Van den Brande 1986; Prader 1992; Borer 1995; Malina 2000).

Consequences of delayed skeletal growth and maturation 17.19

Reduced final height may or may not be a problem for an athlete. Ultimately, what is important is a positive body image. Athletes and their parents should be aware that elite training, in conjunction with a diet that is in negative energy balance, might compromise the attainment of final height (Mansfield & Emans 1993). Another issue to be considered in girls is that delayed menarche is a risk factor for menstrual dysfunction (secondary amenorrhea), and that in some athletes menstrual dysfunction results in low peak bone density (see Chapter 9). Athletes who are involved in high-volume, low-impact sports and have low BM are at risk of menstrual dysfunction and low bone density that may be irreversible (Keen & Drinkwater 1997; Micklesfield et al. 1998). In contrast, it has been reported that athletes who are involved in high-impact sports, particularly during growth, have high bone density despite menstrual dysfunction (Lindholm et al. 1995; Robinson et al. 1995; Bass et al. 1998).

Summary of growth and maturational issues in young athletes 17.20

Growth and maturation are complex processes and the effect of intense exercise and diet on these processes cannot be discerned easily. While some young athletes who are involved in intense training and consume low-energy diets may have intrinsically short stature and familial delayed growth, the prospect of intense training influencing the temporal pattern of growth and maturation (attenuated growth and delayed maturation) should not be dismissed. If growth rate is reduced and maturation is delayed, catch-up growth may occur (if training intensity is reduced and energy intake is increased). Total catch-up growth may be compromised if the delay in maturation is severe. Some individuals may be more at risk of attenuated growth patterns than others; therefore the growth and maturation of young athletes should be monitored to identify those individuals who are at risk (particularly those with severe and prolonged energy-restricted diets, and who are participating in long-term intense training programs). The following annual assessments are recommended: anthropometric measures, pubertal stage, bone age, nutritional status, symptoms of eating disorders and measures of body image. These parameters should be monitored regularly in young athletes committed to long-term training programs (e.g. ballet dancers and gymnasts). Finally, it is important that these athletes and their parents are in a position to make informed choices about their participation in elite sports. Athletes, parents, coaches and dietitians need to be informed and recognize the benefits, potential risks and outcomes associated with the participation of young athletes in intense physical activity, especially when combined with low-energy diets.

17.21 Nutrient and energy requirements for young elite athletes

There is little research specifically relating to the macro- and micronutrient requirements of young elite athletes. In the absence of such specific data, the nutrient recommendations for young elite athletes are usually based on adult athletes in combination with the cut-offs for population nutrient standards for age and gender. For most young elite athletes, population nutrient standards—Nutrient Reference Values for Australia and New Zealand (NRV) and Dietary Reference Intakes (DRI) for the US/Canada)—can be used. However, adolescent athletes during a growth spurt have higher micronutrient requirements and utilize more energy and fat and less carbohydrate (CHO) than adult athletes at the same workload. There are inadequate data on young athletes for most vitamin and minerals for this age group to make definitive nutrient recommendations (see Chapter 11). There is, however, enough evidence to support higher iron, zinc and calcium requirements during growth periods in elite athletes compared with non-athletes. For the purpose of this section of the chapter, children refers to those aged 5–12 years, and adolescents are those aged 13–18 years (NHMRC 2003).

17.22 Energy

Adequate energy intake during childhood and adolescence is necessary to support normal growth and provide the extra energy needs of training and physical activity (American Dietetic Association 1996c, 1996d; 2004). A negative energy balance may be desirable for weight loss in some situations for overweight athletes; however, severe and prolonged energy-restricted diets are not recommended for young athletes. Chronic negative energy balance during growth results in short stature and delayed puberty, menstrual irregularities, poor bone health (see section 17.11), increased incidence of injuries, and risk of developing eating disorders (Thompson 1998).

Unfortunately, few studies have directly measured the energy expenditure of children and adolescents performing various sports. Estimates are often extrapolated from adult data; however, there are inherent errors associated with this approach. Children are less metabolically efficient than adults (MacDoughall et al. 1979; Girandola et al. 1981), and mechanically more inefficient with motor activities. This means that energy expenditure values extrapolated from adults for use in children are underestimated. For instance, girls have a higher energy cost for walking and running compared with women (Haymes et al. 1974), and children aged 6 to 8 years require 20–30% more oxygen per unit BM than adults when running at similar speeds (Astrand 1952; Daniels 1978). This indicates that children and adolescent athletes have higher energy needs than adults for similar activities. As shown in Table 17.1, there is a large variation in the energy intakes of young athletes that is age-, sport- and gender-specific. More recently, the mean energy intake of twenty-one female gymnasts (aged 11 years) was reported to be only 6106 kJ per day (Bass et al. 2000). This is lower than the intakes reported for other gymnasts in Table 17.1. Despite the under-reporting of energy intakes in dietary survey techniques, these apparently low energy intakes are of concern if consistently lower than energy expenditures.

Protein 17.23

Children and adolescents have higher protein requirements than adults because of the extra protein required for growth. In adult athletes, protein recommendations are slightly higher than the RDI/RDA, especially for athletes involved in endurance and strength sports

TABLE 17.1 SELF-REPORTED ENERGY INTAKES OF YOUNG ATHLETES

					ENERGY INTAKE			
SPORT	NUMBER OF SUBJECTS	AGE (YEARS)	HEIGHT (CM)	WEIGHT (KG)	(KJ/KG)	(KCAL/D)	(KCAL/KG)	(KJ/D)
FEMALES								
Gymnastics	29	7–10	134.9	30.6	6 908	226	1 651	53.9
	240	11–14	146.7	36.8	7 502	203	1 793	48.3
	56	15–18	160.6	51.0	7 485	149	1 789	35.6
Swimming	100	11–14	156.5	47.2	8 657	189	2 069	45.1
	22	15–18	–[a]	58.2	14 950	257	3 573	61.4
Volleyball	26	13–17	–[a]	–[a]	7 527	–[a]	1 799	–[a]
Dance	92	12–17	160.2	46.8	7 908	171	1 890	40.8
MALES								
Swimming	9	11–14	–[a]	56.4	12 853	230	3 072	55.0
	42	15–18	182.0	75.1	18 983	252	4 537	60.2
Running	4	7–10	–[a]	–[a]	8 167	272	1 952	65.0
	14	11–14	–[a]	–[a]	10 632	276	2 541	66.0
	4	15–18	–[a]	–[a]	11 447	209	2 736	50.0
Wrestling	4	7–10	–[a]	–[a]	7 916	272	1 892	64.0
	50	11–14	–[a]	–[a]	10 288	222	2 459	53.0
	20	15–18	–[a]	–[a]	11 309	184	2 703	44.0
Football	46	11–14	–[a]	60.9	10 556	173	2 523	41.4
	88	15–18	–[a]	75.9	14 079	185	3 365	44.3

a = value not reported
Source: Adapted from Thompson 1998

(see Chapter 4). There are insufficient data to make definitive recommendations for protein intakes for children and adolescents involved in similar sports (Thompson 1998); thus we can only speculate that this group of young athletes may similarly have higher protein requirements than normally active children. The 2007 Australian National Children's Nutrition and Physical Activity Survey found that the majority of children and adolescents in all age groups met or exceeded the Estimated Average Requirement (EAR) for protein with boys aged between 14–16 years having the highest protein intakes, as expected (see Table 17.2). Even in sports where athletes were reported to be following low-energy diets, protein intakes still met protein levels of between 1.2 and 2 g/kg BM/d, recommended by Lemon (1998). Lemon suggests that when total energy intake matches energy expenditure, protein needs should easily be met. Protein intakes reported by gymnasts and ballet dancers were between 1.5 and 2 g/kg BM/d (Benson et al. 1985, 1990; Loosli et al. 1986; Benardot et al. 1989), which confirmed Lemon's predictions. Nevertheless some young athletes are still likely to be at risk of suboptimal protein intakes, especially during their growth spurt, when requirements are highest, and particularly in those who are strict vegetarians, or are striving to meet high CHO needs and consume bulky diets.

TABLE 17.2 PROTEIN INTAKES OF AUSTRALIAN CHILDREN AND ADOLESCENTS FROM THE 2007 AUSTRALIAN NATIONAL CHILDREN'S NUTRITION AND PHYSICAL ACTIVITY SURVEY

GROUP	AGE (YEARS)	PROTEIN INTAKE (G/D)	PROTEIN INTAKE (% OF TOTAL ENERGY INTAKES)
Males	4–8	74.3	16.4
	9–13	95.2	16.6
	14–16	121.1	17.6
Females	4–8	65.5	16.0
	9–13	79.5	16.3
	14–16	81.6	16.4

Source: Department of Health and Ageing et al. 2008

17.24 Carbohydrate

The benefits of high-CHO diets for enhancing athletic performance in adults are well documented (see Chapters 12, 13 and 14); however, there are few data on the total daily CHO requirements of young athletes or the recommendations for CHO intakes during prolonged exercise. Findings on twelve young adolescent boys (aged 10–14 years) showed that CHO utilization during exercise was 20% lower than in men, although the oxidation of ingested CHO was considerably higher than in men (Timmons et al. 2003). The authors concluded that boys of this age range had a greater reliance on dietary CHO during exercise than men, which may contribute to preserving endogenous fuel use. In a similar study, the same research group compared the differences in dietary CHO utilization between girls aged 12 and 14 years while cycling for 60 minutes at approximately 70% maximal aerobic power. Interestingly, endogenous CHO oxidation was lower in the younger girls than the older girls. However the oxidation of total CHO from dietary sources during exercise was not different between the younger and older girls (Timmons et al. 2007). The implications of this research for both sexes highlight the importance of providing a CHO source between meals and during exercise in young athletes to help inhibit endogenous CHO production and usage, and potentially promote rapid recovery of liver glycogen reserves. Although data are limited, children and adolescents have a higher reliance on fat than CHO oxidation during moderate intensity exercise and produce lower levels of lactic acid at the same exercise intensity as adults but have a higher lactate threshold or tolerance for lactic acid (Montfort-Steiger & Williams 1997). Hence, their tolerance for short-burst anaerobic exercise is probably better than adults.

In summary, there are no definitive recommendations for total daily CHO intakes for young athletes as there are for adult athletes (see Chapter 14). Until further research is undertaken, total CHO recommendations for young athletes are similar to adult athlete recommendations. Young elite athletes can benefit from consuming CHO (e.g. sports drinks) during prolonged exercise.

Carbohydrate loading 17.25

There are no known data published on the practice, benefits or detrimental effects of CHO loading in children and adolescents, nor are there any data on glycogen resynthesis rates in young athletes. Research on maximum glycogen storage capacity in children and adolescents would enable the determination of recommendations for CHO intake. Until such research is conducted, if at all feasible because of its invasive nature, Bar-Or and colleagues (1997) suggest that nutrition advice about CHO intakes provided to young athletes be based on each individual's response and tolerance and that CHO loading be avoided because of potential adverse effects (see section 12.7).

Carbohydrate intakes and dental caries 17.26

While a high-CHO diet may be beneficial for training and performance, there are concerns about the effect of some types of CHO on dental health. Dental caries or tooth decay is the result of repeated acid attacks by bacteria on dental plaque. Fermentable CHOs present in foods and beverages provide the necessary substrates for enhancing acid production (Sank 1999). Eating or drinking sugary foods and beverages between meals, without regular teeth cleaning, promotes dental caries.

The rate of cariogenicity of a food is associated with several risk factors: the amount of fermentable CHO consumed, the physical form of the CHO, the concentration of sugars in the foods consumed, the length of time the teeth are exposed to the acid, the frequency of meals and snacks, and the proximity of eating before bedtime (Sank 1999). Foods known to promote dental erosion are citrus fruits and juices, carbonated and uncarbonated sugary drinks, acidic herbal teas, vinegar and vinegar products, confectionery and acidic medications (such as vitamin C tablets and syrups) (Sank 1999). Although little research has been conducted about eating habits in athletes and dental caries (Murray & Drummond 1996), anecdotal information suggests that providing preventive advice to athletes is warranted, especially in relation to consumption of sports drinks during training.

The potential cariogenicity of fermentable CHO-containing foods or fluids (including sports drinks) is reduced by water rinsing, eating casein-containing food (preferably low-fat), or chewing gum (preferably sugar-free) immediately after consumption of these substances (Sank 1999; NHMRC 2003). The erosive potential of foods can also be reduced by minimizing contact time with the teeth by consuming fluids quickly, through a straw or from a squeeze bottle directly into the mouth (Murray & Drummond 1996; Milesovic 1997).

Chilling of drinks is also recommended because the erosive potential (acid dissociation constant) of the acidic fluids is temperature-dependent.

Saliva also offers protection from dental caries and erosion by acting as a buffer. The buffering effect of the saliva may be reduced if the athlete is severely dehydrated (>8% of BM) or has a dry mouth due to excessive mouth-breathing (Murray & Drummond 1996). Proper dental hygiene should be encouraged and for adolescents wearing braces dental hygiene should be a priority. Collaboration between dietetic and dental professionals is recommended for oral health promotion, disease prevention and intervention (American Dietetic Association 1996a).

17.27 Fat

The Australian Dietary Guidelines for Children and Adolescents provide recommendations to lower total fat intake as a public health initiative where fat intake should contribute around 30% of energy to total daily energy intakes, with no more than 10% contribution from saturated fat (NHMRC 2003). While children and adolescent athletes are not usually concerned about the potential negative associations between fat intake and health outcomes in the short- or long-term, they need to recognize that high-fat diets are not necessarily conducive to optimal training performance and recovery, and are all too often accompanied by a low CHO diet.

Compared to adults, both children and adolescents have a preferential capacity to utilize fat (i.e. oxidize fat) as a fuel source during exercise—as evident from high levels of free glycerol, increased fatty acid uptake and lower respiratory exchange ratios observed during physical activity (Macek & Vavra 1981; Delamarche et al. 1992; Martinez & Haymes 1992; Meyer et al. 2007). However, children and adolescents do not need to consume additional dietary fat to enhance fat oxidation (Bar-Or & Unnithan 1994). It is prudent to encourage child and adolescent athletes to consume fat intakes that are consistent with population recommendations.

17.28 Vitamins

If energy intakes meet energy expenditures then it is likely that vitamin needs will also be met. In athletes who restrict energy intakes, vitamin intakes were reported to be below RDAs (Benson et al. 1985). In a study of twenty-six adolescent female athletes consuming low-energy diets, marginal intakes of vitamin A were found, although vitamin C intakes were well above the RDA. In this study, other vitamins were not measured (Perron & Endres 1985). Other studies confirmed that young athletes met most of their RDAs for B vitamins (Benardot et al. 1989; Rankinen et al. 1995; Kopp-Woodroffe et al. 1999) although, in some instances, intakes of vitamin B6 and folate were below RDAs (Loosli et al. 1986; Guilland et al. 1989; Benson et al. 1990). Those athletes likely to follow low-energy diets and hence be at risk of suboptimal intake of vitamins (and other nutrients) include adolescent ballet dancers, female gymnasts and college wrestlers (Moffatt 1984; Benson et al. 1985; Loosli et al. 1986; Steen & McKinney 1986). Benson and colleagues (1985) found that around 60% of ballet dancers aged 12–17 years reported consuming two-thirds of the RDA for folate and in another study 50% of gymnasts of a similar age failed to consume two-thirds of the RDA for vitamin E (Loosli et al. 1986). Thus low-energy diets may place young athletes at risk of inadequacies of some but not all vitamins.

RDIs/RDAs are not actual requirements, but are the estimated levels of intake of essential nutrients that are judged to be adequate to meet the known needs of the majority of healthy people (Sirota 1994). It is unknown whether the RDIs/RDAs and revised DRIs/NRVs (see Chapter 2) are appropriate for child and adolescent athletes who are training at an elite level.

Determining the vitamin status of any individual or group, child, adult or adolescent is difficult because of the difficulties in collecting reliable dietary intake data on usual dietary intake, the high variability in intakes for different vitamins and the insensitivity of biochemical indicators to detect marginal vitamin deficiencies. For more information on interpretation of biochemical indices of vitamin status, see Chapter 11.

Minerals 17.29

Calcium and iron intakes are often reported below population nutrient cut-offs in dietary surveys of children and adolescents, particularly in girls (see Chapters 9 and 10). Suboptimal intakes of zinc are also of concern in young athletes (Bar-Or et al. 1997), because of the role of zinc in energy production as well as growth, sexual maturation and immunity.

Calcium 17.30

Calcium requirements are highest during childhood and adolescence, with the exception of pregnancy and lactation (see Chapter 9). The 2007 Australian National Children's Nutrition and Physical Activity Survey reported that 82–89% of girls aged 12–16 years did not meet the EAR for calcium, so the probability of inadequate intake for this age group is likely to be high (Department of Health and Ageing 2008), despite potential under-reporting, an inherent problem in all dietary surveys. Interestingly, intakes of magnesium in females and males aged 14–16 years were also below the EAR: 56% and 34% respectively (Department of Health and Ageing 2008). This is indicative of changes in food preferences in this age group and possibly linked to suboptimal intakes of vegetables and unrefined cereals, the major suppliers of magnesium in the diet.

Young female athletes who restrict energy intake tend also to restrict dairy products and thus are at high risk of low calcium intakes (Benson et al. 1985, 1990; Perron & Endres 1985; Benardot et al. 1989; Moen et al. 1992; Bass et al. 2000). Dairy products are the predominant source of calcium in the diets of young, healthy, non-athlete children and adolescents (Department of Health and Ageing 2008), so restricting or limiting these foods usually accounts for the low calcium intakes.

Iron 17.31

According to the 2007 Australian National Children's Nutrition and Physical Activity Survey, the majority of children and adolescents met or exceeded the EAR for iron (Department of Health and Ageing 2008). The only group below the EAR was adolescent females aged 14–16 years. However, the EAR represents 50% of the average requirements of a group of healthy females who are not elite athletes or undertaking the levels of physical activity that might be expected in females regularly training at high levels of intensity and endurance. Iron requirements and turnover is highest in adolescent athletes compared with adults, although dietary iron intakes are usually no different from sedentary controls (Fogelholm 1995, 1999). There is sufficient evidence that iron deficiency or at least iron depletion is a problem in adolescent athletes (see Chapter 10). Iron depletion in young athletes, particularly female athletes, is common, with up to 40–50% of adolescent female athletes reported with low iron stores (based on low serum ferritin levels) (Benson et al. 1985, 1990; Perron & Endres 1985; Loosli et al. 1986; Benardot et al. 1989; Rowland 1990).

In summary, adolescent athletes are at high risk of iron depletion/deficiency because of their high iron requirements and turnover, which is associated with rapid pubertal growth, iron loss from menses, suboptimal iron intakes from low-energy diets and, for some athletes, a preference for vegetarianism (Bergstrom et al. 1995). Endurance and high-intensity training can further increase iron loss via hemolysis, gastrointestinal blood loss and excessive sweating (Rowland et al. 1987; Nickerson et al. 1989; Rowland 1990) (see Chapter 10).

Diagnosis of true iron depletion based on serum ferritin alone may be difficult in children and adolescents, as the increased plasma volume associated with any growth spurt and potential training response can present falsely low values. Strategies for detection and treatment of iron depletion in children and adolescents are similar to those suggested for adult athletes (see Chapter 11).

17.32 Zinc

Several studies have reported suboptimal zinc intakes based in levels below the RDA in young female athletes (Benson et al. 1985; Loosli et al. 1986; Rankinen et al. 1995; Wiita & Stomabaugh 1996; Kopp-Woodroffe et al. 1999). Classical symptoms of zinc deficiency are reduced linear growth velocity and delayed development of secondary sexual characteristics (Prasad et al. 1963; Sandstead 1985). The 2007 Australian National Children's Nutrition and Physical Activity Survey reported that while the majority of boys and girls of all age groups met or exceeded the EAR for zinc, for 13% of adolescents aged 14–16 years, reported zinc intakes were below the EAR, which suggests a high probability of inadequate intake. The distribution of nutrient intake data from this survey are not yet available, so it is difficult to determine the possibility of inadequate intake for this representative sample of the population using frequency data of respondents between the EAR and RDI/RDA cut-offs. In the previous national survey of children and adolescents in Australia, the majority of female adolescents did not meet the RDI for zinc (McLennan & Podger 1997), so it is likely that zinc intakes may not meet the needs of some individual adolescents with high zinc requirements or who are vegetarian. As the best dietary sources of bioavailable zinc are from animal products, vegetarian athletes are at high risk of poor zinc status (see Chapter 20).

17.33 Vitamin and mineral supplements

Young athletes take vitamin and mineral supplements for numerous reasons. In a survey of 742 high-school athletes from nine schools in the US, 38% reported taking such supplements—a higher frequency than among non-athlete adolescents (25–30%) (Sobal & Marquart 1994). The most common supplements taken in this study were vitamin C (25%), multivitamins (19%), iron (11%), calcium (9%), vitamin A (9%), B vitamins (8%) and zinc (3%). Wrestlers and gymnasts were the highest users (59% and 40% respectively). While boys took more vitamin A supplements than girls, girls took more iron. Healthy growth was the most frequently reported reason for taking supplements, followed by treating illness. Around 62% of respondents took supplements to improve sports performance. Similar results were reported in another study of 509 high-school athletes aged 14–18 years

(Massad et al. 1995) although for this group the main reason for taking vitamin A supplements was for healthy skin, rather than for overall health. The American Dietetic Association (1996b) advocated that the best strategy to obtain adequate bioavailable nutrients is from a wide variety of food rather than from supplements. This advice has recently assumed more prominence in view of the increased understanding of the other potential health-promoting effects of the non-nutrients in plants. Vitamin and mineral supplements should, therefore, not be necessary for healthy children and adolescent athletes who are consuming adequate energy for their needs and a well-balanced diet. However, young athletes who are on low-energy diets, vegetarian, who are amenorrheic or diagnosed with iron depletion may warrant supplements under supervision. Some vitamins and minerals, if misused, have adverse side effects that may not be reversible. Prescribed doses of multivitamin and multi-mineral supplements taken as directed (although they may not be necessary) are generally considered safe for use.

Performance-enhancing substances

17.34

Performance-enhancing substances have become extremely popular in athletes of all ages. These substances (also known as ergogenic aids) are touted by manufacturers as increasing muscle mass, providing a performance boost and/or providing increased strength (see Chapter 16). Virtually no experimental research on either the ergogenic effects or adverse effects of these substances has been conducted in subjects younger than 18 years (American Academy of Pediatrics 2005). Young athletes are vulnerable to peer pressure and anecdotal stories, often from well-respected and famous sporting heroes, who may support the use of these products. Young athletes should be aware that performance improvement is reliant on many factors—such as growth, physiological and sexual maturation, skill acquisition, and years of training and good nutrition—and that supplements of any kind will not give them a 'quick fix' to performance problems (Eichner et al. 1999).

Performance-enhancing substances frequently used by young male athletes are muscle-building supplements. These include protein powders, creatine, dehydroepiandrosterone (DHEA) and hydroxy-methyl butyrate (HMB). As the short- and long-term effects of these substances on the immature athlete are not known, caution should be used before recommending these products to young athletes (Eichner et al. 1999).

Some ingredients in these products may also be banned and could result in a positive drug test (especially DHEA and androstenedione, which may have steroid-like anabolic properties). To date, creatine seems relatively safe (see Chapter 16); however, as water is transported into the muscles with creatine, large doses may be a hazard in the heat—especially if young athletes take up to 86 g/d of creatine (Eichner et al. 1999). Product purity and quality are also concerns because, in most countries, quality control tests are not necessarily conducted. It is unknown if HMB is effective in adults, and possible adverse effects are unknown. Guidelines on HMB for children and adolescents cannot be made until further research has been conducted. It would be prudent not to recommend these types of ergogenic aids to young athletes until we fully understand their mechanisms of action.

The increasing consumption of energy drinks containing caffeine (not sports drinks) by young athletes could also have adverse effects on performance. A study in more than 400 schoolchildren found that some boys consumed up to five cans of energy drinks before sport in the belief that performance would be boosted (O'Dea & Abraham 2001). Caffeine intakes were estimated for the first time in the 2007 Australian National Children's Nutrition and Physical Activity Survey (Department of Health and Ageing 2008). Estimated caffeine intakes were low in the youngest children, as expected, but increased in those aged 14–16 years to an average of 47 mg/d in males and 36 mg/d in females. Other popular performance-enhancing substances, bicarbonate and colostrum, should not be recommended for young athletes until further research confirms the level of associated risk and possible side effects. Eichner and colleagues (1999) and others (American Academy of Pediatrics 2005) suggest that athletes younger than 18 years should not consume any ergogenic aid because evidence relating to the safety of long term use in younger athletes is scant. The American Academy of Pediatrics (2005) condemns the use of performance-enhancing substances and vigorously endorses efforts to eliminate their use among children and adolescents. Further, the popular belief among young athletes that all supplements available at health food stores have been scientifically tested and are safe needs to be addressed in education programs or in schools (particularly since some supplements have been shown to have harmful effects) (Cowart 1992; Friedl et al. 1992). In one US study, close to half of the young athletes believed this to be the case (Massad et al. 1995).

17.35 Hydration and thermoregulation

Much is known about the fluid and electrolyte requirements of adults involved in physical activity; however, there is less research about these requirements in children and adolescents. Children have less developed and, therefore, less efficient thermoregulatory mechanisms than adults (Bar-Or et al. 1980). Risks of hypothermia in cold environments and hypohydration and hyperthermia in hot environments are higher in young athletes than in adults. Thermogenesis per kilogram of BM is greater in children than in adolescents and adults, but their ability to transfer heat from the centre of the body to the skin by blood is less effective.

17.36 Hyperthermia

The smaller the child, the greater is the excess in heat production (Bar-Or 1989). Children also have a greater surface area to body volume ratio compared with adults. Thus they are exposed to a faster influx of heat when environmental temperature exceeds skin temperature (Bar-Or et al. 1980). These factors make it more difficult to regulate body temperature.

Dissipation of heat from the body occurs through the skin by one or a combination of conduction, convection, radiation or evaporation. Heat is also dissipated through the lungs (Bar-Or 1989). When heat production is high in response to physical activity, the cooling effect of evaporation of sweat from the skin (an endothermic reaction) is the body's physiological mechanism for cooling (Bar-Or 1989). Unfortunately, the sweat response is less efficient in children compared with adults. Children have a lower sweat rate than adults (~2.5 times less), not due to fewer sweat glands, but due to each gland producing less sweat. Prepubescents rarely produce more than 400–500 mL of sweat per m^2/h, whereas adults under the same conditions can produce more than 700–800 mL of sweat per m^2/h (Bar-Or 1989). Further, the sweating threshold (the core temperature when sweating starts) appears to be higher in children compared with adults (Falk 1998). The sweat rate approaches adult levels early in puberty (Falk et al. 1992). Compared to adults, children dissipate less heat through evaporative sweating and more through convection (the loss of heat through the skin) plus radiation (Bar-Or 1989). This is achieved by greater vasodilation.

Children and adolescents exercising in the heat should be monitored closely for signs of heat stress. Those with high levels of body fat and heavy builds are more susceptible to heat stress because they are less efficient in dissipating body heat. It is important that children have adequate fluid consumption and that sunscreens, lightweight clothing and hats are worn when possible.

Hypothermia 17.37

It is also important for children exercising in the cold to be monitored for signs of hypothermia. Young athletes appear to be at greater risk of hypothermia than adult athletes, because in the cold children have lower skin temperatures (due to greater vasoconstriction) and a higher rate of heat loss (due to their greater surface area to mass ratio) (Smolander et al. 1992; Falk 1998). However, children have a higher metabolic rate in the cold, compared with adults, which is advantageous for heat production (Smolander et al. 1992; Falk 1998).

Hypohydration 17.38

Hypohydration refers to a reduction in body water as the body progresses from a normally hydrated (euhydrated) to a dehydrated state. Young athletes who begin exercise in a hypohydrated state are likely to experience adverse effects on cardiovascular function, temperature regulation and exercise performance (Bar-Or 1989). When adults undertake prolonged exercise they rarely drink enough to replenish fluid losses, even when fluid is offered to them at any time (ad libitum) (Bar-Or & Wilk 1996). This is especially evident in hot and humid conditions. A similar pattern has been noted in young athletes (Bar-Or et al. 1980). Like adults, young athletes dehydrate progressively when left to drink ad libitum. However, in children, adolescents and young adults, dehydration is accompanied by a faster rise in core temperature than in older adults (Bar-Or et al. 1980; Bar-Or & Wilk 1996; Thompson 1998). The reasons for this are unclear, but may be due to lower cardiac output and lower evaporative cooling capacity in children (Bar-Or 1989).

Fluid replacement 17.39

Maintaining adequate hydration is crucial for the prevention of heat stress. Thirst is a late indicator of low hydration status; in fact, when thirst is apparent, hypohydration has already begun and may be well advanced. Recommendations for fluid intake for active children and adolescents are listed in Table 17.3 overleaf.

The guidelines in Table 17.3 may need to be reviewed to reflect the popular use of (or change in attitude towards) CHO-electrolyte fluids (sports drinks, sports water and energy drinks). Sports Dietitians Australia (1998) issued a consensus statement for fluid replacement and, although tailored for adult athletes, the principles of type of beverage, frequency of intake and timing (including drinking pre-exercise, during exercise and post-exercise for recovery) can be applied to young athletes (see Chapters 13 and 14).

TABLE 17.3 SPORTS MEDICINE AUSTRALIA GUIDELINES FOR FLUID REPLACEMENT (WATER) FOR CHILDREN AND ADOLESCENTS[a]

AGE (YEARS)	TIME (MINUTES)	VOLUME[a] (Ml)
Approx. 15	45 (before exercise)	300–400
	20 (during exercise)	150–200
	As soon as possible after exercise	Liberal until urination
Approx. 10	45 (before exercise)	150–200
	20 (during exercise)	75–100
	As soon as possible after exercise	Liberal until urination

[a]In hot environments fluid intake may need to be more frequent
Source: Sports Medicine Australia 1997

While water is often described as the best choice of fluid, there are situations when drinks containing CHO are more appropriate. Studies on voluntary drinking habits and flavor preferences in children and adolescents suggest that greater consumption occurs when flavored drinks or sports drinks are offered instead of water (Meyer et al. 1994). During the voluntary rehydration stage, children (aged 9–13 years) who were drinking fluids other than water not only recovered from dehydration, but drank enough to increase their BM above normal (Meyer et al. 1994). These children favored grape and orange flavors compared with apple. While Canadian children of Caucasian descent tend to prefer grape flavor, children of other cultural backgrounds in other climates preferred other flavors (Bar-Or & Wilk 1996). Therefore, to encourage adequate hydration practices, children's taste preferences need to be catered for by offering them a variety of different flavored drinks. While the above study showed adequate consumption of fluid post-exercise, other junior athletes had insufficient fluid intakes during physical activity (Iuliano et al. 1998).

Although children's sweat contains less sodium and chloride compared with adult sweat composition (Meyer et al. 1992), there appears to be no evidence that children's performance improves when given sugary beverages (e.g. soft drink, cordial, sports drinks) more diluted than those dilutions currently recommended for adults. More information is needed to identify the optimal electrolyte and CHO content for sports drinks that will specifically meet the needs of young athletes (Bar-Or 1995). In the interim, similar dilutions (~4–8%) to those recommended for adults are used before, during and after training. The use and effectiveness of sports water (which is essentially purified water that is lightly flavored and may contain added vitamins, minerals and/or electrolytes) has not been studied in young athletes. However, the inclusion of flavoring and sodium in sports waters may help to increase fluid intake (relative to plain water) during exercise and may also help to improve fluid absorption and retention (Australian Institute of Sport 2004).

A guideline for young athletes is to drink periodically 'until you're not thirsty any more, and then another few gulps' (Bar-Or 1995). For a child younger than 10 years, Bar-Or (1995) suggests half a glass (100–125 mL) beyond thirst and for an older child or adolescent a full glass (200–250 mL) beyond thirst.

17.10 Dehydration and competition

Deliberate hypohydration is often practiced to achieve weight goals. Rapid weight reduction through deliberate dehydration (e.g. through fluid restriction, diuretic and laxative abuse, excessive sweating in saunas or exercising in plastic clothes, or vomiting) may be practiced by young athletes who compete in weight-category sports (such as wrestling, weightlifting and sports with specific body-weight demands). It is known that dehydration severely affects performance and can lead to disturbances in thermoregulation, cardiac output, renal function and electrolyte balance. Thus fluid restriction practices are not recommended at any age because of the adverse consequences of dehydration.

Hyponatremia 17.41

Inappropriate fluid replenishment patterns also include replenishing sweat and urinary losses by drinking only water, which contains little or no sodium (Meyer & Bar-Or 1994). This may result in electrolyte insufficiency and lead to hyponatremia (a severe drop in the concentration of sodium in body fluids), which can cause serious illness. One of the outcomes of hyponatremia is muscle cramps during or following exercise. The occurrence of hyponatremia in children and adolescent athletes appears to be extremely rare. Severe hyponatremia may induce apathy, nausea, vomiting, reduced consciousness, seizures and occasionally even death (Bar-Or 2000).

Food habits 17.42

Data on food consumption behavior and influences on food choice in child and adolescent athletes is scarce. Most information about food consumption attitudes and behavior of adolescents comes from selected studies of non-athlete groups. In early national dietary surveys of children in Australia, a decrease in reported consumption of total energy and many nutrients occurred in girls but not in boys in early adolescence (McLennan & Podger 1997; Department of Health and Ageing et al. 2008). In these studies, adolescent boys increased energy and nutrient intakes at levels comparable with their increased requirements. However, in a more recent national survey in Australia conducted in 2007, around 20% of older boys (aged 14–16 years), estimated energy intakes did not meet the lower end of the range for EER (Estimated Energy Requirements) (Department of Health and Ageing et al. 2008). An even greater proportion (38–50%) of adolescent females (aged 13–16 years) did not meet the cut-off at the lower end of the range. Despite the potential for under-reporting, this high proportion is still of concern if these data are representative of usual fairly low energy intakes. Several studies suggest that adolescent girls involved in elite or recreational sports also reported similar or even lower energy intakes compared to population data, despite extra energy requirements needed to support training programs.

Adolescents, generally, have different eating habits from children and adults. Adolescents are regular breakfast eaters, with 78.9% of those aged 12–15 years and 67.6% of those aged 16–18 years eating breakfast five or more times per week (McLennan & Podger 1997). With increasing age, however, there was an apparent increase in the number of breakfast skippers, particularly girls (McLennan & Podger 1997). In one study, one in five Australian children and one in three adolescents did not eat breakfast (O'Dea 2003). However, comparable data on current food habits in the 2007 Australian National Children's Nutrition and Physical Activity Survey are not yet available to compare current eating habits.

Children and young adolescents rely heavily on snacking, which contributes substantially to the nutrient density of their daily intakes. The 1995 National Nutrition Survey of Australia reported that 63.2% of young adolescents aged 12–15 years ate five to six times per day. Older adolescents snacked less often, with only 47.8% of those aged 16–18 years snacking this frequently, and only 37% snacking between two and four times per day. Boys ate the most frequently, with 20% of those aged 16–18 years eating seven or more times a day compared with only 7% of girls. Forty-four percent of girls at this age ate only two to four times per day compared with only 3% of boys (McLennan & Podger 1997).

In this same survey, cereals and cereal products were the major source of energy for adolescents. Males ate larger quantities than females and had a higher mean daily intake of food from all food groups, with the exception of fruit (McLennan & Podger 1997). In another study, adolescent girls were more likely to try to eat well, had better nutrition knowledge and ate fewer high-fat and sugary foods as well as more fruits and vegetables than boys (Nowak & Speare 1996). Older children were more likely to obtain and consume food and beverages away from home. Take-away and other pre-prepared foods formed a larger proportion of their diet than they did for younger children (McLennan & Podger 1997).

In educating and counseling young athletes, it is important to understand their eating habits and attitudes and the factors that influence their food choices. Table 17.4 summarizes the main determinants influencing food choices of adolescents. Convenience and time considerations are major influences, as adolescents want foods that are easy to access, easy to carry and require little preparation time. Taste, appearance and emotional influences are also important (Neumark-Sztainer et al. 1999). Nowak and Speare (1996) found that half the boys ($n = 412$, 12–15 years) in their study and two-thirds of the girls ($n = 379$, 12–15 years) sometimes ate from boredom. One in four children reported eating more when depressed.

Attitudes and beliefs also play a role. In a study of 791 Year 8 students in Australia, more than 80% felt food was important for health (Nowak & Speare 1996), although these beliefs are not necessarily translated into food choice. Adolescents recognize the

TABLE 17.4 FACTORS AFFECTING ADOLESCENT FOOD CHOICE
• Hunger
• Food cravings
• Appeal of food
• Time considerations
• Convenience
• Food availability
• Peer influence
• Parental influence
• Health beliefs
• Mood
• Body image
• Habit
• Cost
• Media

Source: Neumark-Sztainer et al. 1999

importance of food in the prevention of future illness, but see that the link between nutrition and appearance is more important (Nowak & Crawford 1998). Gender differences also start to become apparent during adolescence, with girls more concerned about the nutritional content of foods than boys (Nowak & Speare 1996).

Perception of body image 17.43

Body image is an important issue for many adolescents (Gibbons et al. 1995; O'Dea 1995). With the physical and emotional changes that occur with pubertal maturation, self-consciousness about the body is accentuated (Baum 1998). Concerns about body image start early in both boys and girls. Adolescent males are vulnerable to social pressure to attain a masculine muscular physique (the perceived ideal body image) (McKay et al. 1997), while female adolescents prefer to be small and lean and thin (O'Dea 1995).

These concerns about body image often translate to poor eating practices and disordered eating (O'Dea 1995; Neumark-Sztainer et al. 1999). In one study, as many as 63% of girls and 16% of boys had dieted at least once, and many claimed to have used extreme dieting methods (Gibbons et al. 1995). For adolescent athletes, although body image concerns dominate, other factors also contribute to the development of disordered eating patterns. These include pressure to optimize performance; pressure to meet unrealistic body-weight and fat goals; societal expectations; and established norms for certain sports, which may influence athletes to attain a certain body shape (Van de Loo & Johnson 1995).

Also, athletes who are not overweight often seek to lose weight and resort to unsafe weight-loss techniques that can have adverse effects on their health and performance. These practices were evident in one study of 487 female elite swimmers (9–18 years), where 60.5% of those who were of average weight and 17.9% of those underweight reported trying to lose weight (Van de Loo & Johnson 1995). Various multiple methods of weight loss were used, including skipping meals (62%), eating smaller meals (77%), vomiting (12.7%), using laxatives (2.5%) and using diuretics (1.5%) (Van de Loo & Johnson 1995).

Sources of nutrition information for adolescents 17.44

Adolescents obtain their food and nutrition information from parents, media (mainly television), peers and the school environment and there are clear gender differences from where they derive their information. Twice as many girls as boys obtained nutrition information from magazines, and five times more girls than boys obtain their weight-loss information from magazines (Nowak & Speare 1996). Teachers and doctors were twice as likely to be information sources as dietitians (Nowak & Speare 1996). Therefore it is important that these sources of information are reliable. Athletes are likely to be no different from non-athlete peers in their sources of nutrition information, except that coaches, sports dietitians and other athletes provide an additional input and can be a major influence on athletes' attitudes and food choices.

Healthy eating habits are established early in life and persist in later life (NHMRC 1995; Tuttle & Truswell 1998; Koivisto Hursti 1999). Parents, carers, siblings, peers and coaches act as role models and are the main influences of young children's food choices (Thompson 1995; Koivisto Hursti 1999).

17.45 Summary

No specific recommendations for energy, protein, CHO and fat intakes for children of different ages and stages of maturation participating in different sports have been published. Population reference standards for nutrients (DRIs/NRVs) can be used as guidelines for determining benchmarks for nutrient and energy intakes. Since young athletes expend more energy than their less active peers, their nutritional requirements are slightly higher, especially for energy and CHO, but should still fit within population nutrient standards. Further research is needed to determine minimum macronutrient and micronutrient intakes for groups of young athletes involved in elite sports. Further studies on child and adolescent athletes involved in elite sport are also needed to determine specific protein recommendations, to investigate glycogen resynthesis rates, and to estimate energy demands for different sports.

Reported micronutrient intakes in young athletes are highly variable as expected, with suboptimal intakes reported for calcium, iron and zinc. Young athletes who severely restrict energy intakes (e.g. gymnasts and ballet dancers) are at high risk of suboptimal intakes of micronutrients and delayed maturation and growth. Long-term energy deprivation may be irreversible, although to date it is not possible to detect an individual's susceptibility to permanent effects. Sports dietitians should ensure that these at-risk athletes have well-balanced, nutrient-dense diets and are not in chronic negative energy balance. In most cases, specific vitamin and/or mineral supplements should not be recommended routinely for young athletes, without a clinical diagnosis of depletion or deficiency. Emphasis should be placed on obtaining nutrients from food sources before advocating the use of vitamin and/or mineral supplements.

Performance-enhancing substances including ergogenic aids are probably not suitable and not recommended because of their unknown efficacy, mechanisms of action and potential long-term harmful effects in this age group. The short- and long-term effects of large intakes of energy drinks and potentially high caffeine intakes in children is of concern.

Since children and adolescents are at high risk of heat stress during exercise, practicing appropriate prevention strategies, including fluid replacement during training, is essential. Deliberate dehydration to 'make weight' should be actively discouraged. During hot weather, modifications to training sessions or competitions should be addressed, and in some situations cancellation may be more appropriate.

The external pressure placed on young athletes to conform to stringent BM and body-fat levels is a concern. The importance of identifying the determinants influencing food choice in this age group cannot be underestimated as a means of targeting facilitators to improving behavioral change. Ideally, improved nutrition knowledge, understanding and practice will result in better sporting performance and recovery. The nutritional requirements of young athletes have largely been ignored in the scientific literature. With advancing technology and increased political interest in developing athletic talent from an early age, specific guidelines for nutrient intakes for young athletes may be developed. Sports dietitians need to be concerned not only with the implications of diet for optimal sporting performance, but also for the growth, maturation and short- and long-term health outcomes of the young athlete. A team approach to management of the young athletes is important—the athlete, parent, coach, dietitian and other members of the health care team should work together to ensure the young athlete has the best possible care.

PRACTICE TIPS

KYLIE ANDREW

GETTING STARTED

- Children and adolescents are generally unaware of the role of diet in enhancing athletic performance. It cannot be assumed that their nutrition knowledge is at any particular level, as they may know very little or be misinformed.
- Children and adolescents do not usually present to a dietitian of their own accord. If brought in by parents or coaches they often hide their true feelings for fear of being judged or reprimanded. Follow-up sessions on a one-to-one basis without a parent or coach present make it easier to build rapport and assess the problem from the athlete's perspective.

ASSESSMENT

- Growth should be assessed at regular intervals. Anthropometric measures including height, weight, skinfolds and circumferences are used. Evaluation is best based on relative changes in these variables in the individual, although comparison with population growth charts is useful in children. The reasons for any substantial deviation from the normal growth curve should be investigated. The outcome of prolonged energy restriction could potentially be growth retardation or a delay in maturation. Pubertal stage and bone age are also used to assess growth and maturation and should be assessed annually in high-risk athletes (see Chapter 9).
- Investigating the average time and intensity per week spent undertaking physical activities is needed to estimate energy expenditure. Young athletes are often involved in many different sports including school, club and national or representative sport.
- In clinical practice, a diet history is the usual method for assessing dietary intakes in young athletes. This method quickly reveals if there are erratic or inconsistent eating patterns and gives a comprehensive insight into lifestyle, health and social issues affecting food behavior. Alternatively, for those young athletes who are erratic eaters, food records can be used. Food records, however, require extensive training and substantially distort usual eating behavior (see Chapter 2), but at least provide a starting point, especially for those who are vague or forgetful. Food intake checklists and 24-hour recalls of food are useful for young athletes as they provide a window into eating habits. Short-term recall techniques are likely to be more accurate and revealing about food and lifestyle habits than food records for this age group.
- A thorough nutrition assessment also includes collecting information about medical history, medication, supplement usage and dosage (including use of sports products and foods), and information about who shops and prepares meals and the family situation. Young athletes may have trouble remembering the names of the supplements they take (or are given), so requesting to see all supplements at the next interview is warranted to check safety and dosage. Some supplements may contain banned substances, have adverse side effects if misused, or have questionable quality control checks (see Chapters 11 and 16). Refer to the Australian Sports Anti-Doping Authority (ASADA) at http://www.asada.gov.au/

- Young athletes, especially adolescent girls, are at high risk of iron deficiency. Blood counts and iron status screening are routinely conducted on elite athletes in sports institutes and national squads as preventive measures. Such tests may be warranted in any young athlete with symptoms of fatigue and lethargy who habitually consumes a poor-quality diet (see Chapter 10).
- Any cessation of menses for more than 3 months should be cause for concern, and referred to a sports physician for further assessment.
- Alcohol misuse by adolescents is of concern in the general population, and young athletes, especially those involved in team sports, are likely to be exposed to alcohol and to peer pressure to consume alcohol at an early age, even under-age.
- Changes in eating behavior frequently occur during competition and need to be assessed at interview.
- Asking an athlete to define their sporting, weight and nutrition goals (if any) helps you to provide effective behavioral strategies that are specific to the individual's attitudes and beliefs.

COUNSELING AND EDUCATION

- Repeated advice or regular practical information sessions about how to choose food in different situations, and the reasons these choices are made, are effective in young athletes. Communal cooking nights have also been popular with young athletes in teams and have been used extensively as an education vector at the Australian Institute of Sport and state institutes of sport around Australia. Guidelines for organizing cooking sessions are found in Chapter 25. Use of appropriate language and an understanding of the differences in the eating habits and culture between girls and boys at different ages are invaluable in conducting these sessions and in individual counseling. Dietary strategies and suggestions for change need to be realistic and acceptable. Lunchboxes at high school are 'not cool'.
- Education of other members in the family, particularly the person responsible for cooking, helps improve compliance and promotes permanent changes in habits and food choices in children. Cooking nights for parents of young athletes are also welcomed as an opportunity for a social event for the parent and a platform for the dietitian to address key concerns and issues.
- Most young athletes, especially adolescents, are focused on their body image and weight. A counseling approach that emphasizes sporting performance, but also recognizes and addresses the importance of weight and body image issues, even at very young ages, is critical. Children and adolescents are likely to be more receptive to your advice.
- A positive approach and positive reinforcement is recommended when counseling children and adolescents. Praise for changes made, rather than constant criticism about existing poor practices and policing food intake, has better results.

PRACTICE TIPS

- Children should be encouraged to take some responsibility for their food choices and eating behavior. It is well accepted that children can influence parents' food choice and change the food purchasing patterns of their parents. Food providers, parents and coaches should be discouraged from dictating what children (and adolescents) should and should not be eating. Self-reliance should be encouraged; athletes seem to benefit from direct involvement in assessing their own diets, identifying problems, setting goals and developing their own strategies.

MEETING NUTRITIONAL NEEDS

- Specific recommendations for energy intakes for young athletes do not exist and there is large variability in reported energy intakes of young athletes. Therefore each child or adolescent athlete needs to be individually monitored to ensure their energy intake matches their energy expenditure.
- Chronic negative energy balance is contraindicated in young athletes and, if prolonged, increases the risk of short stature, delayed puberty, menstrual irregularities, poor bone health, increased incidence of injuries and risk of developing eating disorders. At-risk athletes, including gymnasts, dancers, distance runners and those in weight-class sports, should be assessed regularly.
- To meet daily energy and nutrient requirements for training and recovery, young athletes need to eat at least three nutritious meals a day and in-between meal snacks. Providing specific examples of suitable snacks that are convenient, portable and accessible is essential, including appropriate food choices at school canteens or local take-away shops. Suggesting that high-fat, sugary foods should be avoided is too restrictive and promotes cravings for these foods. If large quantities of these foods that particularly appeal to adolescents and children (e.g. soft drink, ice-cream, confectionery, crisps and hot chips) are consumed every day or in place of meals and a well-balanced diet, some limitations need to be implemented.
- Children with high energy expenditures, who find it difficult to maintain energy balance, require low-bulk, high-energy and nutrient-dense foods such as white breads and cereal products, dried and stewed fruits, high-energy muesli and fruit bars, smoothies and milkshakes. Adding extra sugar to foods is a better alternative than adding fat. In contrast, for athletes who put on weight easily, ensure that they are not in chronic negative energy balance and that their diet meets daily nutrient recommendations.
- Protein recommendations are easily met from a mixed diet, but may be difficult to meet in vegetarians, especially those avoiding dairy products.
- Currently there are no specific recommendations for CHO intakes in young athletes. Young athletes appear to use more endogenous sources of CHO as an energy substrate than adults, so encouraging adequate CHO-based snacks between meals is important. Hence CHO food sources in between meals should always be planned and encouraged

(see Chapter 14 for CHO food choices). Practical suggestions for low-fat snack foods and take-aways should also be provided.

- Because of the preferences for high sugar foods in this age group, dental hygiene should also be addressed at interview. Suggestions for improving dental hygiene include:
  - brush and floss teeth frequently
  - drink high-CHO drinks from a squeeze bottle or use a straw
  - drink plenty of milk and other casein-containing foods
  - drink water after eating between meals to rinse the mouth
  - chew sugar-free gum
  - drink fluids chilled
- DRIs/NRVs can be used in young athletes as a benchmark for measuring nutrient adequacy.
- Early detection and intervention of iron depletion is important to prevent iron deficiency. Strategies to increase iron intakes and bioavailability are outlined in Chapter 10.
- Indiscriminate use of vitamin supplements should be discouraged, although they may be necessary in some situations, such as for vegetarians, amenorrheic athletes, iron-deficient athletes and those on restricted-energy diets.
- Performance-enhancing supplements are not recommended for young athletes as the efficacy and safety of these products have not been investigated in children.

FLUID

- Young athletes who train after school may already be hypohydrated. A practical message to give children, suggested by Bar-Or (1995), is 'to drink periodically until you're not thirsty any more, and then another few gulps'. For a child younger than 10 years, this message translates into half a glass (100–125 mL) beyond thirst; and for an older child or adolescent, a full glass (200–250 mL) beyond thirst. Weighing before and after training determines the extent of fluid loss. As a crude guideline, 500 g of weight lost is equivalent to 500 mL fluid.
- Water, diluted fruit juice (by 50%) or very dilute cordial are suitable beverages during training and competition. Sports drinks and sports waters are suitable for child and adolescent athletes and are the best choice in very hot conditions when sweat rates are high. Usually flavored drinks encourage greater fluid consumption.
- The use of caffeine-containing energy drinks by young athletes should be discouraged.
- Guidelines for the pre-competition meal, eating between events and recovery should be provided (see Chapter 14). Young athletes are often reticent to try new foods in strange environments, so a supply of familiar foods packed for such emergencies is good advice and well received.
- Eating immediately or as soon as possible after training and competition (especially when competing on consecutive days or more than once in the one day) promotes rapid recovery of fuel reserves.

PRACTICE TIPS

FOLLOW-UP

- Several consultations are usually needed. One visit is insufficient to fully develop a rapport and influence change in food choice. Behavioral change is a learned response and needs encouragement and support. Shorter, more frequent consultations provide the opportunity to do this, as the concentration span of children and adolescents is usually short and information retention may not be as good as adults.
- Children and adolescents respond well to take-home tasks or activities, such as keeping a fluid balance chart or using a CHO counter to calculate intake. This helps them focus on their goals and practice suggested strategies, as well as providing encouragement and positive reinforcement.

MULTIDISCIPLINARY APPROACH

- A multidisciplinary, team approach has advantages in clinical counseling and education of young athletes. Other members of the medical team, including the sports physician and psychologist, may be involved, and regular communication is essential for coordinating messages and intervention. Coaches are often present at the interview and can either inhibit or enhance communication. It is important that coaches are informed and kept involved, as they are important members of the support team. When counseling and educating children and adolescents, parental involvement is essential for support, but should not interfere with your communication with the individual athlete.

SPECIFIC ISSUES

- Where there is evidence of an eating disorder, a multidisciplinary approach is essential.
- Rapid weight loss is discouraged. Weight maintenance or gradual weight loss (where required) is recommended. Both the child and parents need to understand the dangers of rapid weight loss. Regular monitoring is essential.
- Children and adolescents who have difficulty maintaining their weight may find commercial liquid meal supplements, such as Sustagen Sport™, useful to help meet their energy needs.
- Young athletes wanting to bulk up should be encouraged to eat five to six meals or snacks per day that are energy-dense and high in CHO with adequate protein. High-energy milk-shakes and smoothies made with fortified milk (such as high-calcium milks) and high-energy supplements like sports drinks, bars and liquid meal supplements are well tolerated.
- Vegetarian athletes require instruction about how to meet their nutrient needs.
- Fussy eaters should always be encouraged to try new foods, which can be compiled at each consultation and checked at the next. Initially constructing the list from favored foods, then adding a few new foods at the next consultation and providing positive reinforcement, encourages behavioral change.

Useful websites

http://www.sportsdietitians.com.au/factsheets/
Sports Dietitians Australia

References

American Academy of Pediatrics. Use of performance-enhancing substances. Pediatrics 2005:115; 1103–6.

American Dietetic Association. Position of the American Dietetic Association: oral health and nutrition. J Am Diet Assoc 1996a;96:184–9.

American Dietetic Association. Position of the American Dietetic Association: vitamin and mineral supplementation. J Am Diet Assoc 1996b;96:73–7.

American Dietetic Association. Timely statement of the American Dietetic Association: nutrition guidance for adolescent athletes in organised sports. J Am Diet Assoc 1996c;96:611–12.

American Dietetic Association. Timely statement of the American Dietetic Association: nutrition guidance for child athletes in organised sports. J Am Diet Assoc 1996d;96:610–11.

American Dietetic Association. Position of the American Dietetic Association: Dietary guidance for healthy children ages 2 to 11 years. J Am Diet Assoc 2004;104:660–7.

Astrand P. Experimental studies of physical working capacity in relation to sex and age. Copenhagen: Munskgaard, 1952.

Australian Institute of Sport. Nutrition fact sheets. At http://www.ausport.gov.au/ais/nutrition/factsheets (accessed 12 June 2009).

Bachrach LK, Katzman DK, Litt IF, Guido D, Marcus R. Recovery from osteopenia in adolescent girls with anorexia nervosa. J Clin Endocrinol Metab 1991;72:602–6.

Bailey DA, Wedge JH, McCulloch RG, Martin AD, Bernhardson SC. Epidemiology of fractures of the distal end of the radius in children as associated with growth. J Bone Joint Surg 1989;71A:1225–31.

Bar-Or O. Temperature regulation during exercise in children and adolescents. In: Gisolfi C, Lamb D, eds. Perspectives in exercise science and sports medicine: youth, exercise and sport. Indianapolis: Benchmark Press, 1989:335–67.

Bar-Or O. The young athlete: some physiological considerations. J Sports Sci 1995;13(Suppl):31S–3S.

Bar-Or O. New and old in pediatric exercise physiology. Int J Sports Med 2000;21:S113.

Bar-Or O, Barr S, Bergeron M, et al. Youth in sport: nutritional needs. Sports Science Exchange Roundtable 1997;8:4.

Bar-Or O, Daton R, Inbar O, Rotshtein A, Zonder H. Voluntary hypohydration in 10–12 year-old boys. J App Physiol 1980;48:104–8.

Bar-Or O, Unnithan V. Nutritional requirements of young soccer players. J Sports Sci 1994;12(Suppl): 39S–42S.

Bar-Or O, Wilk B. Water and electrolyte replenishment in the exercising child. Int J Sport Nutr 1996; 6:93–9.

Bass S, Bradney M, Pearce G, et al. Short stature and delayed puberty in gymnasts: influence of selection bias on leg length and the duration of training on trunk length. J Paediatr 2000;136:149–55.

Bass S, Delmas PD, Pearce G, et al. The differing tempo of growth in bone size, mass and density in girls is region-specific. J Clin Invest 1999;104:795–804.

Bass S, Pearce G, Bradney M, et al. Exercise before puberty may confer residual benefits in bone density in adulthood: studies in active prepubertal and retired female gymnasts. J Bone Miner Res 1998;13:500–7.

Baum A. Young females in the athletic arena. Child Adolesc Psychiatr Clin N Am 1998;7:745–55.

Baxter-Jones ADG, Maffulli N, Mirwald R. Does elite competition inhibit growth and delay maturation in some gymnasts? Probably not. Pediatr Exerc Sci 2003;15:373–82.

Benardot D, Schwarz M, Weitzenfeld-Heller D. Nutrient intake in young, highly competitive gymnasts. J Am Diet Assoc 1989;89:401–3.

Benson J, Allemann Y, Thientz G, Howald H. Eating problems and calorie intake levels in Swiss adolescent athletes. Int J Sports Med 1990;11:249–52.

Benson J, Gillian D, Bourdet K, Loosli A. Inadequate nutrition and chronic calorie restriction in adolescent ballerinas. Phys Sports Med 1985;13:79–90.

Bergstrom E, Hernell O, Lonnerdal B, Persson L. Sex differences in iron stores of adolescents: what is normal? J Pediatr Gastroenterol Nutr 1995;20:215–24.

Blethen SL, Gaines S, Weldon V. Comparisons of predicted and adult height in short boys: effect of androgen therapy. Pediatr Rev 1984;18:467–9.

Blimkie CJR, Lefevre J, Beunen GP, et al. Fractures, physical activity, and growth velocity in adolescent Belgian boys. Med Sci Sports Exerc 1993;25:801–8.

Boersma B, Rikken B, Wit JM. Catch-up growth in early treated patients with growth hormone deficiency. Arch Dis Child 1995;72:427–31.

Borer KT. The effects of exercise on growth. Sports Med 1995;20:375–97.

Borms J. The child and exercise: an overview. J Sports Sci 1986;4:3–20.

Bourguignon JP. Linear growth as a function of age at onset of puberty and sex steroid dosage: therapeutic implications. Endoc Rev 1988;9:467–88.

Bradney M, Karlsson M, Duan Y, Stuckey S, Bass S, Seeman E. Heterogeneity in the growth of the axial and appendicular skeleton in boys: implications for the pathogenesis of bone fragility in men. J Bone Miner Res 2000;15:1871–8.

Brooks-Gunn J, Warren MP, Hamilton LH. The relation of eating problems and amenorrhoea in ballet dancers. Med Sci Sports Exerc 1987;19:41–4.

Buckler JM. A longitudinal study of adolescent growth. London: Springer-Verlag, 1990.

Caine D, Bass S, Daly R. Does elite competition inhibit growth and delay maturation in some gymnasts? Quite possibly. Pediatr Exerc Sci 2003;15:360–82.

Caine D, Cochrane B, Caine C, Zemper E. An epidemiological investigation of injuries affecting young competitive female gymnasts. Am J Sports Med 1989;17:811–20.

Caine D, Lewis R, O'Connor P, Howe W, Bass S. Does gymnastic training inhibit growth of females? Clin J Sport Med 2001;11:260–70.

Caine D, Roy S, Singer K, Broekhoff J. Stress changes of the distal radial growth plate: a radiographic survey and review of the literature. Am J Sports Med 1992;20:290–8.

Cara JF. Growth hormone in adolescence, normal and abnormal. Endocrinol Metab Clin North Am 1993;22:533–53.

Constantini NW, Brautber C, Manny N, et al. Differences in growth and maturation in twin athletes. Med Sci Sports Exerc 1997;29(Suppl):150S.

Cooper C, Cawley M, Bhalla A, et al. Childhood growth, physical activity, and peak bone mass in women. J Bone Miner Res 1995;10:940–7.

Cowart V. Dietary supplements: alternatives to anabolic steroids? Phys Sports Med 1992;20:189–98.

Daly R, Caine D, Bass S, Pieter W, Broekhoff J. Is the growth of elite female gymnasts inhibited? J Sports Sci 2003;21:295–6.

Daly R, Caine D, Bass S, Pieter W, Broekhoff J. Growth and anthropometric comparisons of highly versus moderately trained competitive female artistic gymnasts. Med Sci Sports Exerc 2005;37:1053–60.

Daniels J. Differences and changes in VO_2 among runners 10–18 years of age. Med Sci Sports Exerc 1978;10:200–3.

Davies PSW, Feng JY, Crisp JA, et al. Total energy expenditure and physical activity in young Chinese gymnasts. Pediatr Exerc Sci 1997;9:243–52.

Delamarche P, Monnier M, Gratas-Delamarche A, et al. Glucose and free fatty acid utilisation during prolonged exercise in prepubertal boys in relation to catecholamine responses. Eur J Appl Physiol 1992;65:66–72.

Department of Health and Ageing et al. The 2007 Australian children's nutrition and physical activity survey. Commonwealth of Australia, 2008. At http://www.health.gov.au/internet/main/publishing.nsf/Content/phd-nutrition-childrens-survey (accessed 5 May 2009).

Eichner E, King D, Myhal M, Prentice B, Ziegenfuss T. Muscle builder supplements. Sports Science Exchange Roundtable 1999;10:1–5.

English R, Cashel K, Lewis J, Waters A, Bennett S. National dietary survey of school children (aged 10–15 years): 1985. No. 2: Nutrient intakes. Canberra: Australian Government Publishing Service, 1987.

Falk B. Effects of thermal stress during rest and exercise in the pediatric population. Sports Med 1998;25:221–40.

Falk B, Bar-Or O, Calvert R, MacDougall J. Sweat gland response to exercise in the heat among pre-, mid-, and late-pubertal boys. Med Sci Sports Exerc 1992;24:313–19.

Faulkner RA, Bailey DA, Drinkwater DT, et al. Regional and total body bone mineral content, bone mineral density, and total body tissue composition in children 8–16 years of age. Calcif Tissue Int 1993;53:7–12.

Fogelholm M. Indicators of vitamin and mineral status in athletes' blood: a review. Int J Sports Nutr 1995;5:267–84.

Fogelholm M. Micronutrients; interaction between physical activity, intakes and requirements. Public Health Nutr 1999;2:349–56.

Friedl KE, Moore RJ, Marchitelli LJ. Steroid replacers: let the athlete beware. NSCA J 1992;14:14–19.

Frisch RE, Gotz-Welbergen AV, McArthur JW, et al. Delayed menarche and amenorrhoea of college athletes in relation to age of onset of training. JAMA 1981;246:1559–63.

Georgopoulos N, Markou K, Theodoropoulou A, et al. Growth and pubertal development in elite female rhythmic gymnasts. J Clin Endocrinol Metab 1999;84:4525–30.

Gertner JM. Childhood and adolescence. In: Favus MJ, ed. Primer on the metabolic bone diseases and disorders of mineral metabolism. Philadelphia: Lippincott, Williams & Wilkins, 1999:45–9.

Gibbons K, Wertheim E, Paxton S, Petrovich J, Szmukler G. Nutrient intake of adolescents and its relationship to desire for thinness, weight loss behaviours, and bulimic tendencies. Aust J Nutr Diet 1995;52:69–74.

Girandola R, Wuiswell R, Frisch F, Wood K. Metabolic differences during exercise in pre- and post-pubescent girls. Med Sci Sports Exerc 1981;13:110–12.

Gluckman PD. Foetal growth: an endocrine perspective. Acta Paediatr Scand 1989;349(Suppl):21S–5S.

Gluckman PD. The endocrine regulation of foetal growth in late gestation: the role of insulin-like growth factors. J Clin Endocrinol Metab 1996;80:1047–50.

Greulich WW, Pyle SI. Radiographic atlas of skeletal development of the hand and wrist, 2nd edn. Palo Alto, CA: Stanford University Press, 1959.

Grimston SK, Ensberg JR, Kloiber R. Menstrual, calcium, and training history: relationship to bone health in female runners. Clin Sports Med 1990;2:119–28.

Guilland J, Penaranda T, Gallet C, et al. Vitamin status of young athletes including the effects of supplementation. Med Sci Sports Exerc 1989;21:441–9.

Haymes E, Buskirk E, Hodgson J, Lundergren H, Nicholas W. Heat tolerance of exercising lean and heavy prepubertal girls. J App Physiol 1974;36:566–71.

Iuliano S, Naughton G, Collier G, Carlson J. Examination of the self-selected fluid intake practices by junior athletes during a simulated duathlon event. Int J Sport Nutr 1998;8:10–23.

Jahreis G. Influence of intensive exercise on insulin-like growth factor I, thyroid and steroid hormones in female gymnasts. Growth Regulation 1991;1:95–9.

Karlberg J. On the construction of the infancy–childhood–puberty growth standard. Acta Paediatr Scand 1989a;356(Suppl):26S–37S.

Karlberg J. A biologically-oriented mathematical model (ICP) for human growth. Acta Paediatr 1989b;350(Suppl):70S–94S.

Karlberg J. The infancy-childhood growth spurt. Acta Paediatr Scand 1990;367(Suppl):111S–18S.

Keen AD, Drinkwater BL. Irreversible bone loss in former amenorrheic athletes. Osteoporos Int 1997;7:311–15.

Koivisto Hursti U. Factors influencing children's food choice. Ann Med 1999;31(1 Suppl):26S–32S.

Kopp-Woodroffe S, Manore M, Dueck C, Skinner J, Matt K. Energy and nutrient status of amenorrheic athletes participating in a diet and exercise training intervention program. Int J Sport Nutr 1999; 9:70–88.

Largo RH. Catch-up growth during adolescence. Horm Res 1993;39(3 Suppl):41S–8S.

Laron Z, Klinger B. Does intensive sport endanger normal growth and development? New York: Serono Symposia Publications from Raven Press Book Ltd, 1989.

Lemon PW. Effects of exercise on dietary protein requirements. Int J Sport Nutr 1998;8:426–47.

Lindholm C, Hagenfeldt K, Ringertz BM. Pubertal development in elite juvenile gymnasts: effects of physical training. Acta Obstet Gynecol Scand 1994;73:269–73.

Lindholm C, Hagenfeldt K, Ringertz H. Bone mineral content of young female former gymnasts. Acta Paediatr 1995;84:1109–12.

Loosli A, Benson J, Gillien D, Bourdet K. Nutritional habits and knowledge in competitive adolescent female gymnasts. Phys Sports Med 1986;14:118–30.

MacDoughall J, Roche P, Bar-Or O, Moroz J. Oxygen cost of running in children of different ages: maximal aerobic power of Canadian school children. Can J Appl Sports Sci 1979;4(abs):237.

Macek M, Vavra J. Prolonged exercise in 14-year-old girls. Int J Sports Med 1981;2:228–30.

Maffulli N, King JB. Effects of physical activity on some parts of the skeletal system. Sports Med 1992; 13:393–407.

Malina RM. Physical growth and biological maturation of young athletes. Exerc Sport Sci Rev 1994; 22:389–433.

Malina RM. Growth, maturation and performance. In: Garrett W, Kirkendall DT, eds. Exercise and sport science. Philadelphia: Lippincott, Williams & Wilkins, 2000.

Malina RM, Bouchard C. Growth, maturation and physical activity. Champaign, Illinois: Human Kinetics, 1991.

Mandelbaum BR, Bartolozzi AR, Davis CA, Teurlings L, Bragonier B. Wrist pain syndrome in the gymnast. Am J Sports Med 1989;15:305–17.

Mansfield JM, Emans SJ. Editor's column: Growth in female gymnastics: should training decrease during puberty? J Paediatr 1993;122:237–40.

Maresh MM. Linear growth of long bones of extremities from infancy through adolescence. Am J Dis Child 1955;89:725–42.

Martinez L, Haymes E. Substrate utilization during treadmill running in prepubertal girls and women. Med Sci Sports Exerc 1992;24:975–83.

Massad S, Shier N, Koceja D, Ellis N. High school athletes and nutritional supplements: a study of knowledge and use. Int J Sport Nutr 1995;5:232–45.

McKay Parks P, Read M. Adolescent male athletes: body image, diet and exercise. Adolescence 1997; 32:593–602.

McLennan W, Podger A, eds. National nutrition survey, selected highlights, Australia 1995. ABS Catalogue No. 4802.0. Canberra: Australian Bureau of Statistics and the Department of Health and Family Services, 1997.

Meeussen R, Borms J. Gymnastic injuries. Sports Med 1992;13:337–56.

Meyer F, Bar-Or O. Fluid and electrolyte loss during exercise: the pediatric angle. Sports Med 1994; 18:4–9.

Meyer F, Bar-Or O, MacDougall D, Heigenhauser G. Sweat electrolyte loss during exercise in the heat: effects of gender and maturation. Med Sci Sports Exerc 1992;24:776–81.

Meyer F, Bar-Or O, Salsberg A, Passe D. Hypohydration during exercise in children: effect on thirst, drink preferences and rehydration. Int J Sport Nutr 1994;4:22–35.

Meyer F, O'Connor H, Shirreffs SM. Nutrition for the young athlete. J Sports Sci 2007;25(Suppl):73S–82S.

Micheli LJ. Overuse injuries in children's sports: the growth factor. Orthop Clin North Am 1983;14:337–60.

Micklesfield LK, Reyneke L, Fataar A, Myburgh KH. Long-term restoration of deficits in bone mineral density is inadequate in premenopausal women with prior menstrual irregularity. Clin J Sports Med 1998;8:155–3.

Milesovic A. Sports drinks hazard to teeth. Br J Sports Med 1997;31:28–30.

Moen S, Sanborn C, Dimarco N. Dietary habits and body composition in adolescent female runners. Wom Sport Phys Activ J 1992;1:85–95.

Moffatt R. Dietary status of elite female high school gymnasts: inadequacy of vitamin and mineral intake. J Am Diet Assoc 1984;84:1361–3.

Montfort-Steiger V, Williams CA. Carbohydrate intake considerations for young athletes. J Sports Sci Med 2007;6:343–52.

Mosier Jr HD. The control of catch-up growth. Acta Endocrinol (Copenh) 1986;113:1–8.

Mosier HD. Set point for target size in catch-up growth: auxology 88. In: Tanner JM, ed. Perspectives in the science of growth and development. London: Smith-Gordon, 1989:343–51.

Murray R, Drummond B. Are there risks to dental health with frequent use of CHO foods and beverages? Aust J Nutr Diet 1996;53(4 Suppl):47S.

National Health & Medical Research Council (NMHRC). Dietary guidelines for children and adolescents. Canberra: Australian Government Publishing Service, 2003.

Neinstein LS. Menstrual dysfunction in pathological states. West J Med 1985;143:476–84.

Neumark-Sztainer D, Story M, Perry C, Casey M. Factors influencing food choices of adolescents: findings from focus-group discussions with adolescents. J Am Diet Assoc 1999;99:929–37.

Nickerson H, Holubets M, Weiler B, et al. Causes of iron deficiency in adolescent athletes. J Pediatr 1989;114:657–63.

Nowak M, Crawford D. Getting the message across: adolescents' health and concerns and views about the importance of food. Aust J Nutr Diet 1998;55:3–8.

Nowak M, Speare R. Gender differences in food-related concerns, beliefs and behaviours of North Queensland adolescents. J Paediatr Child Health 1996;32:424–7.

O'Dea J. Body image and nutritional status among adolescents and adults—a review of the literature. Aust J Nutr Diet 1995;52:56–67.

O'Dea J. A nutritional study of 5,000 Australian school children. University of Sydney News, May 2003:42–5.

O'Dea J, Abraham S. Knowledge, beliefs, attitudes and behaviors related to weight control, eating disorders, and body image in Australian trainee home economics and physical education teachers. J Nutr Educ 2001;33:332–40.

Perron M, Endres J. Knowledge, attitudes, and dietary practices of female athletes. J Am Diet Assoc 1985;85:573–6.

Prader A. Pubertal growth. Acta Paediatr J 1992;34:222–35.

Prasad A, Miale A, Farid A, Sandstead H, Schulert A. Biochemical studies of dwarfism, hypogonadism and anemia. Arch Intern Med 1963;111:426–30.

Preece M. The development of skeletal sex differences at adolescence. In: Russo P, Gass G, eds. Human adaptation: a workshop on growth and physical activity. Sydney: Department of Biological Sciences, Cumberland College of Health Sciences, 1982:1–13.

Preece MA, Ratcliffe SG. Auxological aspects of male and female puberty. Acta Paediatr 1992;383(Suppl): 11S–13S.

Pugliese MT, Lifshitz F, Grad G, et al. Fear of obesity: a cause of short stature and delayed puberty. N Eng J Med 1983;309:513–18.

Rankinen T, Fogelholm M, Kujala U, Rauramaa R, Uusitupa M. Dietary intake and nutritional status of athletic and non-athletic children in early puberty. Int J Sport Nutr 1995;5:136–50.

Robinson TL, Snow-Harter C, Taaffee DR, et al. Gymnasts exhibit higher bone mass than runners despite similar prevalence of amenorrhoea and oligomenorrhoea. J Bone Miner Res 1995;10:26–35.

Roche AF, Chumlea WC, Thissen D. Assessing the skeletal maturation of the hand-wrist: Fels method. Springfield, Illinois: Charles C Thomas, 1988.

Rogol AD. Growth and growth hormone secretion at puberty in males. In: Blimkie CJR, Bar-Or O. New horizons in pediatric exercise science. Australia: Human Kinetics, 1995:53.

Rowland T. Iron deficiency in the young athlete. Sports Med 1990;37:1153–63.

Rowland T, Black S, Kelleher J. Iron deficiency in adolescent endurance athletes. J Adol Health Care 1987;8:322–6.

Rowland TW. The 'trigger hypothesis' for aerobic trainability: a 14-year follow-up. Pediatr Exerc Science 1997;9:1–9.

Sandstead H. Requirement of zinc in human subjects. J Am Coll Nutr 1985;4:73–82.

Sank L. Dental nutrition. Nutr Iss Abstr 1999;19:1–2.

Sirota L. Vitamin and mineral toxicities: issues related to supplementation practices of athletes. J Health Ed 1994;25:82–8.

Smith DW, Truog W, Rogers JE, et al. Shifting linear growth during infancy: illustration of genetic factors in growth from foetal life through infancy. J Paediatr 1976;89:225–30.

Smith WJ, Underwood L, Clemmons D. Effects of caloric or protein restriction on insulin-like growth factor-1 (IGF-1) and IGF-1 binding proteins in children and adults. J Clin Endocrinol Metab 1995;80:443–9.

Smolander J, Bar-Or O, Korhonen O, Ilmarinen J. Thermoregulation during rest and exercise in the cold in pre- and early pubescent boys and in young men. J App Physiol 1992;72:1589–94.

Sobal J, Marquart L. Vitamin/mineral supplement use among high school athletes. Adol 1994;29:835–43.

Sports Dietitians Australia. Consensus statement on fluid and energy replacement for exercise and sports activities. Victoria: Sports Dietitians Australia, 1998:1–3.

Sports Medicine Australia. Safety guidelines for children in sport and recreation. Canberra: Sports Medicine Australia, 1997.

Steen S, McKinney S. Nutrition assessment of college wrestlers. Phys Sports Med 1986;14:100–16.

Swissa-Sivan A, Simkin A, Leichter I, et al. Effect of swimming on bone growth and development in young rats. Bone Miner 1989;7:91–105.

Tanner JM. Growth at adolescence. London: Blackwell Scientific Publications and Springfield Thomas, 1962.

Tanner JM, Whitehouse RH, Marshall WA, et al. Assessment of skeletal maturity and prediction of adult height. London: Academic Press, 1975.

Tanner JM, Whitehouse RH, et al. Assessment of skeletal maturity and prediction of adult height. Second edition. New York: Academic Press, 1983.

Theintz G, Howald H, Weiss U, Sizonenko P. Evidence for a reduction of growth potential in adolescent female gymnasts. J Paediatr 1993;122:306–13.

Thompson JL. Energy balance in young athletes. Int J Sport Nutr 1998;8:160–74.

Thompson S. A healthy start for kids: building good eating patterns for life. Sydney: Simon & Schuster, 1995.

Timmons BW, Bar-Or O, Riddell MC. Oxidation rate of exogenous carbohydrate during exercise is higher in boys than in men. J Appl Physiol 2003;94:278–84.

Timmons BW, Bar-Or O, Riddell MC. Energy substrate utilization during prolonged exercise with and without carbohydrate intake in preadolescent and adolescent girls. J Appl Physiol 2007;103: 995–1000.

Tonz O, Stronski SM, Gmeiner CYK. Wachstum und Pubertat bei 7-bis 16 jahrigen Kunstturnerinnen: eine prospective studies. Schweiz Med Wochenschr 1990;120:10–19.

Tuttle C, Truswell S. Childhood and adolescence. In: Mann J, Truswell S. Essentials of human nutrition. Oxford: Oxford University Press, 1998:481–90.

Tveit-Milligan P, Spindler AA, Nichols JE. Genes and gymnastics: a case study of triplets. Sports Med Training Rehab 1993;4:47–52.

Van de Loo D, Johnson M. The young female athlete. Clin Sport Med 1995;14:687–707.

Van den Brande JL. Catch-up growth: possible mechanisms. Acta Endocrinol (Copenh) 1986;113:13–24.

Van Erp-Baart M, Fredrix L, Binkhorst RA, et al. Energy intake and energy expenditure in top female gymnasts. In: Binkhorst RA, Kemper HCG, Saris WMH, eds. Children and exercise. Champaign, Illinois: Human Kinetics, 1985:218–23.

Warren M. The effects of under-nutrition on reproductive function in the human. Endocr Rev 1983; 1983:363–77.

Warren MP. The effects of exercise and pubertal progression and reproductive function in girls. J Clin Endocrinol Metab 1980;51:1150–7.

Warren MP, Brooks-Gunn J. Delayed menarche in athletes: the role of low energy intake and eating disorders and their relation to bone density. New York: Serona Symposia Publications from Raven Books Ltd, 1989.

Warren MP, Stiehl AL. Exercise and female adolescents: effects on the reproductive and skeletal systems. JAMA 1999;53:115–20.

Wiita B, Stomabaugh I. Nutrition knowledge, eating practices and health of adolescent female runners: a 3-year longitudinal study. Int J Sport Nutr 1996;6:414–25.

Wollmann HA, Ranke MB. GH treatment in neonates. Acta Paediatr 1996;85:398–400.

Zonderland ML, Claessons AL, Lefevre J, et al. Delayed growth and decreased energy intake in female gymnasts. In: Armstrong N, Kirby B, Welsman J. Children and exercise XIX. London: E & FN Spon, 1997:533–6.

CHAPTER 18

Nutrition issues for the aging athlete

PETER REABURN

Introduction

18.1

In 2002, around 20% of the world's population was over the age of 60 years. By 2025, this figure is estimated to increase to 29% (WHO 2002). In Australia, the number of people aged 65 years and over has increased to 13.5% of the total population of 21.8 million (Australian Bureau of Statistics 2008). During recent decades, the number of older people participating in physical activity and organized sport has substantially increased. This increase is reflected by a fourfold increase in participants in the World Masters Games, from around 8300 in the 2002 games in Melbourne, Australia, to an expected 30 000 participants for the Sydney games in 2009.

This overall increase in physical activity in the general population and in competitive events is likely to be attributed to the strength of evidence confirming the benefits of physical activity in decreasing the risk factors for chronic lifestyle-related diseases and improving health outcomes in older people. (For reviews, see Blair & Brodney 1999; Wahlqvist & Savige 2000; Min Lee et al. 2004; Melzer et al. 2004; Warburton et al. 2006; Kruk 2007; Paterson et al. 2007; Sui et al. 2007). Government policy and media campaigns in most western countries have reinforced these benefits.

Nutrient recommendations and corresponding nutrition intervention for aging athletes are based on:

- the physiological changes associated with aging and their impact on nutrient requirements
- additional nutrient requirements imposed by physical activity
- the presence of any medical condition that requires specific dietary intervention

Specific nutrient requirements and recommendations for 'healthy' aging athletes, particularly in relation to micronutrients, have not been determined and are difficult to estimate because of large differences in the rate of aging between individuals and the many different types of sports undertaken (from lawn bowls to ironman triathlon). In the absence of definitive values, population nutrient references are used as a benchmark for assessing and planning diets. However, these do not necessarily apply to people on medication. Between 14% and 25% of participants in masters sport have reported a pre-existing medical condition (primarily hypertension, asthma and coronary heart disease), with up to 34% taking medication, particularly for treating cardiovascular, respiratory and inflammatory conditions (Farquharson 1990; Reaburn et al. 1995). For these athletes, there may be interference with nutrient absorption or drug-nutrient interaction that may influence nutrient requirements.

This chapter provides an overview of the physiological changes that occur with aging and their impact on nutrient requirements and corresponding nutrient recommendations for aging athletes. Because of the limited research available in older athletes (i.e. >50 years), nutrient recommendations are predominantly based on extrapolation of data from studies on younger athletes in combination with population nutrient reference cut-offs for older age groups. Population nutrient references, termed Nutrient Reference Values (NRV) in Australia and New Zealand, and Dietary Reference Intakes (DRI) in the USA and Canada, are available for most macro- and micronutrients (Institute of Medicine 2002; Commonwealth Department of Health and Ageing et al. 2006).

For an individual and group, the Estimated Average Requirement (EAR) is considered the best estimate of a nutrient requirement (Institute of Medicine 2000b; Murphy & Poos 2002). However, the data used to determine the cut-offs for the DRI/NRV for some nutrients do not necessarily address the requirements of very active individuals. The oldest age group in these recommendations is 51–70 years and, for some nutrients, older than 70 years (Institute of Medicine 2000a, 2002; Commonwealth Department of Health and Ageing et al. 2006). These age ranges are broad and, although they make some allowance for the metabolic and physiological changes that occur during aging, they may need to be adjusted for older athletes undertaking intensive or endurance activity most days of the week. Moreover, the EAR needs to be used with caution as a benchmark for assessing adequacy or planning nutrient intakes when applied to aging individuals who may be on medication for an existing disease. See Chapter 2 for further information on the use of the varying levels of the DRI/NRV and their application in assessing and planning diets for individuals and groups. Most dietary survey studies of athletes or any population group use the Recommended Dietary Allowance (RDA) or Recommended Dietary Intake (RDI) for assessing the 'adequacy' or 'inadequacy' of nutrient intakes in groups of athletes. The EAR is now the accepted cut-off for this purpose (Murphy et al. 2006).

18.2 Physiological changes in aging athletes

The aging process, at least in sedentary individuals, is accompanied by many physiological changes that affect nutrient and energy requirements and food preferences. Substantial loss of lean body mass (muscle mass and bone mass), reduced immunity, gastric atrophy, decreased sensitivity to taste and smell and a reduced thirst sensitivity occur with aging. Whether these declines are a result of the aging process itself, or the inactivity that often accompanies aging, is unknown. In the general population, fat mass (FM) increases with aging to around 50–60 years, then decreases after 70 years (Going et al. 1994). Similar observations are evident in aging male and female endurance runners, although increases in FM are much less than that of the general population (Kohrt et al. 1992; Van Pelt et al. 2001).

The loss of fat-free mass (FFM) and, in particular, muscle mass, is inevitable with aging, despite the potential effect of resistance exercise on increasing muscle mass. Physical activity appears to have little effect on sparing or preventing loss of FFM (Hawkins et al. 2003; Tanaka & Seals 2003, 2008). Despite the stimulatory effects of physical activity, particularly load-bearing activity, in building and maintaining FFM, particularly bone mass, there is still a decrease in muscle mass with aging in both endurance athletes (Klitgaard et al. 1990; Proctor & Joyner 1997), and in those involved in a lifetime of sprint or power training (Reaburn 1994). Whether these declines are the result of the aging process or the low levels of physical activity in older populations remains to be determined.

Furthermore, bone mineral density in postmenopausal athletic women is still lower than in younger athletic women (Nelson et al. 1991). In women, bone loss occurs earlier than in men (around 45 years) and at a faster rate (1% per year) (see Chapter 9). In men, it is estimated that bone loss commences around 50 years and continues at the rate of around 0.3% per year thereafter. Also, because men usually have a larger bone mass than women, they lose less bone and are therefore at a lower risk of degenerative osteoporosis than women of the same age. There is good evidence that exercise can attenuate or retard the rate of bone loss, and in some cases improve the density of trabecular bone, but does not prevent overall total loss of bone mass (see Chapter 9).

The aging athlete is at high risk for heat stress, cold intolerance and hypohydration. As the fine-tuning of the thermoregulatory responses deteriorates with aging, aging athletes are at similar risk of heat loss and overheating as children. The difficulty in regulating temperature homeostasis is in part related to changes in the cardiovascular system. The age-related changes occurring in the functioning of the cardiovascular system are independent of disease (e.g. atherosclerosis) or disease process (e.g. atherogenesis). These changes include a decline in maximal cardiovascular function (associated with a decreased maximal heart rate and decrease in maximal oxygen consumption) and a diminished contractile function of the heart. This lowers cardiac output and diminishes blood flow to the skin, thus reducing the capacity to remove heat. Hence, adequate hydration and cooling during physical activity in the heat is critical to reducing risk of heat stress in the older athlete.

Table 18.1 summarizes the major physiological changes that occur with aging that are likely to affect nutrient requirements. For further reading see Reaburn et al. 1995; Trappe et al. 1996; Pollock et al. 1997; Maharam et al. 1999; Trappe 2001; Hawkins et al. 2003; Tanaka & Seals 2003, 2008; Reaburn & Dascombe 2008, 2009.

TABLE 18.1 MAJOR AGE-RELATED CHANGES THAT MAY INFLUENCE NUTRIENT REQUIREMENTS OF AGING ATHLETES

AGE-RELATED CHANGE	NUTRITIONAL IMPLICATION
Decreased muscle mass	Decreased energy requirements
Decreased aerobic capacity	Decreased energy requirements
Decreased muscle glycogen stores	Decreased energy requirements
Decreased bone density	Increased need for calcium and vitamin D
Decreased immune function	Increased need for vitamins B6 and E and zinc
Decreased gastric acid	Increased need for vitamin B12, folic acid, calcium, iron and zinc
Decreased skin capacity for synthesis	Increased need for vitamin D cholecalciferol

(continued)

TABLE 18.1 (continued)

AGE-RELATED CHANGE	NUTRITIONAL IMPLICATION
Decreased calcium bioavailability	Increased need for calcium and vitamin D
Decreased hepatic uptake of retinol	Decreased need for vitamin A
Decreased efficiency in metabolic use of pyridoxal	Increased need for vitamin B6
Increased oxidative stress status	Increased need for carotenoids and vitamins C and E
Increased levels of homocysteine	Increased need for folate and vitamins B6 and B12
Decreased thirst perception	Increased fluid needs
Decreased kidney function	Increased fluid needs

Source: Holick 2004

18.3 Nutrient and energy recommendations for aging athletes

Population nutrient standards (NRV in Australia and New Zealand and DRI in the USA and Canada) have been released for essential macro- and micronutrients for different age groups (Institute of Medicine 1997, 2000a, 2002; Commonwealth Department of Health and Ageing et al. 2006). Recommendations for protein, vitamin D and calcium are slightly higher in men and women over 70 years than between 51 and 70 years (Institute of Medicine 1997). Recommendations for other nutrients are no different than in younger adults, except for energy. However, these age ranges are wide and do not necessarily account for the additional metabolic and physiological changes imposed by athletic training of high intensity or duration. These population standards may not be appropriate for assessing the nutrient adequacy of an aging person or group undertaking athletic training. For reviews of nutrient recommendations for the aging athlete, see Sachek and Roubenoff (1999) and more recent publications by Rivlin (2007) and Rosenbloom and Dunaway (2007).

Several studies have been published on dietary intakes of aging athletes (Rock 1991; Butterworth et al. 1993; Hallfrisch et al. 1994; Sykes 1994; Chatard et al. 1998; Maharam et al. 1999) and their supplementary practices (Striegel et al. 2005). The results of these studies suggest that older men and women who are aerobically fit tend to consume a more nutrient-dense diet that is closer to the RDA/RDI than their less-fit peers (Brodney et al. 2001; Van Pelt et al. 2001; Roberts & Rosenberg 2006).

18.4 Energy recommendations for aging athletes

Estimates of energy expenditure are used to determine energy requirements in any population group. Daily energy requirements decrease with aging because of:

- decreases in energy expenditure required for physical activity and resting metabolic rate (RMR) (Elia et al. 2000; Wakimoto & Block 2001; Roberts & Dallal 2005; Roberts & Rosenberg 2006)

- decreases in FFM (Going et al. 1994; Horber et al. 1996)
- decreases in physical activity levels and training volume levels (Rising et al. 1994; Starling et al. 1999; Van Pelt et al. 2001; Weir et al. 2002)

Physical training (aerobic and/or resistance training) in previously untrained people increases energy requirements and helps maintain and reduce the rate of loss of metabolically active muscle and bone mass that occurs with aging (Fiatarone Singh 2002; Lucas & Heiss 2005). Aging athletes undertaking regular physical training have reported higher energy intakes than sedentary controls (Butterworth et al. 1993; Hallfrisch et al. 1994; Beshgetoor & Nichols 2003), especially when matched for energy intake per kilogram of BM (Van Pelt et al. 2001). In some studies, reported energy intakes of aging athletes (aged 55–75 years) were much higher than RDAs and ranged from around 10 300 kJ/d (Hallfrisch et al. 1994) to 11 500 kJ/d (Chatard et al. 1998) but were still lower than those reported in younger athletes (Van Erp-Baart et al. 1989; Burke et al. 1991; Hawley et al. 1995). In those aging athletes who maintained high-intensity training, daily energy needs were still higher than sedentary controls, despite declines in RMR and energy expenditures (Van Pelt et al. 2001).

Macronutrients 18.5

In the general population, total macronutrient intakes—carbohydrate (CHO), fat and protein—tend to decrease with aging (Ruiz-Torres et al. 1995; Wakimoto & Block 2001). Dietary surveys of aging athletes (Van Pelt et al. 2001; Beshgetoor & Nichols 2003; Sallinen et al. 2008) and middle-aged highly aerobically fit athletes (Brodney et al. 2001) have found macronutrient intakes close to the population goals. Although using relative percentages of energy from macronutrients to the total energy of the diet is no longer recommended for use in athletes (see Chapter 14), these population targets or Acceptable Macronutrient Distribution Ranges (AMDR) are used as a basis for evaluating dietary balance in epidemiological surveys. In one epidemiological study of over 10 000 men and women (aged 20–87 years) divided into in low, moderately and highly aerobically fit cohorts, Brodney and colleagues (2001) reported significantly higher percent CHO and lower percent fat intakes in both men and women in the highest fit group, compared with the low and moderately fit groups. However in this study, the relative contribution from CHO was still below the CHO target recommended for athletes (American College of Sports Medicine et al. 2009a). More recently, Sallinen and colleagues (2008) reported relatively high fat intakes (36% or total energy) and low CHO intakes (43% of total energy) in male Finnish national level masters strength and power athletes (mean age 52 ± 5 years) but not in the older athletes (72 ± 4 years). These studies suggest that such imbalances may not be conducive to enhancing sports performance and not optimal for promoting better health outcomes.

Carbohydrate 18.6

The rationale for recommending high-CHO diets for training and recovery is described in detail in Chapters 1 and 14. In aging endurance runners, glycogen storage per unit of muscle is lower than in similarly trained younger runners, while glycogen utilization per unit of energy expenditure is higher during submaximal exercise (Meredith et al. 1989). However, following regular endurance training, older individuals are able to increase muscle glycogen storage and recover glycogen stores at similar rates as younger athletes (Meredith et al.

TABLE 18.2 DIETARY GUIDELINES FOR OLDER AUSTRALIANS (UNDER REVIEW)

1.	Enjoy a wide variety of nutritious foods
2.	Keep active to maintain muscle strength and a healthy body weight
3.	Eat plenty of vegetables (including legumes) and fruit
4.	Eat plenty of cereals, breads and pastas
5.	Eat a diet low in saturated fat
6.	Drink adequate amounts of water and/or other fluids
7.	If you drink alcohol, limit your intake
8.	Choose foods low in salt and use salt sparingly
9.	Include foods high in calcium
10.	Use added sugars in moderation
11.	Eat at least three meals every day
12.	Care for your food: prepare and store it correctly

Source: NHMRC 1999

1989; Tarnopolsky et al. 1997). Earlier studies have also confirmed that healthy, previously sedentary older individuals who undertake aerobic exercise training can improve glucose tolerance and the rate of insulin-mediated glucose disposal, and increase skeletal muscle glucose transporter (GLUT-4) activity (Hughes et al. 1993; Kirwan et al. 1993), similar to younger athletes.

Recommendations for the amount of CHO needed for training and recovery in aging athletes are similar to those recommended for younger adult athletes (see Chapter 14), since CHO absorption and utilization is unaffected by aging, in the absence of any disease (Saltzman & Russell 1998; Elahi & Muller 2000). Diets rich in CHO preferably from a mixture of low to moderate glycemic index foods are recommended (FAO 1998; Burke et al. 2004). The dietary guideline for older Australians to 'Eat plenty of cereals, breads and pastas' (see Table 18.2) also provides an excellent message for older athletes to choose those foods that are high in fiber and have a low glycemic index (NHMRC 1999). However, for some susceptible older individuals, very high fiber intakes often exacerbate abdominal discomfort and flatulence. The health and performance benefits of consuming high CHO intakes usually outweigh any discomfort.

18.7 Fat

Dietary guidelines that recommend a reduction of total and saturated fatty acid intakes are also appropriate for the aging athlete. Aging people retain the ability to digest, absorb and utilize fat (Saltzman & Russell 1998; Toth & Tchernof 2000). Some older athletes report consuming relatively high-fat diets compared with population targets and controls (Butterworth et al. 1993; Reaburn & Le Bon 1995; Chatard et al. 1998; Brodney et al. 2001; Beshgetoor & Nichols 2003; Sallinen et al. 2008). Relatively low fat intakes are still important for aging athletes, particularly those involved in endurance training, so that more energy can be derived from CHO and protein (Economos et al. 1993), which may be related to high energy intakes. Very low fat intakes (i.e. less than 20% of energy from fat) may compromise the intake of fat-soluble vitamins (A, D, E and K) and decrease satiety between meals.

Protein

The DRI/NRV for protein suggest that older adults (>53 years) need 25% higher protein requirements than younger adults to maintain protein balance (Institute of Medicine 2002; Commonwealth Department of Health and Ageing et al. 2006). This increase is reflected in even older adults where the revised RDA/RDI for men (>70 years) is 1.1 g protein/kg BM, compared to 0.84 g protein/kg BM for younger men. Females have slightly lower cut-offs than this (Commonwealth Department of Health and Ageing et al. 2006).

In adult athletes, protein turnover and hence requirements are slightly higher than population reference cut-offs (see Chapter 4). Aging athletes (mainly endurance and power athletes) may have slightly lower protein requirements than younger adult athletes because of:

- a decline in muscle mass with aging (Klitgaard et al. 1990; Reaburn 1994; Proctor & Joyner 1997)
- a decrease in whole-body protein turnover and decreased protein synthesis with aging (Nair 1995; Morais et al. 1997)
- a decrease in use of protein as a fuel because of reduced training intensity and/or volume reported in aging athletes (Trappe et al. 1995; Weir et al. 2002)
- possible age-related reduction in the absorptive capacity of the gut for amino acids and peptides (Saltzman & Russell 1998)

Although further research is needed before definitive recommendations can be made for aging athletes, protein intakes of 0.8–1.0 g/kg BM/d (Sachek & Roubenoff 1999) or even higher intakes for athletes >70 years of 1.0–1.25 g/kg BM/d (Evans 1995, 2004) have been suggested to maintain a positive nitrogen balance. More recently, an extensive review of protein needs in older athletes suggested that master athletes undertaking resistance training should consume 1.0–1.2 g/kg BM/d of protein with around 50% from protein-rich foods with high biological value such as meat, fish, egg whites and milk (Tarnopolsky 2008). Moreover, immediately following resistance training (within 30 minutes), the early provision of CHO and protein can maximize muscle and strength development (Tarnopolsky 2008). These values are well above the Australian RDI of 0.86 g protein/kg BM/d for males older than 70 years (Commonwealth Department of Health and Ageing et al. 2006) but lower than the protein recommendations for younger adult athletes engaged in similar training programs (American College of Sports Medicine et al. 2009a).

Dietary surveys of aging athletes suggest that protein recommendations are easily met when athletes consume adequate energy intake and a variety of high-quality protein sources (dairy, meats, eggs and fish) (Lemon 2000; Van Pelt et al. 2001; Tarnopolsky 2008). Protein intakes of 1.25–1.45 g/kg BM/d reported in dietary surveys of aging athletes from a variety of training backgrounds confirm adequate intakes (Chatard et al. 1998; Starling et al. 1999; Van Pelt et al. 2001; Beshgetoor & Nichols 2003; Sallinen et al. 2008). However, older athletes in heavy training, particularly those involved with strength and power sports, may require slightly higher protein intakes (Lemon 1998, 2000; Tarnopolsky 2008) since resistance exercise increases muscle protein synthesis in both elderly and young individuals (Yarasheski et al. 1993; Campbell et al. 2001).

Do high protein intakes negate losses of fat-free mass in aging athletes?

Studies on the effects of high-protein diets as a means of stimulating protein synthesis and preventing losses of FFM or lean body mass that occurs with aging have been equivocal

(Volpi et al. 1998; Welle & Thornton 1998). The consensus is that high-protein diets (above nutrient reference standards—RDI/RDA) do not provide a significant increase in protein synthesis or conserve muscle mass (Starling et al. 1999; Campbell et al. 2001).

Potential adverse effects of very high protein intakes include impaired kidney function, increased calcium loss, atherogenic effects and increased urinary calcium excretion. These outcomes may be a risk for people with a genetic predisposition to these conditions. Protein supplements and high-salt diets increase excretion of urinary calcium, which can also increase risk of kidney stones in susceptible people. For most people, there is no convincing evidence that the additional nitrogen and possibly calcium excretion that accompanies a high-protein diet cannot be handled by a normally functioning kidney (Lemon 1998, 2000).

In summary, the beneficial effects of high-protein intakes appear to outweigh the possible adverse effects. Protein intakes in older persons of 1.0–1.3 g/kg BM/d, in combination with adequate calcium intake, could be beneficial for bone health (Lucas & Heiss 2005). Lemon (1998, 2000) has confirmed that protein intake of 1.2–1.7 g/kg BM/d will not adversely affect cardiovascular health.

18.9 Micronutrients

The requirements for and effects of micronutrients (i.e. vitamins and trace minerals) on performance in adult and adolescent athletes are reviewed in Chapter 11.

Dietary surveys of older endurance athletes have reported intakes of calcium, iron, zinc, magnesium and vitamins D and E below the RDA, despite adequate energy intakes (Butterworth et al. 1993; Hallfrisch et al. 1994; Reaburn & Le Bon 1995; Chatard et al. 1998; Beshgetoor & Nichols 2003; American College of Sports Medicine et al. 2009a) (see Table 18.3). Intakes below the RDA/RDI but greater than the EAR suggest a possibility of inadequate intake but do not confirm a deficiency. Usually when energy intakes are met, micronutrient intakes are satisfactory. With prolonged low energy intakes, body stores of some micronutrients diminish (Clarkson & Haymes 1994) resulting in a depleted or deficiency state that can negatively affect performance (Campbell & Anderson 1987; McDonald & Keen 1988; Chen 2000). Furthermore, in aging athletes, risks of micronutrient deficiencies may be compounded by chronic medical conditions, use of medications or changes in gut function that impair nutrient absorption (McCabe 2004).

Irrespective of age, athletes have slightly increased requirements and losses of several vitamins and minerals compared to non-athletes (Haymes & Lamanca 1989), especially endurance athletes (Lukaski 1995; Chen 2000).

Aging athletes are at higher risk of micronutrient deficiencies than younger athletes for several reasons:

- an age-related decrease in nutrient absorption reported for several micronutrients (vitamins B6, B12, D and calcium) (Institute of Medicine 1997; Saltzmann & Russell 1998)
- the wide variation in nutrient requirements between individuals (Commonwealth Department of Health & Ageing et al. 2006)
- the use of medications that interfere with nutrient absorption or utilization (Reaburn et al. 1995; McCabe 2004; Pronsky 2008)
- the presence of chronic disease states (Reaburn et al. 1995)

TABLE 18.3 SUMMARY TABLE OF STUDIES EXAMINING DIETARY INTAKES OF AGING ATHLETES

STUDY	AGE (YEARS)	SAMPLE		COMPARED TO RESULTS
Beshgetoor et al. 2000	49.6 ± 7.9	Female endurance	RDA	↓ Calcium (Ca)
Beshgetoor & Nichols 2003	48.4 ± 2.4	Female endurance (non-supplement users)	RDA	↓ Vitamin E ↓ Calcium (Ca)
Butterworth et al. 1993	72.5 ± 1.8	Female endurance (*n* = 12)	RDA	↓ Calcium (Ca) ↓ Energy intake
Butterworth et al. 1993	72.5 ± 1.8	Female endurance (*n* = 12)	Age-matched, healthy controls	↓ Energy intake ↑ CHO, fat, protein ↑ Fiber ↑ Vitamins B6, E, folate ↑ Riboflavin, thiamin, niacin ↑ Ca, Ph, Mg, Fe, Zn, Na, K, Cu
Chatard et al. 1998	63 ± 4.5	Male endurance (*n* = 18)	RDA	↓ Mg, vitamin D, Ca ↑ Energy intake ↑ CHO, fat, protein ↑ Fe, vitamins A, B1, B12, C, E
Hallfrisch et al. 1994	66.6 ± 1.3	Male endurance (*n* = 16)	Age-matched, healthy controls	↑ Energy intake ↑ CHO, protein
Reaburn & Le Bon 1995	50.6 ± 4.2	Male endurance (*n* = 14) Female runners (*n* = 15)	RDA	↑ Protein (M & F), fat (M & F) ↑ Riboflavin, niacin, thiamine (M & F) ↑ Vitamins A, C (M & F) ↑ Na, K (M & F) ↓ Ca (F), Fe (F), Zn (M & F), Mg (M & F)

M = male, F = female
Source: Institute of Medicine 1997

Supplementation with vitamins and minerals is common in athletes (Maughan et al. 2004) and also in the older population (McCabe 2004), which may reflect aggressive marketing by the supplement industry. While marketing claims suggest the benefits of micronutrient supplementation in later life, extensive reviews of large, randomized, controlled trials do not support the use of anti-oxidant vitamin or mineral supplements as preventive therapy in well-nourished populations such as masters athletes (Dangour et al. 2004; Shenkin 2006). Indeed, there is growing evidence of possible adverse effects of micronutrient supplementation in an older population with a healthy and adequate dietary intake (Dangour et al. 2004; Shenkin 2006).

In the US, more than 50% of the general population (>65 years) reported using five or more prescribed medications (McCabe 2004). In surveys of master athletes, around 34% reported taking prescribed medications with between 14% and 25% reporting an existing medical condition (Farquharson 1990; Reaburn et al. 1995). The following sections examine the available evidence on dietary intakes of micronutrients in aging athletes; because of the limited evidence about the micronutrient requirements of aging athletes, recommendations are based on extrapolated data from studies of aging sedentary populations.

18.10 Vitamins

Vitamin A

In a healthy aging population, the clearance of vitamin A is decreased by about 50% compared to younger adults. This suggests that the RDI/RDA cut-offs for vitamin A (or retinol equivalents) for people aged 52–70 years are well in excess of requirements and are therefore likely to easily meet the needs of aging athletes (see Chapter 11 and Commentary B). Dietary surveys of this age group, in combination with biochemical indices (high serum retinol values) have confirmed adequate vitamin A status in the general population (Kivela et al. 1989; Saito & Itoh 1991). Nevertheless, aging athletes may experiment with supplements of vitamin A (or other anti-oxidants) because of their potential role in reducing oxidative stress induced by exercise, and their link with reducing risk of many chronic degenerative disease including atherosclerosis, diabetes and some cancers (Frei 1991; Jacques & Chylack 1991; Simon et al. 1998). Misuse of vitamin A supplements, particularly pre-formed vitamin A—the fat soluble form—is associated with vitamin A toxicity (Krasinski et al. 1990; Fortes et al. 1998). As suggested in Chapter 11 and elsewhere (NHMRC 1999), increasing vitamin A-rich foods from dietary sources for this age group is more appropriate than from supplements and avoids the potential pro-oxidative effects associated with this supplement that can potentially damage cells and tissues (see Chapter 11).

Vitamin B6

Requirements for vitamin B6 increase as the intake of protein increases, which corresponds to the role of B6 in amino acid metabolism (Miller & Linkswiler 1967). The EAR for vitamin B6 is slightly higher for older people (>51 years) than younger adults (31–50 years) (Commonwealth Department of Health and Ageing et al. 2006). However, previous dietary surveys of the general population have reported that vitamin B6 intakes in many elderly people do not always meet the RDI/RDA cut-offs, which suggests a possibility of inadequacy for some people (Russell & Suter 1993; CSIRO 1996). Furthermore, evidence from depletion and repletion studies suggests that the amount of vitamin B6 needed to obtain balance in older persons may be greater than these RDA cut-offs (Ribaya-Mercado et al. 1991).

Older athletes, similar to younger athletes, lose vitamin B6 through urinary 4-PA excretion (Manore 2000), thus suggesting increased turnover. Furthermore, serum concentrations of vitamin B6 decrease with aging and high intakes may be needed to support immune system functioning (Meydani et al. 1990, 1991). This increase is reflected in the EARs for men and women over 51 years (Commonwealth Department of Health and Ageing et al. 2006).

Vitamin B12

Vitamin B12 intakes from dietary surveys of aging athletes consuming a mixed diet have demonstrated that vitamin B12 intakes easily met or exceeded RDA cut-offs, which were used for assessing nutrient adequacy in these studies (Chatard et al. 1998; Beshgetoor & Nichols 2003). In contrast, in one prospective survey of Australian adults, 3–10% of men and 10–17% of women consumed less than the RDI cut-off for vitamin B12 (CSIRO 1996). Moreover, vegans are at risk of vitamin B12 deficiency because it is only found in animal food sources, so aging vegan athletes, or athletes who only occasionally eat meat or dairy products, are likely to be at even higher risk from possibly years of deficit or suboptimal intakes.

Recommended requirements (i.e. EAR) for vitamin B12 for individuals also increase with aging for both males and females. This increase is linked to the age-related atrophic gastritis seen in approximately 30% of those over 60 years (Krasinski et al. 1986), which decreases gastric and intrinsic factor secretion needed for B12 absorption (Russell 1992). The incidence of pernicious anemia as a result of malabsorption and deficiency of B12 increases in aging individuals. Estimated requirements for vitamin B12 for aging athletes who are vegetarians or have atrophic gastritis may be slightly higher than non-athletes (Sachek & Roubenoff 1999). From an athlete perspective, vitamin B12 deficiency can lead to pernicious anemia and reduced endurance performance (American College of Sports Medicine et al. 2009a).

Vitamin C

There is no evidence to suggest that vitamin C absorption or utilization is impaired with aging (Blanchard et al. 1990). Dietary surveys of an aging sedentary population and aging athletes have indicated that vitamin C intakes easily meet or exceed population reference intakes (Butterworth et al. 1993; Hallfrisch et al. 1994; Reaburn & Le Bon 1995; Chatard et al. 1998; Beshgetoor & Nichols 2003). Although vitamin C requirements are slightly increased in cigarette smokers and in people living in hot climates, in heavy pollution or undertaking physical activity, vitamin C supplements are not warranted (Russell & Suter 1993; Sachek & Roubenoff 1999). For those athletes engaged in strenuous and prolonged exercise, the American College of Sports Medicine and colleagues (2009a) suggest an intake of 10–1000 mg/d, which is much higher than the EAR cut-offs. For some athletes, a vitamin C supplement may be warranted. However, for susceptible people, high doses of vitamin C supplements (>1000 mg/d) can increase the risk of kidney stones and gout and potentially impair copper absorption (Herbert et al. 1977; Alhadeff et al. 1984). These doses have also been associated with 'runner's diarrhea' (Hoyt 1980).

Vitamin D

Apart from small amounts of dietary sources of vitamin D (from fortified cereals and margarines, and eggs) most vitamin D is manufactured in the liver and, to a lesser extent, the kidney, by the action of ultraviolet light on a vitamin D precursor in the skin.

Adequate intakes of vitamin D are crucial for older individuals given its importance in maintaining bone integrity and the potential decrease in endogenous production observed with aging. Aging reduces the capacity of the skin to synthesize vitamin D precursors (MacLaughlin & Holick 1985) and decreases renal production of activated vitamin D3 (Tsai et al. 1984). Sedentary aging populations report consuming less vitamin D than younger people (Saltzmann & Russell 1998). Similar suboptimal intakes (i.e. less than the RDA/RDI) were reported in national dietary surveys in the US (National Research Council 1989) and in Australia (McLennan & Podger 1997). To date, no epidemiological data for vitamin D intake or vitamin D status are available on aging athletes.

Slightly higher vitamin D recommendations for older people (51–70 years) are reflected in the population nutrient reference values (Institute of Medicine 1997; Commonwealth Department of Health and Ageing et al. 2006) and until further research is available, these can be recommended for athletes in this age group. Vitamin D supplements may only be warranted in older people, including athletes, who have little exposure to sunlight.

Vitamin E

Vitamin E is another anti-oxidant like vitamins C and A that has a potential protective role against the damaging effects of free oxygen radicals or reactive oxygen species (ROS) induced by prolonged or eccentric exercise such as running, cycling, weight training (Packer 1991; Rokitzki et al. 1994). Free oxygen radicals, which are associated with oxidative stress and an increase in lipid peroxidation (a normal by-product of mitochondrial metabolism), can exert repetitive damage to individual cells, promoting an increase in disease prevalence and aging (Vivekananthan et al. 2003).

Studies on younger adult athletes have not supported the hypothesis that vitamin E supplementation attenuates exercise-induced muscle damage (Dekkers et al. 1996; Kaikkonen et al. 1998). In a critical review, Viitala and Newhouse (2004) concluded that well-designed studies do not support the hypothesis that vitamin E alone attenuates lipid peroxidation induced by strenuous exercise, so supplements are not warranted for this purpose. Whether vitamin E supplements are worthwhile for other reasons in aging athletes is still questionable, although in a review of nutrient requirements for elderly exercisers, Sachek and Roubenoff (1999) suggested that those people with cardiovascular disease undertaking endurance training may consider vitamin E supplements of 100–200 mg tocopherol equivalents/day. Certainly there have been reported benefits from recommended doses of vitamin E supplementation for improving immune function (Meydani et al. 1990a) and reducing incidence of cataracts (Robertson et al. 1989), cancers (Knekt et al. 1991) and cardiovascular disease (Rimm et al. 1993) for elderly people. In contrast to these earlier studies of the protective effects of single anti-oxidant supplements including vitamin E, several more recent meta-analyses actually revealed unfavorable health outcomes at high doses (Vivekananthan et al. 2003; Miller et al. 2005). The second meta-analysis revealed an increase in all-cause mortality when vitamin E was supplemented at high doses (>400 IU/d for at least 1 year) (Miller et al. 2005). In dose-response analyses, all-cause mortality progressively increased when vitamin E dosage exceeded 150 IU/d, but at dosages less than this mortality was decreased (Miller et al. 2005), so there appears to be a threshold level.

In another recent well-designed controlled trial in forty healthy young men with no existing disease, a significant decrease in glucose infusion rates into muscle cells and a decrease in insulin sensitivity with high dosage of both vitamin C and E supplements was reported (Ristow et al. 2009). A combination of daily ingestion of vitamin C and vitamin E supplements (1000 mg/d and 400 IU/d, respectively) taken over 4 weeks actually blocked the beneficial effects of exercise on enhancing insulin sensitivity in both pre-trained and untrained controls. It is well known that physical exercise, even short-term exercise, increases reactive oxygen species (ROS) and insulin sensitivity and can potentially reduce the progression of metabolic syndrome into type 2 diabetes (Pan et al. 1997). However, when these high-dose supplements were taken concurrently in this study, the formation of ROS was inhibited and hence the capacity of ROS to counteract insulin resistance was suppressed. According to the authors, the outcome of supplement use with exercise may actually increase the risk of type 2 diabetes rather than decrease it, which has implications for an older population with existing risk factors (Ristow et al. 2009). This is new research and controversial, although there is some evidence that anti-oxidant use in type 2 diabetes has been linked to increased prevalence of hypertension (Ward et al. 2007) and overall mortality (Bjelakovic et al. 2007). Based on this preliminary evidence, use of anti-oxidants as supplements in people with risk factors for type 2 diabetes or with diagnosed diabetes may counteract the beneficial effects of exercise on increasing insulin sensitivity. Further research on at-risk and older age groups is required to test the long-term consequences of this effect.

In summary, the results from the Ristow study and several meta-analyses of intervention trials investigating the effects of short-term, high-dose vitamin E and other anti-oxidant supplements on health outcomes have not supported their widespread use. Habitual supplementation with high-dose vitamin E and other anti-oxidants in athletes or in any population may therefore be inappropriate.

Riboflavin

Aging athletes who are following low-energy diets or have a sudden increase in training volume or intensity may have higher riboflavin requirements than suggested by population reference standards (Manore 2000). However, the few surveys undertaken indicated adequate riboflavin intakes using RDA cut-offs (Beshgetoor & Nichols 2003), with one exception. In one study of fourteen women (50–67 years) undertaking an exercise program, riboflavin intakes met the RDA, although urinary riboflavin excretion was significantly lower than controls, which may be indicative of riboflavin depletion (Winters et al. 1992). In other studies, low riboflavin intakes have been reported in people who limit dairy products (Russell & Suter 1993) so athletes who also avoid or limit dairy foods for any reason may be at risk of suboptimal riboflavin intakes.

Population reference standards (i.e. EAR) for riboflavin for people aged 51–70 years are the same as for younger adults but slightly higher for people over 70 years (Commonwealth Department of Health and Ageing et al. 2006). These are likely to be applicable to aging athletes as a benchmark for assessing the probability of adequate or inadequate intake.

Folate

In aging athletes with gastric atrophy, which is common in elderly persons (Krasinski et al. 1986), the associated decrease in stomach acid production may lead to decreased folate absorption (Rosenberg & Miller 1992). Otherwise in healthy aging athletes, population nutrient recommendations are likely to meet requirements. Sachek and Roubenoff (1999) suggested that aging athletes should consume at least 200 μg/d of folate, as long as vitamin B12 intakes were adequate, since high levels of folate can mask vitamin B12 deficiency. Major sources of folic acid in the diet include milk, green leafy vegetables, fortified cereals, mushrooms, peas, asparagus, peas and beetroot.

18.11 Minerals

Calcium

Although weight-bearing exercise promotes bone density, aging athletes who already have low bone density and possibly long-standing suboptimal calcium intakes and estrogen insufficiency are likely to be at high risk of stress fractures when undertaking repetitive impact activities (Myburgh et al. 1990; Heaney 2001). Repetitive impact activities such as running—particularly in hot, humid conditions—are associated with substantial calcium loss from sweat (Krebs et al. 1988). Thus, adequate calcium intakes are important in aging athletes, particularly perimenopausal and postmenopausal women, to help maintain bone health (see Chapter 9).

Calcium absorption and vitamin D activity decrease with aging in both sexes. Calcium bioavailability is further affected in people with atrophic gastritis, a common problem in older persons resulting in a decrease in gastric acid production (Eastell et al. 1991). Vitamin D status, according to biochemical markers as suggested earlier, may also be suboptimal in older people. Deterioration in kidney function, where active vitamin D is manufactured, has been attributed to the age-related decrease in circulating active vitamin D and thus further compromises calcium absorption.

In one Australian study, calcium intakes were below the RDI in 18–32% of men and 32–58% of women (CSIRO 1996). Similar results have been found in more recent studies from industrialized countries (Wakimoto & Block 2001; Bates et al. 2002; Marriott & Buttress 2003). In aging athletes, dietary intake studies also suggest that many athletes are either not meeting the RDA or are eating less calcium compared with controls (see Table 18.3).

The RDA/RDI for calcium for both women aged greater than 51 years and men aged greater than 70 years is 1300 mg/d, which is the same as for boys and girls aged 12–18 years. For men aged 51–70 years the RDI is 1000 mg/d (Institute of Medicine 1997; Commonwealth Department of Health and Ageing et al. 2006). The cut-offs which, by definition, meet the needs of 97.5% of healthy people, are still higher than for younger adults and compensate for the degenerative bone loss and reduced absorptive capacity that accompanies aging.

Calcium supplements may be needed in those people who have difficulty meeting calcium requirements, including those who are lactose intolerant, dislike milk and dairy products, or are allergic to milk. The American College of Sports Medicine and colleagues' (2009a) guidelines for younger athletes recommend that supplementation with both calcium and vitamin D is determined after nutrition assessment. They further suggest that athletes with disordered eating or amenorrhea, who are at risk of osteopenia, take a combined supplement of calcium and vitamin D at dosages of 1500 mg/d of elemental calcium and 400–800 IU/d of vitamin D. This combination has been shown to reduce bone loss and fractures (National Institute of Health 2006).

Supplements of calcium citrate malate are better absorbed than calcium carbonate supplements, at least in studies of postmenopausal women with low dietary intakes of calcium, and appear more effective than calcium carbonate in reducing bone demineralization and lowering bone fracture rates in this age group (Dawson-Hughes et al. 1990; Reid et al. 1995). Indeed, Lewis and Modlesky (1998) have suggested that additional calcium supplementation (~1000 mg/d) given to premenopausal and late postmenopausal women who are already consuming a relatively high calcium intake (i.e. 70–1000 mg/d) can reduce bone loss.

Iron

In athletes of any age, particularly those involved with endurance exercise, iron is an integral component of the oxygen-carrying capacity of both hemoglobin in the blood and myoglobin within muscle. Moreover, iron is also found within the mitochondrial cytochrome complex and thus is involved in aerobic metabolism.

Iron deficiency anemia reduces performance capacity and maximal aerobic power in athletes and in animal studies (Celsing et al. 1986). Weight-bearing endurance athletes such as runners are at high risk of reducing iron stores since iron losses occur with excessive sweating (Waller & Haymes 1996), gastrointestinal bleeding (Stewart et al. 1984) and hemolysis (Hunding et al. 1981). Suboptimal dietary iron intakes exacerbate risk and low intakes are not uncommon in female athletes of all ages (see Chapter 10). Although losses of iron in endurance athletes such as younger adults and adolescents may be as high as 18 mg/d (Haymes & Lamanca 1989), iron losses have not been studied in aging athletes undertaking similar levels of physical activity. Iron absorption from non-heme food sources (mainly plants) is also affected by atrophic gastritis, which impairs vitamin B12, calcium and zinc absorption. Additionally, the presence of inhibitors naturally occurring in foods, especially tea, when consumed with iron-rich meals, binds non-heme iron, and further reduces its bioavailability (see Chapter 10).

Iron stores usually increase with aging in both males and females (Casale et al. 1981). Older people, therefore, usually need less dietary iron than younger people. In contrast, dietary iron deficiency is rare in older populations of men and anemia is most commonly associated with the anemia of chronic illness or inflammation (Yip & Dallman 1988).

Nevertheless, our unpublished observations found that the dietary iron intakes in many aging Australian male and female endurance athletes were below RDIs (Reaburn & Le Bon 1995), although a recent study of twenty-five middle-aged female endurance cyclists and runners in the US showed iron intake to more than adequately meet nutrient reference standards (Beshgetoor & Nichols 2003). Decreased iron intake with age appears a consistent finding in different cultures, particularly in women (Wakimoto & Block 2001; Martins et al. 2002; Marriott & Buttress 2003) so iron depletion rather than anemia may still be a problem in older female athletes.

The population reference values for iron are 1.3–1.7 times higher for athletes, and 1.8 times higher for vegetarians (non-athletes) to account for the low bioavailability of iron from vegetarian diets (Institute of Medicine 2000a). The cut-offs for older adults (51–70 years) are no different from younger adults.

Zinc

Dietary zinc is involved in tissue repair and immune function, which is particularly applicable to the aging athlete who is susceptible to tissue damage (Chandra 2004). Zinc is also a cofactor in the synthesis and degradation of CHO, fats, proteins and nucleic acids (Sandstrom 1997). Most zinc losses occur through urine, feces and sweating (Anderson et al. 1984; Couzy et al. 1990) and because of these losses, requirements may be high in an athlete of any age training in hot, humid climates. Interestingly, the turnover of zinc is increased in anaerobic exercise, which is likely to be linked to its metabolic role in glycolysis (Krotkiewski et al. 1982; Lukaski 1995). These functions might suggest a high zinc requirement, particularly for aging athletes undertaking high-intensity interval training. However, there is no evidence to suggest that zinc balance is different between younger and older adult populations on a similar type of diet. While zinc absorption decreases with aging, its excretion diminishes, so zinc balance is better maintained in older people, compared with younger adults (Turnland et al. 1986).

Nevertheless, many older people including older athletes may not be eating enough zinc in their diets, particularly if they are limiting meat intake. In the 1995 National Nutrition Survey in Australia, average zinc intakes of both males and females (>65 years) were just below the RDI for males and much lower than the RDI for females (McLennan & Podger 1998). In another study in the US, 75% of women aged 50–69 years and 90% of men aged greater than 70 years did not meet the RDA for zinc (Wakimoto & Block 2001). Suboptimal or borderline intakes of zinc have also been reported in aging athletes (Reaburn & Le Bon 1995; Beshgetoor & Nichols 2003). Zinc absorption from meals can be further reduced by the presence of naturally occurring inhibitors in food such as phytates (found in whole grain cereals, soy, peanut) and also by calcium and iron supplements taken with a meal (Wood & Zheng 1997). Thus, aging athletes on high-CHO diets (e.g. vegetarians), or who eat only small amounts of meat or seafood (good sources of zinc), may be at risk of zinc deficiency and may warrant zinc supplements. The EAR for zinc for vegetarians can be as much as 50% higher than for meat eaters, particularly strict vegetarians whose main staples are grains and legumes, because of the inhibitory effects of phytates on zinc absorption (Institute of Medicine 2002; Commonwealth Department of Health and Ageing et al. 2006).

In summary, aging athletes may be at risk of zinc depletion if they have high sweat losses, or consume high-CHO or vegetarian-style diets with a high phytate content or routinely take calcium or iron supplements with meals, which inhibit zinc absorption. See Chapter 10, Table 10.9 for the phytate content of foods.

18.12 Water

For an athlete of any age, even modest fluid losses (<2% BW) can impair athletic performance (Barr 1999; American College of Sports Medicine 2009a). Physiologically, aging athletes are more susceptible than younger athletes to hypohydration and heat stress for several reasons:

- a decrease in total body water with aging and subsequent decrease in plasma volume thereby increasing the risk of heat stress (Schoeller 1989)
- reduced efficiency of renal anti-diuretic hormone receptors, which increases urinary excretion rate leading to increased loss of fluid (Rolls & Phillips 1990), thereby increasing the risk of hypohydration
- reduced thirst sensation, caused by a decrease in osmoreceptors that are sensitive to blood concentrations of fluid-regulating hormones and electrolytes (Rolls & Phillips 1990)—hence the potential for a decrease in fluid intake
- decreased ability to regulate temperature homeostasis associated with a diminished contractile function of the heart; the resultant lowering of cardiac output diminishes blood flow to the skin thus reducing the removal of heat and increasing the risk of heat stress
- decrease in sweat production with aging (Kenney & Fowler 1988), together with a delay in the onset of the sweat response, which decreases the cooling effect of vaporization of sweat from skin (Silver et al. 1964; Catania et al. 1980)

Buono (1991), however, reported that lifelong aerobic exercise retarded the decrease in peripheral sweat production normally associated with aging. Other factors, however, exacerbate risk of hypohydration and heat stress in aging athletes, especially if thirst sensors are unreliable. In one study, older people (56 ± 3 years) undertaking strenuous hill-walking of between 10 and 35 km/d over 10 consecutive days became progressively hypohydrated, compared with younger walkers (24 ± 3 years). This was evident from a twofold increase in urine osmolarity, which is the method used to measure fluid balance (Ainslie et al. 2002). The reasons for inadequate fluid intake were not assessed in this study so linking this outcome to reduced thirst was not confirmed. In another study, reduced thirst was confirmed in older 'average fit' males (~60 years) who were progressively hypohydrated and rated themselves less thirsty than younger controls (~20 years) (Meischer & Fortney 1989).

Guidelines recommended for fluid intake before, during and after competition for younger adult athletes can also be applied to aging athletes (see Chapters 12, 13 and 14 and section 18.9) but perhaps need to be applied more aggressively in aging athletes undertaking prolonged physical activity in the heat. Older as well as younger athletes including children consume more fluid when offered sports drinks compared with water. This response was confirmed during a contrived cycling protocol under laboratory conditions where twenty-seven older male and female recreational exercisers (aged 54–70 years) consumed more fluid and restored plasma volume faster when offered a sports drink than those offered only water (Baker et al. 2005). In situations where hypohydration and heat stress are a risk, beverages containing 6–8% CHO (e.g. sports drinks) are the best choice during prolonged exercise (>1 hour), especially in older athletes (Sawka et al. 2007).

Medications: nutrient interactions 18.13

Up to 85% of older persons (>65 years) are estimated to have at least one chronic medical condition (Webster 1990) and up to 34% of masters athletes reported taking medication (Farquharson 1990; Reaburn et al. 1995), which is similar to the prevalence of medication use in the general population (McCabe 2004). Some medications affect nutrient availability and can also affect the normal physiological response to physical activity (e.g. beta blockers blunt heart rate).

Drug–nutrient interactions and adverse effects increase exponentially with aging and with multiple medication use (Stewart & Cooper 1994). While taking medication with a meal is an effective means of improving compliance and may be recommended to help prevent gut irritation, the interaction of food and drug may not maximize ingestion of either (Thomas 1995). For example, anti-cholinergics can change gastrointestinal tract motility, and antacids can decrease gastric acidity and interfere with absorption of calcium, iron and other divalent minerals (Thomas 1995).

Table 18.4 overleaf summarizes the drug–nutrient interactions that can affect nutritional status and the nutrients likely to be affected. Given the complexity of drug–nutrient interactions, it is important that a dietitian works closely with a sports physician to minimize these effects. For a recent review of drug–nutrient interactions, see McCabe (2004).

TABLE 18.4 DRUG–NUTRIENT INTERACTIONS

DRUG	EFFECT	NUTRIENTS AFFECTED
Diuretics (e.g. Aldactone™, Chlotoride™, Lasix™)	Alterations in renal tubular function	Loss of sodium, potassium and magnesium
Antipsychotic/psychoactive	Disinterest in food	Protein and energy intake reduced
Cardiac glycosides (e.g. digoxin)	Anorexia, nausea, vomiting, disinterest in food	Protein and energy intake reduced
Anticonvulsants (e.g. phenytoin, Dilantin™, phenobarbitone)	Induction of liver enzymes Reduced absorption of folic acid	Altered vitamin D metabolism Folic acid
Salicylate (e.g. aspirin, Voltaren™, Nurofen™, Orudis™)	Gastrointestinal blood loss	Iron deficiency
Corticosteroids (e.g. prednisone, prednisolone, cortisone)	Inhibition of calcium absorption, alterations in glucose metabolism and electrolyte imbalance Increased excretion of vitamin C	Calcium imbalance (osteoporosis), hyperglycemia, sodium retention and potassium deficiency Vitamin C
Antacids	Decreased absorption of phosphate	Phosphate
Tetracycline	Increased excretion of vitamin C	Vitamin C
Bile acid sequesters	Malabsorption of fat-soluble vitamins	Vitamins A, D, E and K
Mineral oil laxatives (e.g. Agarol™)	Inhibition of fat-soluble vitamins absorption Depletion of potassium	Vitamins A, D, E and K malabsorption Potassium

18.14 Supplements

Up to 60% of older people in the general population have reported using supplements daily (Houston et al. 1997). Those more likely to take supplements, particularly vitamins, are health conscious and physically active (Kato et al. 1992; Houston et al. 1997). The prevalence of supplement use in aging athletes is similar to population data. In one study of 598 male and female masters athletes, around 61% used supplements. Of these, close to 36% took vitamins and around 30% took minerals (Streigel et al. 2005). The main reasons given for taking these supplements were injuries (25.5%), health reasons (19.9%), success in sports (18.3%), increased endurance and performance (17.3%) and increased strength (10.3%). Supplement users in this study trained more than non-users, which reflects their use of supplements for sports performance. In an earlier study of twenty-five female endurance athletes (mean age 50.4 years), neither supplement users nor non-supplement users met the RDA for calcium and vitamin E, despite meeting energy recommendations (Beshgetoor & Nichols 2003). The authors concluded that at least for the subjects in this study, vitamin and mineral supplements were warranted.

For aging exercisers involved in regular physical training who are considering using micronutrient supplements, a daily multivitamin/mineral supplement that provides no more than 100% of the RDA is suggested (Sachek & Roubenoff 1999). Single-nutrient supplements are not encouraged and should be limited to calcium and vitamins B6, B12, D and E, depending on an individual's risk for certain diseases, existing disease condition and food consumption patterns (Sachek & Roubenoff 1999). As suggested in section 18.10, there may be some disadvantage in taking anti-oxidant supplements for people with metabolic syndrome or type 2 diabetes who are exercising regularly, as these supplements may counteract the beneficial effects of exercise on enhancing insulin sensitivity.

Summary 18.15

There are no specific recommendations for nutrient intakes for aging athletes participating in athletic training. The EAR is considered the best estimate of nutrient requirements for individuals and groups and the recommended targets for CHO and protein for younger athletes are applicable to healthy aging athletes, providing energy requirements are met. The EAR cut-offs account for the physiological changes to nutrient requirements that occur with aging. However, some modifications may be needed to adjust for the presence of chronic disease and/or use of medications that potentially interfere with nutrient bioavailability in those aging athletes who participate in physical activity of high intensity or high volume.

The limited number of dietary intake studies on aging athletes suggests that intakes of several micronutrients (vitamins B6, B12, D and E, folate, calcium, iron and zinc) may be suboptimal or at least below RDA/RDI cut-offs in some groups. RDA/RDIs in isolation are no longer recommended as a cut-off to assess the 'adequacy' or 'inadequacy' of nutrient intakes and may over-estimate true requirements. Nevertheless for those healthy older (and younger) adults who are habitually consuming low micronutrient intakes, improving intake is best achieved through dietary means rather than supplements. If an aging athlete wants to use micronutrient supplements for any reason, a multivitamin–mineral supplement that provides no more than 100% of the RDA/RDI is likely to be both safe and adequate for optimal sports performance.

Dietary guidelines for older people are available in most western countries and provide a basis for advising aging athletes about food choice. With the increased participation in both recreational and competitive sport in the aging population, more studies are needed on aging athletes at different levels of activity to further examine the interactive effects of diet, aging and physical activity, before definitive nutrient recommendations can be made. Epidemiological studies on these interactions in aging athletes are required.

PRACTICE TIPS

VICKI DEAKIN AND GLENN CARDWELL

INTRODUCTION

- Most aging athletes are involved in sport for fun, camaraderie, socializing, fitness and the pure pleasure of being active. Some have a competitive spirit and will seek specific nutrition advice to enhance their sports performance. In many cases, they are as healthy as younger athletes, just a little slower and less flexible. Fortunately, older athletes are likely to have a greater than average interest in all aspects of their health, including their nutritional health. Generally the sports dietitian will be offering healthy eating advice, including tips to improve CHO and protein intake, and strategies to avoid dehydration and reduce risk of heat stress. Older athletes, particularly those aged greater than 50 years, are at higher risk of heat stress than younger athletes.

THIRST AND FLUID INTAKE

- Thirst sensation decreases with aging. This could result in too few fluids being consumed during and after exercise, especially in hot conditions, compromising thermoregulation. An older athlete who has been training or competing for many years may be out-of-date in their knowledge about current practice and have entrenched behaviors about food and fluid requirements for sport. For example, fluids are often avoided because of an outdated belief that dehydration toughens the body or that too much fluid causes cramp. For some older people, fluid may be purposely restricted to minimize night-time urination (although this is probably not effective, as concentrated urine irritates the bladder and encourages more frequent urination). These beliefs in turn increase the risk of chronic low fluid status in the active person. A simple check is the color of the urine. Pale urine suggests adequate hydration and darker-colored urine suggests inadequate hydration (except when vitamin supplements are taken, because some B vitamins darken urine in a well-hydrated person). On the other hand, older athletes participating in endurance events may over-consume fluid and are often at higher risk of hyponatremia than younger athletes if they take a long time to complete an event.
- The most recent fluid replacement guidelines from the American College of Sports Medicine (Sawka et al. 2007) highlight the need to individualize fluid intakes to meet the needs of athletes with very different physical characteristics exercising in a range of environmental conditions. See Chapter 8. There are no fluid guidelines specific for the aging athlete. In the absence of such guidelines, the 2007 guidelines can be applied to aging athletes but may need to be applied more aggressively in those undertaking prolonged physical activity in the heat, particularly in marathon events. In this situation, beverages containing 6–8% CHO and electrolytes (e.g. sports drinks) are recommended for exercise events lasting longer than 1 hour (Sawka et al. 2007).

BONE PROBLEMS

- Although weight-bearing activity, and to a lesser extent resistance exercise, helps to minimize bone loss, an adequate calcium and vitamin D intake is still important because of increased requirement in older people (see section 18.11 and Chapter 10 for information on strategies to meet calcium recommendations). Vitamin D status is mainly determined by exposure to sunlight: 5–10 minutes of mild sunlight on the arms and legs or the hands, arms and face, two or three times a week is enough for adequate endogenous production of vitamin D in a young healthy adult (Holick 2004). In older adults, vitamin D production by this route may be halved (Mahan & Escott-Stump 2008). Adults over the age of 65 years produce four time less vitamin D in the skin compared with adults aged 20–30 years (Institute of Medicine 1997).

- Suboptimal vitamin D status is reported in people who are institutionalized or housebound, actively avoid sunlight exposure and live in climates where there is little daylight in winter months. For older people who are dark-skinned, train indoors in gyms or health clubs, some sun exposure to maintain vitamin D status or activate vitamin D production should be practiced (Working Group of the Australian and New Zealand Bone and Mineral Society et al. 2005). In some cases, a vitamin D supplement may be necessary. A blood test can confirm vitamin D status.
- Good food sources of vitamin D include oily fish (e.g. tuna, sardines and mackerel), cod liver oil, liver, eggs, cheese and margarine. Some foods are fortified with vitamin D (e.g. margarine in Australia and the UK, and milk in the US).

AGING ATHLETES WITH OTHER CHRONIC DISEASES OR RISK FACTORS: ARE SUPPLEMENTS INDICATED?

- An aging athlete may have an existing chronic medical condition such as diabetes, hyperlipidemia, hypertension or an arthritic condition. Older people often have outdated beliefs or are still following advice provided many years ago that is no longer valid. They may avoid entire food groups in the mistaken belief that this will inhibit the progression or even cure the condition, for example, avoiding all dairy foods to lower blood cholesterol levels.
- People with conditions that are generally age-related, such as cancer, heart disease, arthritis, failing eyesight and short-term memory loss, may wish to consume food products and supplements claiming to alleviate symptoms. The role of the dietitian is to assess the value of the product, inform the client of the current thinking, and then allow the individual to decide. The advice given in Chapter 16 on dietary supplements applies to alternative therapies. Many health organizations provide information on their websites about proven and unproven remedies. Some supplements used by older athletes—such as creatine or anti-oxidants—may be based solely on a perceived improvement in sports performance or recovery. Other supplements (multivitamins and herbal supplements) may be taken for general use, unrelated to sport. Recent evidence suggests that supplementing with high doses of the anti-oxidants vitamin C and E counteracts the beneficial effects of exercise on enhancing insulin sensitivity in younger men (Ristow et al. 2009). Short-term, high-dose vitamin E and other anti-oxidant supplements in combination with physical activity may have a disadvantage for those aging athletes who are overweight or obese, with metabolic syndrome or type 2 diabetes, although further studies are required to confirm these effects.

PRACTICE TIPS

SOCIAL FACTORS INFLUENCING FOOD CHOICE IN AGING ATHLETES

- An aging athlete, similar to any older person, may live alone and have very few social support systems. Advise on food preparation for one person, such as the value of making more food than needed for one meal and freezing the extra serves for later. There are cookbooks with recipes for one or two people, although cooking extra and freezing the remainder is potentially more useful. Poor food choices are common in people living alone, especially if they have difficulty shopping, shop infrequently or don't see nutrition as a priority.
- Arthritis in the hands reduces dexterity and affects capacity to prepare food. Some unproven diet regimens for preventing arthritis, if followed rigidly, reduce the variety of foods consumed and increase risk of nutrient depletion. Ask if, and why, any foods or food groups are being avoided and discuss the potential health implications.

CHANGES IN TASTE AND SMELL IN OLDER PEOPLE

- Taste and smell responses diminish with aging, possibly leading to reduced appetite and loss of enjoyment of food. Loss of appetite is also a common physiological response to intense exercise and can last for a long time after cessation. For those older athletes affected by poor appetite, foods such as nuts, peanut butter, dried fruit, avocado, milk shakes, or milk powder added to foods like mashed potato, and meal replacement formulas, are some suggestions to provide energy and nutrient-rich food supplements. Eating almost immediately after exercise, particularly a hard training session, is just as important for the aging athlete as for younger athletes to promote rapid resynthesis of glycogen and promote recovery.

NUTRIENT AND ENERGY REQUIREMENTS IN AGING ATHLETES

- As a person ages, nutrient requirements remain the same as in a younger adult or marginally increase for vitamin B6, B12, D and calcium, while energy requirements usually decrease because of the normal loss of FFM that accompanies aging. In one study of around 3400 Australian adults, higher body mass index levels were still evident in those adults who participated in organized or regular daily exercise but spent the rest of the day in a sedentary occupation or with low levels of incidental activity (Salmon et al. 2000). In this study, subjects who reported watching television more than 4 hr/d were twice as likely to be overweight than those watching 2 hr/d, independent of participation in physical activity. Aging athletes generally consume more food and have higher energy intakes than sedentary controls (see section 18.4). Hence, nutrient-dense foods in combination with a lower energy intake are an important part of healthy eating. For older athletes predisposed to overweight, there may be less room for 'indulgence' foods, particularly when incidental activity is low, despite regular exercise.

- Recommendations for the amount of CHO needed for training and recovery in aging athletes remain the same as younger adult athletes since CHO absorption and utilization is unaffected by aging in a healthy person.
- Recommendations for total daily protein intake for aging athletes, particularly those undertaking resistance exercise, are higher than RDI/RDA cut-offs at 1.0–1.2 g/kg BM/d but still slightly lower than the recommendations for younger athletes undertaking the same type of activity. Consuming protein together with CHO-rich foods immediately following resistance training maximizes muscle and strength development, similar to younger athletes.

GUIDELINES FOR COMMENCING EXERCISE OR PHYSICAL ACTIVITY IN OLDER PEOPLE

- A dietitian is often asked for exercise advice. If an older individual with an existing disease is starting an exercise program after previously being sedentary, consultation and clearance with a physician is important. This clearance is mandatory for membership of gyms and fitness centers. Recent guidelines from the American College of Sports Medicine and the American Heart Association suggest that moderate-intensity aerobic activity, muscle-strengthening activity, reducing sedentary behavior and risk management should be the focus for physical activity and health promotion in older adults (Nelson et al. 2007). These guidelines suggest that:
  - aerobic activity should be undertaken at an intensity that accounts for the older adult's aerobic fitness
  - activities are provided that maintain or increase flexibility
  - balance exercises are included for older adults at risk of falls
- These guidelines further recommended an activity plan for older adults that will eventually achieve the recommended physical activity levels, which integrates both preventive and therapeutic recommendations. For the first time, in March 2009, the Australian Government published physical activity recommendations specifically for older Australians to promote health and positive aging. See http://www.health.gov.au/internet/main/publishing.nsf/Content/phd-physical-choose-health for guidelines on getting started and the types of activities and duration required to achieve positive effects. A Health Monthly Activity Planner to give to clients can be downloaded.

HOW MUCH PHYSICAL ACTIVITY IS REQUIRED TO REDUCE RISK FACTORS?

- Around the same time, the American College of Sports Medicine (2009b) updated its guidelines for the amount and intensity of physical activity required for people to improve health outcomes, prevent transition from overweight to obesity and prevent weight regain after weight loss. Given the increase in obesity and prevalence of other chronic diet/lifestyle-related diseases in many western countries and the rise in obesity

PRACTICE TIPS

in older populations, particularly postmenopausal women, many older adults are either commencing exercise for the first time or increasing the intensity and volume of exercise in the hope of improving health outcomes. These exercise guidelines are summarized in Table 18.5.

- Clearly, this amount of physical activity may be unachievable for most people in terms of time and physical capacity, hence the importance of encouraging greater levels of incidental activity in an individual's daily life, in addition to some structured exercise. For those older adults who are overweight or obese, modest energy restriction and higher total energy expenditure in combination with behavioral therapy is the most effective strategy to improve weight control, reduce other risk factors and potentially improve health outcomes and quality of life (American College of Sports Medicine et al. 2009b).
- In summary, the older a person becomes, the more dissimilar they are from others in their age group, so expect a large variety of fitness levels, personal goals and nutrition knowledge. For the more competitive aging athlete, providing a list of contacts with local and or national sporting organizations, other allied health professionals who are knowledgeable in masters sport and the specific issues experienced by older athletes with existing medical conditions is helpful.

TABLE 18.5 PREVENTIVE AND THERAPEUTIC AMOUNTS AND INTENSITY OF EXERCISE REQUIRED TO REDUCE RISK FACTORS AND CONTROL WEIGHT

OBJECTIVE	FREQUENCY AND INTENSITY	DURATION
To increase cardiovascular fitness and decrease risk factors for cardiovascular disease, hypertension, osteoporosis and type 2 diabetes and falls in older adults	Aerobic: a minimum of 5 d/wk for moderate aerobic intensity or a minimum 3 d/wk of vigorous intensity	30 min/d – moderate intensity 20 min/d – vigorous activity
	Muscle strengthening: at least 2 d/wk	8–10 exercises involving major muscle groups with 10–15 repetitions
	Flexibility and balance: at least 2 d/wk for those at risk of falls, include exercises that maintain and improve balance	
To lose weight in adults	Most days of the week: moderate to vigorous	>250 min/wk to achieve clinically significant weight loss
To prevent the transition from overweight to obesity in adults	Most days of the week: moderate to vigorous	150–250 min/wk
To prevent weight regain after weight loss in obese adults	Most days of the week: moderate to vigorous	>250 min/wk but insufficient evidence to judge the effectiveness of physical activity alone

Moderate intensity = physical activity at a level that causes the heart to beat faster and some shortness of breath, but that you can still talk comfortably while doing; Vigorous intensity = physical activity at a level that causes your heart to beat a lot faster and makes talking more difficult between breaths.

Sources: Adapted from Saris et al. 2003; Nelson et al. 2007; American College of Sports Medicine et al. 2009b

References

Ainslie PN, Campbell IT, Frayn KN, Humphreys SM, et al. Energy balance, metabolism, hydration, and performance during strenuous hill walking: the effect of age. J Appl Physiol 2002;93:714–23.

Alhadeff L, Gualtiery CT, Lipton M. Toxic effects of water-soluble vitamins. Nutr Rev 1984;42:33–40.

American College of Sports Medicine, American Dietetic Association and Dieticians of Canada. Joint Position Statement. Nutrition and athletic performance. Med Sci Sports Exerc 2009a;41:759–71.

American College of Sports Medicine. Position stand. Appropriate physical activity intervention strategies for weight loss and prevention of weigh regain for adults. Med Sci Sports Exerc 2009b;41:709–31.

Anderson RA, Polansky MM, Bryden NA. Strenuous running: acute effects on chromium, copper, zinc, and selected clinical variables in urine and serum of male runners. Biol Trace Elem Res 1984;6:327–36.

Australian Bureau of Statistics 2008. Population by age and sex, Australian States and Territories. Cat. No. 3201.0. Canberra: Australian Bureau of Statistics, 2008. At http://www.abs.gov.au/Ausstats/abs@.nsf/mf/3201.0 (accessed 10 June 2009).

Baker LB, Munce TA, Kenney WL. Sex differences in voluntary fluid intake by older adults during exercise. Med Sci Sports Exerc 2005;37:789–96.

Barr SI. Effects of dehydration on exercise performance. Can J Appl Physiol 1999;24:164.

Bates CJ, Benton D, Biesalski, HK, et al. Nutrition and aging: a consensus statement. J Nutr Health Aging 2002;6:103–16.

Beshgetoor D, Nichols JF. Dietary intake and supplement use in female master cyclists and runners. Int J Sports Nutr Exerc Metab 2003;13:166–72.

Beshgetoor D, Nichols JF, Rego I. Effect of training mode and calcium intake on bone mineral density in female master cyclist, runners, and non-athletes. Int J Sport Nutr Exerc Metab 2000 10:290–301.

Bjelakovic G, Nikolova D, Gluud L, et al. Mortality in randomized trials of antioxidant supplements for primary and secondary prevention: systematic review and meta analysis. J Am Med Assoc 2007;297:842–57.

Blair SN, Brodney S. Effects of physical inactivity and obesity on morbidity and mortality: current evidence and research issues. Med Sci Sports 1999;31(Suppl):646S–62S.

Blanchard J, Conrad KA, Mead RA, Garry PJ. Vitamin C disposition in young and elderly men. Am J Clin Nutr 1990;51:837–45.

Brodney S, McPherson RS, Carpenter RA, Welten D, Blair SN. Nutrient intake of physically fit and unfit men and women. Med Sci Sports Exerc 2001;33:459–67.

Buono MJ, McKenzie BK, Kasch FW. Effects of ageing and physical training on the peripheral sweat production of the human eccrine sweat gland. Age Ageing 1991;20:439–41.

Burke LM, Gollan RA, Read RS. Dietary intakes and food use of groups of elite Australian male athletes. Int J Sport Nutr 1991;1:378–94.

Burke LM, Kiens B, Ivy JL. Carbohydrates and fat for training and recovery. J Sports Sci 2004;22:15–30.

Butterworth DE, Nieman DC, Perkins R, et al. Exercise training and nutrient intake in elderly women. J Am Diet Assoc 1993;93:653–7.

Campbell WW, Anderson RA. Effect of aerobic exercise and training on the trace minerals chromium, zinc, and copper. Sport Med 1987;4:9–18.

Campbell WW, Trappe TA, Wolfe RR, Evans WJ. The recommended dietary allowance for protein may not be adequate for older people to maintain skeletal muscle. J Gerentol 2001;56:6:M373–M380.

Casale G, Bonora C, Migliavacca A, et al. Serum ferritin and ageing. Age Ageing 1981;10:119–22.

Catania J, Thompson JW, Michalewski HA, et al. Comparison of sweat gland counts, electrodermal activity and habituation behavior in young and old groups of subjects. Psychophysiology 1980;17:146–52.

Celsing F, Blomstrand W, Werner B, et al. Effects of iron deficiency on endurance and muscle enzyme activity in man. Med Sci Sports Exerc 1986;18:156–61.

Chandra RK. Impact of nutritional status and nutrient supplements on immune responses and incidence of infection in older individuals. Ageing Res Rev 2004;3:91–104.

Chatard JC, Boutet C, Tourny C, et al. Nutritional status and physical fitness of elderly sportsmen. Eur J Appl Physiol 1998;77:157–63.

Chen J. Vitamins: effects of exercise on requirements. In: Maughan RJ, ed. Nutrition in sport. The encyclopedia of sports medicine. Volume VII. London: Blackwell Science, 2000:281.

Clarkson PM, Haymes EM. Trace mineral requirements for athletes. Int J Sport Nutr 1994;4:104–19.

Commonwealth Department of Health and Ageing, Ministry of Health, National Health and Medical Research Council. Nutrient reference values for Australia and New Zealand. Canberra: NHMRC, 2006.

Couzy F, Lafargue P, Guezennec CY. Zinc metabolism in the athlete: influence of training nutrition and other factors. Int J Sports Med 1990;11:263–6.

CSIRO Division of Human Nutrition. Food and nutrition in Australia–does five years make a difference? Results from the CSIRO Australian Food and Nutrition Surveys 1988 and 1993. Adelaide: Commonwealth Scientific and Industrial Research Organisation (CSIRO) Division of Food and Nutrition, 1996.

Dangour AD, Sibson VL, Fletcher AE. Micronutrient supplementation in later life: limited evidence for benefit. J Gerontol (Biol Sci) 2004;59A:659–73.

Dawson-Hughes B, Dallal GE, Kraall EA, et al. A controlled trial of the effect of calcium supplementation on bone density in post-menopausal women. N Engl J Med 1990;323:878–83.

Dekkers JC, van Doornen JP, Kemper HCG. The role of antioxidant vitamins and enzymes in the prevention of exercise-induced muscle damage. Sports Med 1996;21:213–38.

Eastell R, Yergey AL, Vieira NE, et al. Interrelationship among vitamin D metabolism, true calcium absorption, parathyroid function, and age in women: evidence of an age-related intestinal resistance to 1-25-dihydroxyvitamin D action. J Bone Miner Res 1991;6:125–32.

Economos CD, Bortz SS, Nelson ME. Nutritional practices of elite athletes: practical recommendations. Sports Med 1993;16:381–99.

Elahi D, Muller DC. Carbohydrate metabolism in the elderly. Eur J Clin Nutr 2000;54(3 Suppl): 112S–120S.

Elia M, Ritz P, Stubbs RJ. Total energy expenditure in the elderly. Eur J Clin Nutr 2000;53(3 Suppl): 92S–103S.

Evans WJ. Exercise, nutrition, and aging. Clin Geriatr Med 1995;11:725–34.

Evans, WJ. Protein nutrition, exercise and aging. J Am Coll Nutr 2004;23(Suppl):601S–9S.

Farquharson T. Masters medicine—SA style. Report to Sports Medicine Australia, Canberra, 1990.

Fiatarone Singh MA. Benefits of exercise and dietary measures to optimize shifts in body composition with age. Asia Pacific J Clin Nutr 2002;11(Suppl):642S–52S.

Food and Agriculture Organization (FAO). Carbohydrate in human nutrition. Report of a joint FAO/WHO expert consultation. FAO Food and Nutrition Paper No. 66. Rome: FAO, 1998.

Fortes C, Forastiere F, Agabiti N, et al. The effect of zinc and vitamin A supplementation on immune response in an older population. J Am Geriatr Soc 1998;46:19–26.

Frei B. Ascorbic acid protects lipids in human plasma and low-density lipoprotein against oxidative damage. Am J Clin Nutr 1991;54(Suppl):1113S–18S.

Going SB, Williams DP, Lohman TG, Hewitt MJ. Aging, body composition, and physical activity: a review. J Aging Phys Activ 1994;2:38–66.

Hallfrisch J, Drinkwater DT, Muler DC, et al. Physical conditioning status and dietary intake in active and sedentary older men. Nutr Res 1994;14:817–27.

Hawkins SA, Wiswell RA, Marcell TJ. Exercise and the masters athlete—a model of successful aging? J Gerentol 2003;58A:1009–11.

Hawley JA, Dennis SC, Lindsay FH, Noakes TD. Nutritional practices of athletes: are they sub-optimal? J Sports Sci 1995;13(Suppl):75S–81S.

Haymes EM, Lamanca JJ. Iron loss in runners during exercise: implications and recommendations made for athletes. Sports Med 1989;7:277.

Heaney RP. Calcium needs of the elderly to reduce fracture risk. J Am Coll Nutr 2001;20(2 Suppl): 192S–7S.

Herbert V, Jacob E, Wong KT. Destruction of vitamin B12 by vitamin C (letter). Am J Clin Nutr 1977;30:297–9.

Holick, M. Sunlight and vitamin D for bone health and prevention of autoimmune diseases, cancers and cardiovascular disease. Amer J Clin Nutr 2004;80(6 Suppl):1678S.

Horber FF, Kohler SA, Lippuner K, Jaeger P. Effect of regular physical training on age-associated alteration of body composition in men. Eur J Clin Invest 1996;26:279–85.

Houston DK, Johnson M, Daniel TD, et al. Health and dietary characteristics of supplement users in an elderly population. Int J Vitam Nutr Res 1997;67:183–91.

Hoyt CJ. Diarrhea from vitamin C. JAMA 1980;244:1674.

Hughes VA, Fiatarone MA, Fielding RA, et al. Exercise increases muscle GLUT-4 levels and insulin action in subjects with impaired glucose tolerance. Am J Physiol 1993;264:E855–E62.

Hunding A, Jordal R, Paulev PE. Runner's anemia and iron deficiency. Acta Med Scand 1981;209:315–18.

Institute of Medicine. Dietary reference intakes for calcium, phosphorus, magnesium, vitamin D and fluoride. Washington DC: National Academies Press, 1997.

Institute of Medicine, Food and Nutrition Board. Dietary reference intakes for vitamin A, vitamin K, arsenic, boron, chromium, copper, iodine, iron, manganese, molybdenum, nickel, silicon, vanadium and zinc. Washington DC: National Academies Press, 2000a.

Institute of Medicine. Dietary Reference Intakes: applications in dietary assessment. A report of the subcommittee on interpretation and uses of Dietary Reference Intakes and the Standing Committee on the Scientific Evaluation of Dietary Reference Intakes. Food and Nutrition Board, Washington DC: National Academies Press, 2000b.

Institute of Medicine of the National Academies. Dietary reference intakes for energy, carbohydrate, fiber, fat, fatty acids, cholesterol, protein and amino acids (macronutrients). Washington DC: National Academies Press, 2002.

Jacques PF, Chylack LT. Epidemiologic evidence of a role for the antioxidant vitamins and carotenoids in cataract prevention. Am J Clin Nutr 1991;53(Suppl):352S–5S.

Kaikkonen J, Kosonen L, Nyyssönen K, et al. Effect of combined coenzyme Q10 and d-alpha-tocopheryol acetate supplementation on exercise-induced lipid peroxidation and muscular damage: a placebo-controlled double-blind study in marathon runners. Free Radic Res 1998;29:85–92.

Kato I, Nomura AM, Stemmerman GN, Chyou PH. Vitamin supplement use and its correlates among elderly Japanese men residing in Oahu, HI. Pub Health Report 1992;6:712–17.

Kenney WL, Fowler SR. Methylcholine-activated eccrine sweat gland density and output as a function of age. J Appl Physiol 1988;65:1082–6.

Kirwan JP, Kohrt WM, Wojta DM, et al. Endurance exercise training reduces glucose-stimulated insulin levels in 60- to 70-year-old men and women. J Gerontol 1993;48:M84–M90.

Kivela SL, Maenpaa P, Nissinen A, et al. Vitamin A, vitamin E and selenium status in an aged Finnish male population. Int J Vit Nutr Res 1989;59:373–80.

Klitgaard H, Mantoni M, Schiaffino S, et al. Function, morphology and protein expression of ageing skeletal muscle: a cross-sectional study of elderly men with different training backgrounds. Acta Physiol Scand 1990;140:41–54.

Knekt P, Aromaa A, Maatela J, et al. Vitamin E and cancer prevention. Am J Clin Nutr 1991;53(Suppl): 283S–6S.

Kohrt WM, Malley MT, Dalsky GP, Holloszy JO. Body composition of healthy sedentary and trained, young and older men and women. Med Sci Sports Exerc 1992;24:7:832–7.

Krasinski SD, Cohn JS, Schaefer EJ, et al. Postprandial plasma retinyl ester response is greater in older subjects compared with younger subjects. J Clin Invest 1990;85:883.

Krasinski SD, Russell RM, Samloff IM, et al. Fundic atrophic gastritis in an elderly population: effect on hemoglobin and several serum nutritional indicators. J Am Geriatr Soc 1986;34:800–6.

Krebs J, Schneider V, Smith J, et al. Sweat calcium loss during running. FASEB J 1988;2:A1099.

Krotkiewski M, Gudmundsson M, Backstrom P, Mandroukas K. Zinc and muscle strength and endurance. Acta Physiol Scand 1982;116:309–11.

Kruk J. Physical activity in the prevention of the most frequent chronic diseases: an analysis of the recent evidence. Asia Pac J Cancer Prev 2007;8:325–38.

Lemon PWR. Effects of exercise on dietary protein requirements. Int J Sport Nutr 1998;8:426–47.

Lemon PWR. Beyond the zone: protein needs of active individuals. J Am Coll Nutr 2000; 19(Suppl):513S.

Lewis RD, Modlesky CM. Nutrition, physical activity, and bone health in women. Int J of Sport Nutr 1998;8:250–84.

Lucas M, Heiss CJ. Protein needs of older adults engaged in resistance training: a review. J Aging Phys Act 2005;13:223–36.

Lukaski HC. Micronutrients (magnesium, zinc, and copper): are mineral supplements needed for athletes? Int J Sport Nutr 1995;5(Suppl):74S–83S.

MacLaughlin J, Holick MF. Aging decreased the capacity of human skin to produce vitamin D3. J Clin Invest 1985;76:1536.

Mahan K, Escott-Stump S. Food, nutrition and diet therapy. Eleventh edition. New York: Saunders Publishing Company, 2004.

Maharam LG, Bauman PA, Kalman D, et al. Masters athletes—factors affecting performance. Sports Med 1999;28:273–85.

Manore MM. Effects of physical activity on thiamine, riboflavin, and vitamin B-6 requirements. Am J Clin Nutr 2000;72(Suppl):598S–606S.

Marriott H, Buttress J. Key points from the National Diet and Nutrition Survey of adults aged 19–64 years. Nutr Bull 2003;28:355–63.

Martins I, Dantas A, Guiomar S, Amorim Cruz JA. Vitamin and mineral intakes in elderly. J Nutr Health Aging 2002;6:63–5.

Maughan RJ, King DS. Lea T. Dietary supplements. In: Food, nutrition and sports performance II. The International Olympic Committee Consensus Conference on Sports Nutrition. 2004:153–85.

McCabe B. Prevention of food-drug interactions with special emphasis on older adults. Curr Opin Clin Nutr Metab Care 2004;7:21–26.

McDonald R, Keen CL. Iron, zinc and magnesium nutrition and athletic performance. Sports Med 1988;5:171–84.

McLennan W, Podger A, eds. National Nutrition Survey: selected highlights Australia, Cat. No. 4802.0. Canberra: Australian Bureau of Statistics and Department of Health and Family Services, 1997.

McLennan W, Podger A, eds. National Nutrition Survey: nutrient intakes and physical measurements. Australia, Cat. No. 4805.0. Canberra: Australian Bureau of Statistics and Department of Health and Family Services, 1998.

Meischer E, Fortney SM. Responses to dehydration and rehydration during heat exposure in young and older men. Am J Physiol 1989;257:R1050–R6.

Melzer K, Kayser B, Pichard C. Physical activity: the health benefits outweigh the risks. Curr Opin Clin Nutr Metab Care 2004;7:641–7.

Meredith CN, Frontera WR, Fisher EC, et al. Peripheral effects of endurance training in young and old subjects. J Appl Physiol 1989;66:2844–9.

Meydani SN, Barklund MP, Liu S, et al. Vitamin E supplementation enhances cell-mediated immunity in healthy elderly subjects. Am J Clin Nutr 1990a;52:557–63.

Meydani SN, Meydani M, Blumbery JB, et al. Assessment of the safety of supplementation with different amounts of vitamin E in healthy older adults. Am J Clin Nutr 1998;68:311–18.

Meydani SN, Ribaya-Mercado JD, Russell RM, et al. The effect of vitamin B6 on immune response in healthy elderly. Ann NY Acad Sci 1990;587:303–6.

Meydani SN, Ribaya-Mercado JD, Russell RM, et al. Vitamin B-6 deficiency impairs interleukin 2 production and lymphocyte proliferation in elderly adults. Am J Clin Nutr 1991;53:1275–80.

Miller LT, Linkswiler H. Effect of protein intake on the development of abnormal tryptophan metabolism by men during vitamin B6 depletion. J Nutr 1967;93:53–9.

Miller 3rd ER, Pastor-Barriuso R, Dalal D, Riemersma RA, Appel LJ, Guallar E. Meta-analysis: high-dosage vitamin E supplementation may increase all-cause mortality. Ann Intern Med 2005;142:37–46.

Min Lee I, Sesso HD, Oguma Y, Paffenbarger Jr RS. The 'weekend warrior' and risk of mortality. Am J Epidem 2004;160:636–41.

Morais JA, Gougeon R, Pencharz PB, et al. Whole-body protein turnover in the healthy elderly. Am J Clin Nutr 1997;66:880–9.

Murphy S, Guenther P, Kretsch M. Using the dietary reference intakes to assess intakes of groups: pitfalls to avoid. J Amer Diet Assoc 2006;October:1550–3.

Murphy SP, Poos MI. Dietary Reference Intakes. Summary of applications in dietary assessment. Pub Health Nutr 2002;5:843–9.

Myburgh KH, Hutchins J, Fataar AB, et al. Low bone density is an etiologic factor for stress fractures in athletes. Ann Intern Med 1990;113:754–9.

Nair KS. Muscle protein turnover: methodological issues and the effect of aging. J Germ Series A 1995;50A(special issue):107–12.

National Institute of Health State-of-the-Science Conference Statement: Multivitamin/mineral supplements and chronic disease prevention. Ann Intern Med 2006;145:364–71.

Nelson ME, Fisher EC, Dilmanian RA, et al. A 1 year walking program and increased dietary calcium in postmenopausal women: effects on bone. Am J Clin Nutr 1991;53:1304–11.

Nelson ME, Rejeski WJ, Blair SN, et al. Physical activity and public health in older adults: recommendation from the American College of Sports Medicine and the American Heart Association. Med Sci Sports Exerc 2007;39:1435–45.

National Health and Medical Research Council (NHMRC). Dietary guidelines for older Australians. Canberra: NHMRC, 1999.

National Research Council. Recommended Dietary Allowances. Tenth edition. Washington, DC: National Academy Press, 1989.

Packer L. Protective role of vitamin E in biological systems. Am J Clin Nutr 1991;53 (Suppl):1050S–5S.

Pan XR, Li GW, Hu YH, Wang JX et al. Effects of diet and exercise in preventing NIDDM in people with impaired glucose tolerance. The Da Qing IGT and diabetes study. Diabetes Care 1997;20:537–44.

Paterson DH, Jones GR, Rice CL. Ageing and physical activity: evidence to develop exercise recommendations for older adults. Can J Public Health 2007;98(2 Suppl):69S–108S.

Pollock ML, Mengelkoch LJ, Graves JE, et al. Twenty-year follow-up of aerobic power and body composition of older track athletes. J Appl Physiol 1997;82:1508–16.

Proctor DN, Joyner MJ. Skeletal muscle mass and the reduction of $VO_{2\ max}$ in trained older subjects. Am Physiol Soc 1997;1411.

Pronsky ZM. Food-medication interactions handbook. Birchrunville, PA: Food-Medication Interactions, 2008.

Reaburn P, Dascombe B. Endurance performance in masters athletes. Eur Rev Aging Phys Act 2008; 5:31–42.

Reaburn P, Dascombe B. Anaerobic performance in masters athletes. Eur Rev Aging Phys Act 2009; 6:39–53.

Reaburn PRJ. The lifetime athlete—physical work capacities and skeletal muscle characteristics. Unpublished PhD thesis. University of Queensland, 1994.

Reaburn PRJ, Gillespie A, Lowe J, Balanda K. The World Masters Games (1994) injury study. Report to Australian Sports Commission, 1995.

Reaburn PRJ, Le Bon C. Unpublished observations. 1995.

Reid IR, Ames RW, Evans MC, et al. Long-term effects of calcium supplementation on bone loss and fractures in postmenopausal women: a randomized controlled trial. Am J Med 1995;98:331–5.

Ribaya-Mercado JD, Russell RM, Sahyoun N, et al. Vitamin B6 requirements of elderly men and women. J Nutr 1991;121:1062–74.

Rimm E, Stampfer M, Ascherio A, et al. Vitamin E consumption and the risk of coronary heart disease in men. N Engl J Med 1993;328:1450–6.

Rising R, Harper IT, Fontvielle AM, Ferraro RT, et al. Determinants of total daily energy expenditure: variability in physical activity. Am J Clin Nutr 1994;59:800–4.

Ristow M, Zarse K, Oberbach A, et al. Antioxidants prevent health-promoting effects of physical exercise in humans. Proc National Acad Sci Early Edition, 2009. At http://www.pnas.org/cgi/doi/10.1073/pnas.0903485106 (accessed 25 May 2009).

Rivlin RS. Keeping the young-elderly healthy: is it too late to improve our health through nutrition? Am J Clin Nutr 2007;86(Suppl):1572S–6S.

Roberts SB, Dallal GE. Energy requirements and aging. Pub Health Nutr 2005;8:1028–36.

Roberts SB, Rosenberg I. Nutrition and aging: changes in the regulation of energy metabolism with aging. Physiol Rev 2006;86:651–67.

Robertson JM, Donner AP, Trevithick JR. Vitamin E intake and risk of cataracts in humans. Ann NY Acad Sci 1989;570:372–82.

Rock CL. Nutrition of the older athlete. Clin Sports Med 1991;10:445–57.

Rokitzki L, Logemann E, Sagredos AN, et al. Lipid peroxidation and antioxidative vitamins under extreme endurance stress. Acta Physiol Scand 1994;151:149–58.

Rolls BJ, Phillips RA. Aging and disturbances of thirst and fluid balance. Nutr Rev 1990;48:137–44.

Rosenberg IH, Miller JW. Nutritional factors in physical and cognitive functions of elderly people. Am J Clin Nutr 1992;55(6 Suppl):1237S–43S.

Rosenbloom CA, Dunaway A. Nutrition recommendations for masters athletes. Clin Sports Med 2007;26: 91–100.

Ruiz-Torres A, Gimeno A, Munoz FJ, Vicent D. Are anthropometric changes in healthy adults caused by modifications in dietary habits or by aging? Gerontol 1995;41:243–51.

Russell RM. Micronutrient requirements of the elderly. Nutr Rev 1992;50:463–6.

Russell RM, Suter PM. Vitamin requirements of elderly people: an update. Am J Clin Nutr 1993; 58:4–14.

Sacheck JM, Roubenoff R. Nutrition in the exercising elderly. Clin Sports Med 1999;18:565–77.

Saito, M, Itoh R. Nutritional status of vitamin A in a healthy elderly population in Japan. Int J Vitam Nutr Res 1991;61:105–9.

Sallinen J, Ojanen T, Karavirta L, Ahtiainen JP, Häkkinen K. Muscle mass and strength, body composition and dietary intake in master strength athletes vs untrained men of different ages. J Sports Med Phys Fitness 2008;48:190–6.

Salmon J, Bauman A, Crawford D, Timperio A, Owen N. 2000, The association between television viewing and overweight among Australian adults participating in varying levels of leisure-time physical activity. Int J Obesity 2000;24:600–6.

Saltzman JR, Russell RM. The aging gut: nutritional issues. Gastroenterol Clin North Am 1998;27: 309–24.

Sandstrom B. Bioavailability of zinc. Eur J Clin Nutr 1997;51(1 Suppl):17S–19S.

Saris WHM, Blair SN, van Baak MA, et al. How much physical activity is enough to prevent unhealthy weight gain? Outcome of the IASO first stock conference and consensus statement. Obesity Rev 2003;4:101–6.

Sawka MN, Burke LM, Eichner ER, Maughan RJ, Montain SJ, Stachenfeld NS. Exercise and fluid replacement. Med Sci Sports Exerc 2007;39:377–90.

Schoeller DA. Changes in total body water. Am J Clin Nutr 1989;50:1176–81.

Shenkin A. Micronutrients in health and disease. Postgrad Med J 2006;82:559–67.

Silver A, Montagna W, Karaean I. Age and sex differences in spontaneous adrenergic and cholinergic human sweating. J Invest Dermatol 1964;43:255–6.

Simon JA, Hudes ES, Browner WS. Serum ascorbic acid and cardiovascular disease prevalence in United States adults. Epidemiol 1998;9:316–21.

Starling RD, Ades PA, Poehlman ET. Physical activity, protein intake, and appendicular skeletal muscle mass in older men. Am J Clin Nutr 1999;70:91–6.

Stewart JG, Ahlquist DA, McGill DB, et al. Gastrointestinal blood loss and anemia in runners. Ann Intern Med 1984;100:843–5.

Stewart R, Cooper J. Polypharmacy in the aged. Drugs Ageing 1994;4:449–61.

Streigel H, Simon P, Wurster C, Niess AM, Ulrich R. The use of nutritional supplements among masters athletes. Int J Sport Med 2006;27:236–41.

Sui X, LaMonte MJ, Laditka JN et al. Cardiorespiratory fitness and adiposity as mortality predictors in older adults. JAMA 2007;298:2507–16.

Sykes JC. Women, sports, exercise, and nutrition. In: Harris S, Suominen H, Era P, Harris WS, eds. Toward healthy aging—international perspectives. Part I: Physiological and biomedical aspects. New York: Centre for the Study of Aging 1994:141–5.

Tanaka H, Seals DR. Dynamic exercise performance in masters athletes: insight into the effects of primary human aging on physiological functional capacity. J Appl Physiol 2003;95:2152–62.

Tanaka H, Seals DR. Endurance exercise performance in masters athletes: age-associated changes and underlying physiological mechanisms. J Physiol 2008;586(1):55–63.

Tarnopolsky MA. Nutritional consideration in the aging athlete. Clin J Sport Med 2008;18:531–38.

Tarnopolsky MA, Bosman M, Macdonald JR, et al. Postexercise protein–carbohydrate and carbohydrate supplements increase muscle glycogen in men and women. J Appl Physiol 1997;83:1877–83.

Thomas J. Drug–nutrient interactions. Nutr Rev 1995;53:271–82.

Toth MJ, Tchernof A. Lipid metabolism in the elderly. Eur J Clin Nutr 2000;54(3 Suppl):121S–5S.

Trappe S. Masters athletes. Int J Sports Nut Exer Metab 2001;11(Suppl):196S–207S.

Trappe SW, Costill DL, Fink WJ, Pearson DR. Skeletal muscle characteristics among distance runners: a 20-year follow-up study. J Appl Physiol 1995;78:823–9.

Trappe SW, Costill DL, Vukovich MD, et al. Aging among elite distance runners: a 22-year longitudinal study. J Appl Physiol 1996;80:285–90.

Tsai KS, Heath H, Kumar R, Riggs BL. Impaired vitamin D metabolism with aging women: possible role in pathogenesis of senile osteoporosis. J Clin Invest 1984;73:1668–72.

Turnland JR, Durkin N, Costa F, et al. Stable isotope studies of zinc absorption and retention in young and elderly men. J Nutr 1986;116:1239–47.

Van Erp-Baart AMJ, Saris WHM, Binkhorst RA, et al. Nationwide survey on nutritional habits in elite athletes. Part II: Mineral and vitamin intake. Int J Sports Med 1989;10(Suppl):11S–16S.

Van Pelt RE, Dinneno FA, Seals DR, Jones PP. Age-related decline in RMR in physically active men: relation to exercise volume and energy intake. Am J Physiol Endocrinol Metab 2001;281:E633–9.

Viitala P, Newhouse IJ. Vitamin E supplementation, exercise and lipid peroxidation in human participants. Eur J Appl Physiol 2004;93:108–15.

Vivekananthan DP, Penn MS, Sapp SK, Hsu A, Topol EJ. Use of antioxidant vitamins for the prevention of cardiovascular disease: meta-analysis of randomised trials. Lancet 2003;361:2017–23.

Volpi E, Ferrando A, Yedkel C, et al. Exogenous amino acids stimulate net muscle protein synthesis in the elderly. J Clin Invest 1998;101:2000–7.

Wahlqvist ML, Savige GS. Interventions aimed at dietary and lifestyle changes to promote healthy aging. Eur J Clin Nutr 2000;54(3 Suppl):148S–56S.

Wakimoto P, Block G. Dietary intake, dietary patterns, and changes with age: an epidemiological perspective. J Gerentol 2001;56(A):65–80.

Waller MF, Haymes EM. The effects of heat and exercise on sweat iron loss. Med Sci Sports Exerc 1996;28:197–203.

Warburton DE, Nicol CW, Bredin SS. Health benefits of physical activity: the evidence. Can Med Assoc J 2006;174(6):801–9.

Ward N, et al. The effect of vitamin E on blood pressure in individuals with type 2 diabetes: a randomised double blind controlled, placebo controlled trial. J Hypertens 2007;25:227–34.

Webster L. Key to healthy aging: exercise. J Gerontol Nurs 1990;14:9–15.

Weir PL, Kerr T, Hodges NJ, McKay SM, Starkes JL. Masters swimmers: how are they different from younger elite swimmers? An examination of practice and performance patterns. J Aging Phys Act 2002;10:41–63.

Welle S, Thornton CA. High-protein meals do not enhance myofibrillar synthesis after resistance exercise in 62- to 75-year-old men and women. Am J Physiol 1998;274(4 Part 1):E677–E83.

Working Group of the Australian and New Zealand Bone and Mineral Society, Endocrine Society of Australia, Osteoporosis Australia. Vitamin D and adult bone health in Australia and New Zealand: a position statement. Med J Aust 2005;182:281–5.

World Health Organization (WHO). Keep fit for life: meeting the nutritional needs of older persons. Report of a joint WHO/Tufts University School of Nutrition and Policy expert consultation. Malta: World Health Organization, 2002.

Winters LRT, Yoon JS, Kalkwarf HJ, et al. Riboflavin requirements and exercise adaptation in older women. Am J Clin Nutr 1992;56:526–32.

Wood RJ, Zheng JJ. High dietary calcium intakes reduce zinc absorption and balance in humans. Am J Clin Nutr 1997;65:1803–9.

Yarasheski KE, Zachwieja JJ, Bier DM. Acute effects of resistance exercise on muscle protein synthesis rate in young and elderly men and women. Am J Physiol 1993;265(2 Pt 1):E210–14.

Yip R, Dallman PR. The role of inflammation and iron deficiency as causes of anemia. Am J Clin Nutr 1988;48:1295–300.

CHAPTER 19

Special needs: the athlete with diabetes

VICKI DEAKIN, DENNIS WILSON AND GABRIELLE COOPER

19.1 Introduction

Almost one in four Australians aged 25 years and over has either diabetes or impaired glucose metabolism (i.e. impaired glucose tolerance or impaired fasting hypoglycemia) (Dunstan et al. 2001). The prevalence of diabetes in this age group, using measured blood glucose levels from respondents in the 1999–2000 Australian Diabetes and Lifestyle Survey (AusDiab Survey), the most recent epidemiological survey of the Australian population, was 7.4%, a figure that has more than doubled in the last 20 years (Dunstan et al. 2002). It is estimated that for every known case of diabetes, there is one newly diagnosed case; therefore this figure is conservative (Australian Institute of Health and Welfare 2008). The age-standardized prevalence of diabetes among Indigenous people in Australia is almost three times greater than that of non-Indigenous Australians (Australian Bureau of Statistics 2006).

Diabetes mellitus is a group of metabolic disorders resulting in defects in insulin secretion, insulin action (sensitivity) or both, resulting in abnormalities in carbohydrate, protein and fat metabolism that are life-threatening, if untreated. If poorly controlled or improperly treated blood glucose levels rise to high levels in the acute phase and can cause hyperglycemia (high blood glucose), dehydration, ketosis, weight loss and blurred vision. Long-term complications in poorly controlled diabetes include retinopathy with potential loss of vision; nephropathy leading to renal failure; peripheral neuropathy with risks of foot ulcer and amputation; and autonomic neuropathy causing gastrointestinal, genitourinary and cardiovascular symptoms and sexual dysfunction. People with poorly controlled diabetes also have an increased risk of hypertension, cardiovascular disease and cerebrovascular disease (American Diabetes Association 2009a, 2009b). Hence, the long-term treatment goals, irrespective of the type of diabetes, are to maintain glycemic control, reduce hyperglycemia and the onset and progression of these long-term complications, and ultimately improve quality of life (American Diabetes Association 2009b; Di Piro et al. 2005).

A person with diabetes can become an elite athlete and train and compete at a high level of exercise intensity and endurance. Several renowned athletes with diabetes, including Sir Steven Redgrave, who won five successive gold medals in rowing from

1985 to 2000, and Wasim Akram, the Pakistani fast bowler, provide testament to overcoming any perceived barriers imposed by this condition. As hypoglycemia (low blood glucose) is the most common problem faced by an athlete with diabetes on insulin, certain sports that are solo in nature, take place in mid-air or water or limit an individual's ability to recognize the symptoms of hypoglycemia—which can be masked by exercise—may be contraindicated or undertaken with caution with a training partner. For athletes participating in these types of sports, coaches and training partners need to recognize the symptoms of hypoglycemia and how to treat it.

This chapter focuses on clinical practice guidelines and medical nutrition recommendations for athletes with diabetes, particularly those on insulin, undertaking different levels of physical activity. Although the carbohydrate (CHO) and protein recommendations before, during and after exercise are similar for diabetic and non-diabetic athletes, the metabolic response to exercise in an athlete on insulin is affected by the levels of blood glucose and circulating insulin at the start of exercise. Regular self-monitoring of blood glucose in response to exercise, as well as ongoing consultation with a team of qualified clinicians—including a dietitian with experience in diabetes management, a diabetes educator and a physician—is critical for an athlete with diabetes on insulin—to assist the athlete to fine-tune insulin dosage to match energy requirements for exercise.

Definition and description of diabetes mellitus 19.2

Diabetes mellitus is a group of metabolic disorders resulting in defects in insulin secretion, insulin action (sensitivity) or both (American Diabetes Association 2009a). Most cases of diabetes fall into two broad categories: type 1 and type 2. Type 1 diabetes or immune-mediated diabetes is less common than type 2 diabetes, affecting around 5–10% of people with diabetes. Type 1 diabetes (previously named insulin-dependent diabetes, type I diabetes or juvenile-onset diabetes) mainly affects a younger age group and has an abrupt and often life-threatening onset. It typically involves the autoimmune destruction of pancreatic beta cells, which is the site of insulin production. Management involves lifelong treatment with exogenous insulin, diet modification and self-monitoring of blood glucose levels. There are several other types of diabetes involving genetic defects of the pancreatic beta cells, genetic defects in insulin action, endocrinopathies and drug- or chemical-induced types (American Diabetes Association 2009a).

The most common form is type 2 diabetes (previously named type II diabetes, non-insulin-dependent diabetes or NIDDM, or adult-onset diabetes), which affects around 90–95% of people with diabetes. With this type, individuals have insulin resistance and usually have relative (rather than absolute) insulin deficiency. Type 2 diabetes is a progressive condition, which may take 5–10 years of deteriorating glucose tolerance before being diagnosed (Golberg 1998). An estimated 16.4% of Australians have impaired glucose tolerance (Dunstan et al. 2002) and around 20% more suffer from a clustering of risk factors known as metabolic syndrome (metS) (Dunstan et al. 2002; Ford & Giles 2003). In Australia, the prevalence of type 2 diabetes is highest in older adults, in the Indigenous population, and in several other ethnic groups (South Pacific Islanders, Southern Europeans, and people from Middle Eastern, North African and Southern Asian countries) and, in particular, in people who are overweight or obese (Dunstan et al.

2001; Thow & Waters 2005; Australian Bureau of Statistics 2006; Australian Institute of Health and Welfare 2008). An increased incidence has also been reported in adolescents and children in Australia—a relatively novel occurrence (McMahon et al. 2004). Similar increases around the same time were reported in children and adolescents in the UK (Ehtisham & Hatt Molnár 2004; Ehtisham et al. 2004) and in the US (Alberti et al. 2004) and to a lesser extent in European children (Molnár 2004; Malecka-Tendera et al. 2005).

This increased prevalence at all ages parallels the epidemic of obesity, which is a significant contributor (Dunstan et al. 2001). Obesity is strongly linked to diabetes because it causes some degree of insulin resistance. In the early stages of type 2 diabetes, there are often no symptoms and insulin is not required because autoimmune destruction of the beta cells in the pancreas does not occur (American Diabetes Association 2009a). However, lethargy, polyuria, nocturia and polydipsia, the typical symptoms of hyperglycemia, can occur and usually worsen with progression of the condition. Management for type 2 diabetes is similar to that for type 1 and involves lifestyle changes, diet modification and weight loss, if overweight or obese. For some cases, medication (oral hypoglycemic agents and possibly insulin) is warranted.

19.3 Physiological effects of exercise

For either form of diabetes, regular physical activity including both resistance and at least moderate levels of aerobic activity improves glycemic control, increases insulin sensitivity and reduces associated cardiovascular risk factors (American Diabetes Association 2004a; Sigal et al. 2004). This effect is independent of exercise–related changes in body mass (BM) (Duncan et al. 2003). However, the acute physiological effects of moderate to strenuous levels of physical activity can be risky for an athlete with diabetes and can induce either hypoglycemia (low blood glucose) or hyperglycemia (high blood glucose), especially in an athlete on insulin.

In terms of glucose metabolism, acute exercise is a potent stimulus for glucose uptake and utilization by muscle tissue (Ebeling et al. 1993; Sigal et al. 2004). These mechanisms and the requirements for utilization of fuel for muscular activity are no different from those of an athlete without diabetes. In response to exercise, plasma insulin levels decrease during exercise and that decrease, along with an increase in plasma glucagon and other counter-regulatory hormones, promotes an increase in hepatic glucose production (gluconeogenesis). The amount of glucose produced by gluconeogenesis matches the amount required by the increased metabolic requirements of other physiological systems: the respiratory, neural and cardiovascular systems. As a result, blood glucose levels can remain relatively stable for up to 1–2 hours of continuous exercise without food intake. With no food consumed during exercise and during prolonged moderate- to high-intensity exercise of more than 60–90 minutes duration, blood glucose levels will fall when hepatic glucose production lags behind glucose utilization and liver glycogen becomes depleted (see Chapter 13). For athletes with diabetes (and non-diabetic athletes), there is a substantial benefit from consuming CHO foods during exercise to prevent declines in blood sugar levels and promote recovery for the next training session (Perrone et al. 2005). For reviews about the effects of exercise on glycemic control, see Sigal and colleagues (2004) and the American Diabetes Association (2004a, 2009c).

Effects of long-term physical activity on insulin sensitivity

19.4

Of relevance to a person with diabetes is that repeated aerobic exercise increases insulin sensitivity (Wasserman et al. 2002). Insulin sensitivity can be sustained for 12–15 hours after a single bout of exercise and even longer by regular exercise training (Devlin 1992). The main functions of insulin are to:

- stimulate glucose uptake into most cells of the body
- inhibit glucose release from the liver
- inhibit the release of fatty acids from storage deposits
- facilitate protein synthesis in the body's cells
- stimulate resynthesis of muscle glycogen after exercise

An increase in insulin sensitivity improves these actions, which translates into a reduction in insulin dosage or in other oral medications. See sections 19.21 and 19.37.

Acute effects of exercise in athletes with type I diabetes

19.5

During exercise, insulin 'switches off' and other counter-regulatory hormones (catecholamines, glucagon, growth hormone and cortisol), which regulate glucose metabolism and affect cardiovascular response, body temperature, fluid, and electrolyte homeostasis, 'switch on'.

The magnitude of these metabolic and hormonal effects induced by exercise is determined by the:

- intensity and duration of exercise
- degree of metabolic control before exercise
- type and dose of insulin injected before exercise
- site of insulin injection
- timing of the previous insulin injection
- timing of the previous meal

The primary determinant of the glycemic response to exercise is insulin availability.

Exercise in the presence of hyperinsulinemia

19.6

In athletes with diabetes on insulin, plasma insulin levels may not decrease during exercise. This induces hypoglycemia, as insulin prevents the appropriate rise in hepatic glucose production and accelerates the exercise-induced stimulation of glucose uptake (see Fig. 19.1 overleaf).

Elevated insulin levels also prevent the increase in mobilization of lipids during exercise, leading to a reduced availability of non-esterified fatty acids as a fuel source (Wasserman et al. 1995). Hyperinsulinemia may occur when the usual dose of short-acting insulin (if injected a few hours before exercise) reaches its peak action during exercise. This effect can potentially be exaggerated if the previously injected limb is exercised, which may promote an increase in insulin absorption from the injection site, especially when using an intramuscular site (Koivisto & Felig 1978). Subcutaneous injection, particularly in the

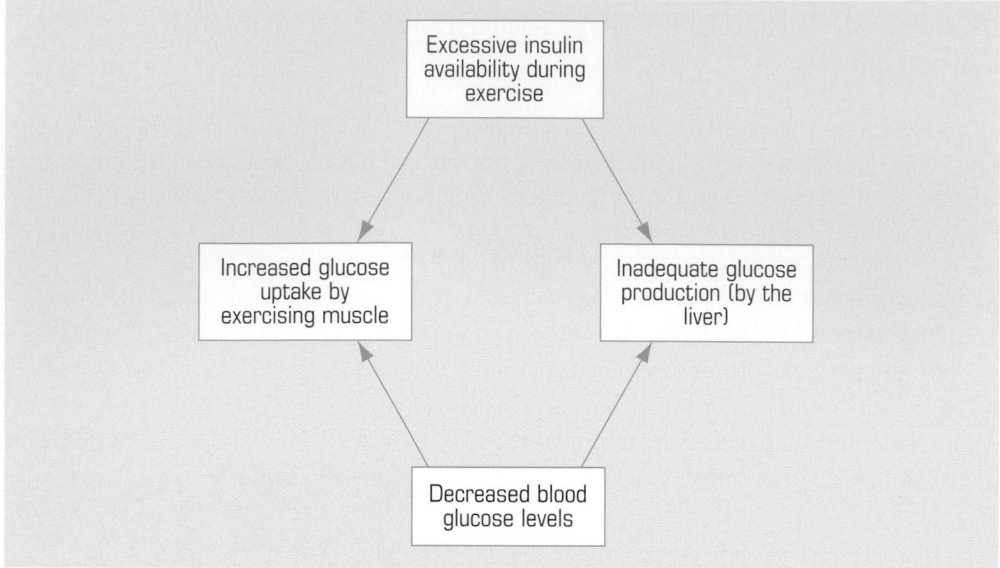

FIGURE 19.1 Metabolic response to exercise in diabetes

abdomen, usually addresses this problem (see section 19.16). If an athlete adjusts both dietary intake and insulin and monitors glycemic response under different training conditions, hyperinsulinemia can be avoided.

19.7 Exercise in the presence of hypoinsulinemia

In this situation, the inhibitory effect of insulin on hepatic glucose production and its stimulating effect on glucose uptake are both reduced. In addition, the counter-regulatory hormone response to exercise is higher than normal during insulin deficiency. These changes substantially increase hepatic glucose production and diminish glucose utilization by the exercising muscle, and result in marked hyperglycemia. During extremely strenuous acute exercise, hyperglycemia can be induced by excessive production of these counter-regulatory hormones, which stimulate a surplus of production of hepatic glucose beyond the limits of peripheral utilization. This can occur in type 1 diabetes even in the presence of insulin.

In a diabetic athlete without adequate insulin, lipid mobilization and ketogenesis induces ketonemia. When both dietary intake and insulin doses are adjusted appropriately, this situation can be avoided.

19.8 Medical nutrition therapy for athletes with type 1 diabetes

In 2006, the American Dietetic Association reaffirmed the critical role of medical nutrition therapy (MNT) in the prevention and treatment of type 2 diabetes and the treatment and management of existing type 1 and type 2 diabetes (Franz & Wylie-Rosett 2007). Nutrition goals for training and competition recommended for athletes with diabetes are no different from those recommended for athletes without diabetes (see Chapter 1) (American Diabetes Association 2004a, 2004b; Dietitians Association of Australia 2006; Franz & Wylie-Rosett 2007). An overall training diet for athletes with diabetes, based on CHO-rich foods (see Chapter 12) and low-fat foods, is compatible with diabetes management and athletic performance. Low-CHO diets are not recommended in the management of diabetes (Dietitians Association of Australia 2006) and are counterproductive to maintaining capacity for athletic performance and recovery.

Athletes with diabetes should be encouraged to adjust insulin dosage according to their lifestyle and training program rather than distorting their eating patterns to suit the insulin dosage. Although it is not necessary to follow a rigid pattern of food intake, a reasonably consistent eating routine facilitates diabetic management. Maintaining consistent training and eating routines day to day also assists in the establishment of insulin dosage and fine-tuning of food intake. A well-trained athlete who regularly exercises at the same time each day will usually need less adjustment to food and insulin than a person who exercises only occasionally (Franz et al. 2002). For athletes with recently diagnosed type 1 diabetes, the stabilization and adjustment phase is usually the first priority and an interruption to training and competition routines may be expected in the short term.

Any individual with type 1 diabetes who participates in regular physical exercise of moderate to high intensity needs to consider:

- the macronutrient content and timing of meals and snacks
- the insulin dose and its predicted peak period of activity in relation to their exercise
- routine monitoring of blood glucose levels to assist with the adjustment of food and insulin to prevent and manage hyperglycemia and hypoglycemia

Type of carbohydrate recommended for athletes with diabetes 19.9

The type of CHO—low or high glycemic index (GI) foods—consumed in the total diet has a minimal effect on achieving glycemic control (Franz & Wylie-Rosett 2007) because of the wide variability in individual responses to CHO-containing foods. Contrary to popular belief, dietary sucrose does not increase blood glucose levels more than isocaloric amounts of starch (Franz & Wylie-Rosett 2007). Glucose polymers—which are the main ingredient in sports drinks—rather than free glucose, do not elevate the blood glucose response (Ivy et al. 1979; Maughan et al. 1987). Although fructose, another 'simple sugar', does not elevate blood glucose levels at the same rate as glucose or sucrose, high concentrations can cause gastrointestinal upset. Sports drinks, which contain a combination of glucose polymer and other sugars, are an ideal fluid and CHO choice during and after prolonged endurance exercise for athletes with diabetes. Nevertheless, for the athlete with type 1 diabetes, high-sugar-containing foods, if consumed in the total diet, should be adequately covered with insulin.

Recommended carbohydrate intakes for athletes with diabetes 19.10

The CHO content in food and the amount consumed, rather than the fat and protein content, remains the cornerstone of glycemic control in an athlete with diabetes. The amount

TABLE 19.1 RECOMMENDED DIETARY CARBOHYDRATE (CHO) INTAKES (G) BEFORE EXERCISE

EXERCISE INTENSITY AND DURATION	BLOOD GLUCOSE (MMOL/L)	DIETARY CHO (G)
Brief high-intensity (<30 minutes) (e.g. weightlifting, sprints)	6–10	No food required
Light (e.g. walking 30 minutes, easy-pace aerobics 60 minutes)	<6 >6	15 No food required
Moderate (<45 minutes) (e.g. swimming, jogging, tennis, basketball)	<6 6–10 10–14 14+	30–45 15 No food required Exercise not advised
Moderate (>60 minutes) (e.g. football, cycling)	10–14 plus reduced insulin dosage >13–14 and ketones 17 (no ketones)	10–15 g/h Exercise contraindicated Exercise not advised
Strenuous (<60 minutes) (e.g. triathlon, marathon, canoeing, kayaking, cross-country skiing, cycling)	<6 6–10 10–14 14+	45 30–45 15–30 Exercise not advised
Strenuous (>60 minutes) (e.g. triathlon, marathon, canoeing, kayaking, cross-country skiing, cycling)	<6 6–10 10–14	50 g/h 25–30 g/h 10–15 g/h

Exercise at any level is contraindicated if ketones are present.
Source: Adapted from Armstrong 1992

of CHO consumed is still the main determinant of post-prandial blood glucose levels. In contrast, proteins in food do not increase blood glucose levels post-prandially. The key strategy for achieving glycemic control is to monitor CHO consumption, either by CHO counting, CHO exchanges or experienced-based estimations (Dietitians Association of Australia 2006; Franz & Wylie-Rosett 2007).

Table 19.1 provides guidelines for the amounts of CHO (in grams) recommended for athletes undertaking exercise of varying intensity and duration. Examples of foods containing 50 g of CHO are found in Chapter 14, Table 14.4. In principle, the recommended CHO intake before, during and after exercise for an athlete with diabetes is no different from that recommended for an athlete without diabetes (see Chapters 12, 13 and 14). These CHO recommendations are derived from laboratory studies of groups of people who are unlikely to be elite athletes and are being tested under contrived experimental conditions. They can be applied to those diabetic athletes who have good metabolic control with usual blood glucose levels between 4 mmol/L and 8 mmol/L (Franz et al. 1994). If blood glucose levels are chronically very high or often low, food choices and/or insulin dosage should be modified.

Adapting these CHO recommendations based on individual responses to exercise of differing intensities and duration is done by trial and error together with blood glucose monitoring. CHO (and protein) recommendations need to be adapted to the individual and to the energy demands of each sporting activity.

Recommendations for carbohydrate intakes for brief, high-intensity sports and light training 19.11

Sprinting, running or swimming less than 1500 m, and other sports involving sudden, intense activity (such as weightlifting), usually require minimal or no adjustment to food intake provided the pre-event blood glucose level is between 5.6 and 10.0 mmol/L (Armstrong 1992; Franz et al. 1994). This is also the case for low-level activity, such as a 30-minute leisurely walk or bike ride.

For a blood glucose level between 10 and 14 mmol/L, there is probably no need for increased food (or CHO) if the exercise is of less than 1 hour duration. If the blood glucose level is above 14 mmol/L, the urine should be tested for ketones. Exercise is contraindicated in the presence of ketones. Blood glucose levels should be below 14 mmol/L before the activity is commenced (Armstrong 1992).

Recommendations for carbohydrate intakes for moderate-intensity exercise of short duration (15–30 minutes) 19.12

A pre-exercise meal 1 to 3 hours before the commencement of exercise is recommended according to the principles of preparation for exercise (see Chapter 12). If insulin action is likely to peak at the time of the event, an additional 10–15 g CHO taken 20–30 minutes beforehand is usually sufficient to prevent hypoglycemia, provided the blood glucose level is between 5.6 and 10.0 mmol/L at the commencement of exercise (Armstrong 1992; Franz et al. 1994). If the blood glucose level is more than 14 mmol/L, postponement of exercise is recommended.

After exercise, 15–30 g CHO food may be required to maintain adequate blood glucose levels, prevent post-exercise hypoglycemia and promote recovery (see Chapter 14).

Recommendations for carbohydrate intakes for moderate- to strenuous-intensity exercise of medium to long duration (<30 minutes) 19.13

A pre-exercise meal of an additional 15 g CHO from foods with a high to moderate GI for each 20 minutes of planned activity should be tried initially. This should be eaten 1 to 3 hours before exercise, with the support of an additional 15 g CHO from high GI foods taken just before competition.

Consuming some type of CHO at around 60–90 minutes or even earlier into a prolonged bout of physical activity helps prevent hypoglycemia during exercise and maintains exercise capacity (Kahn & Vinik 1988; Armstrong 1992). In practice, the form of CHO (solid or liquid) consumed makes no difference to performance outcomes and depends on individual preferences and opportunities for consumption during the activity. The previously held belief that a sugar solution or quickly absorbed CHO food consumed 30–60 minutes before the activity would reduce exercise tolerance is not justified (Maynard 1992; Franz et al. 1994).

For athletes with type 1 diabetes, the American Diabetes Association (2004a) recommends 2–3 mg CHO/kg/min of CHO during moderate levels of physical activity. For more strenuous activity, up to 1 g/CHO/kg body mass (BM) up to a maximum of 60 g CHO/min may be needed (Coyle 1991), although recent evidence suggests that 1.8 g CHO/kg BM improved performance in a cycling trial (Currell & Jeukendrup 2008). For those athletes with type 1 diabetes who do not tolerate solid food, a sports drink is useful during exercise to deliver CHO (Andrade et al. 2005; Perrone et al. 2005). In one study of sixteen adolescent athletes with type 1 diabetes, an average intake of 92 mL sports drink containing 8% CHO maintained blood sugar levels and fluid status during a 60-minute cycle ergometer test at 55–60% VO_{2max} with no change in insulin dosage (Perrone et al. 2005). For four athletes in this study, a sports drink containing 10% CHO during exercise was required to prevent exercise-induced hypoglycemia. The 8% sports drink was not sufficient to prevent hypoglycemia. No gastrointestinal symptoms were reported in this study in any athletes using both concentrations.

19.14 Pre-event carbohydrate loading

Adequate diabetic control is required before an athlete with diabetes should attempt any form of CHO loading.

Dietary and training techniques for CHO loading of glycogen stores for competition are considered in detail in Chapter 12. As CHO loading is dependent on the availability of insulin to store muscle glycogen, this technique should be used with caution in an athlete requiring insulin. The insulin dose should be adjusted to match the changes in diet and the tapering effects of exercise before competition. For the athlete on insulin who has poor diabetic control, stabilizing blood glucose is already difficult and CHO loading can lead to further deterioration in diabetic control.

19.15 Post-exercise re-feeding

CHO should be eaten soon after the completion of exercise (where possible) to promote muscle glycogen resynthesis (see Chapter 14). Around 1.0–1.5 g CHO/kg BM shortly after exercise and again at 60 minutes is recommended to maximize recovery of fuel reserves for the next training session (Armstrong 1992).

19.16 Fluids

Athletes with type 1 diabetes tend to become preoccupied with replacing CHO and forget their requirements for fluid. Thirst is not necessarily a reliable indicator of fluid status in athletes with well-controlled diabetes or without diabetes. Because the thirst mechanism is less sensitive during exercise, it is important to drink water before becoming thirsty. Conversely, excessive thirst could be a sign of hyperglycemia in an athlete with diabetes and not necessarily indicative of fluid balance. Guidelines for the composition and volume of suitable fluids for everyday training and specific competition for an athlete with diabetes are the same as those for non-diabetic athletes (see Chapter 14) and the recently revised fluid replacement guidelines from the American College of Sports Medicine (Sawka et al. 2007).

19.17 Alcohol

Alcohol is a potent inhibitor of hepatic glucose production and may precipitate late and severe hypoglycemia in a person with diabetes on insulin or oral hypoglycemic agents. Excess alcohol also impairs an individual's ability to recognize symptoms of hypoglycemia. For athletes with diabetes, when consuming alcohol, the recommended intakes are

<1 drink/d for women and <2 drinks/d for men as an occasional addition to the regular meal plan (Franz & Wylie-Rosett 2007). When soft drinks are used as mixers with alcohol, or when sweet wines or liqueurs are consumed, the opposite effect—hyperglycemia—can be induced.

Dietary fats and cholesterol 19.18

Recent updates on clinical practice guidelines from the American Diabetes Association (2009c) recommend that average daily intakes of saturated fatty acids are <7% of total energy; dietary cholesterol is <200 mg/d; and trans fatty acid intakes are minimized. It is prudent to modify types of fatty acid intakes at a young age, especially in athletes with type 1 diabetes, so that appropriate food choices and dietary habits become entrenched and hopefully will be sustained into adulthood, to help prevent long-term complications.

The cardiovascular risk for people with diabetes is similar to that for people without diabetes but with pre-existing cardiovascular disease (Franz & Wylie-Rosett 2007). The benefits of decreasing saturated fat and increasing polyunsaturated fats on improving morbidity in people with diabetes are well documented (National Health and Medical Research Council 2005).

Insulin adjustments for athletes with type 1 diabetes 19.19

The main determinant of the glycemic response to exercise is insulin availability. The following regimens are typical of current management of type 1 diabetes.

- *Conventional regimens (split-mixed)* use a combination of short- or ultra-short-acting insulin with intermediate- or long-acting insulin (usually 30% short-acting and 70% intermediate- or long-acting) once or twice daily. If the dosage is split, about two-thirds of the total daily requirement is given before breakfast and the rest before the evening meal.
- *Intensive regimens (basal-bolus)* use bolus injections of short- or ultra-short-acting insulin before each meal, and intermediate- or long-acting insulin once or twice daily (before bedtime and breakfast).
- *Continuous subcutaneous insulin infusion (SCII)* uses a pump that delivers a continuous infusion of short- or ultra-short-acting insulin via a subcutaneous needle with bolus doses activated by patient before meals.

Available insulins 19.20

Available insulin preparations are either purified bovine insulins or human insulins obtained by recombinant DNA technology.

- *Ultra-short and short-acting insulins* are soluble insulins (clear solution); short-acting insulins are the only type that can be given intravenously, for example in diabetic ketoacidosis.

- *Insulin lispro* and *insulin aspart* are insulin analogues obtained by recombinant DNA technology; their ultra-short onset of action allows them to be given immediately before meals.
- *Insulin glargine* is an insulin analogue, which provides basal insulin level that is constantly delivered over 24 hours and allows for once-daily dosing.
- *Intermediate- and long-acting insulins* have a prolonged duration of action resulting from either complexing insulin with a protein such as protamine (isophane insulin) or modifying particle size (e.g. using insulin–zinc suspensions).
- *Mixed insulins* (also called *biphasic insulins*) combine a short- or ultra-short-acting insulin in varying proportions (20–50%) with an intermediate-acting insulin (Rossi 2009).

A few people continue to use bovine or porcine preparations. In recent years, insulin analogues have become available. The short-acting analogue, insulin lispro, is already in clinical use and others, such as insulin aspart, are expected to become available in the near future. Long-acting insulin analogues are also under development. The short-acting analogues have an onset of action within minutes after subcutaneous injection, peak at 1–2 hours and have a duration of approximately 4 hours. The commonly used regular or neutral (clear) insulins have an onset of action of about 30 minutes after subcutaneous injection, peak at 2–3 hours and have a duration of approximately 7 hours. Both kinds of insulin may be given alone, before each meal, using a syringe or a pen injector, or in combination with an intermediate- or long-acting insulin before breakfast and the evening meal. If given alone, they are combined with an injection of an intermediate- or long-acting insulin before bed. The intermediate-acting insulins (Isophane™ or Lente MC™) have an onset of action after 1–2 hours, peak at 6–10 hours and have a duration of 16–20 hours. The long-acting insulin (Ultralente MC™) has an onset of action after 2–3 hours, peaks at 8–14 hours and has a duration of approximately 24 hours. Table 19.2 summarizes the onset and duration of action, and time to peak activity, in these different

TABLE 19.2 TYPES, ONSET, PEAK AND DURATION OF ACTION OF CURRENTLY AVAILABLE INSULINS

INSULIN TYPE	ONSET OF ACTION (HOURS)	TIME TO PEAK ACTIVITY (HOURS)	DURATION OF ACTION (HOURS)
ULTRA-SHORT-ACTING			
Insulin lispro, insulin aspart	0.25	1	4–5
SHORT-ACTING			
Neutral	0.5	2–3	6–8
INTERMEDIATE-ACTING			
Non-mixed	1–2.5	4–12	16–24
Mixed with short-acting insulin	0.5–1	2–12	16–24
Mixed with ultra-short-acting insulin	0.25	1	16–24
LONG-ACTING			
Insulin glargine	1–2	10–20	24
Non-mixed	2–4	10–20	24–36

Source: Adapted from Rossi 2009

types. Pre-mixed preparations of neutral and isophane insulins are also available. The amount of neutral insulin in these preparations varies from 20–50%, with the remainder being isophane insulin.

Site of insulin injection 19.21

The site of injection (subcutaneous or intramuscular) may affect insulin absorption. In one study, intramuscular injection by adults followed by cycle exercise induced a marked increase in insulin absorption and a substantial fall in plasma glucose compared with subcutaneous thigh injection (Frid et al. 1990). No effects of 30 minutes of intense exercise on insulin absorption results were found in a more recent study of thirteen adults using subcutaneous thigh injection of basal-bolus insulin—glargine—on the evening before the study (Peter et al. 2005). Interestingly, in an elaborate crossover study of the effects of moderate exercise in thirteen adults after 30 and 120 minutes from dosage using inhaled human insulin, no change or slightly decreased insulin absorption was reported after 30 minutes of moderate exercise, compared with no exercise, although the glucose uptake at 2 hours post-exercise was substantially increased (Petersen et al. 2007). Thus, people using inhaled insulin may need to adjust insulin dose, independent of time of exercise, and be aware of the possibility of a faster effect when exercising early after dosing. For injected insulin, abdominal bolus subcutaneous injection is the best site for those undertaking exercise and is associated with little to no effects on insulin absorption (American Diabetes Association 2004a).

Insulin adjustment 19.22

The challenge for the management of an individual athlete using bolus injection or these new routes of administration (i.e. inhaled insulin, CSII insulin pump and insulin patch) is to monitor how varying levels of exercise affect blood glucose levels and how to adjust insulin to match (Heiemann et al. 2001).

Smaller total daily insulin dosages are required in athletes with type 1 diabetes who undertake regular physical activity, largely because of an increase in insulin sensitivity associated with exercise. When physical activity is less than 30 minutes' duration, it is usually not necessary to reduce insulin dosage. For more prolonged physical activity, the insulin is adjusted to reduce the insulin operating at the time of the exercise, usually by 15–40%. The exact reduction depends on the intensity and varies considerably between individuals. For physical activity undertaken in the morning, the short-acting insulin dose should be reduced before breakfast by 15–40%. When physical activity is undertaken in the afternoon, intermediate-acting insulin (if used before breakfast) should be reduced. If an athlete is on a combination of short-acting insulin before each meal and intermediate-acting insulin at night, the pre-lunch short-acting dose is reduced for afternoon exercise.

When physical activity is continuous over several hours (e.g. a 3- to 4-hour cycle, or a 2-hour run), then a more substantial reduction in insulin dose is required. In this situation, reducing both morning short-acting (clear) and intermediate-acting (cloudy) doses by up to 50% could be indicated. For some events, such as a marathon or triathlon, insulin has been omitted completely, without adverse effects (Meinders et al. 1988). However, although it is important to avoid the development of hypoglycemia during exercise, an excessive reduction in insulin doses can lead to hypoinsulinemia and result in hyperglycemia, leading to increased fluid loss, possible ketosis and a high risk of dehydration and heat stress.

19.23 Insulin adjustment using a continuous subcutaneous insulin infusion (CSII): insulin pumps

Insulin pumps contain a reservoir or cartridge filled with short-acting insulin analogue. The dose is delivered subcutaneously in the abdomen, buttocks, legs or upper arm through a needle or infusion catheter, which is repositioned every 3 days. This mode of delivery provides adjustable 24-hour insulin as 'basal' delivery with increases in bolus insulin at meal times or when required. The pump can be programmed to accommodate the decreased insulin requirement in response to exercise, so is associated with a lower risk of hypoglycemia, compared to using multiple daily injections (Colberg 2002), which is ideal for athletes. Although expensive, it is estimated that around 20% of people with diabetes in the US are using insulin pumps, whereas in other countries (i.e. the UK and Denmark), usage is only about 1% (Colman 2008). It is likely that CSII use will continue to increase, especially in children and adolescents undertaking sport, because of its advantages in offering more flexibility in dosage and in eating habits. For athletes undertaking non-contact sports, the pump can usually remain connected. Disconnection for up to 1–2 hours is possible in those undertaking water or contact sports (Smart & Morrison 2008).

19.24 Monitoring blood glucose levels

Individuals vary considerably in their metabolic response to physical activity and their diabetic control. It is important to consider the type, intensity and duration of the sports activity (e.g. training or competition) when making decisions about appropriate insulin dosage and how frequently blood glucose is monitored. A management plan based on food requirements after physical activity and corresponding insulin requirement can then be formulated. Once a response pattern is established for a particular individual to a particular type of exercise, it is likely to be similar on future occasions and, therefore, appropriate adjustments can be predicted.

If physical activity is unplanned and insulin has already been administered, then adjustments to CHO intake during or prior to exercise will be needed. Adjustments to insulin doses and food intake after the exercise may still be warranted, if low blood sugar levels are evident.

19.25 Special problems for the athlete with type 1 diabetes

Very low and high blood sugar levels occur from time to time in any individual with diabetes on insulin. Although habitual physical activity improves glycemic control, the acute metabolic effects of exercise, particularly high-intensity exercise, are often disturbed in an athlete on insulin compared to a non-diabetic athlete. During exercise, hypoglycemia or hyperglycemia can occur and late-onset hypoglycemia after exercise is not uncommon, especially in children and adolescents during growth spurts. In individuals with poor metabolic control, blood glucose levels can be extreme. On competition day, further high blood glucose levels may unexpectedly occur, which is attributed to the psychological stress of competition and accompanying increase in circulating catcholamines and other catabolic hormones. For instance, it is not uncommon for an athlete on insulin who is more prone to hypoglycemia on a regular training day to develop hyperglycemia at competition, even though undertaking the same nutritional practices as a training day.

Hypoglycemia 19.26

The most common problem for the athlete with diabetes on insulin is hypoglycemia. Children and adolescents, particularly during growth spurts, are more susceptible to hypoglycemia than adults. Most children and adolescents on insulin who exercise for prolonged period (e.g. >30 minutes) experience a substantial drop in blood glucose levels (Riddell et al. 1999). The associated symptoms—increased sweating, signs of anxiety, nausea and disorientation—are easily confused or masked by the usual physiological effects of exercise. If symptoms of hypoglycemia are not recognized, then severe hypoglycemia can develop. Untreated hypoglycemia, associated with too much insulin or too little food, eventually leads to hypoglycemic coma.

Late hypoglycemia after exercise 19.27

A further problem affecting an athlete on insulin is the occurrence of late hypoglycemia after exercise. This can occur up to 36 hours after exercise and is particularly prevalent in very active children (Shehadeh et al. 1998; Tupola et al. 1998). The onset of delayed hypoglycemia is associated with increased insulin sensitivity for several hours after cessation of exercise (see section 19.2), and possibly incorrect insulin adjustment or inappropriate nutrition intervention (Riddell & Iscoe 2006). If appropriate snacks are used prior to exercise, then reducing the next insulin dose usually avoids this effect. Too much alcohol also precipitates late hypoglycemia and can mask the early symptoms of hypoglycemia and therefore increase the risk of hypoglycemic coma.

Dietary treatment of hypoglycemia 19.28

While foods containing 15 g of quickly absorbed CHO (with a high GI), such as sugar, may relieve the early symptoms of hypoglycemia under normal circumstances, it may be necessary to have two or three times this amount to treat hypoglycemia induced after strenuous exercise (Franz 1991). Dietary treatment must be continued until stable blood glucose levels are achieved.

Hypoglycemic coma 19.29

A 50% dextrose solution is injected intravenously to treat hypoglycemic coma. Fluid or food must not be administered by mouth. If intravenous glucose cannot be given, an intramuscular injection of 1 mg glucagon is used, which induces glucose release from liver glycogen. However, glucagon injections may not work after prolonged exercise if hepatic glycogen stores are depleted, after a marathon or triathlon for example. Rapid medical assistance is crucial for anyone in a diabetic coma.

19.30 Impaired temperature regulation

A further risk associated with hypoglycemia is impaired temperature regulation. If there is risk of hypothermia (in sports such as cross-country skiing) or hyperthermia and potentially hypohydration (in marathon events), then particular care should be taken to maintain fluid balance and glycemic control.

19.31 Hyperglycemia

The usual causes of hyperglycemia are infection, overconsumption of food, inadequate insulin and, in some cases, alcohol consumption (when sweet wines, liqueurs or soft drinks are consumed inappropriately). Exercise is not recommended in individuals with severe hyperglycemia (see section 19.7) as it increases glycogenolysis, leading to even higher blood glucose levels and possibly ketosis. An athlete who exercises with very high blood sugar levels can become confused and disoriented and is at high risk of dehydration from the effects of polyuria. Exercise is contraindicated if ketones are present at the start of exercise.

Hyperglycemia after exercise is likely to be caused by an overconsumption of food (particularly CHO). Often athletes with diabetes who fear the onset of hypoglycemia during exercise consume excess food before or during exercise as a preventative measure. Frequent monitoring of blood glucose levels in this situation is again important (Monk et al. 1995; Franz et al. 2002).

19.32 Long-term complications with poorly controlled diabetes

Poorly controlled diabetes is associated with several long-term complications, which include retinopathy, with potential loss of vision; nephropathy, leading to renal failure; peripheral neuropathy, with risks of foot ulcer and amputation; and autonomic neuropathy, causing gastrointestinal, genitourinary and cardiovascular symptoms and sexual dysfunction. People with poorly controlled diabetes also have an increased risk of hypertension, cardiovascular disease and cerebrovascular disease (American Diabetes Association 2009a, 2009b). These complications increase with aging and with duration of diabetes but can be reduced substantially by improving glycemic control.

19.33 Cardiovascular disease

Poorly controlled diabetes is associated with damage to the large blood vessels, which accelerates atherosclerosis and can damage the capillaries, leading to microvascular disease, peripheral vascular disease and autonomic neuropathy. Any athlete with established type 1 diabetes contemplating a vigorous training program should have a detailed cardiovascular assessment beforehand. With the increased participation in sport by older people, there is an even stronger case for formal cardiac assessment before commencing an exercise program. One of the key findings of the AusDiab study in Australia in 1999–2000 was that about half of the people diagnosed with diabetes did not know they had it (Dunstan et al. 2001). For most people, however, the cardiovascular and psychological benefits of regular physical activity far exceed the risks (Sigal et al. 2004).

19.34 Retinopathy

Another complication of type 1 diabetes, which develops over time, is retinopathy. If this is of a proliferative type, vigorous physical activity and especially non-aerobic activity involving sudden stress, such as weightlifting, should be avoided as the associated rise in blood pressure could increase the chance of a vitreous hemorrhage or risk of retinal detachment.

Peripheral neuropathy 19.35

Many people with type 1 diabetes also develop peripheral neuropathy (damage to nerves in the extremities) over time. This results in loss of sensation in the feet and, in older individuals, is often associated with peripheral vascular disease. This increases the risk of damage to the feet, which is not recognized by the usual symptoms of soreness and pain. Foot ulcers associated with repetitive exercise (pounding on hard surfaces or rubbing of footwear) are a high risk for an athlete with diabetes. Foot ulcers are particularly difficult to heal and often require long hospital admission. The appropriate choice of footwear and advice from a podiatrist are important for all athletes with diabetes involved in weight-bearing exercise (Farrell 2003).

Autonomic neuropathy 19.36

Autonomic neuropathy is an abnormality of the autonomic nervous system and may be induced by long-standing, poorly controlled diabetes; it may result in loss of ability to control heart rate, blood pressure, sweating and bladder function. This complication of diabetes may limit exercise capacity and increase the risk of an adverse cardiovascular event during exercise. Disturbances in blood pressure control that are linked to autonomic neuropathy are more common in people at the start of an exercise program than in those who exercise regularly. A medical assessment to determine the extent of damage from autonomic neuropathy is strongly recommended prior to embarking on an exercise program that involves moderate to strenuous activity.

Physical activity for people with type 2 diabetes 19.37

Physical activity (both aerobic and resistance training, such as weightlifting) is effective in improving glycemic control, reducing HbA_{1c} (glycated hemoglobin), increasing insulin sensitivity and reducing cardiovascular mortality risk in people with type 2 diabetes (Sigal et al. 2004). There is now unequivocal evidence that type 2 diabetes can also be prevented or at least delayed by physical activity (Gill & Cooper 2008; Orozco et al. 2008) and by weight loss in the majority of at-risk people (Nield et al. 2008b). The American Dietetic Association recommends at least 150 minutes of moderate-intensity physical activity a week (50–70% of maximum heart rate), distributed over 3 days and with no more than 2 consecutive days without physical activity to achieve a preventive and treatment effect (Franz & Wylie-Rosett 2007). This level of physical activity is required to improve glucose control, independent of weight loss (Orozco et al. 2008). The risk reduction associated with increased physical activity is greatest in those at increased baseline risk of the disease, such as the obese, those with a positive family history and those with impaired glucose regulation (Gill & Cooper 2008). The prescription for resistance exercise for a risk reduction effect is three times a week using all major muscle groups, progressing to three sets of around 10 repetitions up to a weight that can be managed by the individual (Sigal et al. 2004). Nevertheless, some people do not respond to these interventions. Pooled data from six large-scale diabetes prevention intervention trials involving both physical activity at these levels and weight loss found 2–13% of participants with impaired glucose tolerance that still developed the disease (Gill & Cooper 2008).

A combination of dietary intervention with structured exercise and behavior modification is more effective in improving glycemic control (Boule et al. 2001; Nield et al. 2008a, 2008b), promoting greater weight loss (Wing 2002) and maintaining long-term weight control (Boule et al. 2001; Saris et al. 2003), compared to dietary intervention or physical activity alone. While short-term benefits of diet interventions with no exercise are effective, long-term adherence to diet alone (and maintenance of weight loss) in people with type 2 diabetes is poor (Nield et al. 2008a). Moreover, to maintain weight loss after intervention with exercise alone, a large amount of exercise (up to 7 hr/wk) at moderate to high intensity is required in previously obese people to sustain the weight lost (Saris et al. 2003). Clearly, these targets are unrealistic for most people.

Type 2 diabetes occurs more frequently in older people who have a variety of age-related disabilities that limit the feasibility of exercise. Nevertheless, increasing numbers of the young elderly are participating in regular exercise, and often at competitive levels. For both elderly and young elderly people with type 2 diabetes, a cardiac assessment prior to commencing an exercise program is warranted. This age group is also likely to have some degree of peripheral vascular disease, so care of the feet in impact sports should be addressed. Hypoglycemia can occur in people with type 2 diabetes who use insulin or one of the sulfonylurea medications (which enhance insulin secretion). The dosage of these drugs is reduced in people who undertake regular physical activity. Hypoglycemia is unlikely to occur in individuals using biguanides (e.g. metformin) or insulin-sensitizing agents (e.g. glitazones) or glucosidase inhibitors (e.g. acerbose). As many individuals with type 2 diabetes are overweight or obese, it is usually appropriate to encourage weight reduction and emphasize medication reduction during exercise rather than increasing CHO intake.

19.38 High-risk sports

Individuals with diabetes on treatment with insulin or sulfonylureas are at risk of hypoglycemia and disorientation. Sporting activities that would pose a risk to themselves or to those around them are best avoided. Hypoglycemia may occur in any sporting situation where the individual is alone and does not recognize the symptoms or in a situation where glucose cannot be readily administered as treatment. These situations include hang-gliding, scuba diving, solo yachting or motor car racing. Other activities where there is a lesser element of risk—such as cross-country skiing, surfboard riding or long-distance running—should be undertaken only if the individual is accompanied by someone who is able to recognize and treat hypoglycemia.

19.39 Insulin abuse and sport

Insulin is an anabolic agent, which promotes protein synthesis and inhibits protein breakdown in muscle (Fryburg et al. 1995). It also transports electrolytes and fluid into muscle cells, which makes them swell and gives the muscle a better definition. The misuse and abuse of insulin was reported over 20 years ago in bodybuilders and is still happening today. Use of insulin as an anabolic agent has been claimed in other sports, including cross-country skiing. Deliberately using insulin to produce hypoglycemia to initiate the physiological release of growth hormone has also been claimed. These practices are not without risk, as evidenced in a bodybuilder who developed severe and permanent brain damage after inducing hypoglycemia by using intravenous insulin (Elkin et al. 1997). There are also risks associated with sharing of needles to give insulin. The forms of insulin used for injection can be detected from blood tests. Athletes with diabetes who are prescribed insulin or other diabetic drugs need medical clearance in case of drug testing. Insulin, its analogues and other anabolic agents are banned substances.

Summary 19.40

Athletes with diabetes are able to participate in virtually all sports, apart from a few exceptions that pose a risk because of hypoglycemia. The dietary recommendations for training and competition for athletes with diabetes are similar to those for athletes without diabetes, provided the blood glucose range is within acceptable levels at the commencement of exercise. Older athletes, and those with long-standing diabetes, need to be screened for complications of the condition, such as cardiovascular disease, retinopathy and neuropathy. All athletes need to be properly instructed on strategies to avoid and treat exercise-induced hypoglycemia. Frequent monitoring of blood glucose levels should be encouraged. Exercise should not be undertaken in the presence of hyperglycemia and/or ketosis. Sports coaches of athletes with diabetes should be conversant with the effect of diabetes on athletic performance and, in particular, should be able to recognize and adequately treat hypoglycemia.

PRACTICE TIPS

ELIZABETH BROAD

- Individuals with diabetes come in many ages, sizes and shapes, and their exercise habits may vary from light and infrequent to two or three sessions per day of moderate to high intensity. The management of their overall diet, and prescription around the exercise session, will need to be individualized.
- It is important for the sports dietitian to establish contact and liaise with the athlete's doctor and diabetes educator to provide a coordinated approach to management. It is also important to ensure the coach is aware of the athlete's diabetes and understands the management requirements.

DIETARY ADVICE

- The recommended diet for an athlete with diabetes is no different from that recommended for a non-diabetic athlete (American Diabetes Association 2004a, 2004b; Dietitians Association of Australia 2006). The primary dietary nutrition goal is to meet nutrient and energy requirements to match training needs and body composition goals, and adjust insulin and medications accordingly, rather than distort food intakes to suit insulin or medication doses.
- Maintaining a fairly consistent food intake, and distribution of CHO, at meals and snacks throughout the day can assist glycemic control. In the total diet, moderate to low GI foods improve blood glucose control. However, for those exercising one or more times a day, using a high GI recovery snack within 60 minutes of completing training is advisable for enhanced recovery of muscle glycogen stores. These strategies are similar to those recommended for a non-diabetic athlete.
- Consuming some CHO from food or a sports drink during continuous aerobic exercise lasting longer than 60 minutes is recommended to prevent hypoglycemia and can usually be consumed without requiring extra insulin. Again the same recommendations apply to athletes without diabetes (see Chapters 12 and 13).
- CHO loading, particularly involving a depletion phase, should not be attempted unless good diabetic control has been regularly maintained. Insulin and medication doses require careful adjusting, depending on the method of loading used and the style of exercise tapering practiced before a competition. Even for a diabetic with well-controlled blood glucose, this adjustment is difficult and the glucose response is often erratic. CHO loading is not recommended for children with type 1 diabetes as they are unlikely to be competing in the sort of events that benefit from CHO loading (e.g. marathon or even half-marathon events).
- For any athlete, a fluid intake plan should be put in place to meet the individual's hydration needs according to their own sweat rates. It is important to minimize the risk of dehydration, as well as preventing hyponatremia due to over-zealous fluid consumption.

SPECIAL PROBLEMS

- *Hyperinsulinemia, hypoglycemia and late-onset hypoglycemia*: Repeated physical activity increases insulin sensitivity, so once athletes are adapted to training they will need less total daily insulin than usual levels. To avoid hyperinsulinemia, and potential hypoglycemia, athletes need to reduce their insulin dosage and timing according to their training intensity and duration. Blood glucose should be measured before, during and after physical activity to determine changes to insulin dosages, especially in those involved in endurance training, because of the potential for delayed hypoglycemic reactions, which may occur in the middle of the night or before breakfast the next day or in children up to 36 hours after exercise. Similarly, athletes with type 2 diabetes who are on medication may also need to reduce their dosage. Early in the training program, such adjustments are best made under the supervision of a diabetes specialist to accurately predict and interpret results, with consideration made for variations in training duration, intensity and frequency throughout a training and competition season. Advice about appropriate CHO intakes pre-, during and post-exercise, if training patterns change with little notice (e.g. a session gets cut short or is lengthened), should be included in counseling. Exercise should be delayed if blood glucose is <3.5 mmol/L (National Health and Medical Research Council 2005).

- *Hyperglycemia*: In our experience, athletes with diabetes tend to over-consume food or CHO beverages before or during training or competition to avoid hypoglycemia occurring or to avoid rebound hypoglycemia. They are more frequently hyperglycemic than hypoglycemic and may have poor long-term glucose control. Rather than over-consuming foods to address this fear of hypoglycemia, insulin levels should be adjusted and a CHO intake plan developed that matches estimated requirements (see Table 19.1 for guidelines).
- *Strength training* can induce hyperglycemia due to the hormonal response to training stimulating glycogenolysis. This is usually transient, but athletes should be aware of this and discuss it with their physician and diabetic educator.
- *Physical activity* should be delayed where blood glucose is >13–14 mmol/L or if ketones are present (see Table 19.1) and can induce a further increase in blood glucose concentrations and potential ketoacidosis.
- *Alcohol intake*: Athletes with diabetes on insulin need to be cautious with alcohol consumption. Alcohol inhibits gluconeogenesis and is associated with delayed hypoglycemia, which is responsible for the hangover effect of nausea and light-headedness observed after a drinking binge. This is a normal physiological response to alcohol and the reaction is the same in a person without diabetes. However, in a person with insulin-requiring diabetes, the 'morning-after' effects of alcohol, in combination with insulin, can accelerate a hypoglycemic state into a potentially life-threatening coma.
- *Alcohol* can also induce hyperglycemia in the short term, especially if the alcoholic beverage contains sugar (e.g. spirits mixed with soft drink, juices, sweet wines or liqueurs).
- *Competition*: If the exercise is anaerobic or during heat or competition, an increase in insulin may be required because of risk of hyperglycemia.

PRACTICE TIPS

- *Mixing and administering insulins:* When mixing insulins, short-acting insulin should be drawn up into the syringe first to avoid contaminating the vial with long-acting insulin. Gently rotate vials and cartridges of cloudy insulin in hands before use to ensure re-suspension. Do not mix insulin glargine with other insulins.

MONITORING AN ATHLETE WITH DIABETES

- It is important to encourage athletes to monitor blood glucose levels and corresponding insulin dosage, especially during the training season, and to keep these records to track responses to physical activity or for situations (such as illness) requiring an adjustment to insulin. The availability of insulin pumps may resolve many of these problems. Maintaining relatively even blood glucose concentrations maximizes the benefits of training as opposed to large fluctuations in, or regularly high, blood glucose concentrations. Blood glucose responses to exercise vary substantially between individuals, so alterations to treatments need to be made on a case-by-case basis.
- Athletes with diabetes should be strongly encouraged to take full responsibility for managing their diabetes. This includes always having food readily available (including emergency food in case of hypoglycemia), eating regularly and being responsible for changes to insulin levels during times of physical activity, illness or infection.
- The position statement from the American Diabetes Association for children and adolescents with type 1 diabetes provides current guidelines for clinicians about care and management (Silverstein et al. 2005).

USEFUL WEBSITES

http://www.runsweet.com

UK website specific to diabetes and sport

http://www.diabetes-exercise.org/index.asp

Diabetes, Exercise and Sports Association, formerly the International Diabetic Athletes Association: support site for people with diabetes and health professionals

http://www.glycemicindex.com

Australian site for information about the glycemic index of food and the GI symbol used on Australian food labels

http://www.wada-ama.com/

World Anti-Doping Agency

http://www.diabetes.org

American Diabetes Association: this site contains position statements for all aspects of management of diabetes

http://www.diabetesaustralia.com.au

Diabetes Association of Australia: this site contains the latest national evidence-based guidelines for management of diabetes

References

Alberti G, Zimmet P, Shaw J, Bloomgarden Z, Kaufman F, Silink M. Type 2 diabetes in the young: the evolving epidemic. The International Diabetes Federation Consensus Workshop. Diabetes Care 2004;27:1798–811.

American Diabetes Association. Physical activity/exercise and diabetes. Diabetes Care 2004a; 27(Suppl):S58–62.

American Diabetes Association. Nutrition principles and recommendation in diabetes. Diabetes Care 2004b; 27(Suppl):36S–46S.

American Diabetes Association. Diagnosis and classification of diabetes mellitus. Diabetes Care 2009a; 32(Suppl):62S–7S.

American Diabetes Association. Standards of medical care in diabetes–2009. Diabetes Care 2009b; 32(Suppl):13S–61S.

American Diabetes Association, Summary of revisions for the 2009 clinical practice recommendations. Diabetes Care 2009c;32(Suppl):3S–5S.

Andrade R, Laitano O, Meyer F. Effects of hydration with carbohydrates on the glycemic response in type 1 diabetics during exercise. Rev Brasil Med Esporte 2005;11:61–5.

Armstrong JJ. Overview of diabetes mellitus and exercise. Diabetes Educ 1992;17:1750–8.

Australian Bureau of Statistics, Diabetes in Australia—a snapshot, 2004–5. Cat. No. 4820.0.55.001. At http://www.abs.gov.au/ausstats/abs@.nsf/mf/4820.0.55.001 (accessed 1 May 2009). Australian Institute of Health and Welfare. Diabetes: Australian facts 2008. Canberra: Australian Institute of Health and Welfare, 2008.

Boule N, Haddad E, Kenny G, et al. Effects of exercise on glycemic control and body mass in type 2 diabetes mellitus; a meta-analysis of controlled clinical trials. JAMA 2001;286:1218–27.

Colberg S. Exercising with an insulin pump. Diabetes self management, 2002. At http://www.Diabetesselfmanagment.com (accessed April 2009).

Colman P. Should I go on an insulin pump? DMJ 2008;22:24.

Coyle EF. Timing and method of increased carbohydrate intake to cope with heavy training, competition and recovery. J Sports Sci 1991;9(Suppl):1S–40S.

Currell K, Jeukendrup AE. Superior endurance performance with ingestion of multiple transportable carbohydrates. Med Sci Sports Exerc 2008;40:275–81.

Devlin JT. Effects of exercise on insulin sensitivity in humans. Diabetes Care 1992;11:1690–3.

Dietitians Association of Australia. Evidence-based practice guidelines for the nutritional management of type 2 diabetes mellitus in adults. Canberra: Dietitians Association of Australia, 2006.

Di Piro JT, Talbert RL, Yee GC. Pharmacotherapy. New York: McGraw-Hill Publishing Company, 2005.

Duncan GE, Perri MG, Douglas W, et al. Exercise training, without weight loss, increases insulin sensitivity and postheparin plasma lipase activity in previously sedentary adults. Diabetes Care 2003;26:557–62.

Dunstan DW, Zimmet P, Welborn T, et al. Diabesity and associated disorders in Australia 2000. The accelerating epidemic. Australian Diabetes, Obesity and Lifestyle Study (AusDiab). Melbourne: International Diabetes Institute, 2001.

Dunstan DW, Zimmet PZ, Welborn TA, et al. The rising prevalence of diabetes and impaired glucose tolerance: the Australian Diabetes, Obesity and Lifestyle Study. Diabetes Care 2002;25:829–34.

Ebeling P, Bourney R, Koranyi L, et al. Mechanism of enhanced insulin sensitivity in athletes: increased blood flow, muscle glucose transport protein (GLUT-4) concentration and glycogen synthetase activity. J Clin Invest 1993;92:1623–31.

Ehtisham S, Hatt Molnár D. The prevalence of the metabolic syndrome and type 2 diabetes mellitus in children and adolescents. Int J Obesity 2004;28(Suppl):70S–4S.

Ehtisham S, Hattersley AT, Dunger DB, Barrett TG. First UK survey of paediatric type 2 diabetes and MODY. Arch Dis Child 2004;89:526–9.

Elkin SL, Brady S, Williams JP. Bodybuilders find it easy to obtain insulin to help them in training. BMJ 1997;314:1280.

Farrell PA. Diabetes, exercise and competitive sports. Sports Science Exchange 2003;16:3.

Ford E, Giles W. A comparison of the prevalence of the metabolic syndrome using two proposed definitions. Diabetes Care 2003;26:575–8.

Franz MJ. Exchanges for all occasions. Minnesota: International Diabetes Centre, 1987.

Franz MJ. Nutrition: can it give athletes with diabetes a boost? Diabetes Educ 1991;17:163–4, 166, 168.

Franz MJ, Bantle JP, Beebe CA, et al. Evidence-based nutrition principles and recommendations for the treatment and prevention of diabetes and related complications. Diabetes Care 2002;25:148–98.

Franz MJ, Horton Sr ES, Bantle JP, et al. Nutrition principles for the management of diabetes and related complications. Diabetes Care 1994;17:490–518.

Franz MJ, Wylie-Rosett J. The 2006 American Diabetes Association nutrition recommendation and interventions for the prevention and treatment of diabetes. Diabetes Spectrum 2007;20:49–52.

Frid A, Ostman J, Linde B. Hypoglycemia risk during exercise after intramuscular injection of insulin in thigh in IDDM. Diabetes Care 1990;13:473–7.

Fryburg DA, Jahn LA, Hill SA, Oliveras DM, Barrett EJ, et al. Insulin and insulin-like growth factor 1 enhance human skeletal muscle protein anabolism during hyperaminoacidemia by different mechanisms. J Clin Invest 1995;96:1722–9.

Gill JMR, Cooper AR. Physical activity and prevention of type 2 diabetes mellitus. Sports Med 2008;38:807–24.

Goldberg R. Prevention of type 2 diabetes. Med Clin Nth Amer 1998;82:805–21.

Heiemann L, Pfutzner A, Heise T. Alternative routes of administration as an approach to improved insulin therapy: update on dermal, oral, nasal and pulmonary insulin delivery. Curr Pharm Des 2001;7:1327–51.

Ivy J, Costill DL, Fink WJ, Lower RW. Influence of caffeine and carbohydrate feedings on endurance performance. Med Sci Sports Exerc 1979;11:6–11.

Kahn J, Vinik A. Exercise training in the diabetic patient. Intern Med 1988;9:117–25.

Koivisto VA, Felig P. Effects of leg exercise on insulin absorption in diabetic patients. N Eng J Med 1978;298:79–83.

Malecka-Tendera E, Erhardt É, Molnár D. Type 2 diabetes mellitus in European children and adolescents. Acta Paediat 2005;94:543–6.

Maughan RJ, Fenn CE, Gleeson M, Leiper JB. Metabolic and circulatory responses to the ingestion of glucose polymer and glucose/electrolyte solutions during exercise in man. Eur J Appl Physiol 1987;56:356–2.

Maynard T. Physiological responses to exercise. Diabetes Educ 1992;17:19–20.

McMahon SK, Haymes A, Ratnam N, et al. Increase in type 2 diabetes in children and adolescents in Western Australia. MJA 2004;180:459–61.

Meinders A, Willekens FLA, Heere LP. Metabolic and hormonal changes in IDDM during a long distance run. Diabetes Care 1988;11:1–7.

Molnár D. The prevalence of the metabolic syndrome and type 2 diabetes mellitus in children and adolescents. Int J Obesity 2004;28(Suppl):70S–4S.

Monk A, Barry B, McClark K, Weaver T, Coopa N, Franz MJ, et al. Exercise and the management of diabetes mellitus. J Am Diet Assoc 1995;95:999–1006.

National Health and Medical Research Council. Clinical practice guidelines: Type 1 diabetes in children and adolescents, 2005. At http://www.nhmrc.gov.au/publications/synopses/cp102syn.htm (accessed 24 April 2009).

Nield L, Summerbell C, Hooper L, et al. 2008a. Dietary advice for the prevention of type 2 diabetes mellitus in adults (a review). Cochrane Database of Systematic Reviews. Issue 3. Article No. CD005102 D01: 10.1002/14651858. CD005102.pub2.

Nield L, Summerbell C, Hooper L, et al. 2008b. Dietary advice for the treatment of type 2 diabetes mellitus in adults (a review). Cochrane Database of Systematic Reviews. Issue 3. Article No. CD004097 D01: 10.1002/14651858.CD004097.pub4.

Orozco LJ, Buchleitner AM, Gimenez-Perez G, et al. 2008. Exercise or exercise and diet for preventing type 2 diabetes mellitus. Cochrane Database of Systematic Reviews. Issue 3. Art. No. CD003054. DOI: 10.1002/14651858.CD003054.pub3.

Perrone C, Laitano O, Meyer F. Effect of carbohydrate ingestion on the glycemic response of type 1 diabetic adolescents during exercise. Diabetes Care 2005;28:2537–38.

Peter R, Luzio SD, Dunseath G, et al. Effects of exercise on the absorption of insulin glargine in patients with type 1 diabetes. Diabetes Care 2005;28:560–5.

Petersen AH, Kohler G, Korsatko S, et al. The effect of exercise on the absorption of inhaled human insulin via the AERx insulin diabetes management system in people with type 1 diabetes. Diabetes Care 2007;30:2571–6.

Riddell MC, Bar-Or O, Ayub BV, et al. Glucose ingestion matched with total carbohydrate utilization attenuates hypoglycemia during exercise in adolescents with IDDM. Int J Sport Nutr 1999;9:24–34.

Riddell MC, Iscoe KE. Physical activity, sport, and pediatric diabetes. Pediatr Diabetes 2006;7:60–90.

Rossi, S. ed. Australian medicines handbook, 2008. Adelaide: Australian Medicines Handbook Pty Ltd, 2009.

Saris WHM, Blair SN, van Baak MA, et al. How much physical activity is enough to prevent unhealthy weight gain? Outcome of the IASO 1st stock conference and consensus statement. Obes Rev 2003;4:101–7.

Sawka MN, Burke LM, Eichner, ER, Maughan RJ, Montain SJ, Stachenfeld NS. Exercise and fluid replacement. Med Sci Sports Exerc 2007;39:377–90.

Shehadeh N, Kassem J, Tchaban I, et al. High incidence of hypoglycemic episodes with neurologic manifestations in children with insulin-dependent diabetes mellitus. J Pediatr Endocrinol Metab 1998;11(Suppl 1):183–97.

Sigal RJ, Kenny GP, Wasserman DH, Castaneda-Sceppa C. Physical activity/exercise and type 2 diabetes. Diabetes Care 2004;27:2518–39.

Silverstein J, Klingensmith G, Copeland K, et al. Care of children and adolescents with type 1 diabetes: a statement of the American Diabetes Association. Diabetes Care 2005;28:186–212.

Smart C, Morrison M. Healthy eating on an insulin pump. DMJ 2008;22:4–5.

Thow A, Waters A. Diabetes in culturally and linguistically diverse Australians: identification of communities at high risk. Cat. No. CVD 30. Canberra: Australian Institute of Health and Welfare, 2005.

Tuppola S, Rajantie J, Maenpaa J. Severe hypoglycaemia in children and adolescents during multiple-dose insulin therapy. Diabetes Med 1998;15:695–99.

Wasserman D, Davis S, Zinman B. Fuel metabolism during exercise in health and diabetes. In: Ruderman N. Devlin J, Schnieder S, Kriska A, eds. Handbook of exercise in diabetes. Alexandria, VA: American Diabetes Association, 2002:63–100.

Wasserman DH, O'Doherty RM, Zinker BA. Role of the endocrine pancreas in control of fuel metabolism by the liver during exercise. Int J Obes Relat Metab Disord 1995;19(Suppl):22S–30S.

Wing R. Exercise and weight control. In Ruderman N, Devlin J, Schneider S, Kriska A, eds. Handbook of exercise in diabetes. Second edition. Alexandria, VA: American Diabetes Association, 2002:355–64.

CHAPTER 20

Special needs: the vegetarian athlete

GREG COX

20.1 Introduction

Vegetarian diets are now part of mainstream eating in western countries. Studies of the effects of vegetarian diets have focused on potential short- and long-term health benefits in selected population groups (mainly religious groups) and on nutrient concerns, particularly in children and adolescents. Few studies have been conducted on vegetarian athletes. The main reasons for adopting vegetarian diets reported by the general population include cultural and religious beliefs, ethical beliefs concerning animal rights, health benefits and environmental issues. These reasons vary with age and health status. For athletes, reasons may be similar or extend to the potential of vegetarian diets to enhance performance and meet the high carbohydrate (CHO) demands of their sport or assist in weight control. The popularity of vegetarianism in athletes has been fuelled by the success stories of athletes who are world champions and also vegetarians—Dave Scott (vegan and five-times winner of the Hawaii Ironman Triathlon), Martina Navratilova (tennis), Billie Jean King (tennis), Clare Francis (sailor), Edwin Moses (Olympic hurdler) and many more (see Veggie Sports Associations website at www.veggie.org/).

Although there are no estimates of the prevalence of vegetarianism in athletes, vegetarian diets appear popular with endurance athletes (cyclists, runners and triathletes) and with those athletes continually striving to consume a high-CHO diet and maintain a low body mass. In a national survey of over 9000 American runners, 8% of females and 3% of males reported following a vegetarian diet (Williams 1997). In another study of 209 recreational female athletes from Canada, 37% followed a 'semi-vegetarian' diet (no red meat) and around 2% followed a lacto-ovo-vegetarian diet (Barr 1986).

This chapter describes different types of vegetarian diets and their potential advantages and disadvantages in meeting dietary goals for optimal sports performance. The effects of vegetarian diet on health outcomes, sports performance and nutritional status are discussed. Practical dietary strategies for assessing risks and advising vegetarian athletes are included in the practice tips.

Types of vegetarian diets

Vegetarian diets do not necessarily adhere to the rigid early definitions, which described diets that were based exclusively on plant-based foods and excluded consumption of any animal foods or their products. Today, the term 'vegetarian' is used more broadly than these strict conventions. People who call themselves vegetarian may include some animal foods and their products in their diets. Table 20.1 defines the different styles of vegetarian diets. Of these, the fruitarian and macrobiotic diets are the most restrictive and potentially nutritionally inadequate. A lacto-ovo-vegetarian diet includes, as the name suggests, plant foods as well as eggs and milk and their products.

The term 'vegetarian' is also, according to definition, incorrectly used to describe a diet where red meat is excluded, although poultry and fish are consumed as staple meat options or in comparatively small amounts. Some people, athletes included, describe themselves as vegetarians simply because they avoid eating red meat. This type of vegetarianism has been referred to as 'quasi-', 'semi-', or 'part-time' or—a term coined by Lea and Worsely (2004)—'cognitive' vegetarianism. Rather than defining this style of eating as vegetarian, which it is not, perhaps it is more correctly referred to as 'selective meat-eating'.

People are vegetarian or exclude meat for a wide range of reasons, including beliefs about religion, economics, ethics, politics, the environment and health (Wicks 1999). They may be vegetarian because they dislike the taste, smell or appearance of meat or the way animals are farmed or killed for food, or they believe meat is high in fat and cholesterol (Burke & Read 1987). Although the prevalence of vegetarianism in the Australian population was reported at less than 4%, and around 6% of females between 19 and 24 years (McLennan & Podger 1997), a substantial proportion of females restrict meat (especially red meat) (Baghurst et al. 2000). Restriction of red meat in any population group increases the risk of iron and zinc depletion. For athletes avoiding red meat—especially females, adolescents and endurance athletes, who have high iron requirements—the risk of iron depletion is also high.

TABLE 20.1 CATEGORIES OF VEGETARIAN DIETS

TYPE	COMMENTS
Fruitarian	Consists of raw or dried fruits, nuts, seeds, honey and vegetable oil.
Macrobiotic	Excludes all animal foods, dairy products and eggs. Uses only unprocessed, unrefined, 'natural' and 'organic' cereals, grains and condiments such as miso and seaweed.
Vegan	Excludes all animal foods, dairy products and eggs. In its purest form, excludes all animal products including honey, gelatin, silk, wool, leather, and animal-derived food additives.
Lacto-vegetarian	Excludes all animal foods and eggs. Includes milk and milk products.
Lacto-ovo-vegetarian	Excludes all animal foods. Includes milk, milk products and eggs.

20.3 Effect of vegetarian diets on health outcomes

In the general population, vegetarian diets are associated with a decreased morbidity from chronic lifestyle diseases prevalent in industrialized countries. Lower mortality rates from coronary artery disease and certain forms of cancer, and lower risks for obesity and diabetes, are typical among vegetarian populations, compared with non-vegetarians (Snowdon & Phillips 1985; Levin et al. 1986; Burr & Butland 1988; Burr & Sweetnam 1994; Giovannucci et al. 1994). Lifestyle factors independent of diet partially explain the health differences reported between vegetarians and non-vegetarians (Phillips & Snowdon 1985; Dwyer 1988; Thorogood et al. 1994).

20.4 Effect of vegetarian diets on exercise performance

Despite numerous studies investigating the health benefits of a vegetarian diet, few studies have examined any link between vegetarian diets and performance in well-trained athletes. In theory, if a vegetarian diet was high in CHO and met or exceeded recommendations for other macronutrients, micronutrients and energy, then it would match the ideal or recommended diet for training and recovery. Several reviews have confirmed that vegetarian diets are conducive to maximizing performance (American Dietetic Association 1997; Barr & Rideout 2004) and that nutrient intakes of most vegetarians, with some exceptions, are adequate, compared with recommended nutrient standards or non-vegetarian controls (see Table 20.2).

In the few cross-sectional studies conducted on vegetarian athletes and investigating performance effects, the results have been equivocal. In one study, no differences in aerobic or anaerobic capacities of forty-nine (twenty-nine male, twenty female) lacto-ovo-vegetarian and lacto-vegetarian athletes were detected, compared with non-vegetarian controls (Hanne et al. 1986). Similarly, no differences in maximal oxygen uptake were observed between nine female athletes following a modified vegetarian diet (<100 g of red meat per week), compared with controls on a mixed diet (Synder et al. 1989). In another study of fifty lacto-ovo-vegetarian runners competing in a 1000 km stage foot race, there were also no differences in finishing time or order of finishing the race, compared with the control group consuming a conventional western diet. Both groups in this study consumed diets with the same macronutrient ratio of 60:30:10 (CHO, fat and protein respectively), thereby controlling for any confounding effect that high CHO intakes might have on performance capacity (Nagel et al. 1989).

No differences in endurance performance were also evident in an intervention trial over 12 weeks in eight well-trained male endurance athletes who consumed a lacto-ovo-vegetarian diet for 6 weeks and then a mixed diet for another 6 weeks (Richter et al. 1991; Raben et al. 1992). Diets were isocaloric and formulated to contain similar macronutrient ratios and energy intakes. The results also indicated no differences in other parameters measured (e.g. immune function, strength, muscle glycogen and hormone level), except testosterone, which decreased significantly following the lacto-ovo-vegetarian diet. The

TABLE 20.2 AVERAGE DAILY NUTRIENT AND ENERGY INTAKES FROM DIETARY SURVEYS COMPARING VEGETARIANS TO NON-VEGETARIANS

REFERENCE	TYPE OF DIET	DIET ASSESSMENT	AGE (YEARS)	SEX	N	ENERGY (MJ/D)	CHO (G/D)	P (G/D)	P/KG/DAY (G/KG/D)	FAT (G/D)	Ca^{++} (MG/D)	Fe^{++} (MG/D)	FIBER (G/D)	VIT C (MG/D)
NON-ATHLETES														
Latta & Liebman 1984	MV	2 × 3-day FR	30.6	M	36	10.6[e]	NA	NA	–	–	–	17	7.1[c]	–
	C		30.7	M	18	11.9	NA	NA	–	–	–	18	4.6	–
Marsh et al. 1988	LOV	7-day weighed FR	66.8	F	10	6.74	NA	56	NA	65	898	12.3	5.2	92
	C		64.4	F	10	6.86	NA	68	NA	77	712	13.3	4.7	105
Tylavsky & Anderson 1988	LOV	QFFQ	73.0	F	88	6.41	216[b]	55[c]	0.87	56[c]	823	10.7	5.6[b]	184[b]
	C		78.8	F	28	6.83	188	70	1.16	88	902	10.2	4.2	157
Nieman et al. 1989	LOV	7-day FR	72.3	F	19	5.95	228[c]	44	0.75	49[a]	NA	NA	23.2[b]	NA
	C		69.5	F	12	6.09	186	56	0.88	61	NA	NA	13.3	NA
Pedersen et al. 1991	LOV	3-day FR	35.5	F	34	7.64	264[a]	63[a]	1.08	67	931	20.0	26.0[b]	316
	NV		29.4	F	41	7.14	218	75	1.26	61	873	22.0	15.0	184
Tesar et al. 1992	LOV	6-day semi-weighed FR +24-hour DH	62.9	F	28	6.91	242[b]	63[a]	1.02	56	820	13.0	10.3[b]	143[a]
	C		62.9	F	28	6.94	199	77	1.22	62	863	15.5	7.6	118
Janelle & Barr 1995	V	3-day FR	28.0	F	8	8.04	300	51[a]	0.87	64	578[e]	17.7	35.0[d]	186[d]
	LOV		25.8	F	15	8.46	288	57[a]	0.97	76	875	13.7	24.7	141
	C		27.9	F	22	8.72	284	77	1.24	75	950	15.3	22.4	116

(continued)

TABLE 20.2 *(continued)*

REFERENCE	TYPE OF DIET	DIET ASSESSMENT	AGE (YEARS)	SEX	N	ENERGY (MJ/D)	CHO (G/D)	P (G/D)	P/KG/ DAY (G/ KG/D)	FAT (G/D)	Ca^{++} (MG/D)	Fe^{++} (MG/D)	FIBER (G/D)	VIT C (MG/D)
Ball & Bartlett 1999	LOV	12-day weighed FR	25.3	F	50	6.9	211	54[b]	NA	60	NA	10.7	24.4[c]	150[b]
	C		25.2	F	24	6.9	183	67	NA	65	NA	9.9	17.3	111
Haddad et al. 1999	V	3-day FR + 24-hour DH	36.0	F	15	7.09	NA	52[c]	NA	52[a]	590	17.6	38[c]	230[a]
	NV		33.5	F	10	8.24	NA	74	NA	76	830	15.3	15	115
	V		36.0	M	10	9.29	NA	75	NA	67	715	26.4[c]	48[c]	240[a]
	C		33.5	M	10	9.04	NA	85	NA	80	670	15.0	20	120
Wilson & Ball 1999	MV	12-day semi-weighed FR	33.3	M	39	10.5	357	80[c]	1.13	82[b]	899	20.4[b]	50[c]	218
	V		31.0	M	10	11.6	413	81[b]	1.09	88	911	22.9[c]	64[c]	360[b]
	C		32.7	M	25	11.0	291	108	1.02	98	961	15.8	26	151
ATHLETES														
Synder et al. 1989	MV	3-day FR	37.8	F	9	7.46	229[a]	59[a]	1.05	71	NA	14.7	NA	–
	C		39.2	F	9	6.99	186	73	1.22	71	NA	14.0	NA	–

Diet: V = vegan, LOV = lacto-ovo-vegetarian, MV = modified vegetarian, C = control (non-vegetarian), NA = not available
FR = food record, QFFQ = Quantitative Food Frequency Questionnaire, DH = dietary history
[a,b,c]Mean intake of V, LOV and MV significantly different to C at $p < 0.05$, $p < 0.01$, $p < 0.001$
[d]Significant at $p < 0.05$ compared to LOV and C
[e]Significant at $p < 0.05$ compared to C only

authors suggested that either the sudden switch in diet or high soluble fiber content of the vegetarian diet, which has the capacity to bind cholesterol (a precursor to testosterone synthesis), might influence testosterone reduction (Raben et al. 1992).

Similarly, no differences in performance measures are evident in untrained people on vegetarian diets, despite substantial reductions in risk factors for chronic diseases, compared to controls, even in elderly people. In a small group of untrained, elderly vegetarians (n = 12, mean ages 72.3 ± 1.4 years), no electrocardiographic differences at submaximal or maximal exercise workloads and in maximal oxygen uptake were observed, compared to controls (Nieman et al. 1989). However, in this study, the vegetarian group had significantly lower blood glucose and cholesterol levels, and tended to have less body fat than non-vegetarians.

In theory, the performance advantages of consuming a high-CHO diet, which is achieved more easily with a vegetarian or quasi-vegetarian diet than an omnivorous diet, have been well documented (Simonsen et al. 1991). Athletes who consume vegetarian diets are likely to meet the recommendations for CHO and protein (Nieman 1988) and low fat intakes, as seen in Table 20.2. However, the effect of vegetarian diets on performance capacity in well-trained athletes requires further study.

Diet-related concerns for vegetarian athletes 20.5

It is difficult, if not impossible, to undertake research on vegetarian athletes, particularly elite-level athletes, because of the low numbers of athletes choosing vegetarian diets. Because there are few dietary surveys published on vegetarian athletes, dietary intake data from surveys of vegetarians in the general population will be used as a benchmark for identifying at-risk nutrients in this chapter and then extrapolated to determine the nutrients at risk in an athletic population. Female vegetarians have a higher frequency of suboptimal micronutrient intakes—particularly iron, zinc and calcium—and energy intakes than male vegetarians and omnivorous controls, and female vegetarian athletes are no different in this regard (see Table 20.2).

Recent revisions to population nutrient standards in both the US and Canada have indicated that people consuming vegetarian diets have higher recommendations for zinc, iron and possibly calcium to adjust for the low bioavailability of these nutrients in such diets (Institute of Medicine 2000). For vegetarian athletes, requirements for these nutrients may be even higher than population standards.

Energy 20.6

Vegetarian diets, if very high in fiber and bulk, are associated with low energy intakes because fiber increases satiety. Vegetarian athletes, particularly children and adolescents, may have difficulty maintaining weight and meeting the daily energy requirements of their sport and perhaps growth (Grandjean 1987; Ruud 1990). Legumes, wholegrain cereals and grains, soybeans and many vegetables and fruits are high-fiber, relatively low-fat foods and very filling. For the vegan, incorporating energy-dense foods such as nuts, tofu, tempeh, textured vegetable protein and commercially prepared meat analogues helps increase energy density. For the lacto-vegetarian, the addition of cheese, yoghurt and custard provides energy density. Nathan Pritikin, a strong advocate for improving health outcomes by increasing physical activity and consuming quasi-vegetarian diets, claimed that vegetarian athletes could easily consume sufficient kilojoules on his 'Pritikin' diet, even an individual with high daily energy requirements (Pritikin 1984).

20.7 Protein

It is well documented that protein recommendations for athletes are slightly higher than population nutrient references (see Chapter 4). The ability of vegetarian athletes, in particular vegan athletes, to meet suggested daily protein intakes has been questioned (Grandjean 1987; Ruud 1990). At least in the general population, vegetarians have been found to consume, on average, lower protein intakes than meat eaters, although most protein intakes met population reference standards and the slightly higher sport-specific guidelines for protein of 1.2–1.7 g/kg BM/d (see Table 20.2).

Vegetable or plant proteins may be limiting in one or more indispensable (or essential) amino acids, so food sources need to be combined in such a way to ensure all amino acids are consumed. Provided that the daily total protein intake is adequate and the body is in nitrogen balance, combining different types of plant foods (e.g. legumes and grains together, or legumes and nuts/seeds together) allows low levels of amino acids in one food to be complemented by high levels of amino acids in the other (Young & Pellett 1994). Although some vegetarians believe it is necessary to combine foods in this way at the same meal, this belief is not supported by scientific evidence (American Dietetic Association 1997). Nonetheless, these combinations should be eaten within the same day to ensure the availability of all indispensable amino acids needed to complete protein synthesis (Mahan & Escott-Stump 2008).

In the US and Canadian Dietary Reference Intakes (DRI) and the Nutrient Reference Values for Australia and New Zealand (NRV), a separate recommendation for protein intake was not considered necessary for those vegetarians who consume dairy products or eggs and complementary mixtures of high-quality plant proteins (Institute of Medicine 2002; Commonwealth Department of Health and Ageing et al. 2006). However, for vegetarians avoiding all animal foods, the Institute of Medicine (2000) states that total protein intakes may need to exceed protein recommendations to meet amino acid requirements. This recommendation is largely linked with the low digestibility of vegetable proteins. In summary, vegetarian diets can, for most people and for athletes, provide adequate protein and the complete set of indispensable amino acids without the use of protein supplements or special foods, provided daily energy demands are met (American Dietetic Association 1997).

20.8 Iron

Athletes (especially vegetarian athletes) are at greater risk of low iron stores than untrained people, which may impair performance capacity (see Chapter 10). In the general population, studies have confirmed that vegetarians have lower iron stores than non-vegetarians, despite similar or higher iron intakes (Donovan & Gibson 1995; Haddad et al. 1999; Wilson & Ball 1999; Hua et al. 2001), although the prevalence of iron deficiency anemia is similar (Ball & Bartlett 1999, Haddad et al. 1999). One case study reported iron deficiency anemia in a strict vegetarian male long-distance runner with an estimated habitual iron intake well above the nutrient reference standards (Jacobs & Wilson 1984). The likely cause of the iron deficiency was not reported, but may have been related to low iron bioavailability (which was not directly assessed) and/or high iron turnover (which is expected in athletes undertaking endurance training) (Siegel et al. 1979). In one study conducted on nine female vegetarian athletes who were also endurance runners, no significant difference in average daily intake was found compared to controls, yet iron stores as indicated by serum ferritin were significantly lower in the vegetarian group consuming a modified vegetarian diet (<100 g/wk red meat) (Synder et al. 1989). In another study on fifty male and female ultra-endurance runners (thirty-nine males, eleven females) following a lacto-ovo-vegetarian diet, the mean serum ferritin was also lower than controls, although no effect on performance measures was found in either group (Seiler et al. 1989).

Although in the past the effects of low iron stores without anemia on reducing performance capacity have been equivocal and have leaned towards a minimal impact, well-designed studies on physically active, untrained women with iron depletion, using soluble transferrin receptor (sTfR)—a relatively new and reliable marker of early iron depletion—confirmed that low iron stores reduced endurance capacity and aerobic capacity (Hinton et al. 2000; Brownlie et al. 2002, 2004). Similar findings were observed in iron-depleted recreational athletes after supplementation in one study (Hinton et al. 2007), but no effect was observed on aerobic capacity in another study of female iron-depleted athletes after iron injection (Peeling et al. 2007) (see Chapter 10). Further research is needed to confirm these effects in elite athletes with low iron stores and particularly in high-risk athletes consuming vegetarian diets.

The bioavailability of iron from individual plant foods and from a total vegetarian diet is much lower than in a meat-based diet because of the presence of naturally occurring inhibitors in plants that bind iron from plant sources (that is, non-heme iron) in the gut and reduce its absorption (Hunt 2003). Also, the absence of meat, an enhancer of iron absorption from iron-rich plant sources, further reduces iron bioavailability. This reduced iron bioavailability was confirmed in a group of untrained vegetarian women who had 70% lower iron absorption than non-vegetarian controls (Hunt & Roughead 1999). Although insufficient studies on elite vegetarian athletes have been conducted to confirm a similar response, vegetarian athletes are likely to be at even higher risk of low iron bioavailability, and hence iron depletion, if they consume large amounts of food containing inhibitors (Ruud 1990; Barr & Rideout 2004).

Revisions to the nutrient reference standards in Australia and New Zealand, the US and Canada suggest that the recommended intake—Estimated Average Requirement (EAR)—for iron should be 1.3–1.7 times higher for athletes and 1.8 times higher for vegetarians (non-athletes) to account for the low bioavailability of non-heme iron sources (Institute of Medicine 2000; Commonwealth Department of Health and Ageing et al. 2006). For female vegetarian athletes, the EAR could be additive and more that three times higher than normal EAR values (Institute of Medicine 2000). Such high levels are unlikely to be met by dietary iron intake in this high-risk group, without appropriate dietary planning.

Calcium

20.9

Average daily calcium intakes are often below nutrient reference standards in vegetarians, particular females, avoiding dairy products (Janelle & Barr 1995; Haddad et al. 1999), so some individual vegetarians are at risk of inadequate calcium intakes. In one study, vegan females had significantly lower mean calcium intakes compared to lacto-ovo-vegetarians and omnivores (578, 875 and 950 mg calcium/d respectively as expected) (Janelle & Barr 1995). However, this was not evident in another study of untrained vegans (males and females) where there was no difference in mean daily calcium intakes between vegan males and females compared with non-vegetarian controls (Haddad et al. 1999). Lacto-ovo-vegetarians usually report similar or higher calcium intakes than omnivores (Marsh et al. 1988; Tylavsky & Anderson 1988; Slattery et al. 1991; Tesar et al. 1992) (see Table 20.2).

Apart from dairy products, few foods provide concentrated sources of calcium (Baghurst et al. 1993). In the Australian National Nutrition Survey in 1995, cereal foods were the second supplier of calcium in the average diet (McLennan & Podger 1998). Until recently, individuals who limit or exclude dairy foods have had few other alternative dietary calcium sources except for green leafy vegetables, calcium-fortified tofu and cereal grains as their main sources. Recent modification to the food standards code for vitamins and minerals in Australia (December 2002) has resulted in an increased number of calcium-fortified foods appearing in the marketplace, including commercial breakfast cereals and cereal bars, in addition to calcium-fortified milks, cheeses, yoghurts, dairy desserts and all analogues of meat derived from soy or other legumes. Vegetarians who avoid eating dairy products should increase intake of calcium-fortified foods to help meet daily calcium recommendations (Weaver et al. 1999).

Calcium absorption or bioavailability from vegetable sources, including soy milk and its products, is lower than that from dairy sources, because of the inhibitors naturally present in many plant foods (e.g. phytates found in wholegrain cereals, some vegetables and legumes, including soy) (Weaver & Plawecki 1994; Weaver et al. 1999). See Chapter 10, Table 10.9 for the phytate content of plant foods. Other inhibitors (such as oxalates found in spinach and rhubarb) are found in calcium-rich foods, so that they provide negligible absorbable calcium. Low-oxalate vegetables such as kale, broccoli and bok choy are alternative rich sources of calcium and more readily absorbed. High-salt (sodium) diets and high-protein diets can also influence calcium balance by increasing calcium excretion and may need attention in vegetarian athletes who have difficulty meeting recommended calcium intakes (Weaver et al. 1999). Amenorrheic athletes on vegetarian diets have high calcium losses and need special attention in meeting their high calcium requirements (see Chapter 9).

20.10 Vitamin B12

Clinical vitamin B12 deficiency is uncommon in young people, but increases with aging because of deterioration in gastric acid secretion and intrinsic factors, rather than inadequate B12 consumption (American Dietetic Association 1988). People consuming omnivorous or lacto-ovo-vegetarian diets easily meet vitamin B12 recommendations, because active vitamin B12 is found exclusively in animal foods and their products. No active vitamin B12 is naturally found in any plant foods, including meat analogues or fermented soy products (such as tempeh) or mushrooms, contrary to popular belief (Herbert 1988).

Strict vegetarians following vegan, fruitarian or macrobiotic diets have lower serum vitamin B12 levels than lacto-ovo-vegetarians or those who occasionally eat meat (Obeid et al. 2002) and can slowly develop vitamin B12 deficiency (Herbert 1994). For this group of vegetarians, consuming foods fortified with vitamin B12 (e.g. soy milk and soy products, and vegetable or yeast extracts/spreads) or taking vitamin B12 supplements is essential (American Dietetic Association 1988). Dairy products and eggs provide sufficient vitamin B12 for lacto-ovo-vegetarians.

Zinc

20.11

Meat, particularly red meat, has a higher zinc content than white meat and fish. In the 1995 Australian National Nutrition Survey of adults, the last population nutrition survey in Australia, meat and dairy products were found to provide around 50% of the zinc in the average daily diet of all respondents (McLennan & Podger 1998). For vegetarians, cereal grains and their products are the main zinc suppliers, followed by legumes, nuts, soy products and eggs and finally dairy foods (Gibson 1994). Lower zinc intakes have been reported in dietary surveys of female vegetarians compared to non-vegetarians, which is not unexpected (Janelle & Barr 1995; Haddad et al. 1999). However, in a study of male Australian lacto-ovo-vegetarians, no differences in zinc intakes were found between vegetarians and controls, although in this study a high proportion of all groups (lacto-ovo-vegetarians, vegans and omnivores) had intakes below the zinc RDI of 12 mg/d (Wilson & Ball 1999). For some individuals, zinc intakes and zinc status may be suboptimal.

Zinc absorption is impaired by the concurrent consumption of the same inhibitory components present in food (e.g. phytates, oxalates and tannates) that inhibit iron and calcium absorption. Insoluble dietary fiber can also inhibit calcium absorption (Freeland Graves et al. 1980). Given the high intakes of dietary fiber reported in people on vegetarian diets (Latta & Liebman 1984; Wilson & Ball 1999), zinc absorption may be compromised, so the assessment of zinc status may be warranted in vegetarian athletes with marginal zinc intakes. Unfortunately, biochemical and diagnostic criteria for detecting marginal zinc status are lacking (Hallberg et al. 2000).

Riboflavin

20.12

The major source of riboflavin in the diet of respondents in the Australian National Nutrition Survey was milk and milk products (McLennan & Podger 1998). For the vegan athlete who excludes soy milk and soy-milk products, consuming adequate riboflavin may be difficult as soy is also a good source of riboflavin. Janelle and Barr (1995) reported lower intakes of riboflavin in eight female vegans compared with fifteen lacto-ovo-vegetarians and twenty-two non-vegetarian controls, confirming that riboflavin may be a limiting nutrient in vegetarians who avoid dairy products.

Are creatine supplements of benefit to vegetarian athletes?

20.13

Recent evidence supports the use of creatine supplements (creatine monohydrate) as a means of enhancing the ability of athletes to train and recover more quickly from repeated high-intensity workouts involving isolated muscular efforts followed by a short time to recover between efforts. This effect offers some resistance to fatigue (see Chapter 16).

However, not all athletes respond and there are insufficient data to recommend creatine use in young athletes under 18 years of age (American College of Sports Medicine 2000). The performance-enhancing effects of creatine supplements are greatest when creatine stores are low. Increases of creatine muscle content levels of <20% after supplementation show no performance enhancement (Greenhaff et al. 1994).

The response to creatine supplementation and uptake into muscle are likely to be high in vegetarians who already have low levels of muscle creatine as a consequence of meat avoidance. Creatine is a naturally occurring compound found in meat, where it is stored in muscle tissue and is also produced endogenously from amino acid precursors. Not surprisingly, several studies have demonstrated that vegetarians have lower total creatine (Delange et al. 1989; Shomrat et al. 2000; MacCormick et al. 2004) and lower muscle creatine (Burke et al. 2003) than non-vegetarians, although some studies have shown no difference (Harris et al. 1992). Low muscle creatine stores suggest that vegetarians are not totally compensating from endogenous production or from the lack of dietary creatine intake (Green et al. 1997). Further, switching to a lacto-ovo-vegetarian diet from an omnivorous diet can substantially reduce muscle creatine levels within only 3 weeks (Lukaszuk et al. 2002).

In theory, the potential performance benefits of creatine supplementation in vegetarians with low creatine muscle stores is likely to be more pronounced than in those who eat meat. However, in the few performance studies undertaken on vegetarians, the results have been equivocal. In one study on male vegetarians, no differences in performance tests (3 × 20 s maximal cycling efforts) were found after 6 days of creatine supplementation, when compared to controls (Shomrat et al. 2000). In contrast, in another group of eighteen untrained male vegetarians aged 19–55 years, significant improvements in bench press strength, total work output and increases in lean tissue were found after 8 weeks of creatine supplementation and resistance training, compared to controls on placebo (Burke et al. 2003). These changes correlated with increases in muscle creatine stores. Whether trained athletes who are vegetarian show a similar enhanced uptake of creatine or are more responsive to its performance-enhancing effects is unknown.

20.14 Vegetarian eating and menstrual dysfunction

Several studies have found that the frequency of menstrual irregularity was higher in vegetarian athletes than omnivorous controls (Brooks et al. 1984; Slavin et al. 1984; Pedersen et al. 1991). In a study investigating twenty-six female runners, Brooks and colleagues (1984) reported a higher frequency of secondary amenorrhea in athletes following a modified vegetarian diet (<200 g red meat per week), compared with controls. In another study of eighty-nine females exercising at least twice per week, the frequency of secondary amenorrhea was nearly eight times greater than in controls (Slavin et al. 1984). However, other studies report no difference in menstrual irregularities between female vegetarian and non-vegetarian athletes (Hanne et al. 1986), and between weight-stable, physically active vegetarian females and their non-vegetarian peers (Barr et al. 1994).

For some females, claiming to be vegetarian masks disordered eating behaviors (Martins et al. 1999), and is used as an excuse to disguise inflexibility in food choices, a warning sign of an eating disorder. The association between disordered eating behavior and menstrual dysfunction is described in Chapter 8.

The etiology of menstrual dysfunction in athletes is unclear and multifactorial (see Chapters 8 and 9). No single dietary or lifestyle factor, including vegetarian diets, can account for menstrual irregularities in athletes or non-athletes (Barr 1999; Manore 2002). The effects of vegetarian diets on menstrual status require further study.

Summary

Dietary surveys of vegetarian athletes are scarce; however, several studies have reported nutrient intakes of non-athlete adult populations following lacto-ovo-vegetarian and vegan diets. Given the paucity of research conducted on vegetarian diets among athlete groups, definitive conclusions about the beneficial or adverse effects of a vegetarian diet on athletic performance cannot be made. Further dietary surveys on athlete populations are required to fully understand the influence of a long-term vegetarian diet on exercise performance.

A well-planned lacto-ovo-vegetarian diet and vegan diet appear to be adequate in meeting the nutrient requirements of athletes. A fruitarian-style vegetarian diet, even if well-planned, will not meet nutrient requirements. Vegetarian diets are inherently high in CHO, which is conducive to restoring and maintaining adequate glycogen stores in athletes in hard-training programs. Given that total daily energy requirements are met, plant sources of protein can meet the slightly higher protein requirements of athletes in hard training. Energy-dense plant foods high in protein should be encouraged for athletes with high daily energy and protein requirements.

Although animal foods are good sources of protein, iron, zinc and vitamin B12, and dairy products are rich sources of calcium, alternative plant sources that are either naturally rich or fortified with these nutrients are readily available. Food sources fortified with vitamin B12 should be included in a vegan diet to help meet requirements. Vegetarians, athletes included, appear to be at higher risk of non-anemic iron deficiency. Given the likely effect of iron deficiency on endurance performance, routine assessment of iron status is warranted in vegetarian athletes.

Vegetarians have lower mean muscle creatine stores than non-vegetarians; this may reduce the performance capacity of repeated brief bouts of maximal exercise. As the benefits of creatine supplementation are inversely related to the initial muscle creatine content, vegetarians are likely to experience greater gains in maximal exercise following supplementation with creatine monohydrate than omnivores, although this is yet to be confirmed. Further research is required to gain a better understanding of the effect of a long-term vegetarian diet on menstrual status in female athletes. At present any direct association between menstrual dysfunction and vegetarian diets is unlikely.

PRACTICE TIPS

GREG COX

DIETARY ASSESSMENT

- Clarify why an athlete chooses a vegetarian diet early in the interview. Cultural, ethical, environmental and religious reasons for choosing a vegetarian diet should always be respected. Some vegetarians avoid red meat because of the mistaken belief that it is high in fat, so discussing the fat content in lean cuts is important. Provide ideas for suitable, convenient plant or meat alternatives.
- Determine the type of vegetarian diet followed and assess any potentially limiting nutrients. Vegan diets may be low in vitamin B12, iron and zinc intake. Assess nutrition knowledge and beliefs. An unplanned vegetarian diet is likely to be poorly balanced, as is an unplanned omnivorous diet.

KEY NUTRIENT CONCERNS FOR VEGETARIAN ATHLETES, INCLUDING DIETARY STRATEGIES TO ADDRESS THESE CONCERNS

- If an athlete has recently converted to a vegetarian diet, assess the usual daily energy intake and weight history. It is often difficult for newly converted vegetarian athletes to maintain their usual energy intakes if food choices are predominantly bulky, high-fiber, wholesome CHO foods. Increasing the consumption of high-fiber meat alternatives—for example, legumes and beans—can make it difficult to meet high daily energy requirements and can induce flatulence and abdominal discomfort. Encourage consumption of energy-dense, low-bulk foods to meet high energy requirements with gluten meat alternatives, textured vegetable protein, tempeh, tofu, nuts, peanut or nut butter, fruit juices, dried fruits, honey and jams. For lacto-ovo-vegetarians, low-fat milk, reduced-fat cheese and other low-fat dairy products are also low in bulk and energy-dense. Fortified soy products, including soy milk, soy cheese, soy custard and soy yoghurt, are low-bulk, high-energy alternatives for vegan athletes.
- Examine sources of protein, especially at the midday meal. Lacto-ovo-vegetarians often use cheese in place of meat, whereas vegans may fail to use any protein alternative. Providing examples of convenient meat alternatives for lunch, such as ready-prepared beans (e.g. baked beans) and nut and seed spreads (such as peanut butter, tahini and almond spread), is crucial. Ready-made luncheon meats, derived from wheat gluten, are also an excellent sandwich meat alternative.
- Some dietitians are quick to encourage legumes or tofu as meat alternatives, failing to realize the diverse array of semi-prepared, vegetarian meat alternatives available in supermarkets. Encouraging more regular use of lentils or other dried beans or peas automatically increases the bulkiness and satiety of meals. This is a concern for athletes with high energy requirements, and those who lose their appetites after exercise. Numerous products derived from soy, nut or vegetable protein can provide energy-dense alternatives. Becoming familiar with the taste and method of preparing these foods facilitates more effective counseling.

- Assess usual calcium intakes, particularly in vegans. Determine the types of soy milk consumed, if any, and recommend calcium-fortified varieties. Other suitable non-dairy, calcium-rich alternatives include tofu, soy yoghurts, soy custards, cereals and low-oxalate green vegetables such as broccoli, bok choy and kale.
- Dietary intake of riboflavin may be limited in vegan athletes, particularly those who avoid consuming soy milk and its products. Rich sources of riboflavin for the vegan athlete include fortified breakfast cereals, grains, textured vegetable protein, soy milks, soy yoghurts, soy custards, soy cheeses and yeast extract spreads such as Marmite™ and Vegemite™.
- Assess sources of vitamin B12 in athletes following a vegan diet. Dairy foods and eggs provide sufficient vitamin B12 for lacto-ovo-vegetarians. Vegan athletes should include foods fortified with vitamin B12. In Australia, soy-based products are permitted under food regulations to have added vitamin B12.
- Assessment of total iron intake and iron bioavailability is warranted in all athletes following any type of vegetarian diet and may include biochemical measures of iron status if iron requirements are high (e.g. for endurance athletes and during periods of growth). Excellent dietary iron sources include products fortified with iron (such as breakfast cereals), bread, textured vegetable protein, legumes, dried beans, gluten-based vegetarian meat alternatives, nuts, dried fruits and green leafy vegetables. Chapter 10 provides strategies for improving total dietary iron and optimizing iron bioavailablity. Iron supplements are warranted only where iron depletion or iron deficiency anemia has been diagnosed.
- Vegetarian diets usually provide macronutrients in amounts similar to those recommended for optimal sports performance. Some athletes following a vegetarian diet may have a high fat intake if they consume full-fat dairy products and use large amounts of added fats, oils and salad dressings. Suggestions for low-fat alternatives, low-fat cooking methods and meat alternatives should be made to help meet targets for low-fat diets when required.
- It is not uncommon to see a link between vegetarian diets and disordered eating behavior, particularly in females among whom vegetarian eating may mask restricted eating behavior. Female adolescent athletes are sensitive to weight and body-fat levels, and may disguise a restricted eating pattern by describing their intake as vegetarian.
- Encourage variety in food choice and the consumption of protein-rich and CHO-rich foods at each meal. Vegetarian meat alternatives include lentils, dried beans and peas (ready-to-use products are available), tofu, tempeh, textured vegetable (or soy) protein and ready-made nut, soy or wheat-derived alternatives. Encourage athletes to experiment with new foods and direct them to suitable cookbooks specializing in vegetarian cuisine. The Sanitarium Health Food Company is the largest vegetarian company within Australia and New Zealand, and produces numerous nutrition resources including cookbooks, nutritional product analysis brochures and newsletters. Their current web page address is http://www.sanitarium.com.au.

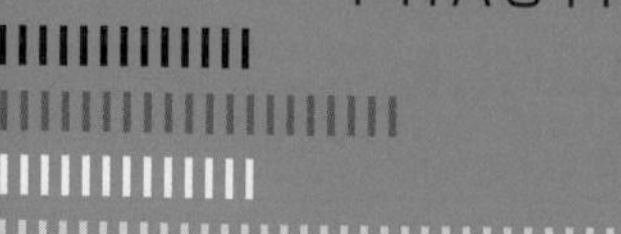

PRACTICE TIPS

PROBLEMS IN NUTRIENT ANALYSIS OF VEGETARIAN DIETS

- Nutrient analysis of vegetarian diets can be difficult, as many commercially available vegetarian meat substitutes are not included in food composition databases. To obtain an accurate nutrient analysis, it may be necessary to obtain nutrient information for food labels or approach the company for nutrient composition of the food. For instance, the Sanitarium Health Food Company produces a range of nutrition analysis brochures for their products. Food labels, however, do not provide a comprehensive nutrient analysis and are not valid for research.

Useful websites

http://www.veg-soc.org

The Australia Vegetarian Society produces a quarterly journal (*New Vegetarian and Natural Health*) and provides recipes, contact with other vegetarians and the locations of restaurants throughout Australia

http://www.ivu.org

The International Vegetarian Union has a comprehensive website providing website addresses for vegetarian societies worldwide

http://www.vrg.org

The Vegetarian Resource Group

http://www.vegansociety.com/html/

The Vegan Society, based in the UK

References

American College of Sports Medicine. Roundtable: The physiological and health effects of oral creatine supplementation. Med Sci Sports Exerc 2000;32:706–17.

American Dietetic Association. Position of the American Dietetic Association: vegetarian diets—technical support paper. J Am Diet Assoc 1988;88:352–5.

American Dietetic Association. Position of the American Dietetic Association: vegetarian diets. J Am Diet Assoc 1997;97:1317–21.

Baghurst K, Record S, Leppard P. Red meat consumption in Australia; intakes, nutrient contribution and changes over time. Aust J Nutr Diet 2000;57(Suppl):3S–36S.

Baghurst K, Record S, Syrette J, et al. What are Australians eating? Results from the 1985 and 1990 Victorian Nutrition Surveys. Adelaide, Australia: CSIRO Division of Human Nutrition, 1993.

Ball MJ, Bartlett MA. Dietary intake and iron status of Australian vegetarian women. Am J Clin Nutr 1999;70:353–8.

Barr SI. Nutrition knowledge and selected nutritional practices of female recreational athletes. J Nutr Ed 1986;18:167–74.

Barr SI. Vegetarianism and menstrual cycle disturbances: is there an association? Am J Clin Nutr 1999;70(Suppl):549S–54S.

Barr SI, Janelle KC, Prior JC. Vegetarian vs non-vegetarian diets, dietary restraint, and sub-clinical ovulatory disturbances: prospective 6-month study. Am J Clin Nutr 1994;60:887.

Barr SI, Rideout CA. Nutritional considerations for vegetarian athletes. Nutrition 2004;20:696–703.

Brooks SM, Sanborn CF, Albrecht BH, Wagner WW. Jr Diet in athletic amenorrhoea. Lancet 1984;1: 559–60.

Brownlie TI, Utermohlen V, Hinton PS, et al. Marginal iron deficiency without anemia impairs aerobic adaptation among previously untrained women. Am J Clin Nutr 2002;75:734–42.

Brownlie TI, Utermohlen V, Hinton PS, Haas JD. Tissue iron deficiency without anemia impairs adaptation in endurance capacity after aerobic training in previously untrained women. Am J Clin Nutr 2004;79:437–43.

Burke DG, Chilibeck PD, Parise G, Candow DG, Mahoney D, Tarnopolsky M. Effect of creatine and weight training on muscle creatine and performance in vegetarians. Med Sci Sports Exerc 2003;35:1946–55.

Burke LM, Read RSD. Diet patterns of elite Australian male triathletes. Phys Sportsmed 1987;15: 140–55.

Burr ML, Butland BK. Heart disease in British vegetarians. Am J Clin Nutr 1988;48:830–2.

Burr ML, Sweetnam PM. Vegetarianism, dietary fiber, and mortality. Am J Clin Nutr 1994;36:873–7.

Commonwealth Department of Health and Ageing (Aust), Ministry of Health (NZ) and National Health and Medical Research Council. Nutrient Reference Values Australia and New Zealand. Canberra: NHMRC, 2006.

Delange J, De Slypere JP, De Buyzere M, Robbrecht J, Wieme R, Vermeulen A. Normal reference values for creatine, creatinine, and carnitine are lower in vegetarians. Clin Chem 1989;35:1802–3.

Donovan UM, Gibson RS. Iron and zinc status of young women aged 14 to 19 years consuming vegetarian and omnivorous diets. J Am Coll Nutr 1995;14:463–72.

Dwyer JT. Health aspects of vegetarian diets. Am J Clin Nutr 1988;48:712–38.

Freeland Graves JH, Bodzy PW, Eppright MA. Zinc status of vegetarians. J Am Diet Assoc 1980;77: 655–61.

Gibson, RS. Content and bioavailability of trace elements in vegetarian diets. Am J Clin Nutr 1994;59(Suppl):1223S–32S.

Giovannucci E, Rimm EB, Stampfer MJ, Colditz GA, Ascherio A, Willett WC. Intake of fat, meat and fiber in relation to risk of colon cancer in men. Cancer Res 1994;54:2390–7.

Grandjean AC. The vegetarian athlete. Phys Sportsmed 1987;15:191–4.

Green AL, McDonald IA, Greenhaff PL. The effects of creatine and carbohydrate on whole body creatine retention in vegetarians. Proc Nutr Soc 1997;56:81A.

Greenhaff PL, Bodin K, Soderlund K, Hultman E. Effect of oral creatine supplementation on skeletal phosphocreatine resynthesis. Am J Physiol Endocrin Metab 1994;266:E725–30.

Haddad EH, Berk LS, Kettering JD, Hubbard RW, Peters WR. Dietary intake and biochemical, hematologic and immune status of vegans compared with non-vegetarians. Am J Clin Nutr 1999;70(Suppl): 586S–93S.

Hallberg L, Sandstrom B, Ralph A, Arthur J. Iron, zinc and other trace elements. In: Garrow JS, James WPT, Ralph A, eds. Human nutrition and dietetics. Tenth edition. London: Churchill-Livingstone, 2000:177–210.

Hanne N, Dlin R, Rotstein A. Physical fitness, anthropometric and metabolic parameters in vegetarian athletes. J Sports Med 1986;26:180–5.

Harris RC, Söderlund K, Hultman E. Elevation of creatine in resting and exercised muscle of normal subjects by creatine supplementation. Clin Sci 1992;83:367–74.

Herbert V. Staging vitamin B-12 (cobalamin) status in vegetarians. Am J Clin Nutr 1994;59(Suppl): 1213S–22S.

Herbert V. Vitamin B-12: plant sources, requirements and assay. Am J Clin Nutr 1988;48:852–8.

Hinton P, Sinclair L. Iron supplementation maintains ventilatory threshold and improves energetic efficiency in iron-deficient nonanemic athletes. Eur J Clin Nutr 2007;61:30–9

Hinton PS, Giordano C, Brownlie T, Hass JD. Iron supplementation improves endurance after training in iron-depleted, nonanemic women. J Appl Physiol 2000;88:1103–11.

Hua NW, Stoohs RA, Facchini FS. Low iron status and enhanced insulin sensitivity in lacto-ovo-vegetarians. Br J Nutr 2001;86:515–19.

Hunt JR. Bioavailability of iron, zinc, and other trace minerals from vegetarian diets. Am J Clin Nutr 2003;78(Suppl):633S–9S.

Hunt JR, Roughead ZK. Nonheme-iron absorption, fecal ferritin excretion, and blood indexes of iron status in women consuming controlled lacto-ovo-vegetarian diets for 8 weeks. Am J Clin Nutr 1999;69:944–52.

Institute of Medicine, Food and Nutrition Board. Dietary Reference Intakes for energy, carbohydrate, fiber, fat, fatty acids, cholesterol, protein, and amino acids. Washington, DC: National Academy Press, 2002.

Institute of Medicine, Food and Nutrition Board. Dietary Reference Intakes for vitamin A, vitamin K, arsenic, boron, chromium, copper, iodine, iron, manganese, molybdenum, nickel, silicon, vanadium and zinc. Washington: National Academy Press, 2000.

Jacobs MB, Wilson W. Iron deficiency anemia in a vegetarian runner. JAMA 1984;252:481–2.

Janelle KC, Barr SI. Nutrient intakes and eating behaviour scores of vegetarian and non-vegetarian women. J Am Diet Assoc 1995;95:180–6, 189.

Latta D, Liebman M. Iron and zinc status of vegetarian and non-vegetarian males. Nutr Rep Int 1984;30:141–9.

Lea E, Worsley A. What proportion of South Australian adult non-vegetarians hold similar beliefs to vegetarians? Nutr Diet 2004;61:11–21.

Levin N, Rattan J, Gilat T. Energy intake and body weight in ovo-lacto-vegetarians. J Clin Gastroenterol 1986;8:451–3.

Lukaszuk JM, Robertson RJ, Arch JE, et al. Effect of creatine supplementation and a lacto-ovo-vegetarian diet on muscle creatine concentration. Int J Sport Nutr Exerc Metab 2002;12:336–48.

MacCormick VM, Hill LM, MacNeil L, Burke DG, Smith-Palmer T. Elevation of creatine in red blood cells in vegetarians and nonvegetarians after creatine supplementation. Can J Appl Physiol 2004;29:704–13.

Mahan LK, Escott-Stump S. Krause's food, nutrition and diet therapy. Twelfth edition. Philadelphia, Pennsylvania: WB Saunders, 2008.

Manore MM. Dietary recommendations and athletic menstrual dysfunction. Sports Med 2002;32: 887–901.

Marsh AG, Sanchez TV, Michelsen O, Chaffee FL, Fagal SM. Vegetarian lifestyle and bone mineral density. Am J Clin Nutr 1988;48:837–41.

Martins Y, Pliner P, O'Connor R. Restrained eating among vegetarians: does a vegetarian eating style mask concerns about weight? Appetite 1999:32:145–54.

McLennan W, Podger A, eds. National Nutrition Survey: nutrient intakes and physical measurements, Australia 1995. ABS Catalogue No. 4805.0. Canberra, Australia: Australian Bureau of Statistics, 1998.

McLennan W, Podger A, eds. National Nutrition Survey: selected highlights Australia 1995. ABS Catalogue No. 4802.0. Canberra, Australia: Australian Bureau of Statistics, 1997.

Nagel D, Seiler D, Franz H, Leitzmann C, Jung K. Effects of an ultra-long-distance (1000 km) race on lipid metabolism. Eur J Appl Physiol 1989;59:16–20.

Nieman DC. Vegetarian dietary practices and endurance performance. Am J Clin Nutr 1988;48:754–61.

Nieman DC, Sherman KM, Arabatzis K, et al. Hematological, anthropometric and metabolic comparisons between vegetarian and non-vegetarian elderly women. Int J Sport Med 1989;10:243–50.

Obeid R, Geisel J, Schorr H, Hübner U, Herrmann W. The impact of vegetarianism on some haematological parameters. Eur J Haematol 2002:69:275–9.

Pedersen AB, Bartholomew MJ, Dolence LA, Aljadir LP, Netteburg KL, Lloyd T. Menstrual differences due to vegetarian and non-vegetarian diets. Am J Clin Nutr 1991;53:879–85.

Peeling P, Blee T, Goodman C, et al. Effect of iron injections on aerobic-exercise performance of iron-depleted female athletes. Int J Sport Nutr Exerc Metabol 2007;17:221–31.

Phillips RL, Snowdon DA. Dietary relationships with fatal colorectal cancer among Seventh-Day Adventists. J Nat Cancer Inst 1985;74:307–17.

Pritikin N. The brave soldiers in the ironman army travel on their stomachs. Runner's World 1984;Feb:129.

Raben A, Kiens B, Richter EA, et al. Serum sex hormones and endurance performance after a lacto-ovo-vegetarian and a mixed diet. Med Sci Sports Exerc 1992;24:1290–7.

Richter EA, Kiens B, Raben A, Tvede N, Pedersen BK. Immune parameters in male athletes after a lacto-ovo-vegetarian diet and a mixed western diet. Med Sci Sports Exerc 1991;23:517–21.

Ruud JS. Vegetarianism—implications for athletes. Omaha: International Center for Sports Nutrition, 1990.

Seiler D, Nagel D, Franz H, Hellstern P, Leitzmann C, Jung K. Effects of long-distance running on iron metabolism and hematological parameters. Int J Sports Med 1989;10:357–62.

Shomrat A, Weinstein Y, Katz A. Effect of creatine feeding on maximal exercise performance in vegetarians. Eur J Appl Physiol 2000;82:321–5.

Siegel AJ, Hennekens CH, Solomon HS, Van Boeckel B. Exercise-related hematuria: findings in a group of marathon runners. JAMA 1979;241:391–2.

Simonsen JC, Sherman WM, Lamb DR, Dernbach AR, Doyle JA, Strauss R. Dietary CHO, muscle glycogen, and power output during rowing training. J Appl Physiol 1991;70:1500–5.

Slattery ML, DR, Jacobs Hilner Jr JE, et al. Meat consumption and its associations with other diet and health factors in young adults: the Cardia study. Am J Clin Nutr 1991;54:930–5.

Slavin J, Lutter J, Cushman S. Amenorrhoea in vegetarian athletes. Lancet 1984;1:1474–5.

Snowdon DA, Phillips RL. Does a vegetarian diet reduce the occurrence of diabetes? Am J Public Health 1985;75:507–12.

Synder AC, Dvorak LL, Roepke JB. Influence of dietary iron source on measures of iron status among female runners. Med Sci Sports Exerc 1989;21:7–10.

Tesar R, Notelovitz M, Shim E, Kauwell G, Brown J. Axial and peripheral bone density and nutrient intakes of postmenopausal vegetarian and omnivorous women. Am J Clin Nutr 1992;56:699–704.

Thorogood M, Mann J, Appleby P, McPherson K. Risk of death from cancer and ischaemic heart disease in meat and non-meat eaters. BMJ 1994;308:1667–70.

Tylavsky FA, Anderson JJB. Dietary factors in bone health of elderly lacto-ovo-vegetarian and omnivorous women. Am J Clin Nutr 1988;48:842–9.

Weaver CM, Plawecki KL. Dietary calcium: adequacy of a vegetarian diet. Am J Clin Nutr 1994;59(Suppl):1238S–41S.

Weaver CM, Proulx WR, Heaney R. Choices for achieving adequate dietary calcium with a vegetarian diet. Am J Clin Nutr 1999;70(Suppl):543S–8S.

Wicks D. Human, food and other animals. The vegetarian option. In: Germov J, Williams L, eds. A sociology of food and nutrition. The social appetite. Melbourne: Oxford University Press, 1999.

Williams PT. Interactive effects of exercise, alcohol and vegetarian diet on coronary artery disease risk factors in 9242 runners: the national runners' health study. Am J Clin Nutr 1997;66:1197–206.

Wilson AK, Ball MJ. Nutrient intake and iron status of Australian male vegetarians. Eur J Clin Nutr 1999;53:189–94.

Young VR, Pellett PL. Plant proteins in relation to human protein and amino acid nutrition. Am J Clin Nutr 1994;59(Suppl):1203S–12S.

CHAPTER 21

Athletes with gastrointestinal disorders

KIERAN FALLON

21.1 Introduction

Gastrointestinal (GI) problems are common reasons for presentation to medical practitioners, but little is known about their prevalence in the athlete population. A number of studies have reported both upper- and lower-GI symptoms during exercise (Brouns et al. 1987; Riddoch & Trinick 1988); however, there is little to no investigation of the cause of these symptoms, or confirmation of similar symptoms at rest. It is recognized that exercise, particularly at high intensities, leads to GI symptoms and may exacerbate existing GI conditions.

21.2 Upper gastrointestinal tract

Major upper-GI problems include gastro-esophageal reflux disease, gastritis, peptic ulcer and functional dyspepsia.

21.3 Gastro-esophageal reflux disease

Gastro-esophageal reflux disease (GERD) is a common disorder, with about one-third of adults experiencing heartburn once a month and 5–10% of adults experiencing heartburn each day. Many patients experience accompanying regurgitation of gastric contents into the mouth. The majority of cases are recurrent, but overeating may induce an acute, isolated episode.

The major factor preventing GERD is normal functioning of the lower-esophageal sphincter; however, delayed gastric emptying, with its attendant maintenance of an elevated gastric volume, and the presence of a sliding hiatus hernia are also important in the pathogenesis of this condition (De Carle 1998). High pressure in the gut lumen keeps the esophageal sphincter closed, preventing stomach contents from entering the esophagus. Until recently, it was thought that the pressure holding the esophageal sphincter closed was persistently low in GERD sufferers, but it now appears that most patients have frequent transient relaxations of the sphincter at inappropriate times, such as after a meal. This relaxation allows acid to enter the esophagus and induce a chemical burn. The primary cause of abnormal function of the lower-esophageal sphincter is unknown, but adult-onset GERD may be a familial condition. Fortunately, only about 10% of cases of GERD are associated with chronic inflammation of the esophagus.

Several forms of exercise can induce gastro-esophageal reflux (GER), which may be asymptomatic. GER increases with intensity of exercise and is more common in endurance athletes. It is more likely to occur with exercise in those who have GER at rest. Yazaki and colleagues (1996) compared the incidence of GER in normally asymptomatic athletes involved in rowing and running, by measurement of intra-esophageal pH, before, during and after rowing, fasted running and post-prandial running. While GER was demonstrated in two out of seventeen athletes prior to exercise, it was induced by exercise in 70% of rowers, in 45% of fasted runners and in 90% of runners who had just eaten. This study indicated that athletes with a history of GER should avoid even small meals close to the time of exercise. Fortunately, GER and GERD are easily treated in the majority of cases. Medical management generally involves:

- avoidance of aggravating factors such as eating large meals, lying down soon after eating and ingestion of alcohol, some of which may be specific to the individual
- weight loss, if overweight
- antacids or medications to reduce acid secretion (e.g. H_2 receptor antagonists, proton pump inhibitors)
- prokinetic agents, which increase the rate of gastric emptying

Factors that reduce the muscle tone in the lower-esophageal sphincter, and hence lower-esophageal sphincter pressure, include cigarette smoking and the use of various classes of medication including anticholinergics, theophylline, progesterone, calcium channel blockers, diazepam, $beta_2$ agonists and alpha adrenergic antagonists (Hughes 1997). Also, athletes with established reflux esophagitis should avoid drugs that are directly damaging to the esophageal mucosa, including non-steroidal anti-inflammatory drugs (NSAIDs) and iron supplements.

Specific dietary factors that decrease lower-esophageal sphincter pressure and/or increase gastric acid secretion include caffeine, fat, chocolate, alcohol and peppermint. Although the effectiveness of avoiding these foods is not evidence-based, avoidance, especially on an empty stomach, does provide relief for some people. When compared with caffeinated coffee, decaffeinated coffee has been demonstrated to reduce the period of abnormally low esophageal pH in some reflux patients (Pehl et al. 1997). Decaffeinated coffee, therefore, may be a useful alternative for coffee drinkers. Tomatoes, citrus juices and spicy foods have been implicated as direct esophageal mucosal irritants. However, some people experience no symptoms eating these foods. Most people with reflux can identify the foods that give them symptoms. Ingestion of large meals and eating just before bed can also exacerbate reflux because a large volume of food/or beverage (e.g. alcohol) stimulate a corresponding high secretion of gastric acid.

Functional dyspepsia

21.4

Functional dyspepsia is defined as chronic or recurrent pain or discomfort in the upper abdomen, with no clinical or endoscopic evidence of known organic disease. It is a common but poorly understood condition.

TABLE 21.1 SUBGROUPS OF FUNCTIONAL DYSPEPSIA, INCLUDING SYMPTOMS

SUBGROUP	SYMPTOMS
Ulcer-like dyspepsia	Nausea, vomiting, epigastric pain. More severe cases may be accompanied by severe pain and hematemesis.
Reflux-like dyspepsia	Heartburn, reflux of stomach contents into the mouth.
Dysmotility-like dyspepsia	Early satiety, post-prandial fullness, nausea, retching and/or vomiting that is recurrent, bloating in the upper abdomen (not accompanied by visible distension), upper abdominal discomfort, often aggravated by food.
Unspecified dyspepsia	Symptoms do not fill the criteria of other categories.

Source: Talley et al. 1991

The symptoms are varied, but four subgroups have been identified, as seen in Table 21.1.

The diagnosis of functional dyspepsia should only be made following clinical evaluation and, ideally, an upper-GI endoscopy. This excludes other disorders, including peptic ulceration, reflux esophagitis, and malignancy.

In view of the uncertain etiology of this condition, management is difficult. The placebo response in dyspepsia is between 30% and 60% and only a few of the large number of drugs tested for this condition have shown benefit in properly conducted clinical trials (Hu & Talley 1998). Despite this poor response, medications used to reduce acid secretion, enhance motility or eradicate *Helicobacter pylori* are commonly tried in clinical practice. As up to 50% of patients with functional dyspepsia have delayed gastric emptying and antral dysmotility (Waldron et al. 1991), it is appropriate to advise avoidance of foods known to retard gastric emptying (such as fatty meals). As in GERD, specific foods may be related to symptoms in some patients, and a formal diet diary recording the relationship of food ingestion to symptoms may be useful. Small, low-fat meals may be useful in some patients (Talley 1996).

Despite the high incidence of this condition in the general population, its incidence in the athlete population has not been studied, but the condition is often seen in sports medicine practice.

21.5 Gastritis and peptic ulcer

Gastritis refers to inflammation of the mucosa of the stomach, which may be acute or chronic. Acute gastritis is associated with severe illness, where it is termed 'acute erosive gastritis' or 'stress-induced gastritis'. In the athlete population or those suffering from rheumatological disorders, direct irritants such as aspirin, NSAIDs and alcohol can induce gastritis. Acute gastritis is also associated with infection by the bacterium *Helicobacter pylori*. In milder cases, which occur most frequently, symptoms include nausea, vomiting and epigastric pain. Severe pain and hematemesis occur in more advanced cases. Chronic gastritis is most often associated with *Helicobacter pylori* infection, with active inflammation apparent in about 30–50% of *Helicobacter pylori* infections.

Management of most acute cases involves avoidance of further irritation and the prescription of antacids or medications that inhibit acid secretion. Those cases associated with *Helicobacter pylori* infection are treated by the above-mentioned measures, with the addition of antibiotics.

Peptic ulcer is a generic term for a common condition, which includes both duodenal and gastric ulcers. The etiology is multifactorial, but involves the action of acid and digestive enzymes, reduction of mucosal defenses and infection by *Helicobacter pylori*. *Helicobacter pylori* infection is found in 80% of cases of duodenal ulcers and 70% of gastric ulcers. NSAIDs are responsible for large numbers of gastric ulcers. Diagnosis is based on clinical history and examination and is usually confirmed by endoscopy. The typical symptom is recurrent epigastric pain, commonly described as sharp, burning or gnawing, which may be relieved by eating food or the ingestion of antacids. The pain recurs several hours after eating and is common at night. Complications include perforation, peritonitis and hematemesis (bleeding and vomiting blood). There is some evidence from a cross-sectional study that the prevalence of duodenal ulcers is significantly lower in males who walk or run more than 10 miles (22 km) per week (Cheng et al. 2000).

Treatment involves eradication of *Helicobacter pylori* (Dev & Lambert 1998), if present, with antibiotics and other medications that inhibit acid secretion, such as the proton pump inhibitors. NSAIDs, aspirin and smoking should be avoided. There is no evidence that bland diets reduce gastric acid secretion, promote healing or relieve the symptoms of duodenal ulcer (McGuigan 1994). Although milk and other dairy products are often tried for early symptomatic relief, they do not assist in healing. The relatively low acidity of milk can actually lead to a large production of gastric acid, which promotes more pain and discomfort later on. Caffeine also increases gastric acid secretion and should be avoided, especially on an empty stomach. Otherwise, sufferers can eat the diet of their choice.

Gastroenteritis

21.6

Probably the most common GI disease in athletes, and indeed in the general population, is acute viral gastroenteritis. While rotavirus is the most common causative agent in children, adults are more likely to develop symptoms following infection by Norwalk and related enteric caliciviruses. Such infections alter small intestinal microarchitecture and function, and are associated with mild steatorrhea, carbohydrate (CHO) malabsorption and decreased levels of enzymes in the brush border of the intestinal villi (Greenberg 1994).

The symptoms are well known and include nausea, vomiting, diarrhea and abdominal pain, in some cases accompanied by headache, mild fever and malaise. No laboratory investigations are usually required, but bloody diarrhea suggests an invasive pathogen. A stool culture and microscopy is warranted if this is present.

Treatment for uncomplicated viral cases is usually by oral rehydration therapy as well as anti-emetic and antidiarrheal medications. When a specific bacterial pathogen is suspected or identified, antibiotics such as ciprofloxacin are useful and, in these cases, anti-diarrheal medications are usually avoided.

Adequate volumes of fluids that contain optimum amounts of sodium and CHO are recommended for management of chronic and acute cases. Sports drinks may be useful in this situation, but should be diluted to one-third the normal concentration. In case of the possibility of transient lactose intolerance, a short period of abstinence from milk and dairy products is often advisable. Conventional advice suggests avoidance of fatty or fried foods for a short period.

21.7 Lower gastrointestinal tract

21.8 Inflammatory bowel disease

The term 'inflammatory bowel disease' includes ulcerative colitis and Crohn's disease, both of which are chronic relapsing diseases of the intestine. The main relevance to the sporting population lies in the age distribution of both diseases. While the prevalence is low in the general population (5–8 per 100 000 for ulcerative colitis and 2–4 per 100 000 for Crohn's disease), the peak incidence for both diseases occurs between the ages of 15 and 35 years (Glickman 1994). The prevalence in the athletic population is not known.

The cause of inflammatory bowel disease is unknown, but both genetic and environmental factors are implicated. Tobacco smokers are twice as likely to develop Crohn's disease as non-smokers, but only half as likely to develop ulcerative colitis. Users of the oral contraceptive pill have about double the risk of developing Crohn's disease (Timmer et al. 1998).

Crohn's disease has multiple presentations, including intermittent abdominal discomfort with periods of diarrhea and constipation, an appendicitis-like illness with right-sided abdominal pain, low-grade fever and tenderness, bloody diarrhea, chronic diarrhea or perianal disease. Management usually involves aggressive therapy early in the course of the disease with a recent shift from corticosteroids and mesalazine to immunosuppressive agents such as azathioprine and methotrexate, biological agents such as infliximab, and antibiotics. More than 50% of patients require surgery at some time.

Ulcerative colitis most commonly presents as proctitis with rectal bleeding and mild diarrhea; as colitis of mild to moderate degree with bloody diarrhea; or as severe colitis with severe bloody diarrhea, abdominal pain, fever, weight loss and anemia. Pharmacological management is based upon mesalazine (5-amino-salicylic acid), which can be delivered as tablets (Salazopyrin™, Dipentum™), suppository (Pentasa™), foam (Salofalk™) or enema. Corticosteroids via the rectal or oral route are potent remission-inducing agents.

Dietary management involves correction of nutrient deficiencies, which are common when the disease is active. These are usually due to reduced food intake, but extensive involvement of the terminal ileum in Crohn's disease may significantly impair vitamin B12 absorption. The most commonly encountered nutrient deficiencies in moderate to severe cases are protein, zinc, magnesium, selenium and a number of vitamins. In the acute phase, a low-residue diet is recommended. Seeds, skins, corn and large intakes of fiber may lead to complications in cases where small bowel stenosis is present, and should be avoided. If fat malabsorption is present, high oxalate foods may lead to the production of oxalate stones (Gibson & Anderson 1998). The meticulous use of elemental and polymeric diets has been shown to be as effective as oral prednisone in leading to remissions of small bowel Crohn's disease (Ferguson et al. 1998). Problems with long-term compliance, cost and acceptability preclude the use of elemental diets, except in severe cases.

21.9 Irritable colon syndrome

Irritable colon syndrome (ICS) is a condition characterized by abdominal pain and altered bowel habit in the absence of any abnormality on radiological, endoscopic or laboratory investigations. Approximately one-third of patients have constipation, one-third diarrhea and one-third alternate between these symptoms. All have abdominal pain. ICS is the most common chronic gastroenterological disorder and has a prevalence of 15–25% in females and 5–20% in males in the general population (Malcolm & Kellow 1998). It is more common in the young and, therefore may be frequently found in the young active population, although the prevalence in this age group has not been studied.

The cause is unknown, but involves abnormalities in intestinal motor function, intestinal sensory function and central nervous system–enteric nervous system regulation. Infection and psychological factors have been implicated in triggering ICS and in determining which patients present for treatment. True allergic or immunologically mediated responses to foods have little role in the etiology of ICS. Food intolerance, however, may play a role, with dairy products and grains implicated as common precipitants of symptoms (Nanda et al. 1989).

Management involves exclusion of serious intestinal disease, education (particularly in relation to trigger factors) and reassurance. Medication choice depends on the dominant symptoms and includes antidiarrheals, laxatives, antispasmodics and anticholinergics. Amitryptaline in low dose (10–20 mg) at night may assist with pain and tegaserod is of value in cases where bloating and constipation are predominant. There is little evidence for the use of probiotics in this condition.

Possible dietary interventions include gradual increases in fiber intake, which can be equally useful in cases with constipation or diarrhea, and reduction of intake of caffeine, alcohol and cigarettes, which may contribute to loose bowel motions. Some patients complain of bloating and flatulence and, for these people, lentils, beans, broccoli and leafy vegetables, carbonated drinks, large amounts of simple sugars and complex CHOs may need to be limited. Limiting intakes of CHO will be difficult in most athletes, so any restriction of these foods should be done on an individual basis in response to offending foods. Bloating and flatulence are also linked to swallowing air, thus advice on methods to reduce aerophagy, including eating slowly, avoidance of gulping fluid and food (a commonly observed behavior in athletes) and abstinence from chewing gum is often useful.

Celiac disease

21.10

Celiac disease, also known as gluten-sensitive enteropathy, is an inflammatory disease of the small intestine. It is caused by the ingestion of a specific protein (gliadin) found in oats, barley, wheat, rye and hybrid grains of these cereals. Most frequently seen in those of Celtic extraction, the prevalence in Australia and New Zealand is estimated to be as high as one in 84 people (Celiac Society of Australia 2005) and in twice as many females as males (Pham & Barr 1996). Many patients have minimal to no symptoms so the prevalence may be much greater than estimated figures suggest.

The common clinical features in adults are abdominal pain, bloating, fatigue, weight loss, mild diarrhea and steatorrhea. Mouth ulcers, glossitis and stomatitis may also be present and, in cases that are more chronic, osteomalacia, osteoporosis, anemia due to iron and/or folate deficiency, and hypoalbuminemia are also seen.

Screening for this disease is through measurement of total serum IgA, anti-transglutaminase IgA and anti-endomysial IgA. These tests are more sensitive and specific than the previously used antigliadin antibody test. A positive antibody test should be followed by small-bowel biopsy, which generally reveals variable chronic inflammation, short villi and crypt hyperplasia, which confirms the diagnosis.

Permanent withdrawal of gluten from the diet is standard treatment. Most patients have a rapid response, showing improvement in a few weeks. Wheat, barley and rye cereals and their products are excluded (Feighery 1999) and the assistance of a dietitian and a local celiac society is invaluable. Oats, which were previously excluded, can be added to the diet of adults with celiac disease without adverse effects (Janatuinen et al. 1995). Supplementation of calcium and vitamin D is recommended. Although withdrawal of gluten is important in terms of alleviating symptoms and general nutrition, it is also important in the prevention of malignancy. Celiac disease is classically associated with T-cell lymphoma of the small intestine, but also with cancer of the pharynx and esophagus. A strict gluten-free diet is protective against these malignancies (Holmes et al. 1989).

Dietary adherence to a gluten-free diet can be monitored by serial tests for anti-transglutaminase and anti-endomysial antibodies as well as by nutritional status measurements (see Chapter 2). Serology should normalize within 9 months of commencing a strict gluten-free diet.

21.11 Lactose intolerance

Lactose intolerance is caused by lactase deficiency. Lactose is the principal CHO contained in milk and milk products; therefore, the typical symptoms of abdominal cramps (such as bloating and perhaps diarrhea) follow the ingestion of milk and some dairy products. Lactose is not digested or absorbed and its presence in the gut leads to fluid shift into the intestinal lumen. Osmotic diarrhea can occur after the ingestion of large quantities of milk. Primary lactose intolerance, while having a hereditary basis, often does not become clinically apparent until adolescence, and is irreversible. Secondary lactase deficiency, which is transitory, is usually associated with intestinal mucosal damage. It is most commonly seen following viral gastroenteritis, but may also be present in association with giardiasis, celiac disease or inflammatory bowel disease.

Management is simple. Avoidance of products containing lactose leads to absence of symptoms. Most people with lactose intolerance can consume small amounts of milk at a time (around 100 mL) with no adverse effects.

21.12 Hemochromatosis

Hemochromatosis, an iron storage disease characterized by excessive mucosal absorption of iron, is an autosomal recessive disorder. Deposition of excess iron occurs in the liver, heart, pancreas, joints and other organs. The most common clinical manifestations are skin pigmentation, diabetes and arthropathy. Presenting symptoms include lethargy, polyuria and excessive thirst, arthralgia and loss of libido.

Very commonly, the diagnosis is suggested from routine screening of iron status measures, or during investigation of persistent fatigue in athletes. If the transferrin saturation is above 45%, and/or the serum ferritin is above the normal range and the athlete is not on iron supplementation, the test should be repeated. If these iron status measures remain at abnormal levels, a nucleic acid amplification gene test is required. Serum ferritin is an acute phase reactant and may be elevated following prolonged endurance exercise (Fallon et al. 1999), which can mask its true value. If such an elevation is suspected, the repeat test should be conducted 48–72 hours after exercise. Although phenotypic expression is dependent upon age and gender, overall, two-thirds of those homozygous for the most common mutation (C282Y) have increased iron stores. Many of these do not develop clinical manifestations.

Management of early cases involves low dietary iron intake and measures to decrease iron absorption. More established cases, characterized by very high ferritin levels, require repeated phlebotomy.

Hemochromatosis highlights the need for correct diagnosis of iron deficiency in athletes prior to recommendation of iron supplementation (which would clearly be contraindicated should this condition be present).

The effect of exercise on the gastrointestinal system: disorders specifically related to exercise 21.13

Gastrointestinal motility and blood-flow 21.14

Exercise is associated with a decrease in lower-esophageal sphincter pressure (Peters et al. 1988). A reduction in duration, frequency and amplitude of esophageal contractions is also observed with exercise intensities above 60% $VO_{2\,max}$ (Soffer et al. 1993).

The effect of exercise on gastric emptying has been addressed elsewhere (see Chapter 14). At exercise intensities up to 70% $VO_{2\,max}$, the gastric emptying rate is usually not influenced by exercise, but is controlled by other physiological and neural factors, and the nutrient composition of foods present (Fordtran & Salting 1967).

The majority of studies indicate that physical activity delays the transit time of food in the small bowel, most likely the result of decreased propulsion (Brouns & Beckers 1993). In contrast, hard physical activity speeds up the transit time of fecal contents in the colon, probably because of increased mucosal secretion, which dilutes colonic contents. As the majority of intestinal transit time of fecal waste occurs in the colon, the overall effect of physical activity on total GI transit time is a reduction.

Disturbances of GI function, including abdominal pain, diarrhea and bleeding, may be related to reduction in local blood-flow. During exercise, splanchnic vasoconstriction occurs, allowing increased blood to be shunted to muscle and skin for oxygen and substrate transport, and thermoregulation, respectively. Both the splanchnic and celiac circulations experience decreased blood-flow. Rowell and colleagues (1964) studied subjects working at 70% $VO_{2\,max}$ and observed a 60–70% decrease in splanchnic blood-flow. This suggested a relationship between increasing exercise intensity and reduction in blood-flow. At $VO_{2\,max}$ splanchnic flow has been shown to be reduced by as much as 70–80%. The reductions in blood-flow are worsened by concomitant dehydration. Blood-flow improves in the trained athlete and when exercise intensity is reduced (Clausen 1977). Hence, there may be some adaptation operating in highly trained athletes.

Diarrhea and other gastrointestinal disturbances during competition 21.15

GI symptoms are common in athletes and have been extensively studied in marathon runners and triathletes (Sullivan 1981, 1986; Keeffe et al. 1984; Worobetz & Gerrard 1985; Halvorsen et al. 1990). Riddoch and Trinick (1988) summarized the findings of four surveys of recreational and competitive runners, marathon runners and triathletes, and presented their own survey data from marathon runners. They reported the incidence of the following GI symptoms during or immediately after running: loss of appetite 28–50%, heartburn 9.5–24%, nausea 6–20%, vomiting 4–6%, abdominal cramps 19.3–39%, urge for a bowel movement 30–42% and diarrhea 14–27%. These authors found that both upper- and lower-GI symptoms were more likely to occur during a hard run than an easy run and were as frequent during as after running. Lower-GI symptoms were more common than upper-GI symptoms and this is consistent with previous surveys. The most common strategies used to minimize symptoms were to run in a fasted state and to have a bowel movement prior to running.

Rehrer and colleagues (1992) studied dietary intake in relation to GI complaints in fifty-five male triathletes in a half-ironman distance triathlon. In these athletes, hyperosmotic beverage consumption during competition was associated with increased incidence of severe GI symptoms. Dietary fiber ingestion before competition increased the likelihood of GI symptoms. The ingestion of fat and protein in a pre-race meal was thought to increase the risk of upper-GI distress in some athletes.

Brouns and colleagues (1987), based on an extensive review of the literature, suggested the recommendations in Table 21.2 for minimization of exercise-related GI symptoms.

21.16 Gastrointestinal blood loss

GI bleeding, although fairly uncommon, is a dramatic GI symptom that may occur in response to hard physical activity. It is most frequently described in long-distance runners (Sullivan 1986). In one study, up to 22% of runners had evidence of GI bleeding based on a positive test for fecal occult blood following a marathon (Schwartz et al. 1990) and almost 85% showed a positive test following an ultramarathon (Baska et al. 1990). Bleeding, again based on the same test, has also been reported in twelve competitive cyclists, with 8.4% of 310 stool samples collected intermittently over 1 year being positive (Dobbs et al. 1988). Yet other studies have reported much lower incidences of blood in the stools of athletes. None out of sixty-three runners reported blood in the stool following a marathon (Halvorsen et al. 1990) and only 6% out of 125 runners reported blood in the stool in another marathon

TABLE 21.2 RECOMMENDATIONS FOR MINIMIZING EXERCISE-RELATED GI SYMPTOMS DURING TRAINING OR COMPETITION

- Solid food should be avoided during the last 3 hours prior to exercise.
- Liquid foods can be taken as a pre-competition meal and also during exercise.
- Whenever fluid is of first priority, drinks should be low in CHO.
- When maximum intakes of both CHO and water are desired, the optimal concentration should be in the range of isotonicity (e.g. sports drinks).
- Athletes suffering frequently from diarrhea or the urge to defecate during exercise may benefit from liquid meal supplements (low in fiber content) during the last day preceding competition.
- Drinking during exercise should be part of the training program.
- In addition, high-fiber foods and caffeine should be avoided prior to exercise.

Source: Adapted from Brouns et al. 1987

(McCabe et al. 1986). These reports were based on self-observation rather than laboratory testing and may have been under-estimations, as the presence of blood in the stool may not be readily apparent by visual examination.

Bleeding is most likely related to GI ischemia, but early studies suggested that mechanical trauma to the gut could be the cause (Porter 1982). The site of bleeding has been assessed by endoscopy in two studies. Gaudin and colleagues (1990) assessed seven runners by upper-GI endoscopy before and after training runs of between 12 and 30 miles. All had gastric mucosal lesions consistent with ischemia following the run, but only four had normal examinations prior to exercise. All had previous GI symptoms, which make conclusions from this study uncertain. Schwartz and colleagues (1990) examined seven runners who had occult blood loss following a marathon by esophago-gastro-duodenoscopy and colonoscopy. Three runners were examined within 48 hours of the race; two of these runners had gastric antral erosions. The third had erosion of the mucosa at the splenic flexure. The other four runners, examined between 4 and 30 days following the run, had normal results. The authors concluded that ischemia was the causative factor in mucosal lesions. Risk of bleeding correlates well with intensity of exercise, but not with use of aspirin or NSAIDs (McMahon et al. 1984). Occasional cases of severe intestinal ischemia leading to bowel resection have been described (Moses 2005). This uncommon complication should be considered in cases of persistent pain and diarrhea.

The cause of macroscopic bleeding should be elucidated by thorough investigation, even in young athletes. The extent of investigation required for microscopic bleeding associated with exercise is age-dependent, with those aged over 40 years requiring full investigation.

Preventive strategies include gradual increases in training, careful hydration and, in cases of recurrent upper-GI bleeding, medication. Use of H_2 receptor antagonists can significantly lower the rate of bleeding (Baska et al. 1990).

Summary 21.17

Although acute intensive exercise can affect gastric emptying and normal gut function in some athletes, this situation is usually transient and unlikely to be linked with chronic GI conditions or problems. These short-term GI symptoms can be minimized by dietary intervention and in some cases with medication. Chronic GI conditions of both the upper- and lower-GI tract can be exacerbated by intensive activity but are not usually caused by it. The dietary and medical treatment of an athlete who has been diagnosed with a GI condition is usually no different from that recommended for a non-athlete.

PRACTICE TIPS

LISA SUTHERLAND AND VICKI DEAKIN

- There is a range of physiological reasons why athletes complain of GI symptoms and might seek advice from a dietitian rather than go directly to their general practitioner. Common complaints including feeling bloated, abdominal discomfort, constipation, flatulence, loss of appetite, vomiting during strenuous exercise, blood in stools, or excessive burping. Some athletes claim they have food allergies, intolerances or GI conditions, but have never been diagnosed. GI symptoms can also be psychological or induced by anxiety or depression, and possibly indicative of disordered eating behaviors.
- Sometimes the cause of these symptoms is obvious and may require minor dietary modifications only. If a medical condition is suspected or the athlete truly believes he or she has a food allergy, intolerance or medical condition, although never diagnosed, referral to a doctor is required for confirmation. The dietary and medical treatment of an athlete who has been diagnosed with a GI condition is usually no different from that recommended for a non-athlete.

GASTRO-ESOPHAGEAL REFLUX DISEASE (GERD)

- The treatment for GERD usually involves a combination of dietary modifications and medication, depending on the cause and severity of the condition. Spacing food intake over the day into small meals and snacks, rather than consuming large meals, which increase gastric acid secretion and exacerbate the condition, and eating slowly and chewing well can reduce symptoms. Reducing the volume of food and fluid consumed just prior to exercise may help. Caffeine and alcohol, especially consumed on an empty stomach, exacerbate the condition by increasing gastric acid secretion and opening the lower esophageal sphincter, so reducing consumption may offer some relief.
- Typical dietary irritants include spicy foods, citrus juices, tomatoes, pineapple and fatty foods, although individuals respond differently and may have no reaction. Providing a food and symptom diary to the athlete and training the athlete to record reactions can identify specific food irritants, which are often difficult to isolate by interview.

FUNCTIONAL DYSPEPSIA

- Reducing meal size, eating snacks between meals and minimizing intake of foods that retard gastric emptying (such as fatty foods) help reduce symptoms.

GASTRITIS

- Chronic use or misuse of anti-inflammatory medications, commonly used for soft tissue or joint injury, can directly damage gastric mucosal cells. Dietary management of gastritis is similar to that for GERD and peptic ulcer, although it is recommended to avoid known irritants.

PEPTIC ULCER

- Peptic ulcers can occur in either the duodenum or stomach. Identification of the cause and treatment with medication is the cornerstone of therapy. Dietary treatment, where required to alleviate symptoms, is the same as that for GERD. Drinking milk to soothe the pain is not recommended. Although milk provides rapid short-term pain relief, it is associated with a delayed increase in gastric acid secretion later on, exacerbating the pain and discomfort (see section 21.5). Bland foods are no longer recommended or necessary.

GASTROENTERITIS

- In the acute phase, anti-emetic and antidiarrheal medications are usually administered. If vomiting or diarrhea are prolonged, the immediate concern is to identify signs and symptoms of dehydration and treat quickly. Iso-osmolar solutions containing both sodium and CHO (available over the counter at pharmacies) should be sipped intermittently rather than consumed as a large bolus to avoid further pain, diarrhea and emesis. Sports drinks are a good alternative. Hyperosmolar beverages (such as soft drink and fruit juices) are contraindicated and induce osmosis and hence osmotic diarrhea. Food should be introduced as soon as possible, with small frequent feedings of low-fiber, low-fat foods (such as dry crackers and toast) that empty quickly from the stomach. Transient lactose intolerance can accompany gastroenteritis so lactose-containing foods should be avoided in the short term until bowel symptoms subside.

INFLAMMATORY BOWEL DISEASES: ULCERATIVE COLITIS AND CROHN'S DISEASE

- When these conditions are not active, no specific dietary intervention is required. When inflammation is active and symptoms are present, low-residue diets (low fat, low-fiber) are indicated for short-term use to rest the bowel and avoid irritation. When inflammation subsides, high-fiber and high-fluid intake are the cornerstones for treatment and prevention. Nutrient deficiency and weight loss are more likely to occur when the conditions are active or chronic because of impaired nutrient absorption and loss of appetite. Vitamin and mineral supplements and high-energy liquids may be warranted in such cases.

IRRITABLE BOWEL SYNDROME

- For this condition, psychological factors often contribute to symptoms, which are variable and often non-specific and range from constipation, bloating, and abdominal discomfort to malaise and lethargy. Reduction of fiber-rich foods can be effective. Some sufferers benefit from reducing caffeine and alcohol. A detailed food and symptom diary helps identify specific food culprits, but often there is no direct link to any particular food or beverage.

PRACTICE TIPS

CELIAC DISEASE

- Avoidance of the specific protein called gliadin, naturally present in some cereal grains (wheat, barley, rye, oats and hybrids of these cereals and their by-products), controls celiac disease. Meeting the requirements for the high CHO diets recommended for athletes is difficult without these food staples, so meticulous dietary planning is needed. Gliadin-free or gluten-free natural CHO sources include rice, corn, legumes, fruit, starchy vegetables and dairy foods. Where lactose intolerance, often seen in the acute stage, is also present, further dietary restrictions are needed (see below). Support groups such as the Coeliac Society of Australia or similar organizations in other countries provide food lists, food product information and recipes, and assist in the adjustment to dietary changes.

LACTOSE INTOLERANCE

- Symptoms of lactose intolerance include abdominal discomfort/pain, bloating, flatulence and sometimes diarrhea or loose stools. Most people with lactose intolerance can tolerate small amounts of lactose (the CHO found naturally in animal milks) and have no problems consuming the amount of milk used on breakfast cereal. Larger volumes of milk are not well tolerated. There are some concerns about low calcium intakes in people with lactose intolerance, if dairy foods are avoided completely. Mature cheeses have minimal lactose and are high in calcium, so dairy foods do not need to be completely eliminated. Recommendations to meet calcium recommendations from low-lactose or lactose-free food sources are discussed in Chapter 9.

GASTROINTESTINAL SYMPTOMS WITH NO KNOWN CAUSE

- Should medical examination reveal no known cause of GI symptoms, taking a detailed dietary and symptom history at an interview to determine any association between particular foods and symptoms is useful, but not always enlightening. Because of the difficulty in accurately recalling food intake and matching symptoms (which are often delayed) to it, dietitians request a detailed food and symptom diary from the athlete. However, thorough training in this technique is essential to get reliable feedback.
- Other potential causes of GI disturbances (such as stress, anxiety, depression and eating disorders) can not be discounted. Referral for stress management may be needed. Table 21.3 provides dietary strategies to help reduce symptoms.

TABLE 21.3 SUGGESTIONS FOR DIETARY INTERVENTION TO HELP AVOID OR TREAT GI DISTURBANCES

PROBLEMS	SOLUTIONS
Any GI pain or discomfort, nausea	Avoid hyperosmolar (e.g. fruit juice and milk) and carbonated beverages (e.g. lemonade) and alcohol. Drink water or sports drink—sip rather than guzzle. Avoid artificial sweeteners, such as those in 'diet' drinks and sugar-free gum. Avoid known irritant foods (such as coffee and alcohol on an empty stomach). During or before physical activity, eat a snack that is emptied quickly from the stomach and well tolerated (e.g. high glycaemic-index, low-fat/protein foods). Practice eating during training. For short events allow sufficient time between eating and the commencement of physical activity.
Urge to defecate during physical activity	Establish a routine of emptying the bowel before physical activity. Consume a low-residue diet (low-fat and low-fiber) before competition.
Diarrhea induced by exercise or loose bowel motions during physical activity	Eat a low-residue diet or diet high in soluble fiber, depending on individual response and the nature of the problem. Avoid hyperosmolar fluids and artificial sweeteners. AND/OR Have anti-diarrheal drug therapy.
Diarrhea or vomiting from an infective agent (e.g. bacteria, virus, parasite)	Cease physical activity. See Chapter 23, Table 23.5 for dietary strategies for treating nausea and vomiting. Give rehydration strategies priority (see Chapter 14, Practice tips). Seek medical advice, if symptoms are prolonged. Gradually re-introduce the usual diet, beginning with small serves of CHO-rich foods.

USEFUL WEBSITES

http://www.coeliacsociety.com.au/
The Coeliac Society of Australia

http://www.celiactravel.com/coeliac-societies.html
Celiac Societies (worldwide)

http://www.gut.nsw.edu.au/
The Gut Foundation (Australia)

REFERENCES

Baska RS, Moses FM, Graeber G, Kearney G. Gastrointestinal bleeding during an ultramarathon. Dig Dis Sci 1990;35:276–9.

Brouns F, Beckers E. Is the gut an athletic organ? Digestion, absorption and exercise. Sports Med 1993;15:242–57.

Brouns F, Saris WHM, Rehrer NJ. Abdominal complaints and gastrointestinal function during long-lasting exercise. Int J Sports Med 1987;8:175–98.

Cheng Y, Macera CA, Davis DR, Blair SN. Physical activity and peptic ulcers. Br J Sports Med 2000;34:116–21.

Clausen JP. Effect of physical training on cardiovascular adjustments to exercise in man. Physiol Rev 1977;57:779–815.

Coeliac Society of Australia. At http://www.coeliac.org.au/coeliac-how- common.htm (accessed 2 September 2005).

De Carle DJ. Gastro-oesophageal reflux disease. Med J Aust 1998;169:549–54.

Dev AT, Lambert JR. Diseases associated with *Helicobacter pylori*. Med J Aust 1998;169:220–5.

Dobbs TW, Atkins M, Ratliff R, Eichner ER. Gastrointestinal bleeding in competitive cyclists. Med Sci Sports Exerc 1988;20:S78.

Fallon KE, Sivyer G, Sivyer K, Dare A. The biochemistry of runners in a 1600 km ultramarathon. Br J Sports Med 1999;33:264–9.

Feighery C. Coeliac disease. BMJ 1999;319:236–9.

Ferguson A, Glen M, Ghosh S. Crohn's disease: nutrition and nutritional therapy. Balliere's Clin Gastroenterol 1998;12:93–114.

Fordtran JS, Salting B. Gastric emptying and intestinal absorption during prolonged severe exercise. J Appl Physiol 1967;23:331–5.

Gaudin C, Zerath E, Guezennac CY. Gastric lesions secondary to long distance running. Dig Dis Sci 1990;35:1239–43.

Gibson PR, Anderson RP. Inflammatory bowel disease. Med J Aust 1998;169:387–94.

Glickman RM. Inflammatory bowel disease. In: Isselbacher KJ, Braunwald E, Wilson JD, et al., eds. Harrison's principles of internal medicine. New York: McGraw-Hill, 1994:1738–52.

Greenberg HB. Viral gastroenteritis. In: Isselbacher KJ, Braunwald E, Wilson JD, et al., eds. Harrison's principles of internal medicine. New York: McGraw-Hill, 1994:819–21.

Halvorsen FA, Lyng J, Glomsaker T, Ritland S. Gastrointestinal disturbances in marathon runners. Br J Sports Med 1990;24:266–8.

Holmes GKT, Prior P, Lane MR, Pope D, Allan RN. Malignancy and coeliac disease—effect of a gluten-free diet. Gut 1989;30:333–8.

Hu WH, Talley NJ. Functional (non-ulcer) dyspepsia: unexplained but not unmanageable. Med J Aust 1998;168:507–12.

Hughes D. Gastroenterology and sport. In: Fields KB, Fricker PA, eds. Medical problems in athletes. Malden: Blackwell Science, 1997:151–69.

Janatuinen EK, Pikkarainen PH, Kamppainen TA, et al. A comparison of diets with and without oats in adults with coeliac disease. N Eng J Med 1995;333:1033–7.

Keeffe E, Lowe D, Goss J, Wayne R. Gastrointestinal symptoms of marathon runners. West J Med 1984;141:481–4.

Malcolm A, Kellow J. Irritable bowel syndrome. Med J Aust 1998;169:274–9.

McCabe ME, Peura DA, Kadakia SC, Bocek Z, Johnson LF. Gastrointestinal blood loss associated with running a marathon. Dig Dis Sci 1986;31:1229–32.

McGuigan JE. Peptic ulcer and gastritis. In: Isselbacher KJ, Braunwald E, Wilson JD, et al., eds. Harrison's principles of internal medicine. New York: McGraw-Hill, 1994:1363–82.

McMahon LF, Ryan MJ, Larson D, Fisher RL. Occult gastrointestinal blood loss in marathon runners. Ann Intern Med 1984;101:846–7.

Moses FM. Exercise-associated intestinal ischaemia. Current Sports Med Reports 2005;4:91–5.

Nanda R, James R, Smith H, Dudley CR, Jewell DP. Food intolerance and the irritable bowel syndrome. Gut 1989;30:1099–104.

Pehl C, Pfeiffer A, Wendl B, Kaess H. The effect of decaffeination of coffee on gastro-oesophageal reflux in patients with reflux disease. Alimentary Pharmacol Ther 1997;11:483–6.

Peters O, Peters P, Clarys JP, et al. Oesophageal motility and exercise. Gastroenterol 1988;94:A351.

Pham TH, Barr GD. Coeliac disease in adults: presentation and management. Aust Fam Phys 1996;25:62–5.

Porter AMW. Marathon running and the caecal slap syndrome. Br J Sports Med 1982;16:178.

Rehrer NJ, van-Kemenade M, Meester W, Brouns F, Saris WHM. Gastrointestinal complaints in relation to dietary intake in triathletes. Int J Sport Nutr 1992;2:48–59.

Riddoch C, Trinick T. Gastrointestinal disturbances in marathon runners. Brit J Sports Med 1988;22:71–4.

Rowell LB, Blackman JR, Bruce RA. Indocyanine green clearance and hepatic blood flow during mild exercise to maximal exercise in upright man. J Clin Invest 1964;43:1766–90.

Schwartz AE, Vanagunas A, Kamel PL. Endoscopy to evaluate gastrointestinal bleeding in marathon runners. Ann Intern Med 1990;113:632–4.

Soffer EE, Merchant RK, Duethman G, et al. Effect of graded exercise on oesophageal motility and gastro-oesophageal reflux in trained subjects. Dig Dis Sci 1993;38:220–4.

Sullivan S. The gastrointestinal symptoms of running. N Eng J Med 1981;304,5:915.

Sullivan SN. Gastrointestinal bleeding in distance runners. Sports Med 1986;3:1–3.

Talley NJ. Modern management of dyspepsia. Aust Fam Phys 1996;25:47–52.

Talley NJ, Colin-Jones D, Koch KL, Nyren O, Stanghellini V. Functional dyspepsia: a classification with guidelines for diagnosis and management. Gastroenterol Int 1991;4:145–60.

Timmer A, Sutherland LR, Bryant HE, Fick G. Oral contraceptive use and smoking are risk factors for relapse in Crohn's disease. Gastroenterol 1998;114:1143–50.

Waldron B, Cullen PT, Kumar R, et al. Evidence for hypomotility in non-ulcer dyspepsia: a prospective multifactorial study. Gut 1991;32:246–51.

Worobetz L, Gerrard D. Exercise associated symptoms in triathletes. Phys Sportsmed 1985;15:105–10.

Yazaki E, Shawdon A, Beasley I, Evans DF. The effect of different types of exercise on gastro-oesophageal reflux. Aust J Sci Med Sport 1996;28:93–6.

CHAPTER 22

Special needs: athletes with disabilities

ELIZABETH BROAD

22.1 Introduction

Sport and exercise have long been recognized as important components in the therapy and rehabilitation of people with disabilities. However, since the inception of the Summer Paralympic Games in 1960 and the Winter Paralympic Games in 1992, the number of individuals with disabilities training and competing at high levels has increased dramatically. Local, national and international competitions are held in summer and winter disciplines throughout the world. Performance standards continue to improve at a rapid rate, such that world records are frequently broken. Even in non-Paralympic sports, athletes with disabilities are accomplishing challenging feats, such as paraplegics swimming the English Channel and completing the Hawaii Ironman Triathlon.

While the participation of athletes with disabilities is large and they participate in many different sports, scientific research about these athletes has failed to match that of their able-bodied counterparts. This chapter covers the known completed research on athletes with disabilities in their own right, and also discusses differences between athletes with disabilities and able-bodied athletes.

22.2 Paralympic sports

There are few sports or activities in which an athlete with a disability cannot compete. At the Paralympic Games, athletes compete in twenty-four disciplines, as shown in Table 22.1. Not all categories of disability are able to compete in each sport. For example, wheelchair rugby is limited to only those athletes who mobilize in a wheelchair and have a disability involving all four limbs and trunk, usually tetraplegia.

The rules governing each sport are outlined on the International Paralympic Committee (IPC) website (http://www.paralympic.org). At times, rules may differ from those of able-bodied sports in order to ensure the safety of competitors.

TABLE 22.1 CURRENT PARALYMPIC SPORTS		
Archery	Goalball	Swimming
Athletics (T & F)	Ice sledge hockey (winter)	Table tennis
Biathlon (winter)	Judo	Volleyball
Boccia	Powerlifting	Wheelchair basketball
Cycling	Rowing	Wheelchair curling (winter)
Equestrian	Sailing	Wheelchair fencing
Football 7-a-side	Shooting	Wheelchair rugby
Football 5-a-side	Skiing (alpine, Nordic) (winter)	Wheelchair tennis

Classification of disabilities

22.3

'Athletes with disabilities' comprises six primary classes (amputees, cerebral palsy, wheelchair/spinal injured, visually impaired, intellectual disability and Les Autres), which are generally grouped together under a functional system for the purpose of competition.

Cerebral palsy (CP) is a group of permanent disabling symptoms primarily affecting voluntary control musculature, resulting from non-progressive damage to the motor control areas of the brain (Winnick 1995). The most common symptoms include impaired muscle coordination, reduced capacity to maintain posture and balance, and reduced ability to perform normal movements and skills. Some athletes with CP will use a wheelchair because their functional ability to walk and undertake general daily activities is greatly restricted. It is acknowledged, however, that walking for short periods of time remains important for improving circulation, bladder control and metabolism.

'Wheelchair/spinal injured' incorporates athletes with traumatic spinal cord (SC) lesions, poliomyelitis and spina bifida. Figure 22.1 overleaf explains the spinal cord segments and likely effects of a disruption along the cord. Traumatic SC lesions generally result from an accident (e.g. sporting or motor vehicle), so the duration of disability will vary between individuals. Spina bifida is a congenital developmental defect of the spinal column in which vertebral arches have failed to fuse, resulting in an abnormal gap in the spinal column (Winnick 1995; Goodman et al. 1996). Since nerve tissue can protrude through this gap, it can become damaged, resulting in varying degrees of paralysis and loss of sensation in the legs and lower trunk. As with traumatic spinal cord injuries, the degree of damage depends on the location of the deformity and the amount of damage to the spinal cord (Winnick 1995). Hence the physiological response of individuals with spina bifida and traumatic spinal lesions are very similar, and for the purposes of this chapter will be grouped as spinal cord injuries (SCI).

The class 'Les Autres' currently includes multiple sclerosis, Freidrich's ataxia, osteoporosis, severe burns, muscular dystrophies, musculo-skeletal or neural pathway damage and lower-limb deformities. People with organ transplants and hearing impairments have their own competitions (such as Deaflympics and Transplant Games).

Each Paralympic sport has its own system or approach to classification, which categorizes athletes according to their physical capability (Buckley 2009). This system helps to ensure that the vast array of those with physical disabilities can compete at the highest

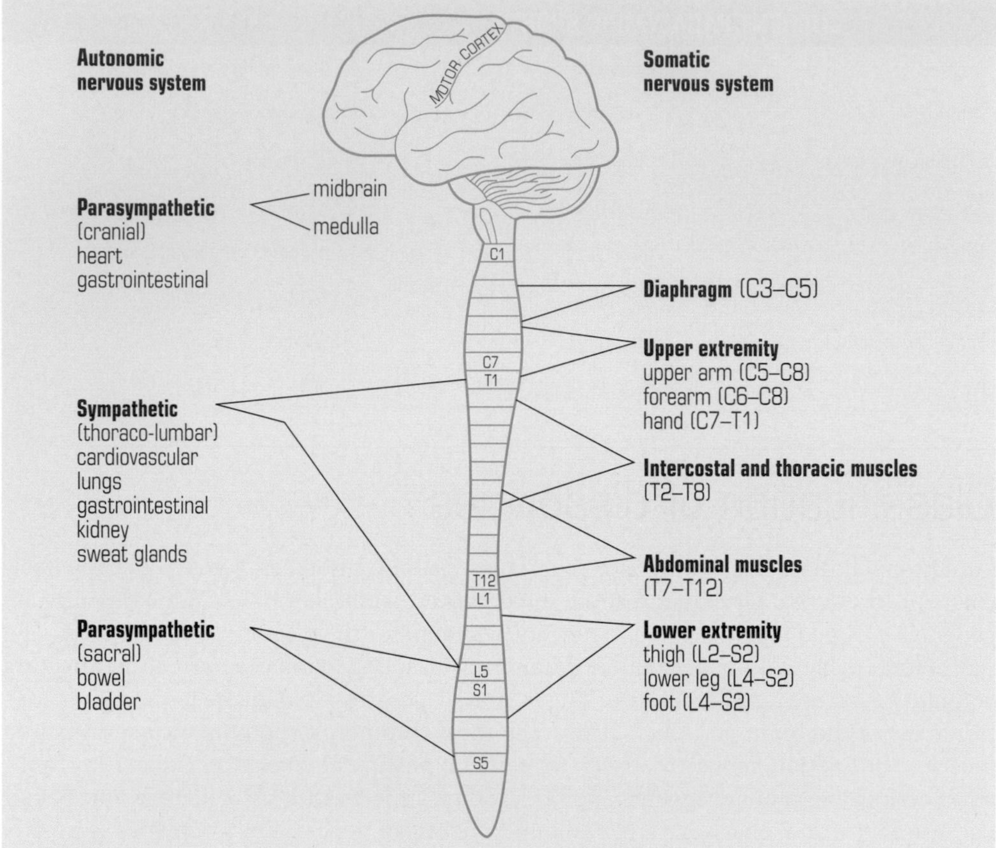

FIGURE 22.1 Spinal cord injury innervation. Adapted from Glaser 1985, p. 269, reprinted with permission

level of which they are capable, with elite competition in mind. All athletes with disabilities must hold an internationally authorized classification to participate in competition. Those athletes whose disability is progressive are reclassified when required. Hence, the running of a competition for athletes with disabilities is far more complex than that for able-bodied athletes as athletes may only compete against similarly classified individuals. The IPC website contains useful information on classification.

22.4 Differences between athletes with disabilities and able-bodied athletes

Research findings are often confusing because of the limited numbers of individuals tested, the large individual variation in functional capacity and the different levels of training undertaken by individual athletes. Most of the existing research about disabled athletes' responses to exercise presented in this section is focused on the physical capabilities of paraplegic and tetraplegic individuals, the outcomes primarily indicating differences that can be explained by relative available muscle mass.

Medical and health-related differences 22.5

As a group, athletes with disabilities have higher incidences of medical problems than other athletes. For example, people confined to wheelchairs have a high risk of pressure sores or infections as a result of wounds, and may have other medical complications depending on the cause of their disability. Amputees also develop wounds around the attachment site of their prosthesis. An individual who has acquired a disability as a result of an accident may have also suffered internal injuries and therefore have a colostomy, ileostomy or other internal problems. Individuals with CP have a higher incidence of epileptic seizures, especially under stress, due to the neurological effects of the disorder. They may also have more feeding difficulties.

Existing medical issues present an additional consideration when working with these athletes, as some disabilities may have been acquired as a result of a medical condition.

Differences in bladder and bowel control 22.6

A common result of SCI is incontinence (lack of bladder and/or bowel control) (Goodman et al. 1996). Therefore many athletes with SCI must consciously schedule visits to the toilet, and require greater control over these bodily functions. Limited mobility as a result of CP, lower-limb amputations or other disorders can also affect normal bowel function. The management of toileting is almost always carefully controlled by the athlete to coincide with the needs of their sport, and may be acutely affected by dietary changes, especially fluid intake.

Use of medications 22.7

Some medications, although necessary for maintaining quality of life and functionality in many athletes with disabilities, have side effects (see Table 22.2 overleaf). It is important for the sports dietitian to be familiar with the medications used, the reason for their use and their potential side effects, as these factors can have an impact on dietary recommendations.

Physiology and metabolism 22.8

While athletes with disabilities may have impaired functional capabilities compared to able-bodied athletes, there is little evidence to suggest that their physiological capabilities differ. Two exceptions to this rule are athletes with some forms of CP and SCI.

Physiological responses to exercise 22.9

The 'normal' physiological response to exercise may be disrupted in people with SCI through a number of mechanisms: ineffective vasoregulation below the SC lesion, increased total peripheral resistance, the inability to increase stroke volume because of blood pooling through the absence of a musculo-skeletal pump from lower limbs, and less total active muscle mass. Hence, individuals with paraplegia, poliomyelitis or spina bifida tend to have dampened peak oxygen uptakes (Shephard 1988) and anaerobic capacity (Van der Woude et al. 1997). As Figure 22.2 overleaf indicates, under normal conditions tetraplegics are unable to raise their maximal heart rates (HR) above 120–130 bpm due to the disruption of their sympathetic nervous system (Wicks et al. 1983; Hjeltnes 1984; Coutts & Stogryn 1987; Bhambhani et al. 1994, 1995). Similarly, their $VO_{2\,peak}$ and lactate levels fall well below those of other athletes undertaking similar work. Even athletes with SC lesions between

TABLE 22.2 FREQUENTLY USED MEDICATIONS AMONG ATHLETES WITH DISABILITIES

PRIMARY CLASSIFICATION	COMMON MEDICATIONS
Bowel management/stool softeners and laxatives	Docusate sodium (Coloxyl™) Sennoside (Senekot™) Enemas (Bisalax™)
Bladder control/antiseptics	Oxybutynin hydrochloride (Ditropan™) Cranberry juice or tablets
Antispasmodics/muscle relaxants	Diazepam (Valium™) Dantrolene sodium (Dantrium™) Gabapentin/Pregabalin Phenobarbitone Baclofen (Clofen™, Lioresal™)
Pain relief/antidepressants	Amitriptyline hydrochloride (Tryptanol™) Carbamazepine (Tegretol™) Gabapentin/Pregabalin Medications containing codeine

Source: Adapted from MIMS Australia 2005

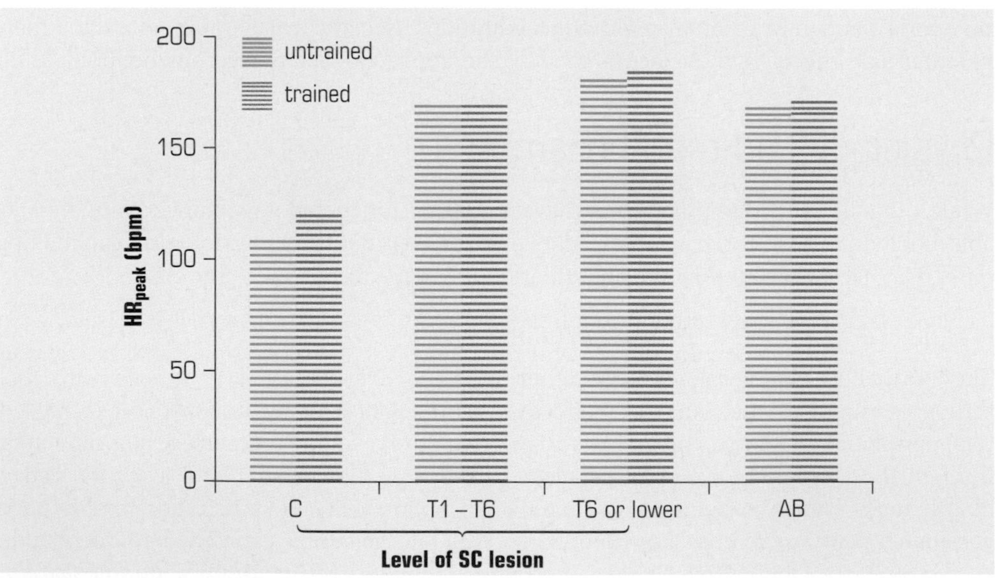

FIGURE 22.2 Comparative peak heart rates in untrained and trained Spinal Cord Injury and able-bodied athletes. Adapted from data by Wicks et al. 1983; Hjeltnes 1984; Coutts & Stogryn 1987; Bhambhani et al. 1994, 1995; Price & Campbell 2003

T1 and T6 tend to have a more restricted peak HR and $VO_{2\ peak}$ relative to able-bodied people and CP (Wicks et al. 1983; Hopman et al. 1993; Barfield et al. 2005). Despite these limitations in absolute exercise capacity, there is no evidence to suggest these athletes' capacity to exercise at a given percentage of maximal capacity is any more restricted than that of an able-bodied athlete.

Individuals with spastic CP exhibited an elevated heart rate response to exercise compared to able-bodied controls, even when gross motor function was considered excellent (Suzuki et al. 2001).

Substrate usage during exercise

22.10

Whether SCI athletes use a different fuel mix to able-bodied athletes during exercise remains uncertain. Only one study has investigated muscle glycogen status in people with SCI. Skrinar and colleagues (1982) took muscle glycogen samples from the deltoid muscle before and after 1 hour of submaximal exercise in four SCI subjects. Although the authors did not control for the effects of pre-exercise diet and used the deltoid muscle (which is not the primary muscle used in wheelchair ambulation), it was interesting to note that the mean pre-exercise glycogen level (92 mmol/kg wet weight) was lower than reported resting glycogen values reported in able-bodied athletes (120–140 mmol/kg wet weight). The mean change over the 1 hour of exercise was 30 mmol/kg wet weight (Skrinar et al. 1982), which was comparable to leg muscle glycogen losses in able-bodied athletes at the same relative exercise intensity (Karlsson & Saltin 1971). The researchers suggested that the lower pre-exercise glycogen levels in the wheelchair athletes could be attributed to a greater dependence on glycogen stores for simple daily ambulation. An alternative explanation could be that upper-body musculature may have a lower capacity to store muscle glycogen compared with that in able-bodied athletes. Clearly, adequate CHO intakes are required for SCI athletes training hard to support glycogen resynthesis.

More recently, Knechtle and colleagues (2003) reported that peak fat oxidation rates occurred at 75% $VO_{2\ peak}$ in both trained SCI athletes undertaking arm ergometry and trained cyclists undertaking cycle ergometry. However, the same group reported lower peak fat oxidation rates (55% $VO_{2\ peak}$) in well-trained SCI athletes undertaking wheelchair ergometry (Knechtle et al. 2004a) and handbike cycling (Knechtle et al. 2004b). Hence, it is apparent that more studies are required to determine fat and CHO oxidation during exercise in SCI athletes.

Energy expenditure

22.11

The typical daily energy expenditure of people with CP varies substantially depending on their mode of ambulation. In a study of non-athletes using doubly-labeled water (used to determine energy expenditure), those individuals who were wheelchair-dependent had lower total energy expenditures (8430 kJ/d) than those who were ambulating (10 360 kJ/d) (Johnson et al. 1997). Regardless of ambulatory status, having athetosis (uncontrollable, jerky movements) increased estimated resting metabolic rate (RMR) (Johnson et al. 1996); however, athetosis also reduced the amount of day-to-day activity undertaken. As a result, total energy expenditure did not differ compared to non-athetotic CP individuals (Johnson et al. 1997). Similarly, amputee athletes may have a higher energy expenditure in ambulation due to the balancing required of prosthetic limbs (Genin et al. 2008) or the lack of limb (for arm amputees) (Yizhar et al. 2008); however, the lesser muscle mass will reduce RMR so overall resting energy expenditure may not differ from that of able-bodied counterparts.

RMRs of SCI individuals have been reported to be up to 30% lower than reference standards (Abel & Platen 2003), primarily because of the reduced active muscle mass (Noreau & Shephard 1995). Consequently, metabolism is relative to the level of SC lesion. Energy expenditure of exercise is also lower than in able-bodied individuals (e.g. 17–27 kJ/min at heart rates ranging 102–145 bpm) (Abel & Platen 2003), due to the smaller absolute muscle mass used. If the use of functional electrical stimulation (FES), which activates lower body muscle groups in people with SCI, becomes more widespread, energy expenditure might also increase.

22.12 Thermoregulation

Due to the neurological interruption of an SC lesion, evaporative cooling from sweating in athletes with SCI is diminished as non-innervated areas cease to release sweat (Hopman et al. 1993; Price 2006). The potential surface area available for cooling (through sweating) is related to the level and completeness of the SC lesion—the higher the lesion, the smaller the surface area (Normell 1974). Although lower sweat rates may appear to be advantageous for minimizing dehydration and slowing the decline in stroke volume in the SCI, such a decrease actually presents a disadvantage for controlling body temperature. In addition, some medications, such as anti-cholinergics (used to control muscle spasms), can also impair thermoregulatory abilities (Kennedy 1995). Finally, the unique body positioning and movements in a wheelchair further limit heat dissipation (Sawka et al. 1984).

In hot conditions, SCI individuals gain heat from the environment, especially those with high-level SC lesions (Petrofsky 1992; Broad 1997). Consequently, the body temperature of an individual with an SCI is more difficult to regulate effectively in the heat (Price & Campbell 2003), even when they are not actively exercising (such as in archery and shooting events) (Broad 1997). The metabolic heat production of exercise exacerbates this heat load, and the ability to manage this depends on the individual's sweating capacity (Price 2006). Active cooling, both before and during exercise, reduces elevations in body temperature and ratings of perceived exertion (Webborn et al. 2005) and results in improved exercise performance (Goosey-Tolfrey et al. 2008a; Webborn et al. 2008). Methods include keeping athletes in the shade as much as possible, spraying them with water and applying cooling devices (e.g. head pieces, neck wraps and cooling jackets) and possibly the use of ice drinks. Cooling needs to be applied regularly, especially when exercising or competing in the heat, as the metabolic heat produced may exceed the cooling potential of the mechanism used (Armstrong et al. 1995; Broad 1997). Whether this maladaptation to exercise in the heat exacerbates CHO usage during exercise has not yet been determined. Fluid intake and total sweat losses should be monitored when active cooling is utilized as it can substantially reduce fluid consumption (Goosey-Tolfrey et al. 2008b) and hence may increase the risk of dehydration.

In cold environments, active heating and heat loss prevention are necessary since the ability to vasoconstrict peripheral blood vessels is usually impaired (Petrofsky 1992), resulting in rapid heat loss in a higher-level SCI athlete. In ambient conditions (20–22°C), there is little difference in the thermoregulatory response to exercise between those with low-level SC lesions and able-bodied individuals, although those with high SC lesions continue to exhibit obvious difficulties controlling body temperature during exercise (Price & Campbell 1999; Price 2006).

Body composition

22.13

In general, the measurement and modification of body composition remain as relevant to athletes with disabilities as they do to any able-bodied athlete. Traditional approaches to measuring body composition may need to be modified for some athletes. For example, the measurement of body mass needs to allow for muscle atrophy and bone resorption in individuals with SCI, spina bifida and severe cases of CP. Furthermore, where muscle atrophy is present, it can be difficult to differentiate the body fat component of skinfold thicknesses (Gass 1988), and other injuries (such as burns) can influence skinfold thickness. Hence, regression equations used in able-bodied athletes to estimate percentage body fat from underwater weighing, bioelectrical impedance, BOD POD and skinfold thicknesses are inappropriate for many athletes with disabilities (see Chapter 3).

It is believed that body mass and sum of skinfolds remain the best practice for assessing and tracking body composition changes for most individual athletes with disabilities (Gass 1988), although modifications in which skinfold sites are used may be required (e.g. sum of four for wheelchair athletes). Waist girth also has been shown to correlate strongly with body fat in wheelchair athletes as assessed by DEXA (Sutton et al. 2009). No normative data have been reported, presumably because of the larger within-sport variability in body shape and size for athletes with disabilities compared with able-bodied athletes.

Bone density

22.14

Bone density of lower limbs in SCI individuals is around 25% lower than that of able-bodied people (Thompson 2000; Miyahara et al. 2008; Sutton et al. 2009), and is negatively correlated with number of years since injury (Miyahara et al. 2008). However, bone density is higher in the arms in wheelchair athletes compared to able-bodied controls (Miyahara et al. 2008; Sutton et al. 2009). Lower bone density is likely in those with CP, if their mobility is more confined.

Dietary issues for athletes with disabilities

22.15

The shortage of information specific to athletes with disabilities means that we can only assume that the nutrient recommendations are the same as those for able-bodied athletes. The main differences are that athletes with disabilities may have lower daily energy requirements, their macronutrient recommendations per kilogram of body mass may require modification, they may have specific hydration issues, and they possibly are more sensitive to dietary changes that affect bowel action than able-bodied athletes. These differences depend on the nature of the disability and the mobility restrictions imposed by the disability.

Current dietary intakes

22.16

Dietary intakes of athletes with disabilities have not been reported in the literature. Some papers have reported dietary intakes of non-athletic SCI individuals with reference to their increased risk of cardiovascular disease. Levine and colleagues (1992) reported that healthy SCI people ate less energy than the average population (7065 kJ for males, 5385 kJ for females). Dietary intakes in this group were relatively higher in fat and lower in CHO than the dietary goals and targets, but were not unlike dietary intakes of the general population. Even considering the extent of under-reporting of energy intake in any dietary survey, low energy intakes make it more difficult to achieve adequate nutrient intakes.

22.17 Fiber, timing of food intake and bowel control

Large bowel (and sometimes small bowel) function can be impaired if mobility is limited and gastrointestinal tract damage has occurred. As a result, frequency of bowel movement and stool formation and consistency can be affected. Some individuals may have a colostomy or ileostomy. Constipation is common and the use of bowel softeners is frequent among wheelchair-confined athletes. Timing and frequency of bowel motions need to be fairly well controlled to occur at a convenient time; therefore the type and amount of dietary fiber may require modification. A consistent dietary and fluid intake in combination with routine training of bowel habits is important for optimal control.

22.18 Fluid intake

While maintaining hydration levels is important for all athletes, the practical consequences of consuming adequate fluid require more attention for many athletes with disabilities. Proximity to appropriate toilet and water facilities and use of urine collection bags require consideration, especially in wheelchair athletes. For athletes with SCI, heat illness is not necessarily a result of insufficient fluid intake or dehydration, but rather is associated with impaired temperature regulation imposed by hot and humid weather conditions. The frequency and types of fluids recommended in Chapter 13 remain appropriate for most athletes with disabilities, provided their gastrointestinal tract is competent, although prescribed volumes may need to be lower. For example, an athlete with an ileostomy may not tolerate the usual prescribed volumes since large volumes can dump into and fill the ileostomy bag too rapidly. Sweat rate estimations, though potentially more difficult to undertake, are likely to be particularly important in athletes with disabilities to guide fluid intake recommendations. Visual assessment of urine output for hydration can also be influenced by medications, hence use of refractometers for urine specific gravity assessment is recommended.

22.19 Body composition management

Extremes of underweight and overfatness are evident in athletes with disabilities. While some body composition issues are related to the disability itself, the genetic background of the athlete is also a contributing factor. Each athlete will need to be considered on an individual basis according to the nature of their disability and any impact their disability may have on their metabolic rate.

People with intellectual disabilities often have body mass control problems for a wide variety of reasons, including poor food choices from lack of insight, food used as a comforter, either limited or excess voluntary activity, and genetic disorders (such as Down syndrome). When working with intellectually disabled athletes, it is imperative to work together with their primary carers to assist in managing the foods provided to the athlete.

Many non-wheelchair-dependent lower-limb amputees or CP athletes appear to have higher energy demands, possibly due to the greater mechanical demand of walking. The impact of using poorly fitting prostheses during exercise, and the resultant damage often incurred, leads to high nutrient requirements to facilitate healing.

The lower energy expenditures of people with SCI may be up-regulated by FES to help muscle activity. If pressure sores are frequent, energy and nutrient requirements will need to be increased to assist with healing. In practice, however, SCI athletes cannot consume high energy intakes to the same levels as able-bodied people without gaining body fat, because of a lower total lean body mass. The focus of their everyday diet should therefore be on nutrient-dense foods (rather than energy-dense foods) that are low in fat, sugar and alcohol.

Nutritional supplements 22.20

The need for nutritional supplements in athletes with disabilities is determined on a case-by-case basis. Vitamin and mineral supplements may be needed if gastrointestinal tract function is disturbed or if athletes have difficulty consuming a balanced diet or sufficient energy to maintain adequate nutrient intakes. Also, some medications compromise the metabolism of some vitamins and minerals (e.g. phenytoin and vitamin D metabolism).

Sports nutrition supplements or sports foods have the potential to improve overall energy intake as well as support performance. A study has shown that paraplegic athletes consuming a sports drink 20 minutes prior to endurance exercise had a similar physiological and metabolic response to that seen in able-bodied individuals (Spendiff & Campbell 2005). However, consumption of a high-fiber sports bar, for example, during exercise may stimulate a bowel movement at an inappropriate time.

Eating difficulties and behaviors observed in some athletes with disabilities 22.21

Regardless of whether you are working with an individual or a group of athletes with disabilities, you should be aware of various aspects of feeding or eating that differ from able-bodied athletes. Examples include but are not limited to the following:

- An amputee or someone with arm deformities may have to eat using their feet; this needs to be accounted for when deciding on accommodation and eating venues.
- People with some forms of CP and classes of 'Les Autres' (see section 22.3) will experience general feeding difficulties, with some athletes known to require enteral feeding to supplement their limited oral intake.
- Athletes with visual impairments generally work on a 'clock' system to locate foods on their plates (e.g. meat at 12 o'clock, peas at 6 o'clock). They frequently use their hands to assist with serving food and eating.
- Athletes with intellectual disabilities can display some 'unusual' responses to food and eating. Examples include unfounded fears of a specific food due to the way it looks, inability to use eating utensils in the customary manner and eating excessive quantities of foods, but not comprehending why such behavior is inappropriate. Resolving these issues takes time, patience and understanding and can challenge a practitioner's imagination, but can be very rewarding.

- When undertaking practical sessions with athletes with disabilities, such as amputations and CP, be conscious of fatigue associated with ambulation in these groups. Chairs should be made available during cooking sessions to enable rest periods, and supermarket tour durations shortened.

22.22 Summary

Working as a health professional with athletes with disabilities is both challenging and rewarding. People with disabilities have often dealt with a lot of discrimination as children and adolescents or may still be adjusting to the disability if received as an adult. They usually have a higher incidence of medical problems than other athletes, and in some cases mental health problems. Traveling away from home to competition is often stressful for athletes with disabilities and poses its own challenges for people leaving familiar surroundings. Most elite athletes with disabilities want to be self-sufficient and treated the same as any athlete without a disability. Therefore the provision of advice, care or management of the disabled elite athlete in both a training and competition situation from any health professional or coach should actively involve the athlete as well as their carers or parents.

PRACTICE TIPS

ELIZABETH BROAD

- While most techniques used to assess nutritional status can be applied to athletes with disabilities (see Chapter 2), additional information—including duration, type, cause and severity of disability, mobility, medications, feeding issues and medical considerations—is required. Sum of skinfolds and girths provide more useful information of body composition than body mass alone.
- General sports nutrition principles apply to athletes with disabilities. While exact macro- and micronutrient requirements have not been determined, they are likely to vary enormously between individuals, highlighting the need for common sense in applying recommendations. Practice similar assessments as you would an able-bodied athlete in terms of determining requirements pre-, during and post-training and the demands of their training and competition loads.
- Be aware of the terminology to use with the athlete and specifically understand the effects that inappropriate language can have on individuals with disabilities. It is also important to understand their specific sport and its rules/requirements, and their classification within the sport (who they compete against).
- Always undertake a medical history to determine other medical issues you may need to consider, including medications and supplements. If you are unsure of any aspects of the disability or associated medical conditions, or how their medication works and its side effects, consult a clinical or sports physician. If the athlete is within the first 12 months of acquiring their disability (e.g. post-trauma), they will still be undergoing many physical and psychological adjustments that can influence energy expenditure, food habits and body composition aside from adjusting to active sports participation.
- Some athletes are always accompanied by a support person or carer, who performs many functions, such as riding the front of a tandem bike for a visually impaired cyclist or assisting an athlete with CP get into position for a throwing event. It is important to respect this relationship and the intimate knowledge carers have about the athlete, and to involve them in discussions.
- Always ask the athlete if they are completely independent or if they require assistance, particularly in lifestyle-management issues; if they do require assistance, ask specifically what they need—they will generally be able to tell you succinctly.
- The energy requirements of some athletes with disabilities may be low, so consuming nutrient-dense foods is a high priority for maintaining nutritional quality. Additional support and advice are important for athletes with disabilities who travel or eat out frequently, since what may appear to some as being small changes in energy intake can have a larger impact on body fat and mass in this population. Conversely, some individuals have high energy requirements, requiring energy supplements in addition to high energy foods and fluids.
- When advising about fluid intake, ask the athlete how they manage their bladder control and the likely effects of increasing fluid intake. Be willing to trial strategies in

PRACTICE TIPS

conjunction with the athlete to come up with the best scenario and look at additional cooling methods for those with SCI.

   – When assessing hydration status, measure urine specific gravity rather than using a visual assessment.

- As with able-bodied athletes, when advising about any changes to the diet or use of sports nutrition supplements, discuss the practical implications and develop ways to practice changes within a 'safe' environment. Athletes with disabilities have misconceptions about food and diet, and similar concerns about body fat control and optimizing performance like any other person, and want to use sports food and supplements. For some athletes with disabilities, the use of these supplements may be inappropriate and unwarranted, especially if they are likely to affect bowel movements/stool consistency or energy intake. For example, dietary fiber intake and regularity of food consumption are important issues for disabled athletes to help control bowel movements and therefore avoid embarrassment and discomfort. Modifications should be made gradually and at a time and place where access to bathroom facilities is relatively easy.
- If working as part of a team, or in an unfamiliar environment for the athletes, you may be required to provide some assistance. For example, visually impaired athletes will generally require assistance in orientation and locating food and utensils at a dining hall when they first arrive. If operating from self-contained units, it is best to room them with sighted athletes with an understanding of how to explain the presentation of food on a plate (such as the clock system). Depending on the disability, assistance with carrying food to their table and cutting up food may be required.

USEFUL WEBSITE

www.paralympic.org

International Paralympic Committee: provides information on events, class of athletes, history of Paralympic sports.

REFERENCES

Abel T, Platen P. Energy expenditure in different sports for individuals with a spinal cord injury. Med Sci Sports Exerc 2003;5(Suppl):300S.

Armstrong LE, Maresh CM, Riebe D, et al. Local cooling in wheelchair athletes during exercise—heat stress. Med Sci Sports Exerc 1995;27:211–16.

Barfield JP, Malone LA, Collins JM, Ruble SB. Disability type influences heart rate response during power wheelchair sport. Med Sci Sports Exerc 2005;37:718–23.

Bhambhani YN, Burnham RS, Wheeler GD, Eriksson P, Holland LJ, Steadward RD. Physiological correlates of simulated wheelchair racing in trained quadriplegics. Can J Appl Physiol 1995;20:65–77.

Bhambhani YN, Holland LJ, Eriksson P, Steadward RD. Physiological responses during wheelchair racing in quadriplegics and paraplegics. Paraplegia 1994;3:253–60.

Broad EM. The effects of heat on performance in wheelchair shooters. Masters thesis. Canberra: University of Canberra, 1997.

Buckley J. Classification and the Games. In: Gilbert K, Schantz O, eds. The Paralympic Games: empowerment or side show? Maidenhead, UK: Meyer & Meyer Sport, 2009:90–102.

Coutts KD, Stogryn JL. Aerobic and anaerobic power of Canadian wheelchair track athletes. Med Sci Sports Exerc 1987;19:62–5.

Gass GC. Physical fitness test procedures for disabled athletes: disabled athlete assessment centre program. Lidcombe, NSW: Cumberland College of Health Sciences, 1988 (unpublished).

Genin JJ, Bastien GJ, Franck B, et al. Effect of speed on the energy cost of walking in unilateral traumatic lower limb amputees. Eur J Appl Physiol 2008;103:655–63.

Glaser RM. Exercise and locomotion for the spinal cord injured. Ex Sports Sc Rev 1985;13:263–303.

Goodman S, Lee K, Heidt F, eds. Coaching wheelchair athletes. Canberra: Australian Sports Commission, 1996.

Goosey-Tolfrey VL, Swainson M, Boyd C, Atkinson G, Tolfrey K. The effectiveness of hand cooling at reducing exercise-induced hyperthermia and improving distance-race performance in wheelchair and able-bodied athletes. J Appl Physiol 2008a;105:37–43.

Goosey-Tolfrey VL, Diaper NJ, Crosland J, Tolfrey K. Fluid intake during wheelchair exercise in the heat: effects of localized cooling garments. Int J Sports Physiol Perform 2008b;3;145–156.

Hjeltnes N. Control of medical rehabilitation of paraplegics and tetraplegics by repeated evaluation of endurance capacity. Int J Sports Med 1984;5(Suppl):171S–4S.

Hopman MTE, Oeseburg B, Binkhorst RA. Cardiovascular responses in persons with paraplegia to prolonged arm exercise and thermal stress. Med Sci Sports Exerc 1993;25:577–83.

Johnson RK, Goran MI, Ferrara MS, Poehlman ET. Athetosis increases resting metabolic rate in adults with cerebral palsy. J Am Diet Assoc 1996;96:145–8.

Johnson RK, Hildreth HG, Contompasis SH, Goran MI. Total energy expenditure in adults with cerebral palsy as assessed by doubly-labeled water. J Am Diet Assoc 1997;97:966–70.

Karlsson J, Saltin B. Diet, muscle glycogen and endurance performance. J Appl Physiol 1971;21:203–6.

Kennedy M. The effect of drugs on heat regulation. In: Sutton JR, Thompson MW, Torode ME, eds. Exercise and thermoregulation. Sydney: The University of Sydney, 1995:223–33.

Knechtle B, Muller G, Willmann F, Eser P, Knecht H. Comparison of fat oxidation in arm cranking in spinal cord-injured people versus ergometry in cyclists. Eur J Appl Physiol 2003;90:614–19.

Knechtle B, Muller G, Willmann F, Eser P, Knecht H. Fat oxidation at different intensities in wheelchair racing. Spinal Cord 2004a;42:24–8.

Knechtle B, Muller G, Knecht H. Optimal exercise intensities for fat metabolism in handbike cycling and cycling. Spinal Cord 2004b;42:564–72.

Levine AM, Nash MS, Green BA, Shea JD, Aronica MJ. An examination of dietary intakes and nutritional status of chronic healthy spinal cord-injured individuals. Paraplegia 1992;30:880–9.

Miyahara K, Wang D, Mori K, Takahashi K, Miyatake N, Wang B, Takigawa T, Takaki J, Ogino K. Effect of sports activity on bone mineral density in wheelchair athletes. J Bone Miner Metab 2008;26:101–6.

MIMS Australia. MIMS annual 2005. Sydney: Medi Media, 2005.

Noreau L, Shephard RJ. Spinal cord injury, exercise and quality of life. Sports Med 1995;20:226–50.

Normell LA. Distribution of impaired cutaneous vasomotor and sudomotor function in paraplegic man. Scand J Clin Lab Invest 1974;33(Suppl):25S–41S.

Petrofsky JS. Thermoregulatory stress during rest and exercise in heat in patients with a spinal cord injury. Eur J Appl Physiol 1992;64:503–7.

Price MJ. Thermoregulation during exercise in individuals with spinal cord injury. Sports Med 2006;36:863–79.

Price MJ, Campbell IG. Thermoregulatory responses of spinal cord injured and able-bodied athletes to prolonged upper body exercise and recovery. Spinal Cord 1999;37:772–9.

Price MJ, Campbell IG. Effects of spinal cord lesion level upon thermoregulation during exercise in the heat. Med Sci Sports Exerc 2003;35:1100–7.

Sawka MN, Gonzalez RR, Drolet LL, Pandolf KB. Heat exchange during upper- and lower-body exercise. J Appl Physiol 1984;57:1050–4.

Shephard RJ. Sports medicine and the wheelchair athlete. Sports Med 1988;4:226–47.

Skrinar GS, Evans WJ, Ornstein LJ, Brown DA. Glycogen utilisation in wheelchair-dependent athletes. Int J Sports Med 1982;3:215–19.

Spendiff O, Campbell IG. Influence of pre-exercise glucose ingestion of two concentrations on paraplegic athletes. J Sport Sci 2005;23:21–30.

Sutton L, Wallace J, Goosey-Tolfrey V, Scott M, Reilly T. Body composition of female wheelchair athletes. Int J Sports Med 2009;30:259–65.

Suzuki N, Oshimi Y, Shinohara T, Kawasumi M, Mita K. Exercise intensity based on heart rate while walking in spastic cerebral palsy. Bull Hosp Jt Dis 2001;60:18–22.

Thompson BA. Comparisons of bone mineral density between elite spinal cord injured athletes and able-bodied individuals. Med Sci Sports Exerc 2000;5(Suppl):355S.

Van der Woude LH, Bakker WH, Elkhuizen JW, Veeger HE, Gwinn T. Anaerobic work capacity in elite wheelchair athletes. Am J Phys Med Rehabil 1997;76:355–65.

Webborn N, Price MJ, Castle PC, Goosey-Tolfrey VL. Effects of two cooling strategies on thermoregulatory responses of tetraplegic athletes during repeated intermittent exercise in the heat. J Appl Physiol 2005;98:2101–7.

Webborn N, Price MJ, Castle PC, Goosey-Tolfrey VL. Cooling strategies improve intermittent sprint performance in the heat of athletes with tetraplegia. Br J Sports Med Online 2008;June 14.

Wicks JR, Oldridge NB, Cameron BJ, Jones NL. Arm cranking and wheelchair ergometry in elite spinal cord-injured athletes. Med Sci Sports Exerc 1983;15:224–31.

Winnick JP, ed. Adapted physical education and sport. Second edition. Champaign, Illinois: Human Kinetics, 1995:167–71, 193–212.

Yizhar Z, Boulos S, Inbar O, Carmeli E. The effect of restricted arm swing on energy expenditure in healthy men. Int J Rehabil Res 2008; Dec 5.

Acknowledgments

The author would like to acknowledge the assistance of Jane Buckley, Chief Classifier (Swimming), Athens 2004 and Beijing 2008 Paralympic Games and Flavia Traven in researching this chapter.

CHAPTER 23

Medical and nutritional issues for the traveling athlete

PETER FRICKER

Introduction 23.1

Today's international athlete is a global traveler and as a result the sports nutritionist is presented with specific nutritional and medical problems. These problems include an increased risk of illness, particularly food- and water-borne illness, jet lag and environmental stress. Early preparation and education is important for prevention. Well before departure, it is the responsibility of the sports medicine team to identify specific problems at the destination and institute strategies for prevention. Such strategies include the planning of vaccination programs (including malarial prophylaxis) and educating athletes and officials about minimizing travel illness and jet lag. This should be done with the help of practitioners who are experienced in the problems of overseas travel, as recommendations vary and are specific to each destination.

Jet lag and jet stress 23.2

International air travel presents the modern phenomena known as jet lag and jet stress. Jet lag refers to problems relating to air travel as a result of the rapid traversal of time zones between countries across the world. It often leads to fatigue, disturbance of the day/night cycle, sleeping difficulties, and mood and bowel disturbances.

Measures to minimize the symptoms of jet lag include setting watches to the destination time on or before departure; avoiding late-night departures; careful planning of flights to maximize appropriate sleep time; and the judicious use of hypnotic drugs, during and immediately after flight. Adopting destination sleep times before departure can also help decrease the effects of jet lag. On arrival, it is important to establish a new sleep/wake cycle as soon as possible, by early exposure to sunlight and physical activity, and avoiding sleep during the daytime.

Jet lag can hinder performance, so adequate time is needed after arrival and before competition to adjust to the new time zone. Adjustments vary among individuals, but usually one full day of acclimatization is required for every (1-hour) time zone crossed (French 1995). Up to three time zones may be crossed, however, before an effect on performance is noticed. Westbound travel tends to cause less jet lag as the body's circadian rhythms are on a 25-hour cycle and traveling west results in a longer day (Manfredini et al. 1998).

Jet stress refers to external problems in transit as a result of air travel and is independent of the number of time zones crossed. The air in the aircraft cabin is relatively dry, so an increased fluid intake is required to counteract increased respiratory fluid losses. Drinks that contain caffeine (such as coffee) were previously thought to contribute to hypohydration, but more recent work has shown that moderate intakes of caffeine by habitual caffeine users do not affect urine losses and hydration status (Armstrong 2002; Armstrong et al. 2005). The effects of alcohol are increased in the pressurized cabin environment so alcohol is best avoided, especially in excessive amounts. Airlines tend to provide a limited variety of foods during travel, but special meals can be arranged in advance. Usually a minimum of 24 hours' notice is required by most airlines for individual catering requests, but a longer period is advised for teams. In general, during long flights athletes should be encouraged to make the flight as comfortable as possible (with bulkhead and aisle seats), use music or literature for relaxation, and carry water bottles and small amounts of carbohydrate-rich foods for consumption during the flight. Careful planning and timing of flights to avoid delays or lengthy periods in transit lounges minimizes the effects of jet stress.

On arrival, adequate time must be allowed for acclimatization to environmental conditions as well as to recover from jet lag. As heat acclimatization may take up to 2 weeks, many athletes can start acclimatizing before departure by exercising in hot environments. However, hypohydration from airline travel itself or from the local climate can negate the adaptive changes of heat acclimatization accomplished at home prior to the journey. In hot and humid countries and sporting venues, sweat rates during physical activity can exceed 2 L/h. Competing athletes may need to increase fluid consumption by up to 10 L/d in such environments to prevent dehydration (Young et al. 1998). Regular monitoring of early morning body weights of individual athletes is useful to determine hydration status. Fluctuations of more than 1–2 kg weight loss during the day, for example, may indicate hypohydration. Indicators of good hydration status from early morning urine samples include color (urine should be light and produced in good volumes) and, where measurements are available, specific gravity or osmolality (Oppliger et al. 2005). This is covered in greater detail in Chapter 14. Drinking large volumes of water, especially during hard exercise, may lower the serum sodium concentration and osmolality in susceptible people. Use of a sports drink that contains low levels of sodium and other sugars such that it is iso-osmolar (the same concentration as solutes in the blood serum) can help to address this potential problem. However, while athletes should be advised to be vigilant about fluid needs, they may also need to be warned against consumption of excessive amounts of fluid such that they become substantially overhydrated.

23.3 Illnesses associated with traveling

All athletes are at risk of acquiring infection from unusual organisms, especially those spread by the feco-oral route and by insect vectors. Travelers' diarrhea affects between 20% and 50% of travelers spending around two weeks in a 'developing' country (O'Kane

& Gottlieb 1996). Most travel-related diarrhea is caused by non-viral pathogens such as enterotoxigenic *Escherichia coli, Salmonella, Shigella, Campylobacter* and *Giardia lamblia*. These pathogens are transmitted in food, water, from other people, from poor sanitary conditions, and from poor personal and food hygiene practices.

Prevention and treatment of diarrhea, nausea and vomiting 23.4

Many of the infections by these pathogens can be prevented by attention to personal hygiene, including washing hands thoroughly with soap before meals, and ensuring that food has been freshly cooked, and that shellfish, unpasteurized milk and unpeeled fruits and vegetables are not consumed. In many countries, the drinking water contains potential pathogenic micro-organisms, which can be transmitted in raw food (such as salads and vegetables) washed in water, in ice cubes and even by brushing the teeth in tap water. Tap water is 'safe' for consumption if boiled for at least five minutes. Water-purifying tablets purchased in pharmacies are another alternative, but are not always effective.

In countries where the risk of travelers' diarrhea is high, it may be appropriate to use prophylactic short-term antibiotics, such as ciprofloxacin (500 mg daily), or doxycycline (100 mg/d), or sulphamethoxazole (800 mg/d) with trimethoprim (100 mg/d). If diarrheal illness does occur, it is wise to consume a bland diet such as dry toast, biscuits, rice and bananas, and avoid alcohol, fat-rich foods and dairy foods until the diarrhea settles. When diarrhea occurs, an increased fluid intake with drinks such as water or electrolyte rehydration salts is required and these should be consumed in small amounts, but often. Antidiarrheal drugs can be used if there is no blood or mucus, but since diarrhea is nature's way of flushing out the pathogens, the illness may be prolonged by their use. If the diarrhea is associated with fever, blood or mucus, antibiotics may be required and a doctor should prescribe these. If low-grade diarrhea persists for more than 3 days, *Giardia lamblia* may be the underlying organism and antibiotics such as metronidazole or tinidazole may be required. Many organisms cause symptoms that may not present until return to the country of origin, and all athletes should be advised to seek medical advice in any case of post-travel illness.

Summary 23.5

With careful preparation, education and appropriate management, most travelers' problems can be prevented.

PRACTICE TIPS

LORNA GARDEN

PRIOR TO DEPARTURE

- Determine all aspects of an athlete's trip (including travel arrangements, accommodation and competition times and venues) well in advance to ensure appropriate and specific practical advice and goal setting can be provided. Table 23.1 provides a checklist of issues to investigate prior to departure.
- Encourage athletes to use a diary to plan and document proposed meal and snack times around travel, training and competition.

TRAVELING LOCALLY

- Where there is an option, staying in self-contained accommodation can provide greater flexibility in food choices and preparation. Discuss portable foods to carry or purchase, as well as cooking utensils (such as a hand-held blender for smoothies, a rice cooker or an electric wok) to bring, where appropriate. Chapter 25 provides additional practical suggestions for self-catering and how to choose foods that meet dietary goals when eating out.
- During road travel carry a small insulated bag with portable snacks (see Table 23.2).
- When traveling by train or bus, check the availability of food en route and the frequency of food stops. Advise athletes to carry snacks to avoid reliance on take-aways and long gaps with nothing to eat.
- For teams traveling to training camps or competitions that last for several days, contact accommodation venues in advance and request 'in-house' menus and offer assistance in menu planning (see Chapter 25). Provide suggestions for food choices and menu plans from the existing menu to catering staff, managers, coaches and athletes prior to departure. Some (but not all) caterers welcome these suggestions and may be receptive to preparing special meals for athletes.

TABLE 23.1 PRE-TRAVEL CHECKLIST
• Vaccinations (where necessary)
• Itinerary, including modes of transport, traveling times and likely breaks in the journey (e.g. meal stops, refueling stops and overnight stopovers)
• Training and competition schedule
• Type of accommodation and meal arrangements
• Trip coordinator/team manager's details
• Familiarity with place of destination (e.g. climate, time zones and food and drink availability)
• Local customs relevant to the athlete (e.g. clothing, language and dietary habits)
• Baggage limits, including equipment
• Food, fluids and supplements (including 'survival kit') to be taken or provided by team management (where applicable)

TABLE 23.2 SUITABLE SNACKS FOR TRAVELING
• Fruit (if traveling locally) or canned fruit
• Dried fruit and nuts
• Rice crackers, pretzels
• Popcorn made with minimum fat/oil
• Muesli and cereal bars, breakfast bars, energy bars (low-fat)
• Dry cereal (in serve-size boxes)
• Low-fat fruit yoghurt or fromage frais
• Low-fat rice pudding
• Sandwiches, rolls, mini bagels, fruit bread, low-fat muffins, pikelets
• Low-fat cheese sticks
• Canned tuna or salmon
• Jelly confectionery (in moderation) and energy bars (low-fat)
• Low-fat flavored or plain milk
• Water, fruit juice, sports drinks, liquid meal supplements (such as Sustagen® Sport or Powerbar Protein Plus®)

TRAVELING OVERSEAS

- Prior to and during overseas travel in countries where the risk of travelers' diarrhea is high, taking probiotic supplements or consuming yoghurts containing probiotic cultures may be useful in reducing the incidence of travelers' diarrhea and assisting recovery (Fedorak & Masden 2004).
- Airlines provide special meal options (such as low-fat, vegetarian and sports meals), which are ordered at time of booking or at least 48 hours prior to departure.
- When traveling to unfamiliar countries where usual foods are unavailable, the athlete should pack a supply of food staples to accompany them on their travels or to be sent to their destination ahead of time. Liquid meal supplements, dried milk powder, breakfast cereals, cereal and sports bars are portable and useful travel items (see Table 23.2). It is worthwhile checking customs regulations before taking or sending any food and drink overseas.
- Prior to departure, athletes can benefit by familiarizing themselves with the food choices and dietary customs of their destination by eating in local restaurants offering similar cuisine.
- Encourage athletes to include a personal first aid and survival kit, especially when traveling overseas. Include the usual first aid items, supplements (e.g. multivitamins/minerals and probiotics), electrolyte-replacement sachets (in case of vomiting and diarrhea), antibacterial wipes for hands (for hygiene) and a food thermometer. This kit is a good idea for domestic travel as well.

PREVENTING JET LAG

Table 23.3 overleaf provides dietary strategies to help minimize jet lag.

PRACTICE TIPS

TABLE 23.3 DIETARY STRATEGIES TO HELP PREVENT JET LAG
• Adapt meal and snack times to destination time 24–48 hours before departure, and during the flight.
• High-carbohydrate, low-protein meals during transit may help induce drowsiness.
• Respiratory fluid losses are increased in the dry environment of a pressurized cabin. Bring a water bottle that can be refilled and sipped continuously to ensure replacement of fluid losses.
• Avoid, or be moderate with, the intake of alcoholic beverages, as the effects of alcohol are exacerbated in the plane environment.
• Pre-arrange special meals that provide carbohydrate and are low in fat.
• Pack portable, high-carbohydrate snacks (including fruit) in your hand luggage.
• Keep a food diary to remind you of when you last ate.
• Bring plenty of activities (e.g. books, games and CDs) to prevent boredom eating.
• Adopt regular meal and snack patterns upon arrival and sustain a higher fluid intake until well hydrated.

PREVENTING FOOD- OR WATER-BORNE ILLNESS

- The risk of food- and water-borne illnesses is minimized in any situation (either at home or away from home) by paying attention to personal hygiene (frequent hand washing), by avoiding foods that are high-risk for contamination, and by adopting hygienic food handling and storage practices (see Table 23.4 for tips).
- High-risk foods for contamination are uncooked fresh foods (meat, fish, vegetables and eggs), unpasteurized dairy products and reheated foods. Cross-contamination of foods also comes from leaving foods uncovered in the refrigerator, and re-using cutting boards, cooking and eating utensils, tea towels and dishcloths.
- Table 23.4 lists practical tips for athletes to raise awareness of food hygiene and food safety issues that can help prevent food-borne illness.

STRATEGIES FOR TREATING DIARRHEA AND VOMITING

- Replacing fluids and electrolytes is the main priority if travelers' diarrhea or vomiting occurs. Low-fat, low-fiber foods can be gradually introduced as tolerated. Table 23.5 provides detailed strategies for dietary treatment of nausea, vomiting and diarrhea.

MEETING DIETARY GOALS

- Regular weight and/or skinfold checks are useful to help prevent substantial body composition changes, a common occurrence observed when athletes are away from home. The easy access to inappropriate food choices at sporting venues, buffet-style eating in restaurants or unfamiliar foods makes it difficult for athletes to maintain weight status or meet their prescribed or usual training diet. Dietary strategies to address this changing environment are best given prior to departure and reinforced by coaches and managers while away (see Chapter 25).
- Monitoring of morning body weight and the characteristics of morning urine samples can be used to gauge the success of hydration strategies (see Chapter 14).

TABLE 23.4 PREVENTING NUTRITION-RELATED ILLNESSES WHEN TRAVELING OVERSEAS
• Wash hands with soap frequently, and for at least 30 seconds, especially before eating. Use a clean towel or air dryer to dry hands.
• If the local water supply is unsafe, boil all drinking water, or preferably drink bottled water. Soft drink is 'safe', but should not be used as a substitute for water.
• Avoid ice in drinks unless you are sure the water is safe for drinking.
• Avoid eating salad or raw vegetables unless the food has been washed in water that is safe for drinking.
• Peel all fruit.
• Avoid other raw foods such as oysters, shellfish and raw fish (as eaten in sushi).
• Avoid buying foods from local stalls and markets where hygiene may be poor.
• If possible, check that cooked food is kept hot (>60°C) and has not been re-warmed or kept warm for more than 2 hours, and that raw food (such as meat) is kept refrigerated.
• Avoid buffet food that is not served very hot or chilled, or which has been sitting for extended periods of time.
• In countries where food hygiene and safety standards are questionable, select foods that have been cooked to order rather than pre-cooked and re-heated.

TABLE 23.5 DIET THERAPY FOR NAUSEA, VOMITING AND DIARRHEA
NAUSEA/VOMITING
• Withhold food in the short term, but maintain fluid intake.
• Consume small, frequent meals (such as dry crackers, plain rice or noodles or dry toast at first, then progress to light, low-fat meals as tolerated).
• Elevate the head, eat slowly.
DIARRHEA
• Maintain a high fluid intake using bottled water and electrolyte replacement drink or sports drink. Avoid milk, caffeine drinks (such as coffee and cola), gaseous drinks (such as soft drinks) and fruit juice.
• In the acute stage, avoid very high-fiber foods and spicy foods and other foods specific to the individual that cause flatulence.
• Avoid fatty foods and high sugar foods.
• Introduce small amounts of low-fiber foods initially (e.g. plain rice, noodles, dry white toast, dry low-fat crackers or canned pears) and, once tolerated, slowly increase dietary fiber intake back to normal.
• Consider taking probiotics and prebiotics to reduce the incidence of diarrhea and help restore natural gut bacteria.

Source: Adapted from Deakin 1998

PRACTICE TIPS

- Daily recording of food intake works well for some athletes (although not many) to control eating behavior while away. It also provides an opportunity to more accurately assess individual food choices and eating behaviors on return, compared to retrospective dietary assessment methods, and allows the dietitian to address any concerns for future travel.
- Regular communication with the athlete living or traveling overseas for extended periods via email or fax is invaluable for providing encouragement, support and preventing diet- and often health-related problems.
- On return, a follow-up appointment with an individual athlete or a group session with a team is invaluable to assist with evaluating any diet-related issues and to check the efficacy of the strategies you provided. This session reinforces dietary goals and helps to better target the dietary intervention strategies for future travel.

USEFUL WEBSITES

http://www.betterhealth.vic.gov.au/bhcv2/bhcarticles.nsf/pages/Travel_health_tips?OpenDocument
Travel health tips (Australian Government site)
http://www.healthinsite.gov.au/topics/Jet_Lag
Minimizing jet lag (Australian Government site)
http://www.cochrane.org/reviews/en/ab001520.html
Melatonin for the prevention and treatment of jet lag

REFERENCES

Armstrong LE. Caffeine, body fluid-electrolyte balance, and exercise performance. Int J Sport Nutr Exerc Metab 2002;12:189–206.

Armstrong LE, Pumerantz AC, Roti MW, Judelson DA, Watson G, Dias JC, Sokmen B, Casa DJ, Maresh CM, Lieberman H, Kellogg M. Fluid, electrolyte, and renal indices of hydration during 11 days of controlled caffeine consumption. Int J Sport Nutr Exerc Metab 2005;15:252–65.

Deakin V. Prevention and treatment of foodborne illness when travelling. Sports Coach 1998;21:15–16.

Fedorak RN, Madsen KL. Probiotics and prebiotics in gastrointestinal disorders. Curr Opin Gastroenterol 2004;20:146–55.

French J. Circadian rhythms, jet lag and the athlete. In: Torg JS, Shephard RJ, eds. Current therapeutics in sports medicine. St Louis: Mosby, 1995:596–600.

Manfredini R, Manfredini F, Fersini C, Conconi F. Circadian rhythms, athletic performance, and jet lag. Br J Sports Med 1998;32:101–6.

O'Kane G, Gottlieb T. Travellers' diarrhoea. Curr Therap 1996;Feb:53–60.

Oppliger RA, Magnes SA, Popowski LA, Gisolfi CV. Accuracy of urine specific gravity and osmolality as indicators of hydration status. Int J Sport Nutr Exerc Metabol 2005;15:236–51.

Young M, Fricker P, Maughan R, MacAuley D. The travelling athlete: issues relating to the Commonwealth Games, Malaysia, 1998. Br J Sports Med 1998;32:77–81.

CHAPTER 24

Nutritional issues for special environments: training and competing at altitude and in hot climates

MARK FEBBRAIO AND DAVID MARTIN

Introduction

24.1

It is fairly common for athletes to train and compete in environmental conditions that can compromise performance. For many endurance athletes, heat and altitude are the most common environmental challenges that have been shown to detrimentally influence endurance performance. In addition to the many known physiological effects of heat and altitude there are other less-well-understood psychological aspects of heat or altitude acclimation training camps that may influence what athletes eat. The purpose of this chapter is to review some of the many interesting aspects of nutrition for athletes training and competing in these unique environmental conditions.

During exercise the conversion of chemical energy into mechanical work is increased several-fold. Given that most chemical energy is derived from the diet, nutritional supplementation and its effect on exercise performance has been an area of scientific interest for over 100 years. In the latter half of the twentieth century, the popularization of the muscle biopsy technique, arteriovenous (a-v) balance measurements and, more recently, the use of isotope tracers as metabolic probes during exercise have made it possible to clearly investigate the role of nutrition in exercise science. Much of the research that has examined the interaction between nutrition and exercise has been conducted at sea level and in comfortable ambient conditions. It is clear, however, that both altitude and environmental temperature are major practical issues that should be considered before advising athletes on the best way to eat and train in these unique environments.

24.2 Nutritional requirements at high altitude

24.3 Substrate utilization at high altitude: acute and chronic exposure

Acute exposure to high altitude results in an increased dependence on blood glucose as a fuel at rest and during exercise (Brooks et al. 1991a, 1991b, 1992; Roberts et al. 1996b). This increase in glucose utilization during exercise does not appear to be accompanied by a concomitant decrease in muscle glycogen use (Green et al. 1989), but rather a decreased reliance on fat as a substrate (Roberts et al. 1996a). Interestingly, after chronic exposure to altitude, the increase in blood glucose disposal is augmented rather than attenuated. Brooks and colleagues (1991b) demonstrated that, upon arrival at altitude (4300 m), glucose disposal during exercise increased by approximately 25%. However, this increase was markedly augmented after 21 days' exposure at this altitude (see Fig. 24.1).

Whether carbohydrate (CHO) oxidation rates are noticeably increased after exposure to moderate altitude, which is more frequently encountered by endurance athletes, is unknown. However, at the Australian Institute of Sport (AIS) we have observed noticeably higher blood lactate concentrations in endurance cyclists exercising at submaximal workloads at about 2500 m (e.g. 6 versus 4 mM @ 250 W), an observation indicative of either increased reliance on glycogen as a fuel source increasing lactate production (Ra) or a decrease in lactate oxidation compromising lactate removal (Rd).

If CHO oxidation is noticeably increased at altitude then athletes exercising at high altitude are presented with a unique challenge, particularly those who are exposed to

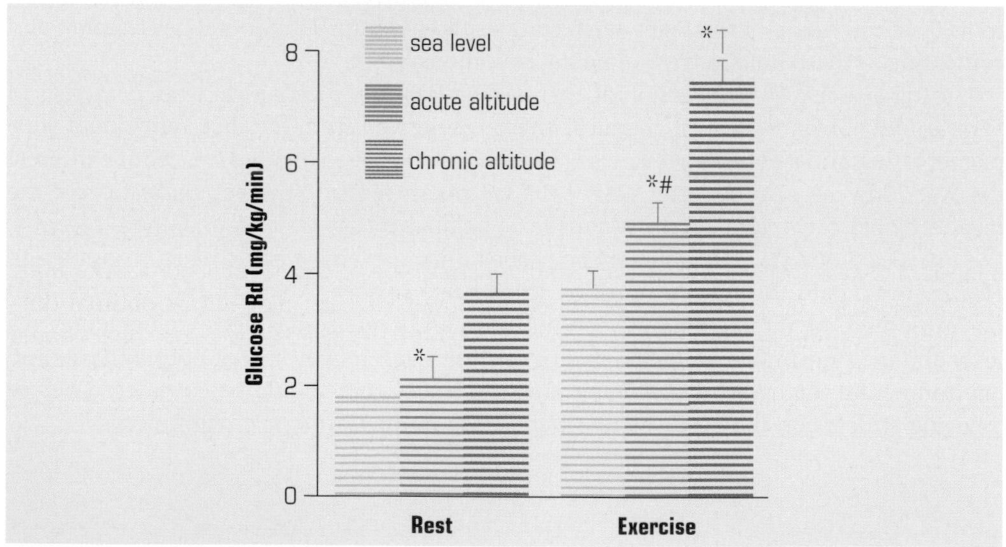

FIGURE 24.1 Rate of glucose disappearance (Rd) at rest and after 45 minutes of exercise at sea level, upon arrival at 4300 m (acute altitude) and after 21 days at 4300 m (chronic altitude). *denotes different ($p < 0.05$) from rest, # denotes different ($p < 0.05$) from sea level, T denotes different ($p < 0.05$) from sea level and acute altitude. Data expressed as mean ± SE ($n = 7$). Adapted from Brooks et al. 1991b

this environment for several days or weeks. The endogenous CHO reserves are limited and there is a heavy reliance on CHO during exercise. As athletes become acclimatized to altitude, physical work capacity is increased (Sutton et al. 1988); therefore, the reliance on endogenous CHO stores is increased. Hence, the reliance on CHO as a substrate increases in both relative and absolute terms.

Energy requirements at high altitude

24.4

It is clear that, upon initial exposure to high altitude, basal metabolic rate (BMR) increases (Kellogg et al. 1957; Moore et al. 1987; Butterfield et al. 1992). This increase may be as high as 28% above that observed at sea level (Butterfield et al. 1992) and, although most studies observe an attenuation in the increase in BMR after 2–3 days of exposure, Butterfield and colleagues (1992) observed this increase to be maintained for up to 3 weeks. Although the exact mechanism for the elevation in BMR has not been fully elucidated, it has been suggested that an increase in stress hormone secretion and/or an inadequate energy intake may be responsible (Butterfield 1999). Both acute and chronic exposure to altitude increases the sympatho-adrenal response during exercise (Mazzeo et al. 1991). However, since glucose appears to be the sole contributor to the increased energy turnover at rest, it is unlikely that an increase in adrenaline mediates this response, since adrenaline infusion reduces, rather than increases, glucose disposal at rest (Bonen et al. 1992). It is more likely that an inadequate energy intake is responsible for the increase in BMR. High altitude exposure greater than 3500 m results in appetite suppression and reduced nutritional intake (Consolazio et al. 1968). Interestingly, when weight is maintained during exposure to altitude the increase in BMR is 7% compared with 28% when subjects ingested food ad libitum (at any time) (Butterfield 1999), suggesting a relationship between BMR and energy balance.

It appears, therefore, that energy intake at high altitude should be greater than that at sea level, even though the appetite is suppressed. Since blood glucose oxidation appears to be increased during exercise at altitude, it would be wise to ingest a diet rich in CHO. In fact, it has been suggested that a CHO-rich diet decreases the symptoms of acute mountain sickness compared with the consumption of a mixed diet (Consolazio et al. 1969). These recommendations assume endurance athletes exercising at moderate altitude respond similarly to the moderately trained individuals who have participated in high altitude research. Whether this assumption is true requires additional study. Also of interest is our observation that many athletes use altitude training camps as an opportunity to reduce body weight and body-fat levels. Since a low-energy/low-CHO diet may not be optimal during altitude training in view of increased energy and CHO needs, the practitioner should always ascertain whether athletes who are attending an altitude training camp are trying to achieve a weight-management goal. Although moderate altitude can reduce absolute exercise intensity, many coaches and athletes select high-volume training programs during altitude camps, a training approach that continues to require high energy expenditure.

Maintaining fluid balance

24.5

One of the major responses to acute altitude exposure is an initial reduction in total body water and plasma volume (Pugh 1964; Hannon et al. 1969). It has been suggested that this fluid loss and resultant hemoconcentration increases the oxygen-carrying capacity of the blood until polycythemia occurs (Grover et al. 1986). In addition, because the air at altitude is dry and cold, water is lost to the environment through breathing. Hence, any fluid loss due to thermoregulation associated with exercise is augmented at altitude. Fluid requirements at rest and during exercise at altitude are thus increased compared with sea level. Given that CHO requirements are increased it would be practical to ingest a sports drink beverage when exposed to altitude. Importantly, commercially available sports drinks contain sodium, potassium and chloride. Although the addition of sodium does not increase glucose or fluid bioavailability during exercise (Hargreaves et al. 1994), such an addition will maintain the drive for drinking, minimize urinary fluid loss during exercise and maintain the extracellular fluid volume space (Maughan & Leiper 1995; Takamata et al. 1995; Nose et al. 1988). Although attention to hydration during exercise cannot be overstated, many athletes concerned with hydration tend to consume excessive amounts of fluids prior to going to sleep. This practice invariably results in a restless night's sleep as the athlete is required to make frequent trips to the toilet. By focusing on hydration issues in the morning and afternoon it is possible to adopt a more moderate approach to fluid consumption during evening meals and pre-bedtime snacks.

24.6 Summary of altitude nutrition issues

In summary, when exposed to altitude both acutely and for a period of time, CHO use is increased and BMR is increased. The alterations are accompanied by a reduced appetite, usually energy imbalance and sometimes cachexia. Therefore, CHO intake should be increased appropriately. Since the appetite is usually suppressed in this environment, it would be prudent to ingest CHO-dense food. Exposure to altitude also results in a decrease in total body water and, therefore, it is important to increase fluid consumption. Of course, it is important to remember that these recommendations are based on studies of high-altitude environments and must be tempered when applied to athletes training at moderate altitude. In such environments, the most important issue may be to advise against reductions in CHO and energy to achieve weight loss.

24.7 Exercise in a hot environment

24.8 Substrate utilization during exercise in the heat

Although there is some conflict in the literature, it is generally accepted that exercise in a hot environment results in a substrate shift towards increased CHO utilization. Muscle glycogenolysis (Fink et al. 1975; Febbraio et al. 1994a, 1994b), liver glucose production (Hargreaves et al. 1996a) and respiratory exchange ratio (RER) (Febbraio et al. 1994a, 1994b; Hargreaves et al. 1996a) are higher during exercise in a hot environment. Furthermore, both muscle (Young et al. 1985; Febbraio et al. 1994a, 1994b) and plasma (Fink et al. 1975; Powers et al. 1985; Young et al. 1985; Yaspelkis et al. 1993; Febbraio et al. 1994a) lactate accumulation are increased in humans during exercise in the heat compared with similar exercise in a cool environment. The increase in CHO utilization at a given workload appears to coincide with a reduced lipid utilization during exercise in the heat. Both plasma-free fatty acid uptake (Gonzalez-Alonso et al. 1999) and intramuscular triglyceride utilization (Fink et al. 1975) are reduced during exercise and thermal stress. These data, along with the consistent observation of an increased RER during exercise and heat stress (Febbraio et al. 1994a, 1994b; Hargreaves et al. 1996a) suggest a substrate shift away from lipid and towards CHO use.

Apart from the increase in CHO use during exercise and heat stress, recent data also suggest that protein degradation may increase during exercise in a hot environment. Mittleman and colleagues (1998) have demonstrated that branched-chain amino acid (BCAA) supplementation increased endurance performance during exercise in the heat. This finding is in contrast with studies conducted during exercise in cooler environments (Van Hall et al. 1995; Madsen et al. 1996). Of note, studies conducted in our laboratory have observed an increase in ammonia (NH_3) accumulation during exercise and heat stress (Snow et al. 1993; Febbraio et al. 1994a). Although a major pathway for NH_3 production during exercise is via the deamination of adenosine 5′-monophosphate to form NH_3 and inosine 5′-monophosphate (IMP), NH_3 can also be formed in skeletal muscle via the oxidation of BCAA. Accordingly, BCAA supplementation augments muscle NH_3 production during exercise (MacLean et al. 1996). In one of our studies (Febbraio et al. 1994b), the augmented muscle NH_3 accumulation, when comparing exercise in the heat with that in a cooler environment, was observed in the absence of any difference in IMP accumulation, suggesting that enhanced BCAA oxidation may have accounted for the increase.

It appears, therefore, that protein requirements may need to be increased when exercise training is undertaken in a hot environment. It should be noted, however, that few studies have examined the relationship between exercise in the heat and protein requirements, and further research is required before definitive recommendations can be made. Another important consideration is that many studies fixed external power output and then evaluated substrate utilization in cool and warm conditions. In reality, athletes tend to self-select lower power output for exercise sessions performed in the heat. For this reason the athlete may self-regulate exercise in such a way that protein needs and CHO needs are not noticeably altered. As previously suggested, additional research is required to establish modifications to nutrient recommendations when exercising in the heat.

Is carbohydrate availability limiting during exercise in the heat? 24.9

During submaximal exercise in comfortable ambient temperatures, the rate of energy utilization is closely matched by rates of energy provision. It is well established that in these circumstances fatigue is often associated with glycogen depletion and/or hypoglycemia (Coyle et al. 1986; Sahlin et al. 1990) and endurance can be increased by providing exogenous CHO during exercise (Coyle et al. 1986; Coggan & Coyle 1987). Since CHO utilization is augmented during exercise in the heat and fatigue often coincides with depletion of this substrate, it is somewhat paradoxical that fatigue during exercise in the heat is often related to factors other than substrate depletion. We (Parkin et al. 1999) and others (Nielsen et al. 1990; Gonzalez-Alonso et al. 1999) have demonstrated that intramuscular glycogen content is approximately 300 $mmol.kg^{-1}$ dry weight (dw) at fatigue when, during exercise in cooler environments, this figure is usually less than 150 $mmol.kg^{-1}$ dw (see Fig. 24.2 overleaf).

This may be because hyperthermia may lead to fatigue prior to CHO stores being compromised. This hypothesis is supported by the observations that, when exercising in the heat to exhaustion, subjects will fatigue at the same body core temperature even if interventions such as acclimatization (Nielsen et al. 1993) or fluid/CHO ingestion (Febbraio et al. 1996b) alter the duration of exercise. There may be circumstances, however, where

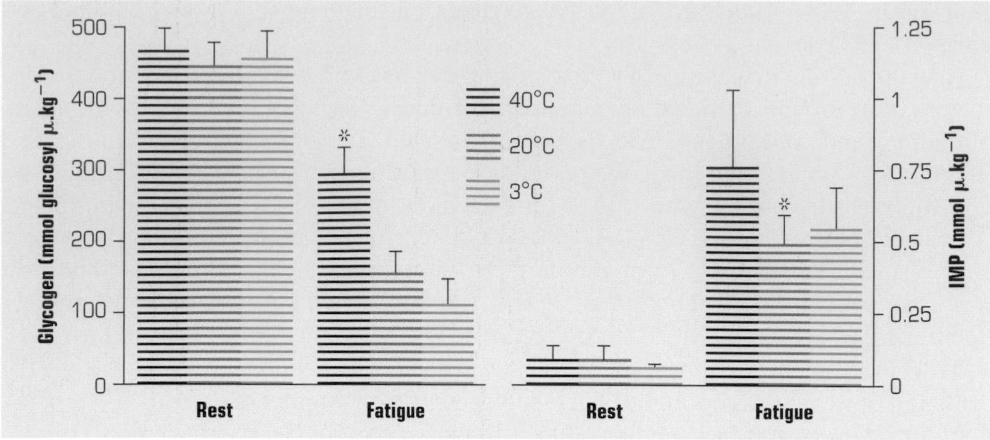

FIGURE 24.2 Glycogen content and inosine 5′-monophosphate (IMP) concentration before (Rest) and after (Fatigue) submaximal exercise to exhaustion in different ambient temperatures. Data expressed as mean ± SE (n = 8). *indicates main effect ($p < 0.05$) for exercise. Adapted from Parkin et al. 1999

CHO may be limiting during exercise in the heat. If the intensity of exercise is moderate, resulting in a relatively low rate of endogenous heat production, or the exercise is intermittent in nature, allowing for effective heat dissipation, CHO may be limiting. Accordingly, CHO ingestion may (Murray et al. 1987; Davis et al. 1988b; Millard-Stafford et al. 1992) or may not (Davis et al. 1988a; Millard-Stafford et al. 1990; Febbraio et al. 1996b) increase exercise performance in the heat.

24.10 Exercise, heat stress and metabolic perturbations

As mentioned previously, glycogen content within human skeletal muscle at the point of fatigue during exercise in the heat is often adequate to maintain energy turnover via oxidative phosphorylation. It is somewhat surprising, therefore, that a marked increase in IMP accumulation at fatigue during exercise and heat stress is observed despite glycogen concentration being adequate to maintain the oxidative potential of the contracting skeletal muscle (see Fig. 24.2) (Parkin et al. 1999). IMP is a marker of inadequate energy turnover via oxidative phosphorylation and is often observed at fatigue during prolonged exercise (Norman et al. 1987; Sahlin et al. 1990; Baldwin et al. 1999) when glycogen stores can no longer provide substrate to maintain oxidative phosphorylation, but not earlier (Norman et al. 1987; Sahlin et al. 1990) when glycogen stores are adequate.

These data suggest, therefore, a disruption to mitochondrial function during exercise and heat stress, and support findings by Mills and colleagues (1996), who observed an increase in plasma concentrations of lipid hydroperoxides, a marker of oxidative stress, in horses exercising in the heat. In addition, when examining the ratio between adenosine diphosphate (ADP) production and mitochondrial oxygen consumption (ADP:O ratio) in isolated rat skeletal muscle mitochondria, Brooks and colleagues (1971) observed a constant ADP:O ratio at temperatures ranging from 25–40°C. Above 40°C, however, the ADP:O ratio declined linearly with an increase in temperature, suggesting that for a given oxygen consumption the increase in ADP rephosphorylation was lower than the rate of adenosine triphosphate (ATP) degradation. Although the data provide only indirect evidence, they suggest that the combination of exercise and heat stress may disrupt cellular function, resulting in oxyradical formation.

Benefits of fluid ingestion

24.11

In circumstances where the endogenous heat production and high environmental temperature result in fatigue prior to CHO stores being compromised, fluid ingestion, irrespective of whether the fluid contains CHO, is of major importance in delaying the rise in body-core temperature. Exercise-induced dehydration is associated with an increase in core temperature (Hamilton et al. 1991; Montain & Coyle 1992), reduced cardiovascular function (Hamilton et al. 1991; Montain & Coyle 1992) and impaired exercise performance (Walsh et al. 1994). These effects are reduced, or indeed prevented, by fluid ingestion (Costill et al. 1970; Hamilton et al. 1991; Montain & Coyle 1992), which also improves exercise performance (Maughan et al. 1989; Walsh et al. 1994; McConell et al. 1997). Fluid ingestion also reduces muscle glycogen use during prolonged exercise (see Fig. 24.3; Hargreaves et al. 1996b; Gonzalez-Alonso et al. 1999).

It is likely that the mechanisms responsible for the attenuated glycogen use during exercise are the reduced circulating adrenaline and decreased muscle temperature that result from fluid ingestion, since muscle temperature (Febbraio et al. 1996a; Starkie et al. 1999) and adrenaline (Febbraio et al. 1998) influence glycogen use. It is clear from these data that fluid ingestion not only attenuates the rise in body core temperature, thereby preventing hyperthermia, but also reduces the likelihood of CHO depletion. Since sweat rate is augmented during exercise in the heat, dehydration progresses more rapidly and,

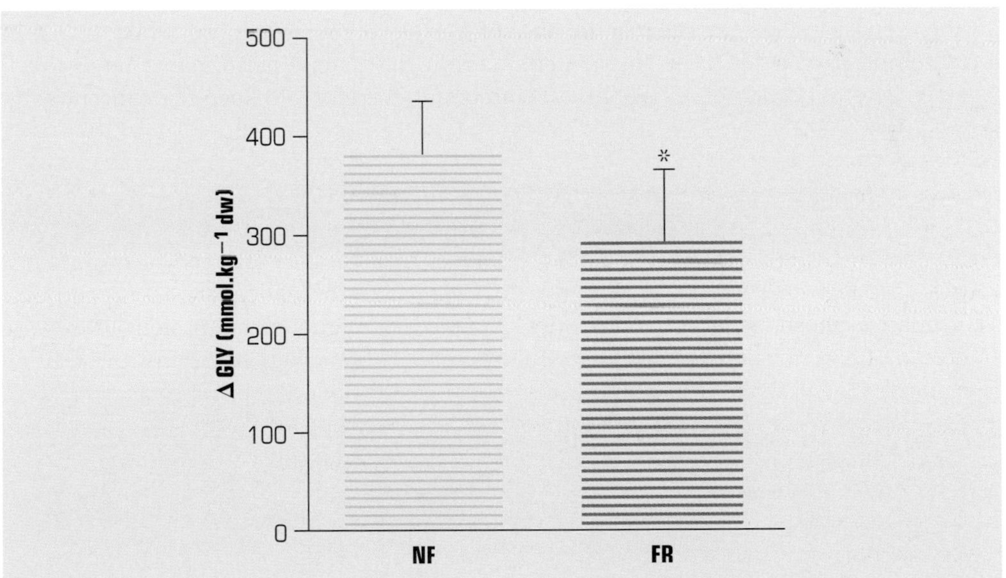

FIGURE 24.3 Net muscle glycogen utilization (Δ GLY; pre- post-exercise) during 120 minutes of exercise in the absence (NF) or presence (FR) of fluid ingestion. * indicates difference ($p < 0.05$) compared with NF. Data expressed as mean ± SE ($n = 5$). From Hargreaves et al. 1996b, used with permission

therefore, the importance of fluid ingestion is increased during exercise in extreme heat. Indeed, Below and colleagues (1995) have demonstrated that fluid ingestion improves exercise performance in a hot environment.

24.12 Nutritional recommendations for exercise in a hot environment

It is clear that both CHO and fluid are very important when making dietary recommendations for those exercising in the heat. Apart from maintaining a CHO-rich diet and remaining euhydrated in the days leading up to exercise, there are strategies that could be employed during exercise, particularly that which lasts for longer than 60 minutes. Athletes should ingest a CHO/fluid/electrolyte beverage frequently during exercise. Since the relative importance of fluid delivery is increased during exercise in the heat, athletes may be tempted to ingest water in these circumstances. This practice, however, is not ideal since the CHO/electrolyte/fluid beverage empties from the gut at the same rate as water (Francis 1979; Owen et al. 1986; Ryan et al. 1989), while it can spare muscle glycogen (Yaspelkis & Ivy 1991) during exercise in the heat. In addition, the relative importance of sodium intake is increased during exercise in the heat, and the addition of sodium in rehydration beverages can replace sweat sodium losses, prevent hyponatremia, promote the maintenance of plasma volume and enhance intestinal absorption of glucose and fluid (for review, see Maughan 1994). The amount of the CHO within a fluid beverage ingested during exercise in the heat appears to have little effect on fluid availability or exercise performance, provided the CHO is not too concentrated. The change in plasma volume and exercise performance in the heat is not different when ingesting beverages containing 0, 4.2 and 7% CHO respectively (Febbraio et al. 1996b). However, when a 14% CHO solution is ingested during exercise in the heat, the maintenance of plasma volume is reduced, while the rise in rectal temperature tends to be augmented. Accordingly, exercise performance tends to fall (see Fig. 24.4) (Febbraio et al. 1996b). It is important, therefore, to keep the concentration

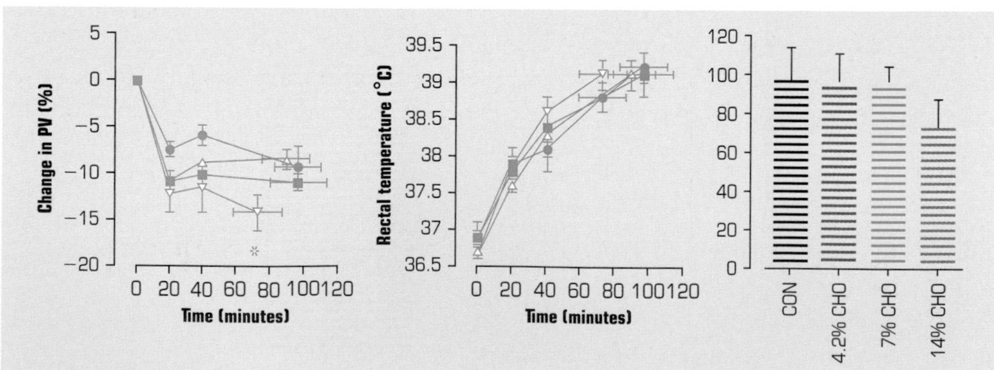

FIGURE 24.4 The change in plasma volume (left), rectal temperature (middle) and time to exhaustion (right), while consuming a placebo (CON, -■-), 4.2% CHO (LCHO, -●-), a 7% CHO (-Δ-) or 14% CHO (HCHO, -∇-) beverage during fatiguing exercise at 70% $VO_{2\,max}$ in 33°C conditions. * denotes difference ($p < 0.05$) from other trials. Data expressed as means ± SE. Adapted from Febbraio et al. 1996b

of CHO within a fluid beverage <~10% during exercise in the heat, even though CHO utilization is augmented in these circumstances. In terms of volume and frequency, a practical recommendation might be 400 mL every 15 minutes. CHO beverage should also be ingested into recovery to replenish intramuscular glycogen stores and promote rehydration, especially when training in a hot environment.

Despite recommendations to increase fluid consumption when exercising in the heat, some athletes fear that rigorous consumption of sport drinks or water will reduce the acute weight loss (sweat loss) that normally accompanies prolonged exercise. This contradicts the desire of cyclists and runners to be as light as possible, especially when they need to run or cycle uphill. As a result, some athletes have adopted a minimalist approach to fluid consumption in races or stages that provide an uphill challenge. In attempts to explore whether it is best to be slightly heavier and hydrated, or lighter and dehydrated, Ebert and colleagues (2005) from the AIS recruited eight male cyclists, who were asked to perform maximal cycling hill climbing efforts on a treadmill. Cyclists rode at 55% of the power output that corresponded to $VO_{2\,max}$ for 2 hours and then performed a maximal duration hill climb at an exercise intensity that was ~105% of lactate threshold power. Cyclists either consumed 1.2 L or 0.2 L per hour during the 2-hour ride and power output was monitored using instrumented power cranks (SRM) during the hill climb. CHO intake during both trials was held constant. Performance time was significantly better during the high fluid intake trial despite the observation that cyclists were nearly 2 kg heavier during this trial. Results from this study highlight the importance of aggressive drinking strategies even when performing endurance events where minimal mass is desired (Ebert et al. 2005).

As previously discussed, there is some evidence to suggest that protein catabolism is increased during exercise in the heat (Snow et al. 1993; Febbraio et al. 1994b; Mittleman et al. 1998), but more research is required before definitive recommendations can be made. Likewise, as discussed, there is some evidence to suggest that oxyradical generation may be increased via the combination of exercise and heat stress (Mills et al. 1996). It may, therefore, be of some benefit to supplement those undertaking repeated exercise in a hot environment with antioxidants such as alpha-tocopherol (vitamin E) and ascorbic acid (vitamin C). This recommendation is speculative, however, since the hypothesis—that such supplementation is advantageous during exercise in the heat—has not been tested. Furthermore, as discussed in Chapter 11 and its accompanying commentary, there may be some disadvantages to chronic supplementation, with individual anti-oxidant vitamins associated with disrupting the complex balance of anti-oxidant defenses or reducing the effectiveness of oxidative signals that underpin the desired adaptations to training.

Special strategies for exercise in the heat: glycerol hyperhydration

24.13

Since the deleterious effects of dehydration during exercise, especially that which is conducted in a hot environment, have been well documented, it would be desirable to hyperhydrate prior to exercise in a hot environment. Glycerol, when ingested with a bolus of water, has been widely reported as an effective hyperhydrating agent by most (Lyons et al. 1990; Freund et al. 1995; Montner et al. 1996; Hitchens et al. 1999; Anderson et al. 2001) but not all (Murray et al. 1991; Latzka et al. 1997) previous researchers.

While it appears that glycerol is an effective hyperhydrating agent, the exact mechanism of fluid retention remains to be elucidated. It has been suggested that glycerol acts via a renal mechanism, due to changes in circulatory osmotic gradients (Freund et al. 1995). In addition, passive diffusion of glycerol across the renal proximal tubule, due to its lipid solubility, may also cause an osmotic gradient for the reabsorption of water. However, no studies have been sufficiently comprehensive to define the mechanism of action clearly. Although most studies observe fluid retention with glycerol ingestion, the consequence of such a change remains equivocal. Glycerol hyperhydration has been demonstrated to reduce thermoregulatory strain and increase sweat rate by some (Lyons et al. 1990) but not all (Latzka et al. 1997) authors. The conflict within the literature may be accounted for by methodological differences such as environmental conditions, exercise intensity and duration, subject population and ingestion protocol. We (Hitchens et al. 1999; Anderson et al. 2001) have demonstrated that glycerol ingestion prior to exercise increases fluid retention, reduces thermoregulatory and cardiovascular strain and enhances exercise performance (see Fig. 24.5).

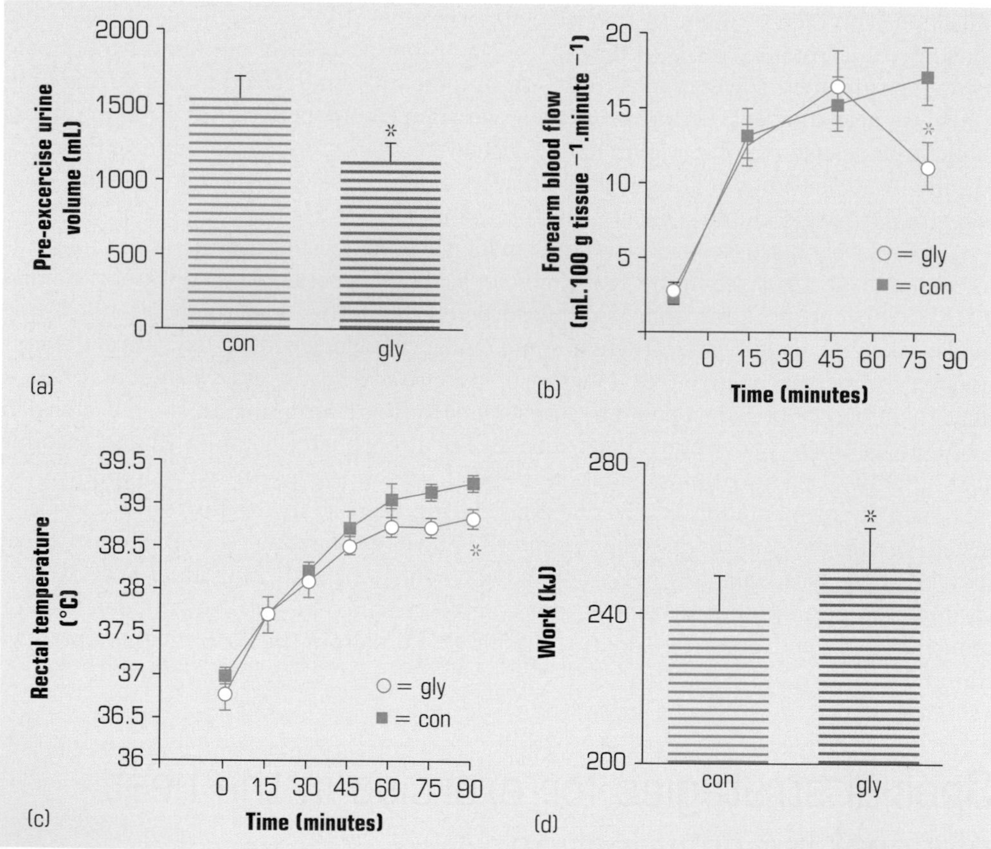

FIGURE 24.5 Pre-exercise urine volume (a), forearm blood flow (b), rectal temperature (c) and exercise performance (d) at rest (a), during 90 minutes of bicycle exercise (b, c) and during a 15-minute cycling time trial following steady state exercise (d) with the ingestion of 1 g.kg^{-1} body weight of glycerol in 20 mL.kg^{-1} body weight dilute cordial (gly, open rectangles and circles) or 20 mL.kg^{-1} body weight dilute cordial (con, solid rectangles and squares). Experiments were conducted at 35°C with a relative humidity of 20%. * indicates difference ($p < 0.05$) compared with con. Data expressed as means ± SE ($n = 6$). Adapted from Anderson et al. 2001

However, during one of our studies, subjects exhibited symptoms of gastrointestinal distress. This may have been due to the high osmolality of the glycerol solution (>600 mosmol/L) resulting in net fluid movement into the gastrointestinal tract. Therefore, athletes must be aware that this practice may have negative repercussions and are advised to test the practice of glycerol hyperhydration in training well before competition. Further discussion on glycerol hyperhydration, including its likely addition to the 2010 World Anti-Doping Agency List of Prohibited Substances can be found in Chapters 12 and 16. Salt loading, involving the consumption of a moderate volume of a high-sodium beverage in the hours prior to exercise in the heat, may offer another strategy to enhance fluid status and capacity for exercise in the heat (Sims et al. 2007a, 2007b).

Summary 24.14

During exercise and heat stress, both intramuscular glycogen use and glycolysis are augmented, whereas lipid utilization appears to decrease. In contrast with submaximal exercise in comfortable ambient temperatures, exercise in the heat does not appear to be limited by CHO availability when the heat stress is severe. However, during mild heat stress it is likely that CHO availability is of critical importance.

With respect to diet, athletes should be advised to (1) consume a diet rich in CHO and (2) maintain hydration levels when preparing for competition in hot environments. Despite the fact that CHO availability does not always appear to be a major limitation to exercise performance in the heat, it is prudent to ingest a 4–8% CHO beverage throughout exercise since such a beverage empties from the gastrointestinal tract as fast as water, but provides extra glucose and electrolytes, which may be required. Importantly, drinking such a beverage may increase ad libitum fluid consumption because of increased palatability. Other dietary practices such as pre-exercise glycerol hyperhydration, BCAA and anti-oxidant supplementation might confer some benefit during exercise in the heat. Although many well-educated endurance athletes probably consume a diet that is more than adequate for supporting their training while at altitude or hot venues, it is possible that some athletes are particularly conscious about their body weight. These athletes may be particularly vulnerable to problems when training and competing at altitude and in the heat because of low energy, protein and fluid intake.

PRACTICE TIPS

LOUISE BURKE

- Special nutrition issues arise from living and/or training in stressful environments such as heat or high altitude. To assess the special requirements or nutritional strategies that will be important in these conditions, it is important to find out more about the duration of exposure to these environments, the purpose of the exposure, and the training or competition goals during this period. It is useful to differentiate between the following situations:
  - The athlete is competing in an important sports competition that has been allocated to a city/country that is at altitude, or experiencing hot/humid weather.
  - The athlete is trekking or climbing at high altitude with the goal of completing a route or conquering a peak.
  - The athlete is undertaking specialized training in a hot climate or at high altitude in order to acclimatize for competition in a similar environment.
  - The athlete is undertaking specialized training in a hot climate or at high altitude to achieve physiological adaptations that may assist performance at sea level or in a cool climate.
  - The athlete is using specialized facilities such as a heat chamber or altitude change/nitrogen house either to undertake training or to sleep in this environment. Exposure to this environment will be limited to certain periods during the day, and the athlete will spend the remainder of the day at lower altitudes or in cooler surroundings. These strategies can be used both to prepare the athlete for competition in the specialized environment and to achieve desirable physiological adaptations.
- Different nutritional approaches may be appropriate for the various situations listed above. For example, an athlete who is climbing or trekking at very high altitudes (>5000 m) may expect to experience greater disturbances to energy balance (increased BMR and suppressed appetite) than an athlete who is training at moderate to high altitudes (2000–3000 m). The nutrition strategies for safety and survival over prolonged periods, particularly when the athlete must transport their own food supplies or prepare meals with minimal facilities, will be different to the goals of the athlete who aims to compete at their best at a single event. Similarly, an athlete who is acclimatizing to compete in a hot or high-altitude environment should aim to practice and fine-tune competition nutrition strategies as an additional requirement to the athlete who is training in such an environment merely for the physiological adaptations. Although athletes should look after fluid and fuel needs in all exercise situations, competition nutrition strategies are more specialized and often more aggressive. The athlete who intends to hyperhydrate with glycerol or consume sports drinks according to a pattern provided by aid stations needs to experiment with these practices during training. Such issues may not be important to the athlete who will not be competing in the special environment.
- Fluid losses are increased both in a hot environment and at hot altitude. Typically, the athlete will not immediately adjust to increased fluid requirements. Behavioral strategies to increase fluid intake should be implemented to complement physiological factors such as increased thirst. This may be especially important for the athlete who is undertaking

intermittent exposure to altitude or heat through specialized chambers. These athletes may incur greater fluid losses during the periods spent at the special environment, but miss cues to increase fluid intake when back in their normal environment. The athlete should target drinking patterns related to exercise sessions (drinking before, during and after a prolonged workout) as well as ensure that additional fluid is consumed with meals and between meals. Monitoring body mass in the morning after visiting the toilet provides a crude measure of hydration status. An acute drop in body mass will signal dehydration, but may become confused with the gradual decrease in body fuel stores (glycogen and body fat) that can accompany inadequate CHO and energy intake. Negative energy balance often occurs at high-altitude environments.

- In hot environments, thermoregulation and dehydration play a greater role in determining performance than they do in a cool environment. Although CHO utilization is increased in the heat, thermoregulation and dehydration are more likely to be limiting than fuel depletion. Therefore, the athlete should prioritize competition nutrition strategies to promote hydration. Strategies include aggressive rehydration after each workout or event to optimize preparation for the next; consideration of hyperhydration strategies such as glycerol loading; and training with fluid intake during exercise, to maximize the fluid volume that can be comfortably and practically consumed. These strategies are not mutually exclusive with practices to promote fuel availability. Athletes should ensure that they have adequately fueled by consuming a high-CHO diet in association with an exercise taper in the days prior to their event. Athletes who compete in prolonged events should also undertake CHO loading strategies. It is uncertain whether the water stored in the glycogen within the muscle becomes available as the glycogen is utilized.
- CHO-containing drinks, especially the commercially produced sports drinks, are suitable for use during exercise in the heat. Although performance during a competitive event undertaken in the heat is more likely to be limited by fluid considerations than CHO availability, it is unlikely that a solution of 4–8% CHO will impair fluid delivery. In fact, the taste of such drinks (containing flavor and electrolytes) has been shown to enhance voluntary intake, providing practical advantages over water. In addition, some studies have shown superior performance following the ingestion of CHO during exercise in the heat, compared to the intake of water. These situations include high-intensity exercise of about 1 hour's duration, in addition to the more traditional endurance exercise tasks. Since fluid losses and CHO utilization during exercise are increased at altitude, sports drinks should also be used during events or workouts in this environment. Again, these drinks offer advantages of promoting additional fluid intake and providing extra fuel.
- Since CHO utilization is increased at altitude and in hot environments, the total fuel requirements of training and/or competition will be increased. Athletes should plan for this by ensuring adequate CHO intake in meals and snacks. High-density CHO foods include dried fruit, grains (rice, noodles and pasta), breakfast cereals, sports bars, sports gels and powdered versions of sports drink/high-CHO sources/liquid meal supplements.

PRACTICE TIPS

These may be useful for athletes who need to carry their own food supplies. These foods may also be appropriate for situations where appetite is suppressed in hot weather or at altitude, since they provide a compact source of fuel. Alternatively, CHO-rich foods that have a high fluid content or require minimal chewing may also appeal to an athlete with a suppressed appetite. These include fruit smoothies and flavored milk drinks, liquid meal supplements, sports gels, flavored yoghurt and ice-cream.

- Although there is some evidence that protein requirements are increased at altitude, there is insufficient research to allow definitive guidelines to be made. Typically, athletes who increase their total energy intake from a variety of nutritious food choices can expect to meet any additional protein requirements. Athletes who might be identified as 'at risk' for inadequate protein intake include athletes who follow energy-restricted diets (e.g. to 'make weight' or to keep body-fat levels artificially low), or athletes who have limited dietary variety. On occasions, athletes may inadvertently reduce their protein intake by becoming over-reliant on foods that are easy to eat rather than nutritionally sound. Athletes who carry limited food supplies or who struggle to find foods to appeal to a suppressed appetite should remember to include some protein and micronutrient-dense foods such as flavored yoghurts, flavored milk drinks and smoothies, and liquid meal supplements.
- There is some evidence that oxidative damage arising from exercise is increased by sudden exposure to a hot environment or high altitude. Although there is no evidence to show performance benefits, it has been suggested that athletes who are training hard in these environments would benefit from taking anti-oxidant supplementation in the form of vitamins E and C for the first 7–10 days of exposure to the new environment. This has not been tested and must be balanced against the emerging evidence that there may be disadvantages in blocking signaling pathways that rely on oxidative mechanisms. On the other hand, it is important that athletes who move to high altitudes have adequate iron status to allow optimal stimulus of red blood cell production. Issues related to iron are summarized in Chapter 10.

References

Anderson, MJ, Cotter JD, Garnham AP, Casley DJ, Febbraio MA. Effect of glycerol-induced hyperhydration on thermoregulation and metabolism in the heat. Int J Sport Nutr Exerc Metab 2001;11:315–33.

Baldwin J, Snow RJ, Carey MF, Febbraio MA. Muscle IMP accumulation during fatiguing submaximal exercise in endurance trained and untrained men. Am J Physiol 1999;277(1 Pt 2):R295–300.

Below PR, Mora-Rodriguez R, Gonzalez-Alonso J, Coyle EF. Fluid and carbohydrate ingestion independently improve performance during 1 hr of intense exercise. Med Sci Sports Exerc 1995;27:200–10.

Bonen A, Megeney LA, McCarthy SC, McDermott JC, Tan MH. Epinephrine administration stimulates GLUT4 translocation but reduces glucose transport in muscle. Biochem Biophys Res Commun 1992;187:685–91.

Brooks GA, Butterfield GE, Wolfe RR, Groves BM, Mazzeo RS, Sutton JR, Wolfel EE, Reeves JT. Increased dependence on blood glucose after acclimatization to 4,300 m. J App Physiol 1991a;70:919–27.

Brooks GA, Butterfield GE, Wolfe RR, Groves BM, Mazzeo RS, Sutton JR, Wolfel EE, Reeves JT. Decreased reliance on lactate after acclimatization to 4,300 m. J App Physiol 1991b;71:333–41.

Brooks GA, Hittleman KJ, Faulkner, JA, Beyer RE. Temperature, skeletal muscle mitochondrial functions, and oxygen debt. Am J Physiol 1971;220:1053–9.

Brooks GA, Wolfel EE, Groves BM, Bender PR, Butterfield GE, Cymerman A, Mazzeo RS, Sutton JR, Wolfe RR, Reeves JT. Muscle accounts for glucose disposal but not blood lactate appearance during exercise after acclimatization to 4,300 m. J App Physiol 1992;72:2435–45.

Butterfield GE. Nutrient requirements at high altitude. Clin Sports Med 1999;18:607–21.

Butterfield GE, Gates J, Fleming S, Brooks GA, Sutton JR, Wolfel EE, Reeves JT. Increased dependence on blood glucose after acclimatization to 4,300 m. J App Physiol 1992;72:1741–8.

Coggan AR, Coyle EF. Reversal of fatigue during prolonged exercise by carbohydrate infusion or ingestion. J Appl Physiol 1987;63:2388–95.

Consolazio CF, Matoush LO, Johnson HL, Krzywicki HJ, Daws TA, Isaac GJ. Effects of high-carbohydrate diets on performance and clinical symptomatology after rapid ascent to high altitude. Fed Proc 1969;28:937–43.

Consolazio CF, Matoush LO, Johnson HL, Krzywicki HJ, Isaac GJ, Witt NF. Metabolic aspects of calorie restriction: nitrogen and mineral balances and vitamin excretion. Am J Clin Nutr 1968;21:803–12.

Costill D, Krammer WF, Fisher, A. Fluid ingestion during distance running. Arch Environ Health 1970;21:520–5.

Coyle EF, Coggan AR, Hemmert MK, Ivy JL. Muscle glycogen utilization during prolonged exercise when fed CHO. J Appl Physiol 1986:61;165–72.

Davis JM, Burgess WA, Slentz CA, Bartoli WP, Pate RR. Effects of ingesting 6% and 12% glucose/electrolyte beverages during prolonged intermittent cycling in the heat. Eur J Appl Physiol 1988a;57:563–9.

Davis JM, Lamb DR, Pate RR, Slentz CA, Burgess WA, Bartoli WP. CHO-electrolyte drinks: effects on endurance cycling in the heat. Am J Clin Nutr 1988b;48:1023–30.

Ebert TR, Martin DT, Bullock N, Quod M, Mujika I, Farthing L, Fallon K, Burke LM, Withera RT. Effect of exercise-induced dehydration on thermoregulation and cycling hill-climbing performance (abst.). Med Sci Sports Exerc 2005(Suppl);37:169S.

Febbraio MA, Carey MF, Snow RJ, Stathis CG, Hargreaves M. Influence of elevated muscle temperature on metabolism during intense, dynamic exercise. Am J Physiol 1996a;271:R1251–5.

Febbraio MA, Murton P, Selig SE, Clark SA, Lambert DL, Angus DJ, Carey MF. Effect of CHO ingestion on exercise metabolism and performance in different ambient temperatures. Med Sci Sports Exerc 1996b;28:1380–7.

Febbraio MA, Lambert DL, Starkie RL, Proietto J, Hargreaves M. Effect of epinephrine on muscle glycogenolysis during exercise in trained men. J Appl Physiol 1998;84:465–70.

Febbraio MA, Snow RJ, Hargreaves M, Stathis CG, Martin IK, Carey MF. Muscle metabolism during exercise and heat stress in trained men: effect of acclimation. J Appl Physiol 1994a;76:589–97.

Febbraio MA, Snow RJ, Stathis CG, Hargreaves M, Carey MF. Effect of heat stress on muscle energy metabolism during exercise. J Appl Physiol 1994b;77:2827–31.

Fink WJ, Costill DL, Van Handel PJ. Leg muscle metabolism during exercise in the heat and cold. Eur J Appl Physiol 1975;34:183–90.

Francis KT. Effect of water and electrolyte replacement during exercise in the heat on biochemical indices of stress and performance. Aviat Space Environ Med 1979;50:115–19.

Freund BJ, Montain SJ, Young AJ, Sawka MN, DeLuca J, Pandolf KB, Valeri CR. Glycerol hyperhydration: hormonal, renal and vascular fluid responses. J Appl Physiol 1995:79:2069–77.

Gonzalez-Alonso J, Calbet JA, Nielsen B. Metabolic and thermodynamic responses to dehydration-induced reductions in muscle blood flow in exercising humans. J Physiol Lond 1999;520:577–89.

Green HJ, Sutton J, Young P, Cymerman A, Houston CS. Operation Everest II: muscle energetics during maximal exhaustive exercise. J Appl Physiol 1989;66:142–50.

Grover RF, Weil JV, Reeves JT. Cardiovascular adaptations to exercise at high altitude. Exerc Sports Sci Rev 1986;14:269–302.

Hamilton MT, Gonzalez-Alonso J, Montain SJ, Coyle EF. Fluid replacement and glucose infusion during exercise prevent cardiovascular drift. J Appl Physiol 1991;1:871–7.

Hannon JP, Chinn SK, Shields JL. Effects of acute high altitude-exposure on body fluids. Fed Proc 1969;28:1178–84.

Hargreaves M, Angus D, Howlett K, Marmy Conus N, Febbraio M. Effect of heat stress on glucose kinetics during exercise. J Appl Physiol 1996a;81:594–7.

Hargreaves M, Costill D, Burke L, McConell G, Febbraio M. Influence of sodium on glucose bioavailability during exercise. Med Sci Sports Exerc 1994;26:365–8.

Hargreaves M, Dillo P, Angus D, Febbraio M. Effect of fluid ingestion on muscle metabolism during prolonged exercise. J Appl Physiol 1996b;80:63–6.

Hitchens S, Martin DT, Burke L, Yates K, Fallon K, Hahn A, Dobson GP. Glycerol hyperhydration improves cycling time trial performance in hot humid conditions. Eur J Appl Physiol 1999;80:494–501.

Kellogg RH, Pace N, Archibald ER. Respiratory response to inspired CO_2 during acclimatization to an altitude of 12,470 feet. J Appl Physiol 1957;11:665–71.

Latzka WA, Sawka MN, Montain SJ, Skrinar GS, Fielding RA, Matott RP, Pandolf KB. Hyperhydration: thermoregulatory effects during compensable exercise-heat stress. J Appl Physiol 1997;83:860–6.

Lyons TP, Riedesel ML, Meuli LE, Chick TW. Effects of glycerol-induced hyperhydration prior to exercise in the heat on sweating and core temperature. Med Sci Sports Exerc 1990;22:477–83.

MacLean DA, Graham TE, Saltin B. Stimulation of muscle ammonia production during exercise following branched-chain amino acid supplements in humans. J Physiol Lond 1996;493:909–22.

Madsen K, MacLean DA, Kiens B, Christensen D. Effects of glucose, glucose plus branched chain amino acids, or placebo on bike performance over 100 km. J Appl Physiol 1996;81:2644–50.

Maughan RJ. Fluid and electrolyte loss and replacement in exercise. In: Harries M, Williams C, Stanish WD, Micheli LJ, eds. Oxford textbook of sports medicine. New York: Oxford University Press, 1994:82–93.

Maughan RJ, Fenn CE, Leiper JB. Effects of fluid, electrolyte and substrate ingestion on endurance capacity. Eur J Appl Physiol 1989;58:481–6.

Maughan RJ, Leiper JB. Sodium intake and post-exercise rehydration in man. Eur J Appl Physiol 1995;71:311–19.

Mazzeo RS, Bender PR, Brooks GA, Butterfield GE, Groves BM, Sutton JR, Wolfel EE, Reeves JT. Arterial catecholamine responses during exercise with acute and chronic high-altitude exposure. Am J Physiol 1991;261(4 Pt 1):E419–24.

McConell GK, Burge CM, Skinner SL, Hargreaves M. Influence of ingested fluid volume on physiological responses during prolonged exercise. Acta Physiol Scand 1997;160:149–56.

Millard-Stafford M, Sparling PB, Rosskopf LB, Dicarlo LJ. CHO-electrolyte replacement improves distance running performance in the heat. Med Sci Sports Exerc 1990;24:934–40.

Millard-Stafford M, Sparling PB, Rosskopf LB, Hinson BT, Dicarlo LJ. CHO-electrolyte replacement during a simulated triathlon in the heat. Med Science Sports Exerc 1992;22:621–8.

Mills PC, Smith NC, Casa I, Harris P, Harris RC, Marlin DJ. Effects of exercise intensity and environmental stress on indices of oxidative stress and iron homeostasis during exercise in the horse. Eur J Appl Physiol 1996;74:60–6.

Mittleman KD, Ricci MR, Bailey SP. Branched-chain amino acids prolong exercise during heat stress in men and women. Med Sci Sports Exerc 1998;30:83–91.

Montain SJ, Coyle EF. Influence of graded dehydration on hyperthermia and cardiovascular drift during exercise. J Appl Physiol 1992;73:1340–50.

Montner P, Stark DM, Riedesel ML, Murata G, Robergs R, Timms M, Chick TW. Pre-exercise glycerol hydration improves cycling endurance time. Int J Sports Med 1996;17:27–33.

Moore LG, Cymerman A, Huang SY, McCullough RE, McCullough RG, Rock PB, Young A, Young P, Weil JV, Reeves JT. Propanolol blocks metabolic rate increase but not ventilatory acclimatization to 4,300 m. Respir Physiol 1987;70:195–205.

Murray R, Eddy DE, Murray TW, Paul GL, Seifert JG, Halaby GA. Physiological responses to glycerol ingestion during exercise. J Appl Physiol 1991;71:144–9.

Murray R, Eddy DE, Murray TW, Seifert JG, Paul GL, Halaby GA. The effect of fluid and CHO feedings during intermittent cycling exercise. Med Sci Sports Exerc 1987;19:597–604.

Nielsen B, Hales JRS, Strange S, Juel C, Christensen N, Warberg J, Saltin B. Human circulatory and thermoregulatory adaptations with heat acclimation and exercise in a hot, dry environment. J Physiol Lond 1993;460:467–85.

Nielsen B, Savard G, Richter EA, Hargreaves M, Saltin B. Muscle blood flow and muscle metabolism during exercise and heat stress. J Appl Physiol 1990;69:1040–6.

Norman B, Sollevi A, Kaijser L, Jansson E. ATP breakdown products in human skeletal muscle during prolonged exercise to exhaustion. Clin Physiol 1987;7:503–10.

Nose H, Mack GW, Shi X, Nadel ER. Role of osmolality and plasma volume during rehydration in humans. J Appl Physiol 1988;65:332–6.

Owen MD, Kregel KC, Wall PT, Gisolfi CV. Effects of ingesting CHO beverages during exercise in the heat. Med Sci Sports Exerc 1986;18:568–75.

Parkin JM, Carey MF, Zhao S, Febbraio MA. Effect of ambient temperature on human skeletal muscle metabolism during fatiguing submaximal exercise. J Appl Physiol 1999;86:902–8.

Powers SK, Howley ET, Cox R. A differential catecholamine response during exercise and passive heating. Med Sci Sports Exerc 1985;14:435–9.

Pugh LGCE. Blood volume and haemoglobin concentrations at altitudes above 14,000 ft (5,500 m). J Physiol Lond 1964;170:344–54.

Roberts AC, Butterfield GE, Cymerman A, Reeves JT, Wolfel EE, Brooks GA. Acclimatization to 4,300-m altitude decreases reliance on fat as a substrate. J Appl Physiol 1996a;81:1762–71.

Roberts AC, Reeves JT, Butterfield GE, Mazzeo RS, Sutton JR, Wolfel EE, Brooks GA. Altitude and β-blockade augment glucose utilization during submaximal exercise. J Appl Physiol 1996b;80: 605–15.

Ryan AJ, Bleiler TL, Carter JE, Gisolfi CV. Gastric emptying during prolonged cycling exercise in the heat. Med Sci Sports Exerc 1989;21:51–8.

Sahlin K, Katz A, Broberg S. Tricarboxylic acid cycle intermediates in humans during prolonged exercise. Am J Physiol 1990;259:C834–41.

Sims ST, Rehrer NJ, Bell ML, Cotter JD. Preexercise sodium loading aids fluid balance and endurance for women exercising in the heat. J Appl Physiol 2007a;103:534–41.

Sims ST, van Vliet L, Cotter JD, Rehrer NJ. Sodium loading aids fluid balance and reduces physiological strain of trained men exercising in the heat. Med Sci Sports Exerc 2007b;39:123–30.

Snow RJ, Febbraio MA, Carey MF, Hargreaves M. Heat stress increases ammonia accumulation during exercise. Exp Physiol 1993;78:847–50.

Starkie RL, Hargreaves M, Lambert DL, Proietto J, Febbraio MA. Effect of temperature on muscle metabolism during submaximal exercise in humans. Exp Physiol 1999;84:775–84.

Sutton JR, Reeves JT, Wagner PD, Groves BM, Cymerman A, Malconian MK, Rock PB, Young PM, Walter SD, Houston CS. Operation Everest II: maximum oxygen uptake at extreme altitude. J Appl Physiol 1988;66:1309–28.

Takamata A, Mack GW, Gillen CM, Jozsi AC, Nadel ER. Osmoregulatory modulation of thermal sweating in humans: reflex effects of drinking. Am J Physiol 1995;268(2 Pt 2):R414–22.

Van Hall G, Raaymakers JSH, Saris WHM, Wagenmakers AJM. Ingestion of branched-chain amino acids and tryptophan during sustained exercise in man: failure to affect performance. J Physiol Lond 1995;486:789–94.

Walsh RM, Noakes TD, Hawley JA, Dennis SC. Impaired high-intensity cycling performance time at low levels of dehydration. Int J Sports Med 1994;15:392–8.

Yaspelkis 3rd BB, Ivy JL. Effect of CHO supplements and water on exercise metabolism in the heat. J Appl Physiol 1991;71:680–7.

Yaspelkis 3rd BB, Scroop GC, Wilmore KM, Ivy JL. CHO metabolism during exercise in hot and thermoneutral environments. Int J Sports Med 1993;14:13–19.

Young AJ, Sawka MN, Levine L, Cadarette BS, Pandolf KB. Skeletal muscle metabolism during exercise is influenced by heat acclimation. J Appl Physiol 1985;59:1929–35.

CHAPTER 25

Providing meals for athletic groups

NICOLA CUMMINGS, FIONA PELLY, VINNI DANG, RUTH CRAWFORD AND MICHELLE CORT

25.1 Introduction

Catering for athletes and providing advice to caterers is an exciting and challenging task. The main role for the dietitian is the design of menus and recipes that meet the nutrient needs of athletic groups and satisfy a wide variety of individual tastes, expectations and cultural preferences. Working directly with caterers provides the opportunity to select suitable foods for consumption and potentially influence the eating behavior of athletes. Unfortunately, sporting venues and institutions that supply food for athletes do not always employ a food-service dietitian or cater adequately for athletes' needs. Usually, the available foods are high in fat, sugar and salt and contradict sports nutrition principles.

This chapter focuses on the processes involved in menu planning and the impact these have on athletes' food choices. The dining hall at the Australian Institute of Sport (AIS) provides an example of a working model of large-scale residential catering for elite athletes. Practical tips and strategies for the self-catering of athletes living away from home are also included (see Table 25.1).

25.2 Influencing the food selection of athletes

Provision of nutrition information in the eating environment influences point-of-choice food selection (Mayer et al. 1989; Seymour et al. 2004). However, determinants of food selection by individuals are complex and influenced by many factors. Eating habits are acquired over a lifetime and dietary change requires a conscious effort, practice and commitment to maintain this change (Nestle et al. 1998).

The most commonly reported influences on food choice are taste, cost, convenience, health and nutrition beliefs, social relationships and food quality (Connor 1994; Furst et al. 1996; Falk et al. 2001). In athletes, health beliefs, performance expectations, concerns over body composition (see Chapter 8) and taste are important determinants of food

TABLE 25.1 TIPS FOR DIETITIANS TO PREPARE ATHLETES FOR SELF-CATERING

- Discuss catering requirements with the athletes/manager/coach.
- Determine the cooking skills of the group. Plan pre-camp cooking sessions if feasible. Alternatively, coordinate the cooking session during the camp, if the dietitian is traveling with the team.
- Determine in advance the cooking equipment, food budget, shop access and cooking facilities available.
- Plan the menu around the length of stay, competition or training program.
- Designate responsibility for shopping and cooking of food among the athletes. Consider contacting the local supermarket and see if they will deliver.
- Develop a list of basic ingredients and cooking equipment that can be taken from home and shared among the team.

PLANNING FOR DINING OUT

- Book a restaurant close to the accommodation rather than dropping in unexpectedly.
- Confirm that the menu provides appropriate and suitable foods for the age, budget and food preferences of the team.
- If a large group of athletes is booked and planning is well in advance, send suitable menu selections.
- For a large group of athletes, arrange a set (à la carte) menu with the option of one or two choices, or a buffet-style servery.
- Inform restaurants of the estimated time of arrival.
- Ensure there is plenty of extra bread served with the meal.
- Ensure water and juices are kept well stocked during the meal.

choice and are linked to consuming low-fat diets (Ryan Smart & Bisogni 2001). In a study of 418 athletes competing at the Commonwealth Games, sensory factors, familiarity and nutrient composition were important determinants of food choice (Pelly et al 2006b). In another study of people eating in an army cafeteria, the main determinants were taste and quality, followed by size of portions (related to cost), length of the serving line, individual cravings, nutrient density of the food, amount of time available to eat, and appetite (Sproul et al. 2003). We have observed similar influences (particularly taste) in athletes living at the AIS residences and eating from a similar cafeteria environment. Several positive outcomes consistently reported by AIS athletes include consuming a diet that is higher in carbohydrate (CHO), fruit and vegetables, and consuming a greater variety of foods compared with their usual consumption at home.

The role of taste in food selection 25.3

Taste is a key determinant of food choice, especially in males (Hess 1997; Buscher et al. 2001; Sproul et al. 2003). High-fat, high-sugar and energy-dense foods have been reported to be associated with feelings of personal satisfaction, reward, free choice and indulgence and hence are high on the taste preference for most people (Nestle et al. 1998). These food preferences are often established in early childhood when high-fat foods are offered in positive contexts associated with celebrations or used as rewards (Nestle et al. 1998).

There are few studies on taste preferences of athletes. In one study, Guinard and colleagues (1995) found no difference in the preferences for fatty animal products (dairy and meat) between male athletes and sedentary controls. In contrast, in another study, female athletes reported a significantly lower preference for high-fat food, compared with sedentary controls (Crystal et al. 1995).

Caterers to athletic groups therefore should consider that taste and other sensory appeal of the food they offer strongly influences food selection, although all too often they are more concerned about cost and minimizing the time and effort that catering staff spend on food preparation (Reichler & Dalton 1998).

25.4 Influence of the food-service setting

Self-serve, buffet-style food service is frequently used when feeding large groups of athletes, to cater for individual needs and food preferences (Modulon & Burke 1997). In this situation, people tend to choose a high-CHO diet with a favorable macronutrient balance (Hickson et al. 1987). Overeating is one disadvantage (Stroebele & De Castro 2004) and this was confirmed in college hockey players, especially when initially exposed to a buffet style of eating (Ryan Smart & Bisogni 2001). Older athletes in this group were less likely to overeat, compared with younger athletes.

Although foods selected from a menu with a wide range of choices may be the first preference for most people, it is not feasible or economical when serving large groups of athletes. A buffet-style self-service is more suitable because it provides readily available food, is cost-effective, allows for bulk cooking and low wastage, and offers flexibility in food choice and serve size.

Athletes living in residence, where buffet-style food is always served, often complain about boredom and lack of menu variety. These complaints are more often voiced by those who consume food from every dish on the buffet, watch what other athletes eat, use the dining hall as a social meeting point and linger over meals, and eat more than necessary.

Some athletes have reported negative attitudes towards eating in an institutionalised environment, which they equate with low quality, limited variety and an unpleasant physical environment (Meiselman et al. 2000; Stroebele & De Castro 2004). Providing a pleasant physical environment (with color and soft lighting) and attractive food presentation can change the perception of the dining experience and alter food selection.

Access to food and beverages also influences food choice. In one study, twice as much water was consumed when placed on the dining table rather than 6 meters away in the same room, or in a different room (Engell et al. 1996). In another study, Meiselman and colleagues (1994) found that intakes of socially desirable foods (e.g. confectionery and potato chips) decreased when located away from the main buffet. Providing easy access to specific foods with limited waiting time also influences food selection.

25.5 Influence of others

Peer acquaintance also influences food choice and volume consumed. People who are less familiar with one another can be self-conscious about communal eating and are often hesitant to overeat (Clendenen et al. 1994). The opposite behavior is observed when food is consumed with friends. In this situation, meal portions were reported to be around 44% larger than when eaten alone (Stroebele & De Castro 2004). People also tend to adapt to the eating behavior of their companions, particularly if they are trying to make an impression. Young athletes are easily influenced by others, particularly their coach, and modify their food intake to either please or impress. This behavior was evident in the younger members of a US college hockey team who were more willing than the more experienced players to try new combinations of foods (Ryan Smart & Bisogni 2001). In a survey of athletes at the 2006 Commonwealth Games, the presence of team-mates and the coach was reported to have a greater influence on food choice for athletes from Asian, African and Caribbean backgrounds than from other regions (Pelly et al 2006b).

Influence of sports

25.6

The type and culture of sport also influences an athlete's food selection. In one study, athletes involved in power/skill sports placed less emphasis on the nutrient content of the food compared to those involved in team, weight-conscious and endurance sports where dietary intake and a lean body composition are perceived to be important to overall performance (Pelly et al. 2006b). Often oversized meals are served to athletes, irrespective of their body mass (BM) or sport because public perceptions about feeding athletes can be distorted. Despite the apparent intensity and duration of physical activity in some sports, energy requirements, and hence food intakes, are not that much greater in athletes than in untrained people (see Chapter 5). Such large meals are quite daunting for those athletes who are watching their BM or skinfolds. For these athletes, foods available need to be nutrient-dense and potentially low-fat so that adequate nutrient intakes can be met from smaller amounts of food. For athletes with large BM (e.g. heavyweight rowers), the serve sizes in restaurants are too small for their energy needs. Providing written guidelines to caterers about serve sizes and meal sizes for different athletes helps address these misconceptions.

Influence of age

25.7

Athletes who travel a lot for competition are faced with the challenge of eating unfamiliar foods and are often reticent to sample unfamiliar foods when away from home. We have noticed that adolescent athletes can be conservative in their food choices and tend to avoid spicy foods and dishes with unusual flavors. For large-scale catering, sufficient basic or plain menu options should be available to accommodate the taste preferences of younger athletes. When feeding a smaller group, meat dishes and their accompanying sauces can be served separately to cater for fussy eaters.

Cultural background

25.8

The home and cultural environment has a major influence on eating habits. Athletes accustomed to western diets encounter difficulties when competing in Asian countries where bread and breakfast cereals are often unavailable. Similarly, difficulties arise when Asians and Africans experience western food. Also, religious beliefs (e.g. kosher and halal), medical problems (e.g. intolerances and allergies) and personal preferences (e.g. vegetarian diets) influence food selection. Traditional Australian eating habits, with the emphasis on meat as the main part of the meal, do not encourage high CHO consumption.

Although it is difficult, if not impossible, for a dietitian to present a menu plan that satisfies every individual in a large group setting, it is possible to offer enough choices to accommodate different types of diets and cultural differences (e.g. vegetarian and non-red-meat eaters). At elite-level competition, where there are a large range of athletes from different cultures, specialist chefs are often employed. At the AIS, vegetarian-style dishes, incorporating either meat alternatives or legumes, are a regular inclusion.

25.9 Gender

Similar responses, based on the influences of smell, visual appeal, familiarity and nutrient composition on food choice, were found between male and female athletes in a study of 418 athletes competing at the Commonwealth Games in Melbourne (Pelly et al. 2006b). Despite this finding, our observations of athletes' eating behavior in a residential environment suggest that food choices are gender-specific for other determinants. Apart from the obvious requirements of larger serve sizes in males, mixed gender groups have different expectations of the type of meal served. Male athletes dining at the AIS prefer a cooked breakfast and hot meals at lunchtime, whereas female athletes prefer cereal and/or toast for breakfast and sandwiches for lunch. Adolescent girls are more adventurous in trying new foods than boys of the same age.

To cater for these apparent differences in food choice between males and females, hot items can easily be incorporated into the breakfast menu by using pre-prepared foods such as tinned spaghetti and baked beans. The difference in food choices between sexes may be a reflection of the influence of different body perceptions reported between male and female adolescents (see Chapter 17).

25.10 Stage of competition

Food choices of athletes also vary with stage of competition and season. During the 2006 Commonwealth Games, athletes rated factors that influenced their sports performance (nutrient composition and stage of competition) much higher than factors related to the sensory appeal of the food (e.g. smell and visual appeal) (Pelly et al. 2006a). In a study of hockey players, the key determinants of food choice during competition were health beliefs and effects of diet on performance, compared with taste during the off-season (Ryan Smart & Bisogni 2001). During tapering, athletes are usually concerned about weight gain, eat much less and often follow extremely low-fat diets. In those athletes in weight-class sports, extreme dieting, fluid restriction and other weight-loss behaviors (e.g. excess time in the sauna and training in plastic clothes) may be practiced (see Chapter 7).

25.11 Strategies to modify food supply in a catering environment

A dietitian working in food service is in an ideal position to modify the foods available for consumption and can directly influence food choice. Common strategies to do this include increasing the availability of healthy foods, increasing access to specific foods, price reduction, changing catering policy, providing point-of-choice nutrition information by using nutrition labels, and encouraging athletes in meal selection. These strategies are effective in changing behavior (Glanz & Hoelscher 2004; Seymour et al. 2004).

Developing a catering policy to standardize the food supply, menus and recipes for athletes is a valuable strategy for quality control and for providing consistent messages about food, and has been used successfully at the AIS, the Olympic and Commonwealth games (Pelly et al. 2006; in press), world championships and International Masters games.

Residential catering for athletic groups 25.12

When catering for elite athletes in a permanent residential environment, the length of the menu cycle is no different from that of any residential facility. However, the type of food offered at each meal, and the availability and type of between-meal snacks, need to take into account the macronutrient balance recommended for elite-level athletes with a focus of menu choices that facilitate a relatively high-CHO diet. Training of catering staff, including chefs and food service staff, about the nutrient requirements of elite athletes provides an opportunity to engage these staff in the nutrition education of athletes and helps to influence athletes' food choices at meal times. The next section provides guidelines and strategies relating to menu design and delivery when catering for athletes in a residential environment. These guidelines can also be adapted for caterers accommodating athletes in short-term residential training camps.

The menu cycle 25.13

The length of the menu cycle is determined by the length of time an athlete spends in residence. A weekly menu cycle is satisfactory for those in residence for less than a month. At elite-level competition such as the Olympic Games residents live in the athletes' village for periods of up to one month. A 10-day menu cycle is common practice to avoid 'menu fatigue' and repetition. For those living in permanent residence, the menu cycle should be much longer. At the AIS, where the athletes are usually in year-long residence, the menu rotation is 4 weeks, including a weekly gourmet café-style Sunday brunch.

Variety and nutritional balance 25.14

Offering a variety of dishes addresses the variable nutrient needs between individuals and allows a wide range of personal choice. At the AIS residence, which caters for approximately 300 residential athletes and up to an additional 300 visiting athletes, the menu options include four choices of hot meals at dinner. The meal choices include two high-CHO dishes, plain meat, a wet dish (e.g. curry or casserole), and a selection of salads, fresh fruit and assorted breads. The four meal choices will also include options for special dietary requirements (e.g. vegetarian and gluten-free food selection). See Table 25.2 for an example of a weekly menu plan.

For a smaller group, one evening meal choice is acceptable, provided that extra CHO-rich foods are offered as an accompaniment. Novelty breads such as focaccia, crusty loaves and Italian-style loaves provide variety. In a small group, individuals with special needs, such as vegetarians, are catered for individually. To increase food diversity and provide visually appealing meals, a variety of meats are offered, using different cooking methods each week (e.g. if roast meat is served each week in a menu cycle, pork, beef, lamb, turkey, chicken and veal are rotated). In addition, legumes are a relatively inexpensive, high-satiety food that can be added to vegetarian or meat dishes to add CHO and protein. The use of different-colored ingredients improves aesthetic appeal and encourages consumption.

TABLE 25.2 WEEKLY MENU PLAN AT THE AUSTRALIAN INSTITUTE OF SPORT DINING HALL

	MONDAY	TUESDAY	WEDNESDAY	THURSDAY	FRIDAY	SATURDAY
BREAKFAST	Pancakes	Baked beans	Pancakes	Muffins	Pancakes	Muffins
	Baked beans	Grilled tomatoes	Tinned spaghetti	Baked beans	Baked beans	Baked beans
	Tinned spaghetti	Stewed fruit	Grilled mushrooms	Tinned spaghetti	Tinned spaghetti	Grilled tomatoes
	Boiled eggs	Poached eggs	Scrambled eggs	French toast	Scrambled eggs	Boiled eggs
		Bircher muesli with tinned berries		Bircher muesli with tinned berries		
LUNCH—GLUTEN-FREE PASTA AVAILABLE EVERY DAY						
Quick hot lunch	Chicken burgers	Pizza supreme	Spicy meatballs with tomato-based sauce	Quiche on fillo pastry	Stir-fried vegetables in oyster sauce with rice noodles	Lamb souvlaki
		Pizza vegetarian		Vegetarian quiche		Vegetarian souvlaki
High CHO	Pasta bake	Pork satay with peanut sauce and pasta	Vegetarian fried rice	Pasta with chicken and aubergine sauce	Pasta bolognese	Pasta al funghi
DINNER—STEAMED RICE AVAILABLE EVERY DAY						
Vegetarian	Vegetable strudel	Vegetable quiche	Mexicana sauce with pasta	Potato pie	Spinach and cheese cannelloni	Stir-fried tofu and vegetables
			BBQ night (served outside)			
High CHO	Pasta carbonara	Chicken stir-fry and noodles	Jacket potatoes with assorted fillings	Alfredo sauce with pasta	Combination chow mein	Tuna pasta
Plain meat	Chicken schnitzel	BBQ pork chops with spicy plum sauce	Roast lamb and gravy	Grilled salmon fillets	Steamed fish with grilled calamari	Roast beef with gravy
Other meat	Beef with black bean sauce with rice	Lamb and sun-dried tomato casserole	Tandoori chicken	Stir-fried chicken and vegetables	Minute steaks in plum sauce with rice	Chicken cacciatore
Hot dessert	Poached pears	Strawberry crêpes	Apple and rhubarb pie	Fruit compote	Banana nut loaf	Chocolate self-saucing pudding
Cold dessert	Lemon meringue pie	Jelly and tinned fruit	Fresh fruit	Hazelnut mousse	Fresh fruit salad	Jelly and tinned fruit
Additional	Vanilla ice-cream	Custard	Chocolate ice-cream	Custard	Vanilla ice-cream	Chocolate custard

Source: Adapted from Australian Institute of Sport dining hall—summer menu plan

Other strategies include incorporating a variety of flavors from different regions of the world (spicy dishes must be balanced against some plain options), and various textures, by offering dishes with differing 'mouth feel' (e.g. if the menu plan has mashed potatoes, the other vegetables can be served al dente). Also, the menu and most recipes should be low in fat and high in CHO to meet the dietary goals of athletes (see the practice tips at the end of the chapter on how to modify fat intake in a recipe).

The menu for large-scale competition events must cater for performance requirements, and cultural and special dietary needs of athletes. The athletes' village contains a large-scale main dining hall that provides a rotational menu consisting of traditional hot and cold items, pizza, pasta, Mediterranean, African and Asian cuisine, and all-day cereal, yoghurt, bread, pastries, fruit, salad, condiments and beverages. A restaurant for 'casual dining' is commonly located elsewhere in the village. The main dining hall is open 24 hours to cater for late night and early morning competition events, and commonly provides an overnight menu ('supper'). Sufficient options need to be available for athletes wanting to choose lower-fat dishes. At least one low-fat alternative for almost every type of traditional/authentic menu item should be offered at each meal period.

Sports dietitians can play a valuable role in ensuring that the menu at large-scale competition events meets the requirements of all athletes. At the Sydney 2000 Olympic Games and the 2006 Commonwealth Games, sports dietitians helped develop and analyze the menus, which resulted in positive feedback from dining hall patrons (Pelly et al. 2006a; in press).

25.15 Cost of food

Cost is a primary concern in menu design. Cost-cutting measures include buying food in bulk at wholesale prices and adapting the menu to incorporate cheaper items, bulking-up casseroles and minced meat dishes using cheaper ingredients including legumes and grains, and cooking meals in bulk and 're-inventing' the dish at a later stage (e.g. bolognese sauce served with pasta can be turned into a spicy bean-based Mexican dish and served with tortillas, jacket potatoes or rice). Leftover foods can also be re-used, provided food safety and hygiene have been addressed (see section 25.18). In addition, self-catering for a group is a cheaper option than eating out.

25.16 Seasonal variations

In winter, athletes prefer hot meals. Thick, hearty soups are an excellent lunchtime option. In summer, lighter dishes including stir-fries, cold meats and salads are popular. To boost CHO intake from salad dishes, rice, couscous, burghul, pasta, potatoes or corn may be added.

25.17 Timing of meals

Offering meals to coincide with training and competition schedules creates problems for catering management and staffing. Some athletes train after school and finish training early while others train after work and may not present for meals until after 8 or even 9 pm. In any catering environment, meal times are usually held within a relatively short timeframe. However, there should be enough flexibility to arrange pre- and post-match meals outside of these times and cater for athletes who regularly eat late. There is often the need for food provision over 24 hours, including options of portable snacks, boxed lunches and recovery snacks.

25.18 Food safety

In a large-scale catering facility, all kitchen staff should be trained in food safety and hygiene practices. A dietitian involved with menu planning can provide training and offer encouragement and adherence to safe food hygiene practices. Food safety issues, including food handling, storage of food, re-use of leftovers and personal hygiene associated with food, are also important for athletes who self-cater. Similar training is also relevant for athletes who travel to countries where the risk of food-borne illness is high.

25.19 Education of food-service staff

Catering staff may not have had experience feeding groups of athletes. Providing written guidelines with menu suggestions and recommended serve sizes encourages appropriate food provision. Suggestions for caterers are serving pasta, rice, potatoes and vegetables at the start of the service point, serving menu items and sauces separately, and ensuring adequate fluid is available on the table. Several recipe books are available for catering for large groups of people and specifically for athletes (see Modulon & Burke 1997). We have found that providing nutrition education sessions to food-service staff makes them feel directly involved as part of the sport service team and more receptive to menu changes and complaints by athletes. An added advantage is that these staff then play an important role in encouraging athletes in food selection, modify food presentation to address any complaints and often change their own dietary habits.

Nutrition education sessions have been successfully conducted for catering staff at the Commonwealth and Olympic games (Pelly et al. 2006a; in press). These should ideally commence one month prior to the dining hall opening to inform chefs about the use of nutrition labels and to reinforce their adherence to recipes.

25.20 Use of nutrition labels

Although the use of nutrition labels in dining halls is a well-established method of providing nutrition information, their success in altering food choice has produced mixed results and has not necessarily translated into increased selection of targeted items (Davis-Chervin et al. 1985; Sproul et al. 2003; Steenhuis et al. 2004a, 2004b). Sites where there are limited food choices available in food outlets have the greatest effect on food choice (Seymour et al. 2004).

Nutrition labels have been used to identify healthy food and menu choices and highlight the energy and nutrient content. Despite using varying means to describe foods—using absolute values or percentages of nutrients present, adjectives or graphics—consumers still have difficulty understanding food labels (Buscher et al. 2001). Appealing labels attract consumer interest, but may not necessarily result in more appropriate food selection (Levy et al. 1992). Graphical formats result in quicker decisions (Balfour et al. 1994) and are preferred by some consumers (Geiger et al. 1991). Furthermore, labeling foods as 'healthy' is often perceived as less tasty (Guthrie et al. 1995; Seymour et al. 2004). Nutrition labels are most effective when adapted for the target audience and when simple messages that include both taste and healthiness are provided (Colby et al. 1987; Holdsworth & Haslam 1998; Buscher et al. 2001). Also, increasing exposure to nutrition information with signs, brochures and nutrition booths, and adding incentives that appeal to other influences on food choice (e.g. price reduction) influence food choice more than labels (Seymour et al. 2004).

Label readers in the general population are predominantly female, tertiary-trained (Guthrie et al. 1995), already eat a healthy diet, health-conscious (Kreuter & Brennan 1997), over 35 years, and less likely to smoke (Neuhouser et al. 1999). Athletes who are also health-conscious and eat a nutrient-dense, low-fat diet read labels more often than non-exercisers (Georgiou et al. 1996). However, label-reading behavior does not necessarily alter food choice, especially in young males (Sproul et al. 2003) and may increase overall energy intake in restrained eaters (Aaron & Mela 1995).

Nutrition labels are now mandatory in the main dining hall at both Olympic and Commonwealth games. A nutrition labeling system was successfully developed for the Sydney 2000 Olympic Games. Each of the menu items was classified according to set criteria for energy and macronutrient content, suitability for special diets and glycemic index. Original icons were developed to represent energy and macronutrients (see Fig. 25.1). Studies conducted at elite-level competition events have found that athletes read the nutrition labels the majority of the time (Pelly et al. 2006a; Pelly, unpublished data, 2007). Figure 25.1 is an example of a nutrition label used for athletes.

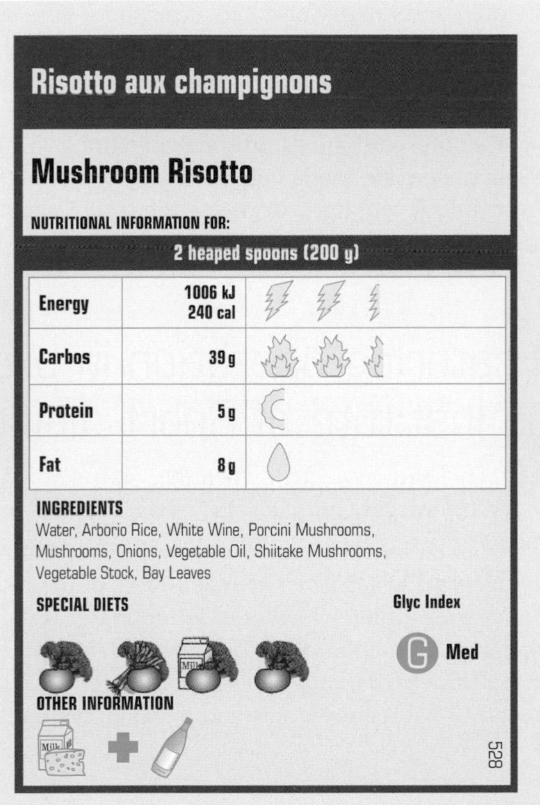

FIGURE 25.1 Example of a nutrition label from the Sydney 2000 Olympic Games. Reproduced with permission from Pelly F & Denyer G, University of Sydney, Australia

25.21 Catering while away from home

25.22 Self-catering while away from home

Dietitians who travel with athletes need to be multi-skilled and offer services other than just menu planning, including shopping, cooking and team management. For example, cooking classes with the team just prior to departure helps instill confidence in those athletes with poor cooking skills and provides an ideal opportunity to plan the menu. Providing guidelines on suitable snacks, meals and recipes is also well received.

Athletes who are unadventurous or inflexible in their eating habits usually resort to poor food choices when away from home. If trips away are frequent (e.g. every weekend), performance capacity and possibly nutritional status can be affected. A supplementary food supply including additional snacks and favorite foods is recommended to help minimize reliance on take-away foods.

25.23 Eating out

Most young athletes have a limited budget and cannot afford restaurant meals, so self-catering is the best option. Restaurant dining or take-away food can provide a convenient meal for athletes who are tired and hungry and a treat for those who self-cater. However, take-away food choices do not always provide a suitable pre-exercise or recovery meal. Restaurant meals also encourage overeating and therefore are more suitable at the end of competition. For some groups, restaurants and take-aways are the only option. Sometimes their accommodation includes pre-paid meals. In these situations, liaison with restaurant staff beforehand can prevent unsuitable foods being offered to athletes. If the timing of the training or competition schedule is very tight, notifying the restaurant ahead of time helps ensure that meals are available soon after the team's arrival.

25.24 A residential catering operation in practice—the Australian Institute of Sport dining hall

The AIS dining hall was opened in 1987 for resident athletes. In 1995, catering was tendered to a private contractor with the proviso that a food-service dietitian be employed as an adviser and overseer of the menu plan. The mission statement in the dining hall is *'Feeding athletes for today, educating them for tomorrow'*. The major tasks of the food-service dietitian are to provide an environment for athletes to choose appropriate foods, develop new recipes, design the menu plan, check on adherence to recipes by chefs and train food-service staff. The dining hall serves a variety of menu options to cater for the wide range of sports, ages, training schedules, nutritional requirements and personal preferences.

25.25 Recipe modification

The food-service dietitian assists chefs in recipe modification by adapting traditional higher-fat recipes to low- or reduced-fat without compromising the flavor, texture or structure of the finished product. The AIS dining hall prides itself on serving traditional 'popular' menu items such as lasagna, schnitzel, and Thai-style curries without the usual high-fat ingredients.

The AIS dining hall is catering for increasing numbers of athletes with special dietary requirements. Recipes are also creatively modified to suit these needs (e.g. vegetarian and gluten-free).

Education of athletes 25.26

Dietitians working at the AIS conduct regular education sessions with residential and visiting athletes. All meals have an accompanying nutrition card highlighting ingredients in the dish and a nutritional analysis per serve. Major food allergens are also declared on the nutrition label.

As an additional education strategy, the food-service dietitian at the AIS is responsible for promoting nutrition education via multiple media. Examples include converting nutrition information into user-friendly terms for the AIS television channel, digital menu screens in the dining hall and weekly newsletters. Planning frequent theme nights encourages athlete participation in menu planning and also helps to alleviate the monotony of eating in the dining hall. This strategy involves groups of athletes planning a themed menu for a specific meal with guidance from the food-service dietitian to ensure a nutritionally balanced menu that includes a few treat items.

Catering for large-scale competition events 25.27

The challenge for catering organizations at large-scale competition events is to develop a menu suitable for thousands of athletes, representing hundreds of nations, who are competing in a wide variety of sports events. The Sydney 2000 Olympic Games was one of the first competition events to provide a comprehensive nutrition service for athletes that included the following:

- review of the dining hall menu for cultural and special dietary needs and sports nutrition requirements by an expert panel of sports dietitians
- nutritional analysis of the dining hall menu and development of nutrition labels
- promotion of the dining hall menu via the development of an interactive website
- promotion of the dining hall menu via a kiosk staffed by members of Sports Dietitians Australia
- education of catering staff

Table 25.3 overleaf provides some indication of the amounts of foods consumed by athletes in the Sydney 2000 Olympic Games dining hall. Around 1.16 million meals were served over 28 days. At its peak, around 49 000 meals were served per day.

Nutrition analysis of the competition menu 25.28

Prior to the Sydney 2000 Olympic Games, we designed a custom database ('Foodweb') to enable dietary analysis of food production data, classify dishes based on macronutrient

TABLE 25.3 CATERING FOR THE SYDNEY 2000 OLYMPIC GAMES
AMOUNTS OF FOODS CONSUMED IN THE MAIN DINING HALL OVER 28 DAYS
27 000 kg pasta
22 000 kg rice
200 000 steaks
53 000 mL milk
700 000 pieces fruit

content and special dietary needs, and create point-of-choice nutrition labels (Pelly, unpublished data, 2007). The Foodweb database was linked to the caterer's recipe database so that the analysis dynamically reflected changes to the preparation of foods. The development of a similar database that can dynamically link recipe and menu development to nutrient analysis and point-of-choice labeling would be of great benefit to both residential and competition events in the future.

25.29 Menu websites

Viewing the menu in advance of elite-level competition can assist athletes with planning their competition diet before arriving at the venue. For the Sydney 2000 Olympic Games, a website was developed for athletes to see the menu and menu cycle well in advance of the games (Pelly, unpublished data, 2007). For people with special requirements, a search could be done for all dishes excluding a certain ingredient (e.g. meat) or for specific dietary needs or religious requirements (e.g. halal). Other features included 'Ask a sports dietitian', sample meal plans and sports nutrition information written by Sports Dietitians Australia.

25.30 The nutrition information centre

A nutrition centre located within the dining hall is a valuable addition to enhance the nutrition service to athletes (Pelly et al. 2006a; in press). The dining hall is the ideal location to assist athletes with appropriate food choice as well as provide advice on specific nutrition issues. Research conducted at the 2006 Commonwealth Games suggested that the nutrition centre served athletes and officials for both sport and clinical nutrition issues (Pelly et al. 2006a). The nutrition centre should be staffed by sports dietitians who can provide athletes with details about the menu, conduct individual dietary assessment, service special dietary requests and answer sports and clinical nutrition enquiries. Sports dietitians can also complete quality assurance checks to ensure that the menu items comply with the analysis on the nutrition labels.

25.31 Special dietary requests

We have found that there are increasing requests by athletes for specialized meals at elite-level competition. At the 2006 Commonwealth Games, the special diet requests were predominately for gluten- and nut-free items, soy and oat milk, garlic, unseasoned food and probiotics (Pelly et al. 2006a).

Since the Sydney 2000 Olympic Games, sports dietitians have had varying levels of involvement with catering at elite-level competition events. Challenges have included the lack of a clearly defined nutrition policy, change in caterers between events and food sponsorship issues. However, several advances have been made in recent years. At the 2006 Commonwealth Games, catering and medical dietetic services combined to provide a comprehensive nutrition support service that was valued highly by athletes (Pelly et al. 2006a). Subsequently, expert panels of international sports dietitians have reviewed the menus for both the Beijing 2008 Summer Olympic Games and the Vancouver 2010 Winter Olympic Games. This collaboration assists with the provision of a suitable menu and dietetic service that can meet the performance, cultural and special dietary needs of all athletes.

Summary 25.32

Menu planning and catering for athletes provide an opportunity to directly influence the food supply and potentially influence food choice. Educational activities including cooking classes and menu design are invaluable in developing athletes' confidence in food selection and preparation. This approach helps to encourage athletes to consume a suitable diet for training and competition.

PRACTICE TIPS

NICOLA CUMMINGS

- Menu planning allows the translation of nutrition principles into real food choices for athletes. Helping athletes select food provides an ideal opportunity to raise awareness of food choice, influence existing beliefs and attitudes and ultimately improve food selection.

THE TASKS OF A DIETITIAN IN FOOD SERVICE

- The primary tasks of a food-service dietitian include development of a menu plan; modification and analysis of recipes provided to athletes; education of athletes, coaches and food-service providers; education and professional development of catering staff; and management of a quality assurance program, which includes evaluation of the menu plan by formal surveys, focus groups and verbal feedback from representative athletes.

MENU PLANNING FOR ATHLETIC GROUPS

- For a menu to be acceptable to athletes, it must meet their nutrient requirements, appeal to their taste preferences and address any special dietary needs for a range of ages and cultural backgrounds. For a menu to be acceptable to an organization, it also has to be cost-effective, minimize wastage and satisfy budgetary constraints, food safety regulations and available cooking facilities.
- When catering for large groups of athletes from differing sports, the preferred option is buffet-style self-service.
- Strategies that enhance CHO intake and improve nutrient balance in a buffet-style servery include offering CHO-rich foods first in the line-up and the meat dishes at the end. This sequence encourages larger serves of CHO and smaller serves of meat, hence improving the macronutrient balance. Placing bread close to soup, for example, and offering a variety of breads, further encourages high CHO choices. Adding legumes to casseroles and soups, thick layers of pasta to lasagne, noodles to salads and soups, and using thick pizza bases further improves the ratio of CHO to other macronutrients. A supply of low-fat snacks, including sandwiches, fruits, yoghurts, cereals and cereal bars, can be provided for in between meals.
- Planning a menu that accommodates several dietary requirements can often create the need for additional recipes. An efficient strategy to minimize this is to modify recipes in such a way that the one recipe suits multiple dietary requirements. For example, using mushroom oyster sauce instead of a regular oyster sauce in a stir-fry has the potential to satisfy a vegetarian option, a gluten-free option and an option that contains no seafood, without compromising the flavor and quality of the original recipe.

RECIPE MODIFICATION FOR CATERERS

- Australian cookbooks written specifically for sportspeople are available in bookshops or newsagents (Inge & Roberts 1996; O'Connor & Hay 1996, 1998; Modulon & Burke 1997; Burke et al. 1999, 2001, 2004). Any low-fat cookbook or recipe is suitable for athletes, although additional CHO-rich foods may need to be added to the final meal. Modifying existing recipes with lower-fat ingredients or alternative ingredients is possible with most recipes, without a large change in texture or flavor.

GUIDELINES FOR ATHLETES WHEN CHOOSING FOODS FROM A BUFFET

- Athletes living and eating in a communal environment frequently overeat, eat suboptimal amounts of one or more food groups (mostly vegetables), or habitually eat a poorly balanced diet when offered food from a buffet service. The disadvantages of a live-in environment are lack of involvement with food, loss of cooking skills and no knowledge of the ingredients in a recipe. These issues are addressed by providing education sessions when athletes arrive, using nutrition cards and involving athletes in menu planning. Table 25.3 provides the information given to athletes at the AIS about developing eating strategies in the dining hall.

EDUCATING CATERING STAFF

- The content and format of education sessions for catering staff need to reflect the particular catering situation and background of the staff involved and can cover standard recipes, service standards, guidelines for healthy eating, special nutrition needs

TABLE 25.3 TIPS PROVIDED TO ATHLETES ABOUT EATING IN THE DINING HALL AT THE AUSTRALIAN INSTITUTE OF SPORT

1. Know clearly your nutritional goals and how to choose foods to achieve these goals most of the time. If you are unsure of how to choose foods to achieve these goals, arrange to see a sports dietitian.
2. Be focused and organized when planning your meal times and snacks. Don't leave it to chance. Stick to this plan—don't try anything new or tricky at or around competition.
3. Treat the dining hall like a restaurant. Look at the menu or do a lap to check out what is on offer. Make a decision as you wait in the queue. Don't just grab!
4. Don't concern yourself with the amount and type of food that other athletes are consuming. The nutritional needs of other athletes may be quite different from your own. Don't be influenced by peer pressure.
5. Don't pile a bit of everything on your plate. This type of eating is haphazard and unbalanced, and you'll probably end up eating more than you need.
6. Eat just what you need from a balanced food selection. Check your plate for mostly high-CHO foods, a protein-rich food, some vegetables or fruit—the more colorful, the more vitamins!
7. Read any nutrition information provided to learn more about your meal choice and to help make other food choices.
8. Relax. There is plenty of food for everyone and menu items will be repeated. If you decide on one item tonight, you can look forward to another choice the next night. This isn't your last meal.
9. Plan for healthy snacks between meals—especially if you have high-energy needs. Good options include sandwiches, yoghurt, fruit and vegetable sticks and dips provided in the dining hall.
10. Don't hang around the dining hall once you have finished your meal. You'll end up eating things that you don't need and don't remember.

Source: Adapted from Modulon & Burke 1997

PRACTICE TIPS

of athletes, menu planning, recipe modification, and food hygiene and safety practices. Aspects of these education programs are easily adapted into written guidelines to give to any caterer. This information is also useful for team managers responsible for organizing meals.

MENU PLANNING FOR SELF-CATERING

- Prior to departure, the dietitian needs to arrange a meeting with the team, coach and manager to determine the catering requirements, competition or training schedules, the food skills of the team and the allocated budget. For most local or national competitions where the athletes are not professional, self-catering is usually the preferred option because of financial constraints. Table 25.4 provides an outline of a suggested intervention strategy for a sports dietitian working with traveling teams.

TABLE 25.4 TIPS FOR DIETITIANS TO PREPARE ATHLETES FOR SELF-CATERING
• Discuss catering requirements with the athletes/manager/coach.
• Determine the cooking skills of the group. Plan pre-camp cooking sessions if feasible. Alternatively coordinate the cooking session during the camp, if the dietitian is traveling with the team.
• Determine in advance the cooking equipment, food budget, shop access and cooking facilities available.
• Plan the menu around the length of stay, competition or training program.
• Designate responsibility for shopping and cooking of food among the athletes. Consider contacting the local supermarket to see if they will deliver.
• Develop a list of basic ingredients and cooking equipment that can be taken from home and shared among the team.
PLANNING FOR DINING OUT
• Book a restaurant in close proximity to the accommodation rather than dropping in unexpectedly.
• Confirm that the menu provides appropriate and suitable foods for the age, budget and food preferences of the team.
• If a large group of athletes is booked and planning is well in advance, send suitable menu selections.
• For a large group of athletes, arrange a set à la carte menu with the option of one or two choices, or a buffet-style servery.
• Inform restaurants of the estimated time of arrival.
• Ensure there is plenty of extra bread served with the meal.
• Ensure water and juices are kept well stocked during the meal.

REFERENCES

Aaron JI, Mela DJ. Paradoxical effect of a nutrition labelling scheme in a student cafeteria. Nutr Res 1995;15:1251–61.

Balfour D, Wise A, Moody R. Visual nutrition information for menu labeling: a study of the decision making process. Hygiene Nutr Foodservice Catering 1994;1:3–12.

Burke L, Bell L, Cort M, Cox G, Crawford R, Minehan M, Wood C. Survival around the world. Sydney: FPC Custom Media, 2004.

Burke L, Cox G, Braakhuis A, Crawford R, Minehan M. Survival from the fittest. Sydney: Murdoch Magazines, 2001.

Burke L, Cox G, Cummings N, et al. Survival for the fittest: the Australian Institute of Sport official cookbook for busy people. Sydney: Murdoch Magazines Pty Ltd, 1999.

Buscher LA, Martin KA, Crocker S. Point-of-purchase messages framed in terms of cost, convenience, taste, and energy improve healthful snack selection in a college foodservice setting. J Am Diet Assoc 2001;101:909–13.

Clendenen VI, Herman CP, Polivy J. Social facilitation of eating among friends and strangers. Appetite 1994;23:1–13.

Colby JL, Elder JP, Peterson G, Knisley PM, Carleton RA. Promoting the selection of healthy food through menu item description in a family-style restaurant. Am J Prev Med 1987;3:171–7.

Connor M. Accounting for gender, age and socioeconomic differences in food choice. Appetite 1994;23:195.

Crystal S, Frye CA, Kanarek RB. Taste preferences and sensory perceptions in female varsity swimmers. Appetite 1995;24:25–36.

Dang V, Crawford R. Survey: habits and knowledge of team athletes eating in the AIS dining hall. 2006 (unpublished).

Davis-Chervin D, Rogers T, Clark M. Influencing food selection with point-of-choice nutrition. Inform J Nutr Educ 1985;17:18–22.

Engell D, Kramer M, Malafi T. Effects of effort and social modelling on drinking in humans. Appetite 1996;26:129.

Falk WL, Sobal J, Bisogni CA, Connors M, Devine CM. Managing healthy eating: definitions, classifications, and strategies. Health Educ Behav 2001;28:425–39.

Furst T, Connors M, Bisogni CA, Sobal J, Falk WL. Food choice: a conceptual model of the process. Appetite 1996;26:247–66.

Geiger CJ, Wyse BW, Parent CRM, Hansen RG. Review of nutrition labeling formats. J Am Diet Assoc 1991;91:808–12.

Georgiou C, Betts N, Hoos T, Glenn M. Young adult exercisers and non-exercisers differ in food attitudes, perceived dietary changes and food choices. Int J Sport Nutr 1996;6:402–13.

Glanz K, Hoelscher D. Increasing fruit and vegetable intake by changing environments, policy and pricing: restaurant-based research, strategies and recommendations. Prev Med 2004;39(Suppl). 88S–93S.

Guinard JX, Seador K, Beard JL, Brown PL. Sensory acceptability of meat and dairy products and dietary fat in male collegiate swimmers. Int J Sport Nutr 1995;5:315–28.

Guthrie JF, Fox JJ, Cleveland LE, Welsh S. Who uses nutrition labelling and what effects does label use have on diet quality? J Nutr Educ 1995;27:163–72.

Hess MA. Taste: the neglected nutritional. J Am Diet Assoc 1997;97(Suppl):205S–7S.

Hickson JF, Johnson CW, Schrader JW, et al. Promotion of athletes' nutritional intake by a university foodservice facility. J Am Diet Assoc 1987;87:926–7.

Holdsworth M, Haslam C. A review of point-of-choice nutrition labelling schemes in the workplace, public eating places and universities. J Hum Nutr Diet 1998;11:423.

Inge K, Roberts C. Food for sport cookbook. Third edition. Melbourne: New Holland Publishers, 1996.

Kreuter MW, Brennan LK. Do nutrition label readers eat healthier diets? Behavioural correlates of adults' use of food labels. Am J Prev Med 1997;13:277–83.

Levy AS, Fein SB, Schucker RE. More effective nutrition label formats are not necessarily preferred. J Am Diet Assoc 1992;92:1230–5.

Mayer JA, Dubbert PM, Elder JP. Promoting nutrition at the point of choice. A review. Health Educ Quart 1989;16:31–43.

Meiselman HL, Hedderley D, Staddon SL, Pierson BJ, Symonds CR. Effect of effort on meal selection and meal acceptability in a student cafeteria. Appetite 1994;23:43–55.

Meiselman HL, Johnson JL, Reeve W, Crouch JE. Demonstrations of the influence of the eating environment on food acceptance. Appetite 2000;35:231–7.

Modulon S, Burke L. Cooking for champions: a guide to healthy large scale cooking for athletes and other active people. Canberra: Australian Sports Commission, 1997.

Nestle M, Wing R, Birch L, et al. Behavioural and social influences on food choice. Nutr Rev 1998;56(Suppl):50S–74S.

Neuhouser ML, Kristal AR, Patterson RE. Use of food nutrition labels is associated with lower fat intake. J Am Diet Assoc 1999;99:45–50.

O'Connor H, Hay D. The taste of fitness. Second edition. Australia: JB Fairfax Creative Cooking, 1996.

O'Connor H, Hay D. Nutrition sports basics. Australia: JB Fairfax Creative Cooking, 1998.

Pelly F. A comprehensive environmental nutrition intervention for athletes competing at the Sydney 2000 Olympic Games. University of Sydney, 2007 (unpublished).

Pelly F, Denyer G, O'Connor H, Caterson I. Nutrition at the Sydney 2000 Olympic Games (abstract). J Sci Med Sport 2004;7:31.

Pelly F, Denyer G, O'Connor H, Caterson I. Catering for the athletes' village at the Sydney 2000 Olympic Games: the role of sports dietitians. Int J Sports Nutr Exerc Metab (in press).

Pelly F, Inge K, King T, O'Connor H. Provision of a nutrition support service at the Melbourne 2006 Commonwealth Games, paper presented at the Second Australian Association for Exercise and Sports Science Conference, Sydney, Australia, 2006a.

Pelly F, King T, O'Connor H. Factors influencing food choice of elite athletes at an international competition dining hall, paper presented at the Second Australian Association for Exercise and Sports Science Conference, Sydney, Australia, 2006b.

Reichler G, Dalton S. Chefs' attitudes towards healthful food preparation are more positive than their food science knowledge and practices. J Am Diet Assoc 1998;98:165.

Ryan Smart L, Bisogni CA. Personal food systems of male college hockey players. Appetite 2001;37: 57–70.

Seymour JD, Yaroch AL, Serdula M, Blanck HM, Khan LK. Impact of nutrition environmental interventions on point-of-purchase behavior in adults: a review. Prev Med 2004;39(Suppl):108S–36S.

Sproul AD, Canter DD, Schmidt JB. Does point-of-purchase nutrition labeling influence meal selections? A test in an army cafeteria. Military Med 2003;168:556–60.

Steenhuis I, Van Assema P, Reubsaett A, Kok G. Process evaluation of two environmental nutrition programmes and an educational nutrition programme conducted at supermarkets and worksite cafeterias in the Netherlands. J Hum Nutr Diet 2004a;17:107–15.

Steenhuis I, Van Assema P, Van Breukelen G, Kok G, De Vries H. The impact of educational and environmental interventions in Dutch worksite cafeterias. Health Prom Int 2004b;19:335–43.

Stroebele N, De Castro JM. Effect of ambience on food intake and food choice. Nutr 2004;20:821–38.

ABBREVIATIONS

3-MH	3-methylhistidine
AA	amino acids
AC	activation co-efficient
ACSM	American College of Sports Medicine
ADP	adenosine diphosphate
AI	Adequate Intake
AIS	Australian Institute of Sport
AMDR	Acceptable Macronutrient Distribution Range
AMP	adenosine monophosphate
AMPK	AMP-activated kinase
AMPK	AMP-activated protein kinase
ASADA	Australian Sports Anti-Doping Authority
AST	aspartate aminotransferase
AT	adaptive thermogenesis
ATP	adenosine triphosphate
a-v	arteriovenous
BCAA	branched-chain amino acid
BCAAT	branched-chain aminotransferase
BCOAD	branched-chain oxo-acid dehydrogenase enzyme
BED	binge-eating disorder
BIA	bioelectrical impedance analysis
BM	body mass
BMC	bone mineral content
BMD	bone mineral density
BMI	body mass index: weight (kg) ÷ height (m^2)
BMR	basal metabolic rate
CAT	carnitine acylcarnitine translocase
CHO	carbohydrate
CHr	reticulocyte hemoglobin content
CPT	carnitine palmityltransferase
CrP	creatine phosphate
CV	coefficient of variation
DHEA	dehydroepiandrosterone
DIT	diet-induced thermogenesis
DLW	doubly labeled water
DRI	Dietary Reference Intake
DXA	dual energy X-ray absorptiometry
E-AC	erythrocyte enzyme activation co-efficient
EAR	Estimated Average Requirement
E-ASTAC	erythrocyte aspartate amino transferase activation co-efficient
EC	excitation–contraction
EDNOS	eating disorders not otherwise specified
EER	Estimated Energy Requirement
E-GRAC	erythrocyte glutathione reductase activation co-efficients
EI	energy intakes
EI:BMR	the ratio of reported energy intakes (EI) to predicted basal metabolic rates (BMR)
eIF2Bepsilon	eukaryotic initiation factor 2B
E_{in}	energy in (energy intake)
EMS	eosinophilic myalgia syndrome
EPOC	excess post-exercise oxygen consumption
E-TKAC	erythrocyte transketolase activation co-efficients
EXOS	exercise-oxidative stress
E_{out}	energy out
FA	fatty acid/s
FBR	fractional breakdown rate
FBR	fractional protein breakdown
FDA	Food and Drug Administration

ABBREVIATIONS

FES	functional electrical stimulation
FFA	free fatty acids
FFM	fat-free mass
FFQ	food frequency questionnaire
FM	fat mass
FSR	fractional synthetic rate
FT	fast twitch
GER	gastro-esophageal reflux
GERD	gastro-esophageal reflux disease
GH	growth hormone
GOT	glutamate oxalacetate transaminase
GR	glutathione reductase
GTF	glucose tolerance factor
HAD	3-hydroxyacyl coenzyme A dehydrogenase
HMB	beta-hydroxy beta-methylbutyrate
HPLC	high pressure liquid chomatography
HSL	hormone-sensitive TG lipase
ICS	irritable colon syndrome
IDA	iron deficiency anemia
IGF-I and IGF-II	insulin-like growth factors I and II
IMP	inosine 5′-monophosphate
IOC	International Olympic Committee
IPC	International Paralympics Committee
ISAK	International Society for the Advancement of Kinanthropometry
LBM	lean body mass
LCFA	long-chain fatty acid
MAP	mean arterial pressure
MAPK	p38 mitogen-activated protein kinase
MCFA	medium-chain fatty acids
MCHC	mean corpuscular hemoglobin concentration
MCT	medium-chain triglyceride
MCV	mean cell volume
MDA	malondialdehyde
MES	minimum effective strain
MNT	medical nutrition therapy
MPS	muscle protein synthesis
mRNA	messenger RNA
MSDS	Materials Safety Data Sheet
mTOR	mammalian target of rapamycin
MVC	maximum voluntary contraction
NBAL	nitrogen balance
NCAA	National Collegiate Athletic Association
NEAT	non-exercise activity thermogenesis
NEFA	non-esterified fatty acid
NHANES	National Health and Nutrition Examination Survey
NHMRC	National Health and Medical Research Council
NO	nitric oxide
NRV	Nutrient Reference Value
NSAID	non-steroidal anti-inflammatory drug
PAL	physical activity level
PDH	pyruvate dehydrogenase
PHV	peak height velocity
PLP	plasma pyridoxal-5-phosphate
PQCT	peripheral quantitative computed tomography
PRPP	phosphoribosyl pyrophosphate
RBC	red blood cells

ABBREVIATIONS

RDA	Recommended Dietary Allowance
RDI	Recommended Dietary Intake
RER	respiratory exchange ratio
RMR	resting metabolic rate
RNI	Recommended Nutrient Intake
ROS	reactive oxygen species
RQ	respiratory quotient
SC	spinal cord
SD	standard deviation
SF	serum ferritin
SMR	sleep metabolic rate
SPA	spontaneous physical activity
SR	sarcoplasmic reticulum
sTfR	serum transferrin receptor
TBARS	thiobarbituric acid reactive substances
TBK	total body potassium
TBW	total body water
TCA	tricarboxylic acid
TEA	thermic effect of activity
TEF	thermic effect of food
TEM	technical error of measurement
TEM	thermic effect of a meal
TfR	transferrin receptors
TG	triacylglycerol
tRNA	transfer RNA
UIL	Upper Intake Level
UL	Upper Level of Intake
URTI	upper respiratory tract infection
UWW	underwater weighing
VLCD	very low calorie diet
VLED	very low energy diet
$\mathbf{VO_{2\,max}}$	maximal oxygen uptake
$\mathbf{VO_{2\,peak}}$	peak oxygen uptake
W	watt
WADA	World Anti-Doping Agency
ww	wet weight

INDEX

INDEX

INDEX

INDEX

INDEX

INDEX

INDEX

INDEX

INDEX

INDEX

INDEX

INDEX

INDEX

INDEX

INDEX

INDEX